Practical Anatomic Pathology

Series Editors

Fan Lin
Geisinger Health System
Danville, PA, USA

Ximing J. Yang
Feinberg School of Medicine
Northwestern University
Chicago, IL, USA

This Book Series is designed to provide a comprehensive, practical and state-of-the-art review and update of the major issues and challenges specific to each subspecialty field of surgical pathology in a question and answer (Q&A) format. Making an accurate diagnosis especially from a limited sample can be quite challenging, yet crucial to patient care. This Book Series, using the most current and evidence-based resources 1) focuses on frequently asked questions in surgical pathology in day-to-day practice; 2) provides quick, accurate, terse, and useful answers to many practical questions encountered in daily practice; 3) emphasizes the importance of a triple test (clinical, radiologic, and histologic correlation); 4) delineates how to appropriately utilize immunohistochemistry, in situ hybridization and molecular tests; and 5) minimizes any potential diagnostic pitfalls in surgical pathology. These books also include highly practical presentations of typical case scenarios seen in an anatomic pathology laboratory. These are in the form of case presentations with step-by-step expert analysis. Sample cases include common but challenging situations, such as evaluation of well-differentiated malignant tumors vs. benign/reactive lesions; distinction of two benign entities; sub-classification of a malignant tumor; identification of newly described tumor and non-tumor entities; workup of a tumor of unknown origin; and implementation of best practice in immunohistochemistry and molecular testing in a difficult case. The Q&A format is well accepted, especially by junior pathologists, for several reasons: 1) this is the most practical and effective way to deliver information to a new generation of pathologists accustomed to using the Internet as a resource and, therefore, comfortable and familiar with a Q&A learning environment; 2) it's impossible to memorialize and digest massive amounts of new information about new entities, new and revised classifications, molecular pathology, diagnostic IHC, and the therapeutic implications of each entity by reading large textbooks; 3) sub-specialization is a very popular practice model highly demanded by many clinicians; and 4) time is very precious for a practicing pathologist because of increasing workloads in recent years following U.S. health care reforms. This Book Series meets all of the above expectations. These books are written by established and recognized experts in their specialty fields and provide a unique and valuable resource in the field of surgical pathology, both for those currently in training and for those already in clinical practice at various skill levels. It does not seek to duplicate or completely replace other large standard textbooks; rather, it is a new, comprehensive yet concise and practical resource on these timely and critical topics.

More information about this series at http://www.springer.com/series/13808

Hanlin L. Wang • Zongming Eric Chen
Editors

Practical Gastrointestinal Pathology

Frequently Asked Questions

Springer

Editors
Hanlin L. Wang
University of California
Los Angeles, CA
USA

Zongming Eric Chen
Mayo Clinic
Rochester, MN
USA

Practical Anatomic Pathology
ISBN 978-3-030-51270-5 ISBN 978-3-030-51268-2 (eBook)
https://doi.org/10.1007/978-3-030-51268-2

This Springer imprint is published by the registered company Springer Nature Switzerland AG
The registered company address is: Gewerbestrasse 11, 6330 Cham, Switzerland

Preface

To most surgical pathologists, gastrointestinal (GI) pathology is part of their bread-and-butter practices. Each day, challenging diagnostic problems constantly emerge and questions regarding best ways of handling individual cases, better known as "best practice," are frequently encountered.

This is particularly true as the field of GI pathology has been advancing quickly in the last few years. Deeper understanding of pathogenesis at molecular, genetic, and genomic levels has driven significant changes in disease nomenclature and classification with emergence of new diagnostic entities. On the other hand, rapid advances in medical technologies including enhanced capabilities of endoscopic and minimally invasive surgical procedures, improved diagnostic imaging modalities, and introduction of new therapeutic agents have dramatically changed clinical management and outcome of patients with many types of GI diseases. Furthermore, with the entire healthcare switching towards personalized medicine, clinical colleagues continue to exert new demands and expectations for histopathologic diagnosis.

Therefore, a comprehensive question and answer (Q&A) book specifically addressing practical issues reflecting the current landscape of GI pathology practice is highly desirable, even in the competitive world of many existing textbooks and online references on the similar subject. For this purpose, we brought together expert diagnosticians in the field and organized the wealthy knowledge and experience of GI pathology practice into a Q&A format to fit the fast-pacing daily life of practicing pathologists. The hope is to provide an easy and quick access to concise, evidence-based, and up-to-date information to aid accurate diagnosis and to ensure best practice in GI pathology.

The book is question driven. There are all together more than 540 questions, addressing difficult, prevailing, and controversial issues in GI pathology that are frequently encountered in daily practice and consultation service. For most questions, answers are straightforward with ample literature support. However, true diagnostic controversies and clinical dilemma cannot be easily resolved with current knowledge and available information. To such challenges, an expert approach regarding how to synthesize complicated topics and clearly communicate the thinking process is valuable to readers and can help guide clinicians making optimal treatment plans for their patients. The latter types of answers are highly enriched throughout the book.

Distinct from other existing GI pathology textbooks, this book is primarily organized according to disease entities and pathological processes instead of specific organs and anatomic locations. Guided by chapter titles and listed questions, readers should be able to look up a disease or a pathological feature and find the most important and relevant diagnostic criteria and pertinent differential diagnoses.

There are also many other important features of this book, some of which are highlighted below:

- In all chapters of GI tumors, new staging systems proposed by the AJCC Cancer Staging Manual 8th Edition and new nomenclatures proposed by the 2019 WHO Classification of Digestive System Tumors are fully incorporated.

- There are more than 1,100 high-quality images to illustrate the characteristic gross, histologic, and immunohistochemical features of various GI diseases. This atlas is extremely useful to configure mental images to formulate diagnosis and differential diagnosis.
- Pediatric pathology is designated as a separate chapter to emphasize its unique clinical setting. This may inevitably create some redundancy with the contents of other chapters. However, it is quite important and helpful to understand similar disease entities from both adult and pediatric perspectives in terms of differential diagnosis.
- Each chapter includes real-life cases in case presentation sections. These carefully selected examples showcase the most useful diagnostic pearls and potential pitfalls in related topics.

In essence, this is a practical reference book to aid surgical pathologists during diagnosis. It is also a useful textbook for pathology trainees and GI clinicians as well as allied health professionals who frequently deal with GI pathology.

We are deeply indebted to all contributing authors who shared their invaluable practice and teaching experience. It is our privilege to work with this group of distinguished contributors in putting together a book which we hope will be of interest to pathologists and clinicians. We are also extremely grateful to Springer's editorial staff for their help. Finally, we would like to thank our families for their unconditional support.

Rochester, MN, USA — Zongming Eric Chen, MD, PhD
Los Angeles, CA, USA — Hanlin L. Wang, MD, PhD

Contents

1 **Gastrointestinal Disorders in the Infant and Child** 1
Heather B. Rytting and Hong Yin

2 **Non-Barrett Esophagitis** 33
Kevin M. Waters, Rifat Mannan, and Elizabeth Montgomery

3 **Barrett Esophagus** 55
Eric Swanson and Bita V. Naini

4 **Nonneoplastic Diseases of the Stomach** 67
Michael Torbenson

5 **Malabsorption Disorders** 89
Rhonda Yantiss and Melanie Johncilla

6 **Inflammatory Bowel Disease** 109
Wenqing Cao and Noam Harpaz

7 **Non-IBD Noninfectious Colitis** 145
Jingmei Lin and Henry D. Appelman

8 **Appendiceal Diseases** 167
Yuna Gong, Hanlin L. Wang, and Sergei Tatishchev

9 **Anal Diseases** 195
Upasana Joneja and Jinru Shia

10 **Infections of the Gastrointestinal Tract** 223
Michael Bachman and Laura W. Lamps

11 **Drug-Induced Gastrointestinal Tract Injury** 267
Rifat Mannan, Kevin M. Waters, and Elizabeth Montgomery

12 **Eosinophilic, Mastocytic, and Histiocytic Diseases of the Gastrointestinal Tract** 289
Michael G. Drage and Amitabh Srivastava

13 **Motility Disorders of the Gastrointestinal Tract** 313
Raffaella Morotti and Dhanpat Jain

14 **Non-syndromic Epithelial Polyps of the Gastrointestinal Tract** 339
Dorina Gui, Hanlin L. Wang, and Kristin A. Olson

15 **Syndromic Epithelial Polyps of the Gastrointestinal Tract** 367
Michael Lee, Zongming Eric Chen, and Hanlin L. Wang

16 **Mesenchymal Lesions Often Presenting as Polyps of the Gastrointestinal Tract** 387
Ari Kassardjian, David Borzik, Aaron W. James, and Sarah M. Dry

17 Neuroendocrine Neoplasms of the Gastrointestinal Tract 409
Brent K. Larson and Deepti Dhall

18 Carcinomas of the Gastrointestinal Tract 427
Eric Swanson, Jolanta Jedrzkiewicz, Hanlin L. Wang, and Wade Samowitz

19 Gastrointestinal Stromal Tumor 473
Karen E. Matsukuma and Zongming Eric Chen

20 Non-GIST Primary Mesenchymal Tumors of the Gastrointestinal Tract 495
Katy Lawson, David Borzik, Aaron W. James, and Sarah M. Dry

21 Lymphomas of the Gastrointestinal Tract 521
Robert S. Ohgami and Ryan M. Gill

22 Transplant-Related Issues in the Gastrointestinal Tract 543
Jamie Koo and Hanlin L. Wang

Index 563

Contributors

Henry D. Appelman, MD University of Michigan Medical School, Ann Arbor, MI, USA

Michael Bachman, MD, PhD University of Michigan Medical School, Ann Arbor, MI, USA

David Borzik, MD Johns Hopkins University School of Medicine, Baltimore, MD, USA

Wenqing Cao, MD New York University Langone Health, New York, NY, USA

Zongming Eric Chen, MD, PhD Mayo Clinic, Rochester, MN, USA

Deepti Dhall, MD University of Alabama at Birmingham School of Medicine,, Birmingham, AL, USA

Michael G. Drage, MD, PhD University of Rochester School of Medicine and Dentistry, Rochester, NY, USA

Sarah M. Dry, MD University of California at Los Angeles David Geffen School of Medicine, Los Angeles, CA, USA

Ryan M. Gill, MD, PhD University of California at San Francisco School of Medicine, San Francisco, CA, USA

Yuna Gong, MD University of Southern California Keck School of Medicine, Los Angeles, CA, USA

Dorina Gui, MD, PhD University of California at Davis School of Medicine, Sacramento, CA, USA

Noam Harpaz, MD, PhD Icahn School of Medicine at Mount Sinai, New York, NY, USA

Dhanpat Jain, MD Yale University School of Medicine, New Haven, CT, USA

Aaron W. James, MD, PhD Johns Hopkins University School of Medicine, Baltimore, MD, USA

Jolanta Jedrzkiewicz, MD University of Utah School of Medicine, Salt Lake City, UT, USA

Melanie Johncilla, MD Cornell University Weill Cornell Medicine, New York, NY, USA

Upasana Joneja, MD Cooper University Hospital, Camden, NJ, USA

Ari Kassardjian, MD, PhD University of California at Los Angeles David Geffen School of Medicine, Los Angeles, CA, USA

Jamie Koo, MD ProPath, Dallas, TX, USA

Laura W. Lamps, MD University of Michigan Medical School, Ann Arbor, MI, USA

Brent K. Larson, DO Cedars-Sinai Medical Center, Los Angeles, CA, USA

Katy Lawson, MD University of California at Los Angeles David Geffen School of Medicine, Los Angeles, CA, USA

Michael Lee, MD Columbia University Vagelos College of Physicians and Surgeons, New York, NY, USA

Jingmei Lin, MD, PhD Indiana University School of Medicine, Indianapolis, IN, USA

Rifat Mannan, MD University of Pennsylvania Perelman School of Medicine, Philadelphia, PA, USA

Karen E. Matsukuma, MD, PhD University of California at Davis School of Medicine, Sacramento, CA, USA

Elizabeth Montgomery, MD University of Miami Leonard M. Miller School of Medicine, Miami, FL, USA

Raffaella Morotti, MD Yale University School of Medicine, New Haven, CT, USA

Bita V. Naini, MD University of California at Los Angeles David Geffen School of Medicine, Los Angeles, CA, USA

Robert S. Ohgami, MD, PhD University of California at San Francisco School of Medicine, Stanford, CA, USA

Kristin A. Olson, MD University of California at Davis School of Medicine, Sacramento, CA, USA

Heather B. Rytting, MD Children's Healthcare of Atlanta, Atlanta, GA, USA

Wade Samowitz, MD University of Utah School of Medicine, Salt Lake City, UT, USA

Jinru Shia, MD Memorial Sloan Kettering Cancer Center, New York, NY, USA

Amitabh Srivastava, MD Harvard Medical School and Brigham and Women's Hospital, Boston, MA, USA

Eric Swanson, MD Scripps Health, La Jolla, CA, USA

Sergei Tatishchev, MD University of Southern California Keck School of Medicine, Los Angeles, CA, USA

Michael Torbenson, MD Mayo Clinic, Rochester, MN, USA

Hanlin L. Wang, MD, PhD University of California at Los Angeles David Geffen School of Medicine, Los Angeles, CA, USA

Kevin M. Waters, MD, PhD Cedars-Sinai Medical Center, Los Angeles, CA, USA

Rhonda Yantiss, MD Cornell University Weill Cornell Medicine, New York, NY, USA

Hong Yin, MD Children's Healthcare of Atlanta, Atlanta, GA, USA

Abbreviations

αSMA	alpha smooth muscle actin
ACG	American College of Gastroenterology
AchE	Acetylcholinesterase
AFAP	Attenuated familial adenomatous polyposis
AFP	Alpha-fetoprotein
AIE	Autoimmune enteropathy
AIN	Anal intraepithelial neoplasia
AJCC	American Joint Committee on Cancer
ALCL	Anaplastic large cell lymphoma
ALT	Atypical lipomatous tumor
AMACR	Alpha-methylacyl-CoA racemase
ANA	Antinuclear antibody
APC	Adenomatous polyposis coli
APECED	Autoimmune polyendocrinopathy-candidiasis-ectodermal dystrophy
APR	Abdominoperineal resection
APS	Autoimmune polyglandular syndrome
ASC-US	Atypical squamous cells of undetermined significance
ATZ	Anal transition zone
AVM	Arteriovenous malformation
BAS	Bile acid sequestrants
BE	Barrett esophagus
BP	Bullous pemphigoid
CAP	College of American Pathologists
CAPN14	Calpain 14
CCS	Clear cell sarcoma
CD	Crohn disease
CFPT/RNFP	Calcifying fibrous pseudotumor/reactive nodular fibrous pseudotumor
CGD	Chronic granulomatous disease
CHRPE	Congenital hypertrophy of retinal pigment epithelium
CI	Confidence interval
CIN	Cervical intraepithelial neoplasia or Chromosomal instability
CMV	Cytomegalovirus
CNS	Central nervous system
CPS	Combined Positive Score
CRC	Colorectal carcinoma
COX	Cyclooxygenase
CVID	Common variable immune deficiency
CTLA-4	Cytotoxic T-lymphocyte antigen-4
DALM	Dysplasia-associated lesion or mass
DDLPS	Dedifferentiated liposarcoma
DEB	Dystrophic epidermolysis bullosa

DIF	Direct immunofluorescence
EAC	Esophageal adenocarcinoma
EBER	Epstein-Barr virus-encoding RNA
EBS	Epidermolysis bullosa simplex
EBV	Epstein-Barr virus
ECD	Erdheim-Chester disease
ECL	Enterochromaffin-like cells
EGE	Eosinophilic gastroenteritis
EGFR	Epidermal growth factor receptor
EGID	Eosinophilic gastrointestinal disease
EHE	Epithelioid hemangioendothelioma
ELISA	Enzyme-linked immunosorbent assay
EM	Electron microscopy
EoE	Eosinophilic esophagitis
EPCAM	Epithelial cell adhesion molecule
ESR	Erythrocyte sedimentation rate
FDC	Follicular dendritic cell
FISH	Fluorescence in situ hybridization
ICC	Interstitial cells of Cajal
IDSA	Infectious Diseases Society of America
IMT	Inflammatory myofibroblastic tumor
5-FU	5-fluorouracil
FAP	Familial adenomatous polyposis
FDA	US Food and Drug Administration
FFPE	Formalin-fixed paraffin-embedded
FGP	Fundic gland polyp
FISH	Fluorescence in situ hybridization
FTA-ABS	Fluorescent treponemal antibody absorption test
FVP	Fibrovascular polyp
GAPPS	Gastric adenocarcinoma and proximal polyposis of the stomach
GAVE	Gastric antral vascular ectasia
GCA	Goblet cell adenocarcinoma
GCBL	Giant condyloma of Buschke-Lowenstein
GCDFP	Gross cystic disease fluid protein
GCHP	Goblet cell-rich hyperplastic polyp
GDH	Glutamate dehydrogenase
GE	Gastroesophageal
GEJ	Gastroesophageal junction
GERD	Gastroesophageal reflux disease
GIST	Gastrointestinal stromal tumor
GJP	Generalized juvenile polyposis
GMS	Grocott methenamine silver
GNET	Gastrointestinal neuroectodermal tumor
GVHD	Graft-versus-host disease
HAART	Highly active anti-retroviral therapy
HAMN	High-grade appendiceal mucinous neoplasm
HCG	Human chorionic gonadotropin
H&E	Hematoxylin and eosin
HD	Hirschsprung disease
H. felix	*Helicobacter felix*
HGD	High-grade dysplasia
H. heilmanni	*Helicobacter heilmanni*
HHT	Hereditary hemorrhagic telangiectasia

HIV	Human immunodeficiency virus
hpf	High-power field
HPV	Human papillomavirus
H. pylori	*Helicobacter pylori*
HRA	High-resolution anoscopy
HSCR	Hirschsprung disease
H. suis	*Helicobacter suis*
HSIL	High-grade squamous intraepithelial lesion
HSV	Herpes simplex virus
IBD	Inflammatory bowel disease
IBS	Irritable bowel syndrome
IEL	Intraepithelial lymphocyte
IFP	Inflammatory fibroid polyp
IgA	Immunoglobulin A
IM	Intestinal metaplasia
IND	Indefinite for dysplasia or Intestinal neuronal dysplasia
IPAA	Ileal pouch-anal anastomosis
IPEX	Immune dysregulation, polyendocrinopathy, enteropathy, X-linked
JEB	Junctional epidermolysis bullosa
JPI	Juvenile polyposis of infancy
JXG	Juvenile xanthogranuloma
LAMN	Low-grade appendiceal mucinous neoplasm
LAST	Lower anogenital squamous terminology
LCH	Langerhans cell histiocytosis
LCNEC	Large-cell neuroendocrine carcinoma
LGD	Low-grade dysplasia
LGV	Lymphogranuloma venereum
LMS	Leiomyosarcoma
LSIL	Low-grade squamous intraepithelial lesion
MAI	*mycobacterium avium-intracellulare complex*
MALT	Mucosa-associated lymphoid tissue
MANEC	Mixed adenoneuroendocrine carcinoma
MEN2	Multiple endocrine neoplasia type 2
MFA	Mycophenolic acid
MiNEN	Mixed neuroendocrine-non-neuroendocrine neoplasm
MMF	Mycophenolate mofetil
MMR	Mismatch repair
MPNST	Malignant peripheral nerve sheath tumor
MSI	Microsatellite instability
MSM	Men who have sex with men
MSTF	U.S. Multi-Society Task Force on Colorectal Cancer
MAP	MUTYH-associated polyposis
MVHP	Microvesicular hyperplastic polyp
NAAT	Nucleic acid amplification test
NCDB	National Cancer Data Base
NEC	Necrotizing enterocolitis or Neuroendocrine carcinoma
NET	Neuroendocrine tumor
NF1	Neurofibromatosis type 1
NFP	Neurofilament protein
NGS	Next generation sequencing
NOS	Not otherwise specified

NSAID	Nonsteroidal anti-inflammatory drug
O&P	Ova and parasite
PAIN	Perianal intraepithelial neoplasia
PAS	Periodic acid–Schiff
PCR	Polymerase chain reaction
PD-L1	Programmed death-ligand 1
PJP	Peutz-Jeghers polyp
PMP	pseudomyxoma peritonei
PPI	Proton pump inhibitor
PPI-REE	Proton pump inhibitor-responsive eosinophilic esophagitis
PSC	Primary sclerosing cholangitis
PSOGI	Peritoneal Surface Oncology Group International
PTEN	Phosphatase and tensin homolog
PV	Pemphigus vulgaris
RPR	Rapid plasma reagin
SCJ	Squamocolumnar junction
SDH	Succinate dehydrogenase
SEER	Surveillance, Epidemiology and End Results
SFT	Solitary fibrous tumor
SIL	Squamous intraepithelial lesion
SLE	Systemic lupus erythematosus
SM	Systemic mastocytosis
SMA	Smooth muscle actin
SSA/P	Sessile serrated adenoma/polyp
SSL	Sessile serrated lesion
SSRI	Selective serotonin reuptake inhibitor
STK	Serine threonine kinase
SWI/SNF	Switch/sucrose-nonfermenting
TA	Tubular adenoma
TACE	Transarterial chemoembolization
TB	Tuberculosis
TNF	Tumor necrosis factor
TNM	Tumor Node Metastasis
TP-PA	*T. pallidum* passive particle agglutination
TPS	Tumor Proportion Score
TSLP	Thymic stromal lymphopoietin
TTG	Tissue-transglutaminase
TVA	Tubulovillous adenoma
UC	Ulcerative colitis
VC	Verrucous carcinoma
VIP	Vasoactive intestinal polypeptide
VDRL	Venereal Disease Research Laboratory
VEOIBD	Very early onset inflammatory bowel disease
WDLPS	Well-differentiated liposarcoma
WHO	World Health Organization

Gastrointestinal Disorders in the Infant and Child

1

Heather B. Rytting and Hong Yin

List of Frequently Asked Questions

Developmental Anomalies

1. What are the most common developmental anomalies of the pediatric gastrointestinal tract that a surgical pathologist may encounter?
2. How do you distinguish omphalomesenteric remnant, gastrointestinal duplication, bronchogenic cyst, and neurenteric cyst?
3. Where are intestinal stenoses and atresias located, and what are their pathologic features? What mutation is associated with familial multiple intestinal atresias? What is an apple-peel atresia?
4. Which disorder may be associated with ileocolonic and colonic atresia?
5. Anorectal malformation repair specimens may be sent for examination. If colonic epithelium, muscularis mucosae and muscular wall are present, what needs to be documented?

Hirschsprung Disease

1. Why should suction rectal biopsy be performed 1 cm or higher above the dentate (pectinate) line? What is the dentate line?
2. In addition to absence of ganglion cells, what are other findings that are useful for the diagnosis of Hirschsprung disease (HD) in a suction rectal biopsy?
3. Does the finding of calretinin positive neurites in the lamina propria rule out HD?
4. What type of biopsy is done at the time of mapping and rectal pull-through procedure? In addition to identifying ganglion cells, what are other factors to consider when analyzing the frozen section biopsy?
5. What is important to document in a pull-through specimen? What is the most reliable feature of a transition zone being present at the proximal margin?
6. How do you diagnose intestinal neuronal dysplasia, hypoganglionosis, hyperganglionosis and ultrashort HD?
7. What is Hirschsprung-associated enterocolitis?

Volvulus, Intussusception, and Necrotizing Enterocolitis

1. How does pediatric volvulus differ from adult volvulus? What is the pathology of pediatric volvulus and intussusception?
2. What are possible pathologic lead points in pediatric intussusception? What is the most common malignancy associated with pediatric intussusception?
3. What are the major histopathologic features of necrotizing enterocolitis?

Tumors and Polyps

1. How is pediatric gastrointestinal stromal tumor different from adult counterpart?
2. What are the major clinicopathologic features of malignant gastrointestinal neuroectodermal tumor?
3. What is the most common pediatric gastrointestinal polyp?
4. What is juvenile polyposis?
5. What is a hamartomatous polyp?
6. What are the pathologic characteristics and clinical behavior of appendiceal carcinoid in children?

H. B. Rytting (✉) · H. Yin
Children's Healthcare of Atlanta, Atlanta, GA, USA
e-mail: heather.rytting@choa.org

H. L. Wang, Z. E. Chen (eds.), *Practical Gastrointestinal Pathology*, Practical Anatomic Pathology,
https://doi.org/10.1007/978-3-030-51268-2_1

Inflammatory Disorders

1. What are the pathologic features of eosinophilic esophageal disease and what is the main clinical differential diagnosis of eosinophils in the esophagus?
2. What is the typical distribution of eosinophils in the pediatric gastrointestinal tract?
3. What is the clinical differential of eosinophilic gastrointestinal disease?
4. When do plasma cells appear in the gastrointestinal tract in infants?
5. What is the differential for a pediatric inflammatory enteropathy? What are the general pathologic features in small intestinal biopsies?
6. What is the significance of heterotopic gastric mucosa in a pediatric esophageal biopsy? What is the significance of small intestinal type mucosa in a pediatric gastric biopsy? Are pediatric patients at risk for Barrett metaplasia?
7. A subset of patients with congenital onset diarrhea and non-inflammatory enteropathy may have diagnostic features on intestinal biopsies. What are they?
8. What is very early onset of inflammatory bowel disease?
9. What are the main differentials for a non-infectious lamina propria histiocytic infiltrate?
10. What are the differentials of granulomatous appendicitis?

Developmental Anomalies

Frequently Asked Questions

1. What are the most common developmental anomalies of the pediatric gastrointestinal tract that a surgical pathologist may encounter?

Omphalomesenteric remnants, duplications, atresias, and stenoses of the small and large intestines and anorectal malformations are the most common. Other malformations such as tracheoesophageal fistula and pyloric stenosis are typically surgically corrected without submission of surgical pathology specimens and are unlikely to be seen outside the perinatal autopsy setting.

2. How do you distinguish omphalomesenteric remnant, gastrointestinal duplication, bronchogenic cyst, and neurenteric cyst?

All are similar histopathologically in that there is heterotopic endodermal tissue. The distinction depends on anatomic location, so correct classification requires correlation with surgical and radiological findings. Duplications are most common in the ileum (Figs. 1.1 and 1.2) but can involve any part of the gastrointestinal tract and are associated with the intestinal wall. They are most often lined by the same type of mucosa as the associated segment, have complete muscular walls often including the myenteric plexus, and may communicate with the segment of the intestine. A broad communication is a diverticulum. Some duplications are solid rather than cystic, and these most often consist of nodules of pancreatic tissue within the gastrointestinal wall (Figs. 1.3 and 1.4). Cystic duplications may be spherical or they may be tubular side-by-side duplications (Fig. 1.5). Pancreatic tissue, heterotopic gastric mucosa, and lymphoid tissue may be present. Esophageal duplications and bronchogenic cysts, being both derived from the foregut, can be histologically identical (Fig. 1.6). Both may be lined by ciliated colum-

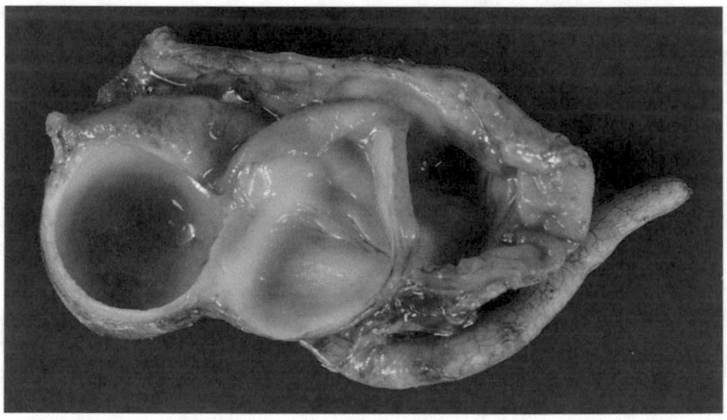

Fig. 1.1 Duplication cyst of the ileum near the ileocecal valve and appendix

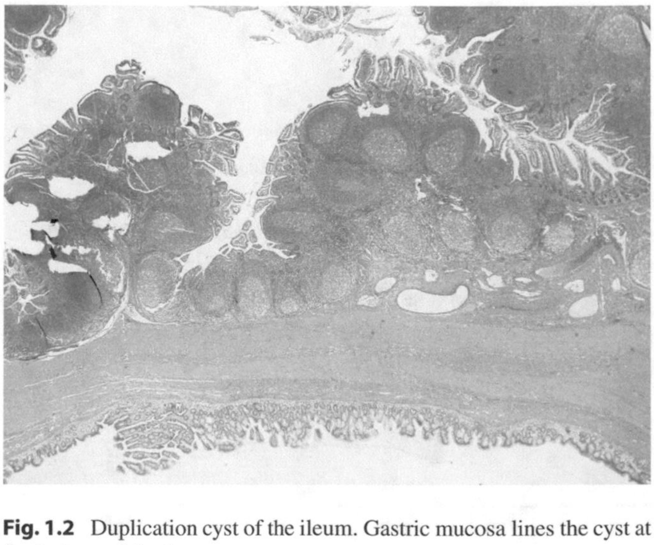

Fig. 1.2 Duplication cyst of the ileum. Gastric mucosa lines the cyst at the bottom of the image

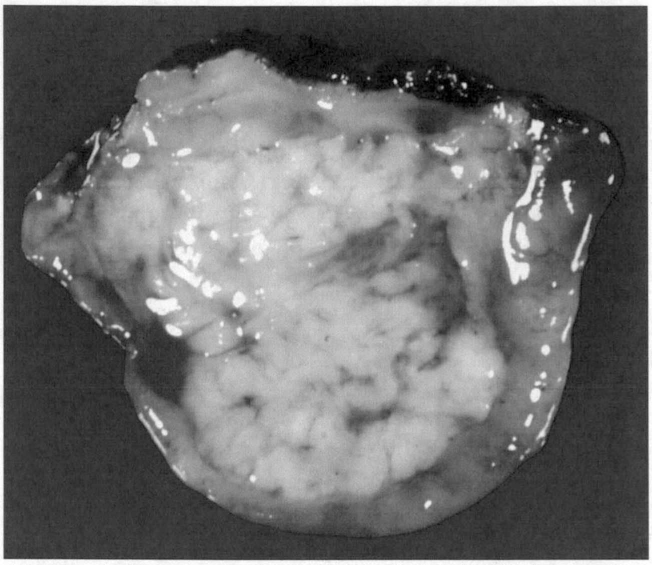

Fig. 1.3 Solid gastric duplication. (Courtesy of Benjamin J. Wilkins, MD, PhD, Children's Hospital of Philadelphia)

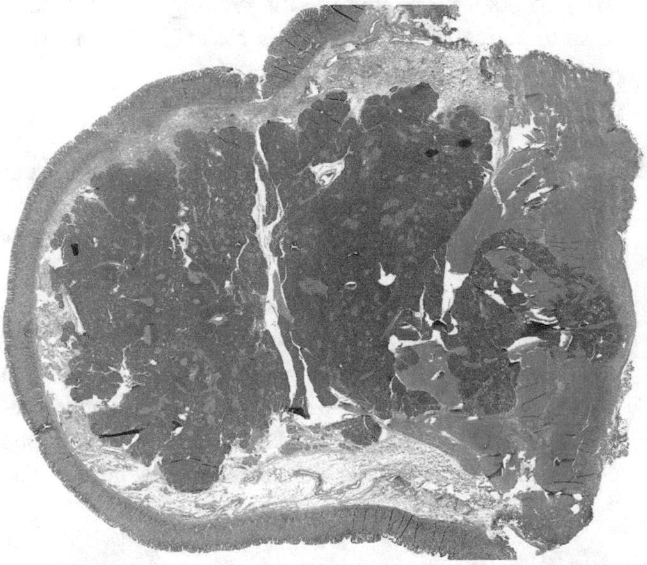

Fig. 1.4 Microphotograph of Fig. 1.3 showing gastric duplication consisting of a solid nodule of pancreatic tissue (Courtesy of Benjamin J. Wilkins, MD, PhD, Children's Hospital of Philadelphia)

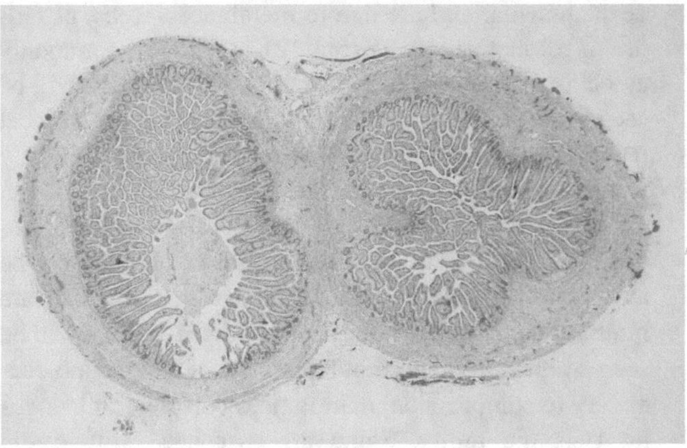

Fig. 1.5 Side-by-side tubular duplication of the small intestine

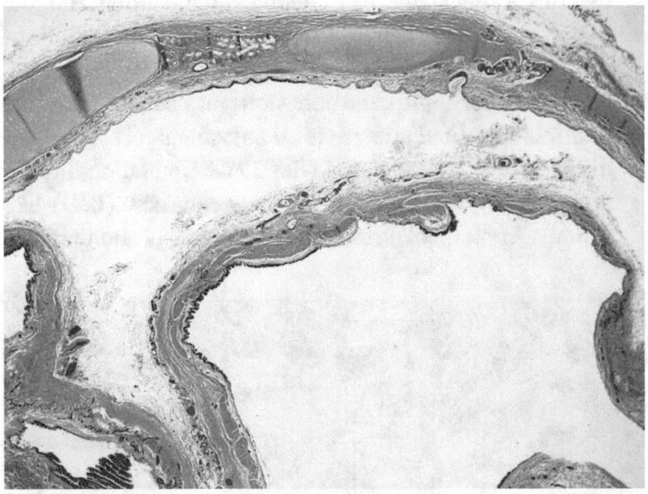

Fig. 1.6 An example of foregut duplication cyst which could be either bronchogenic cyst or esophageal duplication cyst depending on location. This was associated with the esophageal wall, so it is an esophageal duplication cyst

nar epithelium and have cartilage. Again, they are distinguished by location with an esophageal duplication cyst being associated with the wall of the esophagus and a bronchogenic cyst being associated with the tracheobronchial tree. Neurenteric cysts and remnants result from incomplete division of the embryonic ectoderm and endoderm. They are located dorsal to the gastrointestinal tract and may involve the vertebra, spinal cord, and dorsal skin. They may have neural components in addition to endodermal elements. They can be solid or cystic and can communicate with the gastrointestinal tract. Omphalomesenteric remnants are located in the ileum on the antimesenteric aspect. Duplications are located on the mesenteric aspect.

References: [1–3]

3. **Where are intestinal stenoses and atresias located, and what are their pathologic features? What mutation is associated with familial multiple intestinal atresias? What is an apple-peel atresia?**

The location of intestinal atresias and stenoses in order of frequency is duodenal (50%), jejunal-ileal (45%), and colonic (5%). The majority of duodenal atresias occur in the proximal duodenum and are often associated with syndromes or other anomalies. Most of these atresias are developmental and are due to membranes, webs, or failure of recanalization. Trisomy 21 is the most commonly associated syndrome in these cases. These defects will be seen in the perinatal autopsy setting but not in the surgical pathology setting as surgical correction does not typically result in a pathology specimen.

The atresias and stenoses of the distal duodenum, jejunum (Figs. 1.7 and 1.8), ileum, and colon can also be associated with syndromes or malformations, but they are often isolated. Many of these are resected, so they will be seen by the surgical pathologist. These lesions are secondary to compression, malrotation, volvulus, and vascular ischemic injury. Some are associated with cystic fibrosis. Some are post-inflammatory following necrotizing enterocolitis. The pathology of these types of injury is that of varying stages of ischemia and infarction. Remote injury is characterized by luminal and submucosal fibrosis and dystrophic calcification. If perforation occurred, meconium peritonitis and adhesions may be seen. Familial multiple intestinal atresias is an autosomal recessive condition, which is associated with *TTC7A* mutation, immunodeficiency, and inflammatory bowel disease (IBD)-like lesions. Apple-peel atresia is a rare anomaly and the most severe type of jejunal-ileal atresia. It can be familial and is an example which blurs the distinction between malformation and secondary ischemic injury or at least combines the two. Occlusion or maldevelopment of a major mesenteric vessel results in a segmental deficiency of both the mesentery and intestine. A fibrous band connects two abnormally attached blind-ended segments of the intestine, and this allows an apple-peel configured coiling and volvulus.
References: [1, 2]

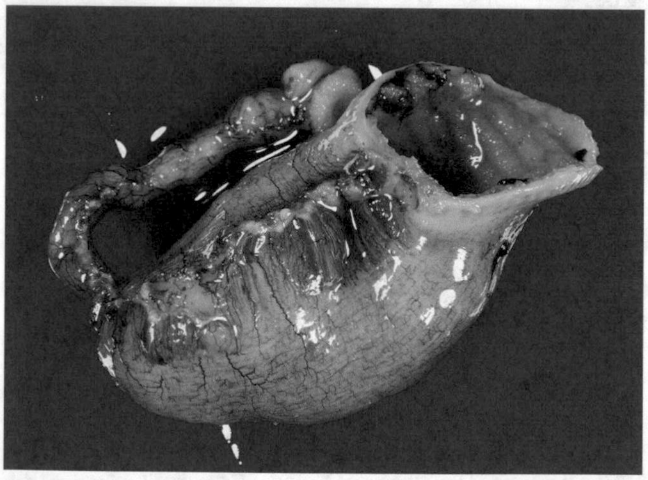

Fig. 1.7 Gross specimen of atresia involving the jejunum

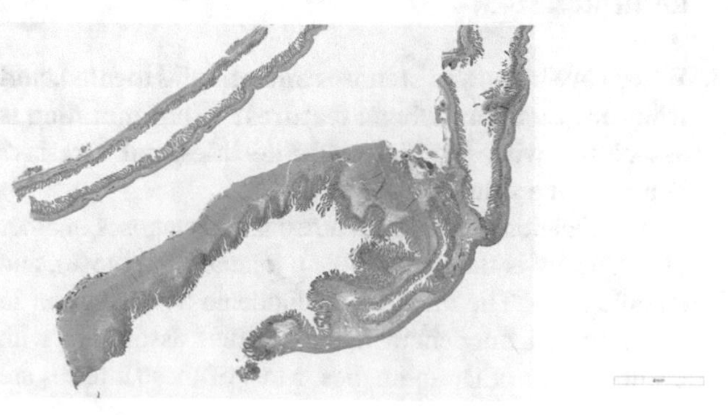

Fig. 1.8 Microphotograph of Fig. 1.7 showing jejunal atresia

4. **Which disorder may be associated with ileocolonic and colonic atresia/stenosis?**

   Atresia at these sites is much less common than the small intestine. When it occurs, there is an association with Hirschsprung disease (HD) so suction rectal biopsy may be warranted. The pathologist should look for ganglion cells in the atretic or stenotic segment (Figs. 1.9 and 1.10). If there are no ganglion cells in the stenotic segment and the rectal biopsy confirms HD, do not assume that the intervening large intestine is automatically aganglionic as rare skip lesions may occur in this setting.
   References: [1, 4]

5. **Anorectal malformation repair specimens may be sent for examination. If colonic epithelium, muscularis mucosae, and muscular wall are present, what needs to be documented?**

   Resected specimens from anorectal malformations of various types may include fistulae or malformed urogenital structures lined by various types of mucosa including transitional, indeterminate, or cloacogenic-type epithelium. If enough well-oriented colonic tissue is present, ganglion cells should be documented as HD

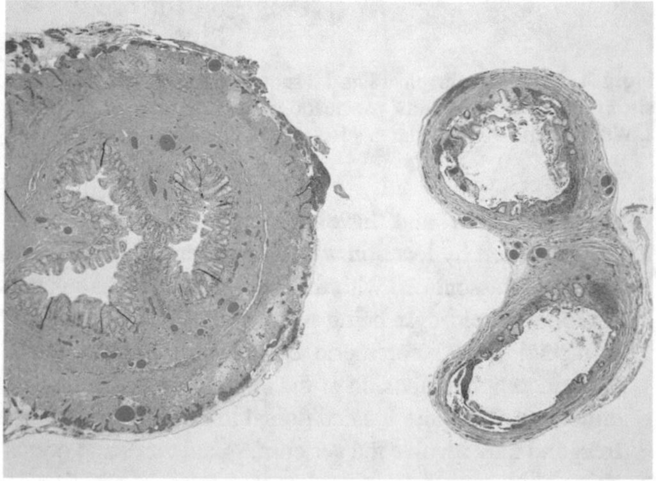

Fig. 1.9 Ileocolonic resection with atresia shown on the right. Ganglion cells were absent in a portion of the resected segment

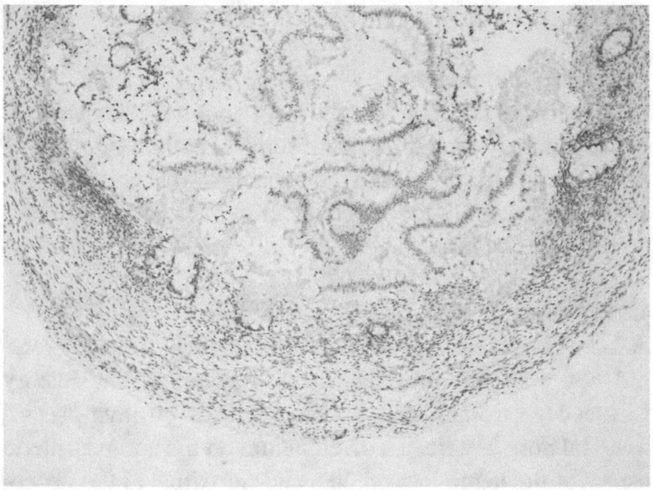

Fig. 1.10 Negative calretinin stain by immunohistochemistry performed on the ileocolonic resection specimen shown in Fig. 1.9. This patient subsequently underwent rectal suction biopsy which was aganglionic, confirming a diagnosis of Hirschsprung disease associated with ileocolonic atresia

may be associated with these malformations. Calretinin staining may aid in identifying ganglion cells and associated mucosal neurites. The presence of ganglion cells or calretinin staining in this setting may not exclude dysmotility or HD, but the absence could indicate HD. There are several case reports where the anorectal malformation is repaired, and the diagnosis of HD is delayed. Anorectal malformation combined with delayed HD diagnosis has been described in Down syndrome.

References: [5]

Case Presentation

Case 1

Learning Objectives

- To understand the gross and histologic findings of a gastrointestinal duplication
- To understand how to correlate pathological and surgical findings in order to classify an anomaly as a gastrointestinal duplication

Case History

A 15-month-old girl presented to the ER with flu symptoms and was found to have an abdominal mass which by ultrasound was 8 cm and cystic. At surgery, one end of the cyst was attached to the greater curvature of the stomach and communicated with the gastric antrum. The opposite end of the cyst was attached to a redundant portion of the pancreas which was attached to the normal pancreas.

Gross Description

A portion of gastric wall contained a cyst which was attached to a portion of tan lobulated pancreatic tissue.

Histologic Findings

The cyst was lined by ulcerated gastric oxyntic mucosa, and the cyst wall had a complete muscularis propria. Pancreatic tissue was confirmed extending from the cyst's muscular wall (Fig. 1.11).

Final Diagnosis

Gastric duplication cyst with accessory pancreatic lobe.

Take-Home Messages and Discussion

- In order to orient and classify this anomaly, review of the surgical findings is necessary.
- The location of the cyst and the intimate association with the gastrointestinal tract make this a gastrointestinal duplication.

Gastric duplications typically involve the greater curvature of the stomach and are uncommon relative to other duplications with approximately 5% being gastric. The associated anomaly of accessory pancreatic lobe is extremely rare.

References: [6]

Case 2

Learning Objectives

- To become familiar with the most common clinical features of neurenteric cyst
- To understand the main pathologic features of neurenteric cyst and be able to distinguish from gastrointestinal duplication cyst

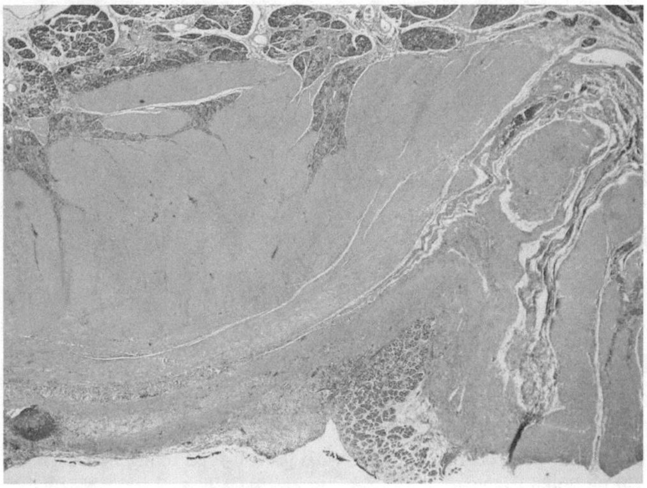

Fig. 1.11 Gastric duplication cyst with ulcerated oxyntic gastric lining (lower) and accessory pancreas (upper)

Case History
An 11-year-old boy was evaluated for back pain. An MRI revealed a 4-cm cystic intradural extramedullary mass anterior to and compressing the spinal cord at level C2–C4.

Gross Description
The resected tissue was dense and fibrous and contained a collapsed cyst. The tissue was 2 cm in maximum dimension.

Histologic Findings
Mucinous columnar epithelium resembling gastric foveolar epithelium lined a cyst wall in which a small amount of glioneuronal tissue was identified (Fig. 1.12).

Final Diagnosis
Neurenteric cyst.

Take-Home Messages and Discussion
- The diagnosis of neurenteric cyst rests on the pathologic findings and correlation with location and surgical findings.
- This case illustrates the features of most neurenteric cysts. Ninety to 95% are intradural and extramedullary and located ventral to the spinal cord. Fifty percent occur in the cervical spine. In children they are more common in males and occur at a mean age of 6.4 years.

Neurenteric cysts are rare congenital anomalies comprising 1% of spinal cord masses. Up to 50% can be associated with vertebral defects. They can extend dorsally to involve the spinal cord and dorsal skin or ventrally to involve the gastrointestinal tract. However, involvement of structures other than vertebrae is not common, occurring in only 10% of cases.
References: [7]

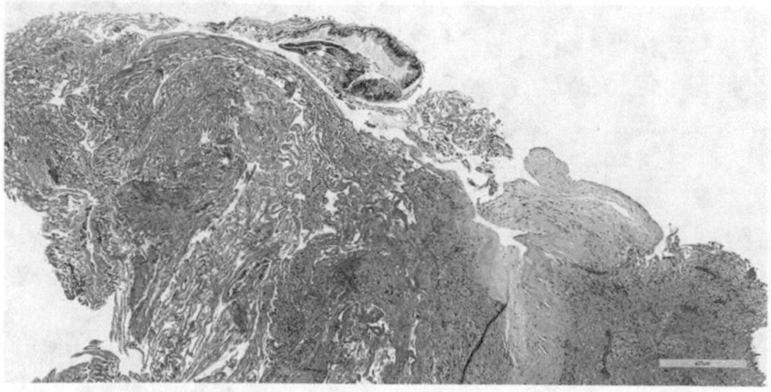

Fig. 1.12 Neurenteric remnant with gastric-type lining and adjacent glioneuronal tissue

Case 3

Learning Objectives
- To become familiar with the most common gastrointestinal anomaly seen in pediatric surgical pathology
- To become familiar with the variants of this anomaly
- To understand important clinical implications of heterotopic gastric tissue

Case History
A 2-cm-length blind-ended intestinal segment from a 2-year-old boy was submitted as "ileum segment." The history included gastrointestinal bleeding with a positive "scan." Surgical note described a diverticulum on the antimesenteric aspect of the ileum located 20 inches proximal to the ileocecal valve.

Gross Description
A blind-ended 2-cm piece of the intestine had a broad opening which was stapled. The mucosa had tan folds (Fig. 1.13) except at the tip where it was lighter yellow and more nodular.

Histologic Findings
The majority of the mucosa was small intestinal. The yellow nodular mucosa at the tip was gastric and included oxyntic glands.

Final Diagnosis
Omphalomesenteric remnant, Meckel diverticulum, with heterotopic gastric mucosa.

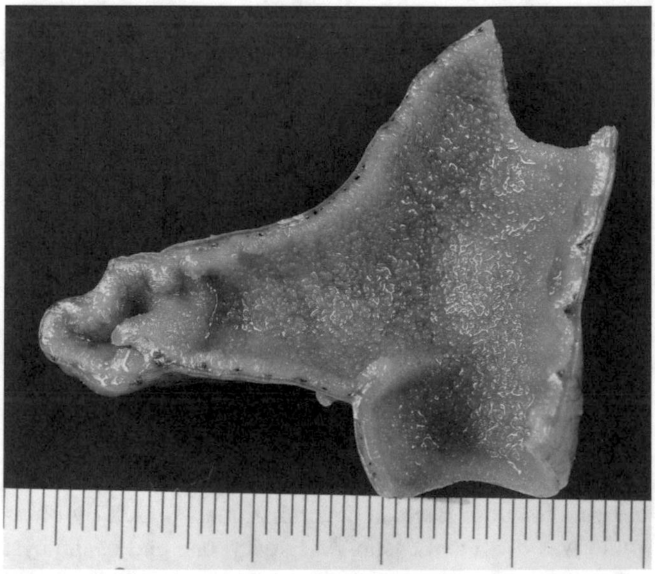

Fig. 1.13 Meckel diverticulum

Take-Home Messages and Discussion

- This is the classic history and site for Meckel diverticulum. It is the most common type of omphalomesenteric duct remnant and is the most common intestinal malformation that the surgical pathologist will encounter. They are found on the antimesenteric aspect of the intestine.
- A preoperative scan is often done to localize gastric mucosa which could account for the bleeding. The pathologist should attempt to confirm the presence of gastric mucosa and particularly the presence of acid-producing oxyntic mucosa (Figs. 1.14 and 1.15). Antral-type mucosa and pancreatic tissue may also be present (Fig. 1.16).

These types of remnants are estimated to occur in 2% of the population. Other less common omphalomesenteric duct remnants include umbilical-enteric fistula (persistent vitelline duct), and fibrous bands attaching the small intestine anteriorly to the umbilicus (vitelline band). Tissue submitted as umbilical polyp or umbilical remnant and containing small intestinal, gastric, or pancreatic tissue is another rare form of omphalomesenteric duct remnant (Fig. 1.17).
References: [1, 2, 8]

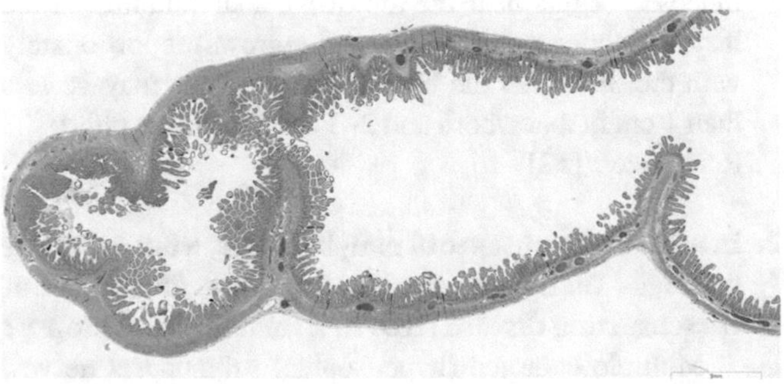

Fig. 1.14 Microphotograph of Fig. 1.13 showing heterotopic gastric mucosa at the tip of the diverticulum (yellow arrows). (Courtesy of Benjamin J. Wilkins, MD, PhD, Children's Hospital of Philadelphia)

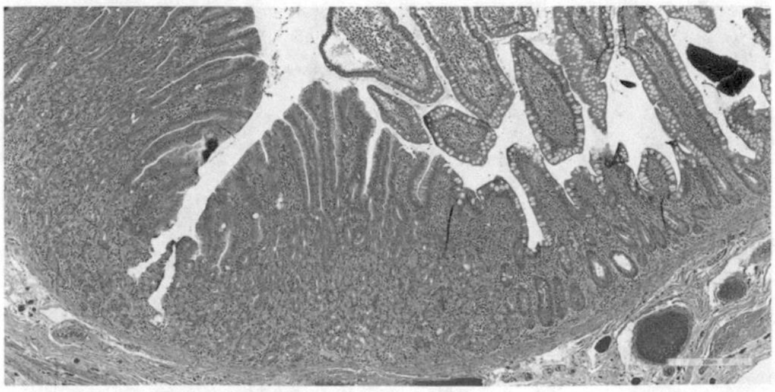

Fig. 1.15 Higher magnification of heterotopic gastric mucosa seen in Fig. 1.14. (Courtesy of Benjamin J. Wilkins, MD, PhD, Children's Hospital of Philadelphia)

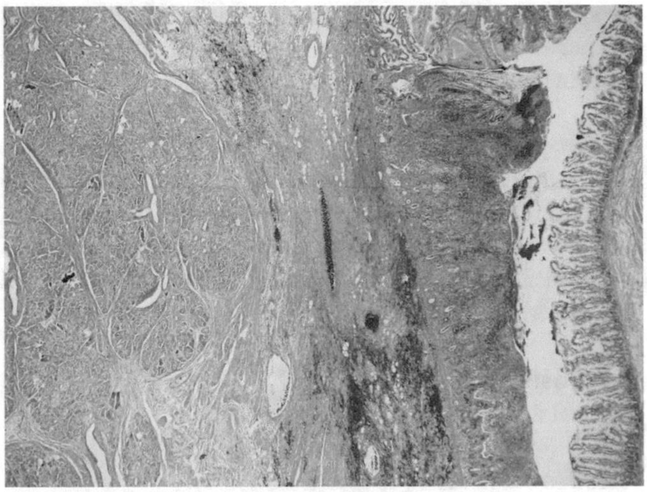

Fig. 1.16 Example of another Meckel diverticulum with pancreatic and gastric heterotopia and ulceration

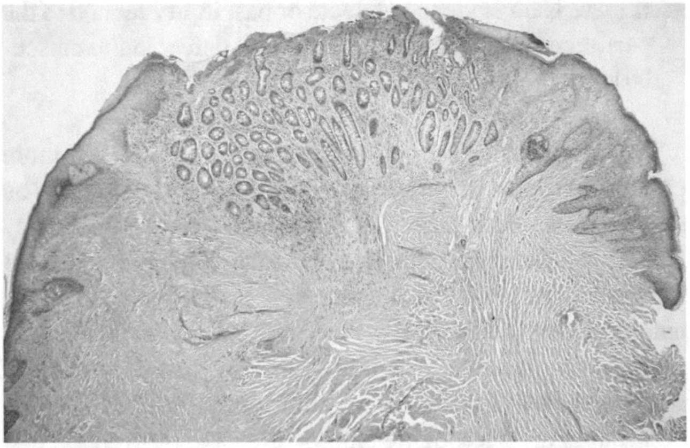

Fig. 1.17 Umbilical polyp with intestinal mucosa

Case 4

Learning Objectives

- To understand the different etiologies of small intestinal perforation in infants
- To understand important gross and histologic features to document in these specimens

Case History

A segment of the small intestine was resected from an infant with history of prematurity, indomethacin treatment for patent ductus arteriosus, and intestinal perforation. Clinical suspicion was necrotizing enterocolitis with perforation.

Gross Description

A 5-cm segment of the intestine had a uniform luminal diameter of 1 cm. A 1 cm wall defect was present in the center of the specimen. The mucosa was tan with folds. The serosa was tan and not dusky or ischemic appearing. The wall had a uniform thickness of 0.2 cm.

Histologic Findings

The mucosa and submucosa were normal-appearing with no histologic evidence of necrotizing enterocolitis or acute ischemic injury. There was no submucosal fibrosis or stricture. The muscularis propria was discontinuous and thin in the area of perforation (Fig. 1.18).

Diagnosis

Segmental absence of intestinal musculature.

Take-Home Messages and Discussion

- Gross examination of resected intestinal segments should document luminal diameter, stenosis, dilatation, atresia, adhesions, and perforation.
- If there is no evidence of acute or past injury related to the perforated area, look for a segmental defect in the muscularis propria.

Some question the causality of this finding, but more cases have been reported recently. The etiology may be remote ischemic injury. The muscle absence or deficiency has been described with and without varying degrees of inflammation. It may also occur as a sequela of necrotizing enterocolitis. Theoretically, the muscularis deficiency is prone to spontaneous perforation. It may also contribute to segmental dysmotility. Other more common etiologies of perforation are necrotizing enterocolitis and obstruction due to stenosis or atresia.
References: [9–11]

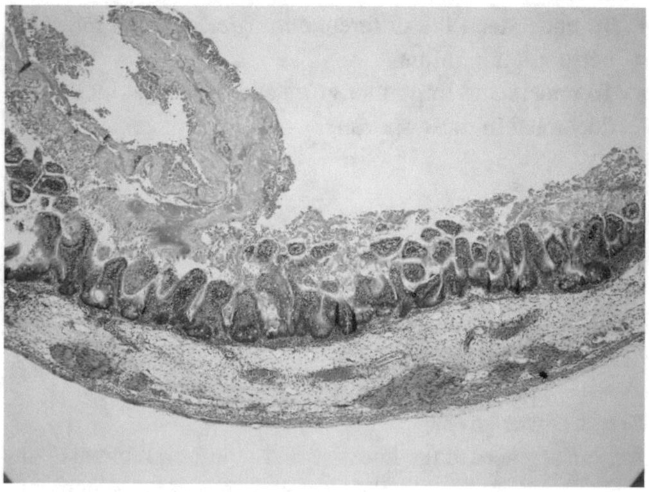

Fig. 1.18 Segmental absence of intestinal muscularis propria showing thin and discontinuous muscularis propria

Hirschsprung Disease

Frequently Asked Questions

1. **Why should suction rectal biopsy be performed 1 cm or higher above the dentate (pectinate) line? What is the dentate line?**

   The physiologic hypoganglionic zone extends approximately 1–2 cm above the dentate line in infants. In children older than 1 year of age, it may be longer. This means that ganglion cells may be sparse or absent in this region, and interpreting biopsies from the hypoganglionic zone has the potential for false-positive diagnosis. Ganglion cells are typically readily identified in biopsies above the hypoganglionic zone. Since the localization of biopsies is estimated and not typically done with direct visualization of the dentate line, biopsies from multiple levels help assure that areas above the hypoganglionic zone are sampled. The dentate line is a gross anatomical landmark at the bottom of the anal columns which roughly corresponds to the histologic transition from squamous mucosa to transitional mucosa. A synonym is pectinate line. In infants, the anal columns are lined by transitional mucosa. Colonic glandular mucosa with muscularis mucosae begins near the top of the anal columns, at the histologic anorectal line. This region grows proportionately with the infant, so the hypoganglionic zone may be less than 1 cm in a newborn and 2–3 cm in an older child.
   References: [12]

2. **In addition to absence of ganglion cells, what are other findings that are useful for the diagnosis of Hirschsprung disease (HD) in a suction rectal biopsy?**

   Multiple enlarged (hypertrophic) submucosal nerves, defined as >40 microns in diameter in an infant younger than 1 year of age (Fig. 1.19), favor HD. It is important to

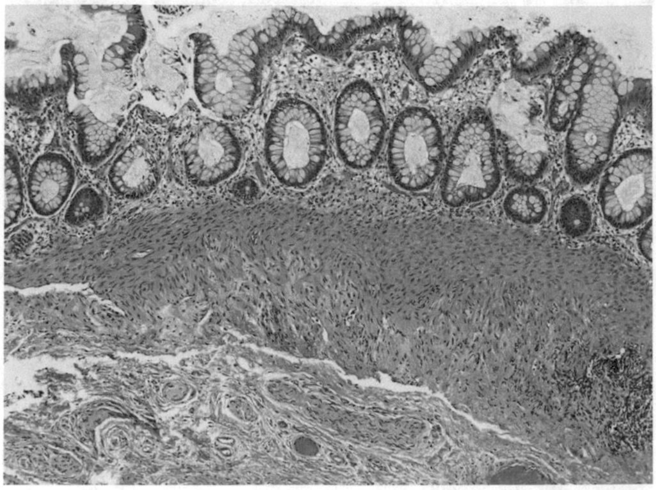

Fig. 1.19 An enlarged submucosal nerve measuring >40 microns in diameter in an infant less than 1 year of age

remember that this feature is neither sensitive nor specific. Number of enlarged nerves, degree of hypertrophy, and patient age are important considerations. Up to one third of patients with HD will not have enlarged submucosal nerves on rectal biopsy. Also, this feature should only be used for primary diagnosis in infants. It is not a reliable feature when examining biopsies in older patients or biopsies from patients being assessed for possible redo or revision operations.

The absence of calretinin-positive mucosal neurites or ganglion cells strongly favors HD (Fig. 1.20). Calretinin immunohistochemistry is an increasingly important adjunct tool in the diagnosis of HD, and its absence has been shown to be at least as good as the absence of ganglion cells. It also appears to be useful in biopsies with limited submucosa and in lower rectal biopsies from the hypoganglionic zone, which are usually considered technically inadequate. It is very important to have adequate control stains for comparison, and mast cells should stain as an important internal positive control. Calretinin immunohistochemistry may not work well on tissue that has been frozen.
References: [13–15]

3. **Does the finding of calretinin-positive neurites in the lamina propria rule out HD?**

The presence of abundant calretinin-positive neurites makes HD unlikely especially when found in the most distal biopsies, but it does not rule out HD completely because the transition zone and proximal aganglionic segment can have calretinin-positive mucosal neurites. The explanation is as follows:

The presence of calretinin-positive neurites in the lamina propria or muscularis mucosae indicates that there is a ganglion cell within approximately 2 cm. Calretinin is a very sensitive marker for the presence of ganglion cells. It appears that the neurites are extensions of ganglion cells themselves, and they seem to be up to 2.5 cm long.

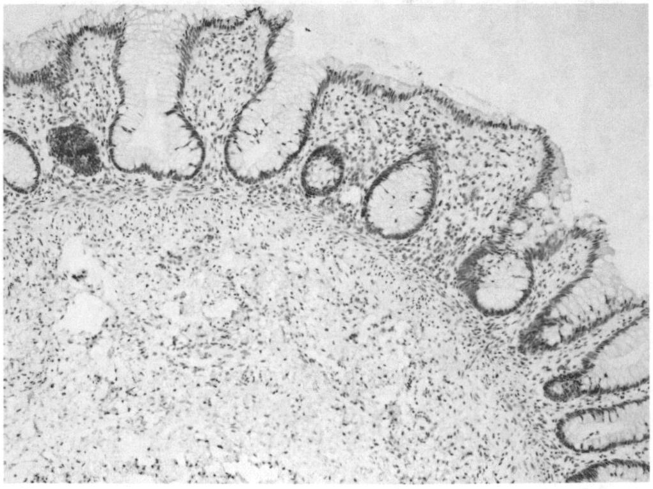

Fig. 1.20 Absence of calretinin-positive mucosal neurites

This is important for two reasons:

First, it means that neurites can extend from the last submucosal ganglion cell for approximately 2 cm. In fact, analysis of pull-through specimens showed that neurites extend distally from the level of the last ganglion cell for 1.5–2.5 cm. Therefore, overly proximal biopsies in very short-segment HD can have positive calretinin staining in the transition zone or the beginning of an aganglionic segment.

Second, it means that detecting calretinin-positive neurites, especially abundant, indicates that ganglion cells are nearby. The lower the biopsy, the shorter the aganglionic segment. Theoretically, if calretinin fibers are detected where the rectal mucosa ends, there may not be a pathologically detectable or clinically significant aganglionic segment. Since biopsies are not usually taken this low, this remains a potential area of investigation.
References: [16, 17]

Key points about calretinin:

- A negative stain with proper internal and external controls is strongly supportive of HD, if not diagnostic.
- A positive stain most often rules out HD but can miss the diagnosis in a small subset of very short-segment HD.

4. **What type of biopsy is done at the time of mapping and rectal pull-through procedure? In addition to identifying ganglion cells, what are other factors to consider when analyzing the frozen section biopsy?**

Seromuscular or full-thickness biopsies are sent for frozen section. Most are seromuscular only. These biopsies need to be oriented on edge on the frozen block to allow visualization of the myenteric plexus. Hopefully, the biopsy will be 4–5 mm long. If the biopsy is large enough, it will form a c-shape which can be oriented on the frozen block so the curve is on edge. The serosa will be located inside the curve (Fig. 1.21). In a well-oriented, 4–5-mm-length, seromuscular biopsy from normally ganglionated colon, ganglia should be readily identified (Fig. 1.22). There are no published data on myenteric ganglion cell density in HE-stained frozen sections, but there are limited data on HE-stained paraffin sections. In infants, average density is ten ganglia per 10 mm of myenteric plexus with two to six neurons per ganglion cell cluster.

The main objective at frozen section is to determine the presence or absence of ganglion cells. Other considerations during frozen section include size of the biopsy, orientation and visualization of the myenteric plexus, obscuring inflammation, and prominent nerves. If the

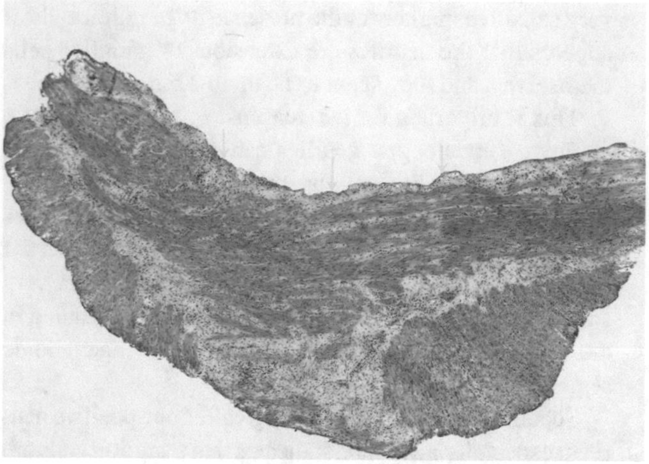

Fig. 1.21 A properly oriented seromuscular biopsy has a C-shape with serosa on the inner curve (yellow arrows). The myenteric plexus is well-visualized

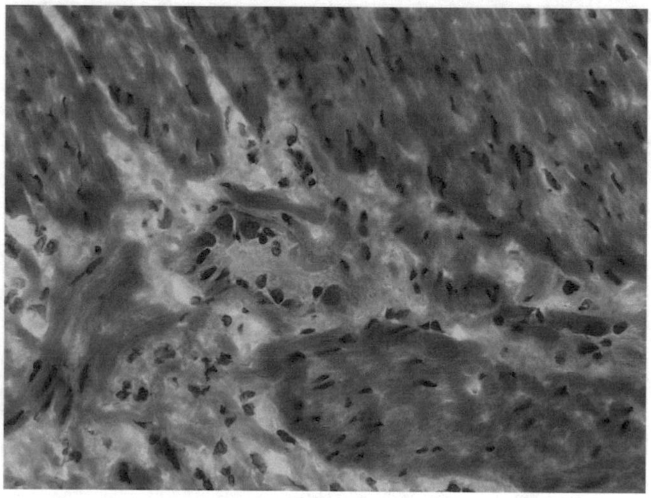

Fig. 1.22 Frozen section showing ganglion cells within myenteric plexus

biopsy is small (e.g., <3 mm) and/or not oriented well, it may not be possible to identify ganglion cells, and more tissue should be requested. Also, qualitative assessment of ganglion cell distribution is not reliable in small biopsies. If enough of the myenteric plexus is well-visualized and it is determined that ganglion cells are decreased, then seeing prominent nerves supports a transition zone area, and this should bc communicated to the surgeon. However, when frequent or normally distributed ganglion cells are seen, the significance of prominent nerves is uncertain. In fact, the significance of hypertrophic nerves (>40 microns in diameter) in ganglionated intestine is not established for certain. Finally, it is not uncommon for inflammatory cells and particularly eosinophils to obscure the myenteric plexus, and this can be a reason for frozen section error, deferral, or additional biopsy request.

After mapping and identifying where the ganglion cells end, the surgeon will resect above this level depending on vascular supply and estimation of the transition zone. The transition zone can measure 2–6 cm in length, and the surgeon will take this into consideration.
References: [16, 18]

5. **What is important to document in a pull-through specimen? What is the most reliable feature of a transition zone being present at the proximal margin?**

First, confirm aganglionosis and its length. Calretinin staining is useful for measuring the length of aganglionic segment. Second, confirm a normal circumferential distribution of ganglion cells in the myenteric plexus at the proximal margin. In order to do these two things, the minimum sectioning includes a complete circumferential donut section of the proximal margin en face and at least one complete longitudinal strip section. The longitudinal strip section can be done similar to a placental membrane roll section (Figs. 1.23 and 1.24) or in separate pieces with proximal and distal ends marked.

In some centers the entire proximal margin is sent for frozen section assessment, and circumferential ganglion cell distribution is assessed before the pull-through is completed. In other centers the circumferential proximal margin is only completely assessed after resection. Surgeons typically allow for transition zone and cut well above where the last ganglion cell is mapped, so the proximal margin is usually normally ganglionated.

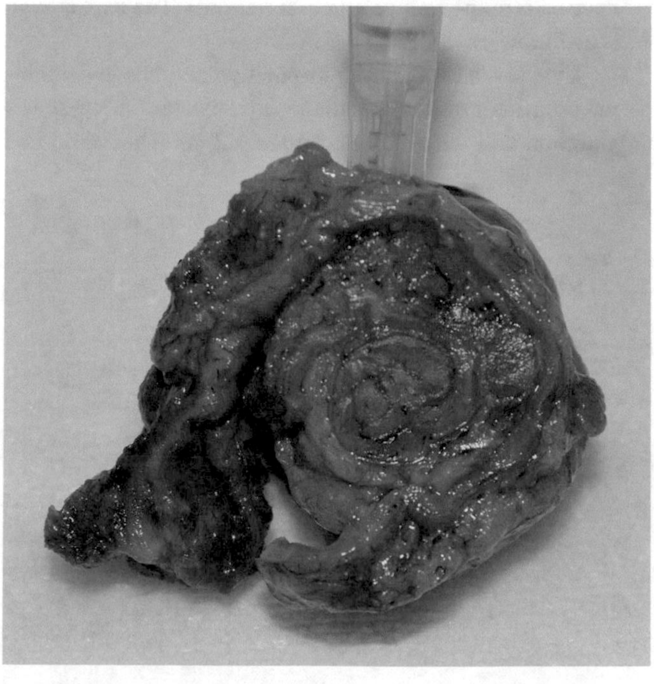

Fig. 1.23 Longitudinal strip section of anorectal pull-through specimen prepared as a roll section after formalin fixation

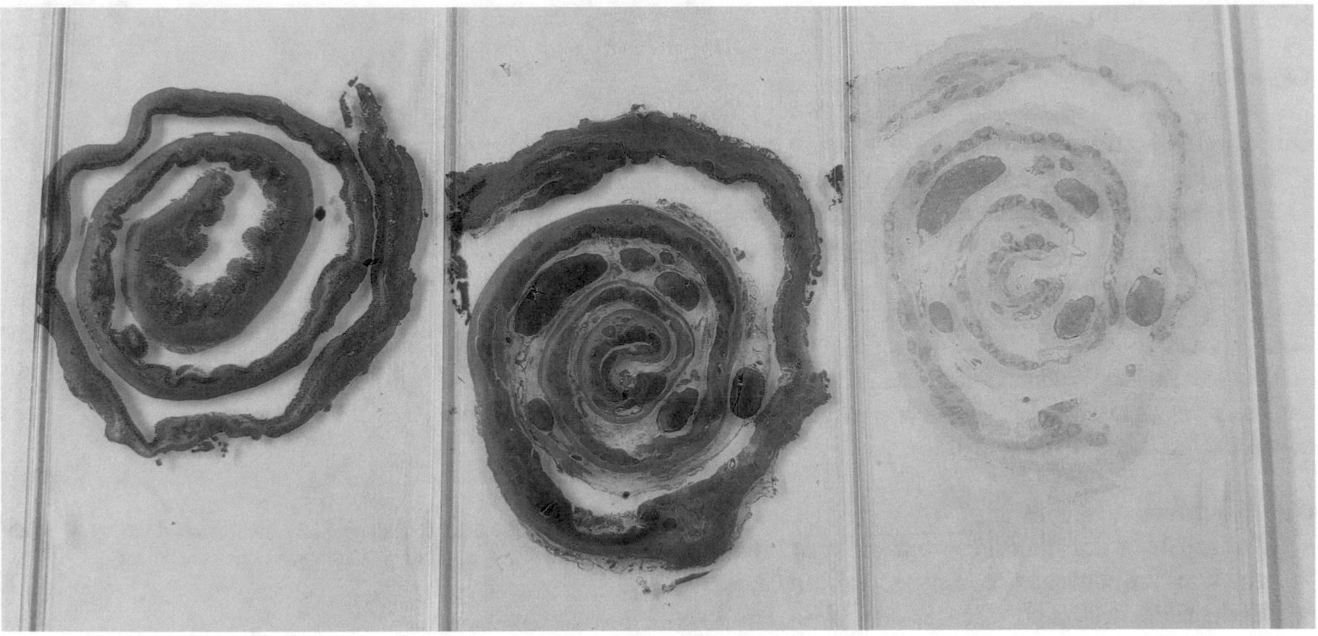

Fig. 1.24 HE and calretinin stains are used to document the length of aganglionosis in a longitudinal roll section

However, transition zone present at the proximal margin is still possible and occasionally encountered. An unequivocal diagnosis of transition zone at the proximal margin requires partial aganglionosis or severe myenteric hypoganglionosis in the proximal margin section. If this is found, then finding prominent nerves is supportive. However, the significance of hypertrophic nerves when there is normal ganglion cell distribution is uncertain, and the finding is not diagnostic of transition zone on its own. Neither is the finding of eosinophilic ganglionitis or other inflammation.

Finally, in small retrospective studies, there is evidence that transition zone at the pull-through proximal margin increases the chance of reocclusion. However it is important to note that not all patients with histologic transition zone at the proximal margin reocclude. The presence or absence of transition zone at the proximal margin does not reliably predict function in each case, but it may increase the chance of reocclusion.

References: [13, 19, 20]

6. **How do you diagnose intestinal neuronal dysplasia, hypoganglionosis, hyperganglionosis, and ultrashort HD?**

Pathologic diagnosis of motility disorders other than HD is an area of needed investigation. Definitions vary for each of these entities. There are not enough well-established criteria for normal versus abnormal neuronal cell density and distribution with clinical correlates for these forms of dysmotility. If these diagnoses are seriously being considered, then a research reference laboratory specializing in the specific disorder might be consulted. Finally, functional dysmotility may not have a current histopathologic correlate.

References: [21]

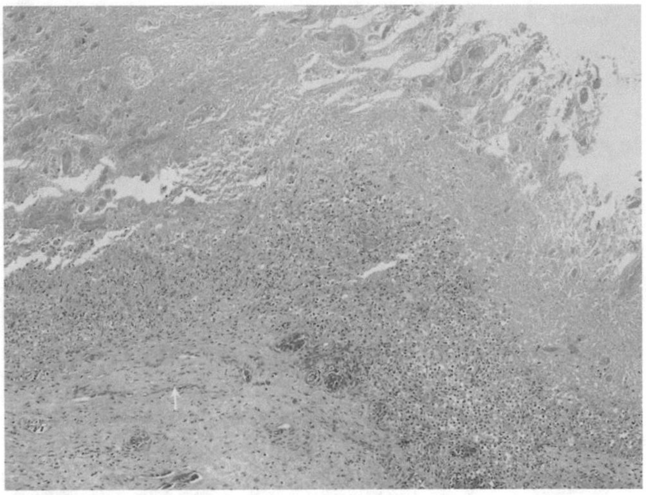

Fig. 1.25 Hirschsprung-associated enterocolitis. Yellow arrow indicates an enlarged submucosal nerve

7. **What is Hirschsprung-associated enterocolitis?**

Hirschsprung-associated enterocolitis is a major and life-threatening complication of HD. It may occur prior to diagnosis or weeks or months after pull-through or ostomy. Trisomy 21 is a risk factor for this complication. The pathology can be acute colitis with or without pseudomembranes or ischemic similar to necrotizing enterocolitis (Fig. 1.25).

References: [22]

Case Presentation

Case 1

Learning Objectives

- To recognize the clinical features of HD
- To understand the requirements of a satisfactory biopsy
- To understand how the suction rectal biopsy is performed and its limitations

Case History

A 3-day-old infant with abdominal distension had not spontaneously passed meconium. Barium enema revealed dilated bowel and rectosigmoid ratio of 1:1.

Questions and Answers

- What should be the clinical concern and what is the next step? What are published specimen recommendations?
- HD should be suspected. When the clinical/surgical diagnosis suggests HD, the next step in most centers is a suction rectal biopsy. Recommendations are one or two biopsies, each measuring approximately 3 mm or greater, taken at two levels, 1–2.5 cm above the dentate line.

Take-Home Messages and Discussion

- The classic history is that of an infant with abdominal distension who does not pass meconium within 24–48 hours of birth. A barium enema may be helpful. A normal rectosigmoid ratio is greater than 1:1.
- Biopsy site is estimated with respect to dentate line. Most centers use a standard suction biopsy device, and exact localization with respect to the dentate line is estimated but not directly visualized. The measurement is often made from the anal opening/verge with biopsies obtained at different levels. For example, biopsies can be obtained 1 cm, 2 cm, 3 cm, and/or 4 cm measured from the anal opening/verge. In infants the dentate line can be 1 mm to 1 cm proximal to the anal verge/opening. So, a 1 cm biopsy could be either too low or 1 cm above the dentate line. A 2 cm biopsy would be approximately 1 to 2 cm above the dentate line and so on. For that reason multiple levels of biopsies are advised.
- In order to look for ganglion cells, sufficient submucosa has to be present. Submucosa should comprise at least one third of a 3-mm specimen or be equal in thickness to the mucosa (Fig. 1.26). Biopsies with squamous or transitional mucosa by definition are within the hypoganglionic zone and too low for identification of ganglion cells.

  References: [21, 23]

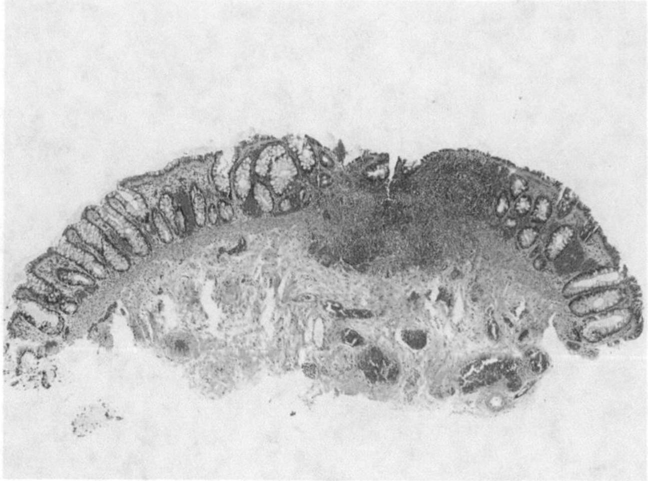

Fig. 1.26 (Case 1). An adequate 3-mm suction rectal biopsy with submucosa thickness equal or greater than mucosal thickness

Case 2

Learning Objectives

- To understand the implications of ileocolonic or colonic atresia in an infant
- To understand the implications of an aganglionic appendix
- To understand what a skip lesion is in HD

Case History

A newborn infant underwent loop ileostomy for ileocecal obstruction and at the same time the appendix was sent for pathology. Suction rectal biopsies were submitted from 2 cm and 4 cm.

Gross Description

The appendix was unremarkable and measured 3 cm in length and 0.4 cm in diameter. Rectal biopsies included two pieces of tissue from each site, with each biopsy measuring 3 mm in greatest dimension.

Histologic Findings

The appendix was aganglionic (Fig. 1.27). The rectal biopsies were without ganglion cells and had submucosal nerves that measured 45–60 microns in diameter.

Ancillary Studies

Immunohistochemistry for calretinin was negative in the appendix and rectal biopsies. There was no staining of mucosal neurites or ganglion cells in any specimens. Mast cells stained positive for calretinin.

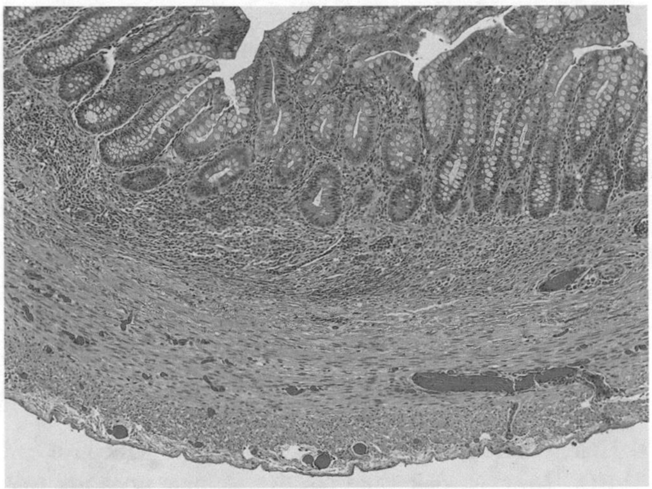

Fig. 1.27 (Case 2). Aganglionic appendix with no ganglion cells in the myenteric plexus

Differential Diagnosis

Total Colonic Hirschsprung Disease vs. Hirschsprung Disease with Skip Lesion

This patient has a rectal biopsy consistent with HD. In order to determine total colonic HD vs. skip lesion, seromuscular biopsy mapping needs to be performed. The appendix, in particular, may be skipped in neuronal migration so there may be normal ganglion cell distribution in the remainder of the gastrointestinal tract even though the appendix is aganglionic. Because this patient presented with ileocolonic obstruction, one should be concerned that the ileocecal region could be aganglionic, not just the appendix.

Follow-Up Seromuscular Biopsy with Pull-through Result

Seromuscular biopsies confirmed aganglionic distal ileum, ileocecal valve, and cecum, ganglionated right colon to splenic flexure, and aganglionic colon from the splenic flexure to the rectum. The infant underwent ileocecectomy and pull-through with preservation of the ganglionated right and transverse colon. Pull-through specimen confirmed aganglionosis involving the rectosigmoid colon to the splenic flexure. Ileocecectomy specimen confirmed aganglionosis of the terminal ileum, cecum, and portion of the ascending colon.

Final Diagnosis

Hirschsprung disease with skip lesion.

Take-Home Messages and Discussion

- This is a rare example of colonic skip lesion defined as two regions of aganglionosis with intervening ganglionated colon.
- Ileocolonic or colonic obstruction related to stenosis or atresia can be associated with HD. Any ileocecal or colon specimen with stenosis should be examined carefully for ganglion cells. Suction rectal biopsy to rule out distal aganglionosis may also need to be done.
- For skip lesion cases, there may be intervening functional colon that can be preserved.
- An aganglionic appendix can be seen without HD, since ganglion cells may skip the appendix during migration. In other words, the skip can be limited to the appendix. References: [13, 24]

Case 3

Learning Objectives

- To understand a typical protocol for processing suction rectal biopsies for HD
- To understand equivocal biopsy findings or how to handle an insufficient biopsy
- To understand calretinin staining in the transition zone or proximal aganglionic segment

Case History

A term newborn infant had abdominal distension and had not passed meconium for 2 days. Barium enema was equivocal. Suction rectal biopsies were received designated as 2 cm and 4 cm above the anal verge.

Gross Description

One specimen consisted of one 3-mm biopsy designated as proximal, 4 cm. A second specimen consisted of one 1-mm biopsy designated as distal, 2 cm.

Histologic Findings

Each piece was embedded separately with 50–100 HE-stained true serial sections examined for each piece. A mid-level section was reserved and stained with calretinin immunohistochemistry. This case was cut with priority and slides were out first the next morning. A single definite submucosal ganglion cell was seen in the 4-cm biopsy sections, and calretinin confirmed it to be a ganglion cell. Some calretinin-positive neurites were seen in the lamina propria and muscularis mucosae (Fig. 1.28). The 2-cm biopsy had mucosa only but without submucosa. Calretinin staining showed only one or two neurites within the muscularis mucosae, and they were difficult to find at high magnification. The lamina propria contained no neurites. Mast cells stained with calretinin (Fig. 1.29).

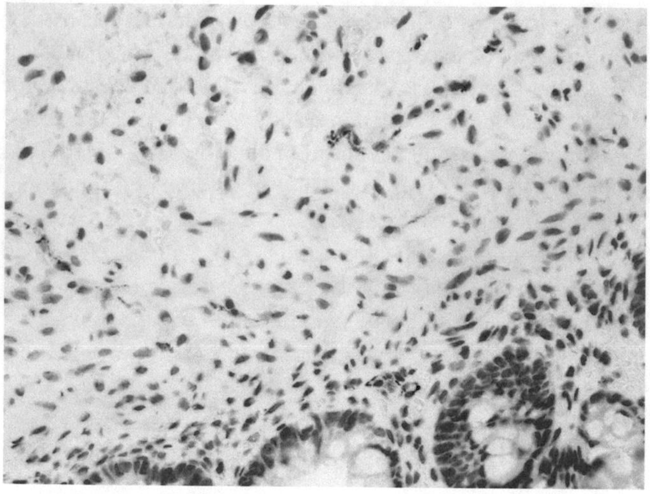

Fig. 1.28 (Case 3). Multiple calretinin-positive neurites in the muscularis mucosae at 4 cm above anal verge

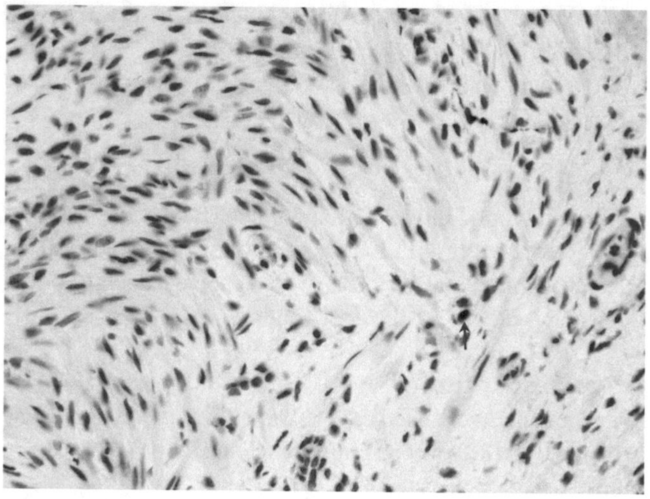

Fig. 1.29 (Case 3). A single calretinin-positive neurite in the muscularis mucosae (yellow arrow) and a positive mast cell as an internal control (red arrow) at 2 cm above anal verge

Differential Diagnosis

Normal vs. Short-Segment Hirschsprung Disease

The findings favor short-segment HD and additional biopsy is recommended. Because short segment seems likely, lower biopsies from 1 cm and 2 cm are requested.

Rebiopsy Findings

The 1 cm and 2 cm biopsies had adequate submucosa with no ganglion cells and no positive calretinin staining. These additional findings were consistent with HD.

Final Diagnosis

Pull-through resection specimen confirmed short-segment Hirschsprung disease with distal aganglionic segment measuring 5 cm.

Take-Home Messages and Discussion

- Extensive serial sectioning of suction rectal biopsies is typical in order to not miss ganglion cells when using HE-stained sections for diagnosis. Examining these sections is time-consuming and having these cases cut as priority limits delay and enables the surgical team to plan for surgery in the event of a HD diagnosis.
- In biopsies with inadequate submucosa or low biopsies with transitional or squamous mucosa adjacent to colonic mucosa, calretinin staining can give some information, but these biopsies are considered technically inadequate, and rebiopsy is typically needed.
- Calretinin-negative staining is highly indicative of HD. However, calretinin-positive staining does not rule out HD. Positive staining can be seen in overly proximal biopsies that sample transition zone or proximal aganglionic segment. These transition zone biopsies can have very few or reduced calretinin fibers.
- In this case, correlating the original set of biopsies to the pull-through specimen with an aganglionic segment, one can see that the original 2-cm and 4-cm biopsies are overly proximal but are within a reasonable estimate of the stated biopsy site. It is important to keep in mind that the biopsy site designations are estimates with respect to the dentate line as the dentate line is not specifically visualized during the biopsy in most cases. The original biopsies are from the transition zone/proximal aganglionic segment explaining why a single ganglion cell is seen at 4 cm and only rare calretinin fibers are seen at 2 cm.

Volvulus, Intussusception, and Necrotizing Enterocolitis

Frequently Asked Questions

1. **How does pediatric volvulus differ from adult volvulus? What is the pathology of pediatric volvulus and intussusception?**

   Pediatric volvulus most commonly involves the small intestine and is associated with malrotation, abnormal mesenteric attachments, or other developmental anomalies such as Meckel diverticulum or duplication. Adult volvulus is more common in the large intestine and is associated with acquired adhesions. Both volvulus and intussusception will have pathologic features of acute hemorrhagic infarction and necrosis. Both may be caused by mass lesions.

   References: [25]

2. What are possible pathologic lead points in pediatric intussusception? What is the most common malignancy associated with pediatric intussusception?

Most pediatric intussusceptions are primary or idiopathic and can be reduced without surgical excision. On occasion a primary intussusception will result in advanced necrosis of the intestinal segment requiring excision (Fig. 1.30). Secondary intussusceptions are those associated with pathologic lead points, and these require surgical excision. A pathologic lead point should be carefully looked for and ruled out in resected segments. In the pediatric age group, pathologic lead points include physiologic lymphoid hyperplasia, hyperplastic Peyer patch lymphoid tissue associated with viral infection, Meckel diverticulum, duplications, lymphatic or vascular lesions, and polyps (Fig. 1.31). If nuclear adenoviral inclusions in epithelial cells are suspected in association with lymphoid hyperplasia, immunohistochemistry is available to confirm. The most common malignant lesion would be lymphoma and in particular Burkitt lymphoma.

References: [26, 27]

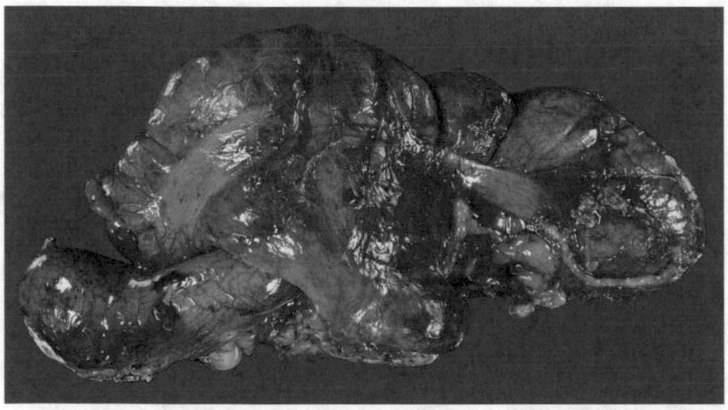

Fig. 1.30 Resected ileocecal intussusception

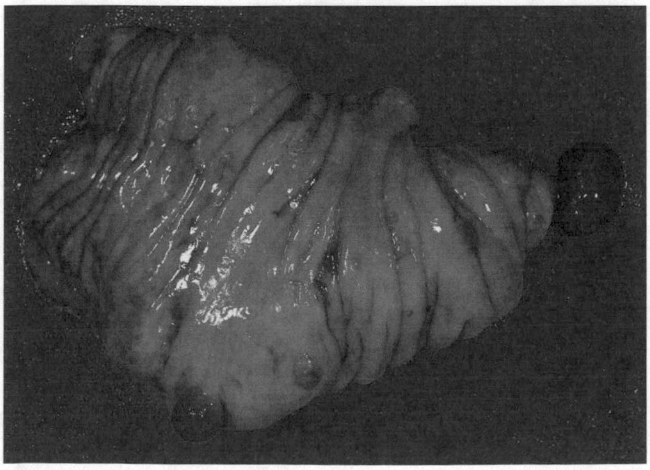

Fig. 1.31 Polyp as pathologic lead point producing intussusception

3. What are the major histopathologic features of necrotizing enterocolitis?

The basic pathology of necrotizing enterocolitis (NEC) is acute ischemic injury with relatively little inflammatory response. Acute hemorrhagic ischemic necrosis, submucosal edema, and infarction are present. There may be air within lymphatics corresponding to pneumatosis intestinalis (Fig. 1.32), which results from bacterial overgrowth and fermentation. The air pockets may involve all layers of the intestine. Vessel thrombosis is often present and thought to be secondary. Histiocytes and pigment in the serosa is evidence of meconium peritonitis (Fig. 1.33) due to perforation. Typically NEC involves the small intestine (Fig. 1.34). The most common area is the ileocecal region, but the process may also involve the large intestine.

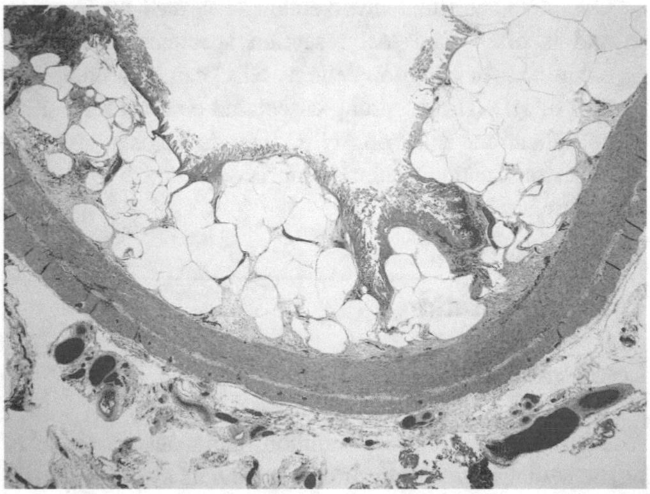

Fig. 1.32 Air-filled spaces of pneumatosis intestinalis dramatically filling the submucosa in necrotizing enterocolitis

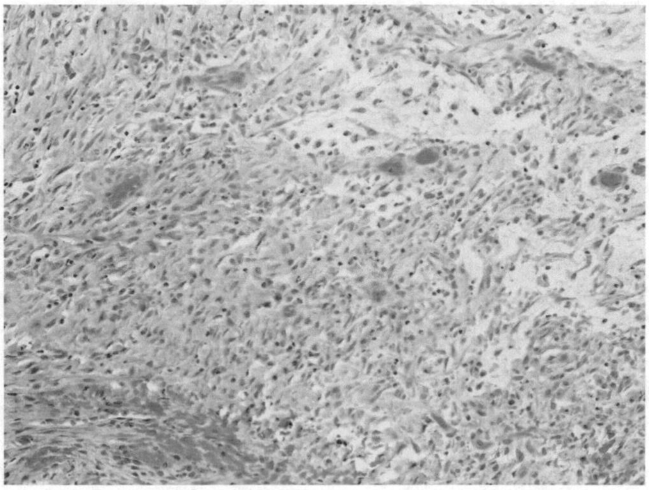

Fig. 1.33 Meconium peritonitis showing numerous brown pigmented macrophages in the serosa

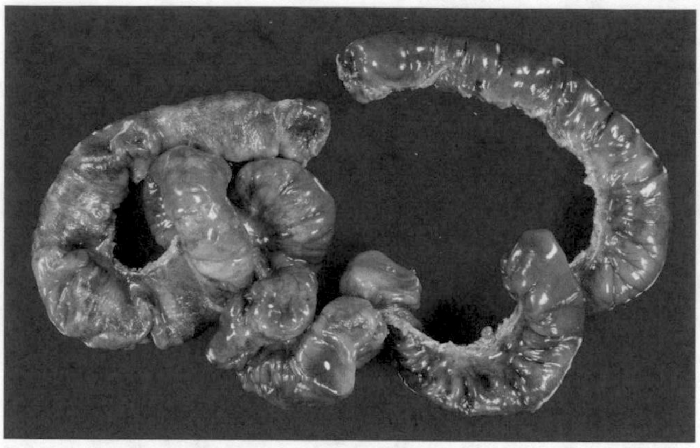

Fig. 1.34 Resected infarcted small intestinal segment with necrotizing enterocolitis. The segment is dull and purple-gray

Complete intestinal involvement is termed NEC totalis and is often fatal. All resection specimens should be examined for ganglion cells as NEC can be a complication of HD (Hirschsprung-associated enterocolitis). Late complications following NEC include fibrosis, stricture, adhesions, and muscularis propria defects.

References: [28]

Case Presentation

Learning Objectives

- To recognize the most common malignant neoplasm of the pediatric gastrointestinal tract and its association with intussusception

Case History

A 12-year-old boy presented with ileocecal intussusception requiring surgical resection for an ileocecal mass.

Gross Description

The gross specimen included an ulcerated mass just proximal to the ileocecal valve (Fig. 1.35). The mass was located primarily within the submucosa and muscular wall.

Histologic Findings

The submucosa contained sheets of discohesive, monomorphic small blue cells with interspersed macrophages, forming a starry sky pattern (Figs. 1.36 and 1.37). The overlying small intestinal mucosa was mostly intact with focal ulceration. Touch preps stained with Diff-Quik also showed discohesive atypical lymphoid cells with deep blue vacuolated cytoplasm.

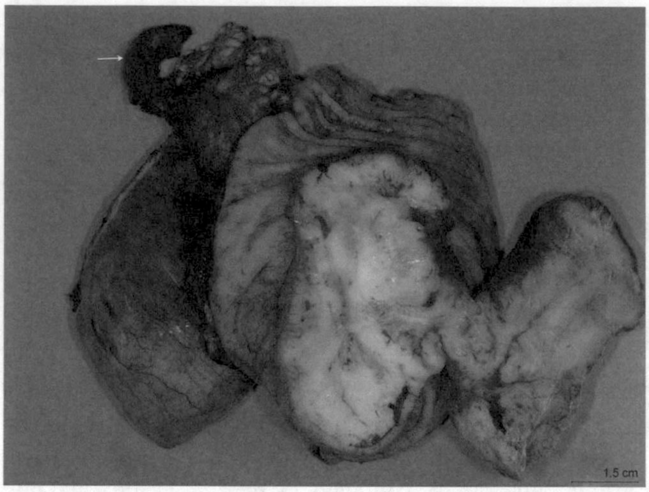

Fig. 1.35 (Case) Resected ileocecal specimen with a lymphoma filling the submucosa. A yellow arrow indicates the appendix

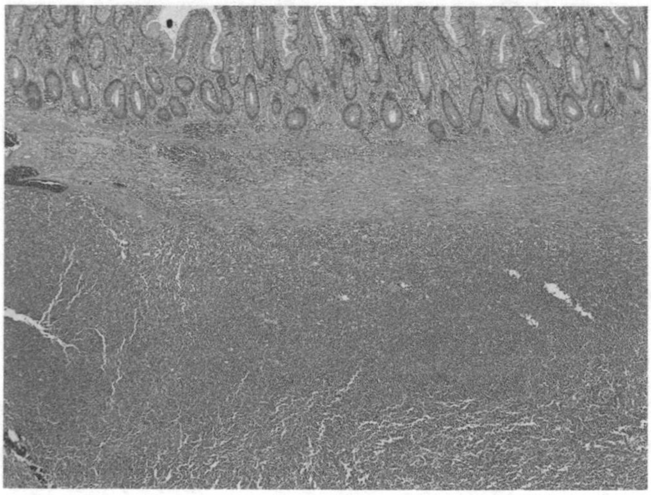

Fig. 1.36 (Case) Low-power view of Burkitt lymphoma involving the ileum

Differential Diagnosis

- Burkitt lymphoma
- Other high-grade lymphomas: diffuse large B-cell lymphoma, Burkitt-like lymphoma with 11q aberration, anaplastic large cell lymphoma
- Small blue cell tumor other than lymphoma: alveolar rhabdomyosarcoma, desmoplastic small round cell tumor

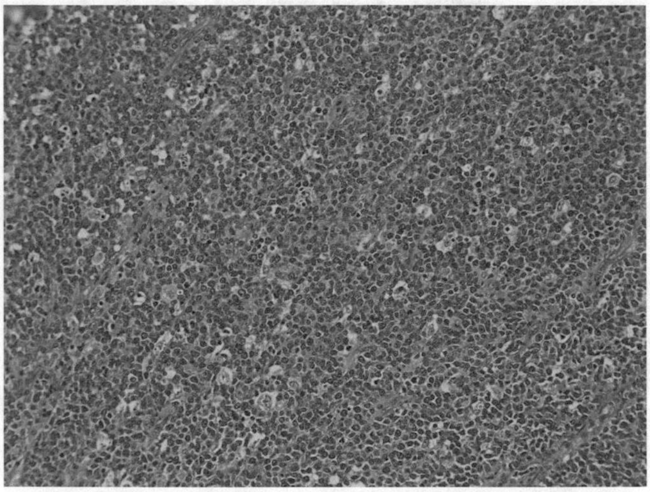

Fig. 1.37 (Case) High-power view showing a starry sky pattern of Burkitt lymphoma

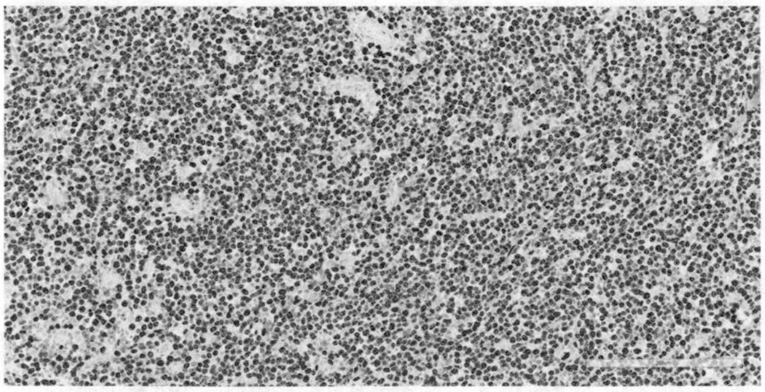

Fig. 1.38 (Case) Near 100% Ki-67 proliferative index in Burkitt lymphoma. (Courtesy of Benjamin J. Wilkins, MD, PhD, Children's Hospital of Philadelphia)

Ancillary Studies

Immunohistochemistry: CD20+, CD10+, BCL6+, BCL2-, TdT-, Ki-67 > 95% (Fig. 1.38).

FISH: 8q24 MYC translocation present.

EBV ISH: negative.

Final Diagnosis

Burkitt lymphoma associated with intussusception.

Take-Home Messages and Discussion

- Lymphoma is the most common malignant tumor of the pediatric gastrointestinal tract. Burkitt lymphoma involving the ileocecal region is the most common of the pediatric gastrointestinal lymphomas.
- Lymphomas in the pediatric gastrointestinal tract are almost always high-grade and typically occur in the older child.
- Pathologic lead points associated with intussusception include lymphoma as well as benign lesions. All intussusception specimens should be examined carefully for pathologic lead points.
  References: [29]

Tumors and Polyps

Frequently Asked Questions

1. **How is pediatric gastrointestinal stromal tumor different from adult counterpart?**

   Gastrointestinal stromal tumor (GIST) is relatively common in adults but extremely rare in children. Most adult tumors have *KIT* or *PDGFRA* mutations, making them candidates for targeted therapy. Most tumors in children lack these mutations, however. Mutations in succinate dehydrogenase complex are more common in pediatric tumors. Immunohistochemistry for SDHB is a sensitive and specific test for picking up these mutations, which can also indicate association with Carney triad (GIST, pulmonary chordoma, paraganglioma) and Carney-Stratakis syndrome (GIST and paragangliomas). SDHB-deficient pediatric GISTs are typically multifocal, occur in the stomach, and have an epithelioid appearance (Figs. 1.39 and 1.40). Another type of pediatric *KIT* and *PDGFRA* wild-type GIST is NF1-associated. These tumors are typically spindled and occur in the small intestine. On the whole, pediatric GISTs are less aggressive than adult tumors, and the adult risk stratification based on size, site, and mitotic rate is not applicable. Like adult tumors, pediatric GISTs are positive for CD117 and/or DOG1 and thought to arise from the interstitial cell of Cajal lineage.

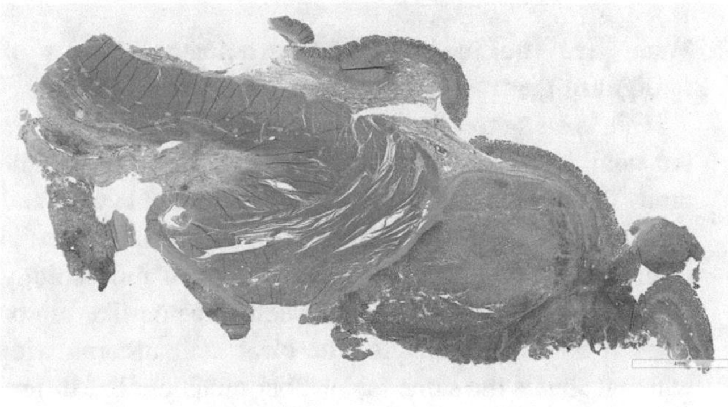

Fig. 1.39 A pediatric gastrointestinal stromal tumor involving the submucosa of the stomach

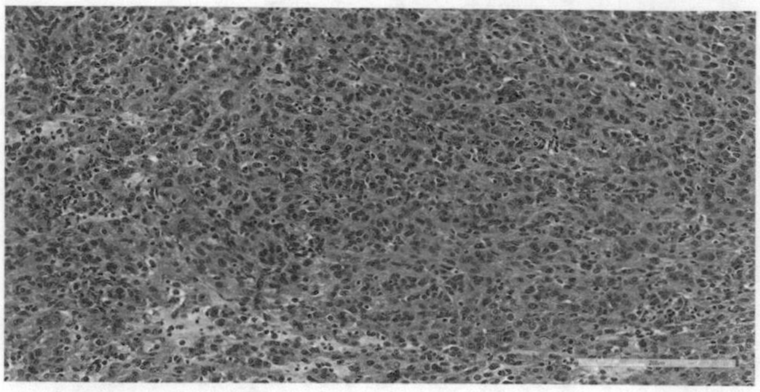

Fig. 1.40 Pediatric gastrointestinal stromal tumor of the stomach showing an epithelioid morphology. (Courtesy of Benjamin J. Wilkins, MD, PhD, Children's Hospital of Philadelphia)

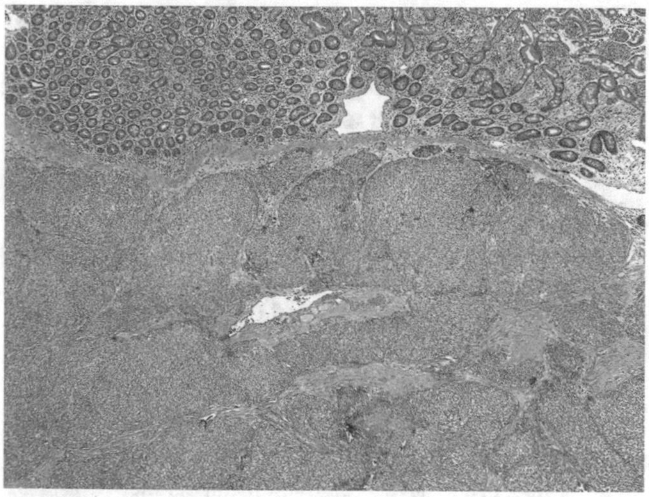

Fig. 1.41 Malignant gastrointestinal neuroectodermal tumor involving the submucosa of the small intestine. Tumor cells are arranged in solid, nested, and pseudoalveolar patterns in fibrous stroma

Other stromal tumors that may rarely involve the gastrointestinal tract include inflammatory myofibroblastic tumor, fibromatosis/myofibromatosis, nerve sheath tumor, and ganglioneuroma. Leiomyoma is also a possibility if GIST is ruled out.
References: [30, 31]

2. **What are the major clinicopathologic features of malignant gastrointestinal neuroectodermal tumor?**

This is an aggressive tumor which most often involves the small intestine of young adults and can occur in children. The tumor mainly involves the muscular wall and submucosa and grows in sheets of undifferentiated cells (Fig. 1.41) with focal or diffuse clear cell morphology (Fig. 1.42). A synonym is clear cell sarcoma-like tumor since it is very similar to true clear cell sarcoma with which it shares the same fusion abnormalities. The difference is that malignant gastrointestinal neuroectodermal tumor does not express melanocytic markers and true clear cell sarcoma does. Like true clear cell sarcoma,

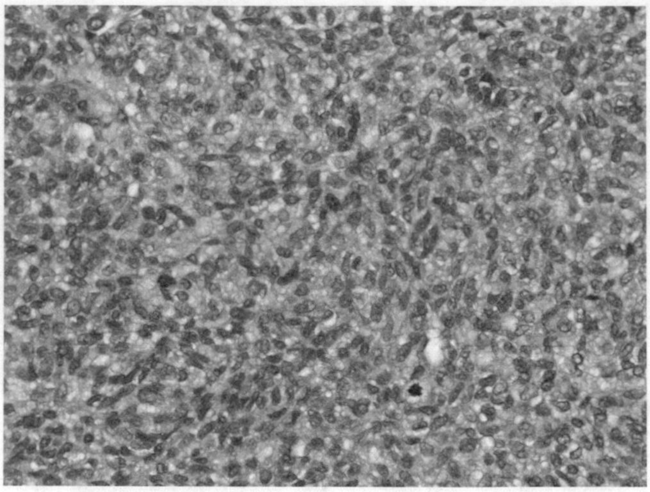

Fig. 1.42 Malignant gastrointestinal neuroectodermal tumor showing small, primitive tumor cells with clear cell sarcoma-like morphology

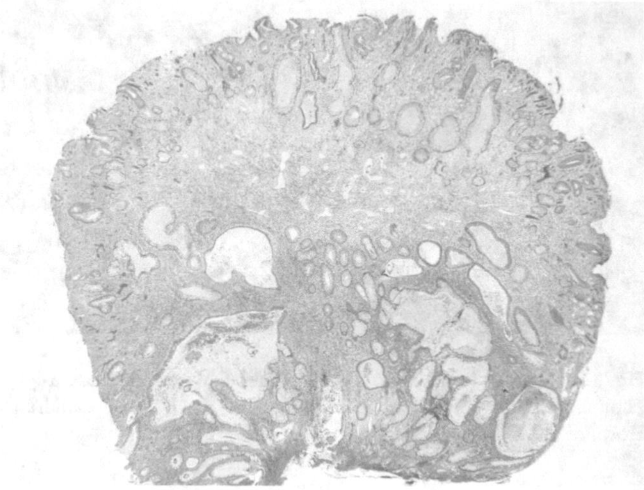

Fig. 1.43 Low-power view of a juvenile polyp

however, the tumor cells are positive for S100 and SOX10 and may have EWSR1-ATF1 or EWSR1-CREB fusions.
References: [32]

3. **What is the most common pediatric gastrointestinal polyp?**

Juvenile polyp is the most common polyp of the pediatric gastrointestinal tract. Sporadic juvenile polyps may affect up to 2% of children under 10, and the vast majority are not associated with any syndrome and do not require additional work-up. The polyp has an inflammatory stroma and disordered cystic mucinous glands and is often eroded/ulcerated. It does not have the smooth muscle or arborizing architecture of a Peutz-Jeghers-type hamartomatous polyp. Most juvenile polyps have straightforward histology (Figs. 1.43 and 1.44). When they occur in adults, they are still termed juvenile polyps. Terms such as inflammatory

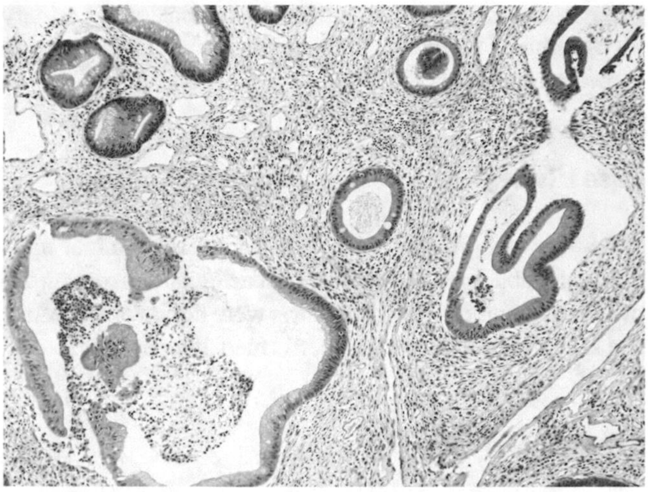

Fig. 1.44 Higher-power view of a juvenile polyp showing dilated glands and inflammatory stroma

polyp, hamartomatous polyp, or retention polyp could result in clinical misinterpretation. One or two isolated polyps in a patient without a family history is considered sporadic and not syndrome-associated. When there are three or more polyps or there is a family history, clinical work-up for a polyposis syndrome should be considered. Since these types of polyps can occur in several syndromes, the work-up may include evaluation for juvenile polyposis as well as other syndromes.
References: [30, 33]

4. What is juvenile polyposis?

This refers to syndromes in which there are multiple gastrointestinal juvenile polyps, specific gene mutations are identified, and/or other syndromes are ruled out by genetic testing. As described in Question 3, patients with three or more juvenile polyps require work-up. Two main forms exist and seem to be variant expressions of one disorder as both forms may occur in the same family. These two forms, juvenile polyposis coli and generalized juvenile polyposis, are autosomal dominant with most having mutations in *SMAD4* or *BMPR1A*. Gastrointestinal carcinoma may arise from adenomatous change within or outside a juvenile polyp in syndromic patients. A third form is rare, occurs in infancy, and is associated with multiple polyps, bleeding, and polyp-associated enteropathy. This form, juvenile polyposis of infancy, often has a poor outcome and is associated with contiguous gene deletions in *SMAD4* and *BMPR1A* on 10q. Please see Chap. 15, Question 12, for additional detail.
References: [33]

5. What is a hamartomatous polyp?

Although hamartomatous polyp is usually referred to as Peutz-Jeghers-type polyp, it is a confusing term because it tends to be used in the clinical literature to include any polyp occurring with a syndrome such as juvenile polyp. Therefore, if the term hamartomatous is used to describe a polyp pathologically, the type of hamartomatous polyp should be specified.

The following list of syndromes each has a major type of associated polyp. The Peutz-Jeghers-type polyps are almost always syndromic. Juvenile and ganglioneuromatous polyps are seen in various syndromes but are more often solitary or sporadic rather than syndromic.

Peutz-Jeghers syndrome: Peutz-Jeghers polyp (Figs. 1.45 and 1.46). These have complex, arborizing glands with prominent smooth muscle cores.

Juvenile polyposis syndromes: juvenile polyps. Inflammatory stroma with disorganized and cystic mucinous glands (Figs. 1.43 and 1.44).

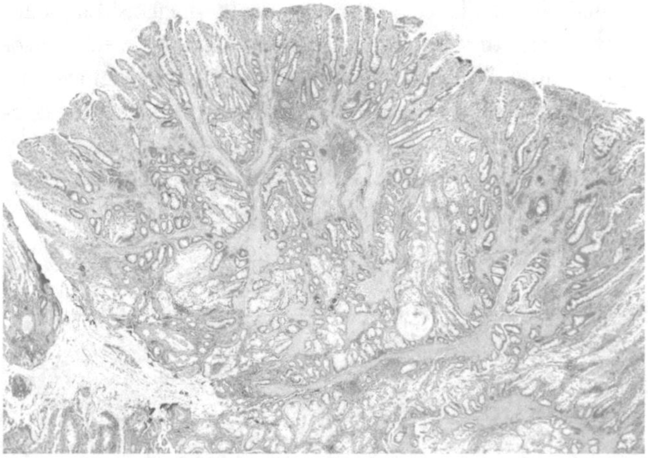

Fig. 1.45 Hamartomatous Peutz-Jeghers-type polyp showing hyperplastic glands separated by prominent smooth muscle bundles into lobules

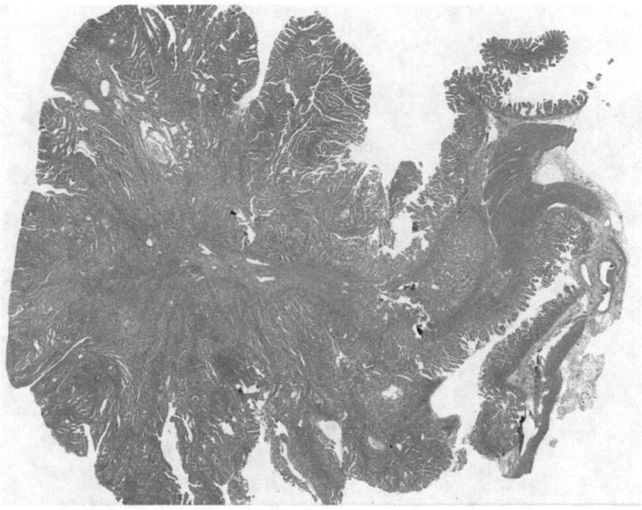

Fig. 1.46 Low-power view of a Peutz-Jeghers-type polyp showing an arborizing architecture. (Courtesy of Benjamin J. Wilkins, MD, PhD, Children's Hospital of Philadelphia)

PTEN-associated Cowden syndrome: Peutz-Jeghers-type polyps, juvenile polyps, lipomatous polyps, ganglioneuromatous polyps, hyperplastic polyps, and inflammatory polyps.

PTEN-associated Bannayan-Riley-Ruvalcaba syndrome: juvenile polyps.

Tuberous sclerosis: Peutz-Jeghers-type polyps.

Cronkhite-Canada syndrome: juvenile polyps.

Neurofibromatosis and MEN2b: ganglioneuromatous polyps (Fig. 1.47). These polyps are composed of Schwann cell stroma and ganglion cells expanding the lamina propria.

References: [30, 33–35] for More Information

6. **What are the pathologic characteristics and clinical behavior of appendiceal carcinoid in children?**

Pediatric appendiceal carcinoids are well-differentiated neuroendocrine tumors typically diagnosed incidentally with or without acute appendicitis. A recent review of nearly 1000 cases found that these tumors behave in a benign fashion even with positive lymph nodes. The conclusion is that, in children, appendectomy and cecectomy is a sufficient treatment for appendiceal carcinoids regardless of size, stage, or lymph node status.

References: [36]

Case Presentation

Learning Objectives

- To understand the differential diagnosis of a small round cell tumor of the abdomen in pediatric pathology
- To know the proper immunohistochemical and ancillary work-up of an intraabdominal small round cell tumor in pediatric patients

Case History

A 14-year-old girl presented with an intraabdominal mass filling the abdomen and pelvis, obscuring and involving the ovaries and mesentery. The kidneys were not involved. A frozen section of the tumor was performed at laparotomy.

Gross Description

The submitted tissue was white and firm and measured 1.5 × 1.0 × 1.0 cm. A representative piece, approximately one third of the biopsy, was frozen for intraoperative consultation.

Histologic Findings

Frozen section showed a neoplasm with fibrous stroma surrounding a monomorphic malignant round cell population. This was confirmed on permanent section (Fig. 1.48).

Differential Diagnosis

Desmoplastic small round cell tumor, translocation-associated sarcoma, lymphoma, blastemal Wilms tumor (less likely), dysgerminoma (less likely).

Ancillary Studies

Flow cytometry: not hematolymphoid.

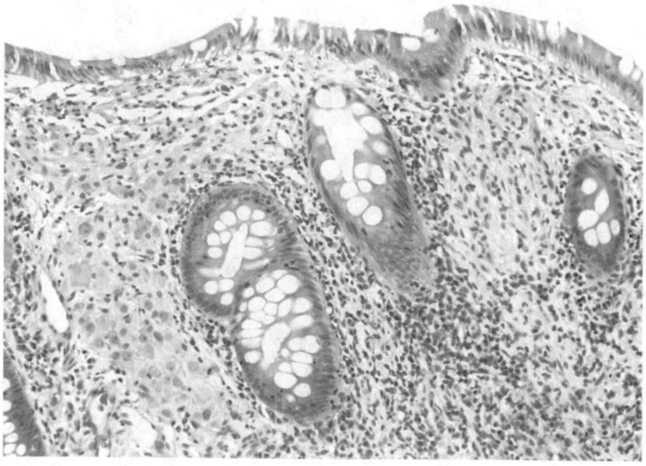

Fig. 1.47 Ganglioneuromatous polyps with ganglion cells and Schwann cell stroma in the lamina propria

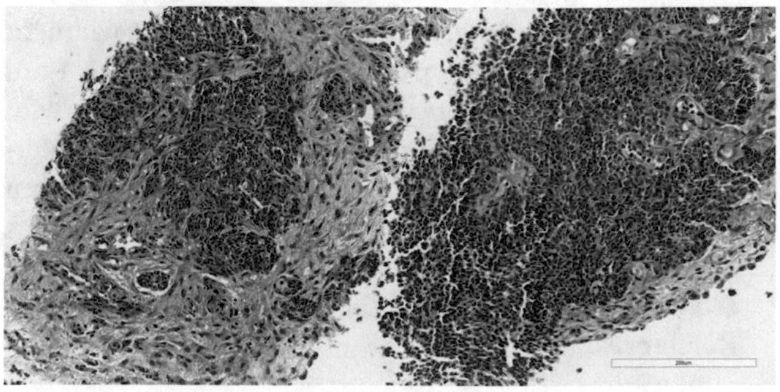

Fig. 1.48 (Case) Clusters of small undifferentiated round tumor cells with desmoplastic stroma proven to be desmoplastic small round cell tumor with EWSR1-WT1 translocation

Immunohistochemistry: WT1 C-terminus stain showed strong and diffuse nuclear positivity. Other stains included WT1 N-terminus negative, desmin positive, CD99 weakly and focally positive, EMA focally positive, myogenin negative, synaptophysin negative, S100 negative, TdT negative, CD45 negative, and OCT3/4 negative.

RT-PCR: t(11:22) (p13:q12) and EWSR1-WT1 positive.

Final Diagnosis

Desmoplastic small round cell tumor.

Take-Home Points and Discussion

- Desmoplastic small round cell tumor is a translocation-associated poorly differentiated tumor of uncertain histogenesis with polyphenotypic expression. Mesentery is a common site and it is most common in pediatric patients.
- There is no diagnostic IHC, although strong nuclear WT1 C-terminus staining is supportive.
- Demonstrating the EWSR1-WT1 translocation is important. This can be done in different ways (RT-PCR, FISH, or targeted gene sequencing) using frozen or paraffin-embedded tissue.

  References: [30, 37]

Inflammatory Disorders

Frequently Asked Questions

1. **What are the pathologic features of eosinophilic esophageal disease, and what is the main clinical differential diagnosis of eosinophils in the esophagus?**

   Eosinophils are absent or rare in the normal esophageal squamous epithelium. When present in a significant number, it is useful to give a maximum count per high-power field. Dense infiltration can be associated with eosinophilic aggregates or microabscesses, prominent degranulation, and surface epithelial sloughing with eosinophilic exudates. Eosinophils may be increased beneath the epithelium in the lamina propria where they can produce fibrosis and stricture. Other features of mucosal damage are typically proportional to the degree of eosinophil infiltration and include spongiosis (intercellular edema), basal layer hyperplasia with elongation of the rete pegs, and vascular ectasia. Intraepithelial lymphocytes may be increased but should not predominate. There may be a few neutrophils, but frequent neutrophils or the presence of ulceration should prompt evaluation for *Candida* or viral infection (Fig. 1.49). In general mild eosinophilic infiltrates (<15 per 400× field) limited to the lower esophagus are thought to represent damage due to gastroesophageal reflux disease. Higher eosinophil counts involving the proximal esophagus are thought to correlate with the allergic eosinophilic esophagitis (Fig. 1.50). However there is significant morphologic, clinical, and treatment response overlap. There may also be situations where both conditions exist, one contributing to the other. In any case the pathologic findings are just one important piece of information needed to aid the clinical diagnosis and to distinguish reflux from allergy or other systemic disorders. Documenting the degree of esophagitis, giving a maximum eosinophil count in a 400x field, and excluding other pathology are the important aspects for pathology report.

   References: [38]

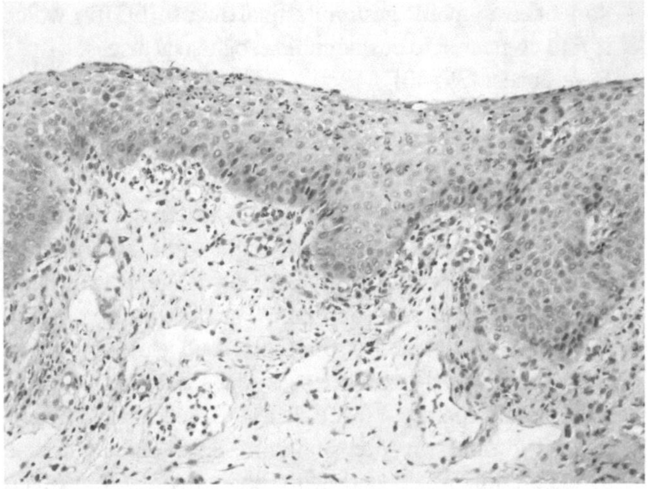

Fig. 1.49 Acute esophagitis with neutrophils requiring exclusion of fungal or viral infection

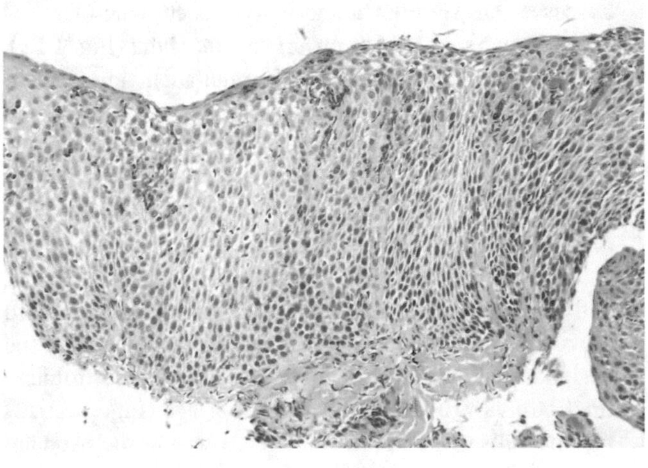

Fig. 1.50 Eosinophilic esophagitis with >50 eosinophils in a concentrated 400× field

2. **What is the typical distribution of eosinophils in the pediatric gastrointestinal tract?**

While rare or absent in the esophageal epithelium, eosinophils are normally present in the lamina propria in the remainder of the gastrointestinal tract. They are not commonly seen within crypt epithelium, however. The cecum and proximal right colon have the highest numbers with up to 50 per high-power field being normal in these regions. Lower numbers are seen in the small intestine and left colon. They are sparse in the stomach and rectum. The presence of mild mucosal eosinophilia limited to the lamina propria should be noted although the significance is not known. The finding is nonspecific and may be seen in many settings including subacute or resolving inflammation, early or treated inflammatory bowel disease, and chronic constipation. Symptomatic eosinophilic predominant infiltrates in the stomach and intestine fall into the broad category of eosinophilic gastrointestinal disease (EGID), which is rare compared to eosinophilic esophageal disease.
References: [39, 40]

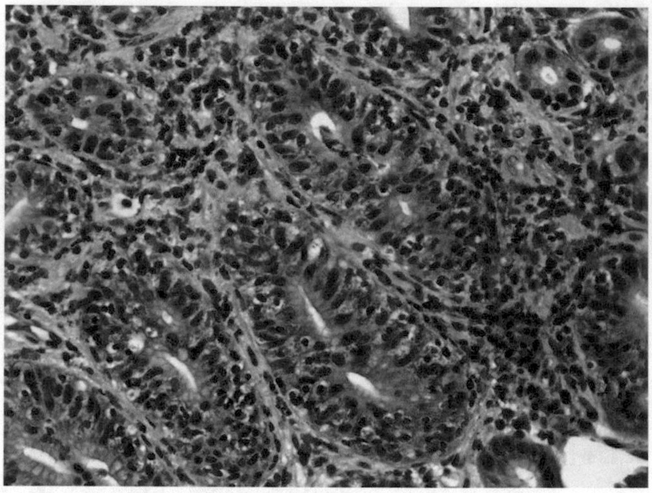

Fig. 1.51 Eosinophilic gastritis showing markedly increased eosinophils in the lamina propria. Epithelial infiltration by eosinophils (eosinophilic cryptitis) is also prominent. The most common etiology is allergy but the clinical differential can be extensive

3. **What is the clinical differential of eosinophilic gastrointestinal disease?**

Some cases are idiopathic with no cause identified. The most common cause is thought to be food allergy. Often patients with allergy-associated EGID have other symptoms of allergy such as eczema or asthma. Some may have peripheral eosinophilia and elevated serum IgE. Other less common secondary causes are parasites, inflammatory bowel disease, medication, hyper-IgE syndrome, hypereosinophilic syndrome, immune dysregulation associated with bone marrow transplant or immunodeficiency, and Churg-Strauss syndrome. The differential is long and requires clinical correlation. Histologically, eosinophils predominate. Aggregates of eosinophils, eosinophilic cryptitis, and eosinophilic crypt abscesses are significant and tend to occur when there is at least moderate lamina propria eosinophilia (Fig. 1.51). Edema, prominent eosinophil degranulation, and reactive epithelial changes may be present.
References: [41]

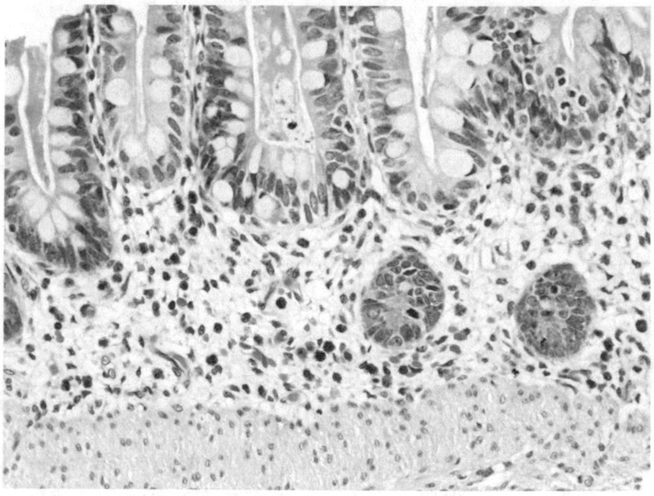

Fig. 1.52 Rectal biopsy from 1-day-old infant. The lamina propria contains no plasma cells which is normal for this age

4. **When do plasma cells appear in the gastrointestinal tract in infants?**

The normal fetus has immature B cell development and circulating plasma cells are not detectable in cord blood. Plasma cells are detected soon after birth in the peripheral blood. They begin to appear in the gastrointestinal lamina propria at 2–4 weeks of age (Fig. 1.52). If plasma cells or germinal centers are seen in the neonate, it suggests abnormal antigenic stimulation in the fetus or fetal infection. However, if plasma cells do not begin to appear by 1 month of age, immunodeficiency should be suggested. For example, two thirds of patients with common variable immunodeficiency (CVID) will have decreased or absent plasma cells in gastrointestinal biopsies (Fig. 1.53). It is thus important to look for plasma cells in gastrointestinal biopsies in children.
References: [42, 43]

5. **What is the differential for a pediatric inflammatory enteropathy? What are the general pathologic features in small intestinal biopsies?**

The major differential is similar to adults and includes celiac disease, infection, allergy, and IBD (particularly Crohn disease). In young children there is a higher chance of immune dysregulation with associated immunodeficiency or autoimmunity. These disorders

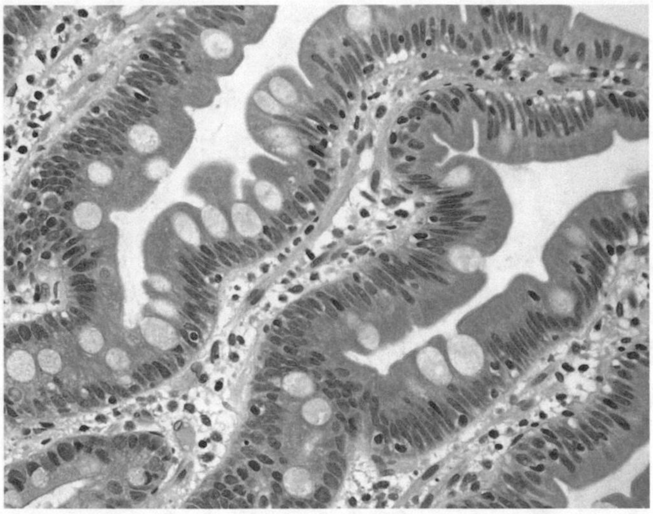

Fig. 1.53 Duodenal biopsy from a young child with common variable immunodeficiency showing complete absence of plasma cells in the lamina propria. Mild intraepithelial lymphocytosis is noted

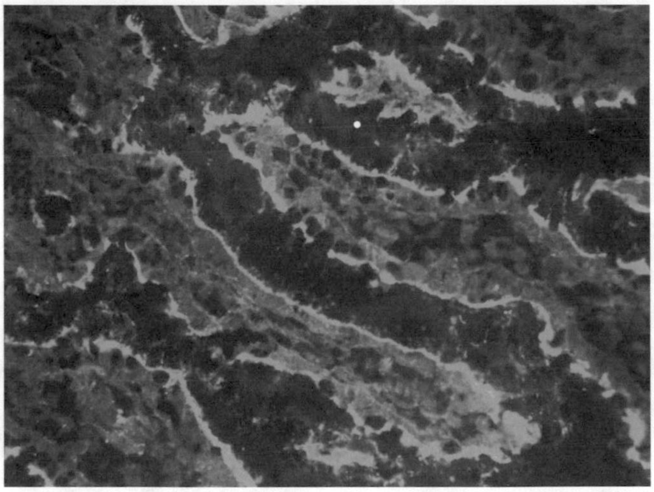

Fig. 1.54 Positive direct immunofluorescent stain for anti-enterocyte antibodies in autoimmune enteropathy. (Courtesy of Benjamin J. Wilkins, MD, PhD, Children's Hospital of Philadelphia)

are rare and the list of immune dysregulation disorders with gastrointestinal manifestations is growing. Some to consider are autoimmune enteropathy (AIE), CVID, and chronic granulomatous disease (CGD). All can have similar pathologic features with considerable morphologic overlap, so clinical work-up and correlation are needed. The general pathologic pattern is villous blunting and varying degrees of chronic active and granulomatous inflammation.

- AIE is often associated with anti-enterocyte or anti-goblet cell antibodies (Fig. 1.54) and is the pattern seen with several immunodeficiency disorders. Syndromic forms of AIE are X-linked immune dysregulation, polyendocrinopathy, and enteropathy (IPEX) and autoimmune polyglandular syndrome (APS). *FOXP3* is mutated in IPEX. AIE can have a celiac disease-type pattern, a chronic active IBD-like pattern, an apoptotic GVHD-like pattern, or a combination of all these patterns. Paneth cells and goblet cells may be decreased or absent (Fig. 1.55). The large intestine and stomach can also be involved. Relative to celiac disease, AIE usually has less prominent intraepithelial lymphocytes, more crypt destruction and apoptosis, and reduced Paneth cells and goblet cells. IBD-like features may extend to the large intestine and stomach in these patients.
- CVID, though uncommon, is an immunodeficiency disorder that is likely to be seen in the setting of pediatric gastrointestinal biopsy. It shares features with IgA deficiency and both disorders may be seen in the same family. There is a B cell maturation defect with reduced or absent plasma cells (Fig. 1.53) and hence decreased immunoglobulins. In addition, duodenal biopsies may show celiac disease-like pattern, IBD-like pattern, nodular lymphoid hyperplasia (Fig. 1.56), granulomatous enteropathy resembling Crohn disease, and increased risk of giardiasis and cryptosporidiosis. Patients may develop multifocal atrophic gastritis with loss of parietal cells and pernicious anemia, but they do not generate anti-parietal cell antibodies. They are at risk for gastrointestinal adenocarcinoma and lymphoma.
- CGD is rare and is an example of primary immunodeficiency that can mimic Crohn disease pathologically, clinically, and endoscopically. It is due to defective NADPH oxidase phagocytosis making the patient prone to bacterial and other infections. Pathologic features are IBD-like pattern with mucosal granulomas (Fig. 1.57). Helpful features on a biopsy include increased pigmented macrophages and numerous epithelioid mucosal granulomas with scant neutrophils.

References: [44–46]

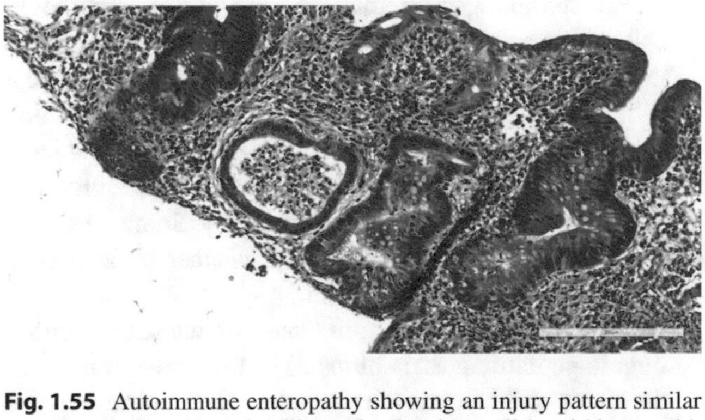

Fig. 1.55 Autoimmune enteropathy showing an injury pattern similar to celiac disease. There is villous blunting in small bowl biopsy with active inflammation, goblet cell depletion, and absence of Paneth cells. (Courtesy of Benjamin J. Wilkins, MD, PhD, Children's Hospital of Philadelphia)

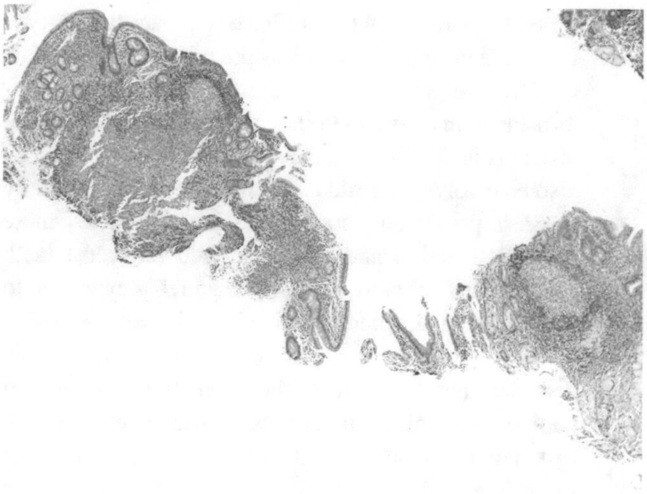

Fig. 1.56 Duodenal biopsy showing prominent lymphoid hyperplasia in common variable immune deficiency

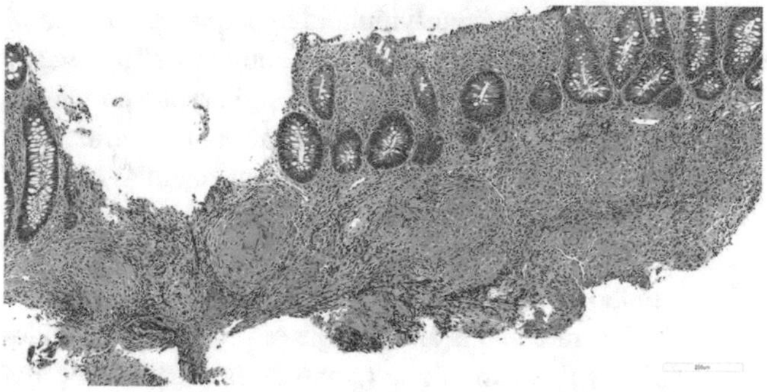

Fig. 1.57 Multiple granulomas in chronic granulomatous disease seen in a colon biopsy. This disease can produce inflammatory enteropathy that mimics Crohn disease. (Courtesy of Benjamin J. Wilkins, MD, PhD, Children's Hospital of Philadelphia)

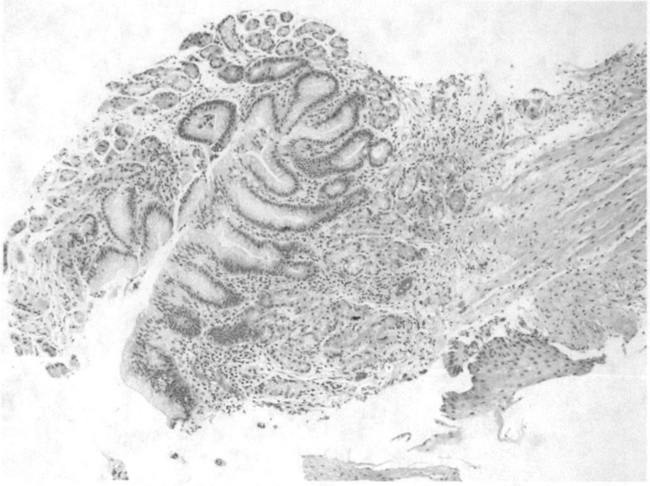

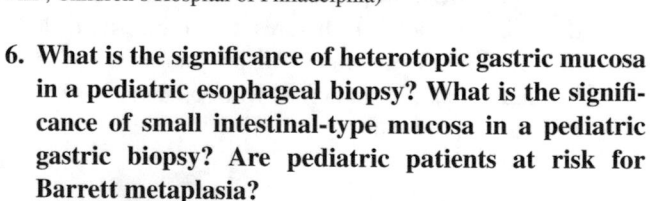

Fig. 1.58 Gastric heterotopia (inlet patch) in the upper esophagus. Note the presence of parietal cells

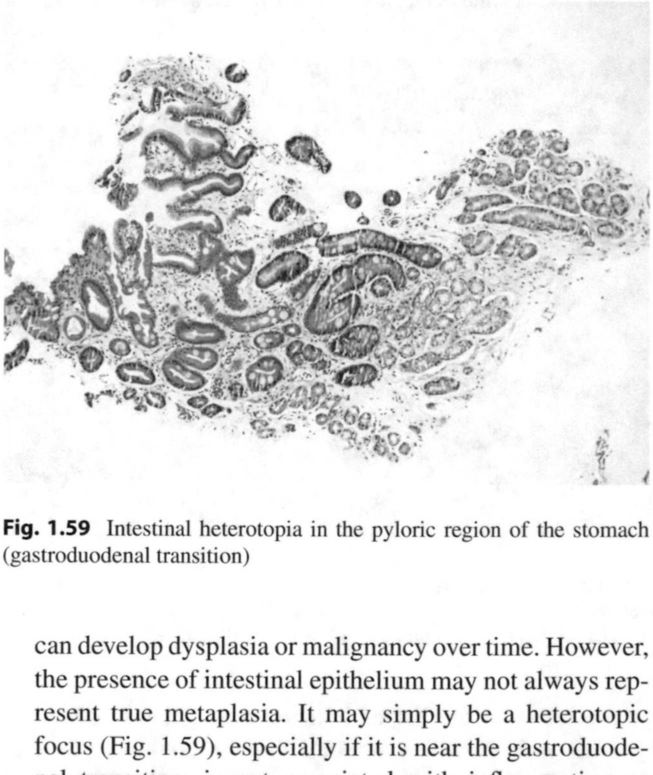

Fig. 1.59 Intestinal heterotopia in the pyloric region of the stomach (gastroduodenal transition)

6. What is the significance of heterotopic gastric mucosa in a pediatric esophageal biopsy? What is the significance of small intestinal-type mucosa in a pediatric gastric biopsy? Are pediatric patients at risk for Barrett metaplasia?

Heterotopic gastric mucosa (Fig. 1.58), commonly called inlet patch, is a congenital anomaly typically found in the cervical esophagus just below the upper esophageal sphincter. It can be symptomatic due to secretions and acid production. It may also become inflamed and infected by *H. pylori*. It rarely undergoes intestinal metaplasia or progresses to dysplasia and malignancy. Some gastroenterologists may request reporting whether parietal cells are present or not in inlet patch.

The incidence and significance of intestinal epithelium in pediatric gastric biopsies is not always certain. In the older child, it may be true metaplasia and may be seen with reactive gastropathy or gastritis. In this situation, it carries the same implication as in adults in that it can develop dysplasia or malignancy over time. However, the presence of intestinal epithelium may not always represent true metaplasia. It may simply be a heterotopic focus (Fig. 1.59), especially if it is near the gastroduodenal transition, is not associated with inflammation or other pathology, and may have associated pancreatic heterotopia (Fig. 1.60) or other anatomical anomalies. The implication of a heterotopia is not the same as true metaplasia.

Barrett metaplasia is rare in pediatric biopsies. It can be seen in older teenage patients with long-standing reflux. Risk factors include family history and early onset of severe reflux. It may also be seen in patients with history of esophageal atresia and fistula.

References: [47–51]

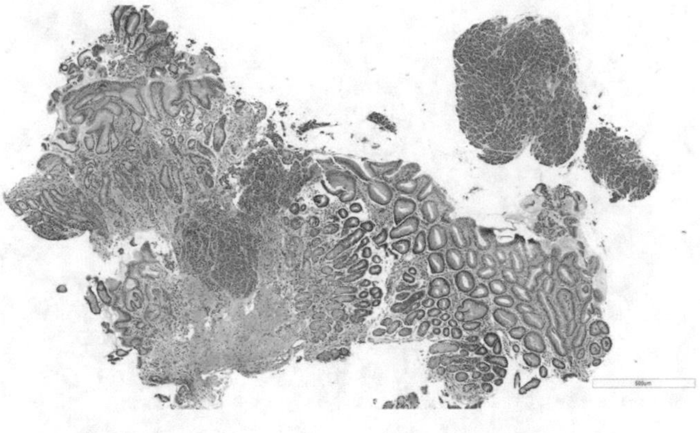

Fig. 1.60 Pancreatic heterotopia in the stomach. (Courtesy of Benjamin J. Wilkins, MD, PhD, Children's Hospital of Philadelphia)

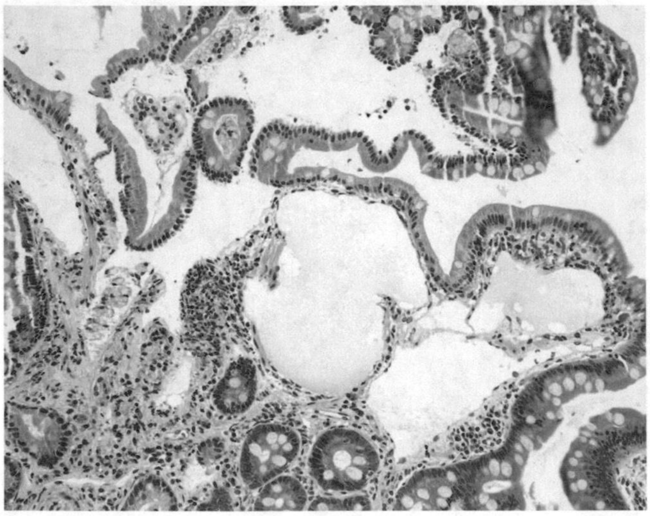

Fig. 1.61 Lymphangiectasia showing dilated lymphatic channels (lacteals) in duodenal villi

7. **A subset of patients with congenital onset diarrhea and non-inflammatory enteropathy may have diagnostic features on intestinal biopsies. What are they?**

Lymphangiectasia: multiple dilated lymphatics (lacteals) seen in the villous tips and lamina propria (Fig. 1.61).

Lipid transport defects (abetalipoproteinemia, hypobetalipoproteinemia, chylomicron retention disease): diffuse vacuolization of the enterocytes due to cytoplasmic accumulation of variable-sized lipid droplets (Fig. 1.62). Involved genes: *MTTP*, *APOB*, *SAR1B*. Diarrhea and fat malabsorption usually develop within the first few weeks of life, with low levels of serum lipids, acanthocytosis, deficiency in fat-soluble vitamins, retinitis pigmentosa, neurologic symptoms, and failure to thrive. It should be mentioned that focal and mild lipid accumulation in enterocytes can be a nonspecific finding in older patients with recent feeding (postprandial endoscopic biopsy).

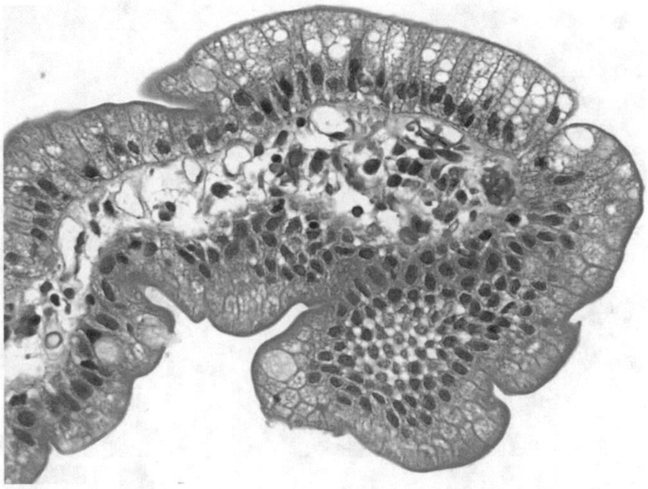

Fig. 1.62 Duodenal biopsy showing cytoplasmic accumulation of lipid droplets seen in a case of hypobetalipoproteinemia

Microvillus inclusion disease: marked villous atrophy, crypt hyperplasia, and absence of brush borders (Fig. 1.63a). Cytoplasmic microvillus inclusion bodies can be seen on electron microscopy (Fig. 1.63d). On PAS (Fig. 1.63b) and CD10 (Fig. 1.63c) stains, disorganized brush borders are demonstrated as an irregular layer of cytoplasmic density in the apex of enterocytes. Involved gene: *MYO5B*.

Tufting enteropathy: crowding of surface enterocytes to form surface aggregates or "tufts" with teardrop-shaped or round enterocytes that tend to shed into the lumens (Fig. 1.64). These abnormalities can be seen in both small and large intestines. Involved gene: *EPCAM*. Immunohistochemistry for EpCAM (epithelial cellular adhesion molecule) may be attempted via a specialized laboratory, which can show decreased EpCAM expression to confirm the diagnosis.

Enteroendocrine dysgenesis: normal morphology on routine HE stain. Chromogranin immunostain shows an absence or marked reduction in enterochromaffin cells in the small bowel and colon. Involved gene: *NEUROG3*. It should be mentioned that loss of endocrine cells may also be seen in the setting of autoimmune enteropathy.

In all of the above conditions, pathologic diagnosis should be done in concert with genetic testing for the disorder if a mutation is known. Genomic sequencing may be necessary.
References: [52–54]

8. **What is very early onset of inflammatory bowel disease?**

In older children, the pathology and pathogenesis of IBD are probably similar to those in adults. However, the

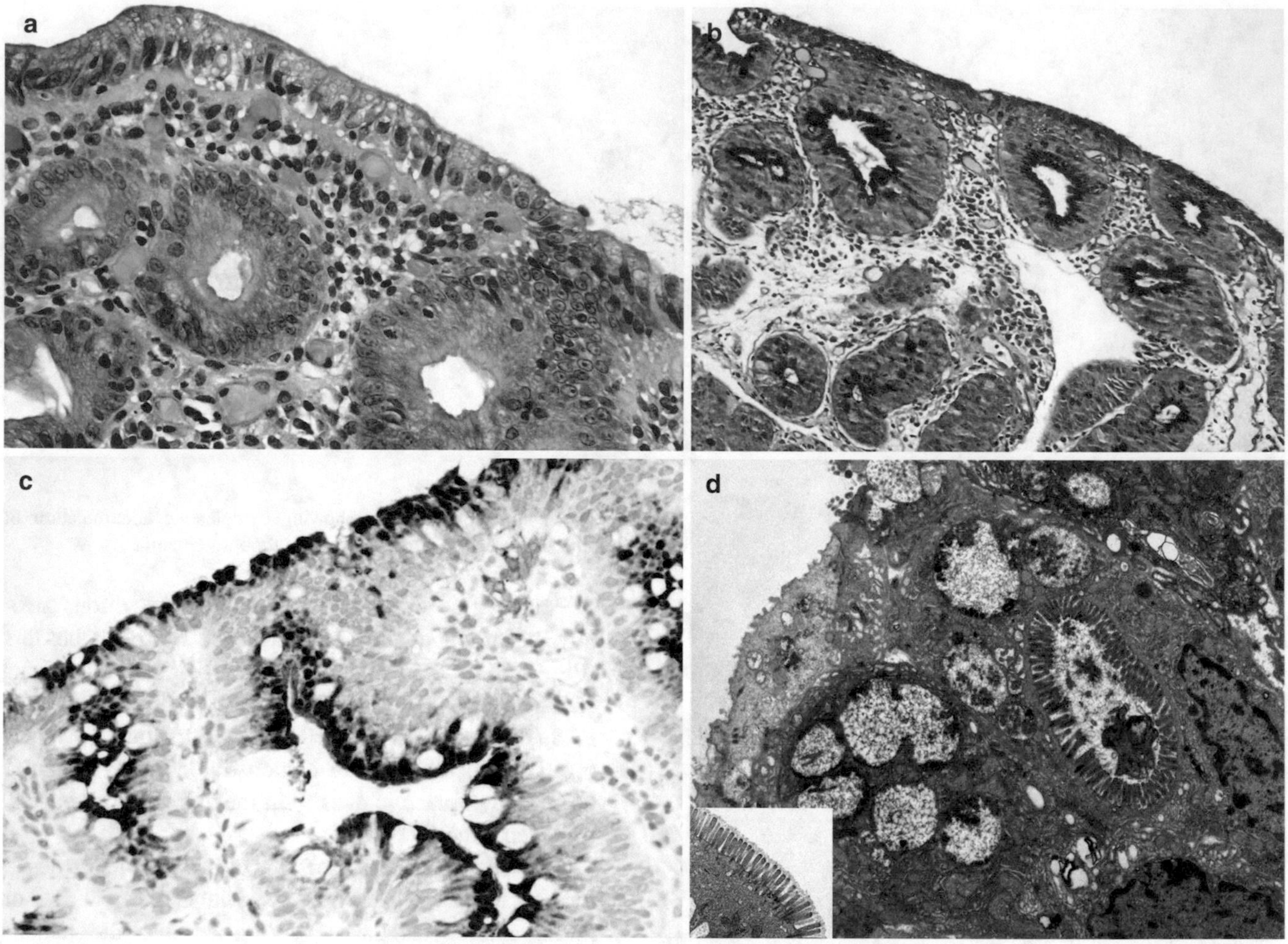

Fig. 1.63 Microvillus inclusion disease seen in a duodenal biopsy showing marked villous blunting, goblet cell depletion, and lack of brushing borders (**a**). Periodic acid-Schiff (PAS) stain (**b**) and CD10 immunostain (**c**) highlight disorganized inclusions arranged in an intracytoplasmic linear density along the apex of enterocytes. Electron microscopy (**d**) showing decreased, disorganized and shortened surface microvilli. Cytoplasmic inclusion of microvilli is seen in the center. Inset is normal surface microvilli. (Courtesy of Eric Wartchow, PhD, Children's Hospital Colorado)

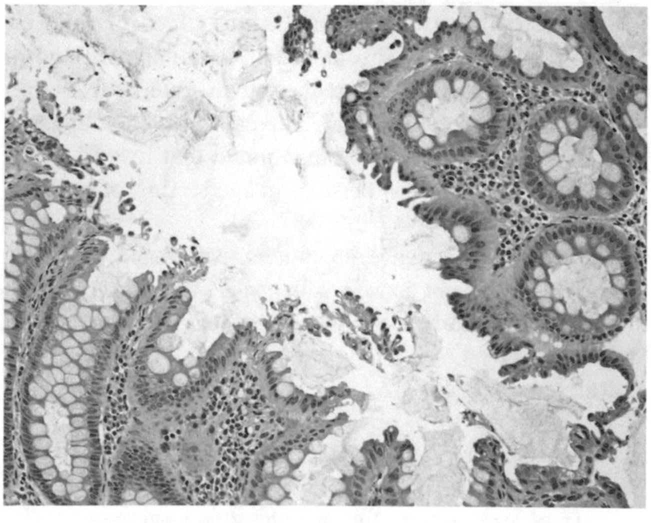

Fig. 1.64 Tufting enteropathy seen in a colon biopsy showing crowded surface enterocytes with teardrop-shaped aggregates shedding into the lumen

younger the patient, the more likely there is an immunodeficiency/disorder or monogenic form of IBD. Very early-onset IBD (VEOIBD) refers to IBD occurring in children younger than 6 years of age (Fig. 1.65). Infantile- and toddler-onset IBD refers to patients younger than 2 years of age. These subsets of patients have pathologic features that are similar to IBD in older children and adults, but the disease is usually more severe and does not respond to conventional IBD therapy. If infection, allergy, and celiac disease are excluded, these patients may need genetic testing, evaluation of extraintestinal manifestations, and evaluation of immunodeficiency to rule out defects that are more common in infants and toddlers, which include IL-10 signaling abnormalities, IPEX syndrome (Fig. 1.66), Wiskott-Aldrich syndrome, and TTC7A mutation (multiple atresias, IBD, and immunodeficiency).

References: [55]

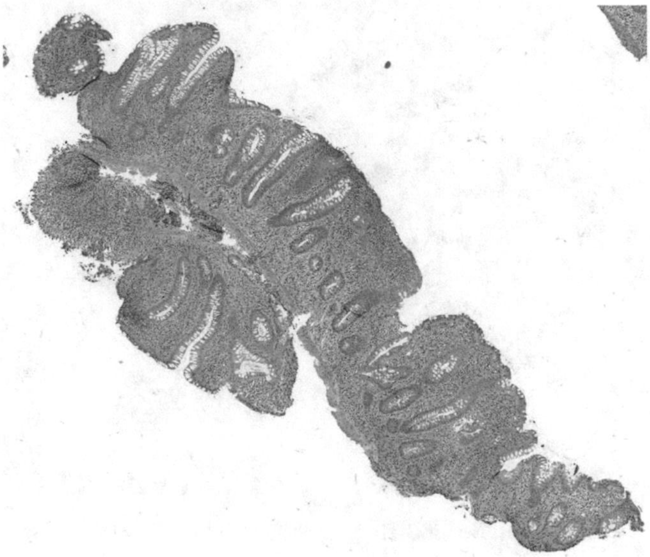

Fig. 1.65 Chronic active colitis seen in a case of very early-onset inflammatory bowel disease. (Courtesy of Benjamin J. Wilkins, MD, PhD, Children's Hospital of Philadelphia)

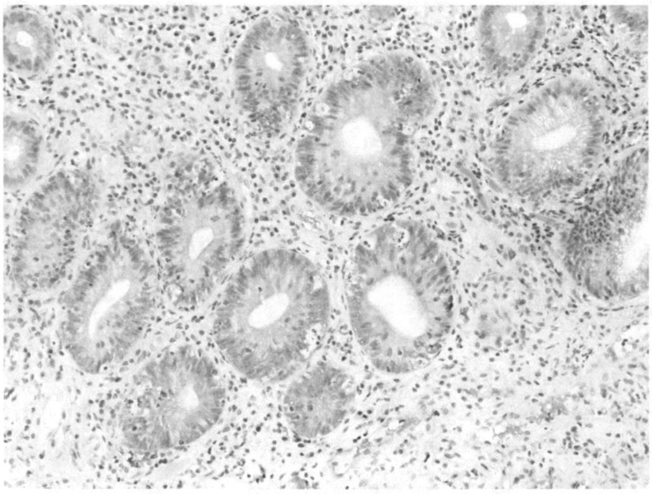

Fig. 1.66 Increased crypt apoptosis in a case of very early-onset inflammatory bowel disease associated with IPEX syndrome

9. **What are the main differentials for a noninfectious lamina propria histiocytic infiltrate?**

   Diffuse infiltration of the lamina propria by histiocytes raises the possibility of histiocytic neoplasm versus metabolic storage disease. Rarely, Rosai-Dorfman disease, Langerhans cell histiocytosis, and juvenile xanthogranuloma can involve the gastrointestinal tract.

   Langerhans cell histiocytosis: CD1a, S100, and langerin-positive Langerhans-type histiocytes (Fig. 1.67a, b).

   Juvenile xanthogranuloma: Factor 13a-positive histiocytes.

   Rosai-Dorfman disease: S100 positive, CD1a variably positive, emperipolesis.

   For metabolic storage disease, electron microscopy can help categorize and localize the abnormal storage material. Mucopolysaccharidoses can cause macrophage accumulation in the lamina propria. Disorders of cholesterol/lipid metabolism (such as Wolman and Tangier diseases) can produce xanthomatous infiltrates of foamy macrophages.

   References: [56, 57]

10. **What are the differentials of granulomatous appendicitis?**

    The appendix is a common pediatric gastrointestinal specimen and > 95% show routine acute appendicitis. Unexpected findings may include *Enterobius vermicularis*, adenoviral inclusions, carcinoid tumor, and granulomas. If granulomatous appendicitis (Fig. 1.68) is encountered, the most common cause may be remote or subacute appendicitis with delayed presentation. Bacterial, parasitic, mycobacterial, and fungal infections are possibilities. The most common infectious cause might be *Yersinia* species. Crohn disease is also a possibility, but isolated granulomatous appendicitis as the preceding manifestation of Crohn disease of the gastrointestinal tract is rare. Most cases are limited to the appendix and appendectomy is curative with no subsequent symptoms of IBD.

    References: [58, 59]

Case Presentation

Learning Objectives

- To recognize clinicopathologic features of immune dysregulation syndromes in patients presenting with gastrointestinal disease
- To understand the pathophysiology of one type of immune dysregulation disorder, CTLA-4 deficiency

Case History

An 11-year-old girl with a history of intermittent diarrhea since infancy was referred to a gastroenterologist for known diagnosis of celiac disease (confirmed by serology and biopsy) with continued gastrointestinal symptoms. Other clinical history included rheumatoid factor-positive juvenile idiopathic arthritis diagnosed at 2 years of age, eczema, vitiligo, and hypothyroidism. Additional laboratory work-up at the time of this visit included elevated immunoglobulin levels, antinuclear antibody (ANA) 1:1280, and elevated erythrocyte sedimentation rate. She underwent upper and lower endoscopic biopsies.

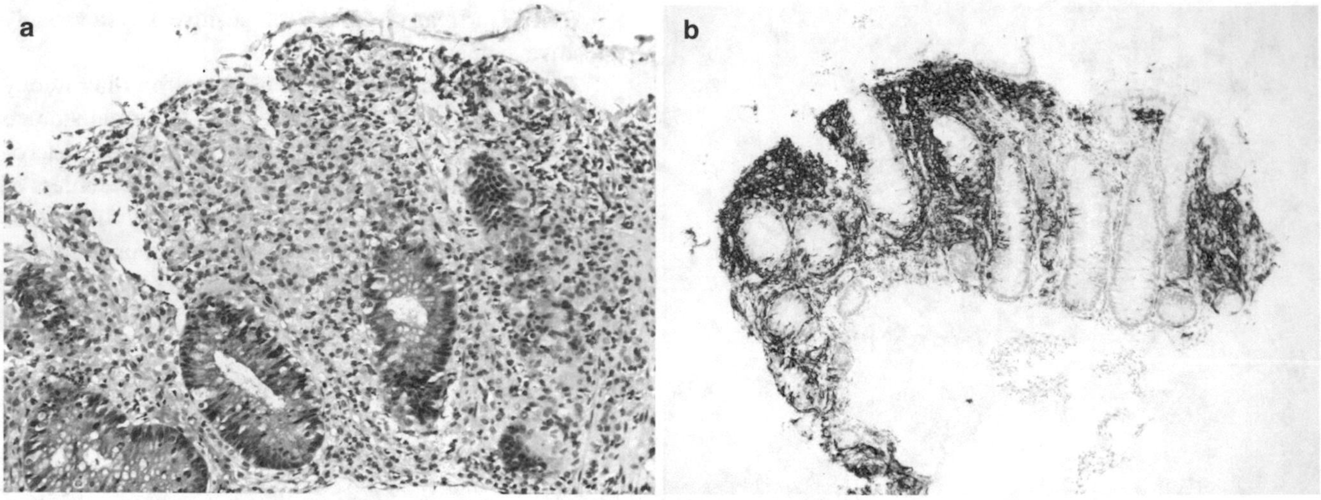

Fig. 1.67 Langerhans cell histiocytosis involving colonic lamina propria (**a**), which is positive for CD1a by immunohistochemistry (**b**)

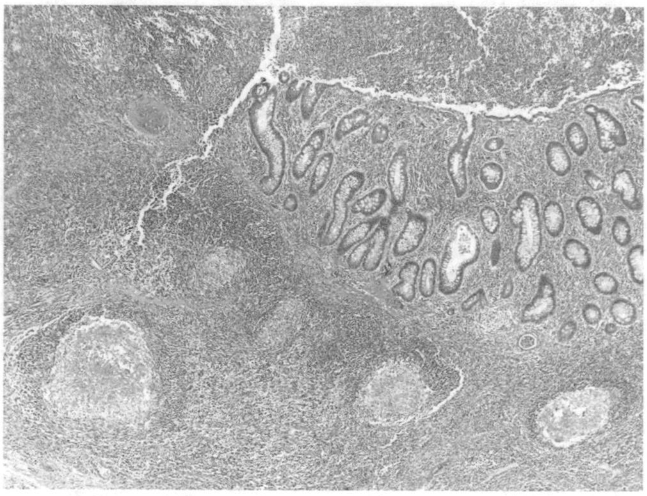

Fig. 1.68 Isolated granulomatous appendicitis seen in an appendectomy specimen

Histologic Findings

Stomach: chronic atrophic gastritis with loss of parietal cells (Fig. 1.69a). *H. pylori* immunohistochemistry was negative.

Duodenum: celiac disease pattern with marked villous blunting (Fig. 1.69b).

Ileum: marked villous blunting (Fig. 1.69c).

Colon: lymphocytic colitis pattern (Fig. 1.69d).

Additional findings in biopsies: no granulomas, no infectious agents. Plasma cells were readily identified. Crypt apoptosis was not increased.

Differential Diagnosis

- Celiac disease
- Inflammatory bowel disease
- Immunodeficiency disorder
- Autoimmune disorder
- Immune dysregulation syndrome

Additional Laboratory Work-Up

Additional testing was positive for anti-parietal cell antibodies. Anti-enterocyte antibodies were negative. Lymphocyte subsets were normal except for increased B cells with increased class-switched B cells. Genetic testing identified a monoallelic mutation in CTLA-4 (cytotoxic T lymphocyte-associated antigen 4/CD152). The patient then received immune modulator therapy, sirolimus and abatacept, with better control of symptoms. Abatacept is a CTLA-4 immunoglobulin fusion protein and functions essentially as CTLA-4 replacement therapy. Monitoring for type 1 diabetes mellitus and bone marrow transplant evaluation was begun.

Final Diagnosis

CTLA-4 deficiency associated with chronic atrophic gastritis, celiac disease, inflammatory enteropathy, and lymphocytic colitis.

Take-Home Messages and Discussion

- Young patients with multiple immunologic symptoms and gastrointestinal pathology should be evaluated for immune dysregulation including immunodeficiency work-up and genetic testing. These patients are often resistant to traditional therapies and more specific therapies may be available.
- CTLA-4 deficiency is one example of immune dysregulation associated with gastrointestinal inflammatory pathology. CTLA-4 deficiency is an autosomal dominant disorder characterized by a pro-inflammatory state with autoimmunity in multiple organ systems. CTLA-4 is an immune checkpoint receptor expressed on T cells after activation by antigen-presenting cells. It helps maintain immune tolerance to self partly through effects on B cell response and antibody production. Celiac disease and

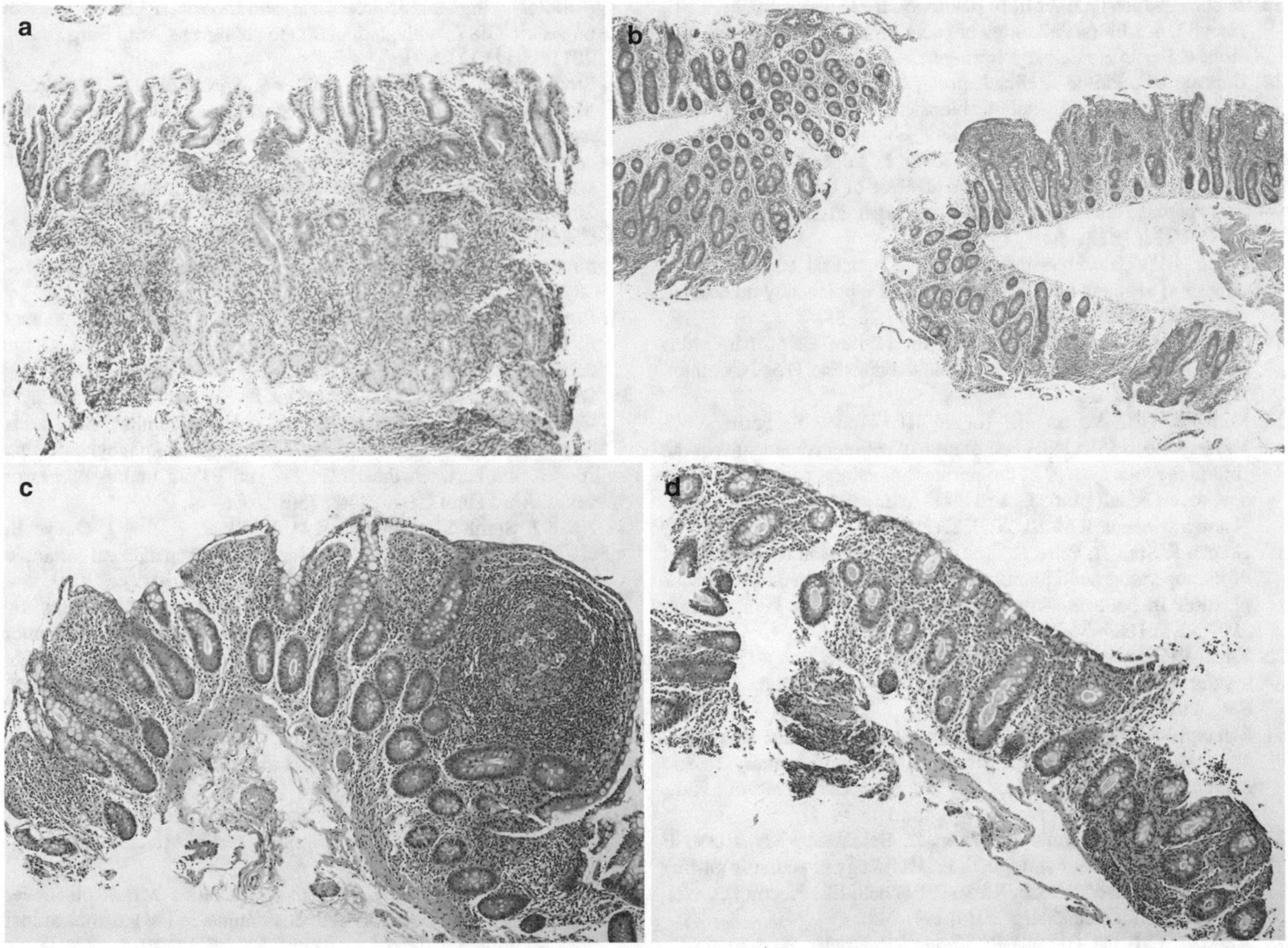

Fig. 1.69 (Case). Atrophic gastritis in CTLA-4 deficiency (**a**). The biopsy was from the gastric body (confirmed by negative gastrin immunostain) and shows complete loss of oxyntic glands. Biopsy from the duodenum showing a celiac disease pattern in CTLA-4 deficiency with marked villous blunting (**b**). Marked villous blunting is also seen in ileal biopsy (**c**). Biopsy from the colon showing lymphocytic pancolitis (**d**)

type 1 diabetes mellitus are strongly associated with this disorder.

References: [60]

References

1. Huff DS. Developmental anatomy and anomalies of the gastrointestinal tract with involvement in major malformative syndromes. In: Russo P, Ruchelli ED, Piccoli DA, editors. Pathology of pediatric gastrointestinal and liver disease. Berlin Heidelberg: Springer; 2014. p. 1–53.
2. Joncilla M, Yantiss RY. Malformations, choristomas and hamartomas of the gastrointestinal tract and pancreas. Semin Diagn Pathol. 2019;36(1):24–38.
3. Hamza AR, Bicaj BX, Kurshumliu FI, Zejnullahu VA, Sada FE, Krasniqi AS. Mesenteric Meckel's diverticulum or intestinal duplication cyst: a case report with review of the literature. Int J Surg Case Rep. 2016;26:50–2.
4. El-Asmar KM, Abdel-Latif M, El-Kassaby AA, Soliman MH, El-Behery MM. Colonic atresia: association with other anomalies. J Neonatal Surg. 2016;5(4):47.
5. Hofmann AD, Puri P. Association of Hirschsprung's disease and anorectal malformation: a systematic review. Pediatr Surg Int. 2013;29(9):913.
6. Jain AS, Patel AM, Jain SR, Thakkar A. Accessory pancreatic lobe with gastric duplication cyst: diagnostic challenges of a rare congenital anomaly. BMJ Case Rep. 2015;2015:bcr2014207751.
7. Savage JJ, Casey JN, McNeill IT, Sherman JH. Neurenteric cysts of the spine. J Craniovertebr Junction Spine. 2010;1(1):58–63.
8. Pacilli M, Sebire NJ, Maritsi D, Kiely EM, Drake DP, Curry JI, et al. Umbilical polyp in infants and children. Eur J Pediatr Surg. 2007;17:397–9.
9. Davis JS, Ryan ML, Shields JM, Sola JE, Perez EA, Neville HL, et al. Segmental absence of intestinal musculature: an increasingly reported pathology. J Pediatr Surg. 2012;47(8):1566–71.
10. Stephens D, Arensman R, Pillai S, Alagiozian-Angelova V. Congenital absence of intestinal smooth muscle: a case report and review of the literature. J Pediatr Surg. 2009;44:2211–5.
11. Hart J, Wilcox W, Weber CR. The gastrointestinal tract. In: Stocker JT, Dehner LP, Husain AN, editors. Stocker and Dehner's pediatric pathology. Philadelphia: Lippincott Williams and Wilkins; 2011. p. 627.
12. Aldridge RT, Campbell PE. Ganglion cell distribution in the normal rectum and anal canal: a basis for the diagnosis of Hirschsprung's disease by anorectal biopsy. J Pediatr Surg. 1968;5(4):475–89.

13. Kapur RP. Intestinal motility disorders. In: Russo P, Ruchelli ED, Piccoli DA, editors. Pathology of pediatric gastrointestinal and liver disease. Berlin Heidelberg: Springer; 2014. p. 249–316.
14. Gonzalo DH, Plesec T. Hirschsprung disease and use of calretinin in inadequate rectal suction biopsies. Arch Pathol Lab Med. 2013;137:1099–102.
15. Narayanan SK, Soundappan SS, Kwan E, Cohen RC, Charlton A, Cass DT. Aganglionosis with the absence of hypertrophied nerve fibers predicts disease proximal to rectosigmoid colon. Pediatr Surg Int. 2016;32(3):221–6.
16. Kapur RP. Calretinin-immunoreactive mucosal innervation in very short segment Hirschsprung disease: a potentially misleading observation. Pediatr Dev Pathol. 2014;17:28–35.
17. Furness JB, Jones C, Nurgali K, Clerc N. Intrinsic primary afferent neurons and nerve circuits within the intestine. Prog Neurobiol. 2004;72(2):143–64.
18. Knowles CH, Veress B, Kapur RP, Wedel T, Farrugia G, Vanderwinden JM, et al. Quantitation of cellular components of the enteric nervous system in the normal human gastrointestinal tract: a report on behalf of the Gastro 2009 International Working Group. Neurogastroenterol Motil. 2011;23(2):115–24.
19. Boman F, Sfeir R, Priso R, Bonnevalle M, Besson R. Advantages of intraoperative semiquantitative evaluation of myenteric nervous plexuses in patients with Hirschsprung disease. J Pediatr Surg. 2007;42(6):1089–94.
20. Kapur RP. Submucosal nerve diameter of greater than 40 μm is not a valid diagnostic index of transition zone pull-through. J Pediatr Surg. 2016;51(10):1585–91.
21. Schappi MG, Staiano A, Milla PJ, Smith VV, Dias JA, Heuschkel R, et al. A practical guide for the diagnosis of primary enteric nervous system disorders. J Pediatr Gastroenterol Nutr. 2013;57(5):677–86.
22. Albenberg LG, Mamula P, Brown K, Baldassano RN, Russo P Colitis in infancy and childhood. In: Pathology of pediatric gastrointestinal and liver disease. Russo P, Ruchelli ED, Piccoli DA, eds. Springer Berlin Heidelberg, 2014; 197–248.
23. Knowles CH, De Giorgio R, Kapur RP, Bruder E, Farrugia G, Geboes K, et al. Gastrointestinal neuromuscular pathology: guidelines for histologic techniques and reporting on behalf of the Gastro 2009 International Working Group. Acta Neuropathol. 2009;118:271–301.
24. Castle S, Suliman A, Shayan K, Kling K, Bickler S, Losasso B. Total colonic aganglionosis with skip lesion: report of a rare case and management. J Pediatr Surg. 2012;47(3):581–4.
25. Kapadia MR. Volvulus of the small bowel and colon. Clin Colon Rectal Surg. 2017;30(1):40–5.
26. Zhao L, Feng S, Wu P, Lai XH, Lv C, Chen G. Clinical characteristics and surgical outcome in children with intussusceptions secondary to pathologic lead points. Pediatr Surg Int. 2019;35(7):807–11.
27. Henning F, Gfroerer S, Rolle U. Systematic review shows that pathologic lead points are important and frequent in intussusception and are not limited to infants. Acta Paediatr. 2016;105(11):1275–9.
28. Albenberg LG, Mamula P, Brown K, Baldassano RN, Russo P. Colitis in infancy and childhood. In: Russo P, Ruchelli ED, Piccoli DA, editors. Pathology of pediatric gastrointestinal and liver disease. Berlin Heidelberg: Springer; 2014. p. 197–248.
29. Pawel BR. Polyps and tumors of the gastrointestinal tract in childhood. In: Russo P, Ruchelli ED, Piccoli DA, editors. Pathology of pediatric gastrointestinal and liver disease. Berlin Heidelberg: Springer; 2014. p. 317–70.
30. Pawel BR. Polyps and tumors of the gastrointestinal tract in childhood. In: Russo P, Ruchelli ED, Piccoli DA, editors. Pathology of pediatric gastrointestinal and liver disease. Berlin Heidelberg: Springer; 2014. p. 317–70.
31. Miettinen M, Wang ZF, Sarlomo-Rikala M, Osuch C, Rutkowski P, Lasota J. Succinate dehydrogenase-deficient GISTs: a clinicopathologic, immunohistochemical, and molecular genetic study of 66 gastric GISTs with predilection to young age. Am J Surg Pathol. 2011;35(11):1712–21.
32. Stockman DL, Miettinen M, Suster S, Spangnolo D, Dominguez-Malagon H, Hornick JL. Malignant gastrointestinal neuroectodermal tumor: clinicopathologic immunohistochemical, ultrastructural, and molecular analysis of 16 cases with a reappraisal of clear cell sarcoma-like tumors of the gastrointestinal tract. Am J Surg Pathol. 2012;36(6):857–68.
33. Cauchin E, Touchefeu Y, Matysiak-Budnik T. Hamartomatous tumors of the gastrointestinal tract. Gastrointest Tumors. 2015;2(2):65–74.
34. Burkart AL, Sheridan T, Lewin M, Fenton H, Ali NJ, Montgomery E. Do sporadic Peutz-Jeghers polyps exist? Experience of a large teaching hospital. Am J Surg Pathol. 2007;31(8):1209–14.
35. Delnatte C, Sanlaville D, Mougenot JF, Vermeesch JR, Houdayer C, Blois MC, et al. Contiguous gene deletion within chromosome arm 10q is associated with juvenile polyposis of infancy, reflecting cooperation between the BMPR1A and PTEN tumor-suppressor genes. Am J Hum Genet. 2006;78(6):1066–74.
36. Njere I, Smith LL, Thurairasa D, Malik R, Jeffrey I, Okoye B, et al. Systematic review and meta-analysis of appendiceal carcinoid tumors in children. Pediatr Blood Cancer. 2018;65(8):e27069.
37. Arnold MA, Schoenfield L, Limketkai BN, Arnold CA. Diagnostic pitfalls of differentiating desmoplastic small round cell tumor (DSRCT) from Wilms tumor (WT): overlapping morphologic and immunohistochemical features. Am J Surg Pathol. 2014;38(9):1220–6.
38. Kia L, Hirano I. Distinguishing GERD from eosinophilic oesophagitis: concepts and controversies. Nat Rev Gastroenterol Hepatol. 2015;12(7):379–86.
39. Lowichik A, Weinberg AG. A quantitative evaluation of mucosal eosinophils in the pediatric gastrointestinal tract. Mod Pathol. 1996;9(2):110–4.
40. Debrosse CW, Case JW, Putnam PE, Collins MH, Rothenberg ME. Quantity and distribution of eosinophils in the gastrointestinal tract of children. Pediatr Dev Pathol. 2006;9(3):210–8.
41. Zhang M, Li Y. Eosinophilic gastroenteritis: a state-of-the-art review. J Gastroenterol Hepatol. 2017;32(1):64–72.
42. Huff DS. Developmental anatomy and anomalies of the gastrointestinal tract with involvement in major malformative syndromes. In: Russo P, Ruchelli ED, Piccoli DA, editors. Pathology of pediatric gastrointestinal and liver disease. Berlin Heidelberg: Springer; 2014. p. 1–53.
43. Blanco E, Pérez-Andrés M, Arriba-Méndez S, Contreras-Sanfeliciano T, Criado I, Pelak O, et al. Age-associated distribution of normal B-cell and plasma cell subsets in peripheral blood. J Allergy Clin Immunol. 2018;141(6):2208–19.
44. Masia R, Peyton S, Lauwers GY, Brown I. Gastrointestinal biopsy findings of autoimmune enteropathy: a review of 25 cases. Am J Surg Pathol. 2014;38(10):1319–29.
45. Agarwal S, Mayer L. Diagnosis and treatment of gastrointestinal disorders in patients with primary immunodeficiency. Clin Gastroenterol Hepatol. 2013;11(9):1050–63.
46. Shi C, Washington MK. Gastrointestinal and hepatic involvement in immunodeficiencies and systemic disease of childhood. In: Russo P, Ruchelli ED, Piccoli DA, editors. Pathology of pediatric gastrointestinal and liver disease. Berlin Heidelberg: Springer; 2014. p. 155–95.
47. Sahin G, Adas G, Koc B, Akcakaya A, Dogan Y, Goksel S, et al. Is cervical inlet patch important clinical problem? Int J Biomed Sci. 2014;10(2):129–35.
48. Camacho-Gomez SM, Bernieh A, Saad AG, Tipnis NA. Non-helicobacter pylori gastric intestinal metaplasia in children: a series of cases and review of the literature. Case Rep Gastrointest Med. 2018;2018:5930415.

49. Weinberg AG. The significance of small intestinal epithelium in gastric antral biopsies in children. Pediatr Dev Pathol. 2012;15(2):101–6.
50. Hsieh H, Frenette A, Michaud L, Krishnan U, Dal-Soglio DB, Gottrand F, et al. Intestinal metaplasia in the esophagus in children with esophageal atresia. J Pediatr Gastroenterol Nutr. 2017;65(1):e1–4.
51. Bakr O, Zhao W, Corley D. Gastroesophageal reflux frequency, severity, age of onset, family history and acid suppressive therapy predict Barrett esophagus in a large population. J Clin Gastroenterol. 2018;52(10):873–9.
52. Ensari A, Kelsen J, Russo P. Newcomers in paediatric GI pathology: childhood enteropathies including very early onset monogenic IBD. Virchows Arch. 2018;472(1):111–23.
53. Thiagarajah JR, Kamin DS, Acra S, Goldsmith JD, Roland JT, Lencer WI, et al. Advances in evaluation of chronic diarrhea in infants. Gastroenterology. 2018;154(8):2045–59.
54. Martin BA, Kerner JA, Hazard FK, Longacre TA. Evaluation of intestinal biopsies for pediatric enteropathy: a proposed immunohistochemical panel approach. Am J Surg Pathol. 2014;38(10):1387–95.
55. Uhlig HH, Schwerd T, Koletzko S, Shah N, Kammermeier J, Elkadri A, et al. The diagnostic approach to monogenic very early onset inflammatory bowel disease. Gastroenterology. 2014;147(5):990–1007.
56. Detlefsen S, Fagerberg CR, Ousager LB, Lindebjerg J, Marcussen N, Nathan T, et al. Histiocytic disorders of the gastrointestinal tract. Hum Pathol. 2013;44(5):683–96.
57. Russo P. Enteropathies associated with chronic diarrhea and malabsorption in childhood. In: Russo P, Ruchelli ED, Piccoli DA, editors. Pathology of pediatric gastrointestinal and liver disease. Berlin Heidelberg: Springer-Verlag; 2014. p. 99–153.
58. Bronner MP. Granulomatous appendicitis and the appendix in idiopathic inflammatory bowel disease. Semin Diagn Pathol. 2004;21(2):98–107.
59. Bischoff A, Gupta A, D'Mello S, Mezoff A, Podberesky D, Barnett S, et al. Crohn's disease limited to the appendix: a case report in a pediatric patient. Pediatr Surg Int. 2010;26(11):1125–8.
60. Verma N, Burns SO, Walker LSK, Sansom DM. Immune deficiency and autoimmunity in patients with CTLA-4 (CD152) mutations. Clin Exp Immunol. 2017;190(1):1–7.

Non-Barrett Esophagitis

2

Kevin M. Waters, Rifat Mannan, and Elizabeth Montgomery

List of Frequently Asked Questions

1. What are the clinicopathologic features seen in gastroesophageal reflux disease (GERD)?
2. What are the clinicopathologic findings in eosinophilic esophagitis (EoE)?
3. How can counting intraepithelial eosinophils add valuable information to a pathology report?
4. Can response to PPI treatment be used to diagnose GERD over EoE?
5. Are eosinophils a necessary component to diagnose GERD?
6. Are increased intraepithelial eosinophils in the esophagus only seen in GERD and EoE?
7. What are the clinical and histologic characteristics of lymphocytic esophagitis pattern?
8. What are the clinicopathologic characteristics of lichenoid esophagitis?
9. What are the causes and long-term implications of corrosive injury to the esophagus?
10. How are the most common types of pill fragments in pill esophagitis histologically distinguished?
11. What other medications cause morphologic changes in the esophagus?
12. What are the features of sloughing esophagitis/esophagitis dissecans?
13. What are the diagnostic features of and the differential diagnosis for pemphigus vulgaris (PV)?
14. How can I figure out the cause of an esophageal ulcer?

K. M. Waters (✉)
Cedars-Sinai Medical Center, Los Angeles, CA, USA
e-mail: kevin.waters@cshs.org

R. Mannan
University of Pennsylvania Perelman School of Medicine, Philadelphia, PA, USA

E. Montgomery
University of Miami Leonard M. Miller School of Medicine, Miami, FL, USA

Esophagitis can be a frustrating diagnostic challenge as the esophagus has a limited number of mechanisms to deal with injury and many causes of esophageal damage create overlapping histologic pictures. While a pathology report may not be able to always offer a specific diagnosis, it is important to both exclude specific treatable conditions and recognize different patterns of injury that can produce a more precise differential diagnosis that, along with clinical history, endoscopic findings, and medication history, can lead a clinician to the proper treatment plan.

Frequently Asked Questions

1. **What are the clinicopathologic features seen in gastroesophageal reflux disease (GERD)?**

   The diagnosis of GERD is multifactorial and is made using a combination of clinical and pathologic findings. Symptoms for GERD are nonspecific but typically consist of burning chest pain that can be worse at night when patients are supine and after eating, chronic cough, difficulty swallowing, and disrupted sleep. GERD is the most commonly diagnosed disorder in the gastrointestinal tract in the United States, and meta-analysis estimates that the prevalence of GERD is between 15 and 20% in North America and Europe. Risk factors for the development of GERD include advancing age, male gender, obesity, smoking, pregnancy, hypothyroidism, scleroderma, poor diet, alcohol, and medications. Endoscopic findings range from normal or mild inflammation to ulceration and stricture. According to the American College of Gastroenterology (ACG) guidelines, a presumptive diagnosis of GERD can be made without biopsy in the setting of typical symptoms of heartburn and regurgitation, and empiric therapy with a proton pump inhibitor (PPI) is instituted. Risk factors for long-term complications of GERD including Barrett esophagus and adenocarcinoma include increased age, Caucasian race, and male sex.

H. L. Wang, Z. E. Chen (eds.), *Practical Gastrointestinal Pathology*, Practical Anatomic Pathology,
https://doi.org/10.1007/978-3-030-51268-2_2

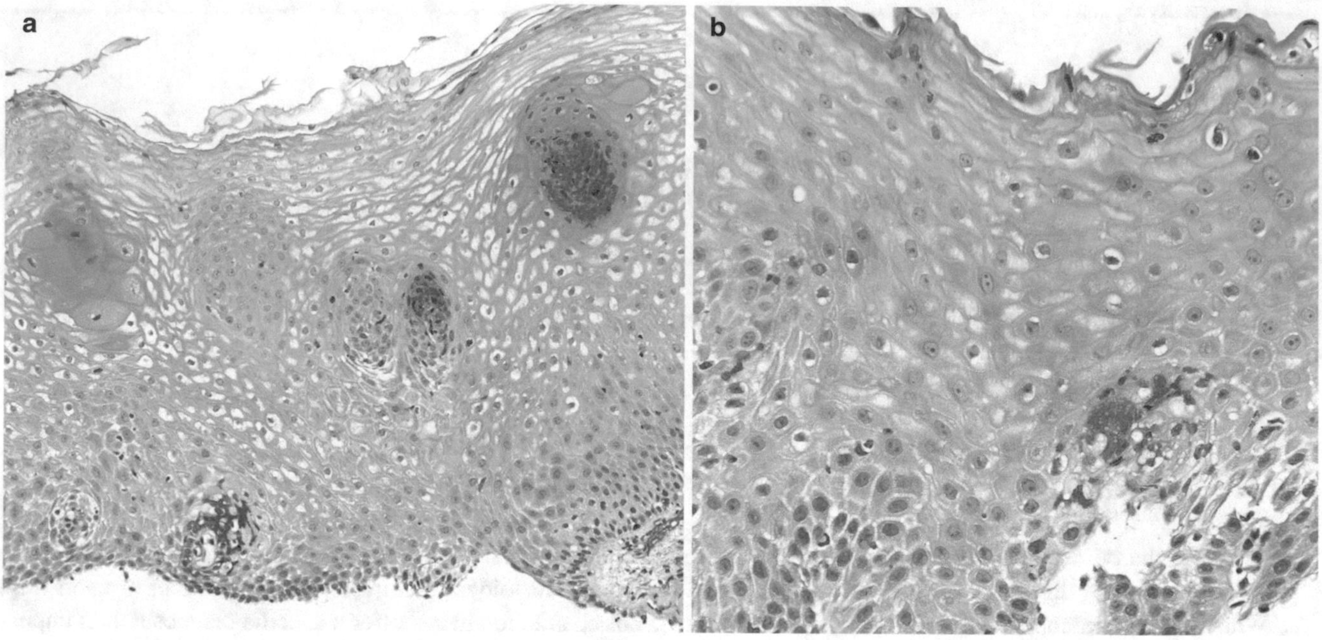

Fig. 2.1 Reflux esophagitis. (**a**) Scattered randomly distributed eosinophils, mild basal layer hyperplasia, elongated papillae, mild intercellular edema, and vascular lakes. (**b**) Additionally shows a superficial layer of parakeratosis

Biopsies of patients with GERD are frequently performed to exclude other types of esophagitis. The histologic features of biopsies in patients with GERD have been well described. These features include elongation of the papillae (>50% of the squamous epithelial thickness), hyperplasia of the basal layer (five to six layers or >15%), mildly increased intraepithelial eosinophils, and dilated intercellular spaces (Fig. 2.1a, b). Increased lymphocytes, keratinocyte vacuolization, vascular lakes, and balloon cells may also be seen. In contrast to eosinophilic esophagitis in which the eosinophils are typically more heavily concentrated near the epithelial surface, the eosinophils in GERD are randomly distributed within the epithelium. A mild parakeratosis at the luminal surface can also be seen. Although it is not practical to measure it in every esophageal biopsy, a recent study also found that increased epithelial thickness was a strong histologic marker for GERD. In the latter study, controls consisted of patients with upper gastrointestinal symptoms, but they did not need to have a different form of esophagitis so it is unclear how the epithelial thickness of GERD compares to that seen in other esophagitides such as eosinophilic or lymphocytic esophagitis. Neutrophils can be seen in more severe reflux esophagitis cases with erosions and ulceration. Unfortunately, these features are seen in other types of esophagitis which need to be excluded both clinically and histologically. Biopsies from the mid- and proximal esophagus can be helpful as these changes are usually concentrated in the distal esophagus in GERD as this is the area most heavily exposed to the refluxed gastroduodenal contents.

References: [1–10]

2. **What are the clinicopathologic findings in eosinophilic esophagitis (EoE)?**

The mechanism of disease in EoE is not fully understood, but it is currently defined as an immune- or antigen-mediated disease with esophageal dysfunction and eosinophil-predominant inflammation. EoE patients are more likely to have a history of allergic disease, and many EoE patients respond to dietary elimination of an offending food group. Seasonal variation in symptoms of EoE that mirrors that seen in allergic disease is further evidence of an association. EoE is relatively rare (1–5 per 10,000 persons in the United States and Europe), has a male gender predilection, and mostly has an onset between childhood and early to mid-adulthood. Symptoms of EoE typically include dysphagia and food impaction in adults and also include failure to thrive, heartburn, and difficulty eating in children. On endoscopy, EoE is classically described with esophageal furrowing or felinization (transverse folds in the esophagus) with possible vascular markings, rings, white exudates, and strictures, but these features are not entirely specific and biopsy is needed to confirm the diagnosis. In addition to biopsy, lack of response to PPI therapy (see question 4) and normal acid exposure on esophageal pH monitoring can aid in the diagnosis. Recent consensus recommendations first published in 2007 and updated in 2011 have aided in creating more uniformity in using both clinical and histologic criteria for making the diagnosis of EoE.

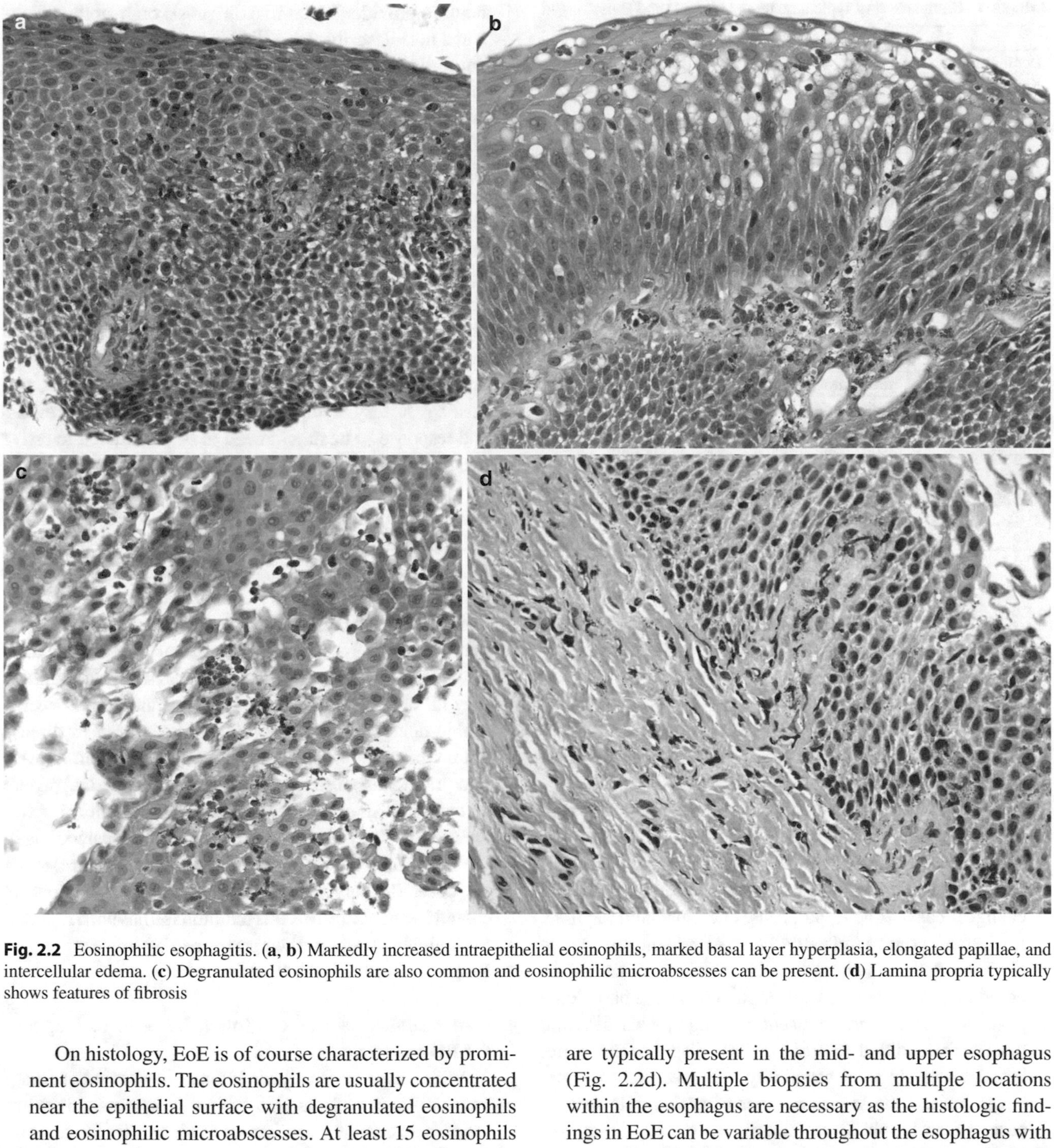

Fig. 2.2 Eosinophilic esophagitis. (**a**, **b**) Markedly increased intraepithelial eosinophils, marked basal layer hyperplasia, elongated papillae, and intercellular edema. (**c**) Degranulated eosinophils are also common and eosinophilic microabscesses can be present. (**d**) Lamina propria typically shows features of fibrosis

On histology, EoE is of course characterized by prominent eosinophils. The eosinophils are usually concentrated near the epithelial surface with degranulated eosinophils and eosinophilic microabscesses. At least 15 eosinophils in a high-power field are required for the diagnosis, but we will discuss eosinophil counts further in question 3. Biopsies also show marked reactive epithelial changes with a desquamated surface, pronounced basal cell hyperplasia, and elongation of the papillae (Fig. 2.2a–c). In contrast to GERD, eosinophil microabscesses and degranulation are common features, the basal cell hyperplasia is typically more pronounced (more than 50% of the epithelium compared to less than 25% in GERD), lamina propria fibrosis is more common, and histologic findings are typically present in the mid- and upper esophagus (Fig. 2.2d). Multiple biopsies from multiple locations within the esophagus are necessary as the histologic findings in EoE can be variable throughout the esophagus with biopsy fragments from a single location in the same patient showing both severe and mild to no disease. Biopsies from other sites in the gastrointestinal tract are important to exclude that the findings in the esophagus are isolated and not a portion of eosinophilic gastroenteritis. Recently, a composite histologic scoring system has been developed to aid in the diagnosis that is reported to outperform a simple eosinophil count. Table 2.1 compares the clinical and pathologic findings in GERD and EoE.

References: [11–18]

Table 2.1 Comparison of typical features of GERD and EoE

	GERD	EoE
Demographic		
Age	Older adults	Children and young adults
Sex	More common in males	More common in males
Main risk factor	Central adiposity	Allergic disease
Overlapping histologic factors	Intraepithelial eosinophils	Intraepithelial eosinophils
	Elongation of papillae	Elongation of papillae
	Basal layer hyperplasia	Basal layer hyperplasia
	Intercellular edema	Intercellular edema
	Parakeratosis	Parakeratosis
Distinguishing histologic features	Findings most pronounced in the distal esophagus	Findings in the mid- and upper esophagus with variation in findings across and within biopsies
	<15 eosinophils in a high-power field	>15 eosinophils in a high-power field
	No eosinophilic microabscesses	Eosinophilic microabscesses often seen
	Evenly distributed eosinophils throughout the epithelium	Eosinophils concentrated in the upper portion of the epithelium

3. **How can counting intraepithelial eosinophils add valuable information to a pathology report?**

The most common setting for which an eosinophil count is helpful is aiding in the differential diagnosis between reflux esophagitis and EoE. This can be a difficult distinction as both diseases feature reactive epithelial changes, basal zone hyperplasia, and elongated papillae. Eosinophil count is usually the most reliable manner to distinguish these two entities on histology. It should be noted that most reported eosinophil counts are based on a peak count in the most concentrated high-power field and that the threshold of 15 eosinophils to diagnose EoE is not based on established sensitivity and specificity testing, but is instead the lowest number of eosinophils seen in cases of eosinophilic esophagitis. One study from colleagues in Germany comparing the histologic features of these entities found that there was a mean of 55 (95% confidence interval (CI) 44–66) eosinophils in a high-power field compared to 9 (95% CI 5–13) in GERD. Cases with eosinophil counts in the middle of these ranges (10–20 eosinophils in a high-power field) can be a diagnostic challenge as they could represent severe GERD or mild EoE. Indeed the above referenced study found that 17% (4/24) of GERD cases had eosinophil counts of at least 15 in a high-power field. In these scenarios, it is difficult to provide a definitive diagnosis on histology alone and a note describing the diagnostic difficulty is prudent, but a diagnosis can be favored using other softer histologic features. As mentioned previously, GERD typically affects the distal portion of the esophagus, while EoE affects the mid- to upper esophagus. Additional samples from the mid- and upper esophagus can be helpful if they are not included in the initial set of biopsies. The eosinophils in GERD are usually randomly distributed throughout the epithelium, whereas the intraepithelial eosinophils in EoE are most concentrated in the upper portion of the epithelium. Eosinophil degranulation, eosinophil microabscesses, and basal zone hyperplasia are also increased in EoE compared to GERD. Biopsy findings are only one portion of the diagnostic puzzle, and the patient age, sex, medical history, symptomatology, ancillary test results, and response to treatment need to be considered to arrive at an appropriate diagnosis.

In addition to making the diagnosis of EoE, pathologists are frequently asked to provide an eosinophil count in known cases of EoE as a marker of disease severity or treatment response. We typically provide a count in the densest high-power field without additional comment. Comparison to prior biopsies should be taken with care as the size of microscopic fields can vary between microscopes and variably thick fragments of rectangular tissue may fill different quantities of area within a round microscopic field. Known variability in the severity of disease within the esophagus should also prompt caution in over-interpreting response to treatment in any individual patient as there still may be severe disease in unsampled areas. One recent study found that the number of eosinophils in the initial biopsy was inversely correlated with treatment response. Readers who work with resident and fellows should be encouraged as this tedious task has been reported to be highly accurate when performed by trainees.

References: [12, 16, 17, 19–21]

4. **Can response to PPI treatment be used to diagnose GERD over EoE?**

While response to empiric PPI treatment is used to diagnose GERD in patients with typical symptoms, this delineation between the two diseases is blurred by the recently described "proton pump inhibitor-responsive eosinophilic esophagitis" (PPI-REE). Patient's with PPI-REE have clinical and histologic features that overlap EoE but achieve clinical and histologic remission on PPI therapy. Endoscopic findings have also proven unreliable in distinguishing EoE from PPI-REE. Studies have additionally found that a portion of EoE patients who have responded to traditional EoE therapies (corticosteroids and/or dietary restriction) respond to PPIs and patients with PPI-REE also respond to traditional EoE therapies. Since EoE and PPI-REE cannot

be distinguished clinically, endoscopically, histologically, or by treatment response, many experts believe that they should all fall under the umbrella of EoE and that PPIs should be considered a possible treatment for EoE. To summarize the answer to the original question, response to PPI treatment likely leads to the incorrect diagnosis of GERD in some patients who actually have EoE, but this does not create a major clinical problem as these patients are effectively treated by the PPI.
References: [6, 22–27]

5. **Are eosinophils a necessary component to diagnose GERD?**

No, while scattered eosinophils aid in the diagnosis of GERD, they are not a sensitive marker and their absence does not exclude the diagnosis. This may especially be the case in acute GERD. Reflux esophagitis is damage to the esophagus caused by the backflow of gastric contents through the gastroesophageal junction into the esophagus. Historically, the damage has thought to have been as a result of mucosal irritation/chemical injury of the hydrochloric acid on the esophageal luminal surface. However, recent studies in both mice and in humans have provided evidence that the damage may be cytokine-mediated. In particular, they have found that biopsies in patients with acute GERD (taken 1 week or 2 weeks after discontinuing PPIs) have increased intraepithelial lymphocytes (mostly T cells). There were very few to no eosinophils or neutrophils in these biopsies of acute GERD.
References: [2, 7–10, 28]

6. **Are increased intraepithelial eosinophils in the esophagus only seen in GERD and EoE?**

Of course not. Like almost everything else in the esophagus, eosinophils are etiologically nonspecific and can be associated with many different entities. Duodenum and stomach biopsies should be examined to ensure that the biopsy does not represent esophageal involvement of eosinophilic gastroenteritis. Scattered eosinophils can also reflect Crohn disease and collagen vascular disease and as a reaction to medication (Table 2.2). Unfortunately, cases with these complicated systemic diseases are often impossible to parse out. The esophageal changes could be due to the disease itself, medications for the disease, and reflux esophagitis related to decreased motility from the systemic disease, and of course people with systemic diseases can also have GERD just like anyone else. Lastly, large eosinophilic abscesses should raise suspicion for parasites and additional levels should be obtained to exclude their presence.
Reference: [29]

7. **What are the clinical and histologic characteristics of lymphocytic esophagitis pattern?**

Biopsies from patients with a lymphocytic esophagitis pattern have numerous intraepithelial lymphocytes randomly distributed throughout the epithelium or exhibiting a predilection of peripapillary distribution (Fig. 2.3a–c). As for other forms of esophagitis, reactive epithelial changes are seen with edema and squamous hyperplasia. Rare to no neutrophils or eosinophils should be present. No count of the lymphocytes needs to be performed as the diagnosis is based on the pathologist's opinion that there are too many. The changes are most commonly seen in the distal esopha-

Table 2.2 Entities where intraepithelial eosinophils can be seen

Reflux disease
Eosinophilic esophagitis
Systemic eosinophilic gastroenteritis
Crohn disease
Medication effect
Collagen vascular disease
Parasite (eosinophilic abscess)

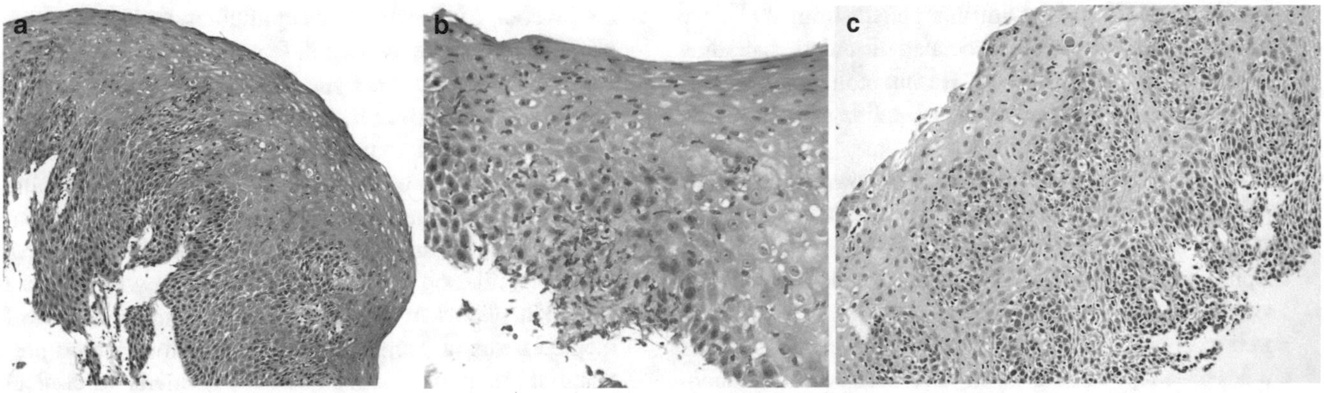

Fig. 2.3 Lymphocytic esophagitis patterns. (**a**, **b**) Squamous epithelium with increased intraepithelial lymphocytes scattered throughout the epithelium, basal layer hyperplasia, and increased papillae height. (**c**) Characteristic peripapillary distribution of intraepithelial lymphocytes can also be seen

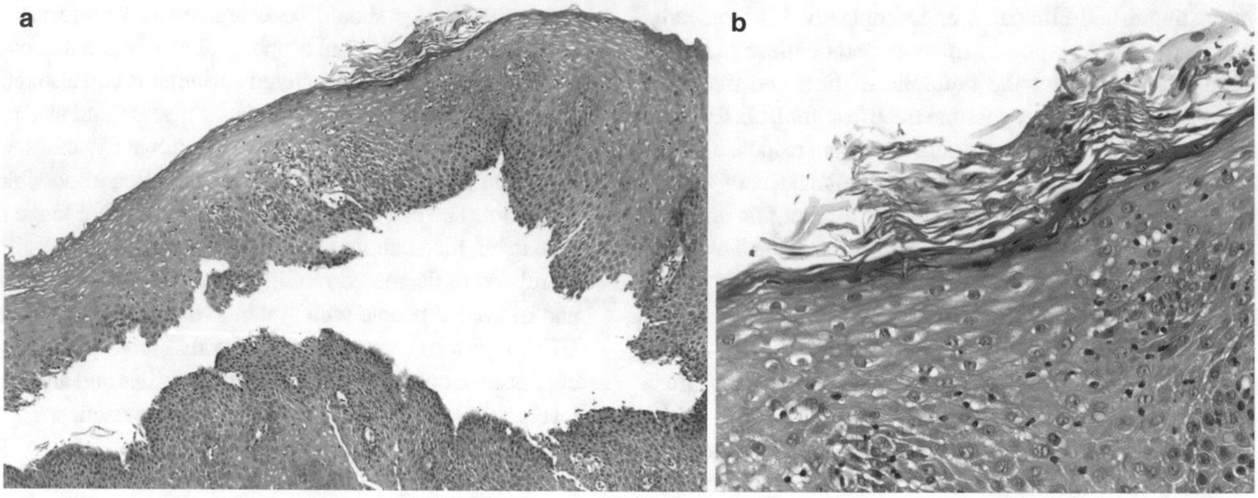

Fig. 2.4 *Candida* esophagitis. (**a**) Focal area of parakeratosis that should raise suspicion for *Candida* infection. (**b**) High-power view showing fungal pseudohyphae mixed with keratin debris compatible with *Candida*

gus but can also affect the mid- and proximal portions. As this is a nonspecific pattern, other more specific forms of esophagitis should be considered. Reflux esophagitis can be lymphocyte-predominant and cannot be excluded on histologic grounds alone. Acid pH monitoring and response to PPI therapy can be used to exclude this possibility. *Candida* esophagitis should also be considered, but it typically has a superficial neutrophilic infiltrate with sloughed off keratin debris with intermixed fungal forms (Fig. 2.4a, b). A range of endoscopic findings can be seen. The esophagus can appear normal or just have mild erythema, but it can also have plaques, rings, strictures, or furrows. The pattern is rare as it was diagnosed in approximately 0.1% of biopsies in one large study of adults. The median age of the patients with lymphocytic esophagitis was 63 and 60% were women. The pattern was more common in a study from a pediatric medical center where it was seen in just over 5% (31/545) of patients. The most common symptoms are dysphagia and reflux symptoms. In the original description of 20 cases with this pattern from 2006, the patients had a range of associated disorders including reflux disease, Crohn disease, Hashimoto thyroiditis, cirrhosis, gastroduodenitis and ulcer, celiac disease, carcinoma, and hiatal hernia, and some patients were asymptomatic. Later studies have also shown a wide range of associations but the majority of cases are idiopathic. Crohn disease has been associated with lymphocytic esophagitis in children, but this is not reproduced in adults. Lymphocytic esophagitis pattern was not increased compared to controls in patients with ulcerative colitis. Some studies have reported this pattern in association with esophageal motility disorders and in Barrett esophagus patients with high-grade dysplasia after ablation therapy.

References: [30–40]

8. **What are the clinicopathologic characteristics of lichenoid esophagitis?**

A lichenoid esophagitis pattern consists of a dense T-cell-rich lymphocytic infiltrate concentrated at the junction of the squamous epithelium and lamina propria with degeneration of the basal epithelium. Scattered degenerated squamous cells with bright eosinophilic cytoplasm can be seen that are akin to Civatte bodies in lichen planus of the skin (Fig. 2.5a, b). As opposed to lichen planus of the skin, which shows hypergranulosis and orthokeratosis, lichenoid esophagitis typically shows parakeratosis and lacks hypergranulosis since the normal esophageal epithelium lacks a granular layer. Also, rather than being acanthotic, lichenoid esophagitis is usually atrophic but can show areas of either atrophy or acanthosis. Esophageal involvement by lichen planus can be differentiated from lichenoid esophagitis pattern through clinical history of mucocutaneous lichen planus or through direct immunofluorescence (DIF). DIF shows round deposits of IgM at the junction of the squamous epithelium and lamina propria. There is some overlap in features between lichenoid esophagitis and lymphocytic esophagitis. While the distinction can be difficult, Civatte bodies have not been described in lymphocytic esophagitis, and it also typically lacks striking apoptosis and band-like inflammation at the junction of the squamous epithelium and lamina propria. The upper, mid-, and lower esophagus can all be affected.

Lichenoid esophagitis is a pattern of injury that is akin to lichen planus in the skin. This pattern does in fact include cases of esophageal involvement of lichen planus, but this pattern is also seen in a variety of clinical settings in the esophagus. Lichen planus is a mucocutaneous inflammatory disease that can affect the skin, nails, oral and genital mucosa, and the esophagus. The mecha-

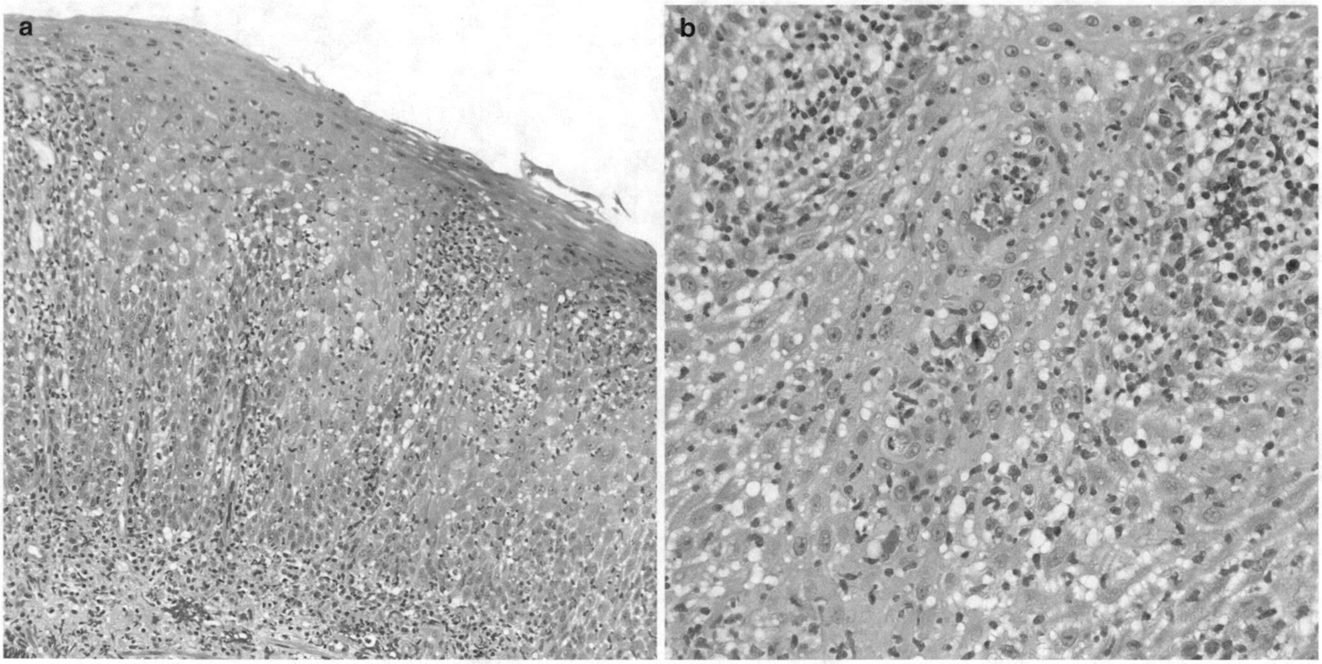

Fig. 2.5 Lichenoid esophagitis pattern. (**a**) Markedly increased lymphocytes most concentrated at the junction of the base of the epithelium and lamina propria. There are also basal layer hyperplasia and intercellular edema. (**b**) Highlights a dyskeratotic cell compatible with a Civatte body

nism of disease is not fully understood, but it can be triggered by allergic disease and hepatitis C viral infection. The condition consists of purplish, flat bumps on the skin that can form blisters that can crust or scab. White plaques can form on mucosal surfaces. Patients with esophageal disease can present with dysphagia and strictures. Endoscopic findings can include stricture and peeling, friable mucosa that can be difficult to distinguish from eosinophilic esophagitis. A large case series of 88 specimens from 65 patients with lichenoid esophagitis pattern was conducted at Johns Hopkins Hospital. These patients were predominantly females in their 50s or 60s. About a third (32%) of the patients had confirmed lichen planus. Of the patients without lichen planus, 59% were taking at least four medications, 23% had a chronic viral disease (HIV or viral hepatitis), 11% had an associated rheumatologic disorder, and 7% progressed to dysplasia or carcinoma. Patients with lichen planus were more likely to have a stricture than those without (38% versus 9%). Table 2.3 details a comparison between lymphocytic and lichenoid esophagitis patterns.
References: [41–44]

Table 2.3 Clinicopathologic comparison of lymphocytic and lichenoid esophagitis patterns

	Lymphocytic esophagitis	Lichenoid esophagitis
Age	60s	50s or 60s
Symptoms	Dysphagia, reflux symptoms, can be asymptomatic	Dysphagia, reflux symptoms, can be asymptomatic
Disease associations	Majority idiopathic, GERD, Crohn, Hashimoto, cirrhosis, celiac disease, gastroduodenitis, carcinoma, esophageal motility disorders, Barrett esophagus s/p ablation for dysplasia	Lichen planus, polypharmacy, chronic viral disease (e.g., viral hepatitis or HIV), rheumatologic disease
Intraepithelial lymphocytes	Randomly distributed throughout epithelium or peripapillary	Concentrated at junction of epithelium and lamina propria
Additional histologic findings	Intercellular edema, squamous hyperplasia, ballooning keratinocytes. Lacks Civatte bodies and apoptosis	Civatte bodies, degeneration of basal epithelium with apoptosis, parakeratosis, atrophic or acanthotic
Location	Distal most common, but can also affect mid and proximal	All levels

9. **What are the causes and long-term implications of corrosive injury to the esophagus?**

Corrosive injury of the esophagus is injury that occurs due to ingestion of lye or another caustic substance. These injuries are very sad as they most commonly result from either accidental ingestion by a young child or a suicide attempt. Grossly there are necrosis and extensive internal hemorrhage (Fig. 2.6a, b). Patients with acute ingestions are rarely biopsied, but acute inflammation and necrosis are seen in a pattern similar to that seen in sloughing

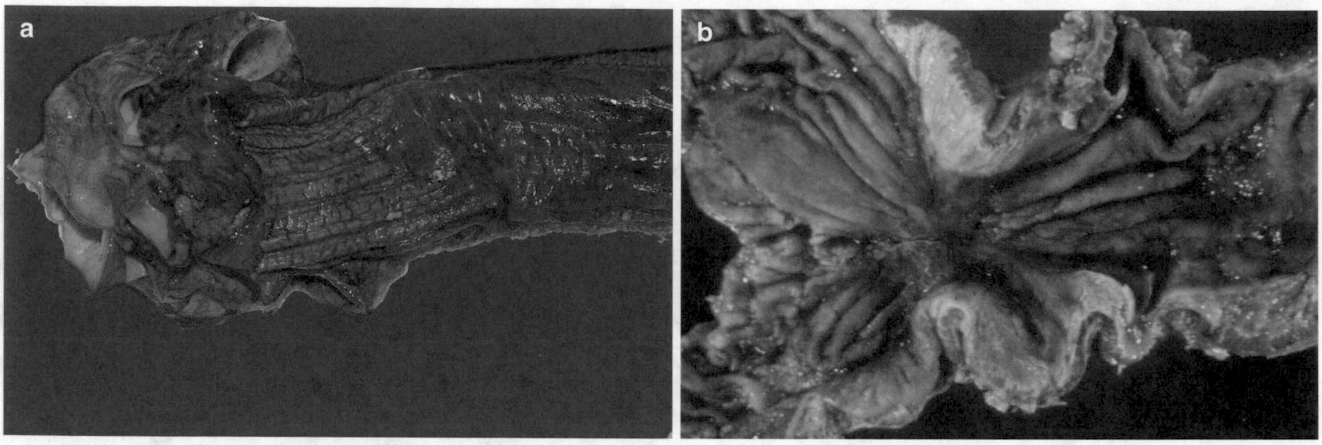

Fig. 2.6 Corrosive ingestion. (**a**) Gross photograph of an esophagus following intentional (suicide) lye ingestion shows diffuse necrosis with extensive internal hemorrhage. (Photograph courtesy of Dr. Priya Banerjee). (**b**) Gross photograph showing ulceration in the stomach following hydrochloric acid ingestion

esophagitis. Chronic lesions typically show full-thickness fibrosis on the esophageal wall that corresponds with an endoscopically apparent stricture and prolonged transit time of food through the esophagus. Importantly, these patients need to undergo lifetime surveillance as they are estimated to have a thousandfold increased lifetime risk of squamous cell carcinoma. Follow-up needs to be long-term as there can be a 40-year latency period before cancer development.

References: [45–49]

10. How are the most common types of pill fragments in pill esophagitis histologically distinguished?

Pill-induced esophagitis is a common cause of injury that refers to injury due to contact between the pills and the esophageal mucosa. It is frequently associated with erosion and ulceration and most commonly affects the mid-esophagus. Oftentimes no pill or just nonspecific polarizable material is seen. The squamous mucosa often shows erosion or ulceration with fibrinopurulent debris. At times, the squamous mucosa can have a sloughing (esophagitis dissecans superficialis) pattern of injury. Marked reactive epithelial and stromal reactive changes can be seen that should not be misdiagnosed as dysplasia or malignancy. Multinucleated squamous giant cells can also be seen. Fungal forms and viral cytopathic effect should be excluded. Treatment includes PPIs, sucralfate, withdrawal of the offending medication, and behavioral modification such as sitting upright while ingesting the medication. In instances for which the biopsy findings are nonspecific, clinical correlation and the establishment of a temporal relationship with the drug are necessary. Among others, NSAIDs, bisphosphonates, and doxycycline are common causes of esophageal injury for which no specific pill fragment is seen. There are, however, certain injurious medications that produce specific microscopic appearances.

Injury due to iron pills is generally seen in the upper gastrointestinal tract, and iron pill esophagitis is not uncommonly seen by practicing pathologists. Iron supplements are most commonly taken in the setting of iron deficiency anemia. They can cause an erosive/ulcerative injury with dark purple or brown-black crystalline material in granulation tissue or fibrinopurulent debris (Fig. 2.7a–d). The iron fragments can be highlighted by iron stain if necessary. The ulceration can cause marked reactive epithelial and stromal changes that should not be mistaken for dysplasia or malignancy.

Pill fragments from three types of resins (kayexalate, sevelamer, and bile acid sequestrants) have been identified in the gastrointestinal tract. While all three are more commonly seen at other sites, they are all rarely identified within the esophagus. Kayexalate (sodium polystyrene sulfonate) is a cation exchange resin used to treat hyperkalemia. It was originally described in the pathology literature as a cause of gastrointestinal injury in a series of five cases of colonic necrosis in 1987. Subsequent case series describing kayexalate effects in the gastrointestinal tract have included cases with active esophagitis, esophageal ulcer, and esophageal squamous carcinoma. Importantly the background squamous epithelium needs to be carefully examined as both series included a patient with herpes esophagitis and another coinfected with *Candida*. While it seems that kayexalate can cause damage to the gastrointestinal tract independent of additional insults, it is unclear whether it potentiates the ulceration caused by herpes simplex virus (HSV) or is a passenger in these situations. In addition to the original descriptions, the morphology of

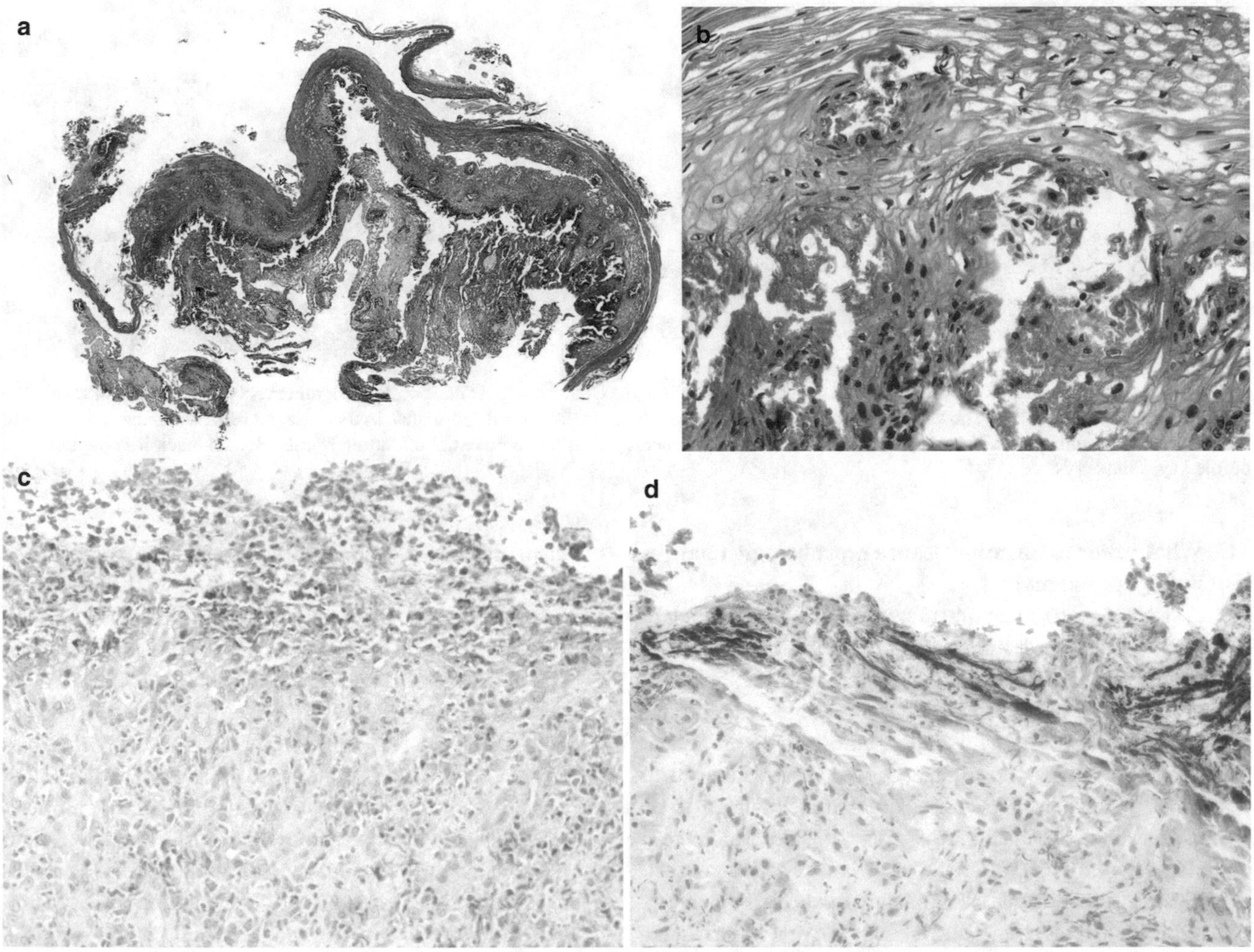

Fig. 2.7 Iron pill esophagitis. (**a**) Low-power view shows reactive squamous mucosa with abundant brown pigment compatible with iron at the base of the epithelium. (**b**) High-power view of light-brown iron pigment crystals at the base of the epithelium. (**c**) Ulcerated esophagus with light-brown iron pigment at the surface. (**d**) Iron stain (blue) confirms the diagnosis of iron pill esophagitis

crystal resins seen in the gastrointestinal tract has been expertly described and compared in great detail in a recent review. Kayexalate crystals are rectangular purple crystals with evenly spaced fish scales (Fig. 2.8a–c). On AFB stain the crystals are black. Confirmation with clinical history is vital as these histologic features can vary depending on the site within the gastrointestinal tract and the various crystals can be mistaken for other types of pill fragments or even dystrophic calcifications.

Sevelamer (Renagel, Renvela) is an anion exchange resin used to decrease phosphate in patients with chronic kidney disease. It was first associated with injury to the gastrointestinal tract in a case series from 2013. One of the seven cases involved the esophagus, which showed extensive circumferential erosions and ulcerations with a thick white exudate. Sevelamer crystals are typically rectangular and "two-toned" in color with bright-pink center and background rusty-yellow edges. One should take caution in relying on color as it can be variable and even look purple like kayexalate. The fish scales in sevelamer crystals are typically wide and irregularly distributed. On AFB stain, sevelamer crystals are magenta. Again, a clinical history can be invaluable to confirming their identity.

Bile acid sequestrants (BAS; including cholestyramine, colesevelam, and colestipol) are used to treat hypercholesterolemia and hyperlipidemia. One large case series of pill fragments in the gastrointestinal tract found them in the esophagus in just 1 of the 25 cases. They can be found in the lumen and within the tissue. Their association with mucosal injury is not well established. The three bile acid sequestrants are histologically indistinguishable. They are polygonal with a homogenous pink color and lack the fish scales seen in kayexalate and sevelamer fragments. On AFB stain they are pale yellow in color.

References: [50–60]

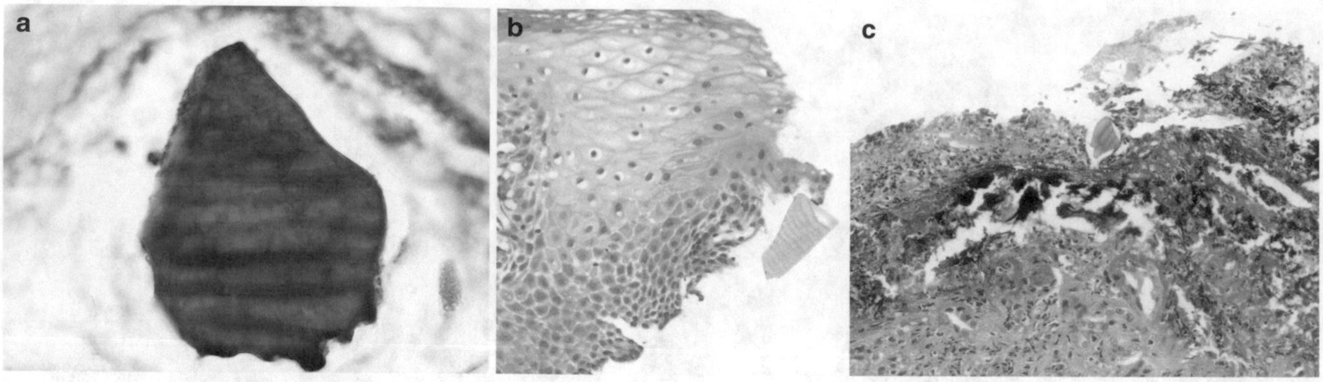

Fig. 2.8 Kayexalate. (**a**) High-power view of a kayexalate crystal with the classic homogenous purple color and evenly distributed fish scales. (**b**) Kayexalate crystal on the right shows homogenous pale purple color and even distributed fish scales. In this case the resin was detached and there was no associated injury in the esophagus. (**c**) A case of erosive esophagitis with two potential offending agents. Brown-black iron pigment and purple kayexalate crystals

11. What other medications cause morphologic changes in the esophagus?

Taxanes are chemotherapeutic agents that bind to microtubules and inhibit depolymerization. They are commonly used to treat carcinoma of the esophagus, breast, and lungs. Marked mucosal changes with prominent mitotic arrest with ringed mitoses and prominent apoptotic bodies due to taxanes were first described in the esophagus in 1989 during initial phase I clinical trials of Taxol. A subsequent large case series described these changes in biopsies throughout the gastrointestinal tract. These dramatic epithelial changes can closely mimic high-grade dysplasia. These changes have not been associated with toxicity, and these changes are thought to be manifestations of the drug's intended mechanism of action.

Colchicine is an alkaloid with antimitotic activity used to treat flares of gout and to prevent attacks of abdominal, chest, and joint pains by familial Mediterranean fever. One case series of colchicine effects in the gastrointestinal tract did not include any cases with esophageal findings, but older studies have reported esophageal injury. Symptoms are nonspecific but can entail abdominal pain, diarrhea, and cramping. Endoscopic findings include inflammation and erosion/ulceration. Similar to those seen in association with taxanes, histologic findings include increased metaphase (ringed) mitoses, increased apoptotic bodies, and reactive epithelial changes. Unlike for taxanes, these changes are only seen with clinical toxicity and are not present with therapeutic drug levels.

Mycophenolate (CellCept or Myfortic) can also induce injury to the upper gastrointestinal tract. It is an immunomodulatory drug used in autoimmune diseases such as systemic lupus erythematosus (SLE) and to prevent rejection in organ transplant recipients. Gastrointestinal symptoms include diarrhea, nausea and vomiting, abdominal pain, dysphagia, and gastrointestinal bleeding. In one series, four of the six evaluable biopsies in the esophagus showed increased apoptotic bodies (Fig. 2.9a, b). Additional findings included active inflammation, erosion, and ulceration. Graft-versus-host disease (GVHD) can be difficult to differentiate from mycophenolate toxicity as both feature increased apoptosis. Clinical information is key as GVHD occurs in stem cell transplants, while mycophenolate is most often used in solid organ transplant recipients, but there are times when a stem cell transplant recipient is given mycophenolate. While there are no reliable features to distinguish mycophenolate toxicity from GVHD in the esophagus, increased adjacent eosinophils are more commonly seen with mycophenolate toxicity in other areas of the gastrointestinal tract. Lastly, cytomegalovirus (CMV) infection should also be excluded in this setting as it often features acute inflammation, ulceration, and increased apoptotic bodies and immunocompromised patients are more prone to this opportunistic infection.

Ipilimumab is a monoclonal antibody directed against cytotoxic T-lymphocyte antigen-4 (CTLA-4) that is used to treat various malignancies. It, along with other immune checkpoint inhibitors (PDL-1), has been associated with gastroenteritis with diarrhea. While, to our knowledge, these medications do not typically produce esophageal injury, one anecdotal case seen at Johns Hopkins showed prominent apoptosis, increased intraepithelial lymphocytes, and marked reactive epithelial changes with basal cell hyperplasia, intercellular edema, and keratinocyte vacuolization.
References: [61–71]

12. What are the features of sloughing esophagitis/esophagitis dissecans?

Sloughing esophagitis (esophagitis dissecans superficialis) is a condition in which a superficial portion of the esophageal epithelium sloughs off or splits from the

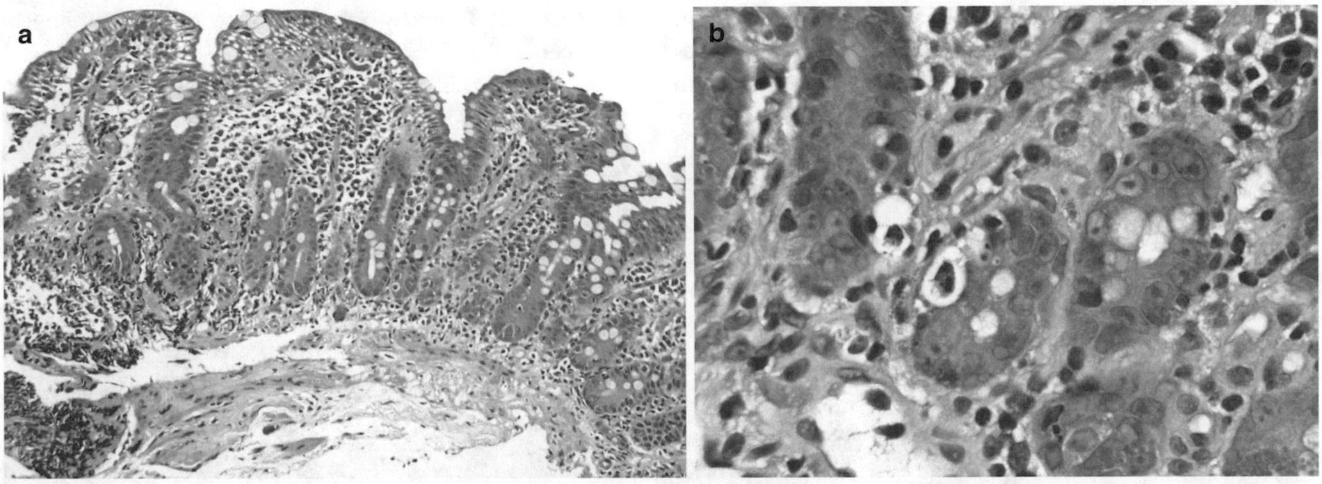

Fig. 2.9 Mycophenolate toxicity. (**a**, **b**) Although these photographs are from the small bowel, they highlight the markedly increased apoptotic bodies, scattered surrounding eosinophils, villous shortening, and epithelial reactive changes that can be seen with mycophenolate toxicity

underlying epithelium. This is seen on endoscopy as single to numerous white patches or a single large white tube of sloughed off mucosa (Fig. 2.10a). This impression is confirmed on histology with a well-delineated, often with splitting above the basal layer, superficial strip of parakeratosis and necrosis (Fig. 2.10b–e). There is typically very little inflammation. Immunohistochemical study has not found any aberration in integrin expression. Immunofluorescence studies have shown no C3 or immunoglobulin deposits. Usually the mid- or distal esophagus is affected. Symptoms can include dysphagia possibly with stricture, gastrointestinal bleeding, weight loss, epigastric pain, and most severely can result in vomiting of tubes of mucosa, but the disease can also be asymptomatic. Like so many other inflammatory conditions in the esophagus, sloughing esophagitis is also a nonspecific pattern of injury. Patients are typically middle-aged to elderly and the pattern of injury is more common in men. Studies have shown an association with some medications including NSAIDs, bisphosphonates, psychoactive medications, and polypharmacy in general. Risk factors include debilitation, immunosuppression, smoking, and physical trauma (e.g., drinking hot beverages).

References: [72–78]

13. What are the diagnostic features of and the differential diagnosis for pemphigus vulgaris (PV)?

Pemphigus vulgaris is a dermatologic condition that, like lichen planus mentioned previously, can affect the esophagus. It is characterized by intraepithelial splitting just above the basal layer (suprabasal) of the squamous epithelium with acantholytic squamous epithelial cells, bullet-shaped nucleoli, and intercellular edema (Fig. 2.11a–d). Direct immunofluorescence (DIF) is key to differentiating the bullous diseases, and an additional request for fresh tissue can be very helpful. In PV, DIF shows homogenous staining of IgG in the intercellular spaces of the perilesional squamous tissue. These antibodies are generally against desmoglein 1 and/or 3. PV is the most common form of pemphigus and most commonly occurs in patients between 30 and 50 years and has no gender predilection. Oral lesions are almost always seen, but any mucosal surface can be affected. Esophageal involvement is almost always found when endoscopy is performed. Dysphagia and odynophagia (painful swallowing) are the most common esophageal symptoms. Once the diagnosis is made, patients are typically treated with steroids and immunomodulatory agents.

Other bullous dermatologic diseases can also less commonly affect the esophagus. Bullous pemphigoid (BP) principally affects the skin in people age 40–70 years old but can rarely affect mucosal surfaces including the esophagus. BP causes a subepidermal split with prominent eosinophils. It is caused by IgG autoantibodies to hemidesmosomal antigens (BP230 and BP180).

Epidermolysis bullosa includes a variety of rare bullous diseases that affect the skin and mucosal surfaces, and the esophagus is among the most common mucosal sites affected. The most common types are dystrophic epidermolysis bullosa (DEB), epidermolysis bullosa simplex (EBS), and junctional epidermolysis bullosa (JEB). The inherited forms of these diseases are caused by mutations to genes encoding structural proteins (type VII collagen, α6βintegrin, cytokeratins 5 and 14, and laminin), while the acquired version has been associated with various viral infections and autoimmune diseases. All forms are characterized by blister formation caused by minor trauma at skin and mucosal locations. Disease severity ranges from minor to severe with ulceration, scarring, strictures, and contractures. Lesions (predominantly described in the skin) show splitting in the dermis (DEB), epidermis (EBS), or dermoepidermal junction (JEB). Table 2.4 highlights clinical and pathologic differences between the bullous entities described above.

References: [79–92]

14. **How can I figure out the cause of an esophageal ulcer?**

The truth is that there are many causes of ulceration that all result in inflamed squamous mucosa with associated granulation tissue and fibrinopurulent debris. As detailed above, some medications can be identified on H&E, but in most cases the pathologist can only report that there is acute erosive esophagitis and maybe sug-

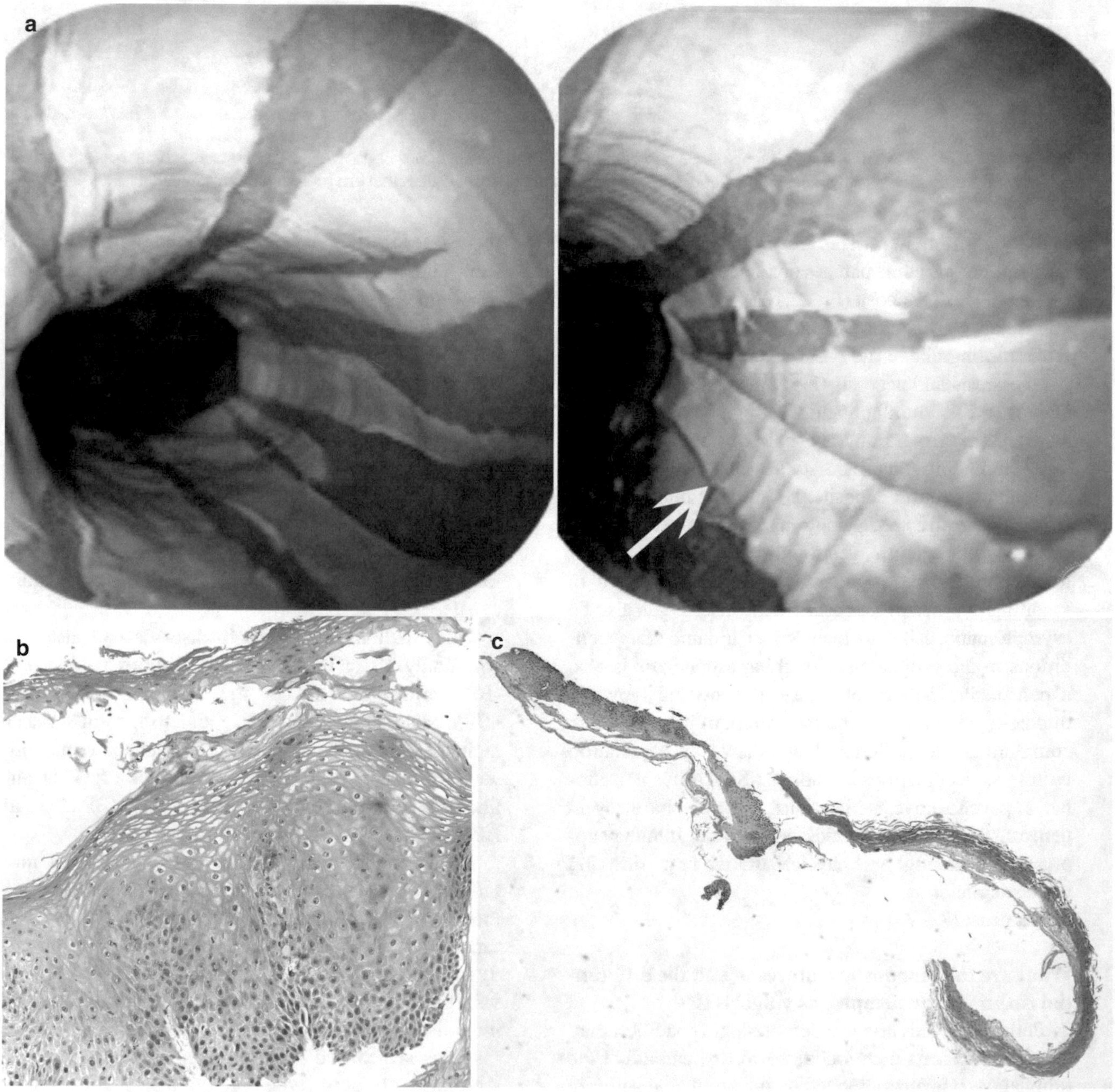

Fig. 2.10 Esophagitis dissecans superficialis. (**a**) Endoscopic examination of the esophagus showing whitish strips of detached squamous epithelium that are dislodged with water spray (white arrow). (**b**, **c**) Medium- and low-power view of squamous mucosa with detached layer of sloughed off superficial epithelium with parakeratosis. (**d**) High-power view of squamous epithelium with distinct superficial layer of parakeratosis with necrosis. Notice the mild acute inflammation. (**e**) High-power view of the classic detached strip of superficial squamous epithelium with parakeratosis, necrosis, and little to no inflammation

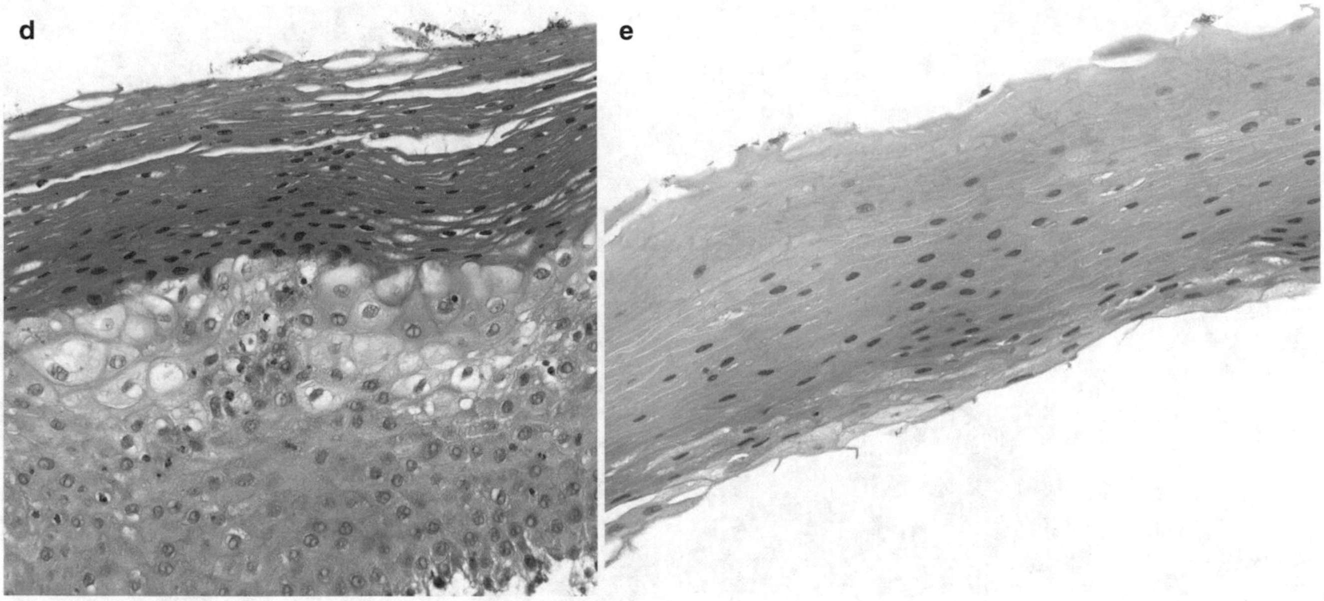

Fig. 2.10 (continued)

gest a cause based on the patient's clinical history and list of medications. The key is actually to exclude causes of ulceration that can either be treated or will drastically change the patient's prognosis and treatment plan.

It is important to exclude malignancy as this diagnosis will have a major impact on the patient. Tumors of the esophagus are covered in detail in a separate chapter, but a neoplastic process should be considered whenever there is ulceration. In addition to primary tumors, metastatic tumors growing up through the muscularis propria can cause ulceration in the overlying mucosa. Even benign tumors like a granular cell tumor in the lamina propria can cause overlying pseudoepitheliomatous hyperplasia or ulceration.

Treatable infections need to also be excluded in esophageal ulceration. HSV only infects epithelial cells, and its inclusions are found in the squamous epithelium immediately adjacent to the ulcer bed and consist of the "three Ms" (multinuclear, margination, and nuclear molding). CMV can infect epithelial cells, endothelial cells, and fibroblasts so its inclusions can be seen both in the epithelium and in the ulcer bed itself. While a careful scan for viral cytopathic effect is prudent in any esophageal ulceration, one should be extra careful in biopsies from immunocompromised patients (e.g., transplant recipients, chemotherapy administration, HIV infection). While not mandatory for each ulceration, immunohistochemical stains for CMV and HSV can be helpful if there are equivocal inclusions on H&E or a strong clinical suspicion. While it often does not cause ulceration, *Candida* esophagitis should also be excluded. Endoscopists are usually quite adept at picking up *Candida* infection as a white plaque, but this may be obscured if there is significant ulceration. The organisms can be visualized as a mixture of pseudohyphae and yeast buds that are most easily picked up in keratin debris of desquamated surface epithelium. Additional histologic findings that should raise suspicion for *Candida* infection are acute inflammation in the squamous epithelium, keratin debris in the luminal space above the epithelium, or lymphocytosis. Again, a careful check should be made in immunocompromised patients, and PAS or GMS special stains can be utilized to help identify organisms.

Case Presentation

Case 1

Learning Objectives

- To learn the differential diagnosis of a large ulcerated lesion
- To exclude identifiable etiologies that are either treatable or confer major prognostic implications
- Two processes and findings can occur simultaneously

Case History

A 71-year-old female with immunosuppression and chronic kidney disease presents with gastrointestinal bleeding.

Endoscopic Findings

Ulcerated necrotic-appearing mass-like area spanning 10 cm of the distal esophagus.

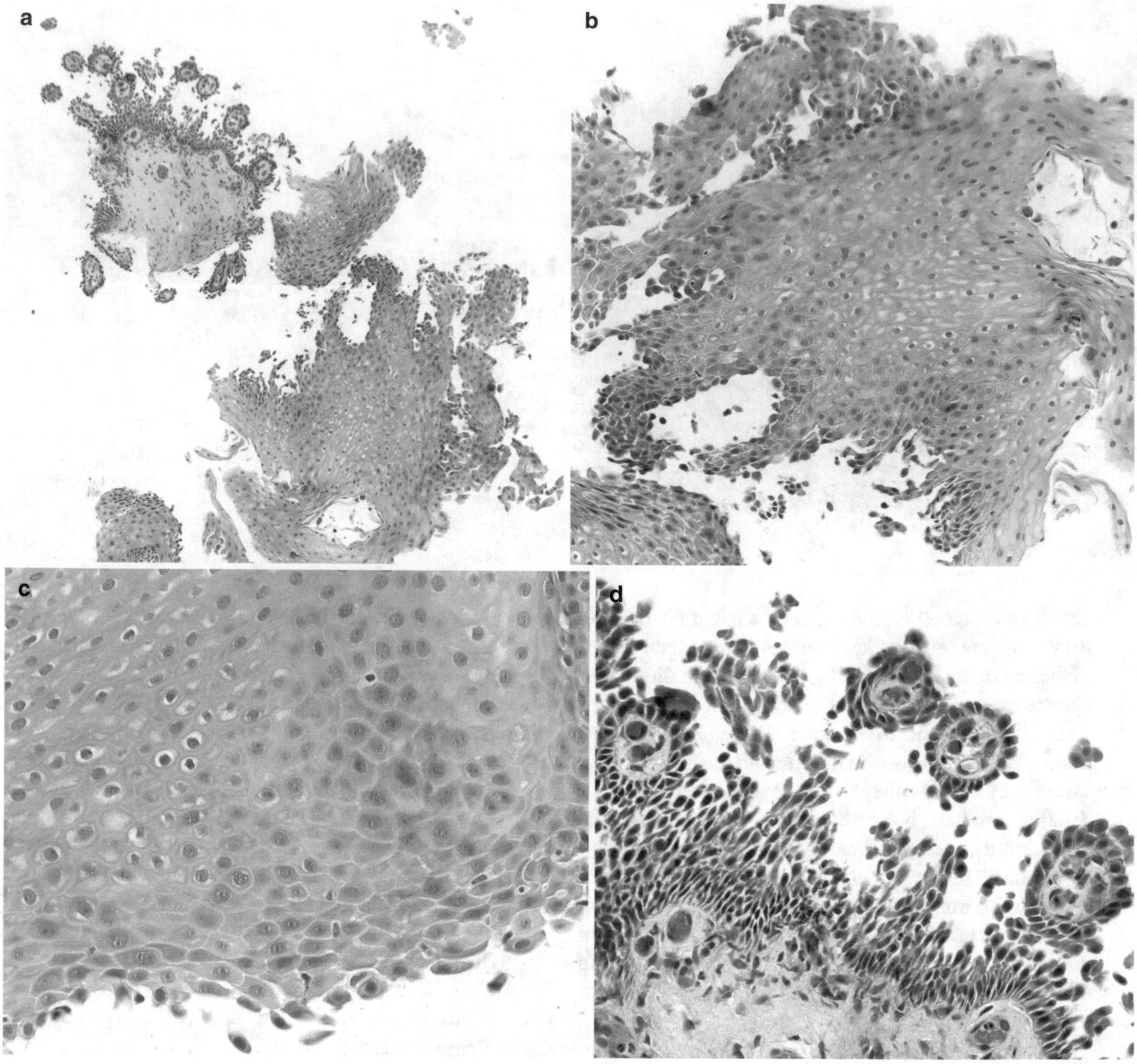

Fig. 2.11 Pemphigus vulgaris. (**a**) Low-power view of a biopsy shows suprabasal clefting of the squamous epithelium. (**b**) Squamous epithelium shows partial loss of the basal layer with acantholysis and mild intercellular edema with little to no inflammation. (**c**) High-power view highlights the "bullet-shaped" nucleoli in the reactive squamous cells. (**d**) Lamina propria and papillae have a layer of remaining basal cells with the hallmark "tombstone" appearance

Differential Diagnosis Prior to Slide Review

- Malignancy
- Virus
- Medication effect
- GERD
- Toxic ingestion

Histologic Findings

- Necroinflammatory debris with numerous pill fragments, bacteria, and foodstuff (Fig. 2.12a, b).
- Numerous crystals with a variety of morphologic appearances. Most were pink with wide irregular fish scales and slightly rust-colored edges. However, some were purple in color, while others lacked fish scales (Fig. 2.12c–e).
- Rare degenerated squamous epithelium with areas where the nuclei were molded with marginated chromatin and multinucleation (Fig. 2.12f).

Differential Diagnosis After Slide Review

- Pill fragments
  - Sevelamer
  - Kayexalate
  - Cholestyramine
  - Others

Table 2.4 Comparison of pemphigus vulgaris with bullous pemphigoid and epidermolysis bullosa

	Pemphigus vulgaris	Bullous pemphigoid	Epidermolysis bullosa
Commonly affects the esophagus	Yes	No	Yes
Esophageal symptoms	Dysphagia, odynophagia	Dysphagia, odynophagia	Dysphagia, odynophagia
Cause	Antibodies to desmoglein 1 and/or 3	Antibodies to hemidesmosomal antigens (BP230 and BP180)	Inherited form: Mutations to structural proteins Acquired form: Viral infection or autoimmune diseases
Level of split	Suprabasal with clinging basal layer with "tombstone" appearance	Subepidermal	Epidermis (EBS) Dermis (DEB) Epidermal/dermal junction (JEB)
Additional histologic findings	Intercellular edema, bullet-shaped nucleoli, mild to no inflammation	Prominent eosinophils	Little to no mixed inflammation
DIF	Intercellular IgG and C3 in lower basal aspect of the epidermis with "chicken-wire" pattern	Linear deposition of IgG and CE at junction	Altered staining pattern at level of molecular defect

- Virus
  - Herpes esophagitis
  - CMV

IHC and Other Ancillary Studies

- Pill fragments are magenta on AFB special stain.
- Degenerated squamous cells are immunoreactive for HSV I immunostain (Fig. 2.12g).

Final Diagnosis

Herpes esophagitis with sevelamer crystals (confirmed by reconciliation with medication list).

Take-Home Messages

- Sevelamer crystals are associated with mucosal injury in the gastrointestinal tract.
- They can have a variable morphologic appearance and be mistaken for other pill types when they have a purple color (kayexalate) or lack fish scales (cholestyramine).
- Underlying viral esophagitis should be carefully examined for and excluded in cases of pill esophagitis.

Case 2

Learning Objectives

- Lichenoid esophagitis is a pattern of injury that is not specific to any single etiology
- A portion of cases are manifestations of lichen planus, but others are associated with viral infections and polypharmacy

Case History

A 51-year-old male with dysphagia and a history of hepatitis B infection.

Endoscopic Findings

Inflammation and scattered ulcers.

Differential Diagnosis Prior to Slide Review

- GERD
- EoE
- Lymphocytic esophagitis
- Lichenoid esophagitis
- Medication effect

Histologic Findings

- Squamous mucosa with dense lymphocyte-predominant inflammation concentrated in band-like pattern at the base of the epithelium and lamina propria (Fig. 2.13a).
- Scattered Civatte bodies (Fig. 2.13b).

Differential Diagnosis After Slide Review

- Lichenoid esophagitis
- Esophageal involvement of lichen planus
- Lymphocytic esophagitis
- GERD

IHC and Other Ancillary Studies

- DIF to rule out lichen planus. Negative for round deposits of IgM at the junction of the squamous epithelium and lamina propria.

Final Diagnosis

Lichenoid esophagitis pattern possibly associated with the patient's viral hepatitis.

Take-Home Messages

- Lichenoid esophagitis pattern of injury can be associated with esophageal involvement of lichen planus, viral infection, polypharmacy, and rheumatologic diseases.

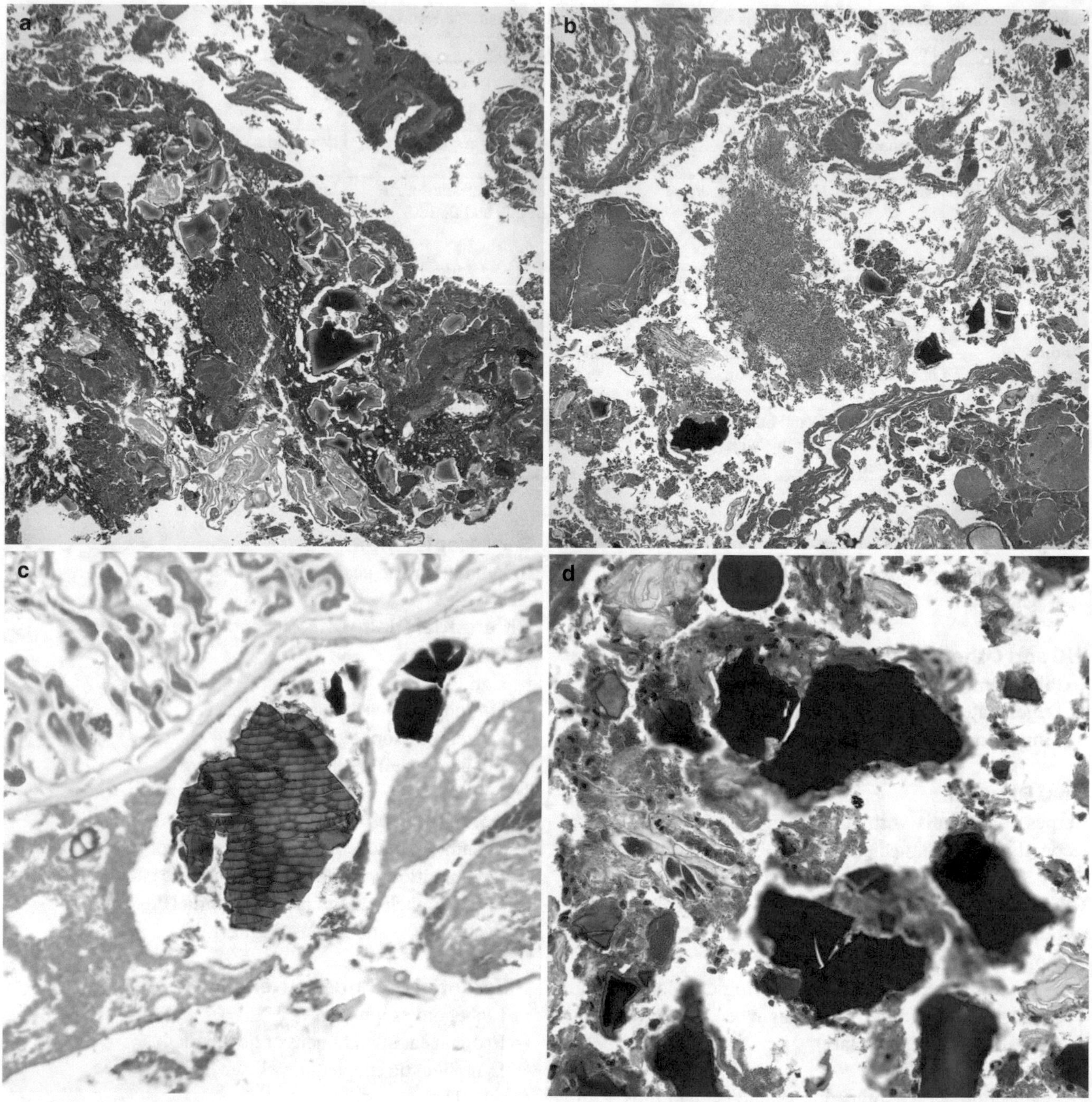

Fig. 2.12 Case 1. (**a**, **b**) Numerous sevelamer crystals mixed in a background of necroinflammatory debris, bacterial colonies, and foodstuff. The crystals show variable morphology throughout the material with some showing (**c**) the typical pink color with rust-colored edges and wide irregular fish scales, while others (**d**) are purple in color raising the differential of kayexalate, and others (**e**) lack fish scales. (**f**) Mixed in the debris are detached degenerated squamous cells showing multinucleation, nuclear molding, and chromatin margination compatible with herpes viral cytopathic effect. (**g**) An HSV I immunohistochemical stain clinched the diagnosis

- While difficult to distinguish from lymphocytic esophagitis, lichenoid esophagitis is more likely to feature band-like inflammation centered at the junction of the base of the epithelium and lamina propria and Civatte bodies.

Case 3

Learning Objectives

- Intraepithelial eosinophils are not limited to reflux esophagitis and eosinophilic esophagitis

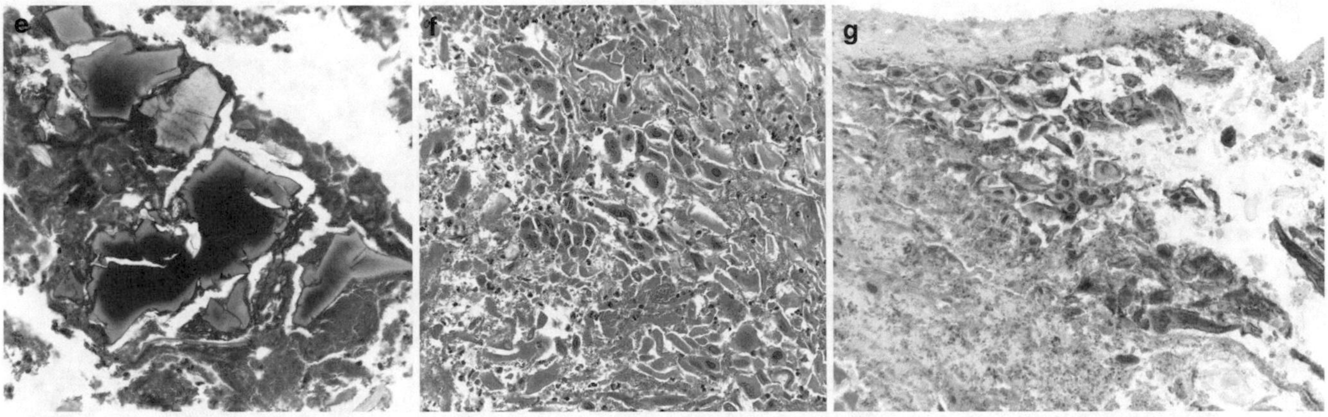

Fig. 2.12 (continued)

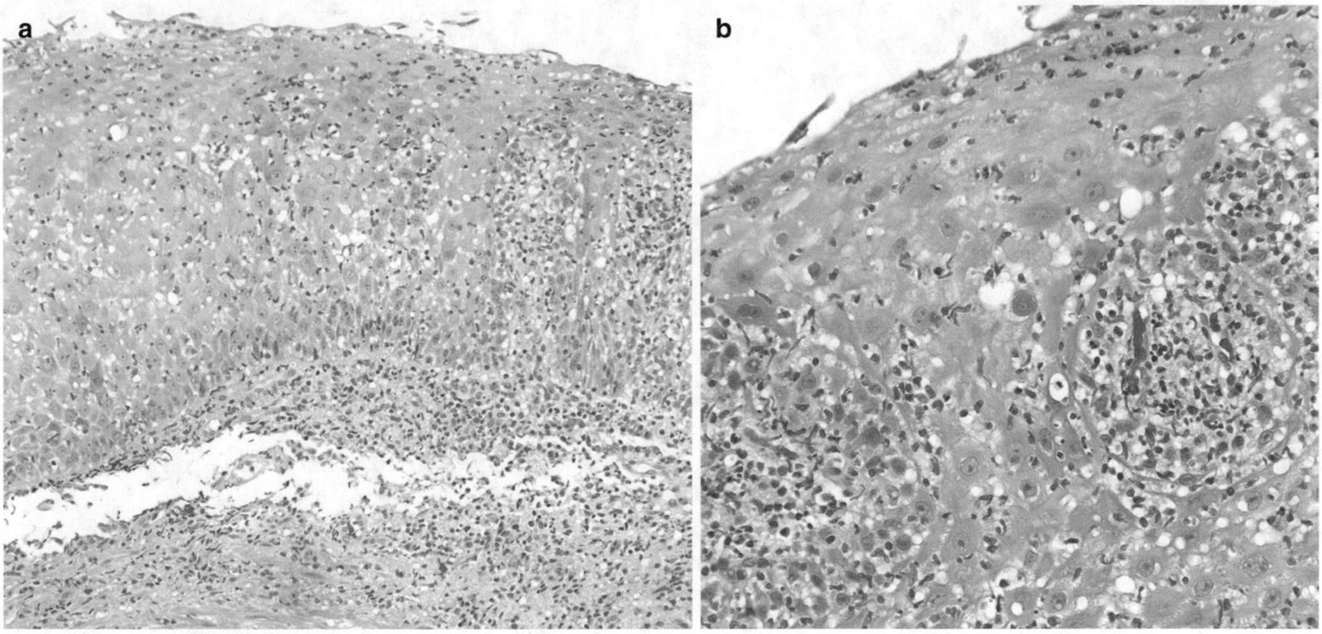

Fig. 2.13 Case 2. (**a**) Dense band-like lymphocytic inflammation most concentrated at the base of the epithelium and lamina propria. (**b**) There are scattered Civatte bodies. Overall, the case is compatible with lichenoid esophagitis pattern. Review of the patient history revealed that it may be associated with hepatitis B infection

- Clinical correlation is required to arrive at a diagnosis

Case History

A 26-year-old female with epigastric pain and history Crohn disease.

Endoscopic Finding

Mild esophageal erythema.

Differential Diagnosis Prior to Slide Review

- Upper tract involvement of Crohn disease
- Medication effect
- Lymphocytic esophagitis
- GERD
- EoE

Histologic Findings

Squamous mucosa with reactive epithelial changes (elongated papillae, mild basal layer hyperplasia) and areas with scattered intraepithelial eosinophils (Fig. 2.14a) and other areas with scattered intraepithelial lymphocytes (Fig. 2.14b).

Differential Diagnosis After Slide Review

- Upper tract involvement of Crohn disease

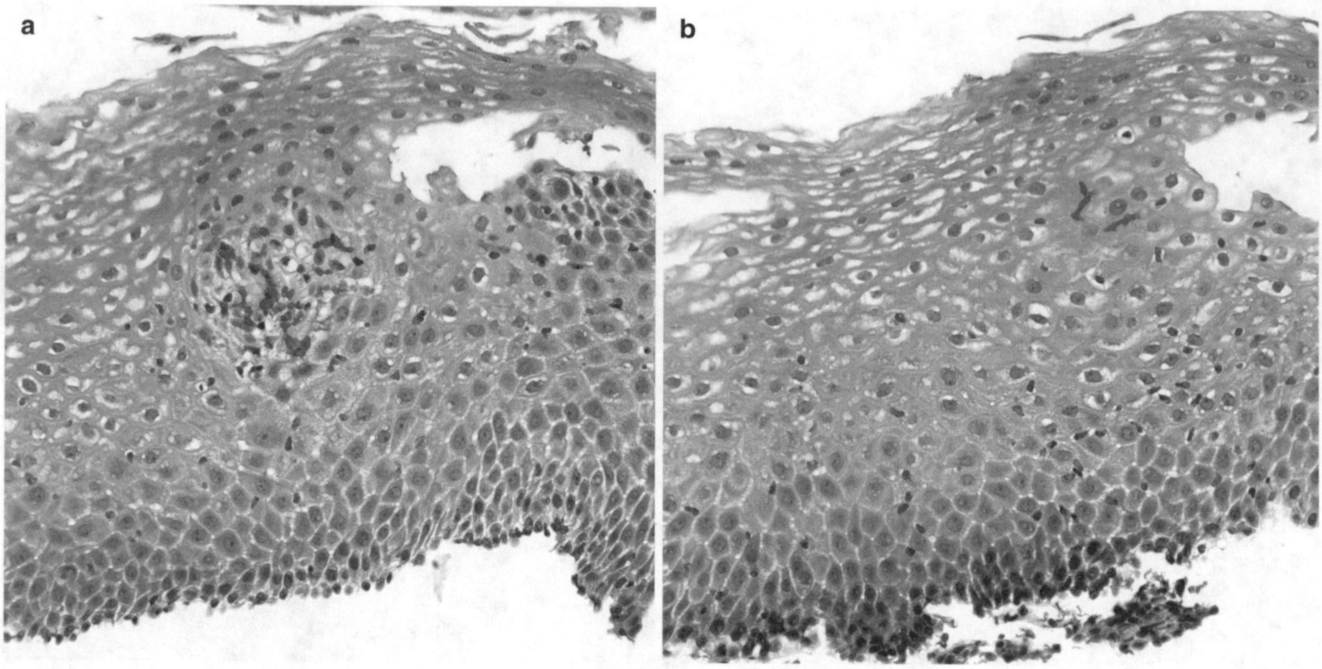

Fig. 2.14 Case 3. Squamous mucosa with mild reactive epithelial changes and scattered intraepithelial (**a**) eosinophils and (**b**) lymphocytes in a patient with a history of Crohn disease

- Medication effect
- Lymphocytic esophagitis
- GERD

IHC and Other Ancillary Studies

None.

Final Diagnosis

Squamous mucosa with reactive epithelial changes and scattered intraepithelial eosinophils and lymphocytes.

- Given the clinical history, these findings could represent upper tract involvement of Crohn disease, but medication effect and reflux esophagitis cannot be entirely excluded.

Take-Home Messages

- In addition to reflux esophagitis and eosinophilic esophagitis, Crohn disease, medication effect, and collagen vascular disease can have intraepithelial eosinophils.
- Often clinical correlation is necessary to arrive at the optimal diagnosis and treatment plan.

Case 4

Learning Objectives

- Bullous disease of the esophagus can be difficult to diagnose, but the clinical features, level of split, and DIF can aid in the diagnosis

Case History

A 42-year-old female with odynophagia. Bullae, blisters, and erosions of the oral mucosa.

Endoscopic Finding

Sheets of sloughed mucosa and erosions on withdrawal of the endoscope.

Differential Diagnosis Prior to Slide Review

- Pemphigus vulgaris
- Esophagitis dissecans superficialis (sloughing esophagitis)
- Bullous pemphigoid
- Epidermolysis bullosa
- Herpes esophagitis
- CMV esophagitis
- *Candida* esophagitis

Histologic Findings

Suprabasal split of the squamous mucosa with acantholytic cells (Fig. 2.15a). Detached squamous epithelium shows loss basal layer, elongated papillae, and intercellular edema with little inflammation (Fig. 2.15b). Lamina propria with irregular papillae and clinging basal layer of epithelium with the so-called "tombstone" appearance (Fig. 2.15c).

Differential Diagnosis After Slide Review

- Pemphigus vulgaris
- Bullous pemphigoid
- Epidermolysis bullosa

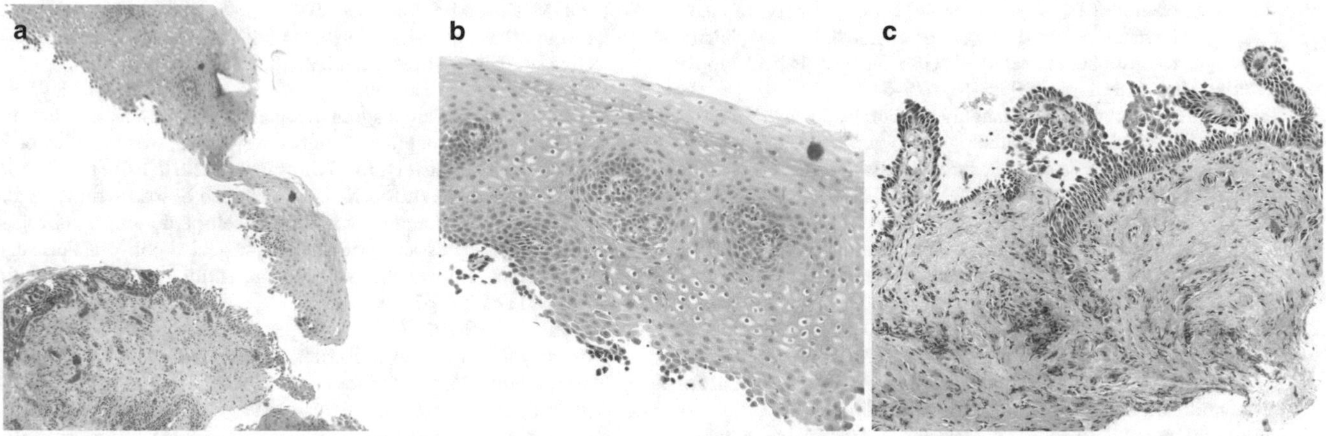

Fig. 2.15 Case 4. (**a**) Suprabasal splitting of the squamous epithelium with scattered acantholytic cells. (**b**) The detached squamous epithelium shows mild reactive epithelial changes with little inflammation. (**c**) The lamina propria with papillae highlights a clinging basal layer in the typical "tombstone" pattern of pemphigus vulgaris

- Herpes esophagitis
- Esophagitis dissecans

IHC and Other Ancillary Studies

- DIF shows intercellular IgG and C3.
- Indirect immunofluorescence is positive for PV antibodies.

Final Diagnosis

Pemphigus vulgaris.

Take-Home Messages

- Pemphigus vulgaris is a bullous disease that often affects the esophagus.
- It is characterized histologically by a suprabasal split with a tombstone appearance of the basal layer clinging to the lamina propria.
- DIF can aid in differentiating bullous diseases.

References

1. Vakil N, van Zanten SV, Kahrilas P, Dent J, Jones R, Global Consensus Group. The Montreal definition and classification of gastroesophageal reflux disease: a global evidence-based consensus. Am J Gastroenterol. 2006;101(8):1900–20; quiz 1943
2. Fiocca R, Mastracci L, Riddell R, Takubo K, Vieth M, Yerian L, et al. Development of consensus guidelines for the histologic recognition of microscopic esophagitis in patients with gastroesophageal reflux disease: the Esohisto project. Hum Pathol. 2010;41(2):223–31.
3. El-Serag HB, Sweet S, Winchester CC, Dent J. Update on the epidemiology of gastro-oesophageal reflux disease: a systematic review. Gut. 2014;63(6):871–80.
4. Rubenstein JH, Chen JW. Epidemiology of gastroesophageal reflux disease. Gastroenterol Clin N Am. 2014;43(1):1–14.
5. Lundell LR, Dent J, Bennett JR, Blum AL, Armstrong D, Galmiche JP, et al. Endoscopic assessment of oesophagitis: clinical and functional correlates and further validation of the Los Angeles classification. Gut. 1999;45(2):172–80.
6. Katz PO, Gerson LB, Vela MF. Guidelines for the diagnosis and management of gastroesophageal reflux disease. Am J Gastroenterol. 2013;108(3):308–28; quiz 329
7. Eastwood GL. Histologic changes in gastroesophageal reflux. J Clin Gastroenterol. 1986;8(Suppl 1):45–51.
8. Frierson HF. Histology in the diagnosis of reflux esophagitis. Gastroenterol Clin N Am. 1990;19(3):631–44.
9. Dunbar KB, Agoston AT, Odze RD, Huo X, Pham TH, Cipher DJ, et al. Association of acute gastroesophageal reflux disease with esophageal histologic changes. JAMA. 2016;315(19):2104–12.
10. Vieth M, Mastracci L, Vakil N, Dent J, Wernersson B, Baldycheva I, et al. Epithelial thickness is a marker of gastroesophageal reflux disease. Clin Gastroenterol Hepatol. 2016;14(11):1544–1551.e1.
11. Shaheen JN, Mukkada V, Eichinger C, Schofield H, Todorova L, Falk G. Natural history of eosinophilic esophagitis: a systematic review of epidemiology and disease course. Dis Esophagus. 2018;31:doy015.
12. Furuta GT, Katzka DA. Eosinophilic esophagitis. N Engl J Med. 2015;373(17):1640–8.
13. Hill DA, Grundmeier RW, Ramos M, Spergel JM. Eosinophilic esophagitis is a late manifestation of the allergic march. J Allergy Clin Immunol Pract. 2018;6:1528.
14. Moawad FJ, Veerappan GR, Lake JM, Maydonovitch CL, Haymore BR, Kosisky SE, et al. Correlation between eosinophilic oesophagitis and aeroallergens. Aliment Pharmacol Ther. 2010;31(4):509–15.
15. Kim HP, Vance RB, Shaheen NJ, Dellon ES. The prevalence and diagnostic utility of endoscopic features of eosinophilic esophagitis: a meta-analysis. Clin Gastroenterol Hepatol. 2012;10(9):988–996.e5.
16. Liacouras CA, Furuta GT, Hirano I, Atkins D, Attwood SE, Bonis PA, et al. Eosinophilic esophagitis: updated consensus recommendations for children and adults. J Allergy Clin Immunol. 2011;128(1):3–20.e6; quiz 21–2
17. Dellon ES, Speck O, Woodward K, Covey S, Rusin S, Shaheen NJ, et al. Distribution and variability of esophageal eosinophilia in patients undergoing upper endoscopy. Mod Pathol. 2015;28(3):383–90.
18. Collins MH, Martin LJ, Alexander ES, Boyd JT, Sheridan R, He H, et al. Newly developed and validated eosinophilic esophagitis histology scoring system and evidence that it outperforms peak eosinophil count for disease diagnosis and monitoring. Dis Esophagus. 2017;30(3):1–8.

19. Mueller S, Neureiter D, Aigner T, Stolte M. Comparison of histological parameters for the diagnosis of eosinophilic oesophagitis versus gastro-oesophageal reflux disease on oesophageal biopsy material. Histopathology. 2008;53(6):676–84.
20. Siddique AS, Corney DC, Mangray S, Lombardo KA, Chen S, Marwaha AS, et al. Clinicopathologic and gene expression analysis of initial biopsies from patients with eosinophilic esophagitis refractory to therapy. Hum Pathol. 2017;68:79–86.
21. Rusin S, Covey S, Perjar I, Hollyfield J, Speck O, Woodward K, et al. Determination of esophageal eosinophil counts and other histologic features of eosinophilic esophagitis by pathology trainees is highly accurate. Hum Pathol. 2017;62:50–5.
22. Molina-Infante J, Bredenoord AJ, Cheng E, Dellon ES, Furuta GT, Gupta SK, et al. Proton pump inhibitor-responsive oesophageal eosinophilia: an entity challenging current diagnostic criteria for eosinophilic oesophagitis. Gut. 2016;65(3):524–31.
23. Molina-Infante J, Rivas MD, Hernandez-Alonso M, Vinagre-Rodríguez G, Mateos-Rodríguez JM, Dueñas-Sadornil C, et al. Proton pump inhibitor-responsive oesophageal eosinophilia correlates with downregulation of eotaxin-3 and Th2 cytokines overexpression. Aliment Pharmacol Ther. 2014;40(8):955–65.
24. Dellon ES, Speck O, Woodward K, Gebhart JH, Madanick RD, Levinson S, et al. Clinical and endoscopic characteristics do not reliably differentiate PPI-responsive esophageal eosinophilia and eosinophilic esophagitis in patients undergoing upper endoscopy: a prospective cohort study. Am J Gastroenterol. 2013;108(12):1854–60.
25. Warners MJ, van Rhijn BD, Curvers WL, Smout AJPM, Bredenoord AJ. PPI-responsive esophageal eosinophilia cannot be distinguished from eosinophilic esophagitis by endoscopic signs. Eur J Gastroenterol Hepatol. 2015;27(5):506–11.
26. Lucendo AJ, Arias Á, González-Cervera J, Olalla JM, Molina-Infante J. Dual response to dietary/topical steroid and proton pump inhibitor therapy in adult patients with eosinophilic esophagitis. J Allergy Clin Immunol. 2016;137(3):931–934.e2.
27. Sodikoff J, Hirano I. Proton pump inhibitor-responsive esophageal eosinophilia does not preclude food-responsive eosinophilic esophagitis. J Allergy Clin Immunol. 2016;137(2):631–3.
28. Souza RF, Huo X, Mittal V, Schuler CM, Carmack SW, Zhang HY, et al. Gastroesophageal reflux might cause esophagitis through a cytokine-mediated mechanism rather than caustic acid injury. Gastroenterology. 2009;137(5):1776–84.
29. De Felice KM, Katzka DA, Raffals LE. Crohn's disease of the esophagus: clinical features and treatment outcomes in the biologic era. Inflamm Bowel Dis. 2015;21(9):2106–13.
30. Rubio CA, Sjödahl K, Lagergren J. Lymphocytic esophagitis: a histologic subset of chronic esophagitis. Am J Clin Pathol. 2006;125(3):432–7.
31. Purdy JK, Appelman HD, Golembeski CP, McKenna BJ. Lymphocytic esophagitis: a chronic or recurring pattern of esophagitis resembling allergic contact dermatitis. Am J Clin Pathol. 2008;130(4):508–13.
32. Haque S, Genta RM. Lymphocytic oesophagitis: clinicopathological aspects of an emerging condition. Gut. 2012;61(8):1108–14.
33. Cohen S, Saxena A, Waljee AK, Piraka C, Purdy J, Appelman H, et al. Lymphocytic esophagitis: a diagnosis of increasing frequency. J Clin Gastroenterol. 2012;46(10):828–32.
34. Sutton LM, Heintz DD, Patel AS, Weinberg AG. Lymphocytic esophagitis in children. Inflamm Bowel Dis. 2014;20(8):1324–8.
35. Nguyen AD, Dunbar KB. How to approach lymphocytic esophagitis. Curr Gastroenterol Rep. 2017;19(6):24.
36. Ebach DR, Vanderheyden AD, Ellison JM, Jensen CS. Lymphocytic esophagitis: a possible manifestation of pediatric upper gastrointestinal Crohn's disease. Inflamm Bowel Dis. 2011;17(1):45–9.
37. Lin J, McKenna BJ, Appelman HD. Morphologic findings in upper gastrointestinal biopsies of patients with ulcerative colitis: a controlled study. Am J Surg Pathol. 2010;34(11):1672–7.
38. Putra J, Muller KE, Hussain ZH, Parker S, Gabbard S, Brickley EB, et al. Lymphocytic esophagitis in nonachalasia primary esophageal motility disorders: improved criteria, prevalence, strength of association, and natural history. Am J Surg Pathol. 2016;40(12):1679–85.
39. Xue Y, Suriawinata A, Liu X, Li Z, Gabbard S, Rothstein R, et al. Lymphocytic esophagitis with CD4 T-cell-predominant intraepithelial lymphocytes and primary esophageal motility abnormalities: a potential novel clinicopathologic entity. Am J Surg Pathol. 2015;39(11):1558–67.
40. Kissiedu J, Thota PN, Gohel T, Lopez R, Gordon IO. Post-ablation lymphocytic esophagitis in Barrett esophagus with high grade dysplasia or intramucosal carcinoma. Mod Pathol. 2016;29(6):599–606.
41. Salaria SN, Abu Alfa AK, Cruise MW, Wood LD, Montgomery EA. Lichenoid esophagitis: clinicopathologic overlap with established esophageal lichen planus. Am J Surg Pathol. 2013;37(12):1889–94.
42. Abraham SC, Ravich WJ, Anhalt GJ, Yardley JH, Wu TT. Esophageal lichen planus: case report and review of the literature. Am J Surg Pathol. 2000;24(12):1678–82.
43. Chryssostalis A, Gaudric M, Terris B, Coriat R, Prat F, Chaussade S. Esophageal lichen planus: a series of eight cases including a patient with esophageal verrucous carcinoma. A case series. Endoscopy. 2008;40(9):764–8.
44. Harewood GC, Murray JA, Cameron AJ. Esophageal lichen planus: the Mayo Clinic experience. Dis Esophagus. 1999;12(4):309–11.
45. Riffat F, Cheng A. Pediatric caustic ingestion: 50 consecutive cases and a review of the literature. Dis Esophagus. 2009;22(1):89–94.
46. de Jong AL, Macdonald R, Ein S, Forte V, Turner A. Corrosive esophagitis in children: a 30-year review. Int J Pediatr Otorhinolaryngol. 2001;57(3):203–11.
47. Kochhar R, Sethy PK, Kochhar S, Nagi B, Gupta NM. Corrosive induced carcinoma of esophagus: report of three patients and review of literature. J Gastroenterol Hepatol. 2006;21(4):777–80.
48. Appelqvist P, Salmo M. Lye corrosion carcinoma of the esophagus: a review of 63 cases. Cancer. 1980;45(10):2655–8.
49. Ramasamy K, Gumaste VV. Corrosive ingestion in adults. J Clin Gastroenterol. 2003;37(2):119–24.
50. Voltaggio L, Lam-Himlin D, Limketkai BN, Singhi AD, Arnold CA. Message in a bottle: decoding medication injury patterns in the gastrointestinal tract. J Clin Pathol. 2014;67(10):903–12.
51. Seminerio J, McGrath K, Arnold CA, Voltaggio L, Singhi AD. Medication-associated lesions of the GI tract. Gastrointest Endosc. 2014;79(1):140–50.
52. Abraham SC, Cruz-Correa M, Lee LA, Yardley JH, Wu TT. Alendronate-associated esophageal injury: pathologic and endoscopic features. Mod Pathol. 1999;12(12):1152–7.
53. Abraham SC, Yardley JH, Wu TT. Erosive injury to the upper gastrointestinal tract in patients receiving iron medication: an underrecognized entity. Am J Surg Pathol. 1999;23(10):1241–7.
54. Haig A, Driman DK. Iron-induced mucosal injury to the upper gastrointestinal tract. Histopathology. 2006;48(7):808–12.
55. Lillemoe KD, Romolo JL, Hamilton SR, Pennington LR, Burdick JF, Williams GM. Intestinal necrosis due to sodium polystyrene (Kayexalate) in sorbitol enemas: clinical and experimental support for the hypothesis. Surgery. 1987;101(3):267–72.
56. Rashid A, Hamilton SR. Necrosis of the gastrointestinal tract in uremic patients as a result of sodium polystyrene sulfonate (Kayexalate) in sorbitol: an underrecognized condition. Am J Surg Pathol. 1997;21(1):60–9.
57. Abraham SC, Bhagavan BS, Lee LA, Rashid A, Wu TT. Upper gastrointestinal tract injury in patients receiving kayexalate (sodium polystyrene sulfonate) in sorbitol: clinical, endoscopic, and histopathologic findings. Am J Surg Pathol. 2001;25(5):637–44.

58. Gonzalez RS, Lagana SM, Szeto O, Arnold CA. Challenges in diagnosing medication resins in surgical pathology specimens: a crystal-clear review guide. Arch Pathol Lab Med. 2017;141(9):1276–82.
59. Swanson BJ, Limketkai BN, Liu T-C, Montgomery E, Nazari K, Park JY, et al. Sevelamer crystals in the gastrointestinal tract (GIT): a new entity associated with mucosal injury. Am J Surg Pathol. 2013;37(11):1686–93.
60. Arnold MA, Swanson BJ, Crowder CD, Frankel WL, Lam-Himlin D, Singhi AD, et al. Colesevelam and colestipol: novel medication resins in the gastrointestinal tract. Am J Surg Pathol. 2014;38(11):1530–7.
61. Hruban RH, Yardley JH, Donehower RC, Boitnott JK. Taxol toxicity. Epithelial necrosis in the gastrointestinal tract associated with polymerized microtubule accumulation and mitotic arrest. Cancer. 1989;63(10):1944–50.
62. Daniels JA, Gibson MK, Xu L, Sun S, Canto MI, Heath E, et al. Gastrointestinal tract epithelial changes associated with taxanes: marker of drug toxicity versus effect. Am J Surg Pathol. 2008;32(3):473–7.
63. Iacobuzio-Donahue CA, Lee EL, Abraham SC, Yardley JH, Wu TT. Colchicine toxicity: distinct morphologic findings in gastrointestinal biopsies. Am J Surg Pathol. 2001;25(8):1067–73.
64. Stemmermann G, Hayashi T. Colchicine intoxication: a reappraisal of its pathology, based on a study of three fatal cases. Hum Pathol. 1972;2:321–31.
65. Finger JE, Headington JT. Colchicine-induced epithelial atypia. Am J Clin Pathol. 1963;40:605–9.
66. Brown W, Seed L. Effect of colchicine on human tissues. Am J Clin Pathol. 1945;15:189–95.
67. Parfitt JR, Jayakumar S, Driman DK. Mycophenolate mofetil-related gastrointestinal mucosal injury: variable injury patterns, including graft-versus-host disease-like changes. Am J Surg Pathol. 2008;32(9):1367–72.
68. Nguyen T, Park JY, Scudiere JR, Montgomery E. Mycophenolic acid (cellcept and myofortic) induced injury of the upper GI tract. Am J Surg Pathol. 2009;33(9):1355–63.
69. Star KV, Ho VT, Wang HH, Odze RD. Histologic features in colon biopsies can discriminate mycophenolate from GVHD-induced colitis. Am J Surg Pathol. 2013;37(9):1319–28.
70. Karamchandani DM, Chetty R. Immune checkpoint inhibitor-induced gastrointestinal and hepatic injury: pathologists' perspective. J Clin Pathol. 2018;71(8):665–71.
71. Chen JH, Pezhouh MK, Lauwers GY, Masia R. Histopathologic features of colitis due to immunotherapy with anti-PD-1 antibodies. Am J Surg Pathol. 2017;41(5):643–54.
72. Carmack SW, Vemulapalli R, Spechler SJ, Genta RM. Esophagitis dissecans superficialis ("sloughing esophagitis"): a clinicopathologic study of 12 cases. Am J Surg Pathol. 2009;33(12):1789–94.
73. Coppola D, Lu L, Boyce HW. Chronic esophagitis dissecans presenting with esophageal strictures: a case report. Hum Pathol. 2000;31(10):1313–7.
74. Moawad FJ, Appleman HD. Sloughing esophagitis: a spectacular histologic and endoscopic disease without a uniform clinical correlation. Ann N Y Acad Sci. 2016;1380(1):178–82.
75. Purdy JK, Appelman HD, McKenna BJ. Sloughing esophagitis is associated with chronic debilitation and medications that injure the esophageal mucosa. Mod Pathol. 2012;25(5):767–75.
76. Ponsot P, Molas G, Scoazec JY, Ruszniewski P, Hénin D, Bernades P. Chronic esophagitis dissecans: an unrecognized clinicopathologic entity? Gastrointest Endosc. 1997;45(1):38–45.
77. Hart PA, Romano RC, Moreira RK, Ravi K, Sweetser S. Esophagitis dissecans superficialis: clinical, endoscopic, and histologic features. Dig Dis Sci. 2015;60(7):2049–57.
78. Hokama A, Ihama Y, Nakamoto M, Kinjo N, Kinjo F, Fujita J. Esophagitis dissecans superficialis associated with bisphosphonates. Endoscopy. 2007;39 Suppl 1:E91.
79. Gomi H, Akiyama M, Yakabi K, Nakamura T, Matsuo I. Oesophageal involvement in pemphigus vulgaris. Lancet. 1999;354(9192):1794.
80. Mignogna MD, Lo Muzio L, Galloro G, Satriano RA, Ruocco V, Bucci E. Oral pemphigus: clinical significance of esophageal involvement: report of eight cases. Oral Surg Oral Med Oral Pathol Oral Radiol Endod. 1997;84(2):179–84.
81. Trattner A, Lurie R, Leiser A, David M, Hazaz B, Kadish U, et al. Esophageal involvement in pemphigus vulgaris: a clinical, histologic, and immunopathologic study. J Am Acad Dermatol. 1991;24(2 Pt 1):223–6.
82. Chang S, Park SJ, Kim SW, Jin M-N, Lee J-H, Kim HJ, et al. Esophageal involvement of pemphigus vulgaris associated with upper gastrointestinal bleeding. Clin Endosc. 2014;47(5):452–4.
83. Mohan P, Srinivas CR, Leelakrishnan V. A rare initial presentation of esophageal involvement in pemphigus. Dis Esophagus. 2013;26(3):351.
84. Coelho LK, Troncon LE, Roselino AM, Campos MS, Módena JL. Esophageal Nikolsky's sign in pemphigus vulgaris. Endoscopy. 1997;29(7):S35.
85. Kershenovich R, Hodak E, Mimouni D. Diagnosis and classification of pemphigus and bullous pemphigoid. Autoimmun Rev. 2014;13(4–5):477–81.
86. Isolauri J, Airo I. Benign mucous membrane pemphigoid involving the esophagus: a report of two cases treated with dilation. Gastrointest Endosc. 1989;35(6):569–71.
87. Popovici Z, Deac M, Rotaru M, Veştemeanu P, Vărgatu V. Stenosis of the esophagus in cicatricial pemphigoid resolved by colon interposition: report of a case. Surg Today. 1997;27(3):234–7.
88. Mönkemüller K, Neumann H, Fry LC. Esophageal blebs and blisters. Gastroenterology. 2010;138(2):e3–4.
89. Fine J-D, Johnson LB, Weiner M, Suchindran C. Gastrointestinal complications of inherited epidermolysis bullosa: cumulative experience of the National Epidermolysis Bullosa Registry. J Pediatr Gastroenterol Nutr. 2008;46(2):147–58.
90. Fine J-D, Eady RAJ, Bauer EA, Bauer JW, Bruckner-Tuderman L, Heagerty A, et al. The classification of inherited epidermolysis bullosa (EB): report of the third international consensus meeting on diagnosis and classification of EB. J Am Acad Dermatol. 2008;58(6):931–50.
91. Tishler JM, Han SY, Helman CA. Esophageal involvement in epidermolysis bullosa dystrophica. AJR Am J Roentgenol. 1983;141(6):1283–6.
92. Ergun GA, Lin AN, Dannenberg AJ, Carter DM. Gastrointestinal manifestations of epidermolysis bullosa. A study of 101 patients. Medicine (Baltimore). 1992;71(3):121–7.

Barrett Esophagus

3

Eric Swanson and Bita V. Naini

List of Frequently Asked Questions

1. What is the normal anatomy and histology of distal esophagus, gastroesophageal junction (GEJ), Z-line, and cardia?
2. What is Barrett esophagus (BE)?
3. What are the endoscopic findings in BE?
4. What are the diagnostic criteria for BE and how does it differ worldwide?
5. Is there a required length of columnar mucosa for a diagnosis of BE?
6. What are pseudo-goblet cells and how are they distinguished from true goblets cells?
7. What is the best way to distinguish true versus pseudo-goblet cells, and are special stains such as periodic-acid-Schiff (PAS) and/or Alcian blue helpful in this distinction?
8. Are immunostains indicated to aid in diagnosis of BE?
9. What is the goal of screening and surveillance in patients with BE?
10. How should GEJ biopsies be evaluated, and should patients with intestinal metaplasia of GEJ undergo endoscopic surveillance?
11. What is the significance of basal crypt atypia in BE?
12. In what situations should you diagnose BE with epithelial alterations indefinite for dysplasia?
13. How do you determine reactive atypia versus dysplasia in BE?
14. What are the histologic features of low-grade dysplasia in BE?
15. What are the histologic features of high-grade dysplasia in BE?
16. How do you distinguish high-grade dysplasia from intramucosal adenocarcinoma in BE?
17. How do you identify submucosally invasive adenocarcinoma?
18. What are the described types of nonconventional dysplasia and how are they identified?
19. Is ancillary testing recommended in identifying dysplasia associated with BE or those at risk of progression?
20. What are the possible treatment modalities when a diagnosis of dysplastic BE is rendered?
21. Is evaluation of BE dysplasia reproducible between pathologists?

Frequently Asked Questions

1. What is the normal anatomy and histology of distal esophagus, gastroesophageal junction (GEJ), Z-line, and cardia?

- The esophagus is lined by stratified squamous epithelium and contains scattered submucosal salivary gland-like mucous glands.
- Endoscopically/grossly, the stomach begins at the most proximal aspect of the gastric folds. The gastric cardia is an extremely short segment of proximal stomach that is typically composed of surface foveolar columnar epithelium and either pure mucous or a mixture of mucous and oxyntic glands. The gastroesophageal junction (GEJ) is defined as the point where the distal esophagus meets the proximal stomach (cardia).
- Normally, the anatomic GEJ should correspond to the histologic transition point between the esophageal squamous epithelium and the gastric columnar epithelium, the so-called "Z-line" or squamocolumnar junctional (SCJ) mucosa. In response to injury from physiologic or pathologic gastroesophageal reflux disease (GERD), metaplastic columnar epithelium

E. Swanson
Scripps Health, La Jolla, CA, USA

B. V. Naini (✉)
University of California at Los Angeles David Geffen School of Medicine, Los Angeles, CA, USA
e-mail: BNaini@mednet.ucla.edu

H. L. Wang, Z. E. Chen (eds.), *Practical Gastrointestinal Pathology*, Practical Anatomic Pathology,
https://doi.org/10.1007/978-3-030-51268-2_3

develops which extends proximally above the level of anatomic GEJ into the distal esophagus. Therefore, many adults have a proximally displaced or irregular Z-line with the SCJ located above the anatomic GEJ.

Reference: [1]

2. **What is Barrett esophagus (BE)?**
   - Barrett esophagus (BE) is a condition that develops secondary to chronic injury from GERD. In patients with BE, metaplastic columnar epithelium that predisposes to the development of esophageal cancer replaces the stratified squamous epithelium that normally lines the distal esophagus.

   Reference: [2]

3. **What are the endoscopic findings in BE?**
   - Endoscopically, the GEJ is identified as the most proximal extent of the gastric folds. BE is recognized as salmon-colored columnar mucosa that extends in tongue-shaped projections above the GEJ and into the grayish squamous mucosa of the distal esophagus.

   References: [3, 4]

4. **What are the diagnostic criteria for BE and how does it differ worldwide?**
   - The diagnosis of BE requires endoscopic evidence that columnar mucosa extends above the GEJ into the distal esophagus, in addition to esophageal biopsy results that confirm the presence of columnar metaplasia. However, the criteria used to diagnose BE vary worldwide, and the main difference is in regard to the histologic type of columnar mucosa that establishes a diagnosis of BE. The metaplastic columnar epithelium may consist of a variety of cell types, including gastric-type non-goblet mucinous cells as well as intestinal-type goblet cells with variable enterocytes, Paneth cells, and endocrine cells (Fig. 3.1).
   - In the United States and part of Europe, the presence of intestinal metaplasia (IM) with goblet cells within metaplastic columnar mucosa is required for diagnosis of BE, whereas in the United Kingdom and Japan, only the presence of columnar mucosa is required, and there is no need for the presence of IM (i.e., goblet cells). This difference is attributed to the difference in cancer risk between these two types of mucosal changes. Currently in the United States, intestinal-type epithelium with goblet cells is the only type of metaplastic columnar epithelium that is clearly shown to be associated with significant cancer risk and hence the current requirement for histologic confirmation of the presence of goblet cells.
   - According to the 2016 criteria of American College of Gastroenterology (ACG), "BE should be diagnosed when there is extension of salmon-colored mucosa into the tubular esophagus extending ≥1cm proximal to the GEJ with biopsy confirmation of intestinal metaplasia."

   References: [4–7]

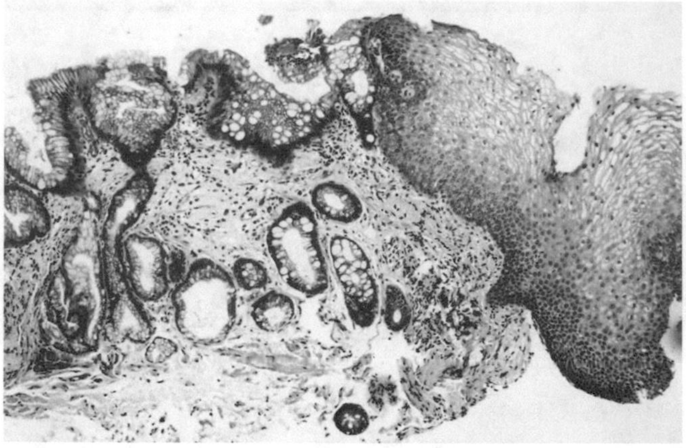

Fig. 3.1 Barrett esophagus. BE represents metaplastic conversion of normal squamous epithelium of the distal esophagus to columnar epithelium composed of those normally seen in the stomach (i.e., mucinous cells) as well as intestine (i.e., goblet cells and less frequently enterocytes, endocrine cells, and Paneth cells). The crypts show slight architectural irregularity and budding. The lamina propria shows a minimal lymphoplasmacytic infiltrate

5. **Is there a required length of columnar mucosa for a diagnosis of BE?**
   - Yes, the recent definition of BE (2016 ACG) adds a required length of columnar/intestinal-type mucosa (≥1 cm proximal to the GEJ) which was not present in previous definitions. The reason for this change is due to very low risk of esophageal adenocarcinoma in patients that have IM limited to the GEJ as well as high interobserver variability among gastroenterologists in detecting the GEJ.

   Reference: [4]

6. **What are pseudo-goblet cells and how are they distinguished from true goblets cells?**
   - Presence of true goblet cells is required for a diagnosis of IM and therefore BE in the United States. Pseudo-goblet cells are foveolar epithelial cells that have distended cytoplasm due to abundant cytoplasmic mucin and can be mistaken for true goblet cells. Pseudo-goblet cells are typically found in clusters and linear rows at the superficial part of the epithelium, whereas true goblet cells are more sparsely distributed among intervening non-goblet columnar cells. True goblet cells have a distinctive cytoplasmic vacuole that compresses the nucleus and contain acid mucin which imparts a blue hue to the mucin vacuole on H&E stain (Fig. 3.2a, b).

   Reference: [8]

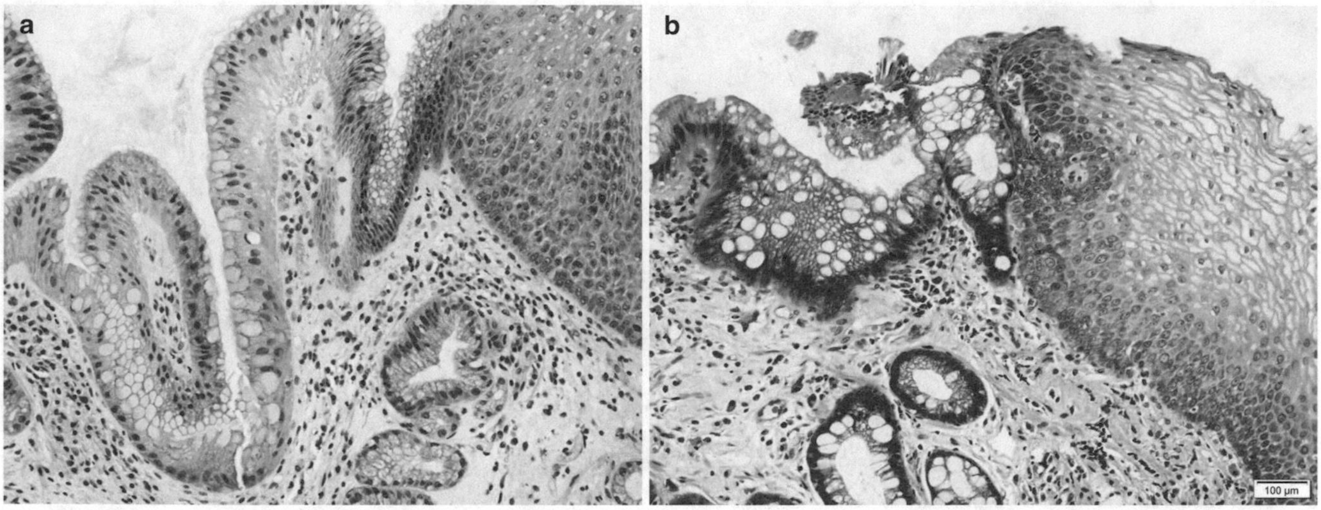

Fig. 3.2 True vs pseudo-goblet cells. In the United States, identification of goblet cells in the metaplastic columnar epithelium is required for the diagnosis of BE. Pseudo-goblet cells (**a**) may be mistaken for true goblet cells (**b**). In contrast to true goblet cells, pseudo-goblet cells are often arranged in clusters and linear rows and show distended cytoplasm without the characteristic triangle-shaped nucleus of true goblet cells

7. **What is the best way to distinguish true versus pseudo-goblet cells, and are special stains such as periodic-acid-Schiff (PAS) and/or Alcian blue helpful in this distinction?**
   - The best way to distinguish true from pseudo-goblet cells is morphology on routine H&E-stained slides. There are no histochemical stains that can reliably distinguish the two and can be used on esophageal biopsies to help diagnose BE. While the acid mucin of true goblet cells stain blue with Alcian blue stain at pH of 2.5, pseudo-goblet cells usually reveal weak positivity as well. Overall, there is insufficient evidence to justify routine use of ancillary histochemical or immunohistochemical studies such as Alcian blue and/or PAS stains to identify goblet cells.

   Reference: [25]

8. **Are immunostains indicated to aid in diagnosis of BE?**
   - Based on the current evidence, the use of intestine-specific mucin glycoprotein immunostains or markers of intestinal differentiation (CDX2, Das-1, villin, Hepar 1, or SOX 9) is not indicated to aid in the diagnosis of BE.

   Reference: [25]

9. **What is the goal of screening and surveillance in patients with BE?**
   - BE is a known precursor and risk factor for the development of esophageal adenocarcinoma (EAC) which evolves through a metaplasia-dysplasia-carcinoma sequence. The goal of endoscopic surveillance in patients with BE is the early detection of neoplasia. At present, the morphologic identification and grade of dysplasia in endoscopic mucosal biopsies is the standard method of detecting patients at increased risk of developing EAC. Systematic four-quadrant surveillance biopsies taken at 1–2 cm intervals are recommended in patients with BE to detect early, treatable neoplasia.

   Reference: [6]

10. **How should GEJ biopsies be evaluated, and should patients with IM of GEJ undergo endoscopic surveillance?**
    - Obtaining biopsy of an irregular GEJ or Z-line is not recommended, if this is the only endoscopic abnormality. However, pathologists continue to receive GEJ biopsies for evaluation to "rule out BE," in patients who have been found to have an "irregular" endoscopic Z-line. Up to 30% of patients develop IM in the GEJ, which can happen secondary to injury from GERD and/or H. pylori infection. In patients who have an irregular Z-line and in whom biopsy samples of the GEJ have been obtained, additional biopsy sampling of mucosa above Z-line and from distal stomach may help interpretation of the etiology of the injury. However, regardless of the presence or absence of IM, these patients are not at significantly increased risk of malignancy, and current guidelines do not recommend surveillance of patients with IM in the GEJ only.

    Reference: [9]

11. **What is the significance of basal crypt atypia in BE?**
    - BE commonly shows atypia of basal crypt epithelium and this should not be misinterpreted as dysplasia. Crypts may show mild crowding at the base with mild pseudostratification of nuclei, hyperchromasia, typical mitotic figures, and mild nuclear enlargement with nuclei that are 1–2 times the size of a lamina

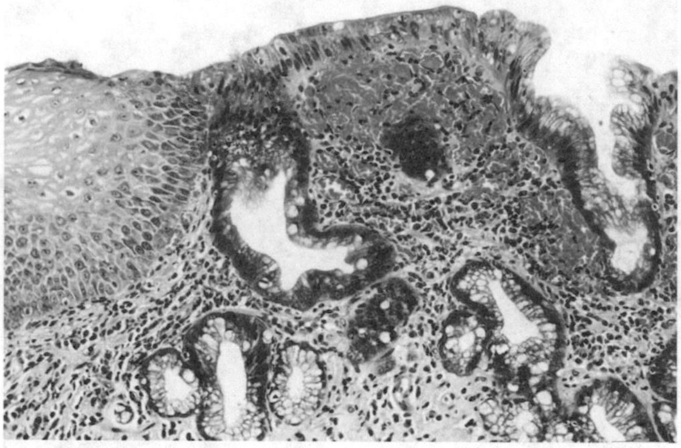

Fig. 3.3 Basal crypt atypia, non-dysplastic (case 1). Basal crypt epithelium is mildly hyperchromatic with enlarged nuclei, nuclear crowding, and pseudostratification. The epithelium matures toward the surface with basally located nuclei and abundant cytoplasm

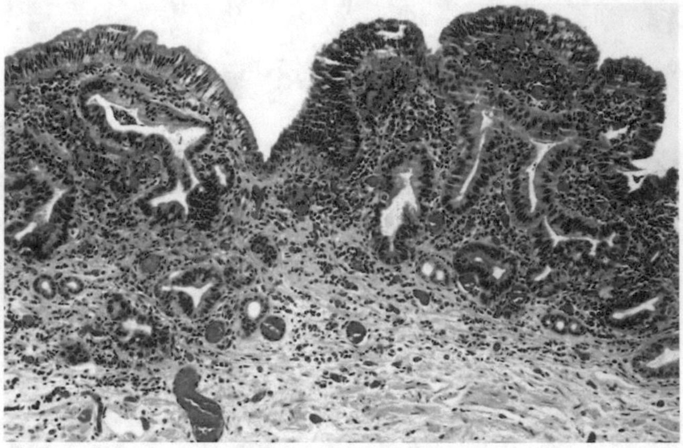

Fig. 3.4 Barrett esophagus, indefinite for dysplasia. In this biopsy, there is atypia of the epithelium with crowded, elongated nuclei that extend to the mucosal surface. The epithelium contains many intraepithelial neutrophils that raise the possibility of reactive epithelial changes. Goblet cells were present in other adjacent areas

propria fibroblast or endothelial cells (Fig. 3.3). However, this atypia is mild and limited to crypt epithelium, and normal "maturation" is seen toward the luminal surface. This maturation is characterized by progressive accumulation of abundant mucinous cytoplasm, with nuclei that are basally located and maintain polarity with respect to the basement membrane and a low nuclear-to-cytoplasmic ratio. The lamina propria is abundant without glandular architectural crowding or complexity.
- In some cases, the atypia of crypt epithelium is more than typically seen in metaplastic epithelium. In these cases, additional levels may be performed to ensure that there is no full-thickness atypia to the epithelium, which would then be considered true dysplasia.

References: [10, 12, 13]

12. In what situations should you diagnose BE with epithelial alterations indefinite for dysplasia?

- In several situations, Barrett epithelium may show cytologic or architectural abnormalities that raise the possibility of neoplasia/dysplasia, but it is difficult to be certain. In these settings, a diagnosis of indefinite for dysplasia is considered appropriate. For example, cytologic abnormalities may be present in the setting of active inflammation or ulceration. These regenerative and inflammatory changes may alter the maturation of the epithelium toward the surface, with cytologic changes including mucin depletion, nuclear hyperchromasia and crowding, and increased mitotic figures. In this setting, a diagnosis of "indefinite for dysplasia" confers uncertainty as to whether the epithelial changes are reactive or neoplastic in nature (Fig. 3.4). Generally, a rebiopsy is performed after the resolution of active inflammation.
- A diagnosis of indefinite for dysplasia may also be used in several other situations when technical difficulties in interpretation of the biopsy are present. Situations in which this may be appropriate include:
  - Tangential sectioning.
  - Poorly oriented tissue fragments.
  - Thick sections, poor staining or fixation, cautery artifact.
  - Significant basal crypt atypia when the surface is not present for evaluation or assessment of maturation is not possible.
- If a diagnosis of "indefinite for dysplasia" is rendered, it is helpful to comment in the pathology report the underlying reason for the indefinite diagnosis as medical therapy may be maximized in cases of ongoing reflux effect/inflammation, and diagnostic yield in subsequent rebiopsy may be optimized.

References: [10, 12]

13. How do you determine reactive atypia versus dysplasia in BE?

- In the presence of active inflammation or ulceration, nonneoplastic epithelium can demonstrate hyperchromasia, mucin loss, and nuclear crowding that can mimic dysplasia.
- A gradual, non-abrupt transition from non-atypical to atypical mucosa favors reactive epithelial changes. A lack of glandular architectural abnormalities such as crowded, cribriform glands also favors reactive changes.
- Reactive cardia-type mucosa demonstrates a "top heavy" distribution of atypia with surface nuclear stratification and bland-appearing cytology in the deeper mucosa.

References: [10, 12, 14]

14. What are the histologic features of low-grade dysplasia in BE?
- Low-grade dysplasia is noninvasive neoplastic epithelium most often resembling intestinal-type dysplasia as seen in adenomas of the colon.
- The epithelium shows full-thickness atypia extending from crypts to surface epithelium. Cytologic features include elongated and crowded nuclei with pseudostratification and hyperchromasia, typically limited to the basal aspect of the cytoplasm (Fig. 3.5). Nuclei generally remain polarized with orientation of the long axis of the nuclei perpendicular to the basement membrane. In general, there is an abrupt transition from non-dysplastic to dysplastic epithelium.
- Goblet cells are typically present but may be depleted.
- The glandular architecture is typically not crowded.
- The histologic features of low-grade dysplasia and non-dysplastic BE mucosa are also summarized in Table 3.1.

References: [10, 12, 16–18]

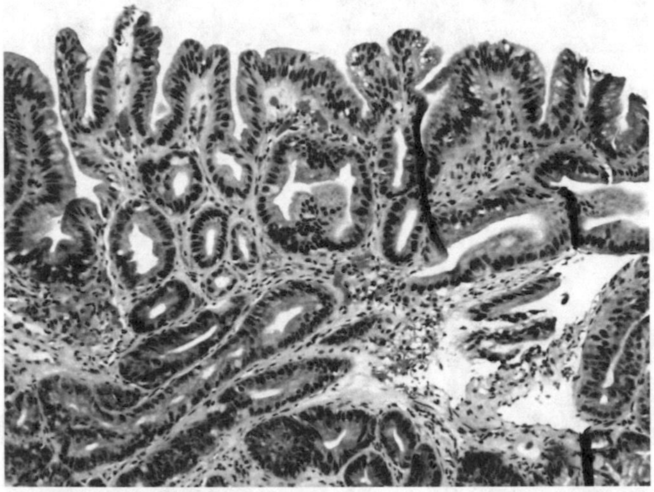

Fig. 3.5 Barrett esophagus with low-grade dysplasia. The epithelium shows full-thickness atypia without surface maturation. The nuclei are enlarged and hyperchromatic but maintain polarity to the basement membrane and retain some apical cytoplasm. There is no significant glandular crowding or complexity

15. What are the histologic features of high-grade dysplasia in BE?
- High-grade dysplasia is noninvasive neoplastic epithelium with high-grade cytologic and/or architectural abnormalities.
- The cytologic atypia is more severe than in low-grade dysplasia, with more pronounced nuclear enlargement, increased nuclear-to-cytoplasmic ratios, loss of nuclear polarity with respect to the basement membrane, and prominent nucleoli (Fig. 3.6).
- Mitotic figures may be seen in the surface epithelium.
- Architectural changes in the epithelium are also present in high-grade dysplasia including villiform morphology, glandular crowding and cribriform glands, intraluminal budding, and branching and lateral budding of crypts.
- Focal glandular intraluminal necrosis may also be present.
- Goblet cells may be depleted.

References: [10–12, 19]

Table 3.1 Histologic features of Barrett mucosa and its progression to intramucosal adenocarcinoma

Barrett esophagus	Non-dysplastic	Low-grade dysplasia	High-grade dysplasia	Intramucosal adenocarcinoma
Cytology	Mild nuclear enlargement and hyperchromasia Scattered crypt mitotic figures	Nuclear enlargement, elongation extending from crypt base to surface Nuclear stratification limited to basal half of cell cytoplasm Increased N/C ratio Preserved or only mild loss of nuclear polarity Increased mitoses, usually limited to crypts	Nuclear enlargement Full-thickness nuclear stratification Mild to marked nuclear pleomorphism Irregular nuclear contours Vesicular chromatin Prominent loss of nuclear polarity Mitoses on surface epithelium Increased number of atypical mitoses	Similar to high-grade dysplasia
Architecture	Preserved	Relatively preserved	Cribriform and crowded glands Irregulary sized and shaped crypts with crypt branching Intraluminal budding Intraluminal necrosis	Single cells in lamina propria Sheets of neoplastic cells Anastomosing pattern of glands Angulated infiltrative glands Intraluminal necrosis

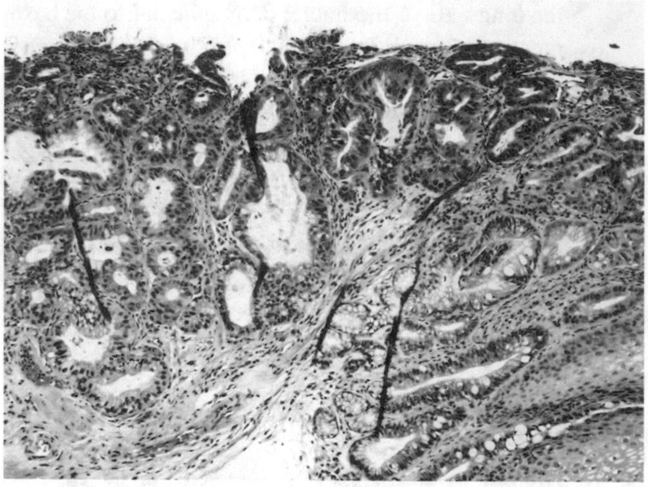

Fig. 3.6 Barrett esophagus with high-grade dysplasia. The epithelium shows full-thickness atypia, with enlarged, round, crowded nuclei with a loss of polarity. There are complex cribriform glandular architecture and glandular crowding. Focal glandular luminal necrosis is present

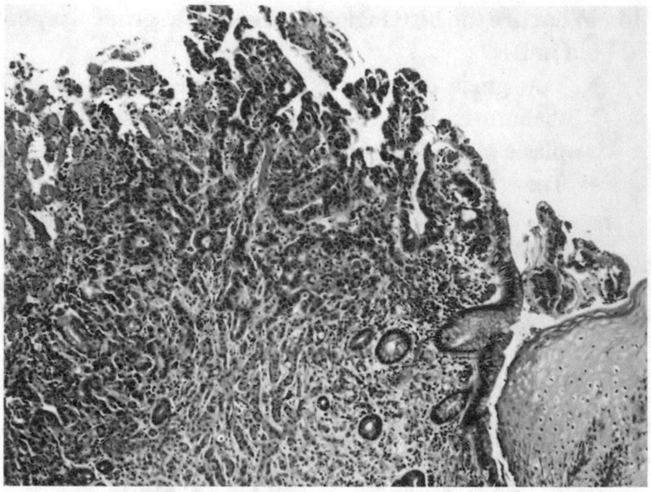

Fig. 3.7 Barrett esophagus with intramucosal adenocarcinoma. The epithelial cells show a never-ending anastomosing glandular pattern and single neoplastic cells within the lamina propria

16. How do you distinguish high-grade dysplasia from intramucosal adenocarcinoma in BE?

- Intramucosal adenocarcinoma describes architectural changes in which neoplastic epithelium has invaded beyond the basement membrane into the lamina propria or muscularis mucosae, but has not penetrated the deep layer of the muscularis mucosa into the submucosa.
- Single-cell invasion into lamina propria (cells that do not have connection to glands), sheets of malignant cells, angulated and infiltrative glands, and a complex "never-ending" anastomosing glandular pattern are architectural features that indicate intramucosal adenocarcinoma (Fig. 3.7).
- Intraluminal necrosis within neoplastic glands and prominent nucleoli are often seen in intramucosal adenocarcinoma.
- The histologic distinction between high-grade dysplasia and intramucosal adenocarcinoma is outlined in Table 3.1.

References: [10, 12, 15, 17, 21]

17. How do you identify submucosally invasive adenocarcinoma?

- Endoscopic biopsy specimens from patients with BE are typically superficial, with sampling of epithelium and lamina propria.
- Most patients with BE have areas of duplicated muscularis mucosae that can lead to the appearance of neoplastic glands invading through the muscularis mucosae, while the glands are actually still within the lamina propria (Fig. 3.8).
- Owing to the superficial nature of biopsies, it is difficult to accurately diagnose submucosally invasive adenocarcinoma in a biopsy specimen. When neoplastic epithelium is present within desmoplastic stroma, this is convincing evidence of submucosal invasion.
- In endoscopic mucosal resection or endoscopic submucosal dissection specimens, the deepest layer of muscularis mucosae may be present, and submucosa

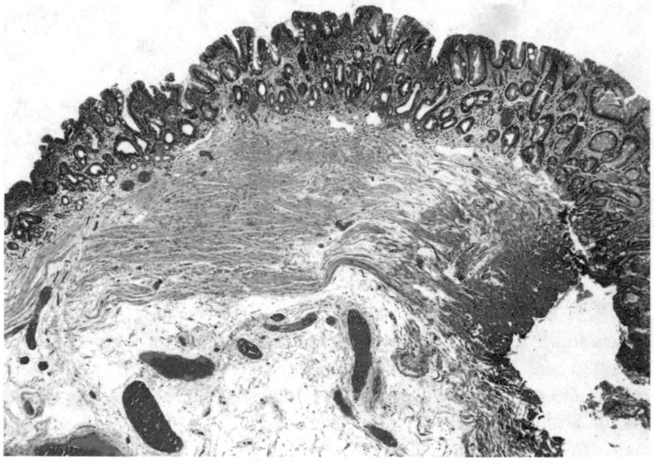

Fig. 3.8 Barrett esophagus with a duplicated muscularis mucosae. This endoscopic mucosal resection specimen shows BE with a thickened and duplicated muscularis mucosae. This muscle layer can be mistaken for muscularis propria, which may lead to overstaging of BE neoplasia

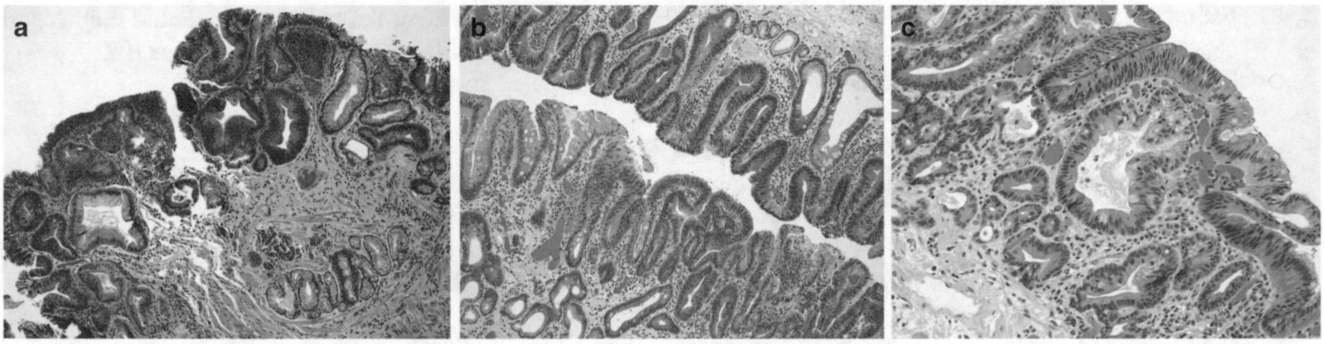

Fig. 3.9 Types of dysplasia seen in Barrett esophagus. (**a**) Intestinal type resembling a tubular adenoma of the colon. (**b, c**) Foveolar type featuring gastric foveolar-type cytoplasm with nuclear dysplastic changes. Note the transition from non-dysplastic BE mucosa (left) to dysplastic mucosa (right) in panel **b**. Panel **c** shows a progression from low-grade (right) to high-grade (left) dysplasia

is more readily identified. In well-oriented tissue profiles, submucosal invasion can be accurately diagnosed and margins assessed.

References: [19, 23, 24]

18. What are the described types of nonconventional dysplasia and how are they identified?

- The most common histologic appearance of dysplasia is intestinal type, which resembles the dysplasia seen in adenomas of the colon (Fig. 3.9a).
- Two additional histologic variants of dysplasia have been described including gastric foveolar dysplasia and serrated dysplasia.
- Gastric foveolar dysplasia (Fig. 3.9b, c) is characterized by mucinous epithelium with gastric foveolar-type cytoplasm and rare goblet cell differentiation. The cells may be cuboidal or low columnar in shape with a single layer of enlarged round nuclei with open chromatin, prominent nucleoli. The epithelium typically shows a crowded glandular architecture (back-to-back glands). Elongated and pseudostratified nuclei can be seen in cases of low-grade dysplasia (Fig. 3.9b, c). A sharp transition from non-dysplastic epithelium can be seen.
- Serrated dysplasia is characterized by architecture similar to serrated polyps of the colon, with a saw-tooth pattern of crypt epithelium when cut longitudinally, or a star-shaped lumen on cross section. The nuclei in serrated dysplasia are oval with open chromatin, while the cytoplasm is typically more eosinophilic.
- Criteria for low- and high-grade dysplasia in gastric foveolar and serrated dysplasia are not well established, but in general, cytologic atypia and architectural complexity are used for the distinction.

References: [21, 22]

19. Is ancillary testing recommended in identifying dysplasia associated with BE or those at risk of progression?

- Morphologic assessment remains the gold standard for identifying dysplasia.
- Recent consensus guidelines from the gastrointestinal pathology society do not recommend ancillary testing at this point in time.
- Some studies have suggested that immunohistochemical staining for p53 is helpful in identifying dysplasia and those at risk of progression. Overall there are insufficient criteria for how to interpret this stain including lack of clarity in the implications of the staining patterns on the presence and grading of dysplasia, as well as the possibility of progression. The overall evidence is not sufficient to recommend this ancillary test for routine use at this point in time.
- Immunohistochemical stains for AMACR, cyclin D1, SOX2, Ki-67, and others have been investigated in the diagnosis of BE dysplasia, with some showing promise for identification of dysplasia or risk of progression. More recent studies have questioned the specificity of some of these markers, and further studies are needed to assess their utility in clinical practice.

Reference: [25]

20. What are the possible treatment modalities when a diagnosis of dysplastic BE is rendered?

- Flat low-grade dysplasia may be treated with surveillance or endoscopic ablation.
- Flat high-grade dysplasia and intramucosal adenocarcinoma are typically managed with endoscopic radiofrequency ablation.
- Nodular lesions are treated by endoscopic mucosal resection/endoscopic submucosal dissection.

Follow-up may include additional radiofrequency ablation.
- If submucosal invasion or presence of unfavorable histology (poor differentiation or lymphovascular invasion) is identified, treatment is discussed with a multidisciplinary oncology group.

Reference: [4]

21. Is evaluation of BE dysplasia reproducible between pathologists?
- There is known interobserver variability among pathologists in the diagnosis of BE dysplasia, even among expert gastrointestinal pathologists. This variability is higher for indefinite and low-grade dysplasia.
- In patients with dysplasia of any grade, it is recommended that the biopsy be reviewed by two pathologists, one of which has expertise in gastrointestinal pathology.

References: [11, 20, 26, 27]

Case Presentation

Case 1

Learning Objectives
1. To understand the diagnostic criteria for BE
2. To understand the implication of evaluating GEJ biopsies

Case History
A 47-year-old male undergoes upper gastrointestinal endoscopy due to dyspepsia. Endoscopically, GEJ appears irregular, but there are no other abnormalities seen. Biopsies of irregular GEJ are obtained to “rule out BE”.

Histologic Findings
Squamous epithelium is seen on the left. There is mucinous columnar epithelium on the right with mild chronic and focal active inflammation. Scattered goblet cells are also present among gastric-type columnar epithelia. The presence of goblet cells indicates IM (Fig. 3.3).

Final Diagnosis
Columnar mucosa with mild chronic active inflammation. IM is present.

Take-Home Messages
- BE is defined as the presence of IM in biopsies taken ≥1 cm above GEJ.
- Presence of IM in GEJ biopsies does not necessarily indicate BE. While theoretically, this could be an extension of more extensive BE, it is not clear based on this biopsy alone, and therefore the pathologists should only report the presence of IM but not designate this as BE.

Case 2

Learning Objectives
1. To understand the clinical and endoscopic presentation of patients with BE
2. To understand the pathologic features of BE with dysplastic epithelium

Case History
A 67-year-old Caucasian male with a long history of reflux symptoms is referred to gastroenterologist by his primary care physician.

Endoscopic Findings
An upper endoscopy shows tongues of salmon-colored mucosa extending 4 cm upward from GEJ into the distal esophagus. Biopsies were obtained in four quadrants every 1–2 cm with jumbo forceps.

Histologic Findings
- Histologic sections demonstrate columnar mucosa with IM (Fig. 3.10a).
- Basal crypt atypia is present, which is expected in BE.
- In some areas, there is an abrupt transition from maturing epithelium to full-thickness cytologic atypia (Fig. 3.10b).
- The nuclei are enlarged and hyperchromatic, with crowding and pseudostratification.
- The long axis of the nuclei remains perpendicular to the basement membrane, and they are located in the basal half of the cytoplasm.
- There is no glandular architectural crowding or complexity.

Differential Diagnosis
- Barrett esophagus
- Barrett esophagus with low-grade dysplasia
- Barrett esophagus with high-grade dysplasia

IHC and Other Ancillary Studies
None.

Final Diagnosis
Barrett esophagus with low-grade dysplasia.

Take-Home Messages
- BE with low-grade dysplasia is characterized by hyperchromatic nuclei that extend from the crypt base to the surface epithelium.

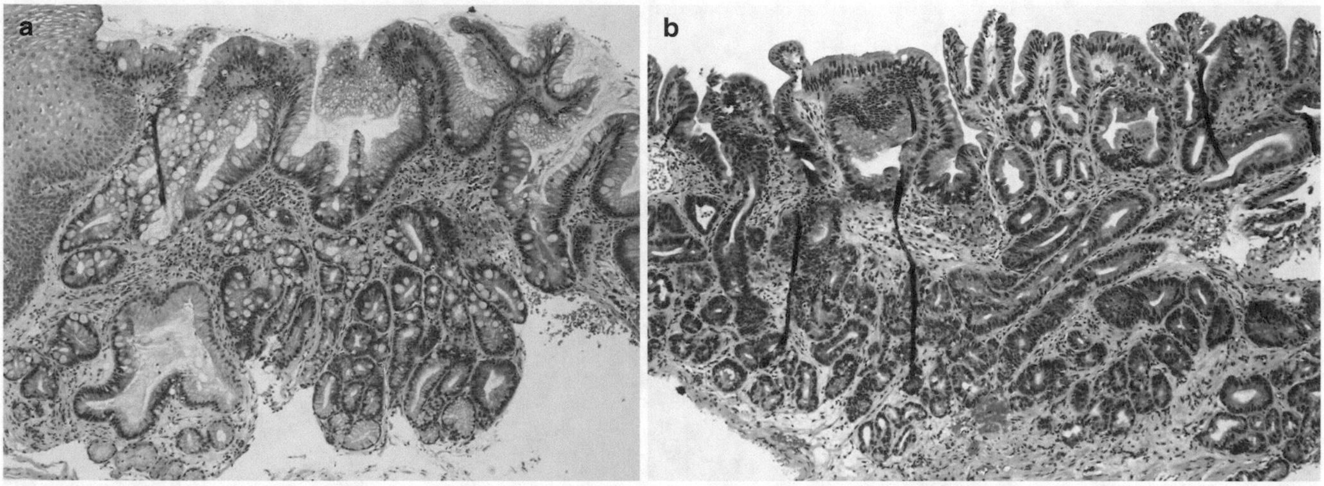

Fig. 3.10 Distal esophageal biopsy (case 2) showing IM (**a**) and areas of full-thickness cytologic atypia (**b**)

- The nuclei maintain polarity with respect to the basement membrane.
- The dysplastic epithelium shows no architectural complexity.

Case 3

Learning Objectives

1. To understand the clinical and endoscopic presentation of patients with BE
2. To understand the pathologic features of BE and dysplastic epithelium

Case History

A 73-year-old Caucasian male presented for follow-up for his known BE. His last endoscopic screening was 3 years prior and biopsies were negative for dysplasia.

Endoscopic Findings

On endoscopic examination, chromoendoscopy noted an irregular/distorted mucosal pattern in the distal esophagus with a small nodule identified. Endoscopic mucosal resection of the nodule was performed.

Histologic Findings

- Histologic sections demonstrate columnar mucosa with focal IM.
- The epithelium shows full-thickness atypia with hyperchromatic, enlarged round nuclei with prominent nucleoli, loss of nuclear polarity, and high nuclear-to-cytoplasmic ratios (Fig. 3.11a).
- The epithelium shows architectural complexity including crowded cribriform glands and a "never-ending" anastomosing glandular pattern (Fig. 3.11b).

Differential Diagnosis

- Barrett esophagus
- Barrett esophagus with low-grade dysplasia
- Barrett esophagus with high-grade dysplasia
- Barrett esophagus with intramucosal adenocarcinoma

IHC and Other Ancillary Studies

None.

Final Diagnosis

Barrett esophagus with intramucosal adenocarcinoma.

Take-Home Messages

- BE with intramucosal adenocarcinoma is characterized by high-grade cytology. Architectural features of intramucosal adenocarcinoma include single cells in the lamina propria or complex, never-ending anastomosed glands.

Case 4

Learning Objectives

1. To understand the diagnostic criteria for IM
2. To understand the difference between true and pseudogoblet cells

Case History

A 58-year-old male presented with reflux symptoms.

Endoscopic Findings

An upper endoscopy revealed an irregular Z-line and a tongue of pink mucosa in the distal esophagus extending ~1.2 cm above the GEJ.

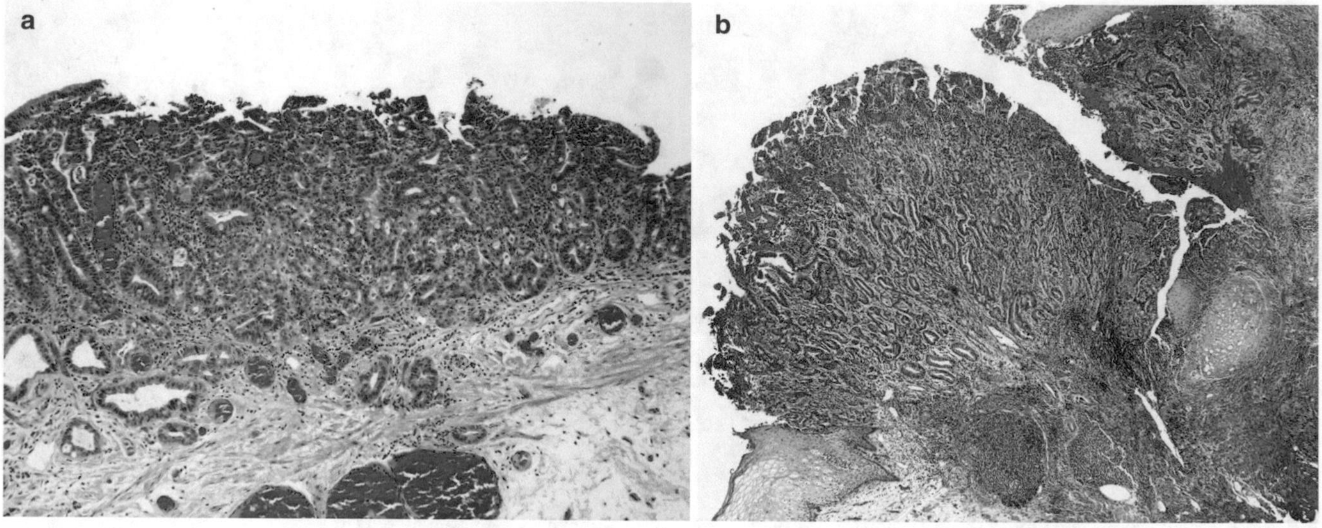

Fig. 3.11 Endoscopic mucosal resection of a small nodular lesion in the distal esophagus from a patient with long-standing history of Barrett esophagus (case 3). Sections show full-thickness epithelial atypia with enlarged round and hyperchromatic nuclei (**a**). There is glandular architectural complexity with a "never-ending" anastomosing pattern (**b**)

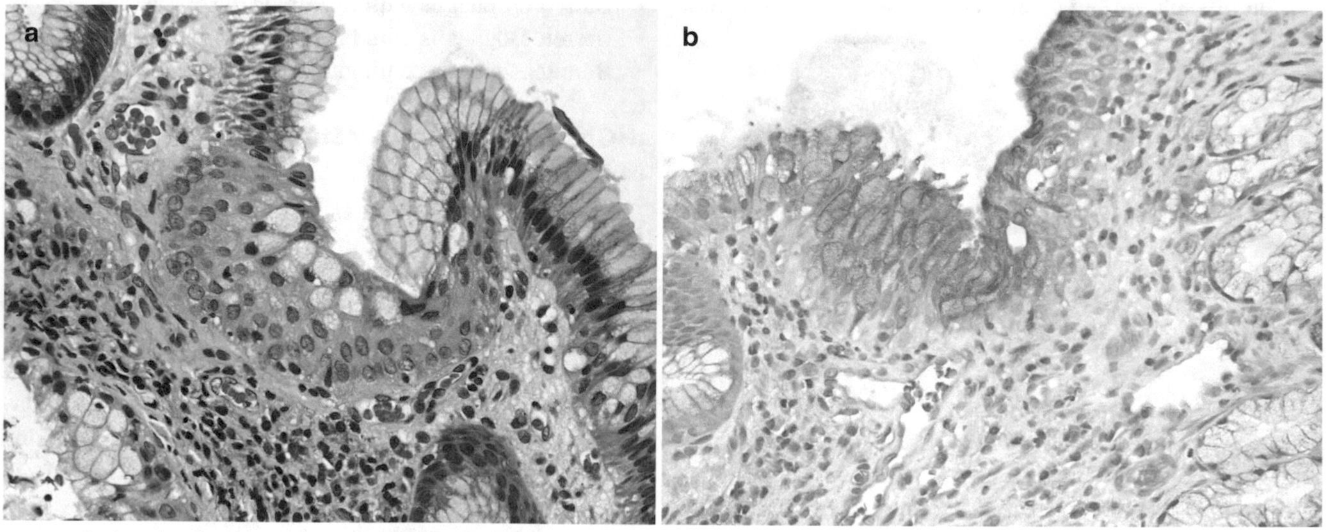

Fig. 3.12 Distal esophageal biopsy (case 4) showing clusters of mucin-containing cells (**a**) that stain blue on Alcian blue at pH 2.5 (**b**)

Histologic Findings

- Histologic sections demonstrate gastric-type columnar mucosa with a small island of multilayered cells.
- Some of the cells have intracytoplasmic mucin vacuoles with a blue hue (Fig. 3.12a).

Differential Diagnosis

- Intestinal metaplasia, consistent with Barrett esophagus
- Pseudo-goblet cells, no support for Barrett esophagus

IHC and Other Ancillary Studies

- Alcian blue stain at pH 2.5 shows "blue mucin" (Fig. 3.12b).

Final Diagnosis

Pseudo-goblet cells, no support for Barrett esophagus.

Take-Home Messages

- Pseudo-goblet cells can have "blue mucin" and even a "goblet" shape.

- Pseudo-goblet cells are typically arranged in clusters or linear rows, whereas true goblet cells are more dispersed among intervening non-goblet columnar cells.
- Alcian blue stain at pH 2.5 stains both true and pseudo-goblet cells blue and is not recommended as a routine stain to help diagnosis.
- True goblet cells are required for BE diagnosis in the United States.

References

1. Odze RD. Unraveling the mystery of the gastroesophageal junction: a pathologist's perspective. Am J Gastroenterol. 2005;100:1853–67.
2. Spechler SJ, Sharma P, Souza RF, et al. American gastroenterological position statement on the management of Barrett's esophagus. Gastroenterology. 2011;140:1084–91.
3. Naini BV, Chak A, Ali Meer A, Odze RD. Barrett's oesophagus diagnostic criteria: endoscopy and histology. Best Pract Res Clin Gastroenterol. 2015;29:77–96.
4. Shaheen NJ, Falk GW, Iyer PG, et al. ACG clinical guideline: diagnosis and management of Barrett esophagus. Am J Gastroenterol. 2016;111:30–50.
5. Fitzgerald RC, di Pietro M, Ragunath K, et al. British Society of Gastroenterology guidelines on the diagnosis and management of Barrett's esophagus. Gut. 2014;63:7–42.
6. Salimian KJ, Waters KM, Eze O, et al. Definition of Barrett esophagus in the United States: support for retention of a requirement for goblet cells. Am J Surg Pathol. 2018;42:264–8.
7. Bhat S, Coleman HG, Yousef F, et al. Risk of malignant progression in Barrett esophagus patients: results from a large population-based study. J Natl Cancer Inst. 2011;103:1049–57.
8. Naini BV, Souza RF, Odze RD. Barrett esophagus; a comprehensive and contemporary review for pathologists. Am J Surg Pathol. 2016;40(5):e45–66.
9. Spechler SJ. Intestinal metaplasia at the gastroesophageal junction. Gastroenterology. 2004;126:567–75.
10. Goldblum JR. Controversies in the diagnosis of Barrett esophagus and Barrett-related dysplasia: one pathologist's perspective. Arch Pathol Lab Med. 2010;134:1479–84.
11. Montgomery E, Bronner MP, Goldblum JR, Greenson JK, Haber MM, Hart J, et al. Reproducibility of the diagnosis of dysplasia in Barrett esophagus: a reaffirmation. Hum Pathol. 2001;32:368–78.
12. Yantiss RK. Diagnostic challenges in the pathologic evaluation of Barrett esophagus. Arch Pathol Lab Med. 2010;134:1589–600.
13. Lomo LC, Blount PL, Sanchez CA, Li X, Galipeau PC, Cowan DS, et al. Crypt dysplasia with surface maturation: a clinical, pathologic, and molecular study of a Barrett's esophagus cohort. Am J Surg Pathol. 2006;30:423–35.
14. Patil DT, Bennett AE, Mahajan D, Bronner MP. Distinguishing Barrett gastric foveolar dysplasia from reactive cardiac mucosa in gastroesophageal reflux disease. Hum Pathol. 2013;44:1146–53.
15. Appelman HD. Adenocarcinoma in Barrett mucosa treated by endoscopic mucosal resection. Arch Pathol Lab Med. 2009;133:1793–7.
16. Skacel M, Petras RE, Gramlich TL, Sigel JE, Richter JE, Goldblum JR. The diagnosis of low grade dysplasia in Barrett's esophagus and its implication for disease progression. Am J Gastroenterol. 2000;95:3383–7.
17. Odze RD. Diagnosis and grading of dysplasia in Barrett's oesophagus. J Clin Pathol. 2006;59:1029–38.
18. Curvers WL, ten Kate FJ, Krishnadath KK, Visser M, Elzer B, Baak LC, et al. Low-grade dysplasia in Barrett's esophagus: overdiagnosed and underestimated. Am J Gastroenterol. 2010;105:1523–30.
19. Takubo K, Vieth M, Aida J, Matsutani T, Hagiwara N, Iwakiri K, et al. Histopathological diagnosis of adenocarcinoma in Barrett's esophagus. Dig Endosc. 2014;26:322–30.
20. Ormsby AH, Petras RE, Henricks WH, Rice TW, Rybicki LA, Richter JE, et al. Observer variation in the diagnosis of superficial oesophageal adenocarcinoma. Gut. 2002;51:671–6.
21. Srivastava A, Sanchez CA, Cowan DS, Odze RD. Foveolar and serrated dysplasia are rare high-risk lesions in Barrett's esophagus: a prospective outcome analysis of 214 patients. Mod Pathol. 2010;23:742A.
22. Mahajan D, Bennett AE, Liu X, Bena J, Bronner MP. Grading of gastric foveolar-type dysplasia in Barrett's esophagus. Mod Pathol. 2010;23:1–11.
23. Abraham SC, Krasinskas AM, Correa AM, Hofstetter WL, Ajani JA, Swisher SG, Wu TT. Duplication of the muscularis mucosae in Barrett esophagus: an underrecognized feature and its implication for staging of adenocarcinoma. Am J Surg Pathol. 2007;31:1719–25.
24. Appelman HD, Streutker C, Vieth M, Neumann H, Neurath MF, Upton MP, Sagaert X, Wang HH, El-Zimaity H, Abraham SC, Bellizzi AM. The esophageal mucosa and submucosa: immunohistology in GERD and Barrett's esophagus. N Y Acad Sci. 2013;1300:144–65.
25. Srivastava A, Appelman H, Goldsmith JD, Davison JM, Hart J, Krasinskas AM. The use of ancillary stains in the diagnosis of Barrett esophagus and Barrett esophagus-associated dysplasia: recommendations from the Rodger C. Haggitt Gastrointestinal Pathology Society. Am J Surg Pathol. 2017;41(5):e8–e21.
26. Kerkhof M, van Dekken H, Steyerberg EW, Meijer GA, Mulder AH, de Bruïne A, et al. Grading of dysplasia in Barrett's oesophagus: substantial interobserver variation between general and gastrointestinal pathologists. Histopathology. 2007;50:920–7.
27. Downs-Kelly E, Mendelin JE, Bennett AE, Castilla E, Henricks WH, Schoenfield L, et al. Poor interobserver agreement in the distinction of high-grade dysplasia and adenocarcinoma in pretreatment Barrett's esophagus biopsies. Am J Gastroenterol. 2008;103:2333–40.

Nonneoplastic Diseases of the Stomach

4

Michael Torbenson

List of Frequently Asked Questions

1. Which types of patients present with acute gastritis?
2. What are the histological findings of acute gastritis?
3. What types of infections cause phlegmonous gastritis?
4. What are the histological features of peptic ulcer disease?
5. What is the difference between an erosion and an ulcer?
6. How do people get infected with *H. pylori*?
7. What laboratory tests are used to detect *H. pylori* infection?
8. Why can't I find *H. pylori* organisms on the biopsy when other tests for *H. pylori* are positive?
9. What does the term environmental metaplastic atrophic gastritis mean?
10. What are the key histological findings in *H. pylori* gastritis?
11. What is the role of histochemical or immunostains for identify *H. pylori* organisms?
12. What is the significance of mucosal atrophy in cases of *H. pylori* gastritis? How should I detect it?
13. What is the significance of metaplasia? How should I detect it?
14. What is the difference between *H. pylori* infection and *Helicobacter heilmanni* (*H. heilmanni*) infection?
15. What is the clinical significance of *H. heilmanni* gastritis?
16. What types of patients have chemical or reactive gastropathy?
17. What clinical symptoms or endoscopic findings are typical for chemical gastropathy?
18. What is the best diagnostic approach in order to get the diagnosis correct?
19. How is reactive gastropathy distinguished from portal hypertensive gastropathy and from the gastric antral vascular ectasia (GAVE) syndrome?
20. What types of patients develop autoimmune gastritis?
21. How is the diagnosis of autoimmune gastritis made?
22. What histological findings suggest autoimmune gastritis?
23. What is the best approach to diagnosis autoimmune gastritis on histology?
24. Why do patients develop ECL hyperplasia and neuroendocrine tumors?
25. What other lesions are patients with autoimmune gastritis at risk for?
26. What causes lymphocytic gastritis?
27. What is the clinical significance of lymphocytic gastritis?
28. What causes collagenous gastritis?
29. How is collagenous gastritis treated?
30. What causes granulomatous gastritis?
31. How is a diagnosis of eosinophilic gastritis made?
32. What causes eosinophilic gastritis?
33. How is the diagnosis of Russell body gastritis made and what is the significance?

Acute Gastritis

In common medical usage, the term *acute gastritis* refers to a clinical presentation with acute symptoms, often severe, that resolve after the underlying injury is removed. This term should not be confused with the histological findings of neutrophilic inflammation, which is properly called *active inflammation*, but is sometimes referred to as *acute inflammation*.

M. Torbenson (✉)
Mayo Clinic, Rochester, MN, USA
e-mail: Torbenson.michael@mayo.edu

H. L. Wang, Z. E. Chen (eds.), *Practical Gastrointestinal Pathology*, Practical Anatomic Pathology,
https://doi.org/10.1007/978-3-030-51268-2_4

Frequently Asked Questions

1. **Which types of patients present with acute gastritis?**
   Overall, most causes of acute gastritis will fall into one of three main categories of injury.
   - The first of these causes results from ischemic injury. The ischemic injury usually results from debilitating illness and hypotension, but sudden acute bleeding can also lead to ischemic injury. Ischemic injury tends to affect the gastric body more than the gastric antrum. As another cause of ischemic injury, embolic beads can escape the liver following transarterial chemoembolization (TACE), get lodged in the stomach, and lead to ischemic injury (Fig. 4.1).
   - A second major cause of acute injury results from ingestion of various industrial chemicals or caustic agents. These agents tend to injure the antrum more than the body. Binge drinking can also lead to an acute gastritis pattern of injury and also tends to be antral predominant.
   - As a third cause, bacterial infection can sometimes lead to acute gastritis, often with extensive necrosis, a pattern called *phlegmonous gastritis* or *suppurative gastritis*. The endoscopic findings vary but commonly show mucosal hemorrhage and necrosis.

2. **What are the histological findings of acute gastritis?**
   The histological findings range from mucosal hemorrhage and edema (Fig. 4.2) to ulcers to frank mucosal necrosis and sometimes to full-thickness wall necrosis. In cases of suppurative gastritis, the stomach shows neutrophil-rich inflammation, often more prominent in the submucosa than the mucosa. In contrast, other forms of acute gastritis generally have sparse to absent inflammation.

3. **What types of infections cause phlegmonous gastritis?**
   Phlegmonous gastritis is essentially always caused by bacterial infections, including *Streptococcus* (most common), *Staphylococcus*, *Enterobacter*, *Escherichia coli*, and *Pneumococcus*.

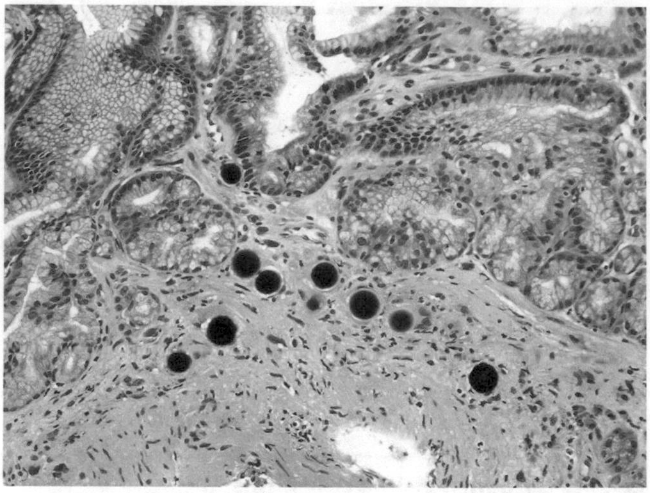

Fig. 4.1 Embolic beads in the stomach. This stomach developed numerous ulcers following TACE for hepatocellular carcinoma. A biopsy shows small embolic beads in the lamina propria

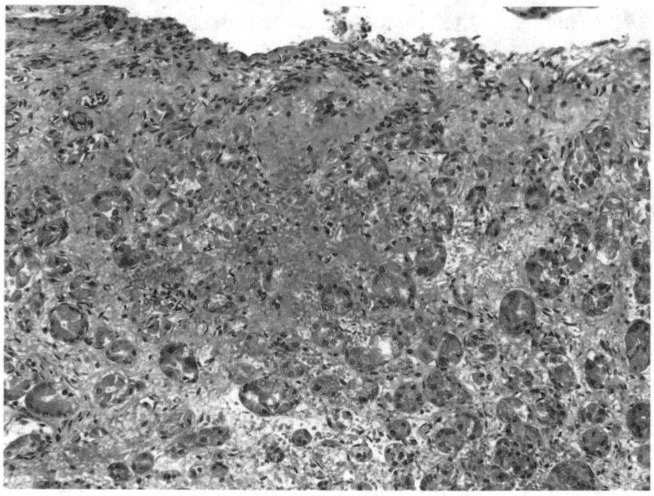

Fig. 4.2 Acute gastritis. This mild case showed lamina propria congestion, hemorrhage, and focal ulcers

Peptic Ulcer Disease

Peptic ulcers are gastric and duodenal ulcers that result from excess gastric acid production or impaired mucosal protection from the gastric acid. The majority of cases (80%) are caused by *Helicobacter pylori (H. pylori)* infection and/or nonsteroidal anti-inflammatory drug (NSAID)/aspirin use. When both risk factors are present, there is an additive risk for peptic ulcer disease. The remaining 20% of peptic ulcer cases are associated with a number of predisposing situations, including high stress.

References: [1–4]

Frequently Asked Questions

4. **What are the histological features of peptic ulcer disease?**
   Peptic ulcers/erosions do not have unique histological findings that allow a histological diagnosis. Instead, the ulcers/erosions are typical of mucosal ulcers in general, with a layer of inflammatory exudate and underling ulceration, often with granulation tissue at the base (Fig. 4.3).

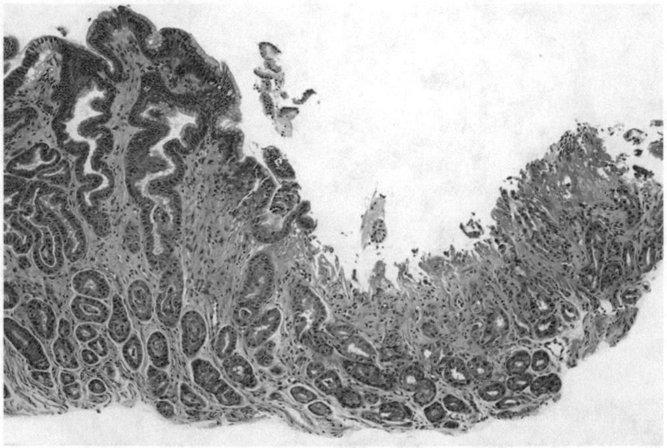

Fig. 4.3 Peptic erosion. The erosion shows relative little inflammation but is otherwise fairly nondescript. This case was associated with heavy NSAID use

- Depending on the cause, the background mucosa often shows *H. pylori* gastritis and/or changes of reactive gastropathy.

5. What is the difference between an erosion and an ulcer?

An erosion shows loss of at least the surface epithelium and can extend to the full thickness of the gastric mucosa but still has an intact muscularis mucosae. Ulcers extend deeper, through the muscularis mucosae.

- Many times these definitions are not strictly followed by pathologists in evaluation of surgical pathology specimens, but using proper terms is encouraged, as it has value in accurately conveying the histological findings.

Helicobacter pylori Gastritis

H. pylori infection leads to a chronic lymphoplasmacytic gastritis of the stomach, typically with at least focal neutrophilic inflammation. Chronic infection is an important cause of peptic ulcers. *H. pylori* is also associated with lymphocytic gastritis. With long-standing infection, the stomach can undergo metaplasia, dysplasia, and carcinoma. Chronic infections also lead to gastric lymphomas, primarily mucosa-associated lymphoid tissue (MALT) lymphomas but also some diffuse large B cell lymphomas.
References: [5, 6]

Frequently Asked Questions

6. How do people get infected with *H. pylori*?

Acute and chronic infections do not have clinical symptoms, so individuals are unaware when they are first infected.

- Infection is by the oral-fecal route. Molecular studies have found that mother to child transmission is the main route of infection and most persons are first infected during their childhood or adolescence.
- Most patients are asymptomatic for the majority of their infection, but some patients can present with chronic anemia and fatigue. If peptic disease develops, then patients can develop additional symptoms.

References: [7–9]

7. What laboratory tests are used to detect *H. pylori* infection?

There are several tests available for managing patients with possible *H. pylori* gastritis.

- First, serology for *H. pylori* is widely available. After infection and subsequent seroconversion, antibodies to *H. pylori* are detectable for many years. Positive serology does not indicate active infection because serology remains positive for years after *H. pylori* clearance, either from treatment or sporadic clearance. Despite this limitation, the test remains clinically valuable because negative serologies make *H. pylori* infection very unlikely.
- A second common clinical test is the urease breath test. This test is based on the observation that *H. pylori* organisms have an enzyme called urease, which breaks down urea. Patients are given an oral solution of urea, after the urea has been first labeled with carbon isotopes ^{13}C or ^{14}C. If there is *H. pylori* gastritis, the bacteria will digest the urea and release the carbon isotopes, which can then be detected in the patient's breath. The urease breath test has excellent clinical sensitivity and specificity, >95% in some studies. A fundamentally similar test is called the rapid urease test. In this office-based test, the endoscopist takes a mucosal biopsy and then adds a labeled urea product to the biopsy specimen. If bacteria are present, they digest the urea and the breakdown products are detected by a color substrate. Of note, prior or ongoing use of antibiotics or proton pump inhibitors, which is very common in most patient settings, will decrease the sensitivity for both of these urease-based tests.
- A third commonly available test is an enzyme-linked immunosorbent assay (ELISA)-based test that detects bacterial antigens in stool. This test does not lose as much sensitivity as the prior tests in patients taking antibiotics or proton pump inhibitors, but has the decided disadvantage of being a home-based fecal test.
- Finally, organisms can also be detected by culture. Cultures are not necessary for routine clinical care but can be helpful if patients have antibiotic-resistant *H. pylori* infections

References: [10, 11]

8. **Why can't I find *H. pylori* organisms on the biopsy when other tests for *H. pylori* are positive?**

A histological diagnosis of *H. pylori* gastritis requires the presence of *H. pylori* organisms on hematoxylin and eosin (H&E) and/or special stains. However, there are a few clinical settings where no organisms are evident on histology, even with immunohistochemistry, but other laboratory tests are positive for *H. pylori* infections, such as the stool antigen test.

- This occurs largely when patients have taken medications, over the counter or otherwise, that substantially suppresses but does not eliminate the bacteria. Examples include the use of proton pump inhibitors, bismuth subsalicylate (Pepto-Bismol), and broad-spectrum antibiotics for other infections.

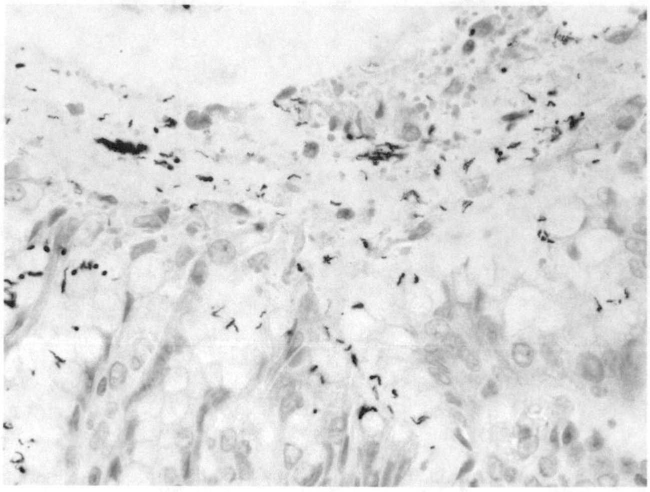

Fig. 4.4 *H. pylori* gastritis, immunostain. Organisms can be seen in the surface mucin layer

9. **What does the term environmental metaplastic atrophic gastritis mean?**

This older term is important for historical reasons but is generally not used in surgical pathology practice today. The current approach is to classify gastritis by etiology. However, before etiologies were widely known, gastritis was classified using the Sydney classification system/updated Sydney classification system, which classified gastritis primarily based on topography and morphology.

- Most cases previously diagnosed as environmental metaplastic atrophic gastritis were cases of *H. pylori* gastritis.

Reference: [12]

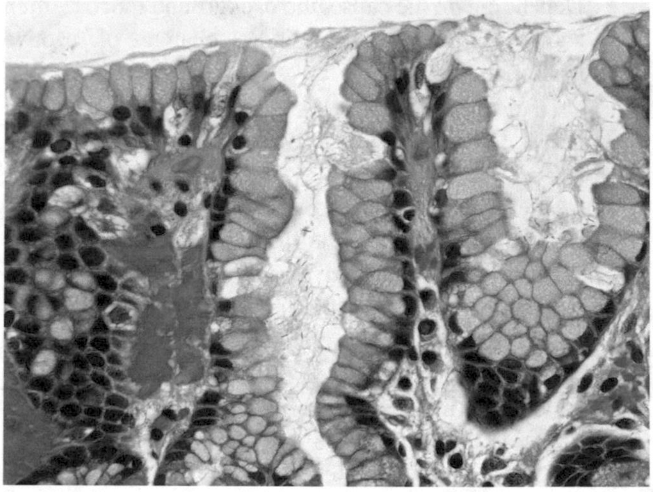

Fig. 4.5 *H. pylori* gastritis. Organisms can be seen in the surface mucin layer and extending into the gastric pits

10. **What are the key histological findings in *H. pylori* gastritis?**

H. pylori organisms are found on the mucosal surface, often in the thick layer of mucin that normally coats the epithelial surface (Fig. 4.4), but are also found in the gastric pits (Fig. 4.5) and sometimes the gastric glands.

- *H. pylori* organisms are shaped as thin and straight to slightly curved rods, sometimes with a broad V or seagull shape. The density of organisms varies from rare and focal to heavy and diffuse. There is no clinical need to indicate the density of organisms in the pathology report. However, if you want to report the density, it is best to use some of standardized reporting tool, such as a visual analog scale.
- Organisms are typically absent or sparse in areas of intestinal metaplasia or right at the edge of an ulcer. In addition, after partial treatment, the organisms can be round in morphology and sparse in numbers (Fig. 4.6).
- In active chronic *H. pylori* gastritis, the mucosa shows chronic inflammation that often is heavier in the superficial half of the mucosa, a finding called a *superficial predominant gastritis pattern* (Fig. 4.7). Of note, however, this pattern of mucosal inflamma-

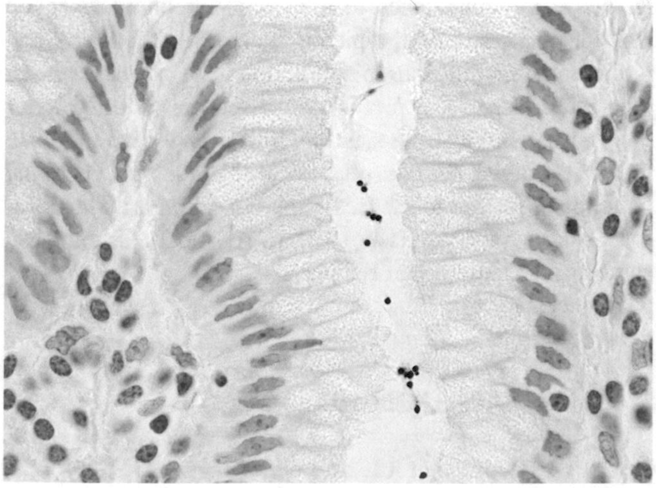

Fig. 4.6 *H. pylori* gastritis following treatment. After treatment, a follow-up biopsy to look for eradication showed residual active chronic gastritis as well as occasional clusters of *H. pylori* that showed a cocci morphology

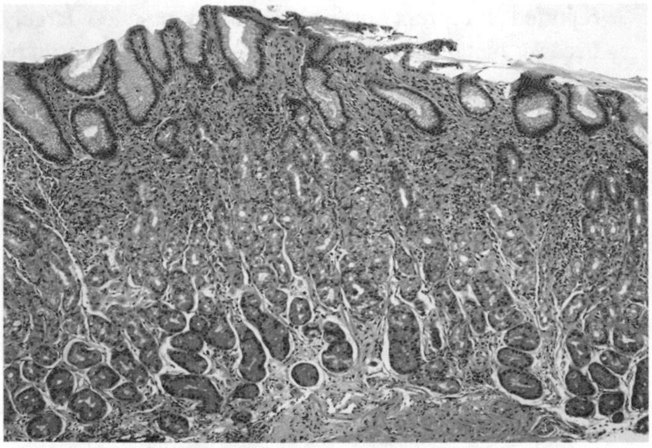

Fig. 4.7 *H. pylori* gastritis, superficial predominant pattern. The gastritis is heavier in the upper half of the mucosa

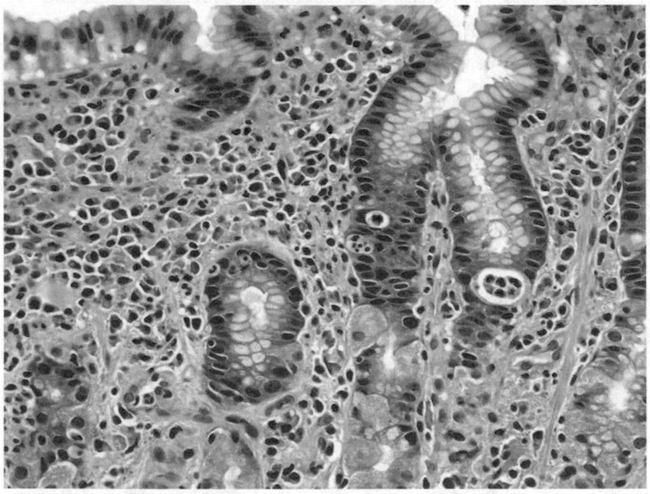

Fig. 4.8 *H. pylori* gastritis, active inflammation. There are neutrophils in the epithelium

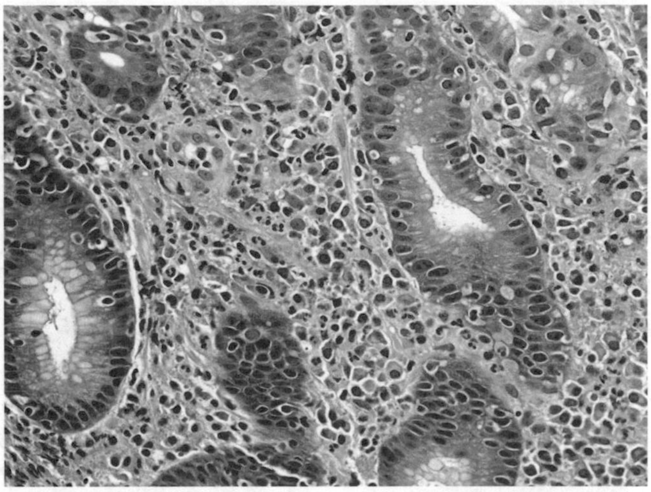

Fig. 4.9 *H. pylori* gastritis, active inflammation. There are neutrophils in the lamina propria

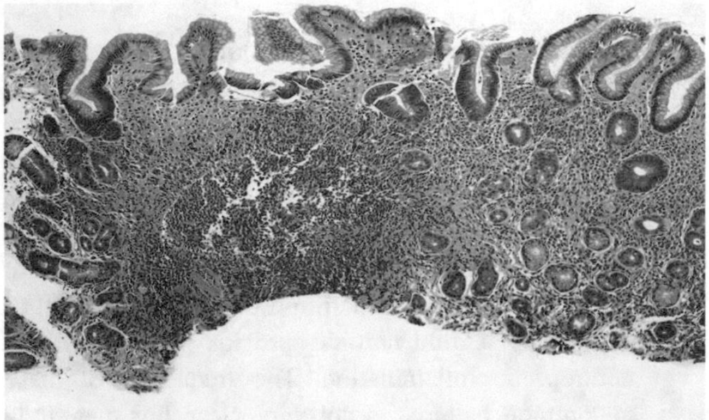

Fig. 4.10 *H. pylori* gastritis, lymphoid aggregate. A prominent lymphoid aggregate is seen in the lamina propria

tion is neither sensitive nor specific for *H. pylori* gastritis, with many cases of *H. pylori* gastritis lacking this pattern and some cases that are negative for *H. pylori* showing this pattern.

- Active (neutrophilic) inflammation is commonly present (Fig. 4.8), but again active chronic gastritis per se is neither very sensitive nor specific for *H. pylori* gastritis. The active chronic gastritis can involve the antrum and/or the body. The active neutrophilic component manifests as neutrophils in the surface epithelium, gastric pits, and sometimes gastric glands. Lamina propria neutrophils are also common (Fig. 4.9).
- The chronic inflammation in the mucosa is mostly lymphocytes, but plasma cells are also present in significant numbers. Lymphoid aggregates are also common (Fig. 4.10). The chronic gastritis can vary in severity from mild to marked. After treatment, the active inflammation disappears quickly, often within days, while the chronic inflammation can linger on, sometimes taking several years to disappear (Fig. 4.11).
- Historically, untreated *H. pylori* was predominately an antral disease, but proton pump inhibitors can modify this pattern, leading to more common and sometimes heavier involvement of the body mucosa.

Reference: [12]

11. **What is the role of histochemical or immunostains for identifying *H. pylori* organisms?**

When *H. pylori* organisms are confidently seen on H&E, then additional stains are not needed.

- If organisms are not clearly present on H&E but the histological or clinical findings are suspicious for infection, then additional stains are warranted, and these can be either histochemical stains like the Diff-Quik stain or the Giemsa stain or can be an *H. pylori* immunostain.
- The recommendations for when to use special stains have changed over the past years because of concerns over cost. In the historically important updated Sydney

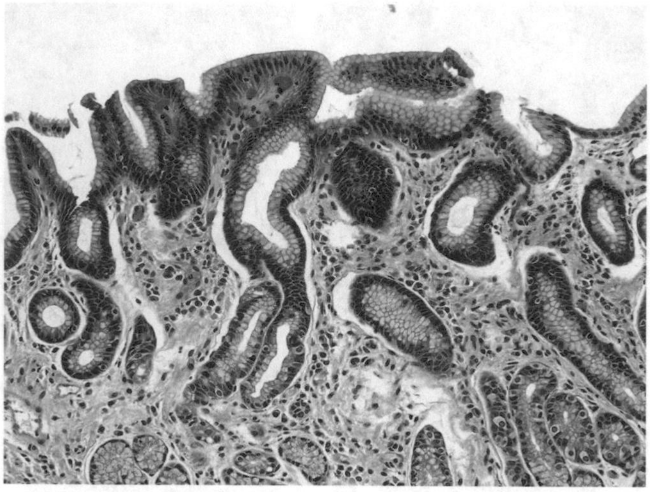

Fig. 4.11 *H. pylori* gastritis, residual chronic inflammation after treatment. This biopsy was taken 1.5 years after successful treatment for *H. pylori* and still showed mild chronic gastritis

classification system, as well as other expert reviews from the same time period, reflex stains were endorsed to identify *H. pylori*. This recommendation was made so as not to miss cases of *H. pylori* gastritis that lacked the typical pattern of active chronic gastritis on H&E. For example, rare cases of *H. pylori* infection can be associated with a reactive gastropathy pattern (presumably from a superimposed chemical insult) or show only a mild chronic gastritis pattern, without neutrophilic inflammation. The frequency of these uncommon patterns is not very clear, but one study found a frequency of 11%.

- Nonetheless, the current recommendations are not in favor of reflex staining because of cost concerns, but instead recommend that special stains be ordered when the H&E is negative for organisms but the histological findings are suspicious for infection (active chronic gastritis pattern or inactive chronic gastritis pattern with moderate or marked inflammation) or when the clinical setting suggests a higher a priori likelihood of *H. pylori* infection (e.g., family history, endoscopic findings, prior treatment for *H. pylori*). Current guidelines do not recommend stains for *H. pylori* in the setting of normal mucosa, chemical gastropathy, or mild chronic inflammation without activity.

References: [10, 12–14]

12. What is the significance of mucosal atrophy in cases of *H. pylori* gastritis? How should I detect it?

Atrophy results from loss of glands, leading to mucosal thinning. However, the atrophy is difficult to reproducibly identify and score by histology. Mucosal atrophy was scored as a separate histological finding in the Sydney classification system, but is not routinely reported in current surgical pathology practice, largely because metaplasia is strongly associated with atrophy, which is more reproducibly identified. In addition, intestinal metaplasia is a potential precursor to carcinoma (see next question).

13. What is the significance of metaplasia? How should I detect it?

Gastric metaplasia is important because it has a low but definite risk of progression through the steps of dysplasia into an adenocarcinoma. Thus, biopsies with metaplasia should also be examined for dysplasia.

- Gastric metaplasia in the antrum can include intestinal metaplasia (Fig. 4.12) or pancreatic acinar cell metaplasia. Intestinal metaplasia has the greatest risk for progression to dysplasia.
- Special stains are not needed to detect metaplasia for clinical purposes; the H&E findings are sufficient.
- During endoscopy, foci of intestinal metaplasia can appear polypoid, especially if the background mucosa shows significant atrophy. In these cases, the specimen can be received labeled as a gastric polyp.
- Research studies have further divided intestinal metaplasia complete metaplasia versus incomplete metaplasia and have found that incomplete intestinal metaplasia has a greater risk of progression to dysplasia and carcinoma. Nonetheless, this classification has not been widely adopted for clinical care.
  - Complete intestinal metaplasia shows numerous goblet cells, and the goblet cells are interspersed with absorptive-type cells with eosinophilic cytoplasm and well-formed brush borders, closely resembling a normal enterocyte (Fig. 4.13).
    - Neuroendocrine cells are also commonly present in cases of complete metaplasia (Fig. 4.14).

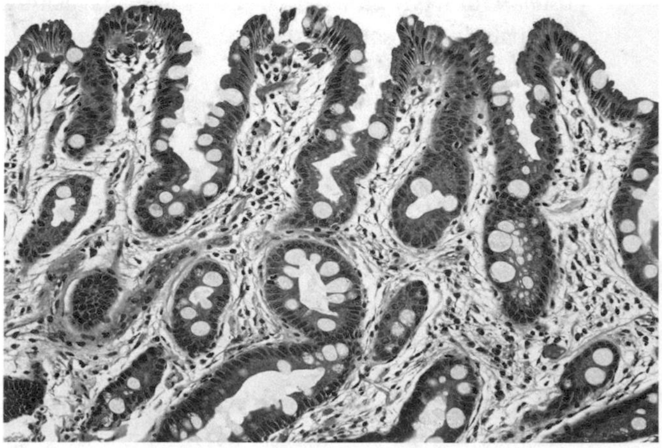

Fig. 4.12 Intestinal metaplasia, complete type. The biopsy shows intestinal metaplasia with goblet cells. The non-goblet cells resemble enterocytes

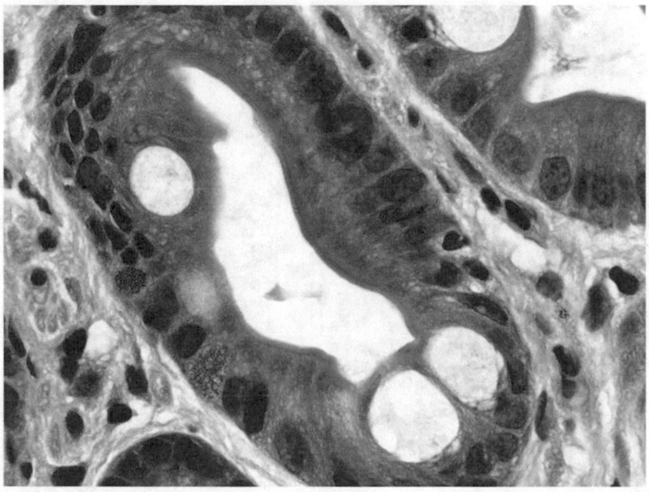

Fig. 4.13 Intestinal metaplasia, complete type. The non-goblet cells have brush borders

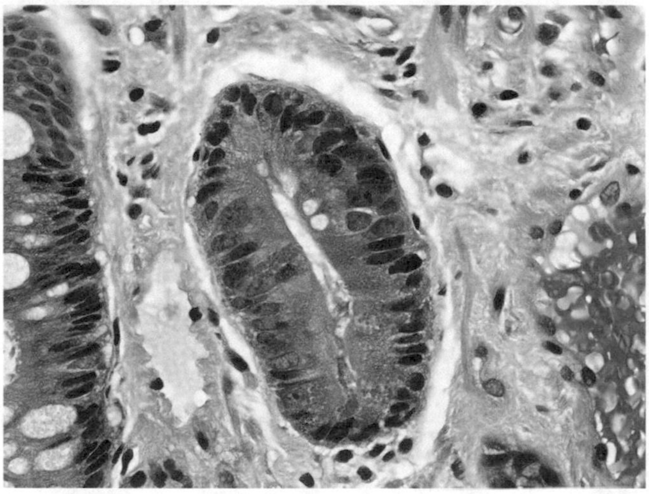

Fig. 4.14 Intestinal metaplasia, complete type. Neuroendocrine cells are present

- In contrast, incomplete metaplasia is defined as mucosa showing occasional to scattered goblet cells that are interspersed with mucin-producing cells (Fig. 4.15). The metaplastic epithelium lacks a well-defined brush border (Fig. 4.16).
- Histochemical and immunostains have been employed for research studies to distinguish complete from incomplete metaplasia. However, for those rare requests by clinicians to subtype the intestinal metaplasia, the decision of incomplete versus complete is adequately made on H&E.

• In the stomach body, metaplasia can also include pyloric metaplasia, a pattern also called *pseudopyloric metaplasia* (Fig. 4.17). By far the most common type of metaplasia in *H. pylori* gastritis is intestinal metaplasia.

References: [15, 16]

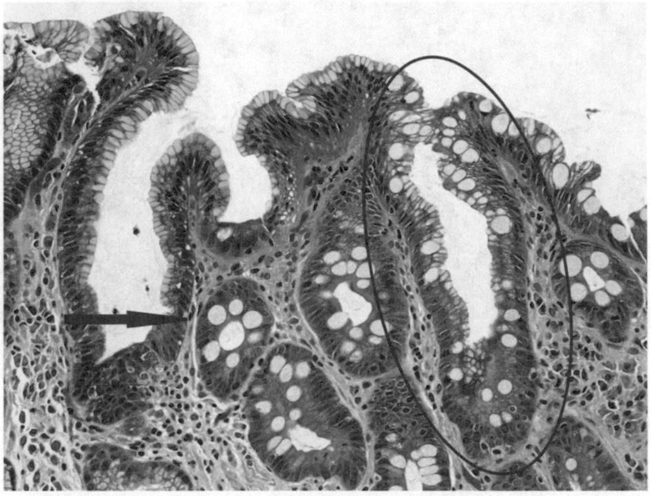

Fig. 4.15 Intestinal metaplasia, incomplete type. The biopsy shows intestinal metaplasia with goblet cells, but many of the intervening cells are mucinous and do not resemble enterocytes (circled). A mixture of complete and incomplete metaplasia is not uncommon, and some of the glands to the left of the circled gland show complete intestinal metaplasia (arrow)

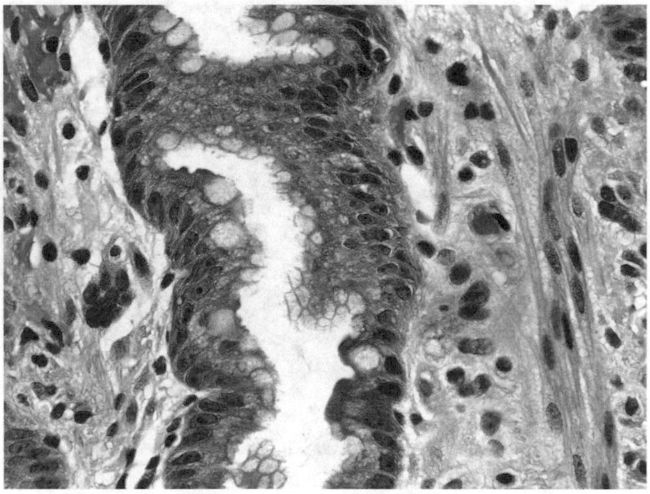

Fig. 4.16 Intestinal metaplasia, incomplete type. The non-goblet cells are mucin producing and not absorptive

14. What is the difference between *H. pylori* infection and *Helicobacter heilmanni* (*H. heilmanni*) infection?

The histological findings in *H. heilmannii* gastritis are generally similar to *H. pylori* gastritis (Fig. 4.18), though the degree of active and chronic inflammation is often milder in *H. heilmannii* gastritis. *H. heilmannii* gastritis is usually acquired from exposure to domestic cats and dogs or farm animals.

• On H&E, *H. heilmannii* organisms are about twice as long as *H. pylori* and on high magnification have distinct spirals (Fig. 4.19). In many cases, the organ-

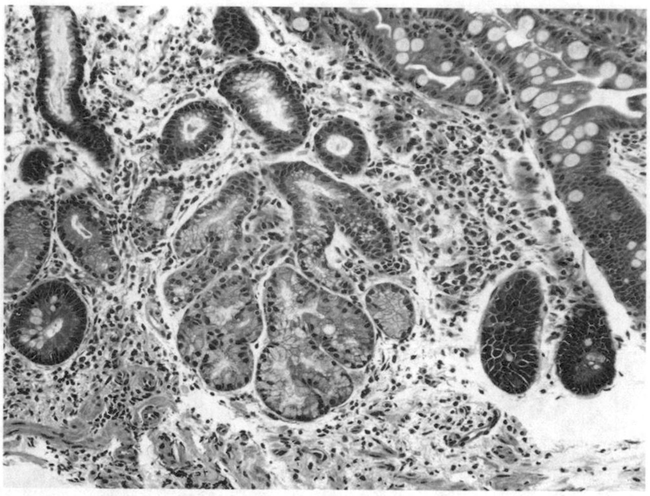

Fig. 4.17 Pyloric metaplasia. This biopsy from the body showed loss of oxyntic glands, which were replaced by glands that resemble antral or pyloric glands

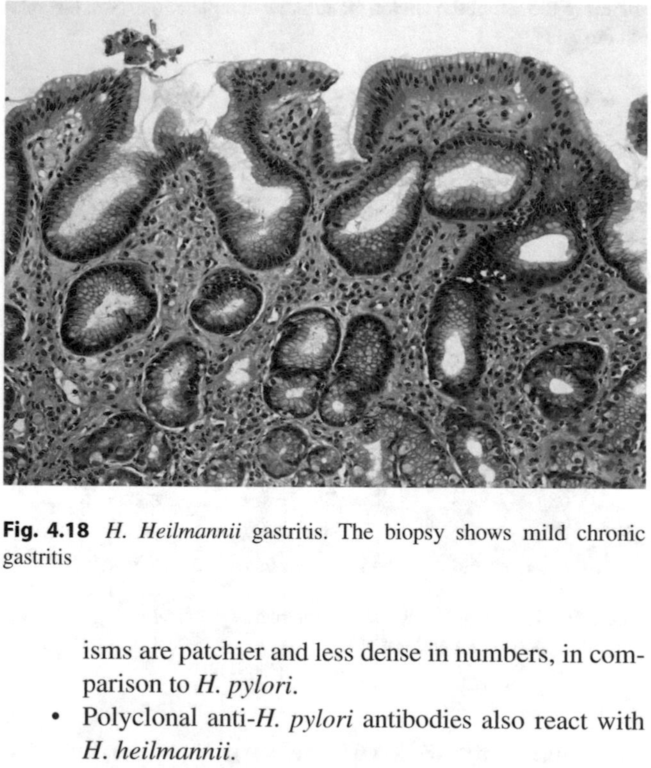

Fig. 4.18 *H. Heilmannii* gastritis. The biopsy shows mild chronic gastritis

isms are patchier and less dense in numbers, in comparison to *H. pylori*.

- Polyclonal anti-*H. pylori* antibodies also react with *H. heilmannii*.
- Of note, *H. heilmannii* is not a single organism, but instead is a group of closely related bacteria that show similar morphology on H&E. The entire group of organisms is generically called *H. heilmannii* when identified solely on H&E or immunohistochemistry, but when cultured or studied by molecular methods, this group is made up of greater than 30 different species, such as *Helicobacter felix* (*H. felix*) or *Helicobacter suis* (*H. suis*). *H. suis* is the most common cause of *H. heilmannii*-associated human gastritis.

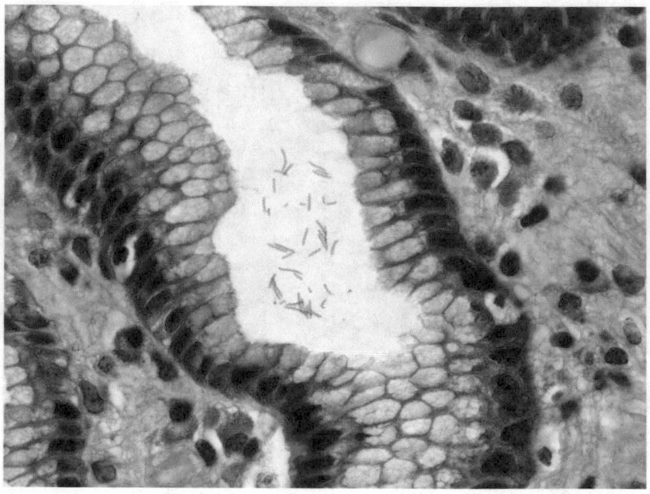

Fig. 4.19 *H. Heilmannii* gastritis. The organisms are spiral and longer and more curvy than *H. pylori*

- The overall prevalence of *H. heilmannii* is much lower than *H. pylori* gastritis, with most studies showing a prevalence of about 0.1%.

References: [17–20]

15. **What is the clinical significance of *H. heilmanni* gastritis?**

    Not too much really, as the clinical treatment options are essentially the same. However, the diagnosis is still fun to make. The source of infection is also different (domesticated animals, mostly).

Reactive Gastropathy

The reactive gastropathy pattern of injury is seen primarily in the antrum, with the body involved only when there is substantial antral disease. The reactive gastropathy pattern of injury is also called *chemical gastropathy* and both terms are equally acceptable. The injury pattern is fundamentally a hyperplastic mucosal response to chronic chemical-type exposures, including medications, bile acids, and alcohol. Inflammation is typically mild or absent.

Frequently Asked Questions

16. **What types of patients have chemical or reactive gastropathy?**

    Chemical gastropathy is rare in children but the frequency increases steadily with age. Overall, a diagnosis of reactive gastropathy is reported in 15–20% of adult biopsy specimens.

    - NSAIDs, other medications, and bile reflux are common causes. Depending on the patient population, alcohol is another important cause. These chemical-type agents chronically irritate the gastric mucosa leading to a hyperplastic mucosa with relatively little inflammation.

References: [21, 22]

17. What clinical symptoms or endoscopic findings are typical for chemical gastropathy?

Clinical symptoms are typically mild and nonspecific, including general complaints of "dyspepsia." In fact, studies have found no consistent correlates between a histological diagnosis of reactive gastropathy and the clinical complaints that initially led to endoscopy. Likewise, the histological diagnosis does not correlate well with endoscopic findings, with endoscopy mostly showing nonspecific findings such as mucosal hyperemia.

- In part, this lack of correlation may result from very loose criteria employed by some pathologists, who diagnose a chemical reactive gastropathy pattern on many biopsies that are essentially normal or have mild nonspecific changes. In fact, it is extraordinarily rare for a pathologist to miss a diagnosis of chemical gastropathy, while overdiagnosis is not uncommon.

Reference: [22]

18. What is the best diagnostic approach in order to get the diagnosis correct?

One helpful point to remember is that the chemical gastropathy pattern should truly be a pattern, having multiple features present, as opposed to a single histological finding. Overdiagnosis usually results from overinterpretation of single nonspecific findings.

- The chemical gastropathy pattern consists of varying degrees of foveolar hyperplasia, reduced surface mucin, and often mild lamina propria edema and congestion.
  - The antral glands and pits are about equal in thickness in normal mucosa, but with foveolar hyperplasia in the setting of a reactive gastropathy, the pits become elongated (Fig. 4.20).
  - The hyperplastic pits often develop a corkscrew appearance, and lamina propria smooth muscle fibers become hyperplastic and more visible, extending into the upper portion of the mucosa (Fig. 4.21). Of note, however, an occasional wisp of smooth muscle in the lamina propria can be seen in normal mucosa.
  - In addition, the foveolar hyperplasia is usually accompanied by some degree of mucin depletion.
  - Cases of reactive gastropathy also can have superficial erosions.
- If the antral mucosa has severe chemical gastropathy, then the body mucosa can also be involved, but a diagnosis of chemical gastropathy restricted to the body is probably a misdiagnosis.
- The chemical gastropathy pattern of injury generally does not lead to mucosal atrophy, but can lead to intestinal metaplasia. In these cases, the metaplasia is typically focal and not as extensive as it can be in some cases of chronic *H. pylori* gastritis. As an exception, stomachs with severe bile reflux that results from prior surgery and loss of the normal pylorus can develop extensive atrophy and extensive metaplasia.

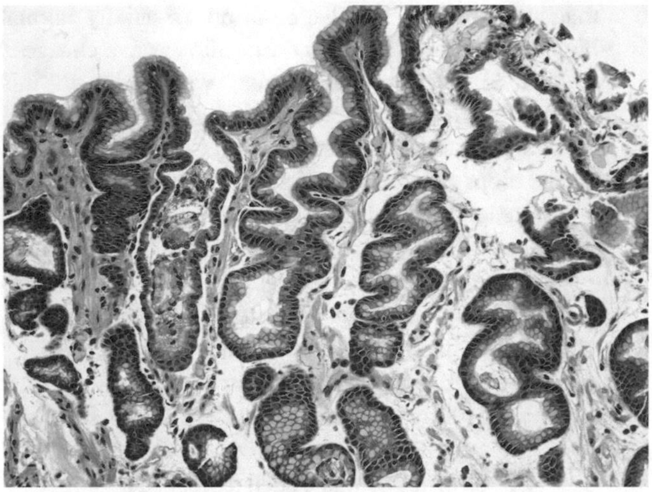

Fig. 4.20 Reactive gastropathy. There is hyperplasia of the upper half of the mucosa, with mucin reduction and a corkscrew appearance to the gastric pits

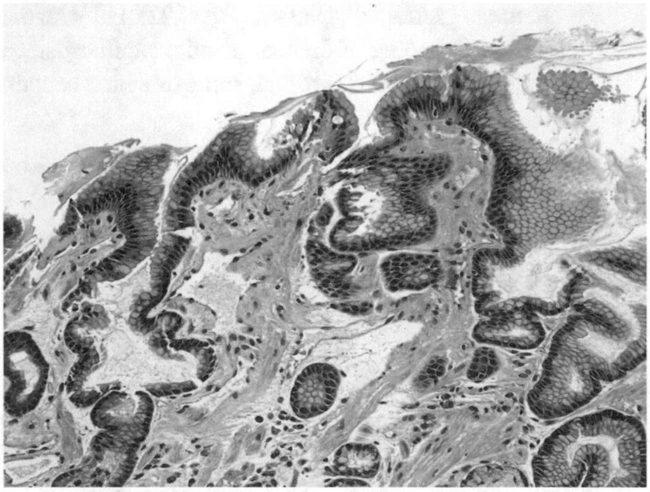

Fig. 4.21 Reactive gastropathy. Slips of smooth muscle in the lamina propria are prominent

19. How is reactive gastropathy distinguished from portal hypertensive gastropathy and from the gastric antral vascular ectasia (GAVE) syndrome?

As noted before, sometimes pathologists use the diagnosis of reactive gastropathy almost as a waste basket diagnosis, making the diagnosis on essentially normal biopsies that have minimal nonspecific reactive changes.

- I once asked a pathologist, who followed this approach, why he did so. His response was that patients who aren't sick don't get endoscopies, so if the biopsy showed no other pattern of injury, then his approach was to diagnose reactive gastropathy. Such an approach is discouraged because it is inaccurate and doesn't advance patient care. Instead, the diagnosis should be made when, and only when, the histological findings warrant the diagnosis.
  - Normal antral biopsies, or essentially normal antral biopsies that are without diagnostic findings, are not uncommon, and a pathologist should not be afraid to make such a diagnosis.
- Other injury patterns in the differential include primarily gastric antral vascular ectasia (GAVE) and portal hypertensive gastropathy. Histologically, the GAVE pattern of injury is fundamentally similar to a chemical gastropathy pattern (Fig. 4.22), but with the additional finding of dilated (ectatic) capillary-sized vessels in the lamina propria, some of which contain small thrombi (Fig. 4.23). Thrombi are needed in order to make the diagnosis. If they are absent, consider portal hypertensive gastropathy. A CD61 immunostain is helpful to identify the small vascular thrombi in GAVE.
  - Endoscopic findings show stripes of erythema that are present in the antrum and converge on the pylorus, resembling the stripes on a watermelon, thus the common endoscopic description of a watermelon stomach.
- The findings in portal hypertensive gastropathy are very similar to that of a chemical gastropathy (Fig. 4.24). There can be subtle differences in some cases, the most noticeable being an increased prominence in dilated capillaries in the lamina propria in portal hypertensive gastropathy. There also can be less mucin reduction than seen in chemical gastropa-

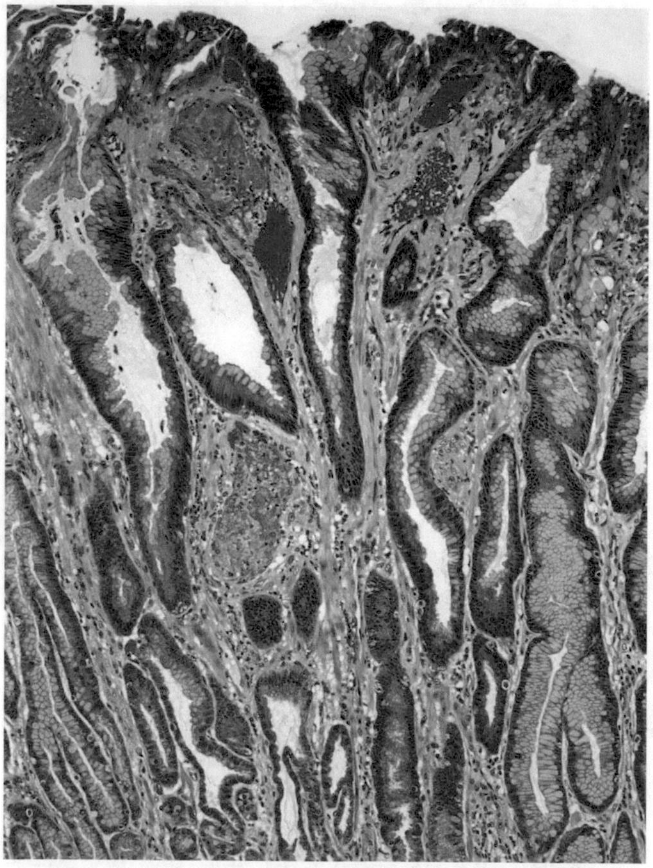

Fig. 4.22 GAVE. The mucosa shows a reactive gastropathy-type pattern, but with ectatic vessels in the superficial mucosa that contain fibrin thrombi

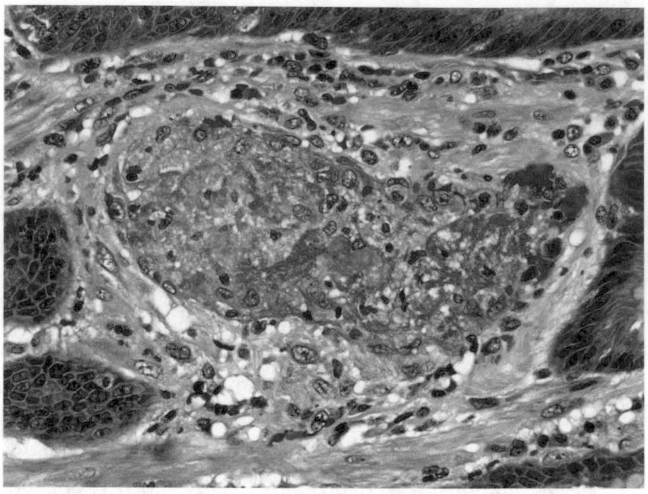

Fig. 4.23 GAVE. A fibrin thrombus is present in one of the dilated vessels in the lamina propria

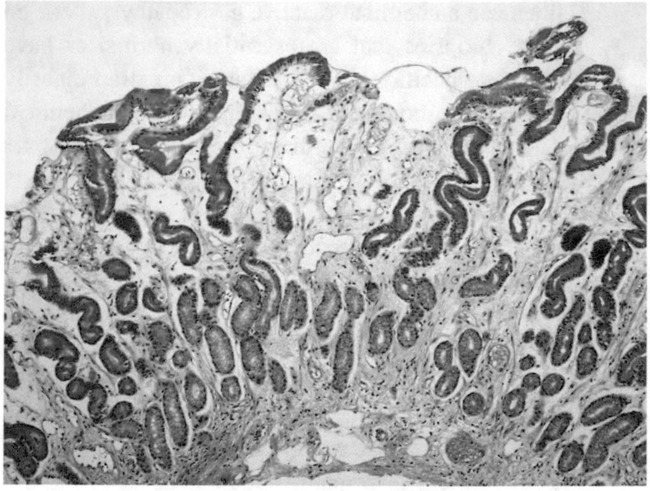

Fig. 4.24 Portal hypertensive gastropathy. The stomach shows a reactive gastropathy pattern with ectatic lamina propria vessels

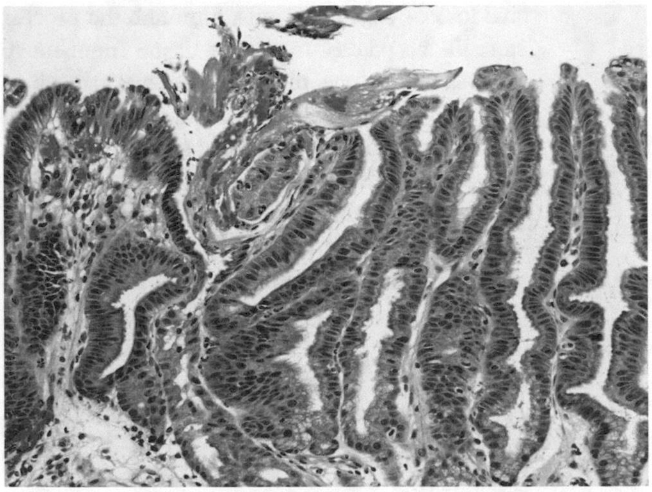

Fig. 4.25 Antrum, edge of an ulcer. The findings resemble reactive gastropathy, but biopsies of the background antral mucosa did not

thy. Nonetheless, there is sufficient overlap that a final diagnosis of portal hypertensive gastropathy requires correlation with clinical findings to ensure the patient has portal hypertension.

- The mucosa right at the edge of an ulcer can also show reactive gastropathy-type changes even when samples away from the ulcer do not (Fig. 4.25).
- Finally, biopsy specimens from the normal pylorus often have mild mucosal hyperplasia and mucin reduction, compared to the antrum, but this is not abnormal for the pylorus.

Reference: [23]

Autoimmune Gastritis

Autoimmune gastritis results from an autoimmune destruction of the oxyntic mucosa, leading to mucosal atrophy and metaplasia, enterochromaffin-like (ECL) cell hyperplasia, and sometimes neuroendocrine tumors. Pernicious anemia also develops if there is substantial loss of the oxyntic mucosa. Older and now discontinued terms for autoimmune gastritis include *type A gastritis* and *autoimmune metaplastic atrophic gastritis*.

Frequently Asked Questions

20. What types of patients develop autoimmune gastritis?

Most patients (70%) are women and the median age at first diagnosis is 55 years. Nonetheless, rare cases occur in children. The prevalence of autoimmune gastritis in surgical pathology specimens is about 2%, though this can vary with factors such as the ethnicity and age of patients.

References: [21, 24, 25]

21. How is the diagnosis of autoimmune gastritis made?

The diagnosis can be made by histological findings (see next question) and/or serological findings. In most cases, both are used to confirm the diagnosis. Individuals with autoimmune gastritis develop serum autoantibodies to parietal cells (~80%) or to intrinsic factor (40%). Overall, intrinsic factor antibodies are more specific (95%) than anti-parietal cell antibodies (70%). Anti-parietal antibodies are directed against the alpha- and beta-subunits of the proton pump H^+/K^+ ATPase located in parietal cells, perhaps because of molecular mimicry from prior but self-cleared *H. pylori* infections.

- Other serological findings can also be helpful, such as elevated serum gastrin and chromogranin A levels, both resulting from the destruction of the parietal cells and subsequent overexpression of gastrin by antral G cells.
- The diagnosis can be made based on histology in patients who are asymptomatic for gastric symptoms or who have mild nonspecific complaints such as dyspepsia. In these cases, the disease tends to be mild, without extensive loss of oxyntic glands.
- On the other hand, symptoms are more common in patients with more advanced disease that has led to extensive loss of body mucosa. These patients commonly have fatigue and anemia at presentation (35%). The anemia can be megaloblastic because of reduced absorption of vitamin B12, but this is somewhat less common today than years ago, because of the widespread use of vitamins and the addition of B12 to foods such as breakfast cereals. Chronic and severe B12 deficiency can sometimes lead to permanent neurological problems.

References: [24, 26, 27]

22. What histological findings suggest autoimmune gastritis?

Autoimmune gastritis is a chronic inflammatory disease that primarily affects the stomach body.

- The antrum can show a variety of mild changes (Fig. 4.26), from minimal nonspecific changes to a reactive gastropathy pattern and to mild nonspecific chronic inflammation. Biopsies are negative for *H. pylori*.
- Biopsies of the gastric body will show a range of changes depending on how far the disease has advanced.
  - Early in the disease, biopsies can show mild patchy lymphoplasmacytic inflammation (Fig. 4.27) with patchy lymphocytosis and damage of oxyntic glands. Neutrophilic inflammation is rare and focal if present.
  - As the disease progresses, there are more diffuse chronic inflammation (Fig. 4.28) and more exten-

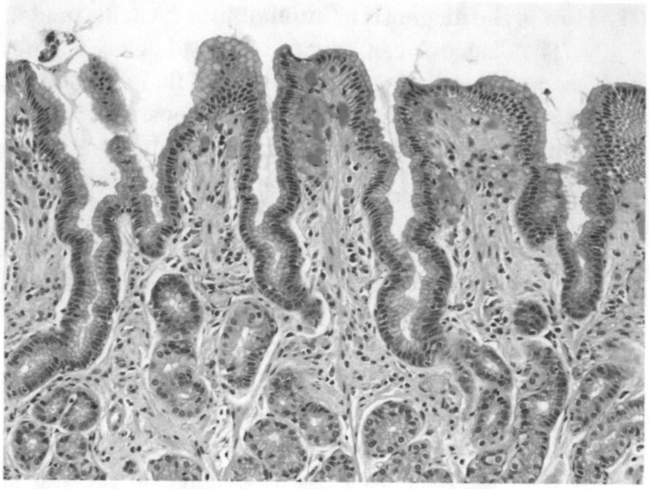

Fig. 4.26 Autoimmune gastritis, antrum. The antrum shows mild nonspecific inflammation and reactive changes

sive loss of oxyntic glands, although the process can still be patchy from one tissue fragment to another, and some biopsy fragments can show intact oxyntic glands. In time, the normal oxyntic glands are gradually destroyed and replaced with metaplastic epithelium.

- The metaplasia can be intestinal, pyloric, or pancreatic (Figs. 4.29 and 4.30). Pancreatic acinar metaplasia is more common in autoimmune gastritis (50% of cases) than in *H. pylori* gastritis, but is not specific for autoimmune gastritis. In most cases, multiple types of metaplasia can be seen.
- The mucosal atrophy and metaplasia is also accompanied by hyperplasia of the ECL cells (Fig. 4.31).

References: [28, 29]

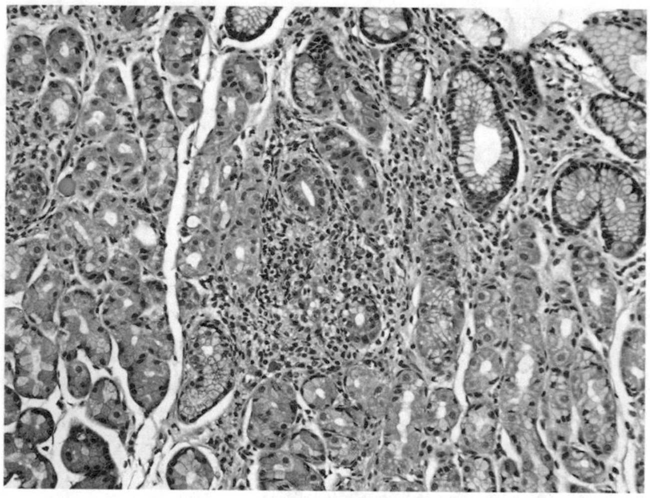

Fig. 4.27 Autoimmune gastritis, body inflammation. The body shows patchy inflammation including focal gland injury

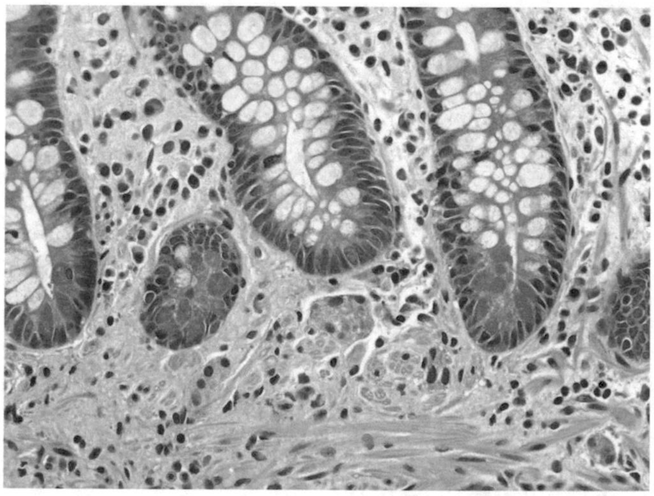

Fig. 4.29 Autoimmune gastritis, intestinal metaplasia. The body mucosa shows intestinal metaplasia

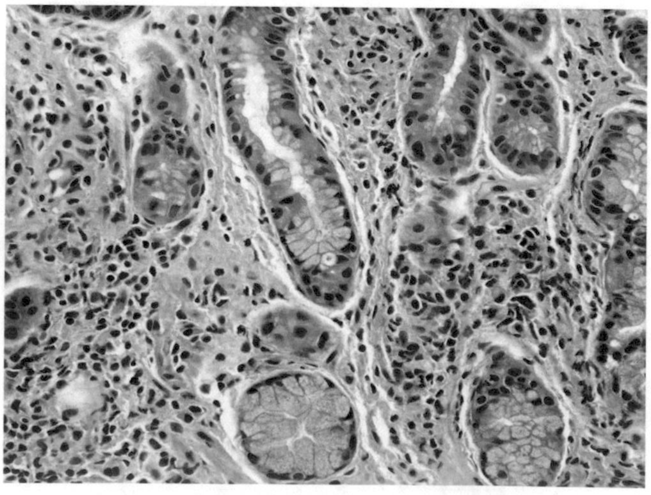

Fig. 4.28 Autoimmune gastritis, body inflammation. The body shows diffuse moderate chronic inflammation with more extensive loss of the oxyntic mucosa

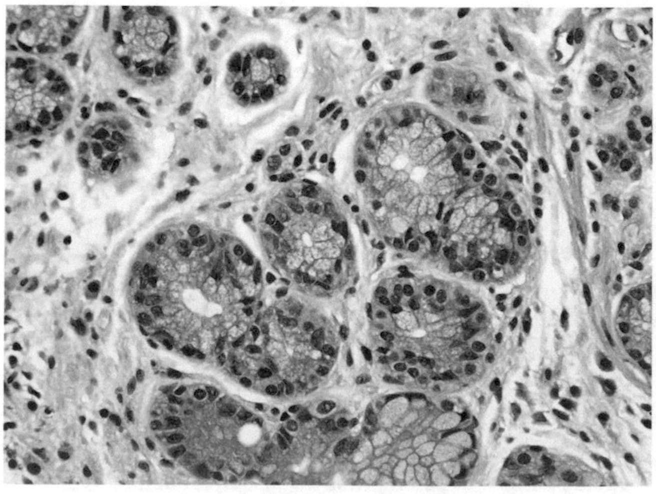

Fig. 4.30 Autoimmune gastritis, body pyloric metaplasia. The normal oxyntic glands of the body have been replaced by glands that resemble antral or pyloric glands

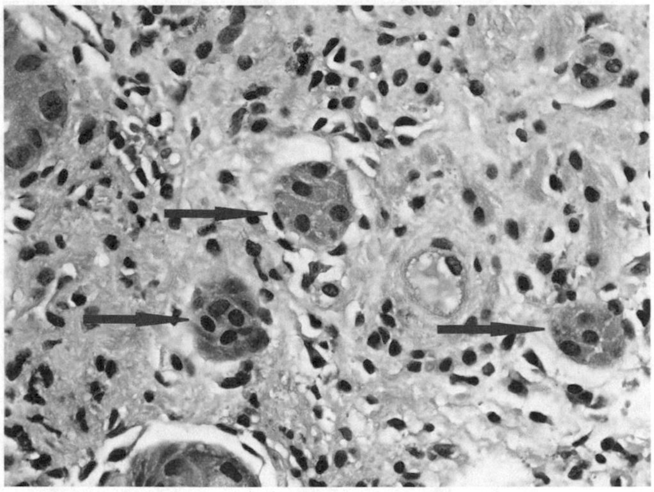

Fig. 4.31 Autoimmune gastritis, ECL cell hyperplasia. Small nodules of ECL cells are seen (arrows)

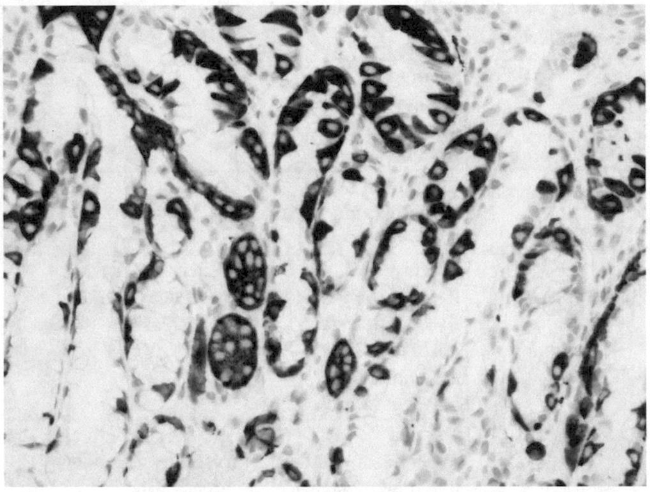

Fig. 4.32 Autoimmune gastritis, ECL cell hyperplasia, chromogranin immunostain. Both linear and nodular ECL cell hyperplasia is present

23. What is the best approach to diagnose autoimmune gastritis on histology?

The histological diagnosis is based on finding a chronic gastritis that is body predominant and is associated with clear ECL. Most cases will also have mucosal metaplasia.

- Currently, it is common for many endoscopists to put samples from the stomach antrum and body in the same container. This can make interpretation challenging because inflamed and metaplastic epithelium could be from the antrum, antral-fundic transition zone, or body. In this situation, stains for gastrin can be very helpful, as gastrin immunostains are positive only in the antrum and antral-fundic transition zone, and staining is retained even if they have metaplasia. Thus, a clearly negative gastrin immunostain indicates that the specimen is from the stomach body.
- Advanced ECL cell hyperplasia can be detected on H&E (Fig. 4.31), but early stages require immunostains for chromogranin or synaptophysin. ECL cell hyperplasia is defined as at least five adjacent cells that are positive for chromogranin or synaptophysin. The ECL cell hyperplasia can be linear in early disease (Fig. 4.32) but in time forms distinct nodules.
  - These ECL nodules can grow slowly, leading to neuroendocrine proliferations (Fig. 4.33) that are classified based on their size (Table 4.1). Most neuroendocrine tumors in the setting of autoimmune gastritis are well differentiated with a World Health Organization (WHO) grade of 1.

Reference: [30]

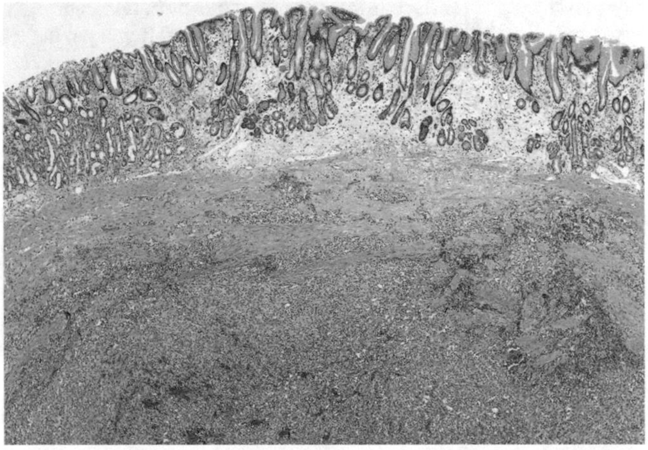

Fig. 4.33 Autoimmune gastritis, neuroendocrine tumor. A neuroendocrine tumor is seen involving the submucosa and the muscularis mucosae, WHO grade 1

24. Why do patients develop ECL hyperplasia and neuroendocrine tumors?

The inflammation in the stomach body over time destroys the parietal cells. Since the parietal cells produce stomach acid, their destruction leads to a hypochloridic gastric lumen. The elevated gastric pH in turn triggers the antral G cells to increase their production of gastrin, since gastrin increases acid production in the remaining but reduced numbers of parietal cells. However, the chronically increased gastrin levels also cause proliferation of ECL cells, which become hyperplastic and, with enough chronic stimulation, can eventually lead to neuroendocrine tumors.

25. What other lesions are patients with autoimmune gastritis at risk for?

- In addition to neuroendocrine tumors, stomachs with autoimmune gastritis can develop pyloric gland adenomas. Overall, pyloric gland adenomas are very rare, making up only 3% of all gastric polyps. However, these polyps are strongly enriched in autoimmune gastritis, with 36% of pyloric gland adenomas occurring in this setting.

Table 4.1 ECL cell proliferations in the stomach body in cases of autoimmune gastritis

Mucosal findings	Finding on chromogranin or synaptophysin immunostain	Notes
Normal	Scattered chromogranin-positive cells	
ECL cell hyperplasia	Linear hyperplasia = at least five immunostain-positive ECL cells that are immediately adjacent to each other	Linear hyperplasia precedes nodular hyperplasia
	Nodular hyperplasia = at least five immunostain-positive ECL cells forming a small nodule	Nodular hyperplasia typically also shows areas of linear hyperplasia. Nodular hyperplasia can often be seen on H&E
Neuroendocrine dysplasia	Nodules composed of ECL cells that are between 150 and 500 microns (0.15–0.5 mm)	This term is used mostly in research studies. If you put it into a pathology report, it is likely to confuse the clinical team
Microcarcinoid	Neuroendocrine nodules that are >0.5 mm but less than 0.5 cm	Involvement of the submucosa also qualifies for microcarcinoid even if the lesion is equal to or less than 0.5 mm
Neuroendocrine tumor	Neuroendocrine nodules that are ≥0.5 cm	Neuroendocrine tumors are graded using standard WHO approach, with Ki-67. Most are WHO grade 1

- Tubular adenomas are less common but have also been reported.
- In addition to true neoplasms, stomachs with autoimmune gastritis can also develop pseudopolyps, including hyperplastic polyps of the antrum and/or body. In addition, relatively preserved islands of mucosa can appear as endoscopic polyps when they are located adjacent to areas with severe mucosal atrophy.

References: [31–33]

Lymphocytic Gastritis

Lymphocytic gastritis is defined by surface epithelial lymphocytosis (Fig. 4.34), often with at least mild epithelial injury. A commonly used formal definition is greater than 25 lymphocytes per 100 surface epithelial cells. The lamina propria often shows chronic inflammation, sometimes with patchy activity. Erosions and ulcers can also develop. In rare cases, the erosions can be located endoscopically on small mucosal nodules, in a background of thickened mucosal folds. This endoscopic pattern is called *varioliform gastritis*, but is not specific for lymphocytic gastritis.

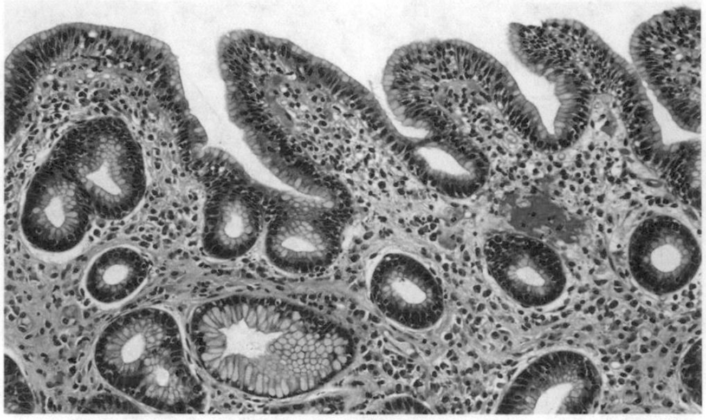

Fig. 4.34 Lymphocytic gastritis. The antral epithelium shows increased intraepithelial lymphocytes. This case was associated with celiac disease

- In some cases, endoscopy shows enlarged mucosal folds, and the endoscopy and histological findings can overlap with Menetrier disease.

Reference: [34]

Frequently Asked Questions

26. **What causes lymphocytic gastritis?**

    The most common etiological associations are with celiac disease (about 40% of patients), *H. pylori* gastritis (about 30%), and idiopathic (about 20% of cases).
    - The remaining 10% of cases are associated with various chronic infections such as HIV or syphilis, various autoimmune conditions such as Crohn disease or common variable immunodeficiency (CVID), or medication usage, including NSAIDs.
    - In cases of celiac disease, the lymphocytic gastritis tends to be more antral predominant. In addition, one study of celiac patients found that the frequency of lymphocytic gastritis increased with the severity of mucosal injury in the duodenum.

    References: [35, 36]

27. **What is the clinical significance of lymphocytic gastritis?**

    Clinically, about 20% of patients present with low albumin levels and/or peripheral edema that results from protein loss. The disease is chronic and is treated by proton pump inhibitors and by addressing any underlying conditions.

    Reference: [37]

Collagenous Gastritis

Collagenous gastritis is defined by thickening of the subepithelial collagen table (Fig. 4.35). For clinical cases, a global assessment is sufficient, and there is no need to measure the

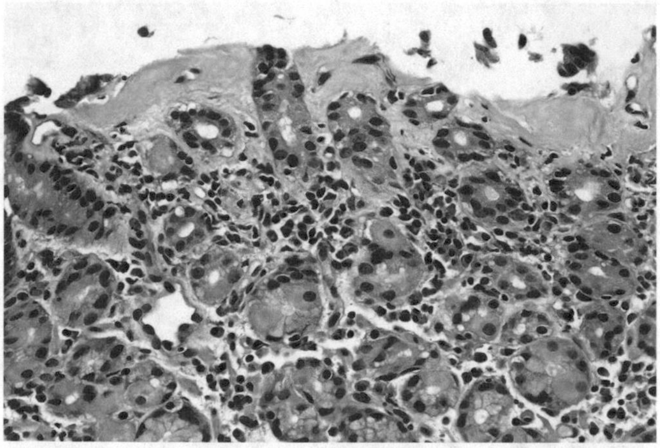

Fig. 4.35 Collagenous gastritis. The subepithelial collagen table is noticeably thickened. Much of the surface epithelium is denuded

thickness of the subepithelial collagen table, but as a point of reference, the normal thickness is up to 10 microns, while collagenous gastritis shows an average thickness of about 40 microns, range 15–120 microns. Of note, there can be considerable variability in the thickness within any given case. The lamina propria shows mild to moderate chronic inflammation, sometimes with patchy activity. Adult cases tend to have more chronic inflammation in the lamina propria than pediatric cases. Mucosal eosinophils can be prominent, especially in pediatric cases.
References: [38, 39]

Frequently Asked Questions

28. What causes collagenous gastritis?

The cause is not known, but there appear to be two largely separate forms, one that occurs in the pediatric population and one that occurs in adults.

- Pediatric patients tend to present with abdominal pain and anemia in their teenage years. Endoscopically, the mucosa often looks nodular, with the nodules representing relatively preserved areas of the mucosa. To date, there have been no strong or consistent links to other disease processes; however, some cases resemble adult pattern disease with associated celiac sprue, collagenous sprue, or collagenous colitis. Pediatric cases can also show prominent eosinophils in the mucosa, with up to 60% of cases showing more than 30 per high-power field (hpf).
- Adults present with chronic watery diarrhea and in most cases have a generalized collagenous disease of the gastrointestinal tract, with collagenous colitis and sometimes collagenous sprue. Endoscopically, the gastric mucosa is more diffusely involved in adults than in children, often lacking the distinctive nodularity that is common in pediatric cases. Adult patients also have a high frequency of concomitant autoimmune disease such as celiac disease and Hashimoto thyroiditis.

References: [38–40]

29. How is collagenous gastritis treated?

To date there is no well-established treatment and therapy instead is focused on symptomatic relief. Proton pump inhibitors and steroids are commonly used. Treatment also focuses on addressing any underlying conditions, such as celiac disease.
Reference: [40]

Granulomatous Gastritis

Granulomatous gastritis is defined by finding numerous granulomas in the mucosa and sometimes the submucosa (Fig. 4.36). Granulomas tend to be more prominent in the antrum than in the body. The granulomas should be a dominate part of the histology and there typically is an associated gastritis, which can be chronic gastritis or active chronic gastritis. Finding a single or rare granuloma by itself does not qualify for the term granulomatous gastritis.
References: [41, 42]

Frequently Asked Questions

30. What causes granulomatous gastritis?

The majority of cases fall into the categories of Crohn disease, sarcoidosis, infectious gastritis, tumor related, or drug reaction, with the first two causes by far the most common. Rare cases are idiopathic. One study found pediatric cases were enriched for patients with Crohn disease, while adults patients were enriched for sarcoid-

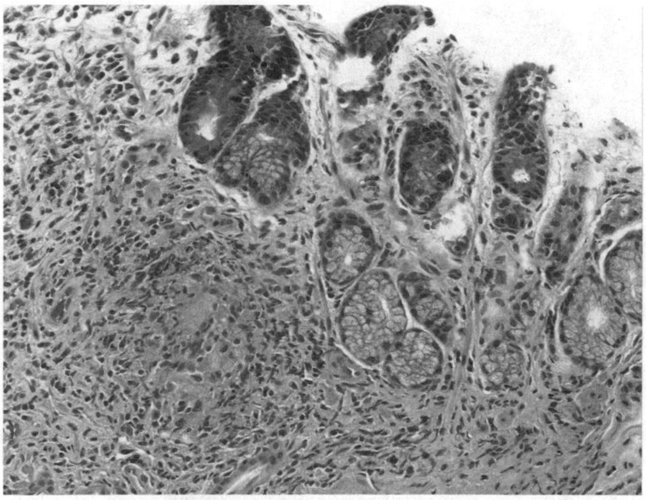

Fig. 4.36 Granulomatous gastritis. This case of granulomatous gastritis resulted from Crohn disease

osis. Studies from the West have consistently found *H. pylori* infection to be a rare association, but a study from South Korea found *H. pylori* in 14 of 18 cases of granulomatous gastritis.
References: [41–45]

Eosinophilic Gastritis

Eosinophilic gastritis is defined by finding a fairly diffuse and prominent enrichment for eosinophils in the lamina propria.

Frequently Asked Questions

31. How is a diagnosis of eosinophilic gastritis made?

Eosinophilic gastritis shows increased eosinophils in the lamina propria (Figs. 4.37 and 4.38). The most commonly accepted formal definition is that eosinophils should be ≥30 per hpf on average. However, some studies use a higher definition to increase specificity. Because of their overall increased density, eosinophils can also be found in the epithelium, forming crypt abbesses, and in the muscularis mucosae. Of note, however, it is the overall increased density that is important for diagnosis, and finding occasional eosinophils in the muscularis mucosae or in the epithelium is not part of the definition of eosinophilic gastritis, being neither sensitive nor specific. Lymphoplasmacytic inflammation is also present and there can be focal active inflammation.

- Increased eosinophils eosinophilic gastritis can also be seen in cases of collagenous gastritis, in which case the primary classification is that of collagenous gastritis.

Reference: [46]

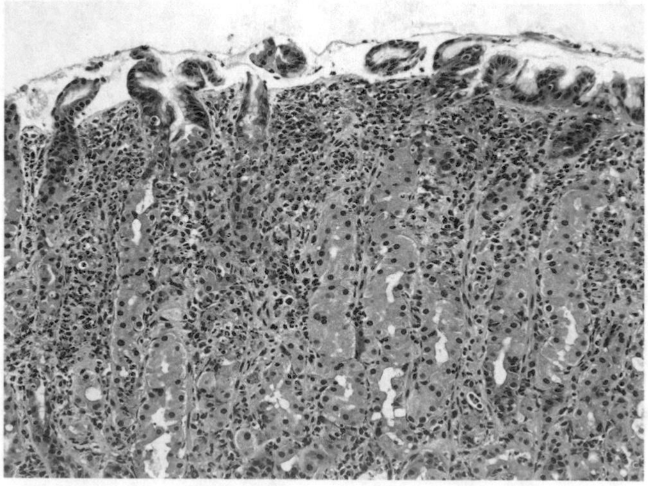

Fig. 4.37 Eosinophilic gastritis, antrum. The antrum and body show diffuse lamina propria eosinophilia

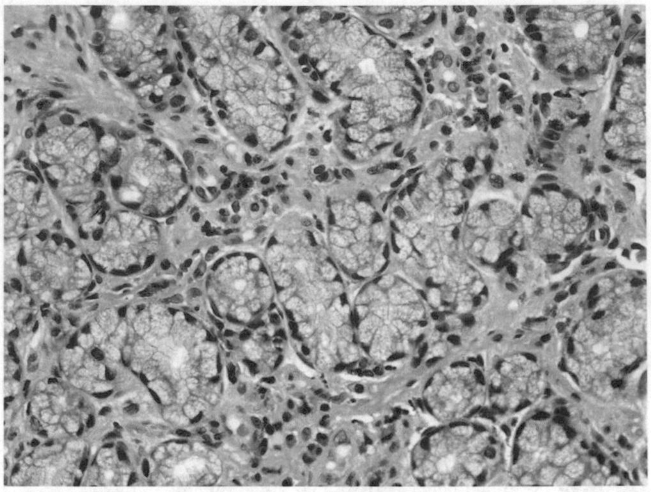

Fig. 4.38 Eosinophilic gastritis. Greater than 30 eosinophils were seen in nearly all high-power fields (40×)

32. What causes eosinophilic gastritis?

Most cases in children are associated with tissue eosinophilia in other parts of the gastrointestinal tract, especially the esophagus, increased blood eosinophil counts, and appear to be related to food allergies, as many children respond to dietary restrictions. In adults, cases are more likely to be idiopathic. Drug reaction and parasitic infestations, such as gastric anisakiasis and strongyloidiasis, can also be associated with gastric eosinophilia.
References: [47, 48]

Russel Body Gastritis

Frequently Asked Question

33. How is the diagnosis of Russell body gastritis made and what is the significance?

Russell body gastritis is a rare form of chronic gastritis that is strongly enriched for Russel bodies in the lamina propria. The lamina propria also usually shows moderate to marked lymphoplasmacytic inflammation, often with patchy activity. In most cases, the Russell bodies are either polytypic or are kappa light chain restricted. About one half of cases are associated with *H. pylori* gastritis. To date, there is no evidence for a risk for progression to lymphoma.
References: [49–51]

Case Presentation

Case 1

Learning Objectives

- Identify the characteristic morphology of *Sarcina ventriculi*

- Identify the clinical relevance of a diagnosis of *Sarcina ventriculi*

Case History

A 42-year-old woman with abdominal pain undergoes upper endoscopy after proton pump inhibitors do not relieve the pain. She has no other known gastrointestinal or systemic disease.

Histological Findings

Biopsies of the antrum and body show mild chronic lymphoplasmacytic inflammation. There is no active inflammation. No *H. pylori* are seen on H&E. However, there are bacterial organisms in the lumen (Fig. 4.39).

Differential Diagnosis

The organisms are clearly bacterial and not fungal, so the differential includes different types of bacteria. Since the organisms are in the lumen and there is no tissue response, the differential would include nonspecific oral contamination from the endoscopic procedure. However, the distinctive tetrads are not typical of oral contamination, and their density is also heavier than seen with oral contamination, which is usually limited to rare organisms.

Immunohistochemistry and Other Ancillary Studies

The bacteria do not have the morphology of *H. pylori*, instead showing coccal forms. However, since partially treated *H. pylori* can develop a cocci morphology, the refereeing pathologist performed a *H. pylori* immunostain, which was negative.

Final Diagnosis

The distinctive tetrad morphology is diagnostic of *Sarcina ventriculi*. This Gram-positive bacterium is not invasive but is associated with delayed gastric emptying, from either physiological or surgical causes. Despite the lack of invasion, *Sarcina ventriculi* can be found in the inflammatory exudate overlying mucosal ulcers or erosions.

Take-Home Messages

- Rarely, other bacterial organisms can be seen in the gastric lumen.
- *Sarcina ventriculi* is not invasive but should be reported in the final pathology report, as patients may require further work-up to identify causes of delayed gastric emptying.

References: [52–54]

Case 2

Learning Objectives

- Identify the characteristic morphology of autoimmune atrophic pangastritis
- Identify the clinical associations with the histological pattern of autoimmune atrophic pangastritis

Case History

A 37-year-old woman with a long history of systemic lupus erythematosus develops chronic abdominal pain and undergoes upper endoscopy.

Histological Findings

Biopsies of both the antrum and body show moderate to marked chronic inflammation with extensive metaplasia (Figs. 4.40 and 4.41). There is patchy mild active inflammation but no *H. pylori* are seen on immunostain.

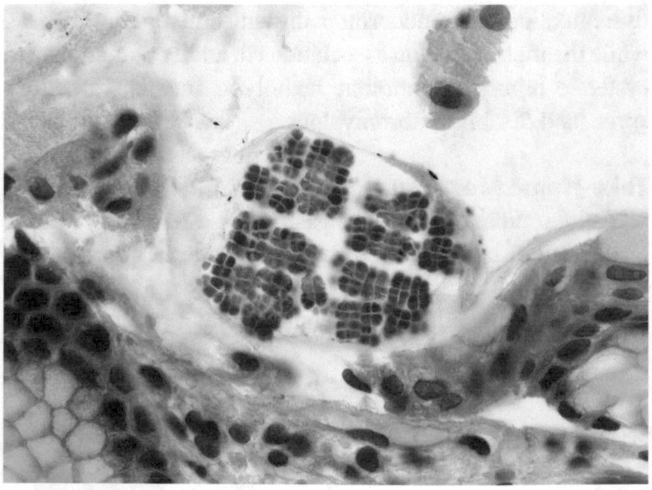

Fig. 4.39 *Sarcina ventriculi*. The organisms are in the gastric lumen and are found in distinctive tetrads

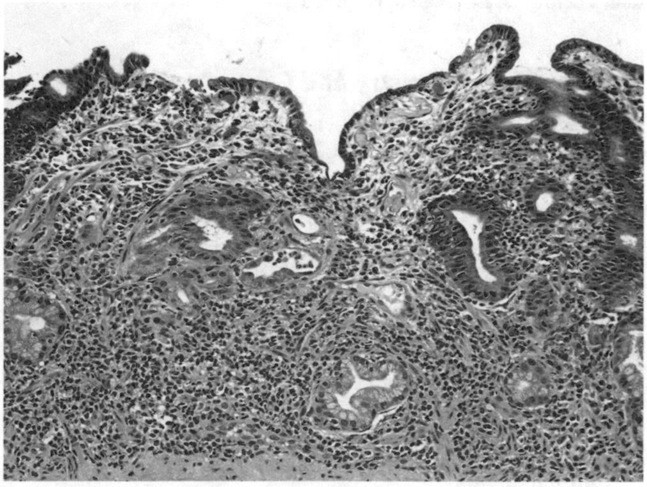

Fig. 4.40 Autoimmune atrophic pangastritis, antrum. The antrum shows marked chronic gastritis with loss of normal mucosal glands

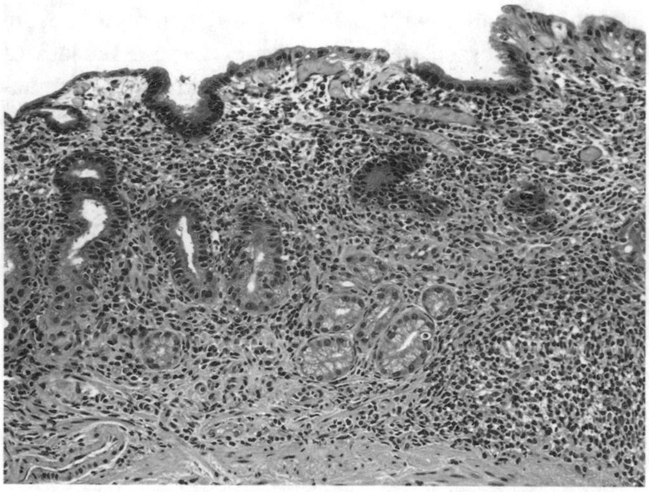

Fig. 4.41 Autoimmune atrophic pangastritis, body. The body also shows marked chronic gastritis with loss of normal mucosal glands

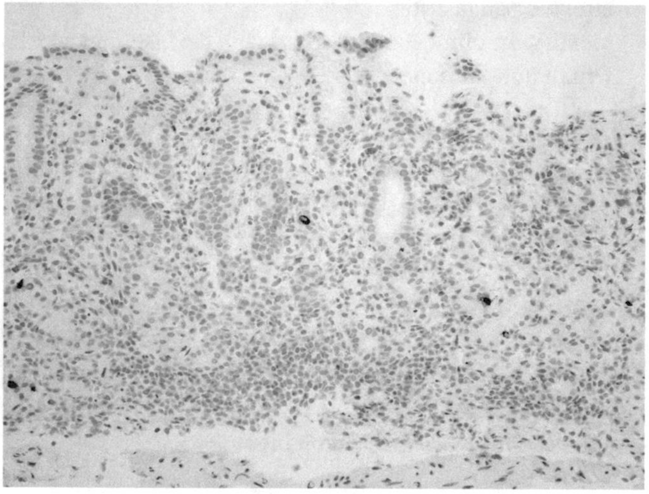

Fig. 4.42 Autoimmune atrophic pangastritis, chromogranin immunostain. There is no ECL cell hyperplasia

Immunohistochemistry and Other Ancillary Studies

A chromogranin shows no ECL cell hyperplasia (Fig. 4.42). A gastrin stain on mucosal biopsies labeled as coming from the antrum shows only rare gastrin-positive cells, clearly diminished from the normal antrum as well as antral specimens in the setting of most chronic disease conditions. A phone call to the endoscopist confirms the antral biopsy was from the antrum.

Differential Diagnosis

- *H. pylori* gastritis. This possibility was excluded by immunostains.
- Autoimmune gastritis. The pattern of both antral and body diseases and the lack of ECL cell hyperplasia exclude typical autoimmune gastritis.

Table 4.2 Classification of common forms of gastritis

Disease	Topographic pattern	Gastrin stains in the antrum	ECL cell hyperplasia in the body
H. pylori gastritis	Antrum≥body	Positive	Absent
Autoimmune gastritis	Body	Positive	Linear or nodular
Autoimmune atrophic pangastritis	Antrum and body	Absent or rare positive cells	Absent

Final Diagnosis

This pattern of injury is diagnosed as autoimmune atrophic pangastritis (Table 4.2). This rare pattern of gastritis is distinct from the usual pattern of autoimmune gastritis because there are chronic inflammation, atrophy, and metaplasia of both the antrum and the body.

In cases of autoimmune atrophic pangastritis, the inflammation is equally dense in both the body and the antrum. The inflammation is predominately lymphoplasmacytic but there can be patchy areas of neutrophilic inflammation. While earlier patterns must exist, by the time of clinical presentation, most cases of autoimmune pangastritis show fairly extensive atrophy and metaplasia of both the antrum and body. The antral G cells are destroyed as part of the antral mucosal destruction, so patients do not have elevated serum gastrin levels and the stomach body does not develop ECL cell hyperplasia.

Clinically, autoimmune atrophic pangastritis affects both pediatric and adult populations. While data is limited because of the rarity of this condition, the current data suggests autoimmune pangastritis generally does not occur as an isolated finding and almost all patients will have concurrent autoimmune conditions that involve other organs. However, the types of concurrent diseases differ, as the most common association in the pediatric population is with autoimmune enterocolitis, including the X-linked syndrome of immune dysregulation, polyendocrinopathy, and enteropathy (IPEX), while the most common associations in adult populations are systemic lupus, autoimmune hemolytic anemia, refractory sprue, and disabling fibromyalgia.

Take-Home Messages

- Autoimmune atrophic pangastritis is a rare autoimmune condition characterized by involvement of both the antrum and body.
- Most patients will have other autoimmune conditions.

Reference: [55]

Case 3

Learning Objectives

- Recognize that some cases of chronic gastritis are idiopathic

- Understand the major diseases that should be excluded
- Unexplained cases of chronic gastritis remain a gap in our knowledge of chronic inflammatory conditions of the stomach

Case History

A 52-year-old man with dyspepsia undergoes upper endoscopy after proton pump inhibitor and Pepto-Bismol therapy do not relieve the pain. He has no other known gastrointestinal or systemic disease.

Histological Findings

Biopsies of the antrum show mild nonspecific changes, while biopsies of the body show a mild chronic gastritis with no activity (Fig. 4.43). There are no gland destruction, no mucosal atrophy, and no metaplasia. No *H. pylori* are seen on H&E.

Differential Diagnosis

- *H. pylori* gastritis
- Early changes of autoimmune gastritis
- Food allergies
- Systemic disease involving the stomach.

IHC and Other Ancillary Studies

An immunostain for *H. pylori* is negative. A chromogranin stain shows no ECL cell hyperplasia. A review of the patient's medical record shows no current medications (besides a proton pump inhibitor and Pepto-Bismol). He has no other known systemic disease.

Final Diagnosis

The final diagnosis was chronic inactive gastritis, with no evidence for *H. pylori* infection or autoimmune gastritis. There are no widely utilized and no well-validated criteria to define a chronic gastritis based on histology alone. Suggested criteria have been put forth, including finding more than five lymphocytes, plasma cells, or macrophages per hpf (40× objective) or finding more than three lymphocytes or plasma cells in the superficial lamina propria. However, these criteria are not validated and are probably too low for routine clinical care. Nonetheless, the pattern of idiopathic chronic gastritis is not rare. For example, one large study found a pattern of *H. pylori*-negative chronic gastritis in 10% of antral biopsies. Another study found 20% of VA patients had idiopathic chronic gastritis, including a subset with active chronic gastritis.

Systemic diseases should be excluded including Crohn disease (Fig. 4.44) and sarcoidosis, even if no granulomas are identified. Food allergies are an important consideration in children. There is no significant body of literature linking cases of chronic gastritis to medication effects, but it seems at least theoretically possible.

Take-Home Messages

- Other rare causes of chronic gastritis include systemic diseases and possibly medications.
- A proportion of cases remains unexplained for etiology, yet shows a definite histological chronic gastritis. The natural history of this pattern of injury remains unclear.

References: [12, 56, 57]

Case 4

Learning Objectives

- Identify the characteristic morphology of Menetrier disease
- Identify the clinical relevance of a diagnosis of Menetrier disease

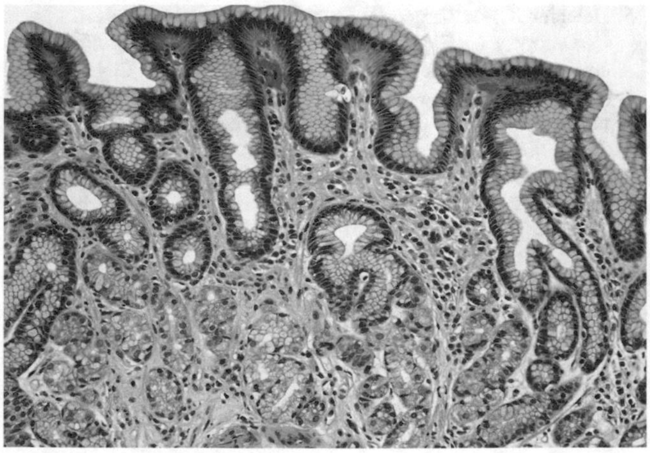

Fig. 4.43 Chronic gastritis, idiopathic. The biopsy shows a chronic gastritis of the antrum and body, but no cause was identified histologically or clinically

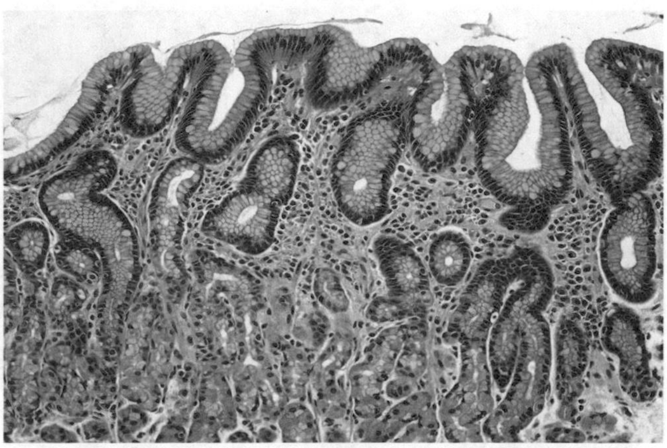

Fig. 4.44 Chronic gastritis, Crohn disease. The biopsy shows a nonspecific chronic gastritis with no active inflammation and no granulomas

Case History

A 38-year-old woman presented with epigastric pain, weight loss, and diarrhea. Endoscopy showed giant rugal folds in the stomach body, with mild nonspecific changes in the antrum.

Histological Findings

Biopsies of the antrum showed mild nonspecific changes. However, biopsies of the body showed atrophy of the oxyntic mucosa with striking foveolar hyperplasia (Figs. 4.45 and 4.46). There were no significant inflammation and no metaplasia. No *H. pylori* were seen on H&E.

Final Diagnosis

These findings are consistent with Menetrier disease. In addition to epigastric pain and weight loss, many patients also present with, or later develop, peripheral edema from protein loss. The cause of Menetrier disease is unknown, but a central path may be overexpression of transforming growth factor alpha. In some cases, there appears to be a genetic cause, while rare pediatric cases have been linked to cytomegalovirus (CMV) infection. Rare adult cases have been associated with *H. pylori* infection.

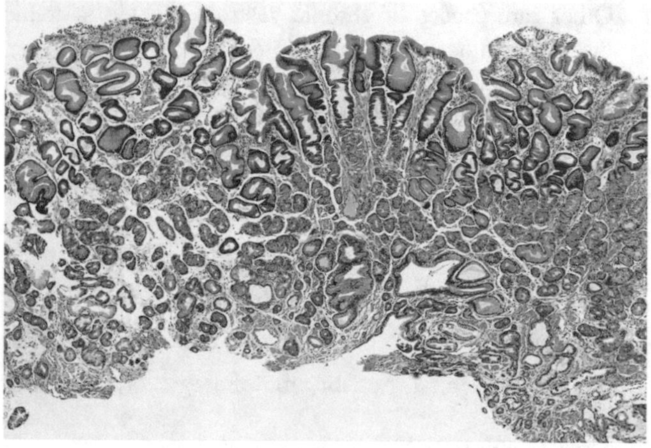

Fig. 4.45 Menetrier disease. At low power, the mucosa shows marked foveolar hyperplasia

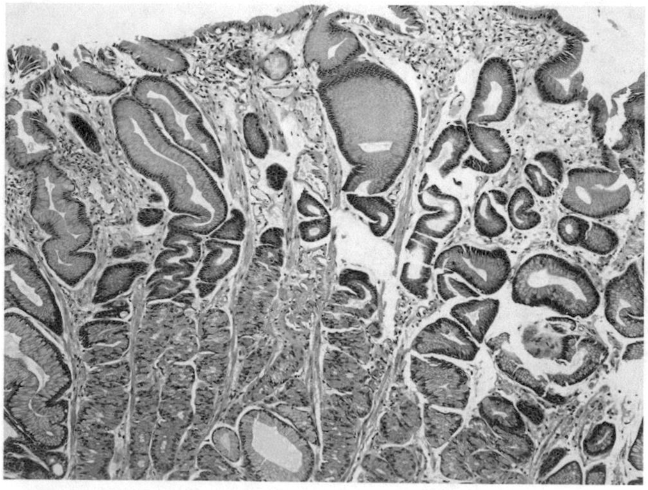

Fig. 4.46 Menetrier disease. At high power, atrophy of the oxyntic glands can also be appreciated

Differential Diagnosis

Atrophy of the body mucosa also occurs in autoimmune gastritis, but Menetrier disease lacks the inflammation and metaplasia. Lymphocytic gastritis can also be associated with some degree of foveolar hyperplasia but generally lacks the massive hyperplasia and edema seen in Menetrier disease.

Take-Home Messages

- Menetrier disease is characterized by giant rugal folds in the stomach body and cardia on endoscopy.
- Histology shows massive foveolar hyperplasia and oxyntic gland atrophy. Edema can also be prominent.
- Most cases are idiopathic, but CMV and *H. pylori* should be excluded.

References: [58–61]

References

1. Yu QQ, Tariq A, Unger SW, Cabello-Inchausti B, Robinson MJ. Phlegmonous gastritis associated with Kaposi sarcoma: a case report and review of the literature. Arch Pathol Lab Med. 2004;128:801–3.
2. Huang JQ, Sridhar S, Hunt RH. Role of Helicobacter pylori infection and non-steroidal anti-inflammatory drugs in peptic-ulcer disease: a meta-analysis. Lancet. 2002;359:14–22.
3. Charpignon C, Lesgourgues B, Pariente A, Nahon S, Pelaquier A, Gatineau-Sailliant G, Roucayrol AM, Courillon-Mallet A. Group de l'Observatoire National des Ulceres de l'Association Nationale des HepatoGastroenterologues des Hopitaux G. Peptic ulcer disease: one in five is related to neither Helicobacter pylori nor aspirin/NSAID intake. Aliment Pharmacol Ther. 2013;38:946–54.
4. Lanas A, Chan FKL. Peptic ulcer disease. Lancet. 2017;390:613–24.
5. Delchier JC, Lamarque D, Levy M, Tkoub EM, Copie-Bergman C, Deforges L, Chaumette MT, Haioun C. Helicobacter pylori and gastric lymphoma: high seroprevalence of CagA in diffuse large B-cell lymphoma but not in low-grade lymphoma of mucosa-associated lymphoid tissue type. Am J Gastroenterol. 2001;96:2324–8.
6. Eck M, Schmausser B, Haas R, Greiner A, Czub S, Muller-Hermelink HK. MALT-type lymphoma of the stomach is associated with Helicobacter pylori strains expressing the CagA protein. Gastroenterology. 1997;112:1482–6.
7. Mamishi S, Eshaghi H, Mahmoudi S, Bahador A, Hosseinpour Sadeghi R, Najafi M, Farahmand F, Khodadad A, Pourakbari B. Intrafamilial transmission of Helicobacter pylori: genotyping of faecal samples. Br J Biomed Sci. 2016;73:38–43.
8. Konno M, Yokota S, Suga T, Takahashi M, Sato K, Fujii N. Predominance of mother-to-child transmission of Helicobacter pylori infection detected by random amplified polymorphic DNA fingerprinting analysis in Japanese families. Pediatr Infect Dis J. 2008;27:999–1003.
9. Demerdash DME, Ibrahim H, Hassan DM, Moustafa H, Tawfik NM. Helicobacter pylori associated to unexplained or refractory

iron deficiency anemia: an Egyptian single-center experience. Hematol Transfus Cell Ther. 2018;40:219–25.
10. Batts KP, Ketover S, Kakar S, Krasinskas AM, Mitchell KA, Wilcox R, Westerhoff M, Rank J, Gibson J, Mattia AR, Cummings OW, Davison JM, Naini BV, Dry SM, Yantiss RK, Rodger CHGPS. Appropriate use of special stains for identifying Helicobacter pylori: recommendations from the Rodger C. Haggitt Gastrointestinal Pathology Society. Am J Surg Pathol. 2013;37:e12–22.
11. Genta RM, Lash RH. Helicobacter pylori-negative gastritis: seek, yet ye shall not always find. Am J Surg Pathol. 2010;34:e25–34.
12. Glickman JN, Noffsinger A, Nevin DT, Ray M, Lash RH, Genta RM. Helicobacter infections with rare bacteria or minimal gastritis: expecting the unexpected. Dig Liver Dis. 2015;47:549–55.
13. Wang YK, Kuo FC, Liu CJ, Wu MC, Shih HY, Wang SS, Wu JY, Kuo CH, Huang YK, Wu DC. Diagnosis of Helicobacter pylori infection: current options and developments. World J Gastroenterol. 2015;21:11221–35.
14. Dixon MF, Genta RM, Yardley JH, Correa P. Classification and grading of gastritis. The updated Sydney System. International Workshop on the Histopathology of Gastritis, Houston 1994. Am J Surg Pathol. 1996;20:1161–81.
15. Pittayanon R, Rerknimitr R, Klaikaew N, Sanpavat A, Chaithongrat S, Mahachai V, Kullavanijaya P, Barkun A. The risk of gastric cancer in patients with gastric intestinal metaplasia in 5-year follow-up. Aliment Pharmacol Ther. 2017;46:40–5.
16. Gonzalez CA, Sanz-Anquela JM, Companioni O, Bonet C, Berdasco M, Lopez C, Mendoza J, Martin-Arranz MD, Rey E, Poves E, Espinosa L, Barrio J, Torres MA, Cuatrecasas M, Elizalde I, Bujanda L, Garmendia M, Ferrandez A, Munoz G, Andreu V, Paules MJ, Lario S, Ramirez MJ. Study g, Gisbert JP. Incomplete type of intestinal metaplasia has the highest risk to progress to gastric cancer: results of the Spanish follow-up multicenter study. J Gastroenterol Hepatol. 2016;31:953–8.
17. Bento-Miranda M, Figueiredo C. Helicobacter heilmanni sensu lato: an overview of the infection in humans. World J Gastroenterol. 2014;20:17779–87.
18. Okiyama Y, Matsuzawa K, Hidaka E, Sano K, Akamatsu T, Ota H. Helicobacter heilmanni infection: clinical, endoscopic and histopathological features in Japanese patients. Pathol Int. 2005;55:398–404.
19. Ierardi E, Monno RA, Gentile A, Francavilla R, Burattini O, Marangi S, Pollice L, Francavilla A. Helicobacter heilmanni gastritis: a histological and immunohistochemical trait. J Clin Pathol. 2001;54:774–7.
20. Joo M, Kwak JE, Chang SH, Kim H, Chi JG, Kim KA, Yang JH, Lee JS, Moon YS, Kim KM. Helicobacter heilmanni-associated gastritis: clinicopathologic findings and comparison with Helicobacter pylori-associated gastritis. J Korean Med Sci. 2007;22:63–9.
21. Wolf EM, Plieschnegger W, Geppert M, Wigginghaus B, Hoss GM, Eherer A, Schneider NI, Hauer A, Rehak P, Vieth M, Langner C. Changing prevalence patterns in endoscopic and histological diagnosis of gastritis? Data from a cross-sectional Central European multicentre study. Dig Liver Dis. 2014;46:412–8.
22. Maguilnik I, Neumann WL, Sonnenberg A, Genta RM. Reactive gastropathy is associated with inflammatory conditions throughout the gastrointestinal tract. Aliment Pharmacol Ther. 2012;36:736–43.
23. Westerhoff M, Tretiakova M, Hovan L, Miller J, Noffsinger A, Hart J. CD61, CD31, and CD34 improve diagnostic accuracy in gastric antral vascular ectasia and portal hypertensive gastropathy: an immunohistochemical and digital morphometric study. Am J Surg Pathol. 2010;34:494–501.
24. Carabotti M, Lahner E, Esposito G, Sacchi MC, Severi C, Annibale B. Upper gastrointestinal symptoms in autoimmune gastritis: a cross-sectional study. Medicine (Baltimore). 2017;96:e5784.
25. Pogoriler J, Kamin D, Goldsmith JD. Pediatric non-Helicobacter pylori atrophic gastritis: a case series. Am J Surg Pathol. 2015;39:786–92.
26. Toh BH, Chan J, Kyaw T, Alderuccio F. Cutting edge issues in autoimmune gastritis. Clin Rev Allergy Immunol. 2012;42:269–78.
27. Miceli E, Padula D, Lenti MV, Gallia A, Albertini R, Di Stefano M, Klersy C, Corazza GR. A laboratory score in the diagnosis of autoimmune atrophic gastritis: a prospective study. J Clin Gastroenterol. 2015;49:e1–5.
28. Torbenson M, Abraham SC, Boitnott J, Yardley JH, Wu TT. Autoimmune gastritis: distinct histological and immunohistochemical findings before complete loss of oxyntic glands. Mod Pathol. 2002;15:102–9.
29. Jhala NC, Montemor M, Jhala D, Lu L, Talley L, Haber MM, Lechago J. Pancreatic acinar cell metaplasia in autoimmune gastritis. Arch Pathol Lab Med. 2003;127:854–7.
30. Lee HE, Mounajjed T, Erickson LA, Wu TT. Sporadic gastric well-differentiated neuroendocrine tumors have a higher Ki-67 proliferative index. Endocr Pathol. 2016;27:259–67.
31. Vieth M, Kushima R, Borchard F, Stolte M. Pyloric gland adenoma: a clinico-pathological analysis of 90 cases. Virchows Arch. 2003;442:317–21.
32. Chlumska A, Boudova L, Benes Z, Zamecnik M. Autoimmune gastritis. A clinicopathologic study of 25 cases. Cesk Patol. 2005;41:137–42.
33. Krasinskas AM, Abraham SC, Metz DC, Furth EE. Oxyntic mucosa pseudopolyps: a presentation of atrophic autoimmune gastritis. Am J Surg Pathol. 2003;27:236–41.
34. Wolber RA, Owen DA, Anderson FH, Freeman HJ. Lymphocytic gastritis and giant gastric folds associated with gastrointestinal protein loss. Mod Pathol. 1991;4:13–5.
35. Wu TT, Hamilton SR. Lymphocytic gastritis: association with etiology and topology. Am J Surg Pathol. 1999;23:153–8.
36. Lebwohl B, Green PH, Genta RM. The coeliac stomach: gastritis in patients with coeliac disease. Aliment Pharmacol Ther. 2015;42:180–7.
37. Perardi S, Todros L, Musso A, David E, Repici A, Rizzetto M. Lymphocytic gastritis and protein-losing gastropathy. Dig Liver Dis. 2000;32:422–5.
38. Leung ST, Chandan VS, Murray JA, Wu TT. Collagenous gastritis: histopathologic features and association with other gastrointestinal diseases. Am J Surg Pathol. 2009;33:788–98.
39. Arnason T, Brown IS, Goldsmith JD, Anderson W, O'Brien BH, Wilson C, Winter H, Lauwers GY. Collagenous gastritis: a morphologic and immunohistochemical study of 40 patients. Mod Pathol. 2015;28:533–44.
40. Kamimura K, Kobayashi M, Sato Y, Aoyagi Y, Terai S. Collagenous gastritis: review. World J Gastrointest Endosc. 2015;7:265–73.
41. Renault M, Goodier A, Subramony C, Hood B, Bishop P, Nowicki M. Age-related differences in granulomatous gastritis: a retrospective, clinicopathological analysis. J Clin Pathol. 2010;63:347–50.
42. Ectors NL, Dixon MF, Geboes KJ, Rutgeerts PJ, Desmet VJ, Vantrappen GR. Granulomatous gastritis: a morphological and diagnostic approach. Histopathology. 1993;23:55–61.
43. Shapiro JL, Goldblum JR, Petras RE. A clinicopathologic study of 42 patients with granulomatous gastritis. Is there really an "idiopathic" granulomatous gastritis? Am J Surg Pathol. 1996;20:462–70.
44. Zuckerman MJ, al-Samman M, Boman DA. Granulomatous gastroenteritis. Case report with comparison to idiopathic isolated granulomatous gastritis. Dig Dis Sci. 1994;39:1649–54.
45. Maeng L, Lee A, Choi K, Kang CS, Kim KM. Granulomatous gastritis: a clinicopathologic analysis of 18 biopsy cases. Am J Surg Pathol. 2004;28:941–5.
46. Lwin T, Melton SD, Genta RM. Eosinophilic gastritis: histopathological characterization and quantification of the normal gastric eosinophil content. Mod Pathol. 2011;24:556–63.

47. Caldwell JM, Collins MH, Stucke EM, Putnam PE, Franciosi JP, Kushner JP, Abonia JP, Rothenberg ME. Histologic eosinophilic gastritis is a systemic disorder associated with blood and extragastric eosinophilia, TH2 immunity, and a unique gastric transcriptome. J Allergy Clin Immunol. 2014;134:1114–24.
48. Ko HM, Morotti RA, Yershov O, Chehade M. Eosinophilic gastritis in children: clinicopathological correlation, disease course, and response to therapy. Am J Gastroenterol. 2014;109:1277–85.
49. Klair JS, Girotra M, Kaur A, Aduli F. Helicobacter pylori-negative Russell body gastritis: does the diagnosis call for screening for plasmacytic malignancies, especially multiple myeloma? BMJ Case Rep. 2014;2014:bcr2013202672.
50. Zhang H, Jin Z, Cui R. Russell body gastritis/duodenitis: a case series and description of immunoglobulin light chain restriction. Clin Res Hepatol Gastroenterol. 2014;38:e89–97.
51. Pizzolitto S, Camilot D, DeMaglio G, Falconieri G. Russell body gastritis: expanding the spectrum of Helicobacter pylori – related diseases? Pathol Res Pract. 2007;203:457–60.
52. Lam-Himlin D, Tsiatis AC, Montgomery E, Pai RK, Brown JA, Razavi M, Lamps L, Eshleman JR, Bhagavan B, Anders RA. Sarcina organisms in the gastrointestinal tract: a clinicopathologic and molecular study. Am J Surg Pathol. 2011;35:1700–5.
53. Ratuapli SK, Lam-Himlin DM, Heigh RI. Sarcina ventriculi of the stomach: a case report. World J Gastroenterol. 2013;19:2282–5.
54. Gaspar BL. The significance of Sarcina in routine surgical pathology practice. APMIS. 2016;124:436–43.
55. Jevremovic D, Torbenson M, Murray JA, Burgart LJ, Abraham SC. Atrophic autoimmune pangastritis: a distinctive form of antral and fundic gastritis associated with systemic autoimmune disease. Am J Surg Pathol. 2006;30:1412–9.
56. Shiota S, Thrift AP, Green L, Shah R, Verstovsek G, Rugge M, Graham DY, El-Serag HB. Clinical manifestations of Helicobacter pylori-negative gastritis. Clin Gastroenterol Hepatol. 2017;15:1037–46 e3.
57. Nordenstedt H, Graham DY, Kramer JR, Rugge M, Verstovsek G, Fitzgerald S, Alsarraj A, Shaib Y, Velez ME, Abraham N, Anand B, Cole R, El-Serag HB. Helicobacter pylori-negative gastritis: prevalence and risk factors. Am J Gastroenterol. 2013;108:65–71.
58. Strisciuglio C, Corleto VD, Brunetti-Pierri N, Piccolo P, Sangermano R, Rindi G, Martini M, D'Armiento FP, Staiano A, Miele E. Autosomal dominant Menetrier-like disease. J Pediatr Gastroenterol Nutr. 2012;55:717–20.
59. Eisenstat DD, Griffiths AM, Cutz E, Petric M, Drumm B. Acute cytomegalovirus infection in a child with Menetrier's disease. Gastroenterology. 1995;109:592–5.
60. Fretzayas A, Moustaki M, Alexopoulou E, Nicolaidou P. Menetrier's disease associated with Helicobacter pylori: three cases with sonographic findings and a literature review. Ann Trop Paediatr. 2011;31:141–7.
61. Wolfsen HC, Carpenter HA, Talley NJ. Menetrier's disease: a form of hypertrophic gastropathy or gastritis? Gastroenterology. 1993;104:1310–9.

Malabsorption Disorders

5

Rhonda Yantiss and Melanie Johncilla

List of Frequently Asked Questions

1. What is an adequate tissue sample for evaluating patients with malabsorptive symptoms?
2. Which artifacts simulate chronic enteritis in biopsy samples?
3. Are there any pitfalls specific to evaluating samples from the duodenal bulb?
4. What is the malabsorptive pattern of small bowel injury?
5. What is the differential diagnosis for a malabsorptive pattern of small bowel injury?
6. What are the environmental and genetic risk factors for celiac disease?
7. How reliable are serologic markers in the evaluation of celiac disease?
8. What are the specific histologic features of celiac disease?
9. Does immunohistochemistry help when assessing intraepithelial lymphocytosis?
10. What are the complications of celiac disease?
11. What is the differential diagnosis of collagenous sprue?
12. What does Crohn disease look like in the proximal small bowel?
13. What are the clinical features of autoimmune enteropathy?
14. What are the histologic features of autoimmune enteropathy?
15. What are the clinical features of common variable immunodeficiency?
16. Which histologic features should lead one to suspect a diagnosis of CVID?
17. How does eosinophilic gastroenteritis manifest in small bowel biopsy samples?
18. Which drugs cause changes that simulate celiac disease?
19. Which features help distinguish gastrointestinal graft-versus-host disease (GVHD) from medication-related injury?
20. Which features should raise suspicion for tropical sprue?
21. What changes suggest bacterial overgrowth in the small bowel biopsy samples?
22. Which types of infection cause intraepithelial lymphocytosis?
23. Which types of disorders cause malabsorptive symptoms in pediatric patients?
24. How should I sign out small bowel biopsy cases that show a malabsorptive pattern?

Frequently Asked Questions

1. **What is an adequate tissue sample for evaluating patients with malabsorptive symptoms?**
   - Small-intestinal biopsy sampling represents the gold standard for patients with malabsorptive symptoms. Many conditions, particularly celiac disease, are patchy or cause variably severe abnormalities at different sites in the proximal small bowel. In fact, inflammatory changes vary from sample to sample at different sites in the duodenum in nearly two-thirds of patients with celiac disease and show a spectrum of villous abnormalities in more than 10% of samples obtained from the same site in the duodenum. Samples obtained from the duodenal bulb can be difficult to interpret due to several reasons, as discussed below, but they can also be the only samples that show diagnostic abnormalities in up to one-third of patients. Thus, the most recent guidelines from the Rodger C. Haggitt Gastrointestinal Pathology Society and North American Association for the Study of Celiac Disease recommend obtaining two tissue sam-

R. Yantiss (✉) · M. Johncilla
Cornell University Weill Cornell Medicine, New York, NY, USA
e-mail: rhy2001@med.cornell.edu

H. L. Wang, Z. E. Chen (eds.), *Practical Gastrointestinal Pathology*, Practical Anatomic Pathology,
https://doi.org/10.1007/978-3-030-51268-2_5

ples from the duodenal bulb and at least four from the distal duodenum when evaluating patients with malabsorptive symptoms.

References: [1–6]

2. **Which artifacts simulate chronic enteritis in biopsy samples?**
   - The normal duodenum features villi that are approximately three times the length of adjacent crypts. They are lined by enterocytes and scattered goblet cells; the crypts contain goblet cells, Paneth cells, and endocrine cells. Villi tend to be longer with broader tips in the jejunum and ileum; the latter features villi with numerous goblet cells. Villi throughout the small intestine tend to be shorter overlying lymphoid aggregates and may appear flattened when tangentially sectioned or stripped (Fig. 5.1). An adequate biopsy sample consists of three to four intact, well-oriented villi in a row. Although some authors advocate placing specimens on porous filter paper or sponges prior to processing, this practice is impractical in many high-volume centers.

   Reference: [7]

3. **Are there any pitfalls specific to evaluating samples from the duodenal bulb?**
   - Villi are shorter overlying Brunner glands, gastric heterotopias, and lymphoid aggregates, all of which are commonly encountered in the duodenal bulb. Epithelium overlying lymphoid aggregates normally contains numerous lymphocytes and occasional granulocytes that should not be interpreted to represent enteritis (Fig. 5.2). Peptic duodenitis in the duodenal bulb causes variable villous abnormalities with intraepithelial lymphocytosis. Neutrophilic infiltrates, Brunner gland hyperplasia, and gastric foveolar metaplasia (also known as gastric surface metaplasia or gastric mucous cell metaplasia) are clues to a diagnosis of peptic injury (Fig. 5.3). It should be emphasized, however, that focal gastric foveolar metaplasia is a common finding in duodenal biopsies, which should not be used as a specific feature for the diagnosis of peptic duodenitis secondary to *Helicobacter pylori (H. pylori)* infection. In fact, it may be found in otherwise unremarkable duodenal mucosa in patients with gastric biopsies showing no *H. pylori* or even unremarkable histology. Its presence may just simply indicate an adaptive response to prior chronic stimulation.

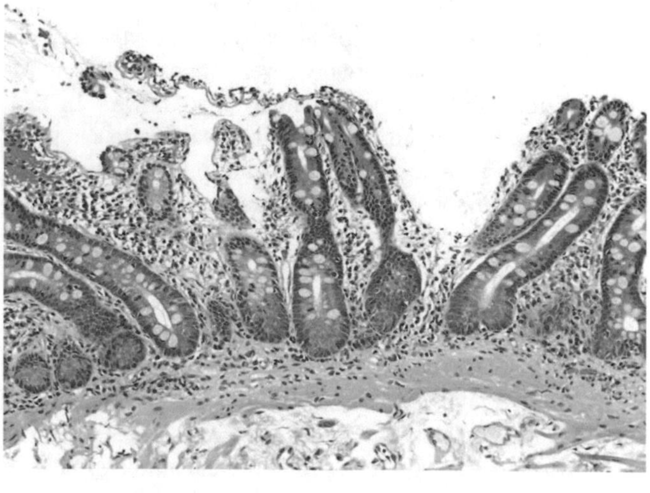

Fig. 5.1 Stripped duodenal villi appear blunted. The absence of any other signs of active or chronic injury is one clue that the changes represent an artifact of processing

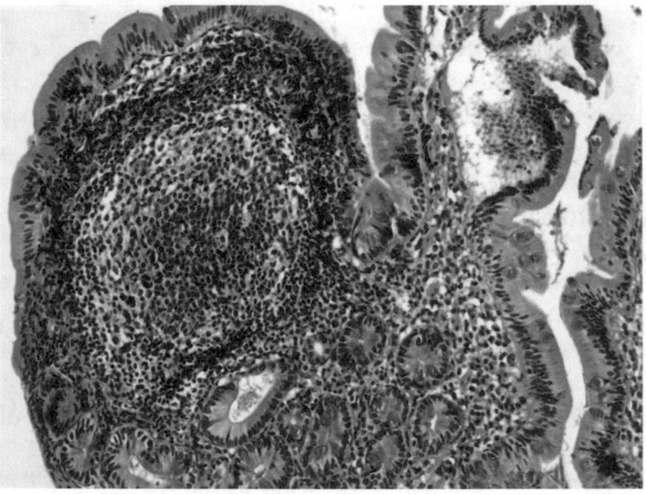

Fig. 5.2 Epithelium overlying lymphoid aggregates may contain increased intraepithelial lymphocytes, which should not be interpreted as a malabsorptive pattern of injury

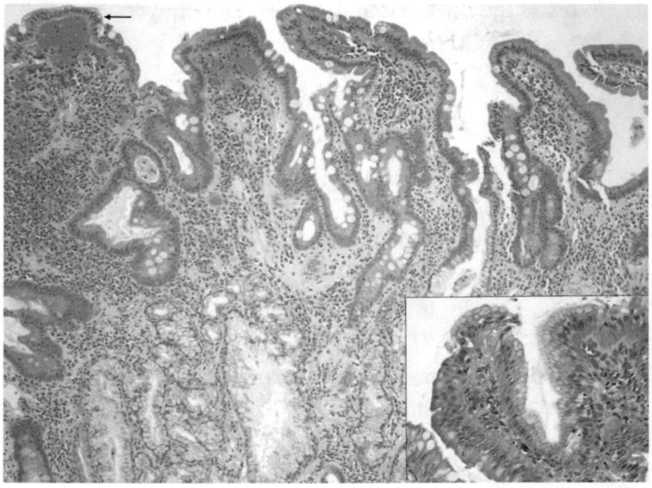

Fig. 5.3 Peptic duodenitis features villous blunting, Brunner gland hyperplasia, and mildly increased plasma cell infiltrates in the duodenal bulb. Gastric foveolar metaplasia is present in the surface epithelium (arrow and inset)

4. **What is the malabsorptive pattern of small bowel injury?**
   - A variety of endoscopic abnormalities can be seen in patients with celiac disease and other inflammatory conditions. The examination can be normal in up to 20% of patients, particularly children. Features that suggest mucosal disease include decreased or absent mucosal folds, effacement of mucosal folds upon insufflation, a mosaic pattern, scalloped folds, nodularity, and increased visibility of the vasculature. Although all of these features have been well-described in patients with celiac disease, they do not reliably distinguish it from other immune-mediated and drug-related injuries that cause a malabsorptive pattern of injury in biopsy samples. These include remodeling of villous architecture, crypt hyperplasia, and expansion of the lamina propria by mononuclear cell-rich inflammation. Additional features, such as intraepithelial lymphocytosis, eosinophilia, crypt abscesses, crypt cell apoptosis, gastric foveolar metaplasia, and plasmacytosis, are variably present. These features can help distinguish between different types of injury, especially when interpreted in light of clinical and laboratory findings.

   Reference: [6]

5. **What is the differential diagnosis for a malabsorptive pattern of small bowel injury?**
   - A variety of medications, immune-mediated disorders, and infections can cause variable villous architectural abnormalities with, or without, intraepithelial inflammation. Peptic injury and *H. pylori* infection cause inflammatory changes that are most pronounced in the duodenal bulb and rapidly diminish in the second part of the duodenum. They do not cause malabsorptive symptoms. On the other hand, entities that cause profound diarrheal illness generally cause severe, diffuse mucosal abnormalities throughout the proximal small bowel. Correct classification requires knowledge of the severity of symptoms, serologic studies, distribution of disease, and endoscopic findings, as enumerated in Table 5.1.

   Reference: [8]

Table 5.1 Key features of disorders that can cause a malabsorptive pattern of duodenal injury in biopsy samples

Entity	Clinical associations	Endoscopic findings	Disease distribution	Distinguishing histologic features
Topical injury				
Peptic duodenitis	*H. pylori* gastritis Zollinger-Ellison syndrome	Ulcers Erythema	Duodenal bulb, periampullary mucosa	Gastric foveolar metaplasia Intraepithelial lymphocytosis is patchy Neutrophils
Altered immunity				
Celiac disease	Dermatitis herpetiformis Anti-TTG and anti-endomysial antibodies	Malabsorptive pattern	Duodenum, proximal jejunum	Surface injury greater than crypt injury Intraepithelial lymphocytosis most prominent in surface epithelium Rare crypt abscesses and granulocytes
Inflammatory bowel disease	Arthralgias Oral aphthous ulcers	Malabsorptive pattern Ulcers, strictures	Gastrointestinal tract	Neutrophilic cryptitis Non-necrotic granulomata Patchy inflammation
Autoimmune enteropathy	IPEX syndrome APECED/APS1 Anti-enterocyte antibodies	Malabsorptive pattern	Gastrointestinal tract	Severe crypt injury compared with surface epithelium Crypt-predominant intraepithelial lymphocytosis Numerous crypt abscesses Apoptotic crypt epithelial cells Decreased Paneth, endocrine, and goblet cells
Common variable immunodeficiency	Hemolytic anemia Recurrent infections	Malabsorptive pattern	Gastrointestinal tract	Crypt injury greater than surface injury Crypt-predominant intraepithelial lymphocytosis Granulocytes and crypt abscesses Apoptotic crypt epithelial cells common Decreased or absent lamina propria plasma cells

Table 5.1 (continued)

Entity	Clinical associations	Endoscopic findings	Disease distribution	Distinguishing histologic features
Eosinophilic gastroenteritis	Atopy	Malabsorptive pattern	Gastrointestinal tract	Lamina propria and intraepithelial eosinophils
Graft versus host disease	Bone marrow or hematopoietic stem cell transplantation	Non-specific	Gastrointestinal tract	Paucicellular lamina propria Apoptotic crypt epithelial cells Sparing of endocrine cells
Food allergies	Atopy	Non-specific	Gastrointestinal tract	Intraepithelial lymphocytes with variable eosinophilia
Protein intolerance	Atopy	Non-specific	Small bowel, colon	Intraepithelial lymphocytes with variable eosinophilia
Morbid obesity		Non-specific	Jejunum	Lymphocytosis with normal villous architecture
Medications				
Immune checkpoint inhibitors/targeted agents		Non-specific	Gastrointestinal tract	Neutrophilic cryptitis Apoptotic crypt epithelial cells common Intraepithelial lymphocytosis
Angiotensin receptor blockers	History of hypertension	Malabsorptive pattern	None	Malabsorptive pattern with apoptosis and neutrophils
NSAIDs	Numerous clinical associations	Occasional ulcers	Gastrointestinal tract	Mild villous blunting Mild intraepithelial lymphocytosis
Infection				
Tropical sprue	Vitamin B12 deficiency	Mild villous flattening	Ileum most affected	Villous abnormalities mild in the duodenum
Bacterial overgrowth	Impaired gut motility	Non-specific	None	Partial villous blunting Intraepithelial lymphocytosis with neutrophils
Viruses		Non-specific	Gastrointestinal tract	Neutrophils frequently present Viral cytopathic changes (CMV, adenovirus)
Parasites		Non-specific	Gastrointestinal tract	Organisms may be detected in samples

TTG tissue-transglutaminase, *IPEX* immune dysregulation, polyendocrinopathy, enteropathy, and X-linked syndrome, *APECED/APS1* autoimmune polyendocrinopathy-candidiasis-ectodermal dystrophy/autoimmune polyglandular syndrome type 1, *NSAIDs* non-steroidal anti-inflammatory drugs

6. **What are the environmental and genetic risk factors for celiac disease?**
   - Celiac disease is the most common inherited malabsorption disorder. It results from an immune-mediated reaction to gliadin, a component of gluten, in genetically susceptible individuals. Virtually all patients with the disease have HLA types DQ2 or DQ8, although there is only a 70% concordance among monozygous twins. It is widely speculated that sensitivity to gliadin is triggered by an environmental exposure to adenovirus or reovirus, both of which share peptide sequences with gliadin.

   References: [9–11]

7. **How reliable are serologic markers in the evaluation of celiac disease?**
   - Patients with celiac disease generally have elevated anti-gliadin, anti-endomysial, and anti-tissue transglutaminase (TTG) antibodies. Assays for TTG immunoglobulin A (IgA) antibodies have the highest sensitivity (74–100%) and specificity (78–100%) for celiac disease, although these tests may be negative in some situations. Approximately 10% of patients with celiac disease have IgA deficiency and lack anti-TTG IgA antibodies; serum IgG antibodies to TTG or deamidated gliadin peptides should be tested in these patients. Anti-endomysial antibody tests are highly specific (98%) for disease but are costly and difficult to interpret. Of note, serologic assays must be performed while patients are exposed to gluten. They are generally negative among patients adherent to a gluten-free diet. All of these assays are less sensitive among patients with minimal or no symptoms, and antibodies can be spuriously elevated in patients with other immune-mediated disorders and malabsorptive conditions.

   References: [6, 12, 13]

8. **What are the specific histologic features of celiac disease?**
   - Characteristic histologic features of celiac disease include variable villous blunting with crypt hyperplasia, plasma cell-rich lamina propria inflammation, and

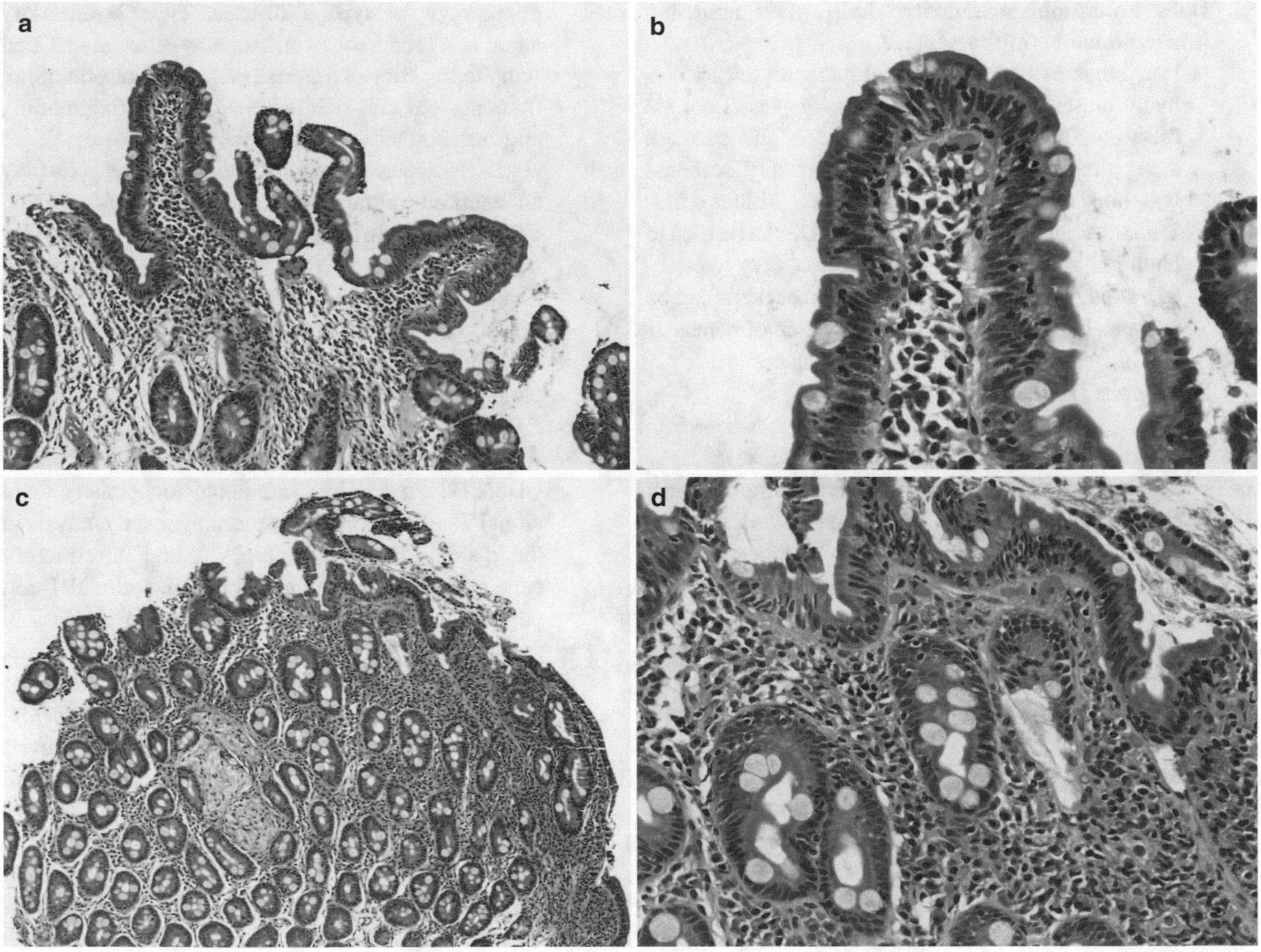

Fig. 5.4 Celiac disease causes variable villous architectural abnormalities accompanied by intraepithelial lymphocytosis. Samples from some symptomatic patients display normal villous architecture without increased lamina propria cellularity (**a**), as well as increased intraepithelial lymphocytes in the villous tips (**b**). Severe villous blunting and crypt hyperplasia are accompanied by plasma cell-rich lamina propria inflammation (**c**). Intraepithelial lymphocytosis is more pronounced in the surface epithelium compared with the crypts (**d**)

increased intraepithelial lymphocytes (Fig. 5.4a–d). Some patients have mild inflammatory changes with minimal or no villous architectural abnormalities and normal or nearly normal lamina propria cellularity. However, intraepithelial lymphocytosis is uniformly present when patients have symptomatic celiac disease. Intraepithelial lymphocytes tend to be dispersed along the sides and tips of the villi and are more numerous in the villous tips. They number >25/100 enterocytes and often exceed 40/100 enterocytes. Injured surface epithelial cells may be cuboidal and contain vacuoles. Some pathologists classify the severity of mucosal injury based on a combination of villous abnormalities and inflammatory changes (such as the Marsh Score System; see Table 5.2). This practice is of limited clinical utility and lacks reproducibility; most authors recommend that classification of histologic features be limited to the research setting.

References: [6, 14–16]

Table 5.2 The modified Marsh score system for celiac disease[a]

Marsh lesion	IEL/100 enterocytes	Crypts	Villi
0	<40	Normal	Normal
1	>40	Normal	Normal
2	>40	Hyperplasia	Normal
3a	>40	Hyperplasia	Mild atrophy
3b	>40	Hyperplasia	Moderate to marked atrophy
3c	>40	Hyperplasia	Complete atrophy (flattened)

IEL intraepithelial lymphocytes

[a]Even if Marsh scores may be demanded by clinicians in clinical practice, the terms Marsh lesion 1 and Marsh lesion 2 are rarely used in pathology reports. This is so because Marsh lesion 1 (intraepithelial lymphocytosis with normal villous architecture) is a nonspecific diagnosis that is not only seen in celiac disease. As discussed in the text, many other conditions can cause intraepithelial lymphocytosis such as tropical sprue, autoimmune enteropathy, inflammatory bowel disease, infections (*H. pylori*, bacterial overgrowth, etc.), medications (olmesartan, NSAIDs, etc.), CVID, and others. Marsh lesion 2 is a challenging diagnosis because of the difficulty to assess crypt hyperplasia

9. **Does immunohistochemistry help when assessing intraepithelial lymphocytosis?**
   - Low numbers of intraepithelial lymphocytes are normally present in duodenal biopsy samples. They are most numerous near the villous bases and decrease along their lateral aspects such that only scattered lymphocytes are present in the villous tips. Immunostains against CD3 and/or CD8 can be used to highlight T-cells, but they are not necessary to establish a diagnosis; intraepithelial lymphocytosis can be adequately assessed based on evaluation of hematoxylin and eosin (H&E)-stained slides alone.

   References: [17, 18]

10. **What are the complications of celiac disease?**
   - Celiac disease can lead to several complications: refractory sprue (refractory celiac disease), collagenous sprue, lymphoma, and adenocarcinoma. Refractory sprue is defined by a combination of features: recurrent malabsorptive symptoms in patients who initially responded to gluten withdrawal for a period of 6–12 months, a malabsorptive pattern of injury in biopsy samples, and exclusion of other etiologies. It occurs in 5–10% of patients with celiac disease and is classified into two groups. Type 1 disease is characterized by villous shortening and intraepithelial lymphocytosis similar to celiac disease. Intraepithelial lymphocytes are immunophenotypically normal and express CD3, CD7, CD103, and TCR-β, often with concomitant CD8 expression. By immunohistochemistry, the number of CD8+ intraepithelial T-cells may be fewer than that of CD3+ cells even for type 1 disease, but the loss of CD8 coexpression is generally <50% in comparison to CD3+ intraepithelial T-cells. T-cell receptor gene rearrangement studies demonstrate a polyclonal population for type 1 disease. Type 2 refractory sprue is a precursor to enteropathy-associated T-cell lymphoma. Biopsy findings include villous blunting, mononuclear cell-rich lamina propria inflammation, and intraepithelial lymphocytosis without cytologic atypia. However, intraepithelial lymphocytes display an aberrant immunophenotype with loss of CD3, CD7, and CD8 in 20% of cells by flow cytometry. By immunohistochemistry, >50% CD3+ intraepithelial T-cells may show loss of CD8 coexpression (Fig. 5.5a–c). Molecular analysis demonstrates intraepithelial T-cells to be monoclonal; 37–50% of patients progress to overt T-cell lymphoma within 5 years.
   - A recent study questioned the reliability of using CD8/CD3 ratio by immunohistochemistry and clonal T-cell receptor gene rearrangement analysis in the distinction between types 1 and 2 refractory celiac disease. The authors found that clonal T-cell populations were present with a similar frequency in patients with type 1 and type 2 refractory sprue, newly diagnosed celiac disease, established celiac disease with follow-up biopsies, and *H. pylori*-associated intraepithelial lymphocytosis. However, no clonal T-cell populations were detected in normal controls. The CD8/CD3 ratios also did not differ significantly among these study groups. The authors thus concluded that T-cell immunophenotyping and clonal analysis appeared insufficient to reliably distinguish between refractory sprue types 1 and 2.
   - Although gluten restriction decreases lymphoma risk among patients with celiac disease, those with longstanding gluten exposure are at increased risk for both B- and T-cell lymphomas, particularly enteropathy-associated T-cell lymphoma (i.e., EATL 1). Enteropathy-associated T-cell lymphoma accounts

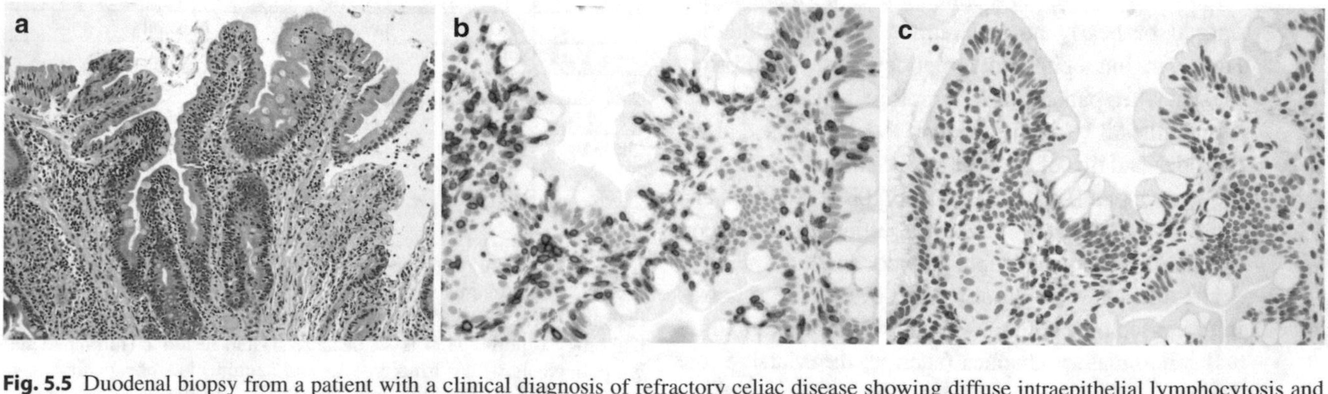

Fig. 5.5 Duodenal biopsy from a patient with a clinical diagnosis of refractory celiac disease showing diffuse intraepithelial lymphocytosis and mild villous blunting (**a**). Immunohistochemical stain for CD3 highlights numerous intraepithelial T-lymphocytes (**b**), which show a near-complete loss of CD8 coexpression (**c**). Note the presence of CD8-positive lymphocytes in the lamina propria. This case also showed clonal T-cell receptor gene rearrangement for the TRG locus by polymerase chain reaction. Though controversial, these findings are thought to be supportive of type 2 refractory sprue

for 10–25% of all primary intestinal lymphomas. Patients may present with refractory symptoms as well as intestinal obstruction and/or perforation in up to 50% of cases. The disease may produce solitary or multifocal ulcers and nodules. In fact, detection of ulcers in a patients with established celiac disease should raise concern for lymphoma development. Tumors consist of pleomorphic medium-to-large neoplastic T-cells admixed with nonneoplastic lymphocytes, plasma cells, and eosinophils that expand the lamina propria or infiltrate the intestinal wall (Fig. 5.6a, b). Features of celiac disease are often present in the adjacent mucosa. Neoplastic cells usually express CD3, CD30, and CD103 and are negative for CD4, CD5, and CD56; immunostains for CD8 show variable staining.

References: [19–24]

11. **What is the differential diagnosis of collagenous sprue?**
    - Collagenous sprue can result from chronic mucosal injury due to a variety of causes. It may explain development of refractory sprue and has been reported in patients with tropical sprue and milk protein intolerance and in association with sartans. Small-intestinal biopsy samples show increased lamina propria inflammation, intraepithelial lymphocytosis, and patchy subepithelial collagen deposition that displays an irregular interface with the lamina propria. The collagen layer may contain entrapped inflammatory cells, capillaries, and fibroblasts but tends to be less pronounced than that of collagenous colitis (Fig. 5.7a, b). Treatment consists of immunomodulatory therapy and is usually met with symptomatic improvement.

References: [25, 26]

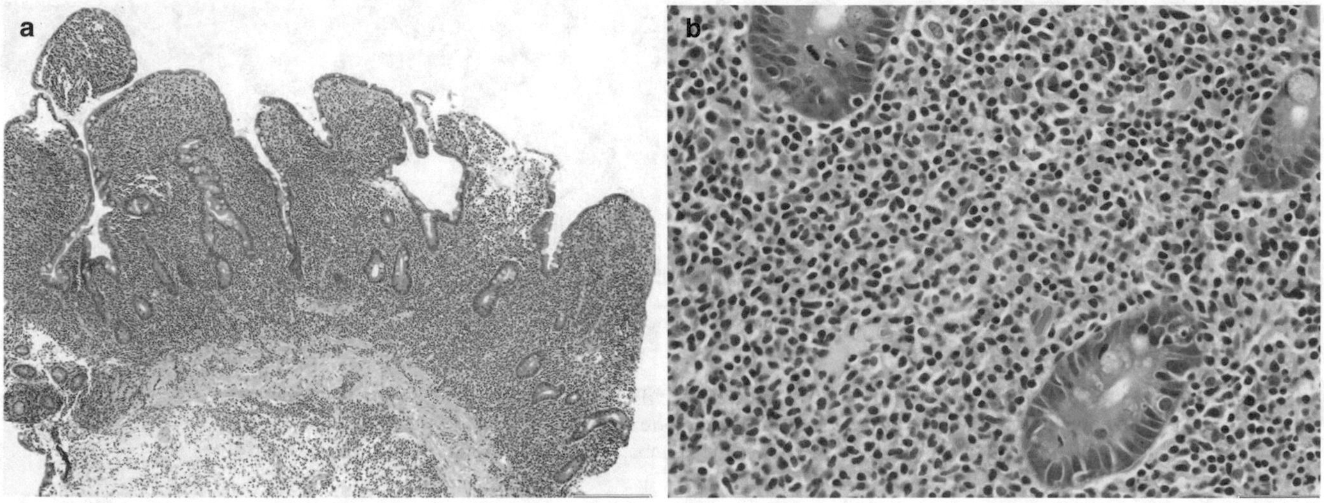

Fig. 5.6 Enteropathy-associated T-cell lymphoma expands the lamina propria and extends through the muscularis mucosae (**a**). The tumor is composed of pleomorphic T-cells admixed with eosinophils and plasma cells (**b**)

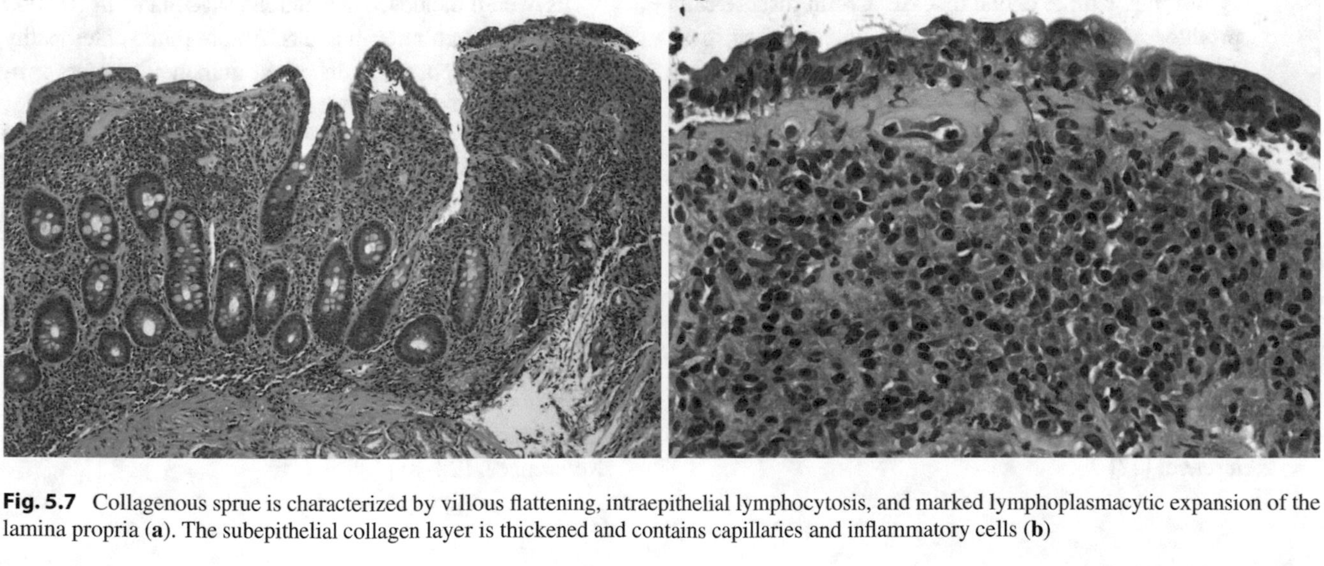

Fig. 5.7 Collagenous sprue is characterized by villous flattening, intraepithelial lymphocytosis, and marked lymphoplasmacytic expansion of the lamina propria (**a**). The subepithelial collagen layer is thickened and contains capillaries and inflammatory cells (**b**)

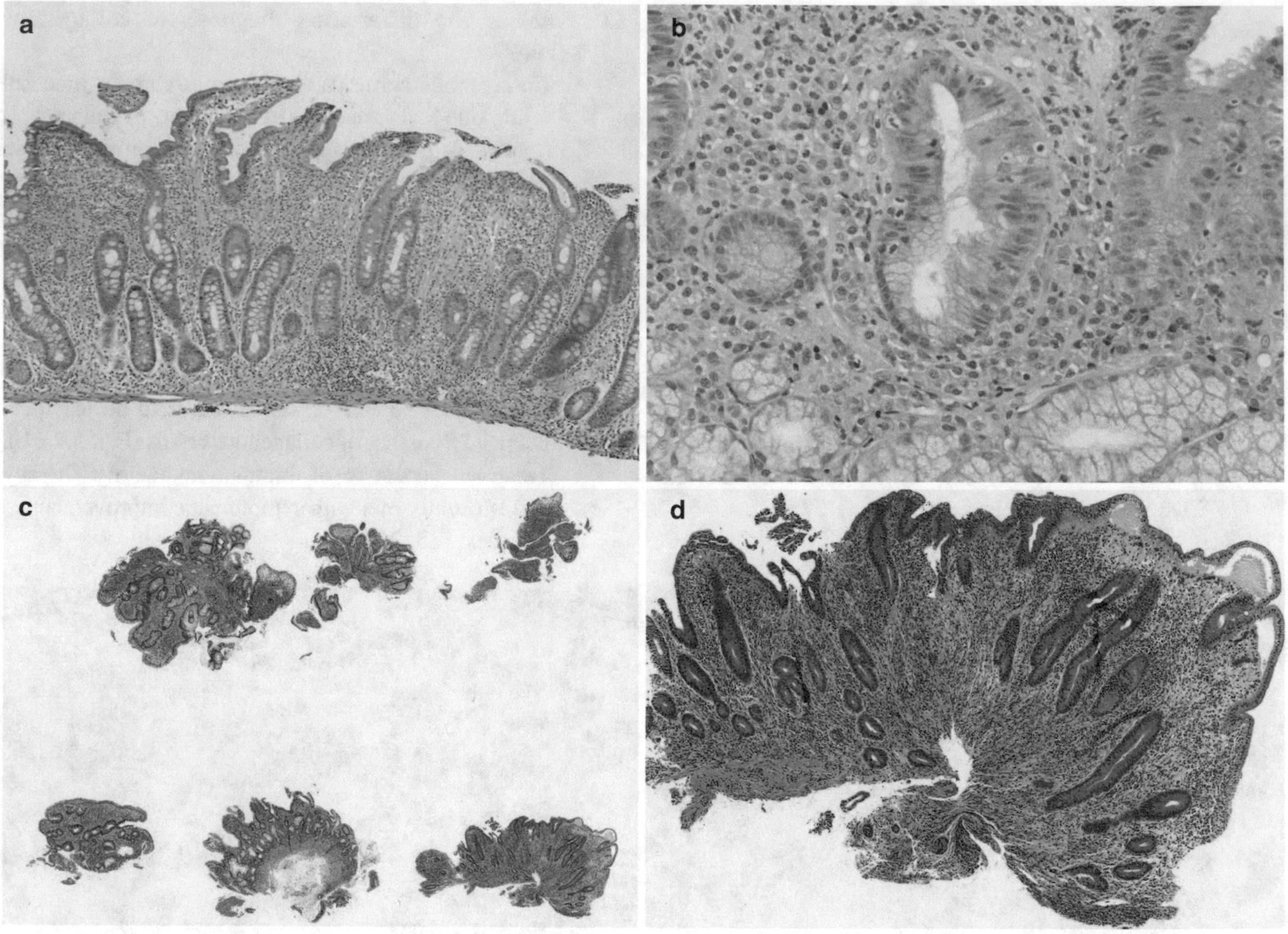

Fig. 5.8 Crohn disease can simulate features of celiac disease. Variable villous shortening is accompanied by lamina propria lymphoplasmacytosis (**a**) and neutrophilic crypt injury (**b**). The distribution of disease is often patchy; each fragment of this small-intestinal biopsy sample shows varying degrees of injury (**c**). One fragment shows more prominent inflammation and villous shortening than the others (**d**)

12. **What does Crohn disease look like in the proximal small bowel?**
    - Patients with Crohn disease can develop flares in the proximal small bowel that cause malabsorptive symptoms. Unlike celiac disease, Crohn disease can produce erythema, erosions, and ulcers, often in a segmental distribution. Plasma cell-rich inflammation in the lamina propria is accompanied by extensive neutrophilic cryptitis and ulcers; granulomata are uncommon (Fig. 5.8a–d). Some patients with Crohn disease have biopsy samples that display normal villous architecture with intraepithelial lymphocytosis and a normocellular lamina propria. Crohn duodenitis is characteristically patchy; multiple tissue samples from the same area often show variably severe injury (Fig. 5.8c). Foci of increased inflammation may even be present in a single tissue fragment.

    Reference: [27]

13. **What are the clinical features of autoimmune enteropathy?**
    - Autoimmune enteropathy is a rare malabsorptive disorder that typically presents in infancy and young children. Its overall incidence in children is less than 1 in 100,000 and it is even rarer in adults. Autoimmune enteropathy is one component of inherited immune disorders syndromes. Immune dysregulation, polyendocrinopathy, enteropathy, X-linked (IPEX) syndrome is caused by mutations in *FOXP3*, a gene responsible for regulatory T-cell function. It is also a component of autoimmune polyendocrinopathy-candidiasis-ectodermal dystrophy (APECED/APS1). This disorder results from mutations in *AIRE*, which regulates autoreactive T-cells. Patients with autoimmune enteropathy often have severe diarrheal symptoms and weight loss that require hospitalization. More than two-thirds have autoantibodies to enterocytes and goblet cells, among others.

    References: [28–31]

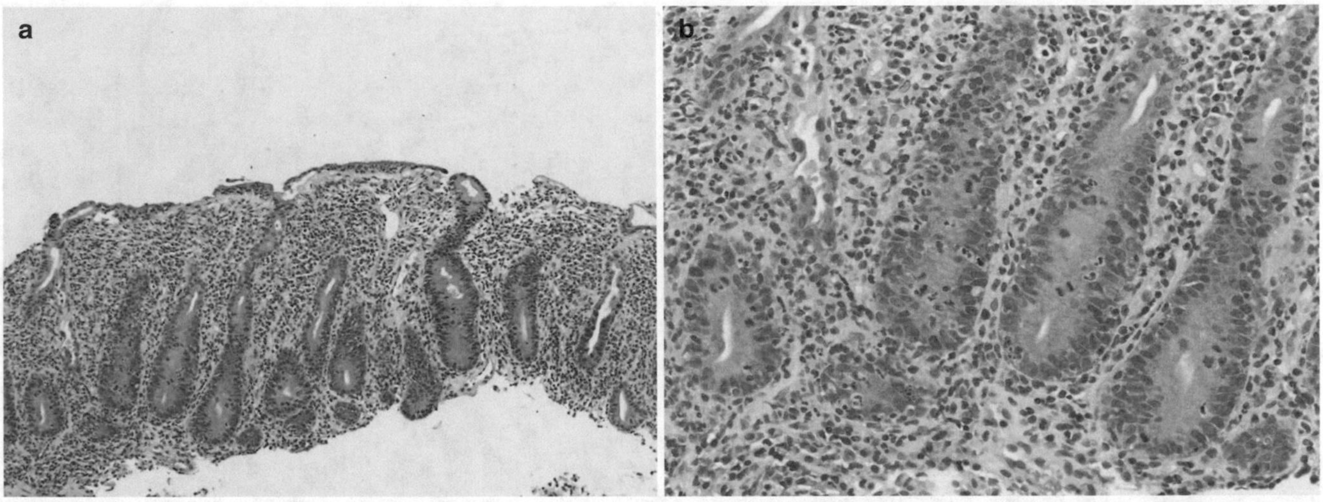

Fig. 5.9 Autoimmune enteropathy produces marked villous flattening accompanied by dense plasma cell-rich lamina propria inflammation (**a**). Patchy neutrophilic cryptitis and apoptotic crypt epithelial cells are present. Note the absence of goblet cells and Paneth cells (**b**)

14. **What are the histologic features of autoimmune enteropathy?**
    - Autoimmune enteropathy causes variable mucosal abnormalities ranging from intraepithelial lymphocytosis and normal villous architecture to villous blunting, crypt hyperplasia, and plasma cell-rich lamina propria inflammation. Intraepithelial lymphocytosis tends to be patchy and more pronounced in crypts than surface epithelium. Neutrophilic cryptitis and apoptotic debris are frequently present. Paneth cells, goblet cells, and endocrine cells are decreased in numbers or absent, but this feature is not uniformly present. Biopsy samples from patients with IPEX syndrome show severe villous abnormalities with crypt epithelial cell apoptosis, intraepithelial lymphocytosis, and loss of goblet cells. Autoimmune enteropathy causes injury throughout the gastrointestinal tract. Both gastric and colonic samples can show chronic active inflammation and apoptotic epithelial cells in the deep mucosa. Prominent neutrophilia and crypt abscesses are commonly present (Fig. 5.9a, b).

    References: [32–34]

15. **What are the clinical features of common variable immunodeficiency?**
    - Common variable immunodeficiency (CVID) affects roughly 1 in 50,000 people and usually presents in the second decade of life. The disorder can result from a number of molecular alterations culminating in failed plasma cell maturation. Affected patients have decreased levels of at least two immunoglobulin serotypes and are at increased risk for infections, particularly mycoplasma, *Haemophilus influenzae*, *Giardia lamblia*, *Salmonella*, *Campylobacter jejuni*, and *Shigella*.

    References: [35–37]

16. **Which histologic features should lead one to suspect a diagnosis of CVID?**
    - The histologic features of CVID simulate changes of celiac disease. Intraepithelial lymphocytosis and variably severe villous blunting are common. The lamina propria may be paucicellular owing to decreased plasma cells or hypercellular due to mononuclear cell-rich inflammation accompanied by macrophages and neutrophils. Additional features include neutrophilic cryptitis, striking crypt cell apoptosis, and lymphoid hyperplasia. The disease can involve the entire gastrointestinal tract. Esophageal, gastric, and colonic samples often show intraepithelial lymphocytosis, chronic active inflammation, and epithelial cell apoptosis in the deep mucosa. Diminished plasma cell infiltrates are highly specific for CVID compared with celiac disease and other immune-mediated disorders. *Giardia lamblia* and CMV infections are common among patients with CVID; detection of either organism in duodenal samples should raise the possibility of CVID, especially when accompanied by lymphoid hyperplasia and inconspicuous plasma cells (Fig. 5.10a–d).

    References: [20, 38]

17. **How does eosinophilic gastroenteritis manifest in small bowel biopsy samples?**
    - Primary eosinophilic gastroenteritis (EGE) is an uncommon hypersensitivity disorder that shows a predilection for boys and young men. Most patients have a history of atopic conditions and present with malabsorptive symptoms secondary to small bowel involvement. Villous abnormalities are accompanied by patchy intraepithelial lymphocytosis simulating the appearance of celiac disease. Clues to the diagno-

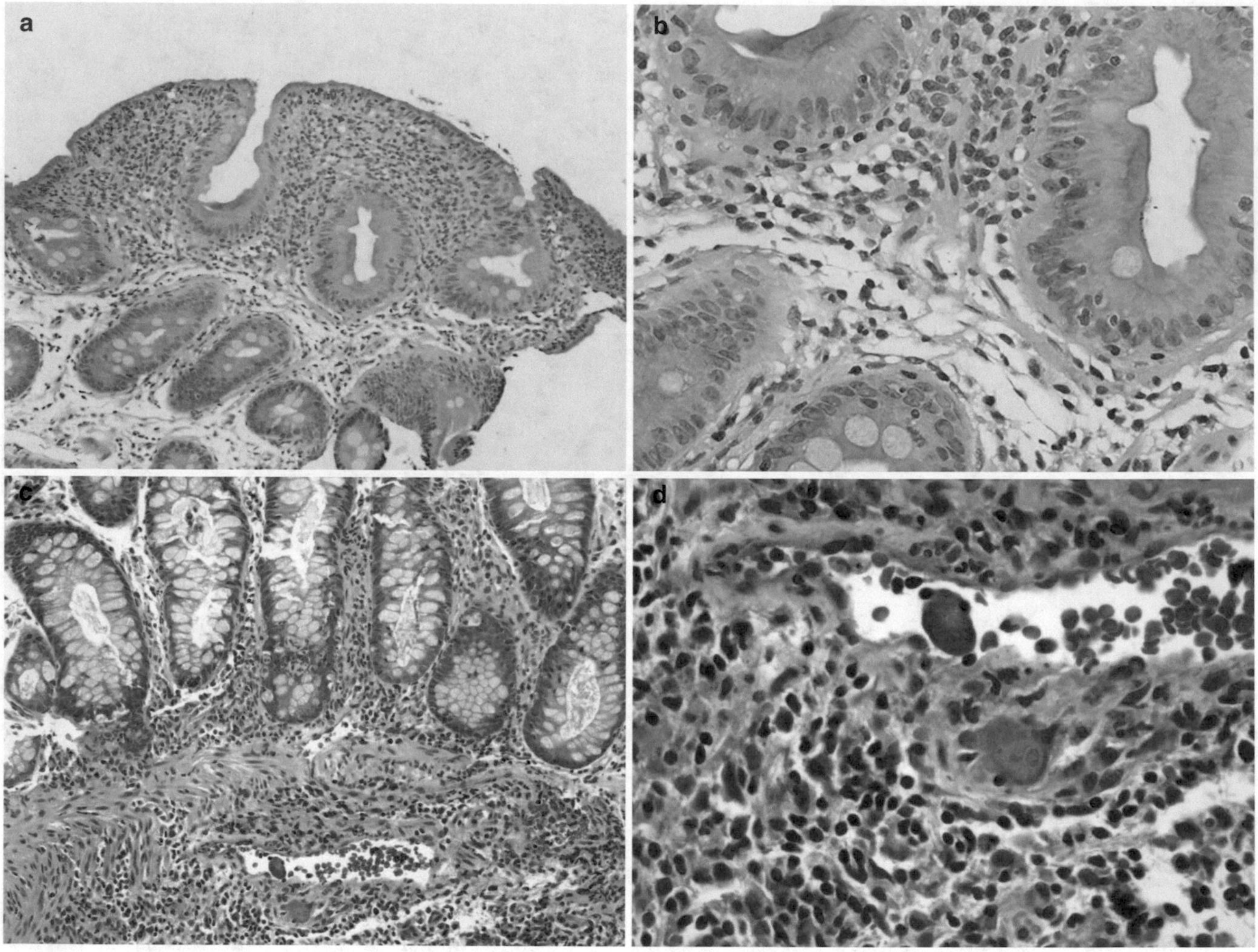

Fig. 5.10 Common variable immunodeficiency produces villous abnormalities with patchy intraepithelial lymphocytosis (**a**). The lamina propria contains a mixed infiltrate with inconspicuous plasma cells (**b**). The disease frequently involves the colon where it causes colitis with crypt distortion that simulates features of inflammatory bowel disease (**c**). Reactivation of CMV is common among patients with CVID (**d**)

sis include expansion of the lamina propria by mixed eosinophil-rich inflammation, single and clustered eosinophils in the epithelium, and eosinophilic crypt abscesses.

18. Which drugs cause changes that simulate celiac disease?

- A variety of medications cause a malabsorptive pattern of injury that simulates features of celiac disease. Nonsteroidal anti-inflammatory drugs (NSAIDs) can cause duodenal ulcers and erythema, as well as mild villous blunting with intraepithelial lymphocytosis. Neutrophils may be numerous, especially in patients with ulcers.
- Olmesartan is a drug in the class of angiotensin II receptor blockers. Olmesartan and related agents can cause severe enteropathy with malabsorptive diarrhea, simulating the endoscopic and histologic features of immune-mediated enteropathy. Anti-TTG serologic studies are usually negative and patients do not respond to gluten withdrawal. Villous blunting and crypt hyperplasia are accompanied by intraepithelial lymphocytosis, plasma cell-rich lamina propria inflammation, and crypt cell apoptosis. Subepithelial collagen deposits are characteristic of sartan-related gastrointestinal injury and can be found in the stomach, small bowel, and colon. Symptoms generally resolve with cessation of therapy, although severely ill patients may require corticosteroid therapy. Resolution of histologic changes may take weeks to months.
- Immune checkpoint inhibitors (e.g., ipilimumab, nivolumab, and pembrolizumab) can cause malabsorptive pattern of injury and diarrhea. Histologic features include villous blunting and intraepithelial lymphocytosis accompanied by occasional neutrophils in crypts and apoptotic crypt epithelial cells. Drug cessation with, or without, corticosteroid treatment reduces or eliminates symptoms.

- Idelalisib is a kinase inhibitor used to treat low-grade B-cell lymphomas. It causes diarrheal symptoms in nearly 50% of treated patients and can be severe enough to warrant drug withdrawal in 20% of cases. Biopsy findings include villous blunting with intraepithelial lymphocytosis and crypt cell apoptosis. Neutrophilic cryptitis is commonly present. Similar findings are often present in colonic biopsy samples. The combination of intraepithelial lymphocytosis, neutrophilic inflammation, and crypt cell apoptosis should prompt careful review of the patient's medication history.

References: [39–44]

19. Which features help distinguish gastrointestinal graft-versus-host disease (GVHD) from medication-related injury?

- Acute GVHD is the most common cause of nausea, diarrhea, and anorexia in patients following bone marrow or hematopoietic stem cell transplant. Gastrointestinal sampling is often necessary to distinguish GVHD from infections and medication-related injury that cause similar symptoms. Seminal features of acute gastrointestinal GVHD include crypt epithelial cell apoptosis associated with a paucicellular lamina propria (Fig. 5.11a–d). Severe injury results in crypt destruction and frank ulcers. Endocrine cells are relatively spared and may appear as residual clusters in the lamina propria.
- Induction chemotherapy during the peritransplant period can produce histologic changes that mimic GVHD, including striking crypt cell apoptosis. For this reason, it is nearly impossible to distinguish between gastrointestinal GVHD and therapy-related injury within 21 days of transplant. Medication-related injury can also simulate GVHD after this period. Mycophenolate mofetil inhibits DNA synthesis in both B- and T-lymphocytes; it is commonly used as an immunosuppressant in stem cell transplant recipients. The drug causes crypt epithelial cell apop-

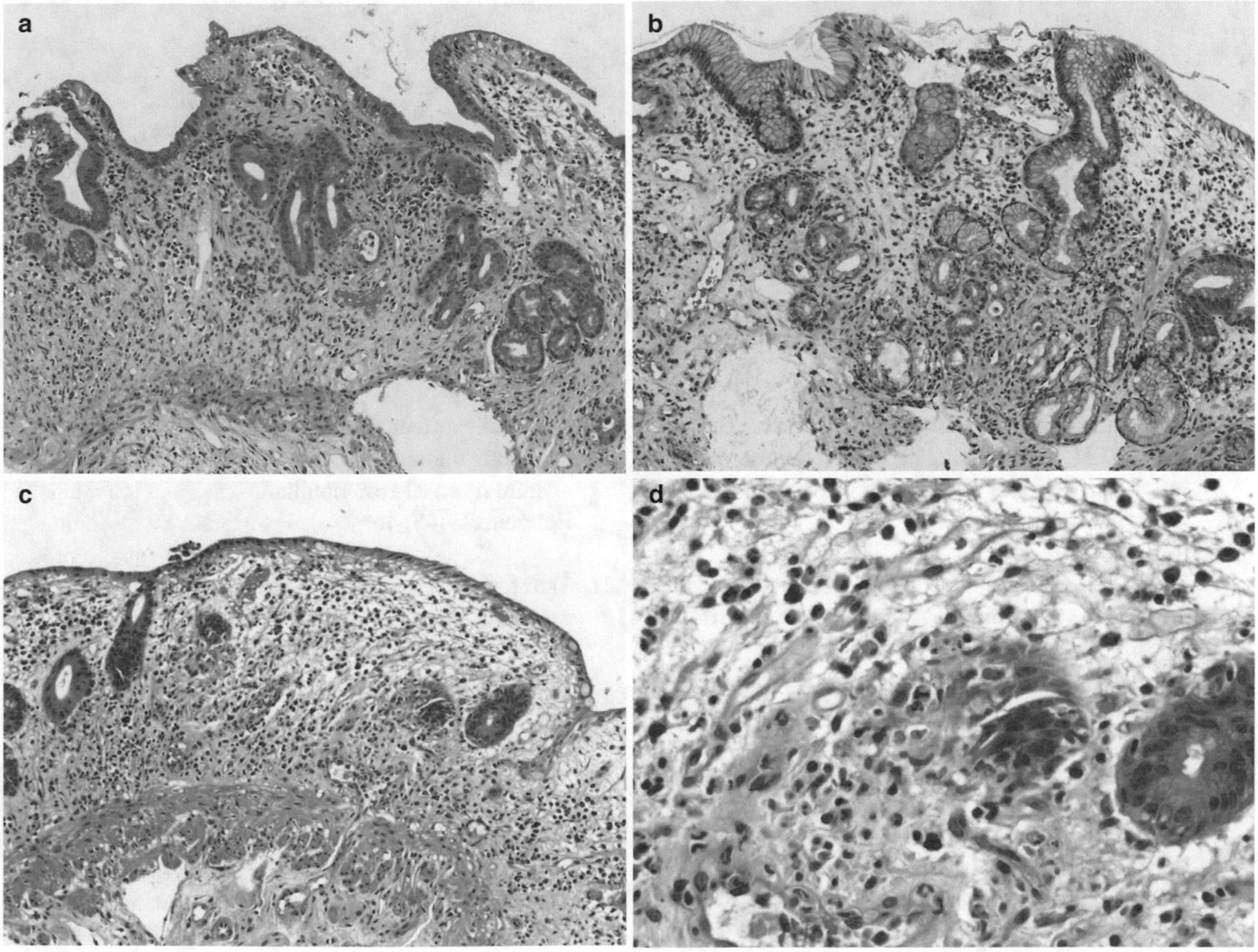

Fig. 5.11 Graft-versus-host disease causes severe crypt injury with apoptotic debris in the duodenum (**a**), as well as scattered necrotic epithelial cells in deep gastric glands (**b**). Severe GVHD manifests with complete or near-complete loss of colonic crypts (**c**) and numerous apoptotic crypt cells (**d**). Note the disproportionately hypocellular lamina propria accompanying destruction of mucosal elements

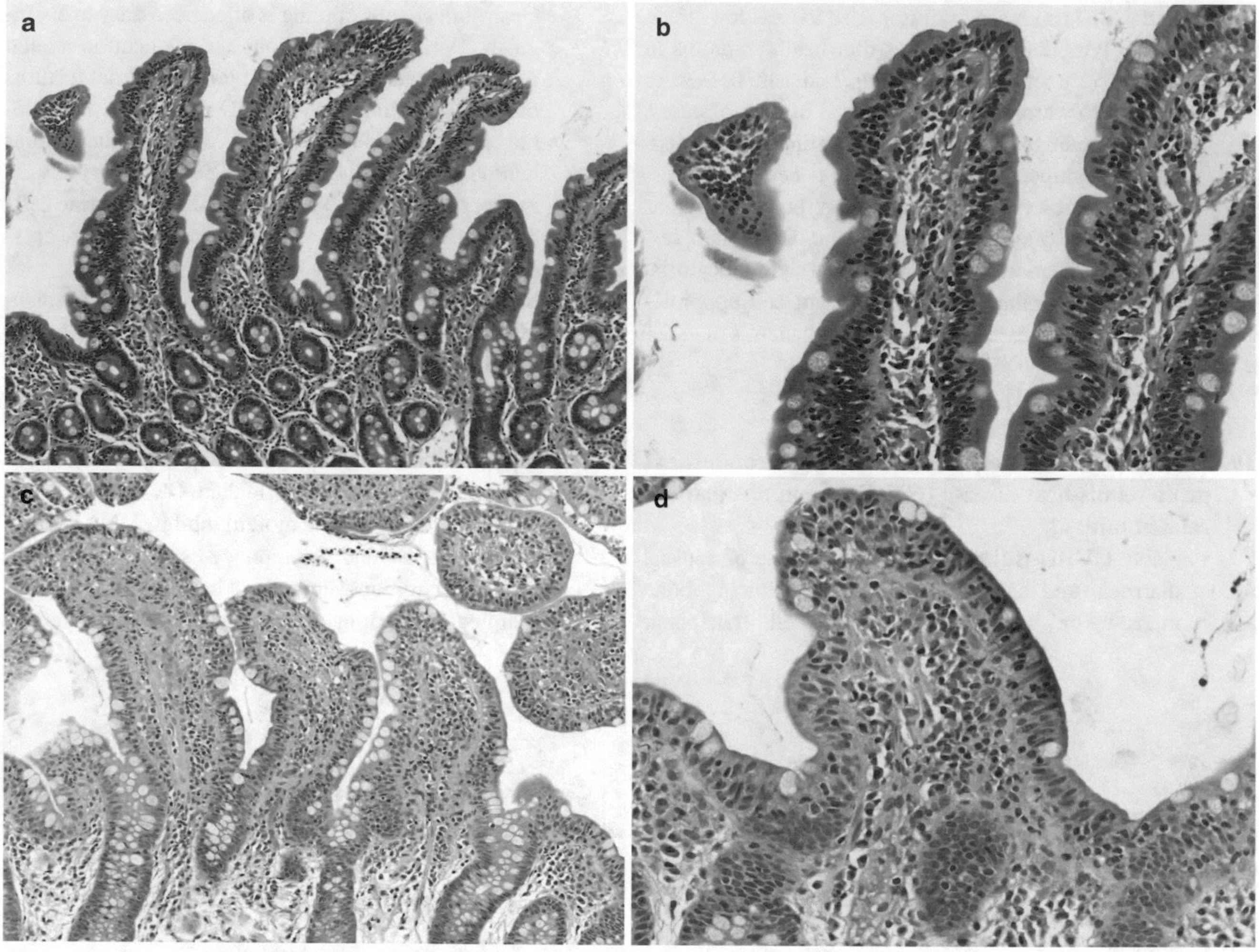

Fig. 5.12 Samples from a patient with tropical sprue show intraepithelial lymphocytosis and normal villous architecture in the duodenum (**a**, **b**); ileal samples display a greater degree of villous blunting (**c**, **d**)

tosis throughout the gastrointestinal tract. In contrast to GVHD, mycophenolate-related injury tends to elicit mucosal eosinophilia and does not spare endocrine cells.

References: [37, 44]

20. Which features should raise suspicion for tropical sprue?

- Tropical sprue is most commonly seen in residents of, and visitors to, tropical regions. Individuals with HLA DQ2/DQ8 haplotypes and those with anti-TTG antibodies are not overrepresented among affected patients. Tropical sprue presumably results from an infection, although no causative organism has been identified. The disease shows a predilection for the distal small bowel, and, thus, patients present with diarrhea and vitamin B12 deficiency. Biopsy samples display intraepithelial lymphocytosis and mild-to-moderate villous blunting that tends to be more severe in the ileum than the duodenum (Fig. 5.12a–d). Complete villous flattening is rare. Tropical sprue may feature mild mucosal eosinophilia.

References: [45, 46]

21. What changes suggest bacterial overgrowth in the small bowel biopsy samples?

- Bacterial overgrowth occurs in patients with impaired gut motility, stricturing Crohn disease, cystic fibrosis, short bowel syndrome, and prior surgical procedures. Alterations in the number and type of bacterial flora result in malabsorptive symptoms. The disorder is under-recognized, particularly among older adults. The diagnosis is established by counting colony-forming units of bacteria in duodenal aspirates. Biopsy findings are nonspecific, showing partial villous blunting and increased inflammation in the lamina propria and surface epithelium (Fig. 5.13a, b). Some patients with symptoms and supportive

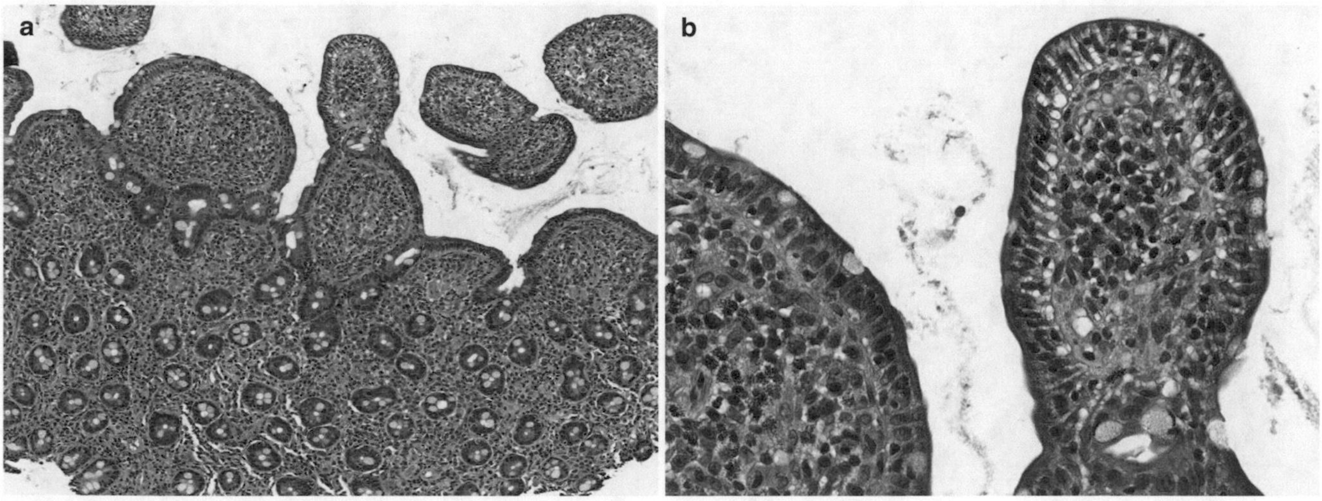

Fig. 5.13 Small-intestinal bacterial overgrowth causes variable villous abnormalities with expansion of the lamina propria by mixed, plasma cell-rich inflammation (**a**). Intraepithelial lymphocytosis is not prominent (**b**)

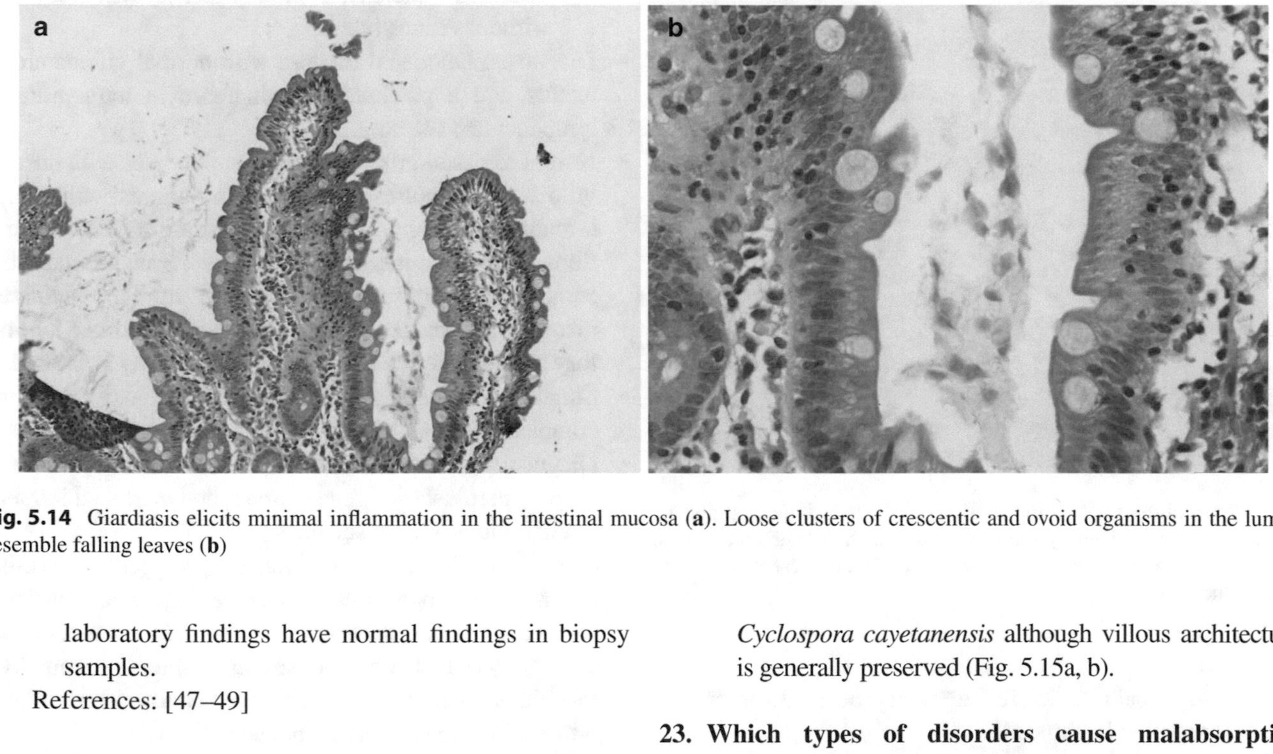

Fig. 5.14 Giardiasis elicits minimal inflammation in the intestinal mucosa (**a**). Loose clusters of crescentic and ovoid organisms in the lumen resemble falling leaves (**b**)

laboratory findings have normal findings in biopsy samples.

References: [47–49]

22. Which types of infection cause intraepithelial lymphocytosis?

- A variety of infectious organisms can cause intraepithelial lymphocytosis in duodenal samples, usually in combination with minimal villous architectural abnormalities. Intraepithelial lymphocytes are mildly increased in the duodenal bulb of patients with *H. pylori*-associated gastritis. Lymphocytosis may be patchy, or absent, in patients with giardiasis (Fig. 5.14a, b). A greater degree of intraepithelial lymphocytosis accompanies infection with *Cryptosporidium*, *Microsporidia*, *Cystoisospora* (*Isospora*), and *Cyclospora cayetanensis* although villous architecture is generally preserved (Fig. 5.15a, b).

23. Which types of disorders cause malabsorptive symptoms in pediatric patients?

- Multiple disorders can cause malabsorptive symptoms in pediatric patients. Inflammatory conditions include celiac disease, autoimmune enteropathy, CVID, and Crohn disease, the features of which have been previously described. Although a number of genetic disorders cause malabsorptive symptoms in this population, only a handful can be diagnosed based upon histologic evaluation. These include abetalipoproteinemia, microvillus inclusion disease, enteroendocrine cell dysgenesis, and tufting enteropathy (Fig. 5.16). A summary of the salient

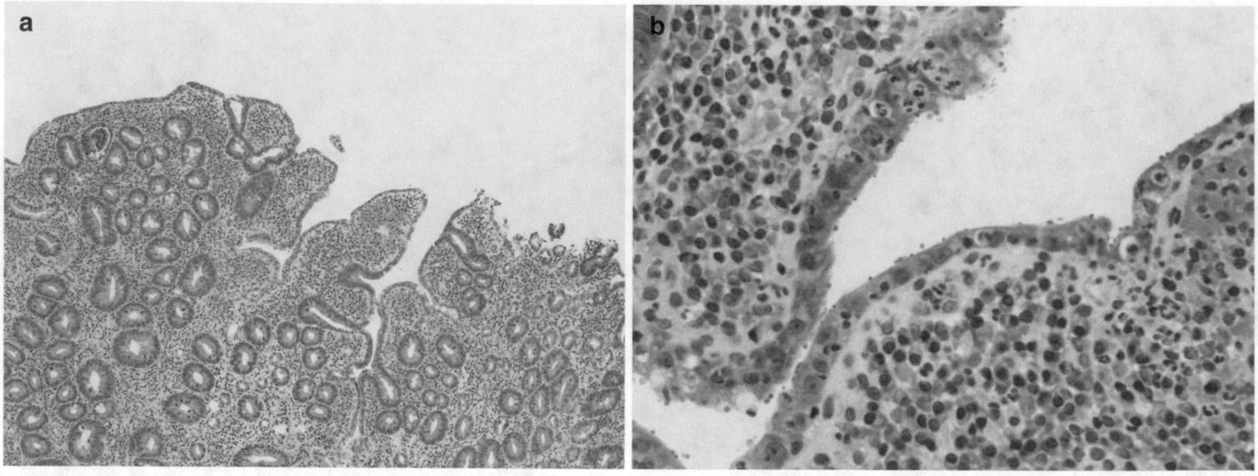

Fig. 5.15 Infection by *Cryptosporidium* causes villous architectural abnormalities and increased lamina propria inflammation (**a**). The surface epithelium contains lymphocytes and granulocytes. Scattered round, basophilic organisms are present at the surface (**b**)

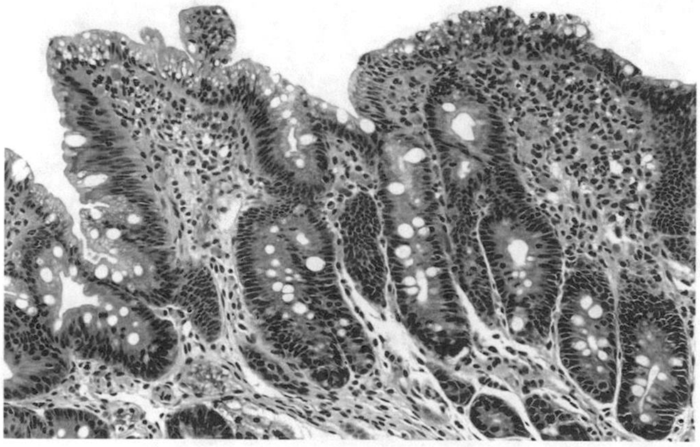

Fig. 5.16 Tufting enteropathy results in villous architectural abnormalities unaccompanied by intraepithelial lymphocytosis and lamina propria inflammation. Characteristic tufts of cells are present in the surface epithelium

clinicopathologic features of these disorders is presented in Table 5.3.

24. **How should I sign out small bowel biopsy cases that show a malabsorptive pattern?**
    - Given the broad differential diagnosis of a malabsorptive histologic pattern, pathologic reporting of duodenal biopsy samples should be tailored to clinical scenarios in the context of serologic and other laboratory data. Unfortunately, adequate information is not always available. In these situations, descriptive diagnoses with comments regarding clinical possibilities may be considered as described below.
      - Situation: Increased intraepithelial lymphocytosis without villous blunting.
    - Diagnosis: Duodenal mucosa with normal villous architecture and a patchy/diffuse increase in intraepithelial lymphocytes; see note.
    - Note: Increased intraepithelial lymphocytes with normal villous architecture can be seen in patients with symptomatic or asymptomatic celiac disease. Other associations include peptic disease, *H. pylori*-related gastritis, some medications, infections, and immune-mediated disorders. Correlation with serologic and other laboratory studies may be considered as clinically indicated.
    - Situation: Intraepithelial lymphocytosis and partial or complete villous blunting.
    - Diagnosis: Chronic enteritis with villous shortening, crypt hyperplasia and regeneration, and increased intraepithelial lymphocytes; see note.
    - Note: This pattern of injury is strongly suggestive of celiac disease in the appropriate clinical setting. Other considerations include non-gluten protein allergies, immune-mediated injury (e.g., Crohn disease, autoimmune enteropathy), infections, peptic injury, and medications, particularly olmesartan and related compounds.

Case Presentation

Case 1

Learning Objectives

1. To develop a differential diagnosis for a malabsorptive pattern of injury
2. To recognize specific histologic features of immune-mediated enteritis

Table 5.3 Clinicopathologic features of pediatric malabsorption disorders

Disorder	Incidence	Gene mutated	Clinical features	Small bowel histology	Ancillary studies
Abetalipoproteinemia	1:100,000	*MTP* (*MTTP*)	Diarrhea Steatorrhea	Diffuse vacuolization of absorptive enterocytes	Recommend genetic testing Correlate with lipoprotein levels
Microvillus inclusion disease	200 cases reported	*MYO5B*, *STX3*	Secretory diarrhea	Loss of brush border	RAB11A, CD10 (IHC): highlight cytoplasmic inclusions
Tufting enteropathy	1:75,000	*EPCAM*	Severe intractable diarrhea	Tufts of detached enterocytes Villous atrophy Minimal to no inflammation	Absent EPCAM expression
Enteroendocrine cell dysgenesis	3 reported cases	*NEUROG3*	Diarrhea Insulin-dependent diabetes	Absence of endocrine cells Villous atrophy with minimal inflammation	Loss of chromogranin A staining

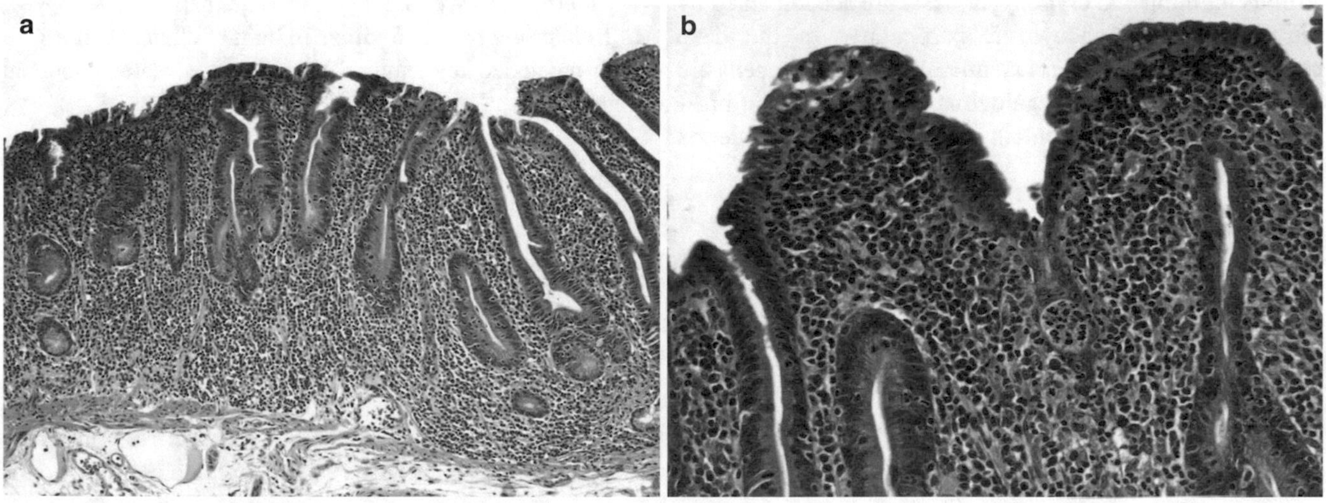

Fig. 5.17 (case 1). The duodenal sample shows increased plasma cell-rich lamina propria inflammation with marked villous blunting. Goblet cells and Paneth cells are conspicuously absent (**a**, **b**)

3. To learn to recognize abnormal features in biopsy samples as well as the absence of findings that should be present

Case History

A 4-year-old boy with malabsorptive diarrhea and failure to thrive underwent upper endoscopic examination and duodenal sampling.

Histologic Findings

Duodenal samples display marked villous blunting with dense plasma cell-rich inflammation in the lamina propria. Neutrophilic cryptitis is prominent. Goblet cells and Paneth cells are conspicuously absent (Fig. 5.17a, b).

Differential Diagnosis

- Celiac disease
- Autoimmune enteropathy
- Crohn disease
- Common variable immunodeficiency

Final Diagnosis

Autoimmune enteropathy.

Take-Home Messages

Severe malabsorptive diarrhea requiring hospitalization does not occur among patients with celiac disease and should prompt consideration of other entities. Villous blunting resulting from celiac disease is always accompanied by intraepithelial lymphocytosis, which is not a striking feature of this case. Crohn disease typically affects the upper gastrointestinal tract in a patchy distribution with severe active inflammation, usually in combination with ileal and colonic disease. Prominent lamina propria inflammation is often present in association with CVID but plasma cells are inconspicuous.

Case 2

Learning Objectives

1. To develop a differential diagnosis for malabsorptive pattern of injury
2. To recognize features suggesting CVID in biopsy samples

Case History

A young girl with diarrhea underwent endoscopy with duodenal sampling.

Histologic Findings

Villous blunting and crypt hyperplasia are accompanied by intraepithelial lymphocytosis, particularly in the deep crypts. The lamina propria is inflamed but plasma cells are inconspicuous. A cytomegalovirus inclusion is also present. Several crypts contain apoptotic luminal debris (Fig. 5.18a, b).

Differential Diagnosis

- Crohn disease
- Autoimmune enteropathy
- Celiac disease
- Common variable immunodeficiency

Final Diagnosis

Common variable immunodeficiency.

Take-Home Message

CVID can cause villous blunting, crypt hyperplasia, and increased intraepithelial lymphocytosis. Unlike celiac disease, however, lymphocytosis is more prominent in the deep crypts and accompanied by conspicuous epithelial cell apoptotic debris and infiltrating neutrophils. Plasma cells are decreased in number or absent, despite the presence of lamina propria infiltrates containing other cell types. Granulomata may be present, particularly in association with ruptured crypts. Lymphoid nodules may be large and multiple. Patients with CVID are prone to a variety of infections, especially CMV and giardiasis.

Case 3

Learning Objectives

1. To develop a differential diagnosis for the malabsorptive pattern in biopsy samples from older patients
2. To interpret biopsy findings in light of clinical history
3. To recognize key features of medication-related duodenal injury

Case History

An 80-year-old female presented with several months of progressively severe malabsorptive diarrhea requiring multiple hospitalizations. Upper endoscopic examination revealed villous flattening. Serologic studies demonstrated an absence of anti-TTG antibodies.

Histologic Findings

The duodenum displays a malabsorptive pattern of injury with intraepithelial lymphocytosis and villous blunting (Fig. 5.19).

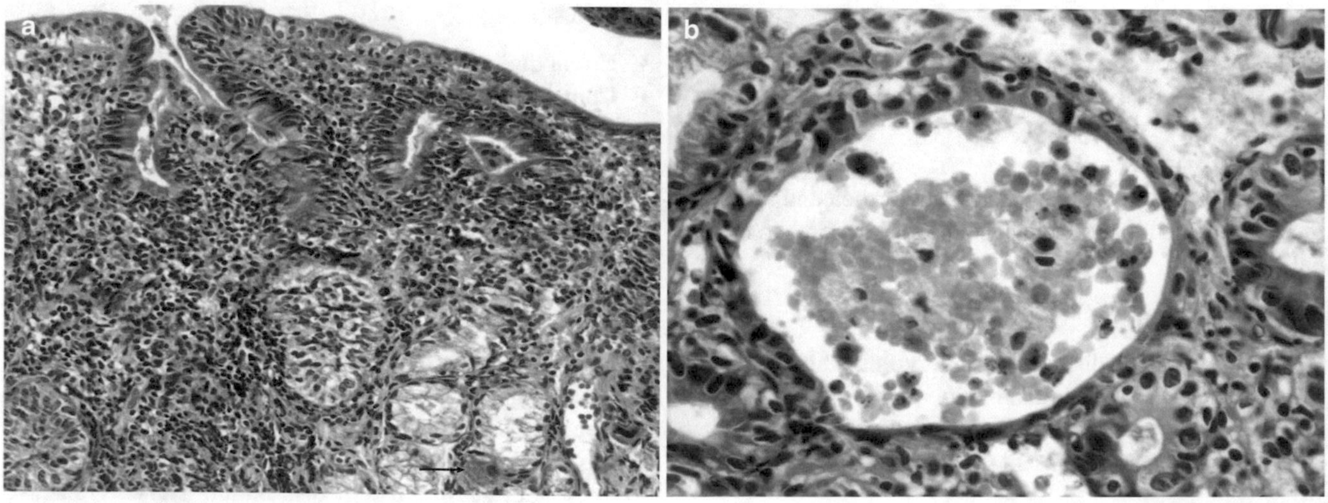

Fig. 5.18 (case 2). A duodenal biopsy shows diffusely flattened villi with intraepithelial lymphocytes that are more numerous in the crypts than surface epithelium, as well as a cytomegalovirus inclusion (bottom right, arrow) in a Brunner gland (**a**). Severe crypt injury with apoptotic luminal debris is associated with increased lamina propria cellularity but plasma cells are lacking (**b**)

Differential Diagnosis

- Celiac disease
- Medication-associated enteropathy
- Autoimmune enteropathy
- CVID

Case History, Continued

Review of the past medical history revealed long-standing hypertension. The patient had been treated with telmisartan, an angiotensin receptor blocker.

Final Diagnosis

Medication (sartan)-associated enteropathy.

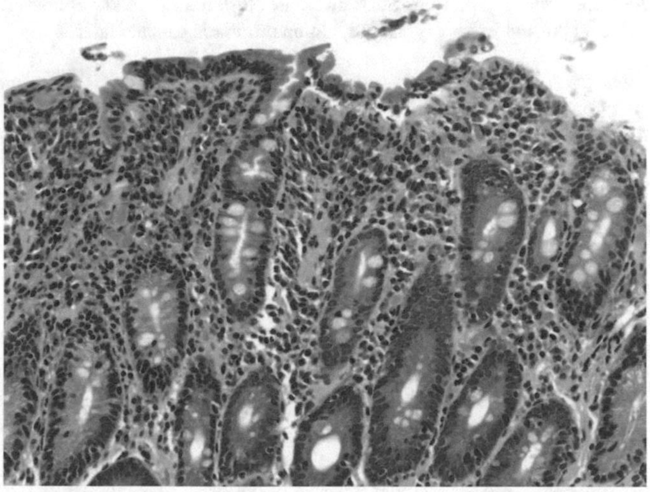

Fig. 5.19 (case 3). A duodenal sample shows complete villous flattening accompanied by intraepithelial lymphocytosis and lamina propria plasmacytosis

Take-Home Messages

Older patients are likely to have comorbidities that require pharmacologic therapy. Hypertension is quite common in this population, and many patients are managed with angiotensin receptor blockers due to their high efficacy. These agents can cause severe enteritis with malabsorptive symptoms months to years after initiation of treatment. Importantly, new-onset celiac disease is uncommon among older individuals, and it rarely causes symptoms serious enough to require hospitalization.

Case 4

Learning Objectives

1. To develop a differential diagnosis for malabsorption in pediatric patients
2. To recognize specific histologic features of abetalipoproteinemia
3. To formulate differential diagnosis for cytoplasmic vacuolization in intestinal epithelial cells

Case History

A 1-year-old female with end-stage renal disease, malnutrition, and failure to thrive underwent upper and lower endoscopic examination, which revealed normal findings. Serologic studies revealed negative anti-TTG and anti-endomysial antibodies and normal immunoglobulin levels. Subsequent testing on this patient revealed normal cholesterol and LDL levels.

Histologic Findings

The superficial intestinal epithelial cells show vacuolization without inflammation (Fig. 5.20a, b).

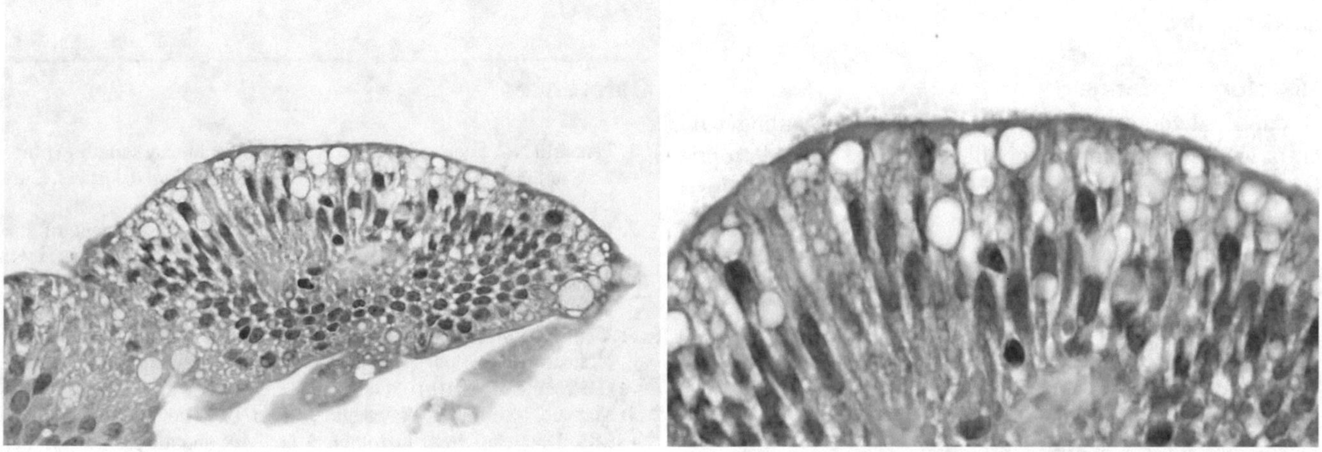

Fig. 5.20 (case 4). Enterocytes contain multiple bubbly cytoplasmic vacuoles unaccompanied by inflammation (**a**, **b**)

Differential Diagnosis
- Abetalipoproteinemia
- Fatty meal
- Malnutrition
- Microvillus inclusion disease

Final Diagnosis
Malnutrition.

Take-Home Message
Enterocyte vacuolization is not specific and can be present in biopsy samples from patients with abetalipoproteinemia, hypobetalipoproteinemia, Anderson disease (chylomicron retention disease), malnutrition and after a fatty meal. The diagnosis of a lipid malabsorption disorder requires correlation between histologic and clinical findings; the presence of normal cholesterol and LDL levels exclude such entities in this case. Microvillus inclusion disease causes variable villous blunting and an absence of the brush border.

Case 5

Learning Objectives
1. To develop a differential diagnosis for severe duodenal injury with crypt destruction
2. To distinguish between GVHD and mycophenolate mofetil
3. To develop a differential diagnosis for prominent epithelial cell apoptosis in the gastrointestinal tract

Case History
A 43-year-old woman with a history of diffuse large B-cell lymphoma presented with diarrhea 2 months after a matched related donor stem cell transplant. Endoscopic examination of the upper gastrointestinal tract revealed erythematous duodenopathy.

Histologic Findings
A duodenal biopsy sample displays villous blunting with crypt loss and apoptotic epithelial cells. The lamina propria is paucicellular and there is no intraepithelial lymphocytosis (Fig. 5.21). No viral cytopathic changes are identified. Immunohistochemical stains for adenovirus and cytomegalovirus are negative.

Differential Diagnosis
- Graft-versus-host disease
- CMV colitis
- Mycophenolate mofetil-associated injury
- Autoimmune enteropathy

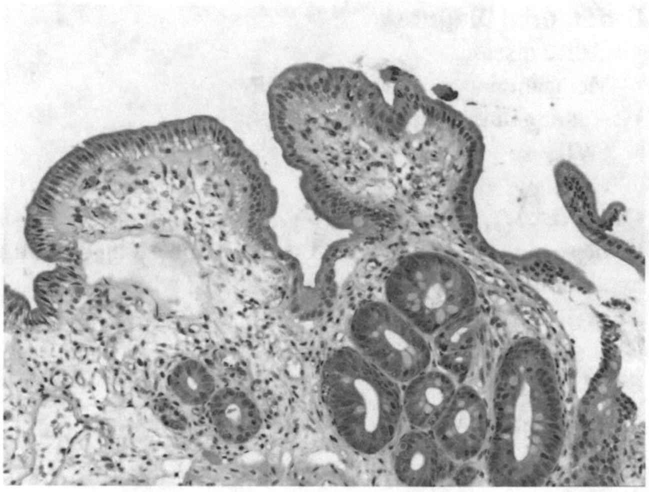

Fig. 5.21 (case 5). A duodenal biopsy shows villous blunting with crypt loss and mucin depletion. Scattered and clustered apoptotic epithelial cells are present in the crypts; the lamina propria is paucicellular

Case History, Continued
A review of the patient's medication reveals that the patient received tacrolimus without any other immunomodulatory therapy.

Final Diagnosis
Graft-versus-host disease.

Take-Home Message
Histologic features of GVHD include apoptotic crypt epithelial cells and crypt destruction with relative preservation of endocrine cells. The lamina propria is often normocellular or shows slightly increased cellularity. Viral infection can cause similar changes, and thus, immunohistochemical stains should be considered in the evaluation of transplant patients with new-onset diarrheal symptoms. Mycophenolate-related injury simulates the features of GVHD but often shows increased mucosal inflammation with eosinophils.

References

1. Panarelli NC, Yantiss RK. The importance of biopsy sampling practices in the pathologic evaluation of gastrointestinal disorders. Curr Opin Gastroenterol. 2016;32(5):374–81.
2. Prasad KK, Thapa BR, Nain CK, Singh K. Assessment of the diagnostic value of duodenal bulb histology in patients with celiac disease, using multiple biopsy sites. J Clin Gastroenterol. 2009;43(4):307–11.
3. Weir DC, Glickman JN, Roiff T, Valim C, Leichtner AM. Variability of histopathological changes in childhood celiac disease. Am J Gastroenterol. 2010;105(1):207–12.
4. Mansfield-Smith S, Savalagi V, Rao N, Thomson M, Cohen MC. Duodenal bulb histological analysis should be standard of care when evaluating celiac disease in children. Pediatr Dev Pathol. 2014;17(5):339–43.

5. Caruso R, Marafini I, Del Vecchio Blanco G, Fina D, Paoluzi OA, Colantoni A, et al. Sampling of proximal and distal duodenal biopsies in the diagnosis and monitoring of celiac disease. Dig Liver Dis. 2014;46(4):323–9.
6. Robert ME, Crowe SE, Burgart L, Yantiss RK, Lebwohl B, Greenson JK, et al. Statement on best practices in the use of pathology as a diagnostic tool for celiac disease: a guide for clinicians and pathologists. Am J Surg Pathol. 2018;42:e44.
7. Bell WC, Young ES, Billings PE, Grizzle WE. The efficient operation of the surgical pathology gross room. Biotech Histochem. 2008;83(2):71–82.
8. Smyrk TC. Practical approach to the flattened duodenal biopsy. Surg Pathol Clin. 2017;10(4):823–39.
9. Fasano A, Berti I, Gerarduzzi T, Not T, Colletti RB, Drago S, et al. Prevalence of celiac disease in at-risk and not-at-risk groups in the United States: a large multicenter study. Arch Intern Med. 2003;163(3):286–92.
10. Fasano A, Catassi C. Clinical practice. Celiac disease. N Engl J Med. 2012;367(25):2419–26.
11. Bouziat R, Hinterleitner R, Brown JJ, Stencel-Baerenwald JE, Ikizler M, Mayassi T, et al. Reovirus infection triggers inflammatory responses to dietary antigens and development of celiac disease. Science. 2017;356(6333):44–50.
12. Thawani SP, Brannagan TH 3rd, Lebwohl B, Green PH, Ludvigsson JF. Risk of neuropathy among 28,232 patients with biopsy-verified celiac disease. JAMA Neurol. 2015;72(7):806–11.
13. Leonard MM, Sapone A, Catassi C, Fasano A. Celiac disease and nonceliac gluten sensitivity: a review. JAMA. 2017;318(7):647–56.
14. Corazza GR, Villanacci V, Zambelli C, Milione M, Luinetti O, Vindigni C, et al. Comparison of the interobserver reproducibility with different histologic criteria used in celiac disease. Clin Gastroenterol Hepatol. 2007;5(7):838–43.
15. Oberhuber G, Granditsch G, Vogelsang H. The histopathology of coeliac disease: time for a standardized report scheme for pathologists. Eur J Gastroenterol Hepatol. 1999;11(10):1185–94.
16. Dickson BC, Streutker CJ, Chetty R. Coeliac disease: an update for pathologists. J Clin Pathol. 2006;59(10):1008–16.
17. Mino M, Lauwers GY. Role of lymphocytic immunophenotyping in the diagnosis of gluten-sensitive enteropathy with preserved villous architecture. Am J Surg Pathol. 2003;27(9):1237–42.
18. Hudacko R, Kathy Zhou X, Yantiss RK. Immunohistochemical stains for CD3 and CD8 do not improve detection of gluten-sensitive enteropathy in duodenal biopsies. Mod Pathol. 2013;26(9):1241–5.
19. Rishi AR, Rubio-Tapia A, Murray JA. Refractory celiac disease. Expert Rev Gastroenterol Hepatol. 2016;10(4):537–46.
20. Malamut G, Verkarre V, Suarez F, Viallard JF, Lascaux AS, Cosnes J, et al. The enteropathy associated with common variable immunodeficiency: the delineated frontiers with celiac disease. Am J Gastroenterol. 2010;105(10):2262–75.
21. Celli R, Hui P, Triscott H, Bogardus S, Gibson J, Hwang M, et al. Clinical insignficance of monoclonal T-cell populations and duodenal intraepithelial T-cell phenotypes in celiac and nonceliac patients. Am J Surg Pathol. 2019;43(2):151–60.
22. Delabie J, Holte H, Vose JM, Ullrich F, Jaffe ES, Savage KJ, et al. Enteropathy-associated T-cell lymphoma: clinical and histological findings from the international peripheral T-cell lymphoma project. Blood. 2011;118(1):148–55.
23. Ondrejka S, Jagadeesh D. Enteropathy-associated T-cell lymphoma. Curr Hematol Malig Rep. 2016;11(6):504–13.
24. Foukas PG, de Leval L. Recent advances in intestinal lymphomas. Histopathology. 2015;66(1):112–36.
25. Vakiani E, Arguelles-Grande C, Mansukhani MM, Lewis SK, Rotterdam H, Green PH, et al. Collagenous sprue is not always associated with dismal outcomes: a clinicopathological study of 19 patients. Mod Pathol. 2010;23(1):12–26.
26. Lan N, Shen B, Yuan L, Liu X. Comparison of clinical features, treatment, and outcomes of collagenous sprue, celiac disease, and collagenous colitis. J Gastroenterol Hepatol. 2017;32(1):120–7.
27. Patterson ER, Shmidt E, Oxentenko AS, Enders FT, Smyrk TC. Normal villous architecture with increased intraepithelial lymphocytes: a duodenal manifestation of Crohn disease. Am J Clin Pathol. 2015;143(3):445–50.
28. Montalto M, D'Onofrio F, Santoro L, Gallo A, Gasbarrini A, Gasbarrini G. Autoimmune enteropathy in children and adults. Scand J Gastroenterol. 2009;44(9):1029–36.
29. Pilarski R, Burt R, Kohlman W, Pho L, Shannon KM, Swisher E. Cowden syndrome and the PTEN hamartoma tumor syndrome: systematic review and revised diagnostic criteria. J Natl Cancer Inst. 2013;105(21):1607–16.
30. Walker-Smith JA, Unsworth DJ, Hutchins P, Phillips AD, Holborow EJ. Autoantibodies against gut epithelium in child with small-intestinal enteropathy. Lancet. 1982;1(8271):566–7.
31. Kobayashi I, Imamura K, Kubota M, Ishikawa S, Yamada M, Tonoki H, et al. Identification of an autoimmune enteropathy-related 75-kilodalton antigen. Gastroenterology. 1999;117(4):823–30.
32. Akram S, Murray JA, Pardi DS, Alexander GL, Schaffner JA, Russo PA, et al. Adult autoimmune enteropathy: Mayo Clinic Rochester experience. Clin Gastroenterol Hepatol. 2007;5(11):1282–90; quiz 1245.
33. Masia R, Peyton S, Lauwers GY, Brown I. Gastrointestinal biopsy findings of autoimmune enteropathy: a review of 25 cases. Am J Surg Pathol. 2014;38(10):1319–29.
34. Patey-Mariaud de Serre N, Canioni D, Ganousse S, Rieux-Laucat F, Goulet O, Ruemmele F, et al. Digestive histopathological presentation of IPEX syndrome. Mod Pathol. 2009;22(1):95–102.
35. Goebel EA, Walsh JC. Heterotopic bone in the distal esophagus. Int J Surg Pathol. 2016;24(5):427.
36. Gushima R, Narita R, Shono T, Naoe H, Yao T, Sasaki Y. Esophageal adenocarcinoma with enteroblastic differentiation arising in ectopic gastric mucosa in the cervical esophagus: a case report and literature review. J Gastrointestin Liver Dis. 2017;26(2):193–7.
37. Sicherer SH, Winkelstein JA. Primary immunodeficiency diseases in adults. JAMA. 1998;279(1):58–61.
38. Park A, Lee JH, Park A, Jung YH, Chu HJ, Bae SS, et al. Prevalence rate and clinical characteristics of esophageal ectopic sebaceous glands in asymptomatic health screen examinees. Dis Esophagus. 2017;30:1):1–5.
39. Rubio-Tapia A, Herman ML, Ludvigsson JF, Kelly DG, Mangan TF, Wu TT, et al. Severe spruelike enteropathy associated with olmesartan. Mayo Clin Proc. 2012;87(8):732–8.
40. Hsieh H, Frenette A, Michaud L, Krishnan U, Dal-Soglio DB, Gottrand F, et al. Intestinal metaplasia of the esophagus in children with esophageal atresia. J Pediatr Gastroenterol Nutr. 2017;65(1):e1–4.
41. Leon F, Olivencia P, Rodriguez-Pena R, Sanchez L, Redondo C, Alvarez I, et al. Clinical and immunological features of adult-onset generalized autoimmune gut disorder. Am J Gastroenterol. 2004;99(8):1563–71.
42. Oble DA, Mino-Kenudson M, Goldsmith J, Hodi FS, Seliem RM, Dranoff G, et al. Alpha-CTLA-4 mAb-associated panenteritis: a histologic and immunohistochemical analysis. Am J Surg Pathol. 2008;32(8):1130–7.
43. Louie CY, DiMaio MA, Matsukuma KE, Coutre SE, Berry GJ, Longacre TA. Idelalisib-associated enterocolitis: clinicopathologic features and distinction from other enterocolitides. Am J Surg Pathol. 2015;39(12):1653–60.
44. Weidner AS, Panarelli NC, Geyer JT, Bhavsar EB, Furman RR, Leonard JP, et al. Idelalisib-associated colitis: histologic findings in 14 patients. Am J Surg Pathol. 2015;39(12):1661–7.

45. Peitz U, Vieth M, Evert M, Arand J, Roessner A, Malfertheiner P. The prevalence of gastric heterotopia of the proximal esophagus is underestimated, but preneoplasia is rare – correlation with Barrett's esophagus. BMC Gastroenterol. 2017;17(1):87. https://doi.org/10.1186/s12876-017-0644-3.
46. Brown IS, Bettington A, Bettington M, Rosty C. Tropical sprue: revisiting an underrecognized disease. Am J Surg Pathol. 2014;38(5):666–72.
47. Lappinga PJ, Abraham SC, Murray JA, Vetter EA, Patel R, Wu TT. Small intestinal bacterial overgrowth: histopathologic features and clinical correlates in an underrecognized entity. Arch Pathol Lab Med. 2010;134(2):264–70.
48. Greenson JK. The biopsy pathology of non-coeliac enteropathy. Histopathology. 2015;66(1):29–36.
49. Elphick HL, Elphick DA, Sanders DS. Small bowel bacterial overgrowth. An underrecognized cause of malnutrition in older adults. Geriatrics. 2006;61(9):21–6.

Inflammatory Bowel Disease

6

Wenqing Cao and Noam Harpaz

List of Frequently Asked Questions

1. What are the characteristic pathologic features of chronic ulcerative colitis in resection specimens?
2. What are the characteristic pathologic features of Crohn colitis in resection specimens?
3. What are common pitfalls in the differential diagnosis between ulcerative and Crohn colitis in resection specimens?
4. When should one render a diagnosis of indeterminate colitis and what are the clinical implications?
5. What are the characteristic histological features of chronic IBD in biopsies?
6. What histological features are most useful in discriminating between ulcerative and Crohn colitis in biopsies and what potential pitfalls should be avoided?
7. How is infectious colitis distinguished from IBD in mucosal biopsies?
8. What drugs and other toxic agents might mimic IBD in colorectal biopsies?
9. How does the pathology of pediatric IBD patients differ from that in adults?
10. What is the differential diagnosis of IBD in biopsies?
11. What are the upper GI manifestations of ulcerative colitis and Crohn disease?
12. What are the main complications of ileoanal pouch surgery for IBD?
13. What are the defining histological characteristics of dysplasia in IBD?
14. What is the spectrum of nonadenomatous dysplasia in IBD?
15. How is dysplasia distinguished from reactive epithelial changes in IBD?
16. What is the value of adjunctive markers in distinguishing dysplasia from reactive epithelial changes in IBD?
17. How are sporadic adenomas distinguished from IBD-associated dysplasia?
18. How is a diagnosis of dysplasia integrated into the clinical management of patients with IBD?
19. Are there distinctive pathological features of colorectal carcinoma in IBD?

Frequently Asked Questions

1. What are the characteristic pathologic features of chronic ulcerative colitis in resection specimens?

Ulcerative colitis (UC) is characterized macroscopically by diffuse, continuous, mucosal-based inflammation that involves the rectum, either alone or in continuity with a variable length of the colon in a retrograde fashion. Patients are classified accordingly as having ulcerative proctitis, proctosigmoiditis, left-sided colitis, extensive colitis (i.e., beyond the splenic flexure), or pancolitis. The transition between the diseased distal mucosa and the proximal normal mucosa may appear gradual or abrupt; however, in some cases, a normal-appearing proximal colon belies the presence of more extensive microscopic involvement (Fig. 6.1).

The pathologic manifestations of UC vary depending on the state of disease activity and the cumulative sequella of prior inflammation. Macroscopically, they include petechia, hyperemia, or ulcerations superimposed on structural mucosal changes such atrophy, granularity, nodularity, or inflammatory polyps (Fig. 6.2). Microscopically, the mucosa is characteristically expanded and the lamina propria is densely infiltrated by plasma cells, lymphocytes, and eosinophils. The infiltrates extend from the surface to the basal lamina propria, separating the crypts from one another and often from the muscularis muco-

W. Cao (✉)
New York University Langone Health, New York, NY, USA
e-mail: wenqing.cao@nyulangone.org

N. Harpaz (✉)
Icahn School of Medicine at Mount Sinai, New York, NY, USA

H. L. Wang, Z. E. Chen (eds.), *Practical Gastrointestinal Pathology*, Practical Anatomic Pathology,
https://doi.org/10.1007/978-3-030-51268-2_6

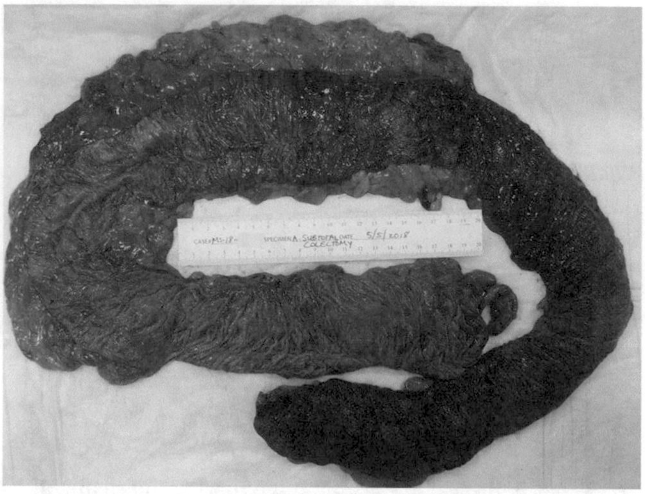

Fig. 6.1 Colectomy specimen showing active ulcerative colitis extending retrograde to the mid-transverse colon. Note the gradual macroscopic transition from the involved to the uninvolved colon

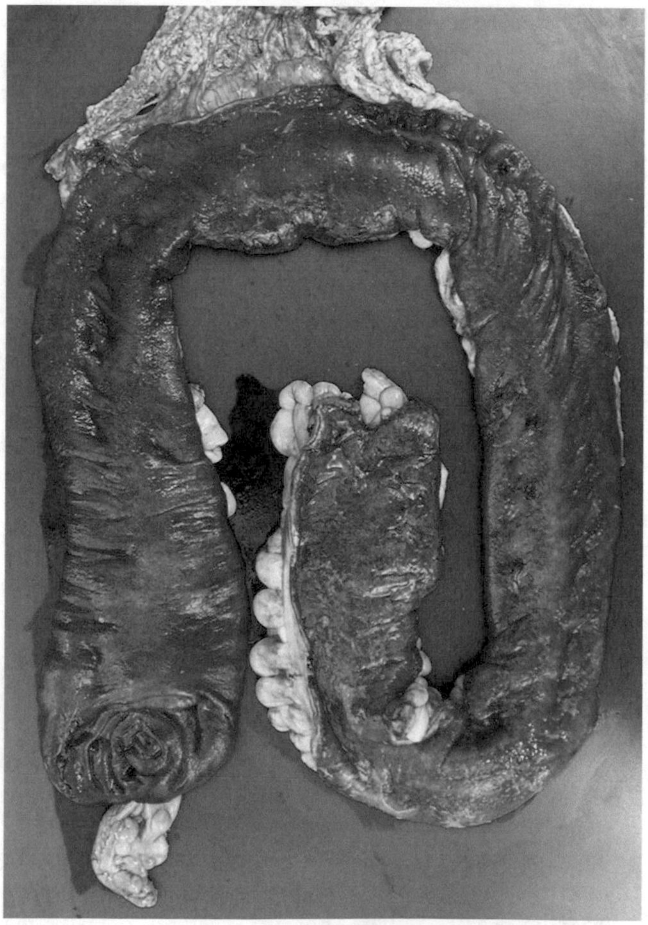

Fig. 6.2 Colectomy specimen showing ulcerative pancolitis featuring diffuse atrophy punctulated by scattered ulcers and inflammatory polyps

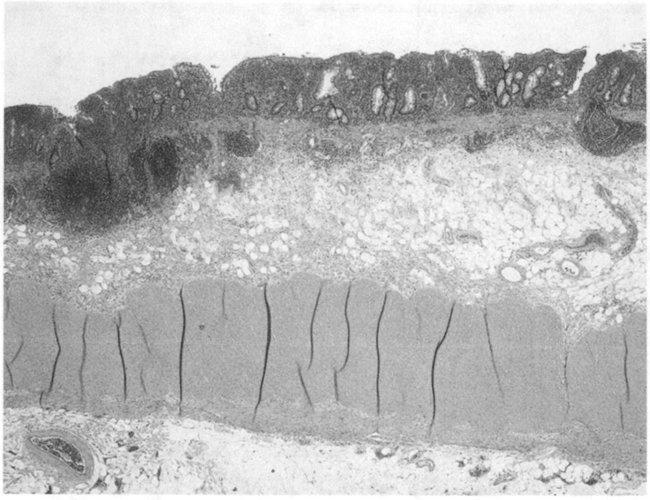

Fig. 6.3 Ulcerative colitis showing diffuse inflammation involving the mucosa and superficial submucosa

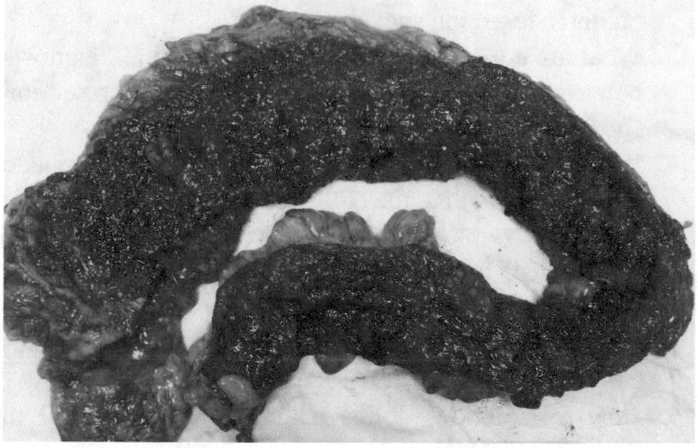

Fig. 6.4 Colectomy specimen showing fulminant ulcerative colitis characterized by extensive ulceration and toxic dilatation of the proximal transverse colon

sae. The mucosal architecture is variably altered, presenting skewed, distorted, and bifurcated crypts (Fig. 6.3). Active disease is characterized by erosions, broad-based ulcers, superficial fissures, cryptitis, neutrophilic crypt abscesses, and damaged crypts. The inflammatory infiltrates are generally limited to the mucosa and superficial submucosa; however, chronic ulcers may be accompanied by underlying regions of intramural and subserosal inflammatory infiltrates. Quiescent colitis is characterized by resolution of the neutrophilic inflammatory infiltrates and diminished lymphoplasmacytosis, but crypt architectural abnormalities resolve slowly if at all.

In fulminant UC, the mucosa is intensely hyperemic and extensively ulcerated or sloughed (Fig. 6.4). It may progress to generalized or segmental dilation culminating in toxic megacolon with thinning of the wall and potential perforation. The transverse colon is affected initially because its superior location in the supine patient permits gas and fluid to accumulate when peristalsis is diminished and its intraperitoneal location permits free expansion. Microscopically, fulminant colitis is characterized by extensively denuded mucosa, penetration of ulcers into the muscularis propria, fissuring ulcers, vascular congestion, and phlegmonous neutrophilic infiltration.

Residual or partially sloughed mucosa and granulation tissue present as inflammatory polyps. They may be widely dispersed or clustered in individual colonic segments and assume diverse shapes, including filiform excrescences, broad-based mounds, or ragged, leaf-like tags.

The colonic wall in UC generally remains thin and pliant even in long-standing disease; however, some patients develop a foreshortened colon with a slightly, but uniformly, thickened wall. Stricturing due to severe localized inflammation is uncommon in UC and should raise concern for an unrecognized tumor or for Crohn disease (CD). References: [1, 2]

2. What are the characteristic pathologic features of Crohn colitis in resection specimens?

The majority of patients with CD have some degree of large intestinal involvement, including isolated colonic involvement in 20–30% and combined ileocolitis in 25–40%. Of these patients, 25–30% have pancolitis and the remainder have segmental disease, usually of the rectum or ileocecal region. Additionally, roughly 1/3 of patients with CD have perianal fistulas, fissures, or abscesses.

The macroscopic hallmarks of Crohn colitis are manifestations of transmural, segmental chronic inflammation (Fig. 6.5). Single or multiple diseased segments occur in any location and are sharply demarcated from adjacent normal segments. In nascent disease, the mucosa features pinpoint aphthous ulcers in a background of normal, edematous, or erythematous mucosa and the wall may show varying degrees of edema. With advancing disease, the ulcers coalesce into larger geographic or longitudinally oriented ulcers, the wall grows increasingly thickened and rigid, and the serosa becomes opacified or encased in creeping fat.

Deep fissuring ulcers, fibrous adhesions, creeping mesenteric fat, fistula tracts, and strictures are all distinctive features of CD (Fig. 6.6). Fusiform strictures occur anywhere, although most frequently in the ileocecal and anorectal regions, and they vary greatly in length. On sectioning the colonic wall, cicatrization obscures or obliterates the mural landmarks and extends into the pericolic fat (Fig. 6.7). As in UC, fulminant Crohn colitis may result in toxic megacolon.

Distinctive patterns of mucosal inflammation in CD include single or multiple parallel longitudinal ulcers with narrow bases ("bear claw" or "garden rake" ulcers) and a cobblestone pattern produced by intersecting longitudinal and transverse ulcers (Fig. 6.8). By contrast, some cases of Crohn colitis resemble UC macroscopically, featuring diffuse inflammation, atrophy, or inflammatory polyposis. Attention to localized thickening or stenosis may suggest the correct diagnosis, but in a subset of cases the distinction from UC depends entirely on histological recognition of Crohn-like characteristics.

Microscopically, colonic segments involved by Crohn colitis are characterized by transmural lymphoid aggregates, chronic inflammatory infiltrates, expansion and

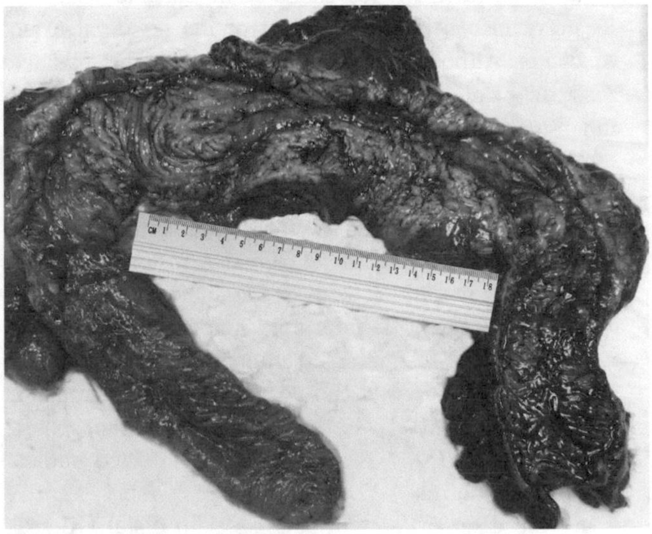

Fig. 6.5 Colonic Crohn disease with massive inflammatory thickening and stricture of the transverse colon

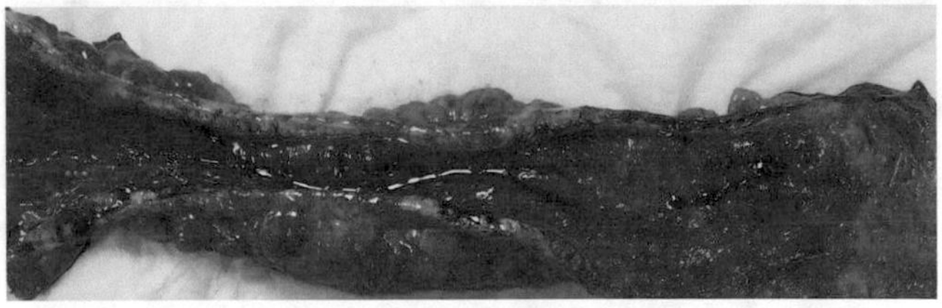

Fig. 6.6 Colonic Crohn disease with stricture resulting from contracture of the colonic wall. Note the corresponding segmental wrapping of mesenteric fat

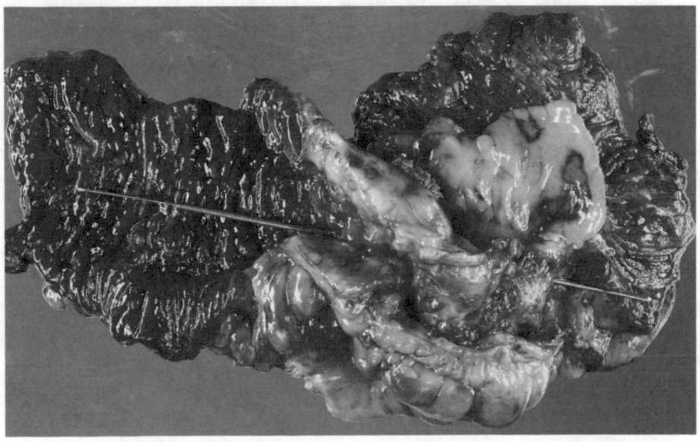

Fig. 6.7 Stricturing Crohn ileocolitis associated with mural thickening, fibrous serosal adhesions, gross deformity, and ileocolic fistula

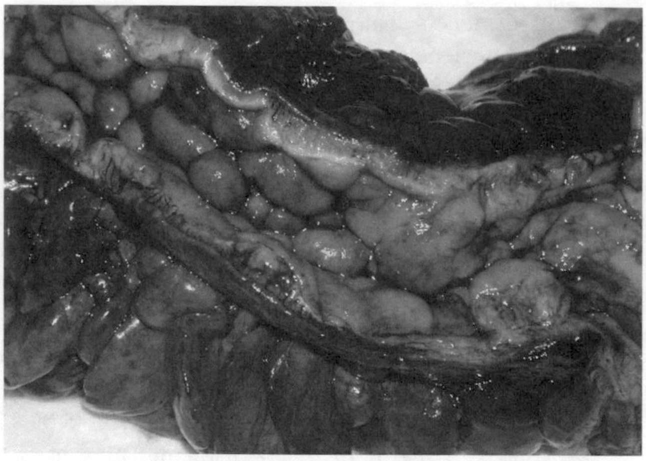

Fig. 6.8 Colonic Crohn disease showing mucosal cobblestoning corresponding to mounds of edematous mucosa surrounded by longitudinally and transversely oriented fissuring ulcers

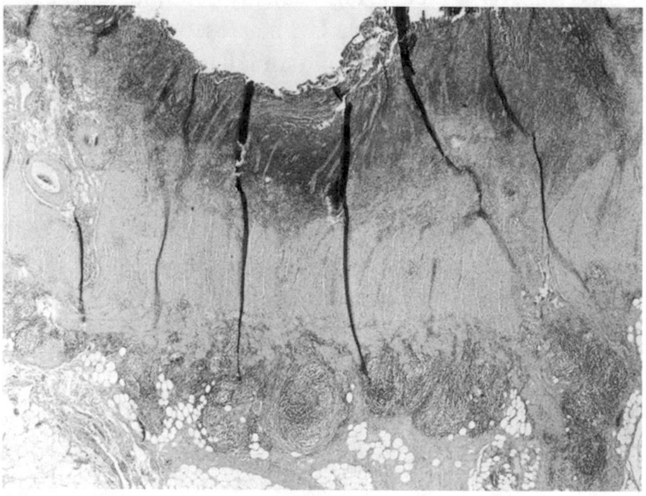

Fig. 6.9 Crohn disease with transmural lymphoid aggregates

splaying of the muscularis mucosae, fibrosis and fatty replacement of the submucosa, neural hypertrophy, deep fissuring ulcers, and fistula tracts (Fig. 6.9). The pericolic fat is fibrotic and chronically inflamed. Nonnecrotizing granulomas occur in approximately 50% of resection specimens and present in all layers of the colonic wall and in the pericolic lymph nodes.

References: [1, 2]

3. **What are common pitfalls in the differential diagnosis between ulcerative and Crohn colitis in resection specimens?**

Rectal Sparing in UC

Rectal involvement is a consistent feature of UC; however, macroscopic inspection may give a false impression of rectal sparing resulting from spontaneous or therapy-induced healing. Rectal sparing does occur, however, in

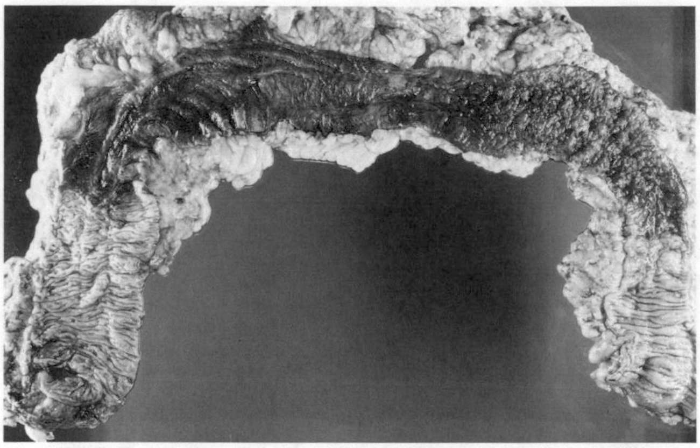

Fig. 6.10 Active ulcerative colitis showing gross sparing of the ascending and distal sigmoid colon. Microscopically, the sigmoid colon was chronically inflamed but the ascending colon was normal. The extent and distribution of inflammatory bowel disease are determined based on the combination of gross and microscopic findings since discrepancies are not uncommon

patients with concomitant primary sclerosing cholangitis (PSC), in whom the colitis often is predominantly right sided and diminishes distally. Rectal sparing or patchy inflammation also occurs frequently in pediatric patients with UC.

Discontinuous Inflammation in UC

Cognizance of exceptions to the typical continuous pattern of inflammation in UC is important to avoid an incorrect diagnosis of CD (Fig. 6.10).

Discontinuous involvement of the cecum, referred to as an isolated cecal patch, occurs in approximately 10% of patients with left-sided or distal UC. The histological characteristics and severity of the cecal inflammation generally mirror those in the remainder of the involved colon.

Ulcerative appendicitis affects 48–85% of nonobliterated appendices in resections from patients with UC, its prevalence being independent of the proximal extent of colitis. Although the appendix appears unremarkable macroscopically, it presents a microscopic mucosal-based inflammation that closely resembles the rest of the colon but remains limited to the mucosa even in severe UC. Unlike Crohn appendicitis, there is no mural expansion, transmural lymphoid aggregates, or granulomas. Endoscopically, the base of the appendicitis in UC often features a tell-tale ring of erythema, which helps distinguish it from CD.

Although patchy microscopic mucosal inflammation is a hallmark of CD, it also occurs at the transition zone between inflamed distal and normal proximal mucosa in UC.

Fulminant Colitis

Severe disease flares in patients with distal UC may result in patches of active inflammation in the previously uninvolved colon, which mimic features of CD

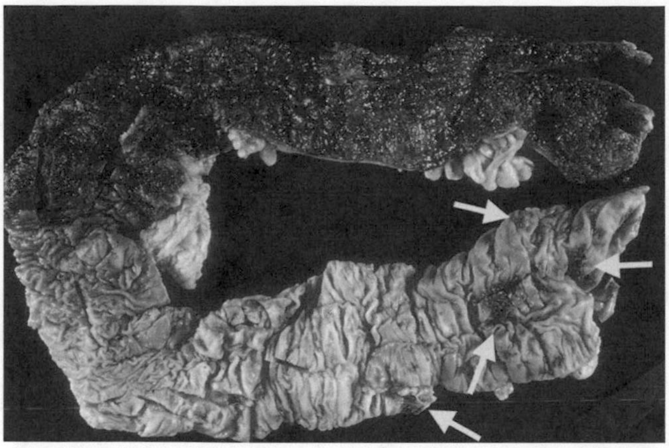

Fig. 6.11 Ulcerative colitis showing discontinuous fulminant colitis. The patient experienced a severe flare, which progressed to fulminant colitis requiring a colectomy. There are multiple foci of discontinuous inflammation in the previously uninvolved proximal colon (arrows)

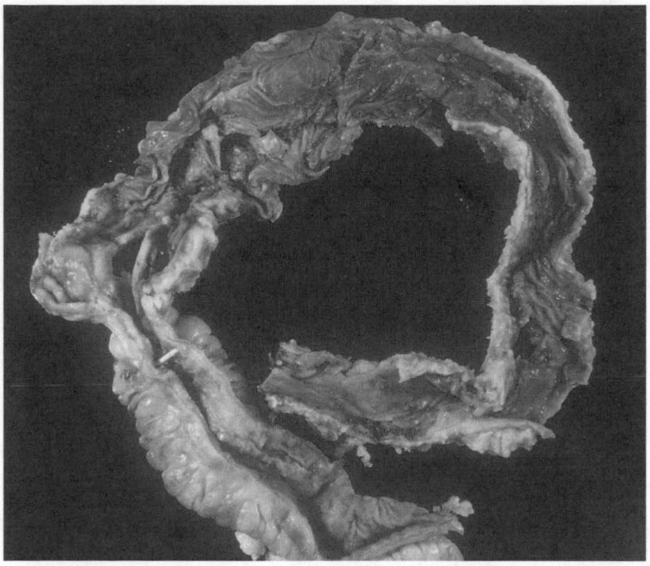

Fig. 6.12 Ileocolic resection with superficial Crohn colitis. The ileal segment exhibits typical features of Crohn ileitis, including fat wrapping and segmental thickening. The colon, in contrast, is thin walled, and the mucosa shows diffuse atrophy

and the severity of which mirrors that of the distal colon (Fig. 6.11). Active UC may also result in superficial fissuring ulcers, which may become deep in fulminant colitis. Their distinction from fissuring ulcers of CD depends on the absence of a granulation tissue lining, recognition of the context of fulminant colitis, and the absence of other classical Crohn features such as granulomas and transmural lymphoid aggregates.

Transmural Inflammation in UC
In UC, the colonic wall directly underlying foci of chronic ulceration may feature deep or even transmural chronic inflammation which is absent beneath the adjoining intact mucosa. Importantly, classical Crohn-like features such as lymphoid aggregates, neural hypertrophy, and lymphatic dilatation are either absent or inconspicuous.

Backwash Ileitis in UC
Backwash ileitis refers to inflammation of a short segment of the distal-most terminal ileum. It affects approximately 10% of resections with pancolitis, mirroring the degree of colonic inflammation in the proximal colon. Unlike Crohn ileitis, it does not result in the thickening of the ileal wall or linear ulceration and does not extend more than a few centimeters proximal to the ileocecal valve.

Granulomas in UC and CD

Although nonnecrotizing granulomas are a hallmark of CD, foreign body granulomas may be elicited by sutures, intraperitoneal contaminants, medications, or parasitic ova. Granulomas may also be associated with lytic crypt abscesses in UC, CD, and other colitides. CD-associated granulomas may contain conchoidal bodies, which are spherical aggregates of basophilic calcium phosphate and refractile crystals of calcium oxalate and are identical to the Schaumann bodies that occur in other systemic granulomatous disorders. They may be mistaken for ova or parasites. Conchoidal bodies are an isolated feature in less than 5% of CD resections but rarely can be numerous.

Superficial Crohn Colitis
Rare patients with CD present with colitis that is diffuse and mucosal based rather than transmural, referred to as superficial or "UC-like" CD (Fig. 6.12). The distinction from UC depends either on the detection of granulomas in sections of the intestinal wall or lymph nodes, which may require numerous histological sections, or on the presence of concomitant Crohn ileitis.

Giant Inflammatory Polyposis
Rarely, segmental agglomerations of inflammatory polyps and entrapped feces in patients with IBD, most frequently UC, may form a tumor-like mass that elicits clinical and radiological signs of stenosis and suspicion of CD or malignancy. Histologically, the underlying colonic wall may contain deep fissures and transmural lymphoid aggregates, reinforcing the impression of CD; however, these are absent in the remainder of the colon. One study of 12 resected cases reported that ten patients were ultimately diagnosed as having UC despite that seven of the ten colectomies had classical Crohn-like transmural inflammation limited to the polyposis segment.
References: [3, 4]

4. **When should one render a diagnosis of indeterminate colitis and what are the clinical implications?**

Indeterminate colitis is diagnosed in up to 15% of colectomy specimens that are pathologically compatible with IBD but resist clear subclassification as UC or CD due to overlapping or ambiguous features. Although the prototype of indeterminate colitis originally referred to fulminant colitis, the term is now applied in a variety of other circumstances where the pattern of inflammation deviates from the classical rules, whether spontaneously or as a result of therapy. For example, the colon may contain foci of transmural chronic inflammation beneath intact mucosa, but the absence of other classical features of CD, such as follicular lymphoid inflammation, neural hypertrophy, or granulomas, might be attributable to incomplete healing of severe UC. Long-standing refractory UC may present submucosal lymphoid aggregates, mild neural proliferation, pericolic fibrosis, or relative sparing of the rectum. Segmental interposition of grossly normal mucosa between segments with otherwise classical features of UC (excluding the isolated cecal patch or appendiceal inflammation) could warrant a diagnosis of indeterminate colitis unless subtle evidence of healed UC is found microscopically.

The term indeterminate colitis is applied to resection specimens only. The term "unclassified colitis," in contrast, is applied to biopsies from patients with clinical, endoscopic, and histological evidence of IBD that lack specific features to permit confident subclassification as UC or CD.

The distinction between UC and CD plays a pivotal role in determining whether or not patients will undergo restorative proctocolectomy with construction of a continent ileal pouch since CD carries substantially higher rates of complications and pouch failure. Follow-up studies of patients diagnosed with indeterminate colitis who elected to have pouch surgery report indices of long-term pouch function and quality of life, which are more similar to their counterparts with UC than CD; however, 6–14% experience serious Crohn-like complications such as fistulas or afferent limb strictures, which may require pouch revision or excision. As a result, many surgeons will be reluctant to perform pouch surgery in the setting of indeterminate colitis.

References: [5–9]

5. **What are the characteristic histological features of chronic IBD in biopsies?**

Endoscopic and pathologic assessments of the colorectal mucosa are essential components of the workup and management of patients with IBD. Adequate endoscopic sampling of the colon and rectum is required to avoid potential errors due to sampling variations. For the initial evaluation of patients with IBD, it is suggested that at least two biopsies be taken from the terminal ileum and at least four from the colon and rectum, including both grossly inflamed and normal-appearing mucosae.

The classical histological features of chronic IBD in biopsies include neutrophil infiltration of the crypt and surface epithelium and associated reactive epithelial changes combined with evidence of chronic mucosal damage such as architectural disarray, basal lymphoplasmacytosis, crypt shortfall, and metaplastic Paneth cells or pyloric glands (Fig. 6.13a–c). Assessment of the distribution of microscopic findings within biopsies (focal, segmental, and continuous) and between sites may provide additional information that would help classify chronic IBD.

The passage of time and therapy may result in alterations in histological features and patterns in follow-up biopsies. In histological remission, neutrophils are absent, goblet cell mucin is restored, and lymphoplasmacytic infiltration may be reduced, but abnormal mucosal architecture and metaplastic changes usually persist (Fig. 6.14a). It should be noted that no single histological feature is diagnostic of chronic IBD; rather, a combina-

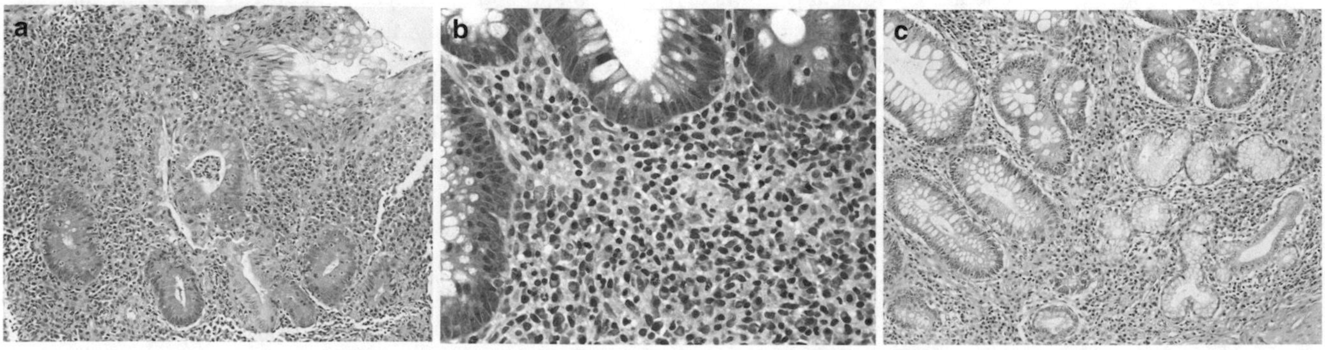

Fig. 6.13 (**a**) The mucosa in inflammatory bowel disease is expanded by a dense lamina propria infiltrate of mononuclear inflammatory cells. The crypts are reduced in number and distributed haphazardly. The crypt epithelium is infiltrated by neutrophils, and goblet cell mucin is markedly reduced. A crypt abscess is seen in the center. Neutrophils in the lamina propria are located mostly in blood vessels. (**b**) Basal lamina propria infiltration by lymphocytes, plasma cells, and eosinophils in a case of Crohn disease. Neutrophils are sparse. A few histiocytes are present in the center, suggestive of a microgranuloma. (**c**) Mildly active Crohn colitis featuring pyloric gland metaplasia

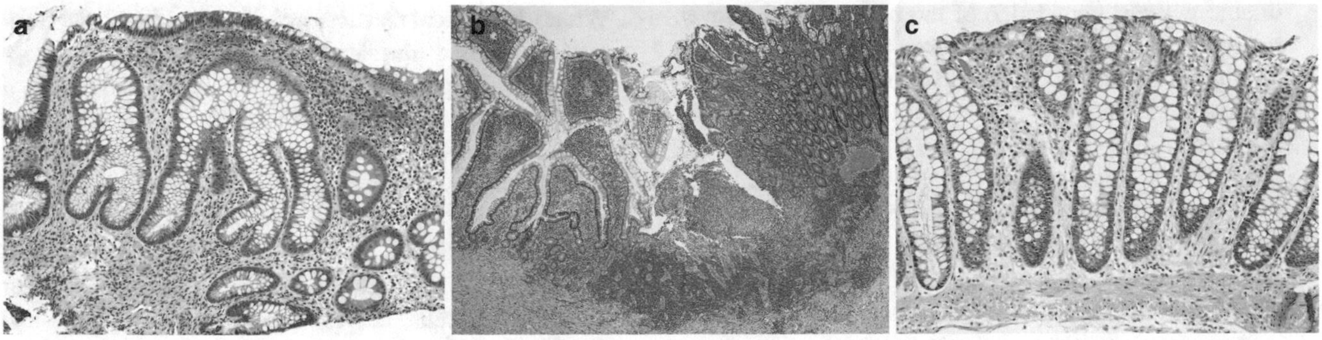

Fig. 6.14 (**a**) Inflammatory bowel disease in remission exhibiting marked crypt architectural distortion. (**b**) Aphthous ulcer in Crohn ileitis characterized by an abrupt mucosal breach filled with acute inflammatory exudate and with underlying lymphoid aggregates. (**c**) Normal colonic mucosa contains parallel crypts of uniform diameter that extend from the surface to the muscularis mucosae and are lined mostly by enterocytes and goblet cells with small basal nuclei. The lamina propria features a top-down gradient of mononuclear inflammatory cells

tion of histological features in conjunction with supportive clinical and endoscopic data is required to reach a definitive diagnosis.

Crypt and Surface Inflammation Active colitis or enterocolitis characterized by cryptitis, crypt abscesses, surface erosions, fissures, or ulcers is commonplace in UC and CD but by no means specific. A more specific feature of IBD is selective neutrophil infiltration of the crypt and surface epithelium combined with relative sparsity of neutrophils within the lamina propria, except areas adjacent to erosions and lysed crypt abscesses (Fig. 6.14b).

Architectural Disarray Normal colorectal crypts are parallel, evenly spaced, uniform in size, and extend from the surface to the muscularis mucosae (Fig. 6.14c). The crypt architecture near the anorectal junction may be irregular. Bifurcated crypts are uncommon except during expansion of the colonic surface area, i.e., in the pediatric age range. Disarray of the crypt architecture occurs in IBD as a result of severe or repeated bouts of inflammatory mucosal injury, producing skewed crypts, branching, budding, and other deviations in shape and size; surface irregularities; and crypt "shortfall," i.e., interposition of fibrous or chronic inflammatory tissue between the crypt bases and the muscularis mucosae. In severe cases, the mucosa becomes dramatically transformed, assuming either a haphazard or villiform appearance on one extreme or an atrophic, pauci-cryptal appearance on the other.

Basal Lymphoplasmacytosis Normal colorectal mucosa includes sparse mononuclear inflammatory cells, most of which are located in the upper third of mucosa, resulting in a top-down inflammatory cell gradient. In chronic inflammatory states, including IBD, the inflammatory cell population becomes dense and expands into the basal region of the lamina propria. Of note, mild basal lymphoplasmacytosis in cecal biopsies is normal.

Mucin Depletion Reduction in the mucin content of goblet cells is a reactive change that is proportionate to the severity of acute inflammation and is therefore a common but nonspecific feature of IBD. Near absence of mucin is characteristic of mucosa during recovery from ulceration. Uniformly reduced surface mucin may also occur in response to bowel preparation.

Granulomas Granulomas in CD range from inconspicuous clusters of a few epithelioid histiocytes, so-called microgranulomas, to compact collections of five or more epithelioid histiocytes, Langhans cells, and intermingled lymphocytes. They occur in 5–20% of biopsies from adult patients and more frequently in children. The differential diagnosis includes granulomatous infections such as lymphogranuloma venereum, tuberculous and nontuberculous mycobacterial colitis, syphilis and parasitoses, and a variety of other systemic granulomatous diseases. The granulomas of CD lack central necrosis or suppurative inflammation, are rarely larger than 0.4 mm, and are usually isolated and discrete rather than confluent. Foreign body granulomas resulting from ruptured crypts (cryptolytic granulomas) can pose a diagnostic pitfall since they occur in UC and other colitides (see question 6). Isolated multinucleated giant cells in the mucosa have no diagnostic significance.

Paneth Cell Metaplasia Paneth cells are a normal constituent of the basal crypts of the small intestinal and proximal colonic mucosa. Paneth cells that occur in mucosa originating beyond the distal transverse colon are considered to be a metaplastic adaptation to chronic mucosal injury and are commonplace in IBD, albeit not specific. The presence of metaplastic Paneth cells in otherwise normal mucosal biopsies is diagnostically useful, providing tell-tale evidence of healed colitis despite histological normalization. The metaplastic cells are usually grouped in their normal basal positions and are not identifiable without knowledge of the biopsy site; however, metaplasia can be recognized even in biopsies from the proximal colon when the Paneth cells are more numerous than usual, are noncontiguous, or proliferate beyond the crypt base.

Pyloric Gland Metaplasia Also referred to as pseudopyloric metaplasia, mucinous gland metaplasia, ulcer-associated cell lineage, and spasmolytic polypeptide-expressing metaplasia, this type of metaplasia is considered to be a ubiquitous response to long-standing chronic mucosal injury in the gastrointestinal tract. Although commonplace in IBD, especially in Crohn enteritis and colitis and in chronic pouchitis, it can occur in UC, in nonsteroidal anti-inflammatory drug (NSAID)-associated colitis, and in other chronic inflammatory disorders.
References: [10–13]

Table 6.1 Characteristic histological features of UC and CD in biopsies

Histological feature	UC	CD
Crypt architectural distortion	Variable	
Basal plasmacytosis	Present	
Distribution of inflammation	Diffuse	Diffuse or patchy
Location of inflammation	Mucosa ± superficial submucosa	Mucosa and deeper layers
Mucin depletion	Proportionate to active inflammation	
Cryptitis, crypt abscess	Variable	
Lamina propria neutrophils	Rare except in blood vessels and adjacent to erosions, ruptured crypts	
Epithelioid granulomas	Absent (except adjacent to damaged crypts)	5–20%
Paneth cell metaplasia	Common	Less common than UC
Pyloric gland metaplasia	Uncommon	Common

6. **What histological features are most useful in discriminating between ulcerative and Crohn colitis in biopsies and what potential pitfalls should be avoided?**

Biopsies are most helpful in the subclassification of IBD when they yield features that are specific for CD. The two most diagnostically significant features are nonnecrotizing epithelioid granulomas and focal inflammation (Table 6.1).

Granulomas should be distinguished from perivascular mesenchymal cells, nerves, smooth muscle bundles and tangential sections of crypts. Most such ambiguities can be resolved by comparing serial histological sections to obtain different views of the lesion. Cryptolytic granulomas elicited by ruptured crypt abscesses are nonspecific but can closely mimic the specific granulomas of CD (Fig. 6.15a). Most occur at the bases of crypts, but the location alone is nondiagnostic. The "missing crypt" sign corresponds to a granuloma that has replaced a lytic crypt abscess that became resorbed (Fig. 6.15b). Other clues that favor cryptolytic over Crohn granulomas include superposition on a partially lytic crypt abscess, the presence of intermingled or clustered neutrophils or eosinophils, a loose rather than compact appearance, pale or foamy histiocytic cytoplasm, and the presence of Touton giant cells (Table 6.2). It is helpful when crypt abscesses and recognizable cryptolytic granulomas are present in the neighboring mucosa. Granulomas that are composed of compact histiocytes with eosinophilic cytoplasm or are located within a lymphoid aggregate are likely related to CD (Fig. 6.15c).

Focal inflammation, i.e., discrete areas of inflammation abutting on otherwise normal mucosa, is suggestive of CD but should be interpreted cautiously (Fig. 6.16a). For example, focal inflammation in UC occurs during the course of healing, during inflammatory flares in patients with previously well-healed colitis, and in the transition zone between involved and uninvolved colonic segments. Crypt inflammation that is limited to only a few crypts, referred to as "focal active colitis," is predictive of CD in

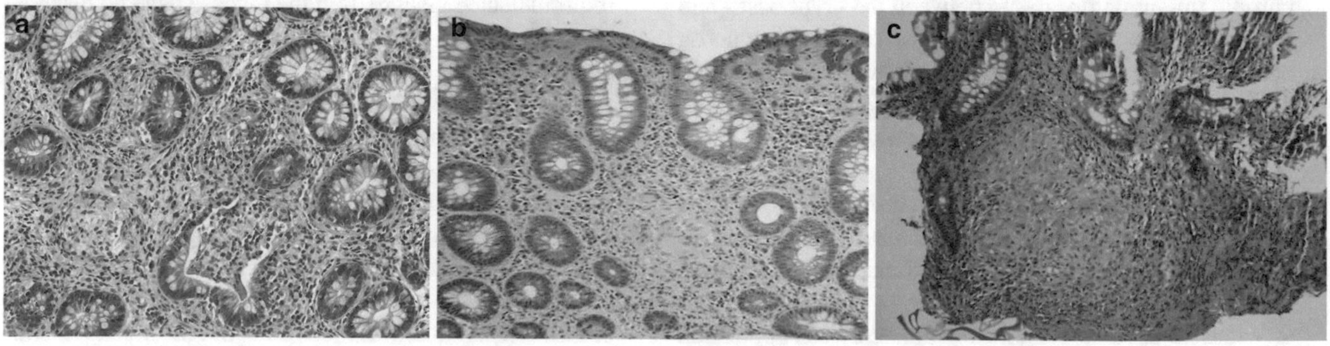

Fig. 6.15 (**a**) Cryptolytic granulomas in inflammatory bowel disease are associated with damaged crypts and are not diagnostic of Crohn disease. In addition to histiocytes and lymphocytes, they often contain neutrophils or eosinophils that originated in ruptured crypt abscesses. (**b**) A cryptolytic granuloma replaces a resorbed crypt abscess. (**c**) A nonnecrotizing granuloma in Crohn disease

children but is seen in adults in the setting of NSAID use, infections, and other conditions.

The presence of chronic submucosal inflammation in biopsies of IBD is not specific for CD since inflammation of the upper region of the submucosa occurs in UC as well (Fig. 6.16b). By the same token, submucosal involvement is not always present in CD. Although a biopsy series that suggests a continuous active colitis without submucosal involvement is more likely to indicate UC than CD, our policy is to avoid subclassification of IBD based on biopsies alone unless they reveal diagnostic features of CD. References: [14, 15]

Table 6.2 Distinguishing features between Crohn-associated and cryptolytic granulomas

	Crohn-associated	Cryptolytic
Location	Anywhere in mucosa	Usually basal mucosa
Boundaries	Well defined	Well or poorly defined
Intragranuloma neutrophils	None	Common, ± microabscesses
Intragranuloma eosinophils	Few	Common, ± microabscesses
Intragranuloma crypt epithelial cells	No	Common
Histiocytes	Lightly to moderately eosinophilic	Pale
Giant cells	Occasional, Langhans type	Occasional, Touton type
Nearby crypt abscesses	Variable	Present
Lymphoid aggregates	Common within lymphoid aggregates	Rare within lymphoid aggregates

7. **How is infectious colitis distinguished from IBD in mucosal biopsies?**

Acute infectious colitis is caused by various foodborne agents, other contaminated environmental sources, and person-to-person or zoonotic transmission. Most cases resolve within 2–4 weeks from the onset of symptoms, but some infections may linger for a month or longer. The pathogens implicated most frequently in immunocompetent patients in the US are *Clostridium difficile*, *Salmonella*, *Shigella*, *Campylobacter*, *Yersinia*, and *Escherichia coli* O157:H7, as well as Norwalk virus, enterovirus, rotavirus, adenovirus, and Coxsackie virus. Conventional laboratory testing fails to identify a specific agent in most cases but is being increasingly supplemented by highly sensitive polymerase chain reaction (PCR)-based stool tests.

Patients with acute colitis symptoms generally do not undergo endoscopic examination unless their presentation is atypical, they have specific risk factors, or they have already failed antibiotic therapy. The endoscopic changes include patchy or diffuse erythema, obscured vasculature, granularity, petechia, erosions, or, in certain cases, pseudomembranes. Certain pathogens, particularly *Yersinia*, *E. coli*, *Campylobacter*, *Salmonella*, and tuberculosis, tend to involve the right colon preferentially.

Biopsies performed during the initial week of symptoms feature edema and neutrophils in the lamina propria, neutrophil infiltration of the surface and crypt epithelium, and preservation of the parallel crypt architecture (Fig. 6.17a). At this stage, the normal top-down mucosal gradient of lymphocytes and plasma cells is maintained. Crypt abscesses are often dilated and lined by low cuboidal or flat epithelium. Ruptured crypts may elicit

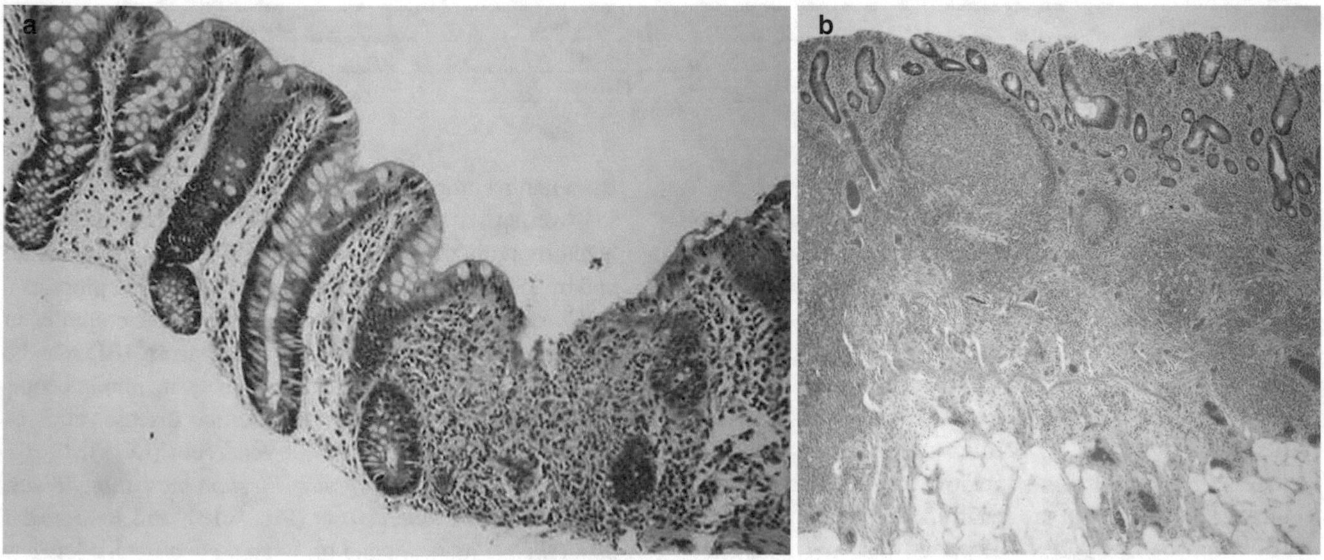

Fig. 6.16 (**a**) Focal colitis is a common feature of biopsies in Crohn disease but can occur in other settings such as reactivation of quiescent ulcerative colitis or in the transition zone of ulcerative colitis. (**b**) Ulcerative colitis with inflammation involving the mucosa and superficial submucosa. Submucosal inflammation in standard-sized biopsies should not be used as a criterion to favor Crohn disease over ulcerative colitis

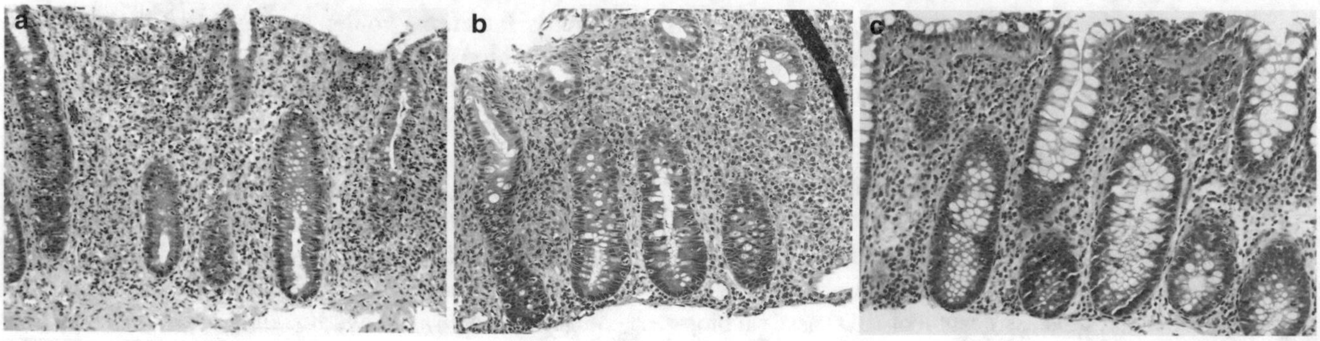

Fig. 6.17 (**a**) Biopsy of a patient with acute infectious colitis featuring preserved crypt architecture, lamina propria edema, and neutrophilic infiltrates involving the lamina propria and the crypt epithelium. (**b** and **c**) Beyond the first week from symptom onset, biopsies of patients with acute infectious colitis feature gradual increases in mononuclear cells and progressive involvement of the basal lamina propria

Table 6.3 Features distinguishing between IBD and acute and chronic infectious colitis

	IBD	Acute infectious colitis	Chronic infectious colitis
Architecture			
Irregular/villiform surface	Common, UC > CD	Uncommon	Uncommon
Crypt architectural distortion	Present	Absent	Mild
Crypt atrophy	Common	Uncommon	Uncommon
Edema	Uncommon	Common, especially in early stage	Variable
Inflammation			
Basal lymphoplasmacytosis, crypt shortfall	Common	Absent	Variable
Top-down mononuclear cell gradient	Absent	Present	Variable
Lamina propria neutrophils	Relative paucity	Present	Present
Cryptitis	Present	Present	Present
Crypt abscesses	Columnar lining epithelium	Cuboidal to flat lining epithelium	Variable
Granulomas	Nonnecrotizing (CD)	Rare, ill-defined (e.g., *Salmonella*)	Necrotizing (TB, fungi), nonnecrotizing (LGV, syphilis)
Epithelium			
Mucin depletion	Common	Common	Common
Paneth cell metaplasia	Common	Absent	Rare
Pyloric gland metaplasia	Present, CD>UC	Absent	Rare

a granulomatous reaction. Infections with *C. difficile*, *Shigella*, enterohemorrhagic strains of Escherichia coli and Klebsiella oxytoca may feature pseudomembranous exudates, lamina propria hemorrhage, or frank ischemic features such as microcystic or withered crypts.

Histologically, IBD contrasts starkly with acute infectious colitis even when biopsied at its inception (Table 6.3). The presence of full-thickness lymphoplasmacytosis, mucosal expansion, crypt disarray, shortfall, columnar-lined crypt abscesses, and relative paucity of neutrophils in the lamina propria are readily identified as features of IBD. Nonetheless, patients suspected of having acute infectious colitis are unlikely to undergo endoscopic biopsies until several weeks after the onset of symptoms, the exclusion of incipient IBD being one of the main indications. At this subacute stage, edema has subsided and mononuclear inflammation becomes dense and gradually occupies the basal lamina propria (Fig. 6.17b and c). Despite the resulting overlap with IBD, subacute infections can be recognized by noting the absence of crypt disarray or shortfall and by the presence of neutrophils in the lamina propria.

Chronic infectious colitis is relatively uncommon in Western countries, and its distinction from IBD can be challenging. The most common agents in immunocompetent patients are sexually transmitted diseases such as syphilis and lymphogranuloma venereum (LGV), *C. difficile*, *Aeromonas hydrophila*, *Plesiomonas shigelloides*, *Mycobacterium tuberculosis* (Fig. 6.18), and *Entamoeba histolytica* (Fig. 6.19a and b). In some geographic locales, IBD may be mimicked by endemic strains of *Salmonella*, *Shigella*, and other enteropathogens as well as by schistosomiasis, but these are infrequently encountered in the US.

Syphilis (Fig. 6.20 and b) and LGV (Fig. 6.21) both involve the anus and rectum and are endoscopic mimics

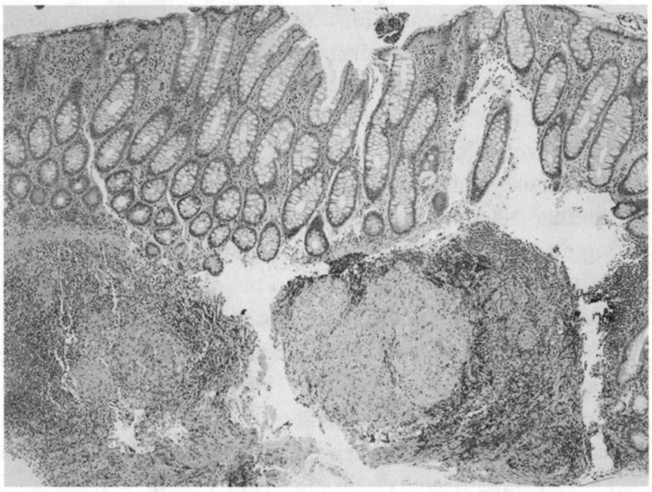

Fig. 6.18 Tuberculous colitis featuring large submucosal granulomas beneath intact mucosa. Early necrosis is seen in the granuloma on the left

of IBD. Histologically, they are characterized by mucosal expansion associated with dense plasmacytosis but only mild crypt architectural distortion. Other features that might suggest the diagnosis include band-like submucosal lymphoplasmahistiocytic infiltration, nonnecrotizing granulomas, and perivascular lymphoplasmacytic cuffing in the submucosa. Immunostaining for *Treponema pallidum* (*T. pallidum*) is diagnostic, but the organisms may be faintly stained and difficult to recognize.

Gastroenteric infections are both risk factors and potential triggers for the development of IBD, often within the first year after the infectious episode. The agents most commonly identified are *Campylobacter*, *Salmonella*, and *Shigella*, but *C. difficile* and *Aeromonas* have also been implicated. Histologically, serial biopsies over the span of a few months may show progression from an acute or subacute infectious pattern to classical IBD.

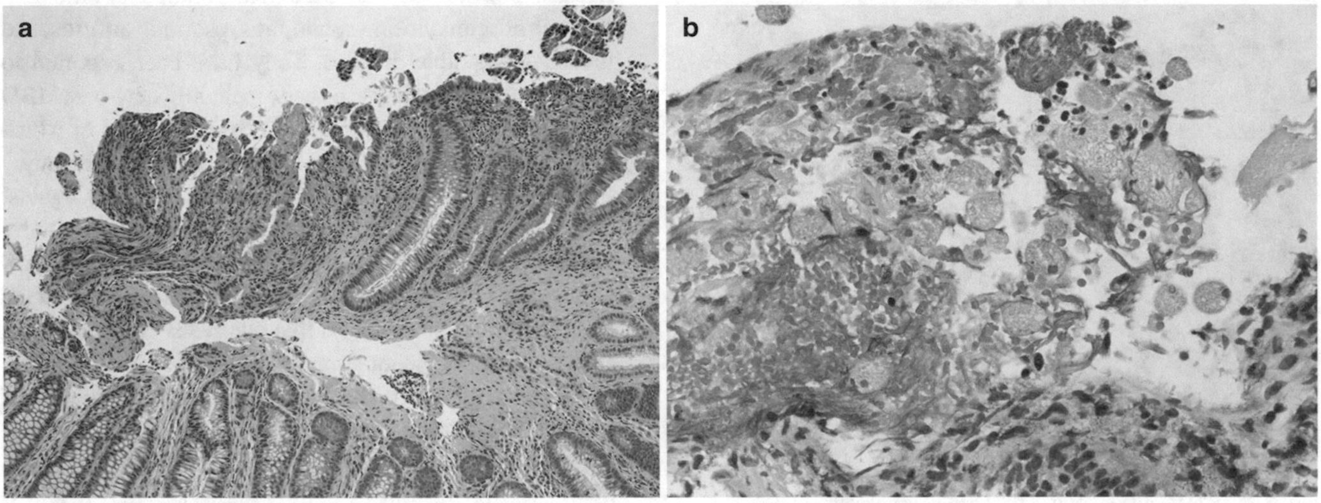

Fig. 6.19 Amebic colitis. (**a**) The mucosa features very mild chronic inflammation and an erosion surrounded by mucin-depleted epithelium. (**b**) Ameba histolytica trophozoites

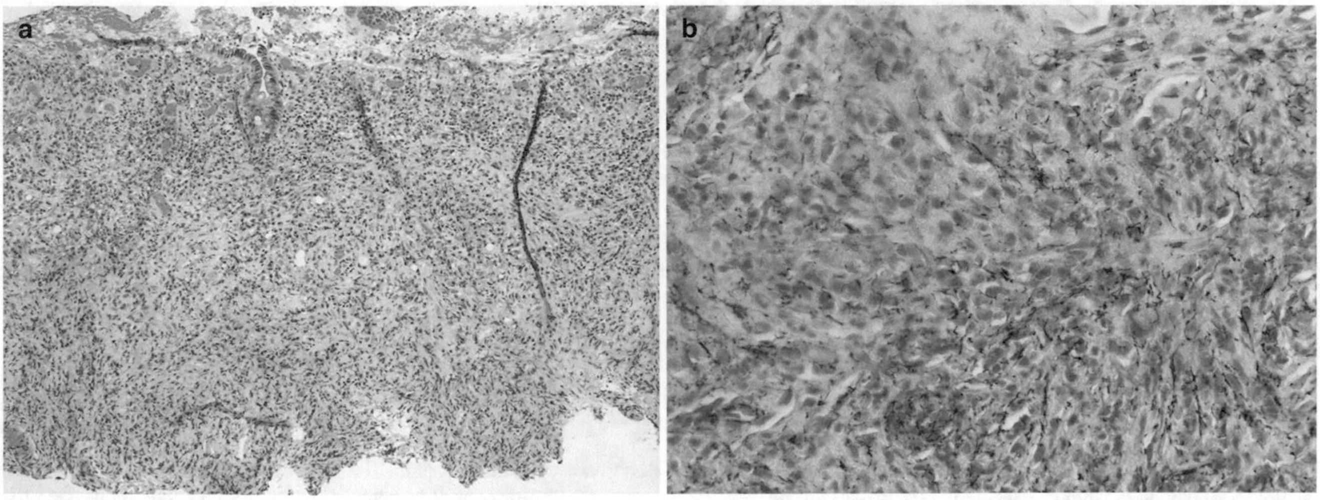

Fig. 6.20 Syphilitic proctitis. (**a**) Dense chronic inflammation in a rectal biopsy. (**b**) A clinical history relating prior anal condylomas elicited immunostaining for spirochetes

References: [13, 16–19]

8. What drugs and other toxic agents might mimic IBD in colorectal biopsies?

Drug-related colitis should always be considered in the differential diagnosis of IBD. The following commonly used drugs are particularly prone to mimic IBD in biopsies.

NSAIDs are cyclooxygenase (COX) inhibitors that are widely administered for a variety of complaints. They cause acute upper and lower gastrointestinal (GI) inflammation, the results of direct topical toxicity and local depletion of prostaglandins, and they elicit diverse histological effects, including reactive epithelial changes, ischemic-type injury, acute inflammation and ulceration, postinflammatory crypt architectural disarray, and pyloric gland metaplasia (Fig. 6.22a). Rarely, long-term NSAID use results in so-called diaphragm disease characterized by concentric protrusions of mucosa and submucosa, which can mimic stricturing CD.

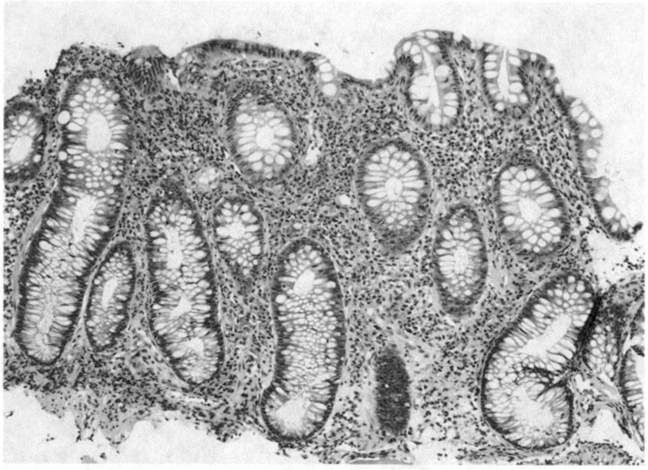

Fig. 6.21 Chlamydia proctitis. The histological features closely resemble those of inflammatory bowel disease, including full-thickness lymphoplasmacytosis and mildly distorted crypt architecture. Clinical data suggesting sexually transmitted disease are essential to the diagnosis

Mycophenolate mofetil (MMF) is an immune suppressant that is commonly used for prophylaxis of organ rejection in renal, cardiac, liver, and stem cell transplantation and for the treatment of autoimmune diseases such as autoimmune hepatitis, lupus nephritis, and autoimmune blistering diseases. GI side effects occur in 30–64% of patients, most commonly during the first 6 months of treatment. The histological effects have been grouped into four patterns: acute infectious-like (16%), ischemia-like (3%), graft-versus-host disease (GVHD)-like (19%), and IBD-like (28%). The latter group is characterized by crypt architectural distortion, acute and chronic inflammation, and dilated crypts with eosinophils and neutrophils (Fig. 6.22b).

Antitumor necrosis factor (TNF) agents include etanercept, a TNF- α inhibitor, and two anti-TNF-α antibodies, infliximab and adalimumab. In addition to the treatment of IBD, TNF-α inhibitors are used in the treatment of rheumatoid arthritis, ankylosing spondylitis, psoriatic arthritis, and juvenile idiopathic arthritis. They have been reported to elicit paradoxical adverse effects, including new-onset IBD or flares of colitis in patients with IBD, the onset of which may occur days to years after the introduction of therapy.

Rituximab is a chimeric monoclonal antibody against CD20, a surface protein on most B lymphocytes. Initially approved for the treatment of non-Hodgkin B-cell lymphoma and later for rheumatoid arthritis, it is also used for other autoimmune disorders that involve B-cell activation, such as lupus, Wegener granulomatosis, dermatomyositis, and steroid refractory UC. New onset and exacerbation of UC-like colitis after rituximab salvage therapy have been reported. GI symptoms occur weeks to months after rituximab exposure. Biopsies mainly show UC-like features, including mixed inflammatory cell infiltrates, ulceration, and cryptitis.

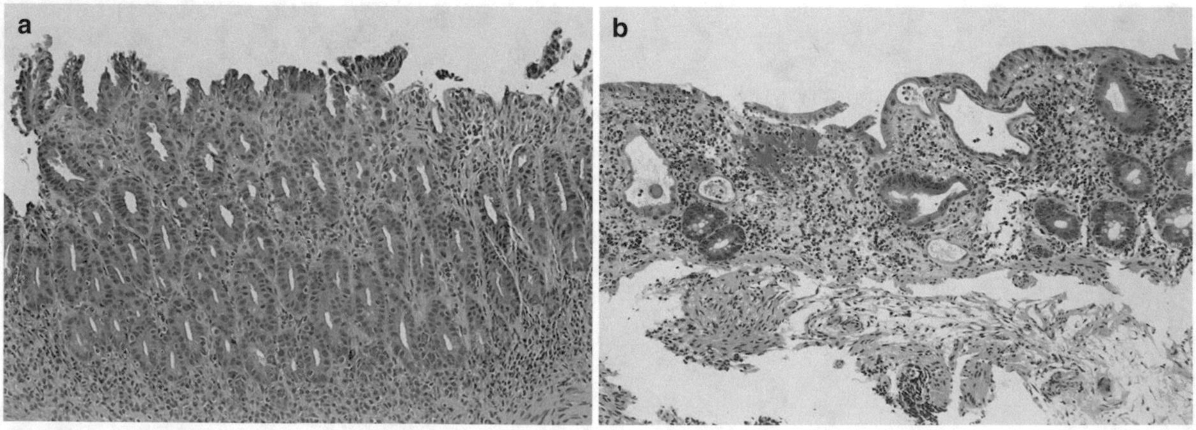

Fig. 6.22 (**a**) Chronic NSAID-associated enteropathy. The villi of the small bowel are blunted/atrophic. The crypt cells contain reactive nuclei, are devoid of goblet cells, and are reduced in size toward the surface, features that are reminiscent of ischemic change. (**b**) Mycophenolate-mofetil-associated colitis featuring damaged crypts lined by attenuated eosinophilic cytoplasm, some containing necrotic debris

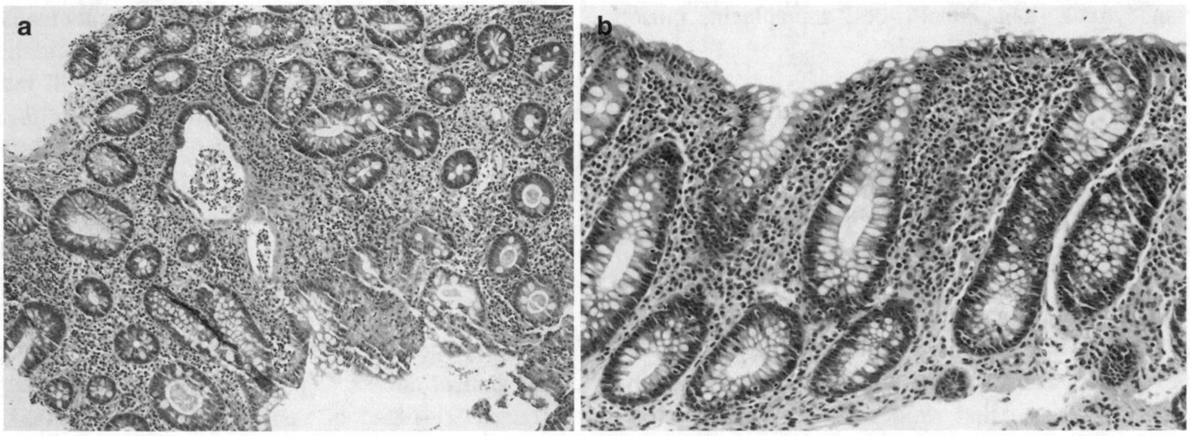

Fig. 6.23 Ipilimumab-associated colitis. (**a**) The dense lymphoplasmacytosis and crypt distortion in this case closely mimic inflammatory bowel disease. (**b**) Another case of ipilimumab-associated colitis in which the histology mimics lymphocytic colitis

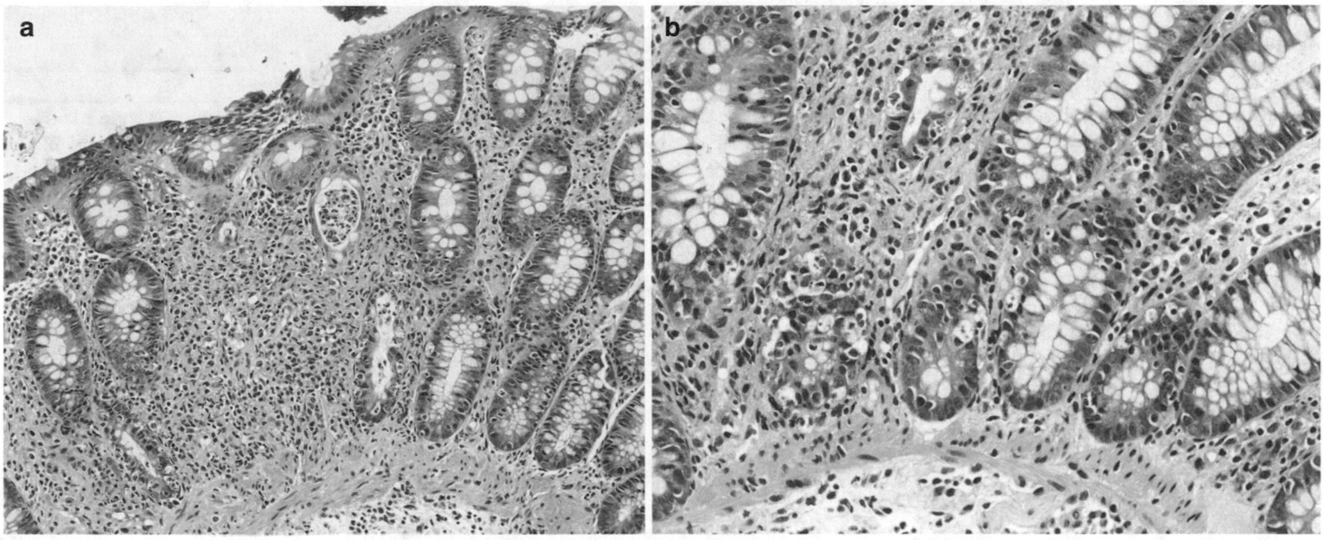

Fig. 6.24 (**a**) PD-1-associated colitis. Full-thickness lymphoplasmacytosis indicates chronicity, but the features in this case are otherwise nonspecific and the diagnosis requires knowledge of the drug history. (**b**) Another case of PD-1 colitis. The numerous crypt apoptotic bodies are consistent with immunotherapy-related drug toxicity

Ipilimumab is an immune checkpoint inhibitor that consists of a monoclonal antibody that targets CTLA-4, a protein receptor that competes with CD28 to bind B7, thereby downregulating T-cell activation. The drug is approved for the treatment of late-stage melanoma and is undergoing trials for the treatment of various other cancers. Treatment is associated with diarrhea in 21–35% of patients. Biopsies reveal marked lamina propria mixed inflammatory cell infiltrates composed of neutrophils, lymphocytes, plasma cells and eosinophils, cryptitis and crypt abscesses, and rarely granulomas (Fig. 6.23a). Intraepithelial lymphocytosis mimicking lymphocytic colitis may be seen (Fig. 6.23b). Life-threatening colitis with perforation has been reported.

Other immune checkpoint inhibitors include the anti-PD-1 agents pembrolizumab and nivolumab and anti-PD-L1 agents such as atezolizumab, which are approved for the treatment of a growing list of malignancies. The drugs act by limiting the effector function of activated T cells; however, disruption of the immune balance results in distinctive toxicity profiles, among them colitis and endocrine dysfunction. Eleven to 20% of patients develop GI symptoms such as diarrhea, abdominal pain, discomfort, and cramping, beginning from weeks to months after treatment onset, and 0.3–2.3% experience morbidity from colitis, including fatalities. Two histological patterns of colitis have been described. One is GVHD-like featuring varying degrees of apoptosis, cryptitis, crypt abscesses, crypt atrophy, and dropout (Fig. 6.24a and b). The other resembles lymphocytic colitis with surface epithelial damage, intraepithelial lymphocytosis, and occasionally apoptosis. Recurrent active anti-PD-1 colitis may result in crypt architectural distortion, basal lymphoplasmacytosis, and Paneth cell metaplasia, closely mimicking IBD.

References: [20–26]

9. How does the pathology of pediatric IBD patients differ from that in adults?

Twenty to 25% of patients with IBD are diagnosed before the age of 20, most during adolescence; 18% before age 10; and 4% before age 5. In contrast with adult UC patients, most of whom present with distal or left-sided disease, up to 90% of pediatric UC patients either present from the outset with pancolitis or have aggressive disease that progresses to pancolitis in a short time. The incidence of pediatric CD is higher than that of UC and is reportedly increasing in Western countries. Children with CD are most likely to present with isolated colitis or ileocolitis, whereas isolated terminal ileitis is increasingly common in adolescents and adults. Up to 15% have proximal small intestinal disease, at least 40% have histological manifestations of CD in the upper gastrointestinal tract, and 15–20% develop perianal disease.

The histological diagnosis of IBD in pediatric patients may be challenging, thereby contributing to the relatively high proportion of pediatric patients, 30% in some studies, who are diagnosed with indeterminate colitis. Rectal sparing and patchiness are more prevalent in pediatric than in adult UC patients, with approximately 30% (range: 21–68%) of new onset pediatric patients having either complete or more frequently relative sparing of the rectosigmoid colon. In patients under 10, initial colonic biopsies reveal less crypt architectural distortion

Table 6.4 IBD differential diagnosis—helpful clinical and pathologic features

Entity	Predisposing conditions	Clinical features	Distinguishing pathologic features
Acute self-limited colitis	Travel, community, or institutional outbreaks; sexual transmission; antibiotic use	Acute onset, diarrhea, fever, dysentery, bleeding per rectum	Neutrophilic infiltration of mucosa, lamina propria edema (first 4–5 days), preserved crypt architecture, necklace-like crypt abscesses with flat epithelium, surface neutrophils with epithelial tufting, lack of basal lymphoplasmacytosis until 2–3 weeks; certain infections feature pseudomembranes and/or right-sided colonic predominance
Ischemic colitis	Elderly, comorbidities, cardiovascular disease, hypovolemic shock, drugs (vasopressors, oral contraceptives), heavy exercise, sickle cell disease	Abdominal pain, bloody diarrhea	Microcystic crypts with surface tapering and few or absent goblet cells, eosinophilic lamina propria, surface necrosis (Fig. 6.25)
Diverticular-disease-associated colitis	Elderly, diverticulosis	Pain, bleeding per rectum	Chronic colitis limited to diverticular colon, rectal sparing, IBD-like histology
Diversion colitis	Colon bypass surgery	Mucous discharge, bleeding	Lymphoid hyperplasia, mild crypt architectural distortion
Drug-associated colitis	Drug use (mycophenolate, immune checkpoint inhibitors, antihypertensives, chemotherapeutic, colchicine, many others)	Variable, diarrhea	Variable depending on drug
GVHD	History of bone marrow or solid organ transplantation	Diarrhea, skin rash, elevated liver enzymes	Glandular apoptotic bodies, crypt dropout (Fig. 6.26)
Lymphocytic colitis and collagenous colitis	Elderly, female (collagenous), celiac disease, and other autoimmune diseases	Insidious or abrupt onset, nonbloody watery diarrhea, fecal incontinence	Preserved crypt architecture, increased lamina propria mononuclear cells ± top-down gradient, increased intraepithelial lymphocytes (variable in collagenous colitis), subepithelial collagen band (collagenous colitis) (Fig. 6.27)
Autoimmune enteropathy	Children, less commonly adults, genetic predisposition (IPEX syndrome, APECED syndrome), posttherapy for hematological malignancies	Intractable diarrhea	Surface and crypt epithelial apoptotic bodies, reduced or absent goblet cells and/or Paneth cells, mononuclear cell infiltration of lamina propria; sometimes little or no histological changes (Fig. 6.28)
CVID	Adults	Variable, recurrent sinonasal respiratory and other infections	Paucity of plasma cells in lamina propria (70%), intraepithelial lymphocytes, follicular lymphoid hyperplasia, apoptotic bodies (Fig. 6.29)
Chronic granulomatous disease	Children, X-linked inheritance	Recurrent bacterial and fungal infections, diarrhea	Pigment-laden macrophages, eosinophilic cryptitis, paucity of neutrophils

GVHD graft-versus-host disease, *IPEX* immune dysregulation, polyendocrinopathy, enteropathy, X-linked, *APECED* autoimmune polyendocrinopathy-candidiasis-ectodermal dystrophy, *CVID* common variable immunodeficiency

and other evidence of chronicity than in adolescents and adults. Atypical features of UC such as backwash ileitis, periappendiceal inflammation, and isolated cecal patch are as common in children as in adults.

Mucosal lesions of CD in children can be subtle and lacking in features of chronicity. Early histological manifestations include aphthous lesions; focal active colitis, i.e., localized neutrophilic and lymphoplasmacytic infiltrates in an otherwise normal background; and increased lamina propria eosinophils. Epithelioid granulomas are more common in children with CD than in adults. Their presence has been linked to more extensive disease and perianal complications. Upper GI inflammation occurs in most children with CD, even in the absence of symptoms and of radiological or endoscopic manifestations, and granulomas are detected in up to 40%. Focally enhanced gastritis featuring a localized mixed neutrophilic and mononuclear inflammatory infiltrate occurs in approximately half of children with CD. This and other patterns of upper GI inflammation also occur in UC, albeit less frequently.

References: [15, 27–31]

10. What is the differential diagnosis of IBD in biopsies?

The major differential diagnoses of IBD in biopsies are listed in Table 6.4, along with associated characteristic clinical and histological features.

References: [16, 32–34]

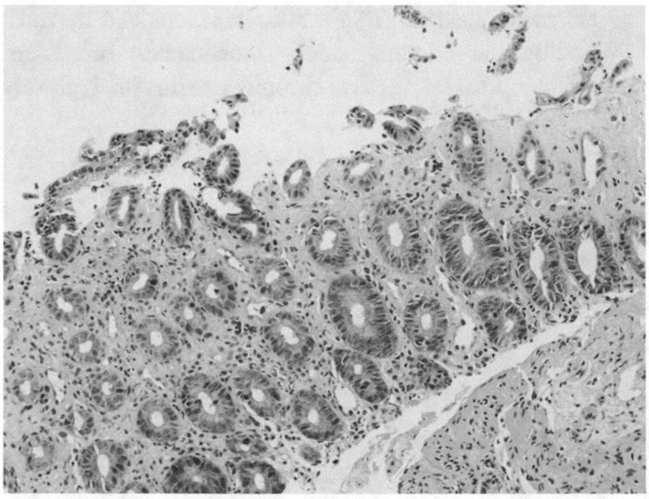

Fig. 6.25 Ischemic colitis characterized by densely eosinophilic hyalinized lamina propria and withering, goblet-cell-depleted crypts near the luminal surface

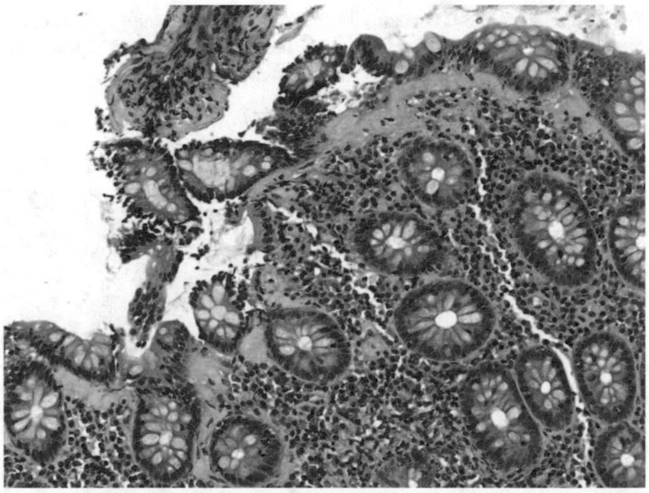

Fig. 6.27 Collagenous colitis featuring preserved crypt architecture, lamina propria expansion due to lymphoplasmacytosis, and a thickened subepithelial collagen band

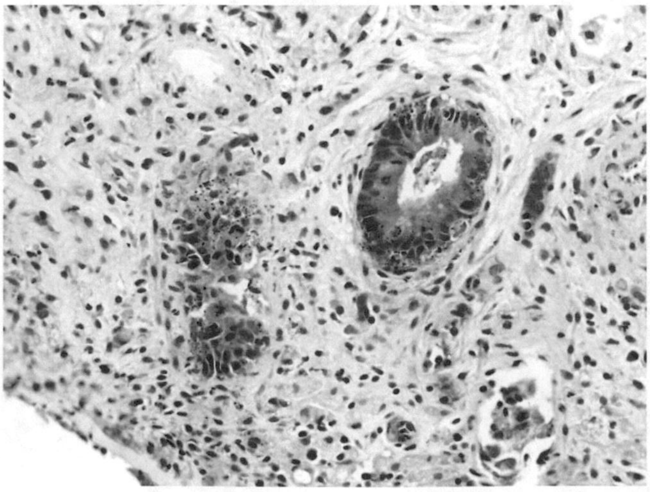

Fig. 6.26 Graft-versus-host-disease characterized by numerous crypt apoptotic bodies, damaged crypts, and crypt dropout

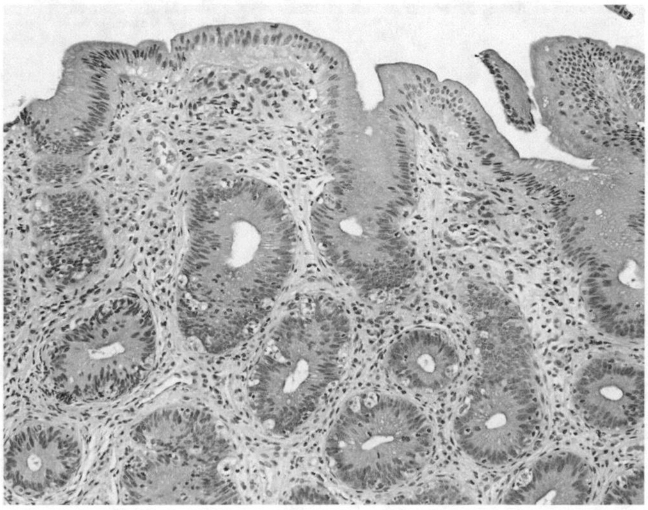

Fig. 6.28 Autoimmune enteropathy featuring complete loss of goblet cells and numerous crypt apoptotic bodies. Paneth cells are absent in many cases

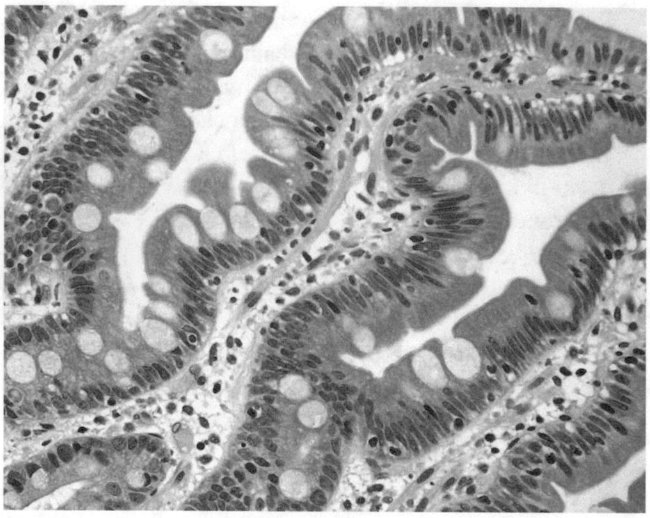

Fig. 6.29 Common variable immunodeficiency usually features a paucicellular lamina propria due to reduced density or absence of plasma cells, as well as surface intraepithelial lymphocytosis and lymphoid hyperplasia

11. **What are the upper GI manifestations of ulcerative colitis and Crohn disease?**

Severe gastroduodenal involvement occurs in approximately 5% of patients with CD; however, routine diagnostic endoscopy identifies macroscopic inflammation in 30–64% and histological inflammation in up to 80% of CD patients when endoscopically visible lesions are targeted. Children with UC are reported to have IBD-like inflammation in the upper GI tract with nearly the same frequency as those with CD.

The prevalence of granulomas in CD is highest in children, approximately 30%, and decreases with age to approximately 15% (Fig. 6.30a). The differential diagnosis includes cryptolytic granulomas, infections, sarcoidosis, chronic granulomatous disease, and malignancy.

Other upper GI manifestations of CD include focally enhanced gastritis (Fig. 6.30b), characterized by focal perifoveolar or periglandular mononuclear or neutrophilic infiltrates, active chronic gastritis that closely

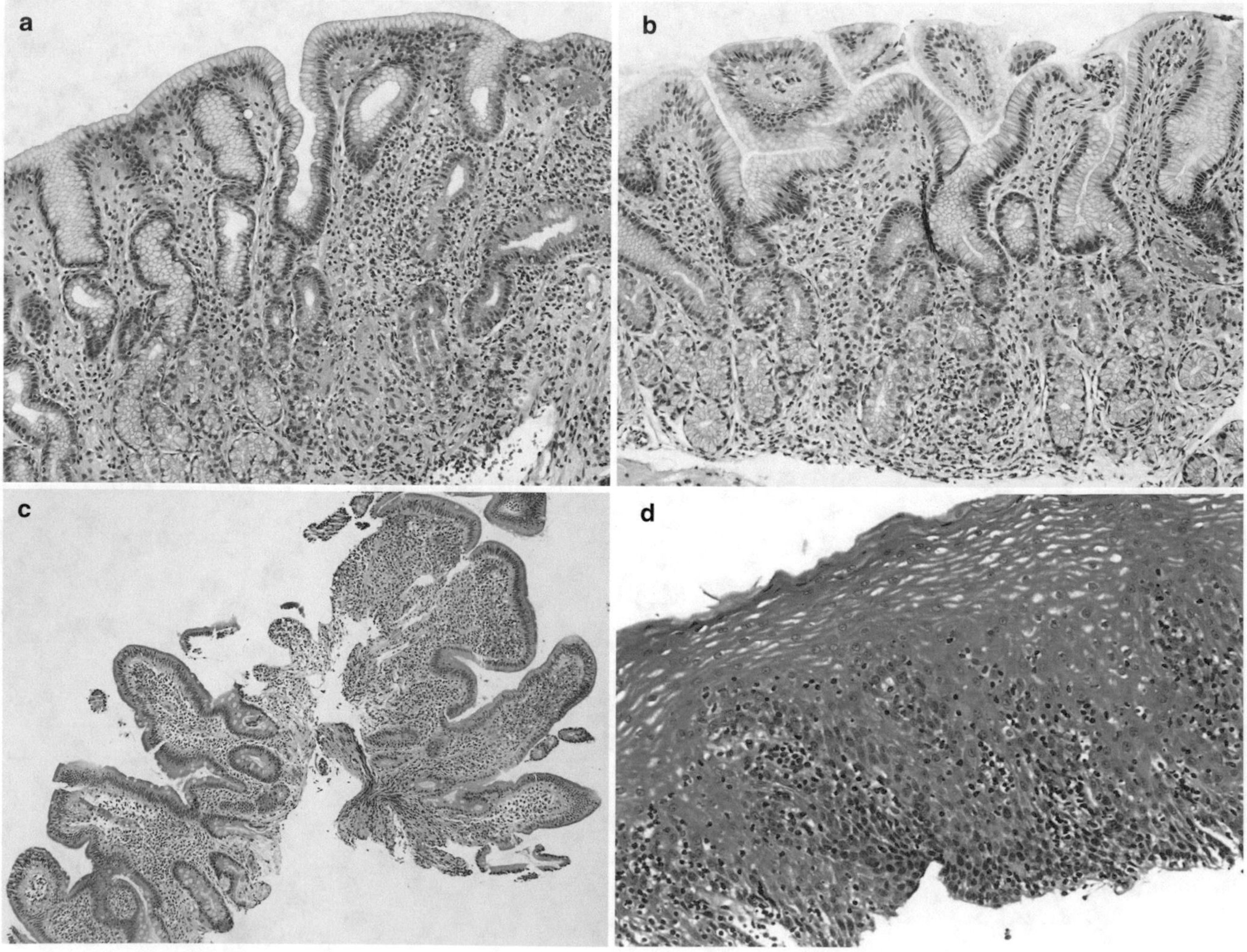

Fig. 6.30 (**a**) Crohn gastritis with an epithelioid granuloma. (**b**) Focally enhanced gastritis in Crohn disease characterized by periglandular neutrophilic and lymphohistiocytic infiltrates. (**c**) Chronic duodenitis in a patient with ulcerative colitis. (**d**) Lymphocytic esophagitis featuring peripapillary lymphocytosis, which can be seen in patients with Crohn disease

mimics *Helicobacter pylori* infection, and intraepithelial lymphocytosis of the small intestine, which may be evident before the diagnosis of IBD has been made. Duodenal ulceration and villous atrophy are reported in UC as well as CD but need to be distinguished from other common etiologies such as peptic duodenitis and NSAID-associated inflammation. IBD-like diffuse chronic duodenitis (Fig. 6.30c) with lamina propria lymphoplasmacytosis has been described as a unique upper GI manifestation of UC that may predict adverse outcomes, including colectomy and pouchitis.

Esophageal inflammation, including "lymphocytic esophagitis" manifested by peripapillary lymphocytosis (Fig. 6.30d), can be attributed to known CD if accompanied by granulomas; however, it does not otherwise discriminate between gastroesophageal reflux disease and other etiologies.

References: [35–39]

12. **What are the main complications of ileoanal pouch surgery for IBD?**

Restorative proctocolectomy with ileal pouch-anal anastomosis (IPAA) is the surgical treatment of choice for medically refractory UC or colitis-associated dysplasia. Although Crohn colitis is considered to be a relative contraindication for IPAA due to the risk of pouch failure and its potentially serious complications, many centers perform the procedure selectively in patients with isolated colitis and no evidence of fistulizing disease. As a result, pouch retention rates exceeding 85% have been reported. The postoperative complications of IPAA include septic complications such as leaks, fistulas, and abscesses; nonseptic complications such as stenosis, pouchitis, and cuffitis; mechanical complications such as prolapse; and the long-term development of dysplasia or cancer.

Pouchitis Pouchitis is the most common complication, affecting nearly half of patients. The risk factors for developing pouchitis include extensive UC, backwash ileitis, risk polymorphisms of NOD2/CARD15, PSC, and use of biologics or NSAIDs. Pouchitis encompasses a spectrum that ranges from acute antibiotic-responsive to antibiotic-dependent to chronic antibiotic refractory disease. Specific causative factors include infections with cytomegalovirus, *Clostridium difficile*, or *Candida*; treatment-associated factors such as radiation and chemotherapy; ischemia; PSC; IgG4-associated disease; and autoimmune pouchopathy.

Histological evaluation has limited value in grading pouchitis compared with endoscopic scoring. Villous blunting, crypt hyperplasia, and mildly increased mononuclear cells in the lamina propria are frequently observed in biopsies from asymptomatic patients and are thought to be adaptive. However, potentially informative findings should be sought, including viral inclusions (CMV), granulomas (infections, drugs, or CD), prominent apoptotic bodies (autoimmune enteritis), IgG4-positive plasma cells, pyloric gland metaplasia (chronic mucosal injury), and dysplasia.

Cuffitis Inflammation of the rectal cuff that interposes between the anastomosis and dentate line is one of the more common complications of IPAA. Patients with symptomatic cuffitis may present with increased frequency, urgency, abdominal or pelvic pain, or rectal bleeding. Cuffitis is generally isolated and attributable to a flare of UC, which can be managed with topical treatments. However, it can present atypically in conjunction with pouchitis, accompanied by stricture or fistula formation, or as de novo CD, all of which are more difficult to manage. The respective origins of pouch and rectal biopsies may be very difficult to distinguish histologically due to inflammatory and adaptive changes, and even the clinician may not be certain as to the location of the anastomosis. The histological features of cuffitis span the gamut of changes of IBD.

CD of the Pouch Secondary CD after IPAA for UC or indeterminate colitis may develop weeks to years after surgery. The reported incidence ranges from 2.7% to 13% but is more typically in the 5–10% range. By analogy with conventional CD, it is classified into inflammatory, fibrostenotic, and penetrating types with their respective histological manifestations. Differentiating CD of the pouch from other inflammatory conditions such as fecal stasis, ischemia, anastomosis-related changes, and NSAID-induced injury can be challenging. The diagnosis is suspected or favored when there is Crohn-like inflammation of the neoterminal ileum, when nonforeign body granulomas are identified in biopsies, and when CD is diagnosed on review of prior resection specimens (Fig. 6.31a–c).

References: [40–46]

13. **What are the defining histological characteristics of dysplasia in IBD?**

Dysplasia in IBD is defined as unequivocal intraepithelial neoplasia of the intestinal epithelium, i.e., neoplasia that is confined to the basement membrane in which it originated. To qualify, the histological abnormalities should not be attributable to reactive or regenerative epithelial changes caused by inflammation.

In most cases, dysplasia in IBD resembles that of conventional adenomatous polyps. The nuclei are characterized by hyperchromatic staining, high nuclear-to-cytoplasmic ratios, crowding, overlapping, and

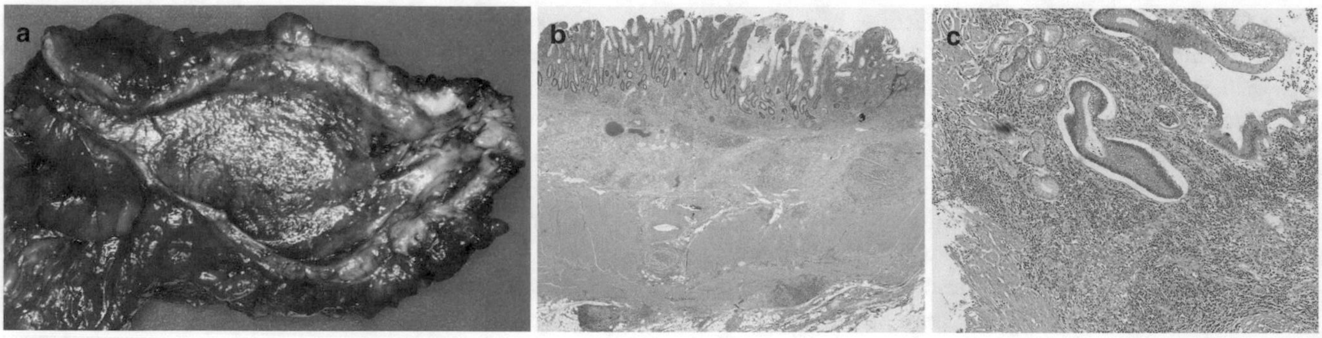

Fig. 6.31 Ileoanal pouch with Crohn disease. (**a**) Resected pouch showing perianal disease, mural thickening, and loss of compliance. (**b**) Histologic sections of the failed pouch show marked mural thickening, transmural lymphoid aggregates, and architectural distortion of the mucosa. (**c**) The mucosa is chronically inflamed, featuring lymphoplasmacytosis, crypt distortion, pyloric metaplasia, and an epithelioid granuloma (bottom center)

anisocytosis. The cytoplasm is characterized by aberrant differentiation (Fig. 6.32a). The differentiation between goblet cells and enterocytes is indistinct, and there may be excessive columnar mucinous cells, goblet cells, dystrophic (upside down) goblet cells, or Paneth cells (Fig. 6.32b). The architectural growth pattern is analogous to that of conventional tubular, villous, or mixed sporadic adenomas, although the microscopic patterns tend to be less uniform. Less frequently, dysplasia assumes serrated or flat growth pattern, as discussed in the next section (question 14).

Dysplasia is graded according to the nomenclature and criteria of the IBD Morphology Study Group. An alternative but mostly analogous Vienna nomenclature is used in some European practices. Grading is based on a three-tier scale comprising low-grade dysplasia (LGD), high-grade dysplasia (HGD), and invasive adenocarcinoma. An additional "indefinite for dysplasia (IND)" category provides a means of classifying mucosa that eludes definitive distinction between reactive and dysplastic or that is uninterpretable for technical reasons. Examples may include cases showing concerning cytological and/or architectural changes in the basal crypts but with surface maturation, worrisome features in the presence of active inflammation or ulceration, tangential sectioning of the specimen with the mucosal surface not well represented, and severe cautery, crushing, or other processing artifact that makes histological assessment difficult.

The distinction between LGD and HGD depends mainly on the degree to which the polarity of the dysplastic epithelium is retained or lost. The nuclei in LGD maintain a parallel orientation and are confined to the basal halves of the epithelial cells. Cytologically, they are typically crowded, ovoid, or penicillate and variably hyperchromatic. Their nuclear membranes are thin, nucleoli are inconspicuous, and mitotic figures are morphologically typical (Fig. 6.32a and b). HGD is characterized by loss of nuclear polarity, which is manifested by skewed or markedly stratified nuclei or by cribriform glandular architecture (Fig. 6.33a and b). The nuclei show high nuclear-to-cytoplasmic ratios, marked anisocytosis, thick or irregular nuclear membranes, prominent nucleoli, or atypical mitotic figures. Since the individual abnormalities in dysplasia lie on a continuum, interobserver variation is unavoidable in some cases.

Dysplasia usually involves the entire length of the crypt with little or no epithelial "maturation" toward the epithelial surface. However, maturation may occur in dysplasia with a villous growth pattern, the atypia of the basal crypt epithelium diminishing or even normalizing within the villous tips. In such lesions, grading is assigned according to the features of the basal epithelium. Surface maturation is less commonly encountered in nonvillous dysplasia and should be interpreted cautiously since it is one of the histological hallmarks of reactive mucosa. References: [47–49]

14. **What is the spectrum of nonadenomatous dysplasia in IBD?**

Most cases of dysplasia in IBD are histologically similar to conventional tubular, villous, or mixed colorectal adenomas; however, other types of dysplasia are recognized based on their distinctive combinations of growth pattern and cellular characteristics. Endoscopically, dysplastic foci may be visible or invisible and can be polypoid or flat.

Sessile Serrated Lesion-Like These lesions are typically elevated (polypoid) and are characterized histologically by a serrated, architecturally irregular growth pattern reminiscent of sporadic sessile serrated lesions; however, they also feature atypical nuclear cytology. The epithelium combines goblet cells and columnar cells with microvesicular cytoplasm (Fig. 6.34a). Analogous lesions without significant nuclear atypia, the so-called serrated epithelial change (also known as

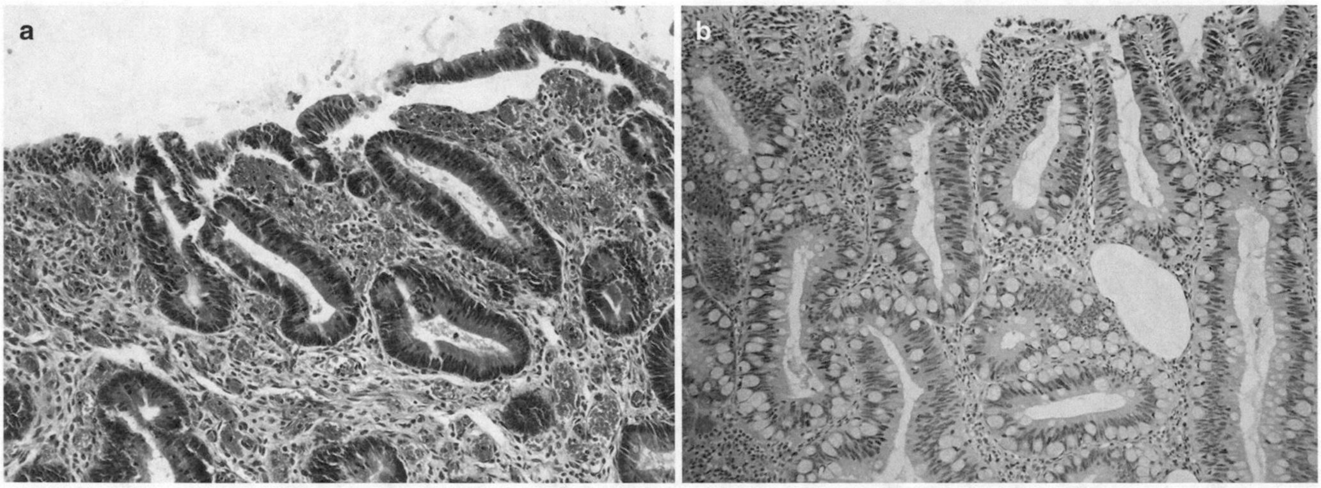

Fig. 6.32 (**a**) Low-grade dysplasia characterized by crypt and surface epithelium with hyperchromatic, enlarged, elliptical nuclei that retain parallel orientation and basal polarity. The cytoplasm is undifferentiated. This type of dysplasia resembles conventional colorectal adenomatous epithelium cytologically but lacks the typical crowded tubular or villous architecture. (**b**) Low-grade dysplasia featuring mildly hyperchromatic, crowded nuclei, and numerous dystrophic goblet cells

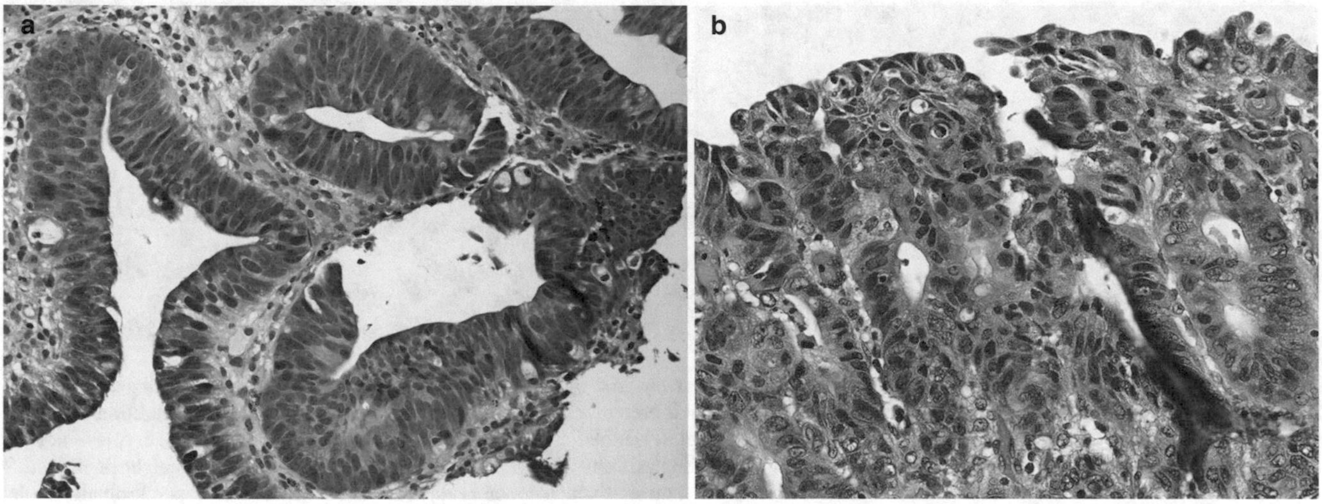

Fig. 6.33 (**a**) High-grade dysplasia characterized by nuclear hyperchromasia, enlargement, and stratification. (**b**) High-grade dysplasia featuring nuclear pleomorphism and disarray, high nuclear-to-cytoplasmic ratios, and partial loss of nuclear polarity

"flat serrated change" or "hyperplastic-like mucosal change") found in random biopsies of flat mucosa from IBD patients, do not seem to pose high risks for the development of cancer.

Traditional Serrated Adenoma-Like These polypoid lesions are characterized by tubulovillous architecture with ectopic crypts and consist of columnar cells with eosinophilic cytoplasm and variable goblet cells. The nuclei are elongated and hyperchromatic and may contain small nucleoli (Fig. 6.34b). Most lesions occur in the left colon and harbor *KRAS* mutations. Clinical follow-up of IBD patients after endoscopic resection of these polyps reportedly has a similar rate of progression to HGD or carcinoma as conventional LGD.

Goblet-Cell-Deficient Dysplasia This type of dysplasia consists of noncrowded tubular crypts lined by nongoblet columnar cells. The crypts are typically similar in height to those in the surrounding mucosa (flat lesion), but elevated lesions and direct progression to carcinoma may occur (Fig. 6.34c). One follow-up study of IBD patients reported a similar rate of progression to HGD and cancer as in those with conventional LGD.

Crypt Cell Dysplasia This uncommon type of dysplasia presents as noncrowded, nonelevated crypts (flat lesion) lined by cytologically atypical but differentiated columnar cells, i.e., goblet cells, enterocytes, basal Paneth cells, and endocrine cells. The nuclei are ovoid, vesicular, or hyperchromatic and extend to the luminal

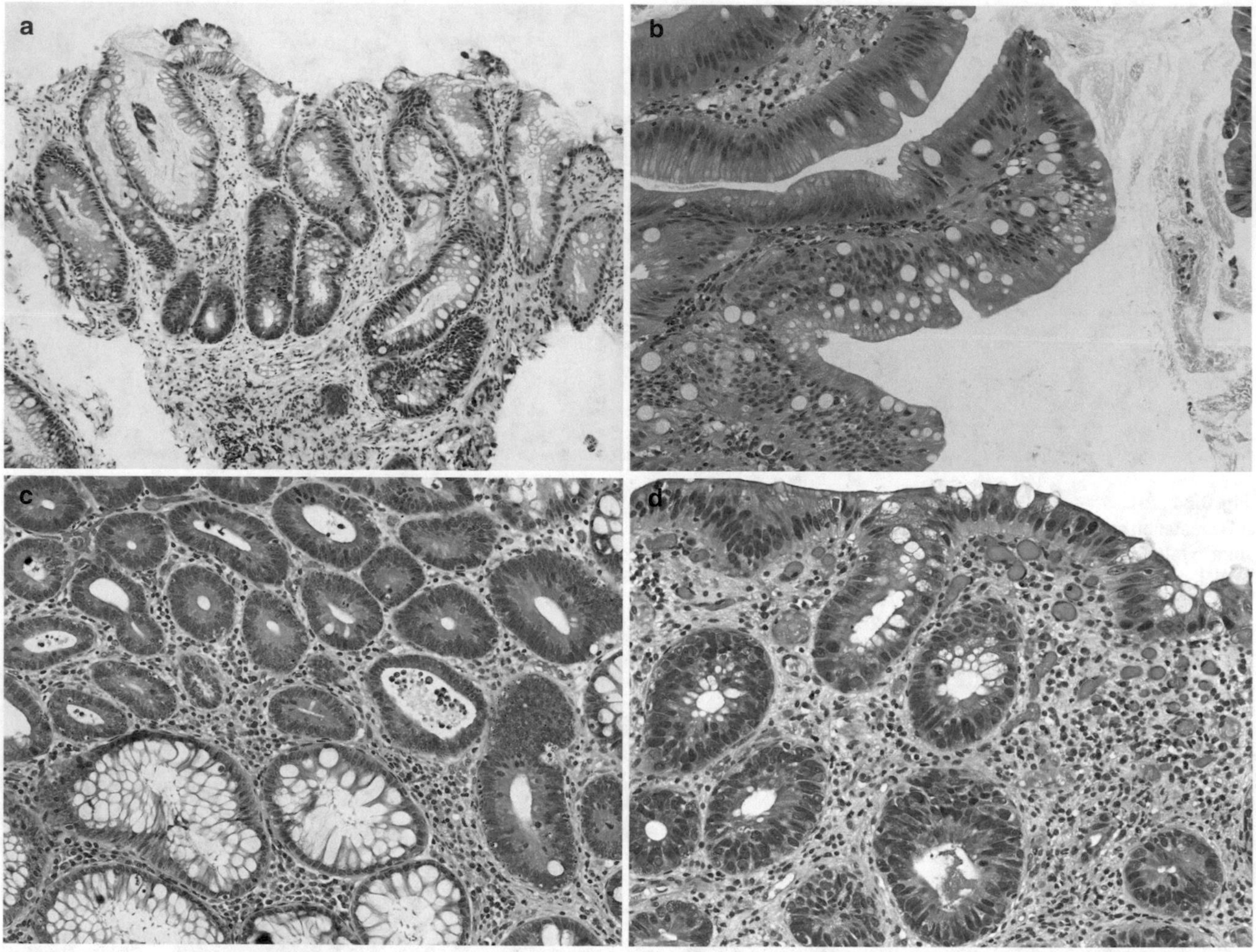

Fig. 6.34 (**a**) Dysplasia reminiscent of a sessile serrated lesion characterized by disorganized serrated growth pattern and mixed goblet and microvesicular columnar cells with atypical nuclei. Surface maturation is present, especially on the left side. (**b**) Dysplasia with traditional serrated adenoma features, such as eosinophilic cytoplasm and pencillate nuclei. (**c**) Goblet-cell-deficient dysplasia featuring noncrowded crypts of normal height lined by uniformly basophilic columnar cells. (**d**) Crypt cell dysplasia characterized by noncrowded crypts of normal height lined by differentiated goblet cells, enterocytes, Paneth cells, and Kulchitsky cells, most of which contain relatively large, vesicular to hyperchromatic nuclei with minimal surface maturation

surface without significant maturation (Fig. 6.34d). In view of its architectural similarity to the surrounding mucosa, it is not surprising that this type of dysplasia accounts for a disproportionate share of dysplasia encountered in nontargeted endoscopic biopsies (flat dysplasia). The distinction from reactive mucosa can be challenging in the setting of active inflammation.

Hypermucinous Dysplasia This is another uncommon type of polypoid dysplasia, which consists of columnar epithelium with a villous, tubulovillous, or serrated growth pattern; gastric-type foveolar-like apical mucin globules; and variable numbers of interspersed goblet cells. Importantly, the nuclear size and degree of atypia decrease toward the luminal surface, and superficial biopsies may belie the presence of deep dysplasia. This type of dysplasia has been variably termed "mucinous dysplasia" or "villous dysplasia" (Fig. 6.35a and b). The biological behavior of this type of dysplasia is currently unknown.

References: [50, 51]

15. **How is dysplasia distinguished from reactive epithelial changes in IBD?**

The distinction between dysplastic and reactive epithelium in IBD is a common and impactful challenge, especially in the setting of active or resolving colitis, but truly problematic cases are the exception rather than the rule (Table 6.5). A hallmark of reactive crypts is the base-to-surface "maturation gradient," which describes the gradual transition from phenotypically undifferentiated, mitotically active basal colonocytes with relatively

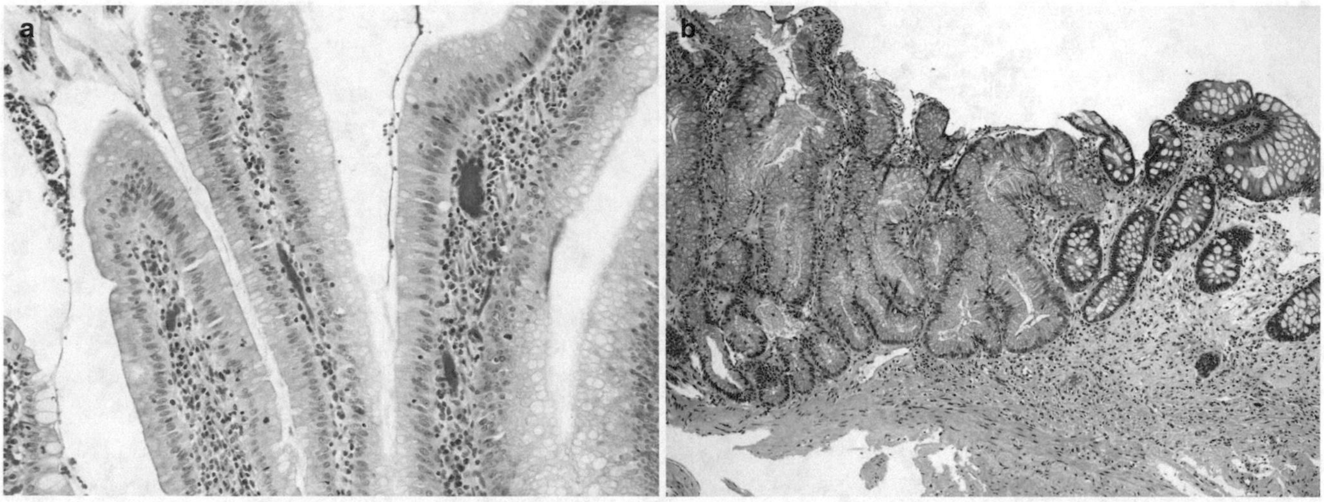

Fig. 6.35 Hypermucinous (villous) dysplasia showing a villous architecture with mixed gastric foveolar and goblet cell features (**a**). The lesion is sharply demarcated from adjacent nondysplastic colonic mucosa in this example (**b**)

Table 6.5 Distinguishing features between reactive and dysplastic epithelium in IBD

Histological feature	Nondysplastic	Dysplastic
Differentiation toward mature epithelium	Yes	None or minimal except certain types, such as villous dysplasia
Sensitivity to inflammatory milieu	Highly sensitive	Relatively insensitive
Transitions between phenotypes	Gradual	Abrupt
Persistence after resolution of active inflammation	Variable	Always

high nuclear-to-cytoplasmic ratios to differentiated surface enterocyte and goblet cell epithelium with small, normochromatic nuclei. In severe inflammation and early regeneration, expansion of the reactive basal epithelium along the crypt axis may resemble dysplasia by displacing the maturation gradient toward the surface (Fig. 6.36a). Nondysplastic epithelium is more responsive than dysplasia to local variations in inflammatory activity. Thus, atypia associated with intense inflamma tion merges gradually with mature colonocytes in adjoining less inflamed mucosa (Fig. 6.36b and c).

In contrast, dysplastic epithelium extends uniformly from the base to the surface with little or no surface maturation (Fig. 6.36d), and its interface with adjacent nondysplastic epithelium is more abrupt. Notable exceptions to this rule are villous and serrated dysplasias in which the surface epithelium is relatively bland and is potentially underdiagnosed if the crypt bases are not sampled. Other features that favor dysplasia are diffuse nuclear hyperchromasia, uniformly prominent or enlarged nucleoli, atypical mitotic figures, loss of nuclear polarity, and dirty intraluminal necrosis. Whenever possible, biopsies should be interpreted in conjunction with clinical history and, in problematic cases, should be reviewed by pathologists with experience in IBD.

References: [48, 52, 53]

16. What is the value of adjunctive markers in distinguishing dysplasia from reactive epithelial changes in IBD?

Immunohistochemical stains may play an adjunctive diagnostic role but do not replace histology as the gold standard. The best studied immunostains involve the aberrant expression of proteins implicated in colorectal carcinogenesis. Alterations of *TP53* are frequent and relatively early events in the inflammation-dysplasia-cancer sequence. Whereas normal synthesis and degradation of wild-type TP53 maintain low homeostatic levels of the nuclear protein, many mutations interfere with degradation and result in nuclear overexpression. Mutations can occur prior to emergence of the histological features of dysplasia, albeit infrequently (<5%), but their prevalence increases progressively in LGD, HGD, and adenocarcinoma. The most widely used reagent is the clone DO-7 antibody. A wild-type expression pattern seen in normal and reactive epithelia presents weak (1+) or occasionally moderate (2+) but heterogenous staining and is typically limited to the lower half of the crypts (Fig. 6.37a and b). Mutant TP53 overexpression presents a pattern of homogeneous strong (2–3+) nuclear expression which spans the entire crypt axis (Fig. 6.38a and b). Alternatively, certain "null" mutations can cause complete absence of TP53 expression. Both overexpression and silencing of TP53 expression are supportive of dysplasia in equivocal cases where the morphology is strongly suggestive but are not diagnostic in themselves.

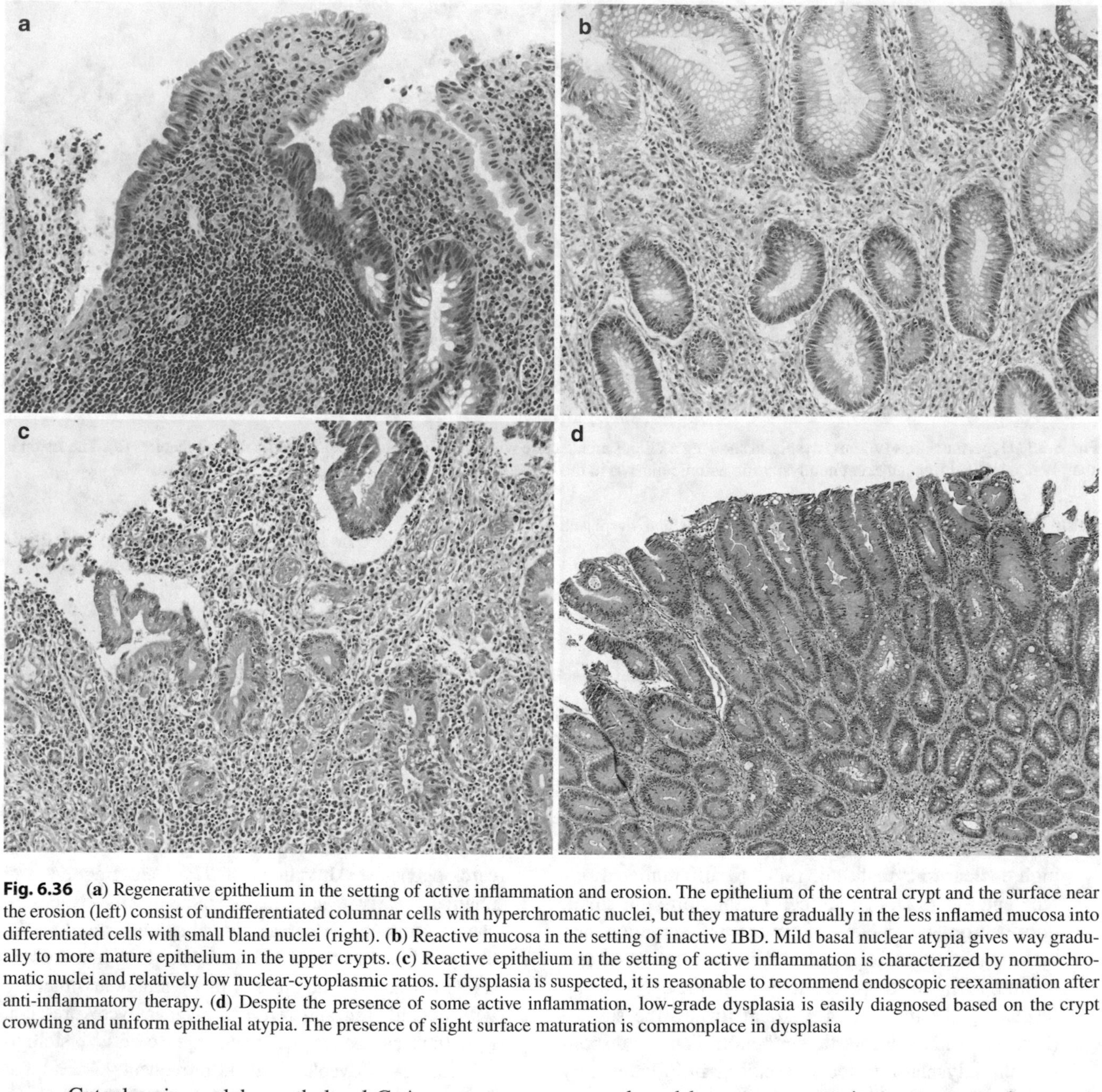

Fig. 6.36 (**a**) Regenerative epithelium in the setting of active inflammation and erosion. The epithelium of the central crypt and the surface near the erosion (left) consist of undifferentiated columnar cells with hyperchromatic nuclei, but they mature gradually in the less inflamed mucosa into differentiated cells with small bland nuclei (right). (**b**) Reactive mucosa in the setting of inactive IBD. Mild basal nuclear atypia gives way gradually to more mature epithelium in the upper crypts. (**c**) Reactive epithelium in the setting of active inflammation is characterized by normochromatic nuclei and relatively low nuclear-cytoplasmic ratios. If dysplasia is suspected, it is reasonable to recommend endoscopic reexamination after anti-inflammatory therapy. (**d**) Despite the presence of some active inflammation, low-grade dysplasia is easily diagnosed based on the crypt crowding and uniform epithelial atypia. The presence of slight surface maturation is commonplace in dysplasia

Cytoplasmic alpha-methylacyl-CoA racemase (AMACR) overexpression has been reported in IBD-related neoplasia. Low-level expression of AMACR in inflamed and normal mucosa limits its diagnostic value, but coexpression with TP53 has a confirmatory role, reportedly occurring in 76% of neoplastic biopsies, 30% of biopsies with indefinite dysplasia, and only 0.6% of nonneoplastic biopsies.

Cytoplasmic expression of CK7 occurs in 61% of dysplastic tissues and less frequently in inflamed mucosa. In one study, combined immunostaining for CK7 and TP53 afforded 95% sensitivity and 82% specificity for dysplasia using carefully adjusted threshold values.

It should be mentioned that using TP53 immunostain to help diagnose dysplasia in IBD is not universally endorsed because regenerating crypts may also potentially show strong TP53 expression. AMACR and CK7 do not appear to be reliable markers for IBD dysplasia and are thus not currently used in practices: [47, 54–57]

17. How are sporadic adenomas distinguished from IBD-associated dysplasia?

Sporadic colorectal adenomas, which are dysplastic by definition, can occur incidentally in patients with IBD, particularly those in the age range where adenomas are prevalent. Experience has shown that the occurrence of adenomas in patients with IBD does not have a significant impact on the risk of developing cancer and that adenomas may be managed by simple polypectomy in the same manner as in non-IBD patients.

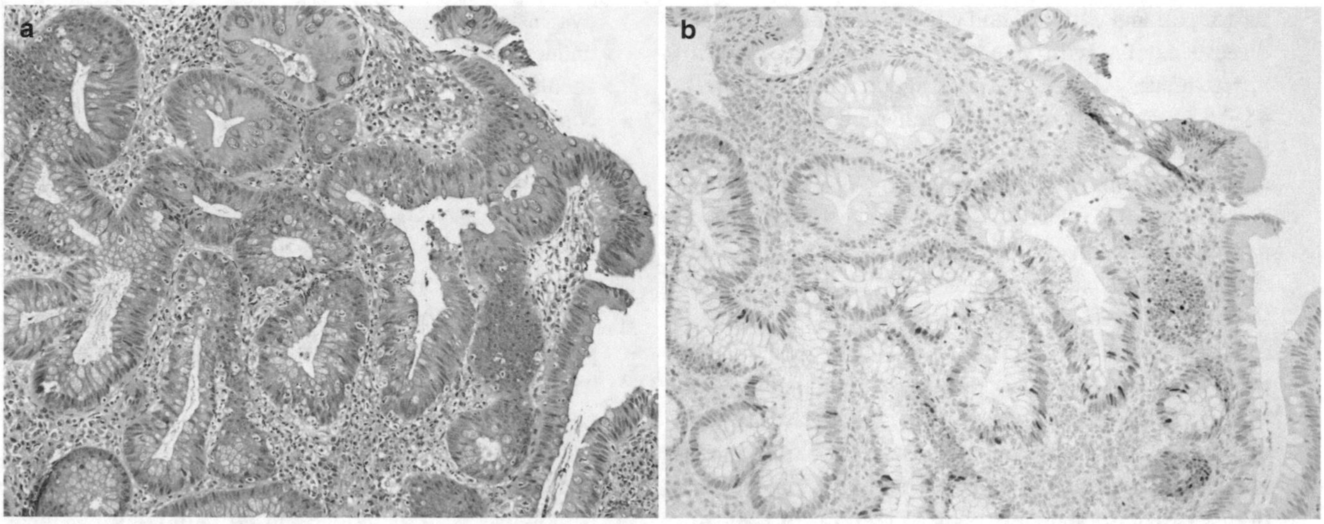

Fig. 6.37 (**a**) A case of active colitis with crypts and surface epithelium on the right showing mildly crowded, hyperchromatic nuclei, which may be interpreted as "indefinite for dysplasia." (**b**) Immunostain reveals a wild-type expression pattern of TP53 expression consisting of heterogenous, mostly 1+ staining limited to the crypts

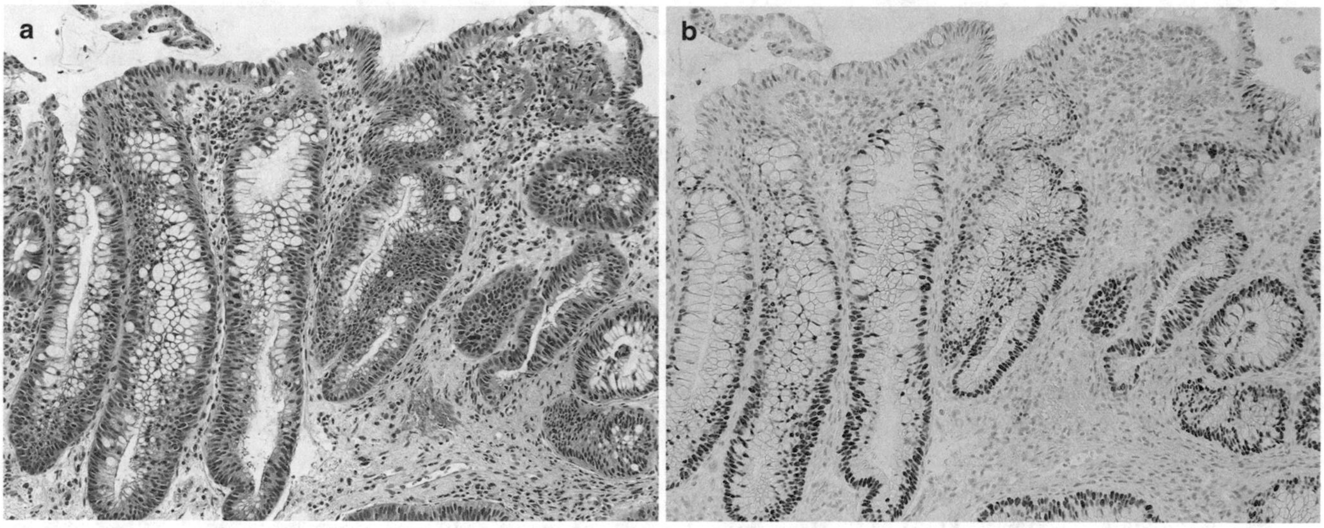

Fig. 6.38 A case of low-grade dysplasia (**a**) showing homogeneous 3+ expression of TP53 in dysplastic crypts (**b**)

Histological criteria, such as sharp circumscription from the surrounding mucosa or a top-down rather than a bottom-up pattern of dysplasia, may support a diagnosis of adenoma, but none have been proven to be definitive.

An adenoma can be diagnosed when the surrounding mucosa is both endoscopically and histologically normal, as in the right side of the colon of patients with left-sided UC. Likewise, pedunculated dysplastic polyps comprising a discrete dysplastic head and nondysplastic pedicle are considered to be sporadic even if the surrounding mucosa is involved by colitis. Studies have shown that patients with IBD who have sessile dysplastic polyps that appear adenoma-like, i.e., endoscopically discrete, dome shaped, and symmetrical, can be managed by simple polypectomy even when they occur in the background of colitis and even if they contain HGD.

Nonetheless, in recent years the pathological distinction between sporadic adenoma and IBD-associated polypoid dysplasia has been rendered largely moot by the use of advanced endoscopic methods for local resection. Following endoscopic resection, biopsy sampling of the immediate adjacent mucosa is advisable and at least one reexamination should be carried out within a few months.

References: [48, 49, 52, 58]

18. **How is a diagnosis of dysplasia integrated into the clinical management of patients with IBD?**

Patients with IBD are predisposed to the development of colorectal cancer. The magnitude of risk is similar for patients with UC and CD of similar duration and disease extent, with standardized incidence ratios of approximately 2–2.5. The peak age of cancer victims is 45–55 years, and nearly 1/3 are under age 40. Patients at the highest risk are those who have concurrent PSC, anatomically extensive disease, long disease duration, persistent disease activity, IBD onset at a young age, and a family history of early colorectal cancer.

Endoscopic examination to detect dysplasia, the earliest recognizable cancer precursor and best predictor of neoplastic progression, plays a key role in prevention by providing a window of opportunity for therapeutic intervention before cancer develops. The standards of care recommended by professional gastroenterology organizations include a screening examination after 8–10 years of disease, or immediately upon a diagnosis of PSC, followed by periodic surveillance examinations entailing careful inspection and biopsy sampling throughout the large intestine. Biopsies are both random and targeted to any suspicious lesions. Because dysplasia in IBD can be flat and indistinct or may be obscured by surrounding inflammatory changes such as inflammatory polyps or strictures, surveillance examinations are best performed with high-resolution optics or with dye spray techniques (chromoendoscopy).

The natural history and management of patients with IBD-associated dysplasia depend on its endoscopic characteristics. A recent international consensus statement (SCENIC: Surveillance for Colorectal Endoscopic Neoplasia Detection and Management of Inflammatory Bowel Disease) has classified dysplastic lesions in IBD as either visible or invisible. Visible dysplasia is subclassified as either polypoid or nonpolypoid and is modified to describe any ulceration and whether the borders are distinct or indistinct. This terminology replaces older terms such adenoma-like polyps and DALM (dysplasia-associated lesion or mass), which are no longer recommended.

Following a biopsy diagnosis of LGD, the cumulative 5-year probability of developing HGD or cancer ranges from 23 to 54%, but the risk can be reduced substantially if the dysplastic lesion can be identified visually and resected. Thus, once polypoid LGD has been resected, the cumulative risk of long-term progression to carcinoma is less than 3% both in UC and CD. Biopsies taken adjacent to the resection site can be used to confirm that complete endoscopic resection has been achieved.

"Invisible" dysplasia refers to randomly detected, i.e., nontargeted lesions, including those that are truly invisible and those that are camouflaged by background inflammatory changes. As expected, visible dysplasia accounts for the great majority of dysplastic biopsies, especially when chromoendoscopy is used. Nevertheless, random biopsies have not been abandoned by most practitioners; in fact, their yields are comparable to those of targeted biopsies in patients diagnosed previously with dysplasia. When invisible dysplasia is encountered under standard white light examination, the patient should be referred for examination by chromoendoscopy or with high-definition optics.

Carcinoma and unresectable dysplasia are indications for colectomy regardless of their endoscopic features. Surgery is also considered when dysplasia is invisible or multifocal, especially if it is high grade, and for patients with inflammatory changes that might limit the effectiveness of endoscopic examination, such as inflammatory polyposis or stenosis. Patients with indefinite dysplasia or with dysplasia that has been removed endoscopically should have close endoscopic follow-up at short intervals.

It is recommended that biopsy diagnoses involving potential dysplasia be confirmed by at least one other pathologist with experience in GI pathology whenever they are likely to impact management decisions.
References: [58, 59]

19. Are there distinctive pathological features of colorectal carcinoma in IBD?

The mean age of patients with IBD who develop colorectal cancer is 10–15 years younger than their sporadic counterparts. Cancers arise in regions of the colon that are chronically inflamed. In UC, most cancers occur in the left side, particularly the rectosigmoid colon, whereas in CD they are more evenly distributed between the left and right sides. Approximately 10% of cancers in IBD are multiple, especially in younger patients.

In resected specimens, cancers in IBD patients present as exophytic or ulcerated masses, plaques, or strictures which often mimic inflammatory lesions (Fig. 6.39a–d). Some deceptively flat, inconspicuous tumors are more easily detected by palpation in the unfixed state than by visual inspection. Compared with sporadic cancers, they are poorly delimited, irregularly shaped, and asymmetrical. Classical round, ulcerated lesions with heaped-up edges and smooth borders are rare in IBD and are likely to be coincidental sporadic cancers.

Most colorectal cancers in IBD have conventional morphology; however, at least 15% are mucinous, compared with ~10% in the general population, and up to 7% comprise signet ring cells, compared with ~1% in the general population. Approximately 10% have extremely well-differentiated, low-grade tubuloglandular features, which are rarely encountered outside the IBD setting (Fig. 6.39e). They consist of individual round or elliptical glands with relatively mild cytological atypia that elicit little or no desmoplastic reaction. Other rare subtypes such as goblet cell, adenosquamous, clear cell, and hepatoid carcinomas have been reported.

Long-standing chronic fistulizing perianal disease in CD predisposes to both adenocarcinoma and squamous cell carcinoma, which can arise within fistula tracts, making them notoriously difficult to diagnose, or near

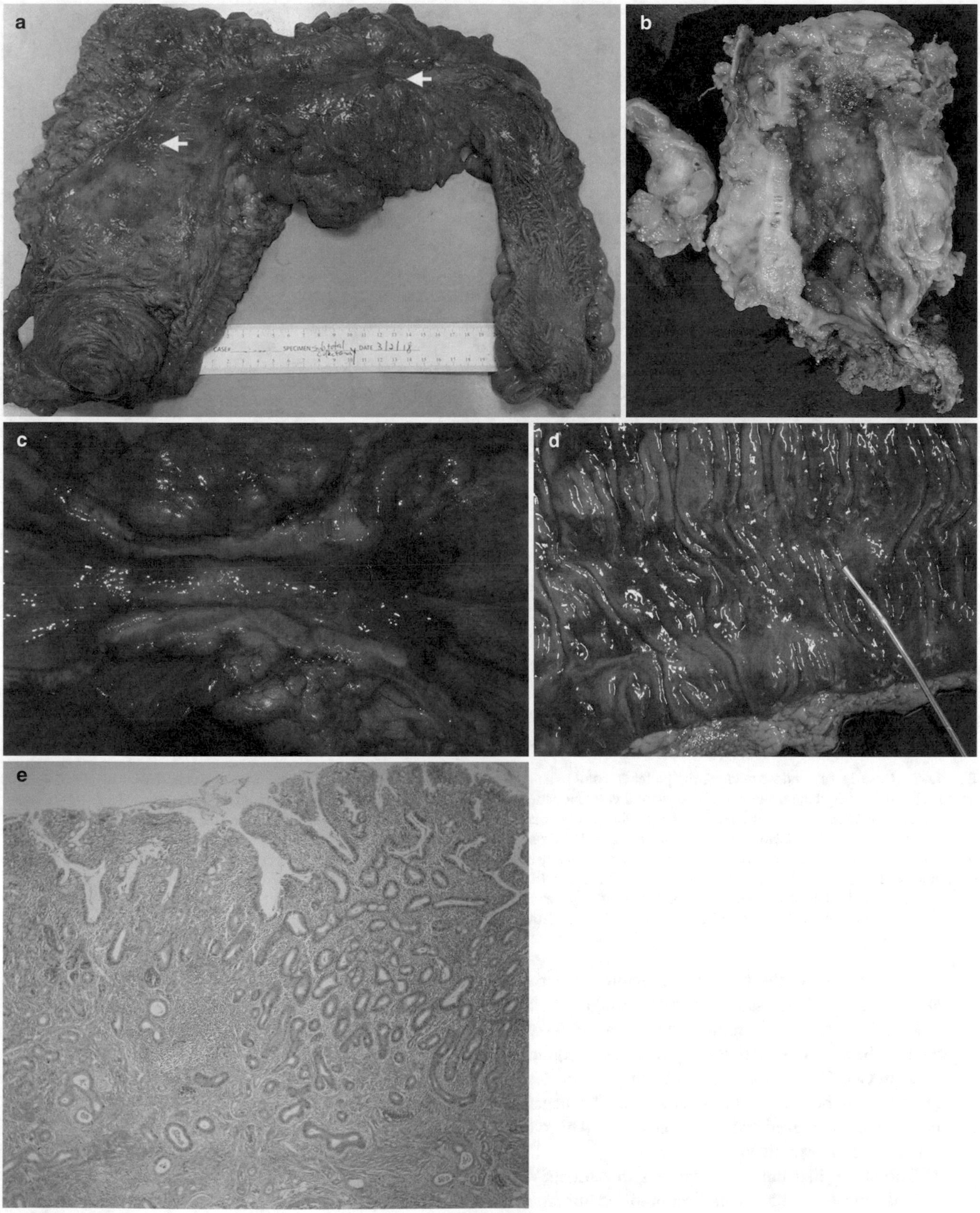

Fig. 6.39 (**a**) Ulcerative colitis with two ulcerated cancers (arrows). Note the absence of distinct borders. (**b**) Proctectomy specimen and lymph nodes showing advanced mucinous adenocarcinoma in the setting of ulcerative colitis. (**c**) Stricturing carcinoma of the transverse colon in a patient with Crohn disease. Microscopic examination revealed signet ring adenocarcinoma. (**d**) Diminutive cancer with ill-defined borders (probe) in a patient with ulcerative colitis. (**e**) Low-grade tubuloglandular adenocarcinoma arising from mucosa with low-grade dysplasia. The infiltrative glands have round profiles and open lumens, and they elicit little or no desmoplastic stromal reaction

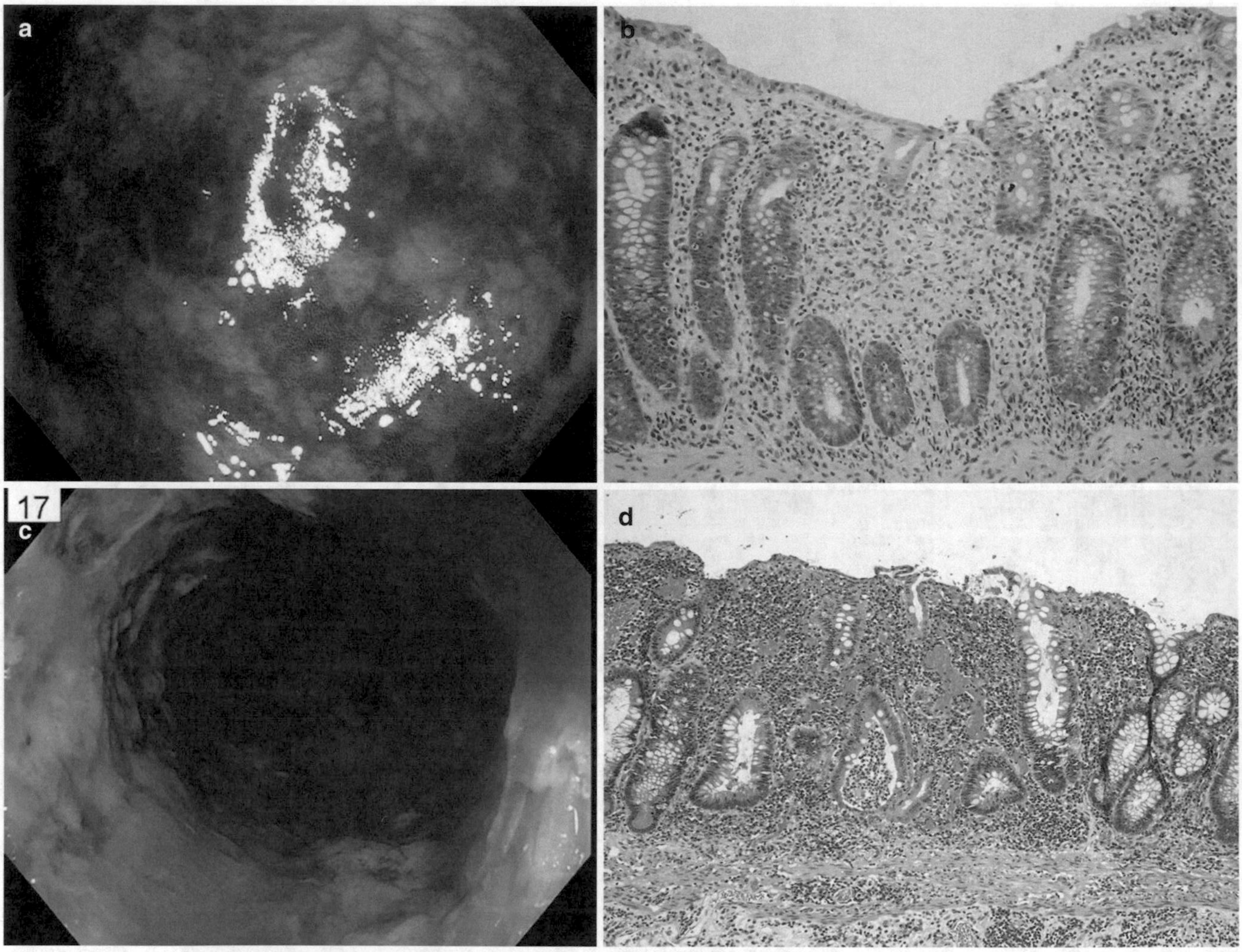

Fig. 6.40 (Case 1). (**a**) Endoscopically, the patient's colonic mucosa at the time of her initial presentation was characterized by slight surface granularity, patchy erythema, and partially obscured vascular pattern. (**b**) Microscopic appearance of acute infectious colitis. The crypts retained their normal caliber and parallel orientation. The lamina propria was edematous and infiltrated by neutrophils, and the crypts exhibited neutrophilic cryptitis and crypt abscesses. Note the incipient basal lymphoplasmacytosis, which typically appears during the second week after symptom onset. (**c**) Four months later, the colon was characterized endoscopically by nodularity, ulcers, and completely obscured vascular pattern, which are typical features of idiopathic chronic inflammatory bowel disease. (**d**) Microscopic features of chronic inflammatory bowel disease include dense, full-thickness infiltration of the lamina propria by mononuclear inflammatory cells; irregularly shaped crypts that fall short of the muscularis mucosae; and neutrophilic cryptitis and crypt abscesses with relatively few neutrophils in the lamina propria

fistula openings in the anal canal, rectum, or perianal skin. Crohn ileitis is associated with a roughly 60-fold risk of ileal adenocarcinoma. The diagnosis is often delayed because obstructive symptoms are so commonplace in CD. The macroscopic presentation may closely mimic that of benign strictures; as a result, the diagnosis may not be recognized by the pathologist until histological sections are examined.

The stage distribution of cancers in patients with IBD is similar to that of their sporadic counterparts. Cancers detected in the course of routine endoscopic surveillance examinations have lower stages than those presenting symptomatically. Published survival data for cancers complicating IBD are too scanty to permit clinical comparisons to patients in the general population.

References: [60–65]

Case Presentation

Case 1

Case History

A 37-year-old woman was admitted to the emergency department with an 8-day history of progressively worsening diarrhea, nausea, abdominal bloating, chills, and light-headedness. She denied recent travel or antibiotic use and had no significant medical conditions, HIV risk factors, or family history of IBD. Flexible sigmoidoscopy revealed mild mucosal erythema and granularity (Fig. 6.40a). A biopsy was performed. A PCR-based stool pathogen test was positive for *Shigella* and enteroinvasive *E. coli*, and she was discharged on azithromycin. A stool culture was positive for *Shigella* and negative for *E. coli* 0157:H7. Telephone follow-up 3 days later disclosed a marked improvement in her symptoms.

Histology

The first biopsy features preserved crypt architecture, neutrophil infiltration of the lamina propria and surface and crypt epithelium, reduced goblet cell mucin, and minimal basal lymphoplasmacytosis (Fig. 6.40b).

Differential Diagnosis

- Subacute infectious colitis
- Incipient inflammatory bowel disease
- Irritable bowel syndrome

The histological features are typical of infectious colitis. The finding of minimal basal lymphoplasmacytosis suggests a duration of infection for at least 1–2 weeks. Features of chronicity would be prominent even in incipient IBD. Irritable bowel syndrome presents little or no histological changes.

Four months later, the woman returned to the emergency department with complaints of bloody diarrhea and abdominal cramps but no nausea or fever. Flexible sigmoidoscopy revealed ulcerations and loss of the colonic folds and vascular markings (Fig. 6.40c). Stool tests were negative for pathogens and *C. difficile* toxins. The second biopsy features full-thickness lymphoplasmacytosis, crypt architectural distortion, crypt shortfall, and crypt abscesses (Fig. 6.40d).

Differential Diagnosis

- Recurrent infectious colitis
- Chronic infectious colitis
- New onset of inflammatory bowel disease

Ancillary Studies

None.

Final Diagnosis

Progression of infectious colitis to inflammatory bowel disease.

Follow-Up

A colonoscopy revealed normal mucosa beyond the splenic flexure, and additional workup disclosed no involvement of the small intestine or other evidence of CD. The patient was diagnosed with left-sided UC, possibly triggered by her earlier infection, and was managed with mesalamine.

Take-Home Messages

- Acute infectious colitis can be diagnosed in biopsies in the setting of supportive clinical data and absence of other causes of colitis (drugs, radiation, etc.).
- Basal lymphoplasmacytosis begins to appear during the second week from onset. Infections that persist beyond 2–3 weeks can gradually evolve histological features of chronicity, resulting in diagnostic ambiguity just when persistent symptoms begin to elicit clinical concerns for IBD.
- IBD presents characteristic histological features, including full-thickness lymphoplasmacytosis, crypt distortion and shortfall, and selective neutrophil infiltration of the crypt epithelium. The combination of these features is histologically quite specific.
- Acute infections are a recognized risk factor for the development of IBD, with hazard ratios of approximately 4.1 during the first year. The most common pathogens are *Salmonella* and *Campylobacter*, but no etiological link has been established with any specific pathogens or commensal organisms. Potential factors include shifts in the host microbiome, stimulation of acute inflammation, and incapacitation of host protective mechanisms.

References: [19, 66, 67]

Case 2

Case History

A 41-year-old woman with long-standing well-controlled UC had been undergoing annual colonoscopic surveillance examinations for the past 10 years with no dysplasia detected.

Endoscopy showed an elevated, broad-based lesion with a villiform surface in the proximal sigmoid colon (Fig. 6.41a). Despite having indistinct boundaries, the lesion was estimated to be 5–6 cm in size. The remainder of the colonic mucosa was flat and atrophic appearing.

Histology

A superficial biopsy of the sigmoid lesion showed villiform mucosa (Fig. 6.41b). The nuclei in some of the villi were enlarged, hyperchromatic, and crowded (Fig. 6.41c), while the nuclei in other areas were small and normochromatic (Fig. 6.41d).

Differential Diagnosis

- Indefinite for dysplasia
- Low-grade dysplasia
- High-grade dysplasia

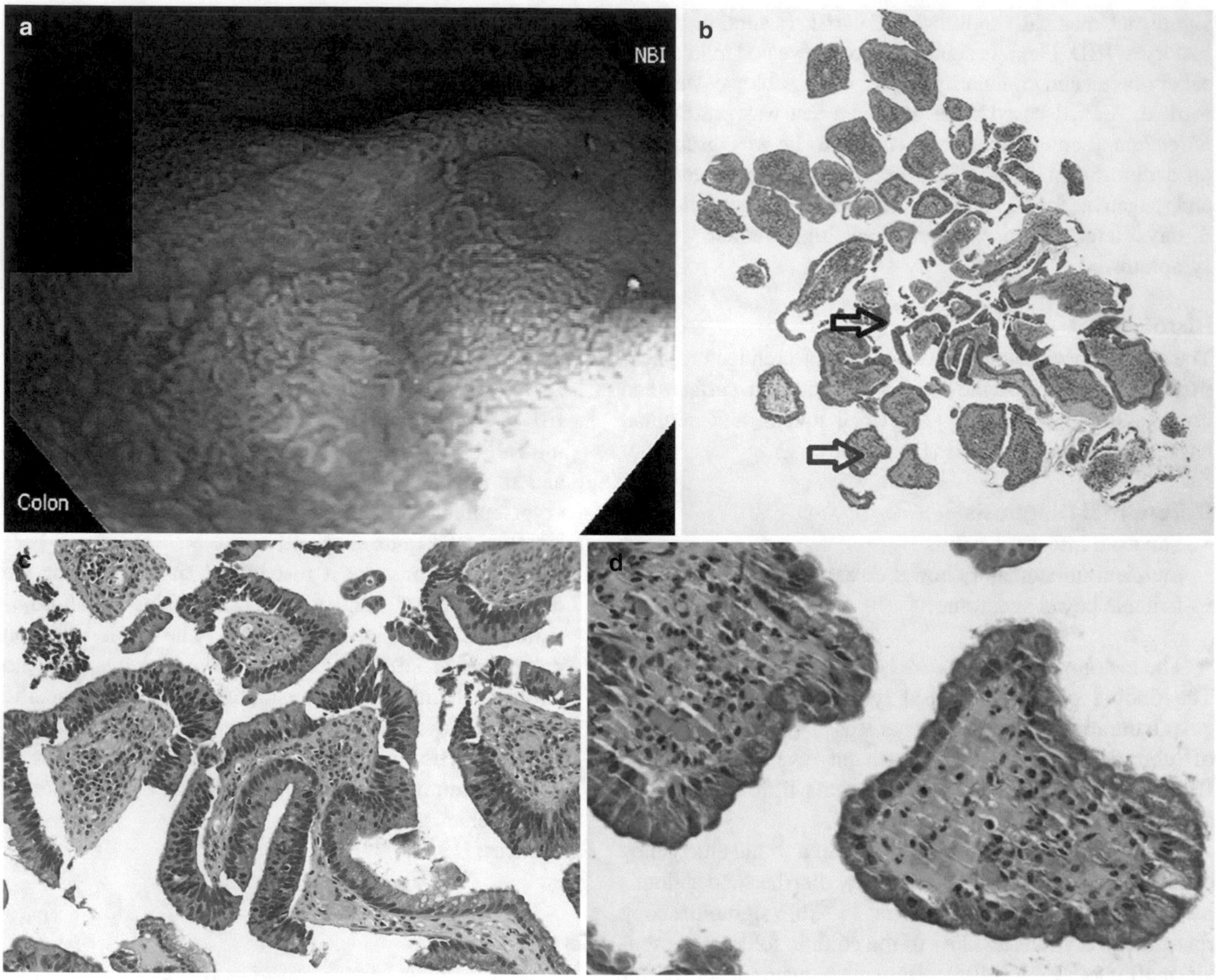

Fig. 6.41 (Case 2). (**a**) Endoscopic appearance of broad-based, slightly elevated lesion with villiform surface. (**b**) Villiform tissue sampled from the surface of the lesion. (**c**) Higher magnification revealed that some of the villi (indicated by a black arrow in **b**) were lined by low-grade dysplastic columnar epithelium characterized by uniformly enlarged, elliptical, hyperchromatic nuclei. (**d**) Other villi (indicated by a red arrow in **b**) were lined by nondysplastic cuboidal epithelium containing small, normochromatic nuclei

Management Options

- Repeat the examination with chromoendoscopy.
- Repeat the examination and biopsies in 3 months.
- Advise the patient to undergo colectomy.

Ancillary Studies

None.

Final Diagnosis and Management

Tentatively LGD based on the most severe changes; however, histological evaluation of the entire lesion is required since it might contain invasive cancer or HGD. The clinical impression was that the size and location of the lesion precluded an endoscopic resection. The patient was therefore advised to undergo a colectomy.

Follow-Up

The patient underwent colectomy (Fig. 6.42a). Complete histological evaluation of the lesion showed areas of LGD and negative for dysplasia in the villi (Fig. 6.42b and c) but revealed HGD at the crypt bases (Fig. 6.42d). No cancer was found.

Take-Home Messages

- Villous dysplasia may exhibit surface maturation that is discordant with findings in the deep crypts.
- Biopsies that contain nondysplastic villous structures should be followed up as potentially significant.
- Colectomy is the standard of care for endoscopically visible, nonresectable dysplasia.

References: [47, 53, 58]

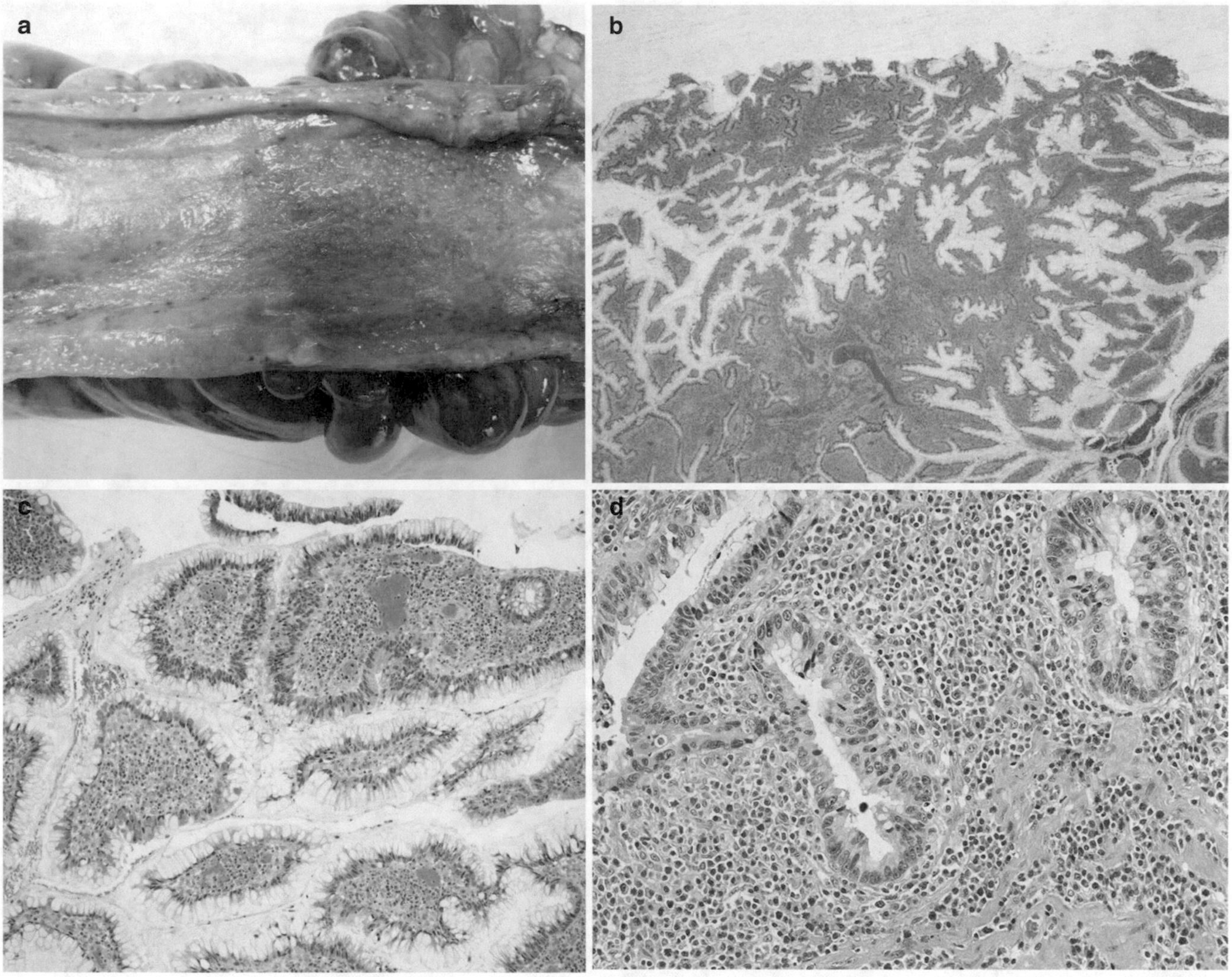

Fig. 6.42 (Case 2). (**a**) Villiform dysplasia in the colectomy specimen. Surgical management was elected over attempted endoscopic mucosal resection due to the large size of the lesion and its lack of well-defined margins. (**b**) Villous dysplasia at low magnification. (**c**) Higher magnification revealed hypermucinous epithelium with low-grade dysplasia involving some of the villi. (**d**) High-grade dysplasia seen in the deep crypts characterized by large, vesicular, variably stratified nuclei

Case 3

Case History

A 48-year-old man with a 15-year history of well-controlled Crohn colitis had undergone annual colonoscopic surveillance examinations with biopsies, by his private gastroenterologist, for the past 7 years. A recent examination disclosed LGD in a single random biopsy of the sigmoid colon, which surprised the gastroenterologist since he had not noted any suspicious findings during the examination and saw none on reviewing his endoscopic photographs. The slides were reviewed by a second pathologist, who confirmed the diagnosis. The patient was referred to a gastroenterologist specializing in IBD, who reexamined the colon with chromoendoscopy under high-definition optics but saw nothing suspicious. Specifically, white-light image of the sigmoid colon mucosa showed slightly obscured mucosal vasculature, a characteristic of quiescent colitis. There was focal black pigmentation from a prior India ink tattoo (Fig. 6.43a). Chromoendoscopy of the sigmoid colon revealed a normal pattern of mucosal pits (Fig. 6.43b).

Histology

A nontargeted biopsy of the sigmoid colon was performed (Fig. 6.43c).

Differential Diagnosis

- Negative for dysplasia
- Indefinite for dysplasia
- Low-grade dysplasia
- High-grade dysplasia

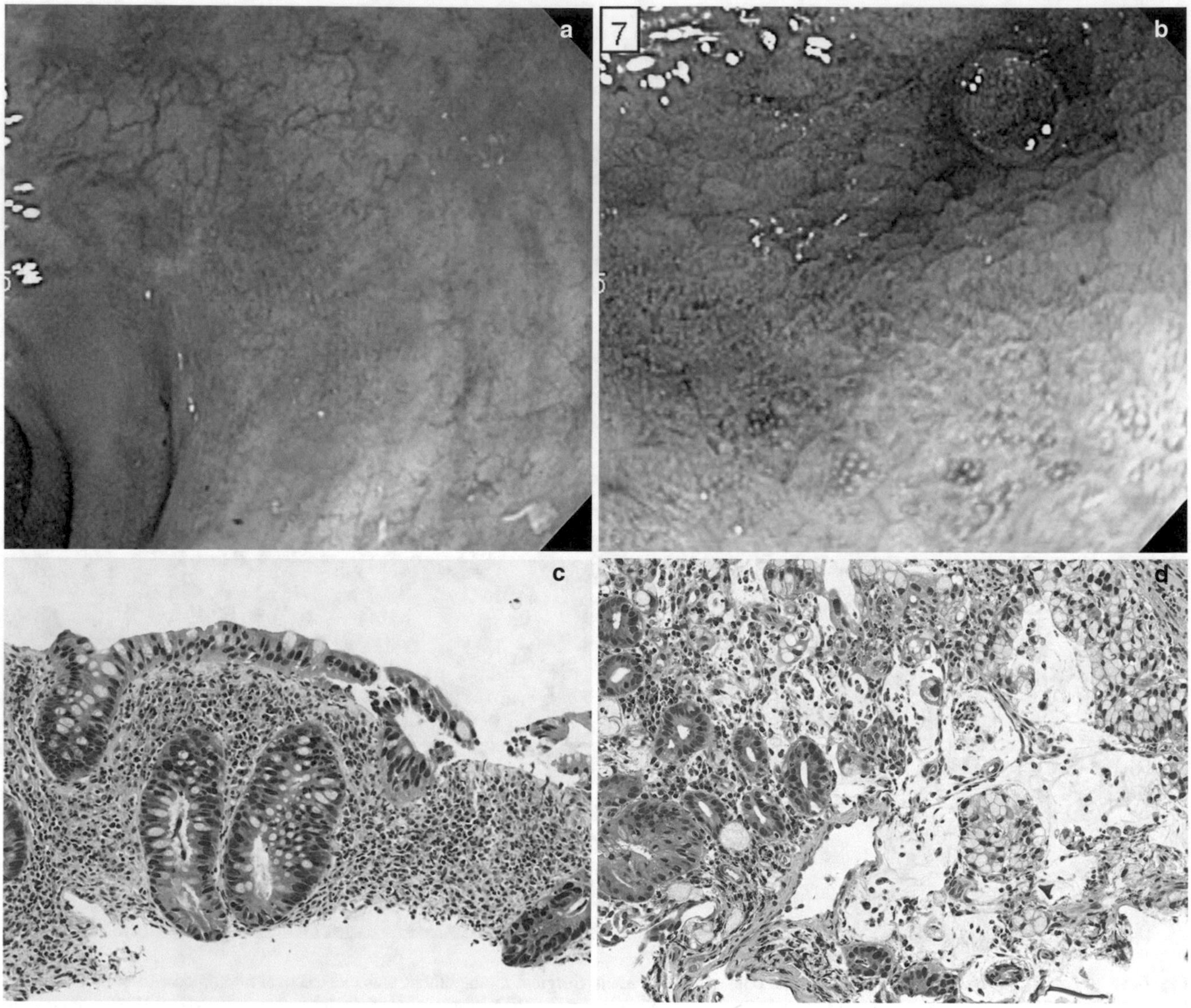

Fig. 6.43 (Case 3). (**a**) Endoscopic appearance of inactive chronic colitis under white-light illumination characterized by slightly obscured mucosal vasculature. An India ink tattoo had been previously administered to mark the location. (**b**) Appearance of the mucosa after spraying with methylene blue revealed a normal mucosal pit pattern. (**c**) Low-grade dysplasia, crypt cell type. The dysplastic epithelial cells had differentiated into enterocytes, goblet cells, and Paneth cells, the latter occupying the crypt bases, mimicking normal colonic mucosa. However, the nuclei are abnormally enlarged and hyperchromatic along the entire crypt axis. (**d**) Poorly differentiated adenocarcinoma identified in the same location as prior biopsies that had featured low-grade crypt cell dysplasia

Ancillary Studies

None.

Final Diagnosis

Low-grade dysplasia (crypt cell type).

The mucosa is flat and chronically inflamed, and the crypts assume an uncrowded tubular growth pattern. The lining epithelium replicates normal crypt epithelium with respect to differentiation into enterocytes, goblet cells, and basal Paneth cells but contains enlarged, hyperchromatic, and moderately pleomorphic nuclei along the length of the crypts and extending to the surface. The dysplasia is classified as low-grade on the basis of its retained cellular polarity and highly differentiated cell phenotypes.

This case exemplifies a distinctive type of dysplasia referred to as crypt cell type. Its flat, uncrowded growth pattern accounts for the lack of a visible lesion at endoscopy under optimal conditions of high-definition optics and chromoendoscopy.

There are few studies in the literature addressing this type of dysplasia. One study published in abstract form reported that crypt cell dysplasia accounted for 48% of 52 nontargeted dysplasia biopsies from 30 patients who underwent surveillance during a period of 44 months.

Follow-Up

Despite being advised to undergo colectomy, the patient elected to continue surveillance on an accelerated schedule and continued to have repeated biopsies showing LGD in the sigmoid colon. On the sixth examination, a small elevation was seen in the sigmoid colon and a biopsy was positive for poorly differentiated adenocarcinoma with signet ring cells (Fig. 6.43d). The colectomy specimen contained a stage III adenocarcinoma.

Take-Home Messages

- Dysplasia in IBD can be endoscopically occult even with optimal endoscopic techniques and is likely to be missed if biopsies are targeted to visible lesions only.
- The natural history and biological characteristics of crypt cell dysplasia warrant further study.
- Nevertheless, any unresectable LGD should be considered a relative indication for colectomy, especially if it is detected repeatedly and the diagnosis is confirmed by a second pathologist.

References: [51, 68]

Case 4

Case History

A 44-year-old male with a 12-year history of UC had been on anti-inflammatory therapy with mesalamine until recently when he began to experience progressive constipation and bloating. Colonoscopic examination revealed active inflammation and multiple mucosal polyps in the sigmoid colon, quiescent colitis with scattered polyps in the descending and transverse colon, and luminal occlusion of the proximal transverse colon, preventing completion of the examination. A subsequent barium study revealed multiple filling defects in the ascending and transverse colon, deep mural fissures, and evidence of pericolic inflammation. The patient underwent an abdominal colectomy.

Gross

Subtotal colectomy specimen showed segmental erythema and mass-like agglomerations of polyps in the ascending, transverse, and sigmoid colon. The polyps had filiform and leaf-like configurations and a soft consistency (Fig. 6.44a).

Histology

The colon was ulcerated and covered by a canopy of congested mucosa with irregular, partially dilated crypt architecture. The wall was punctuated by deep fissuring ulcers surrounded by chronic inflammation. The subserosa showed lymphoid aggregates (Fig. 6.44b), transmural chronic inflammation, and fibrosis (Fig. 6.44c). The remainder of the colon showed diffuse chronic inflammation, which was limited to the mucosa (not shown). No granulomas were identified in any of the colonic sections or pericolic lymph nodes.

Differential Diagnosis

- Crohn colitis
- Indeterminate colitis
- Ulcerative colitis with massive inflammatory polyposis

Ancillary Studies

None.

Final Diagnosis

Ulcerative colitis with massive inflammatory polyposis.

Follow-Up

Six months later, the patient underwent a completion proctectomy and ileoanal pouch anastomosis. Two years later, he was doing well with good pouch function and no manifestations of IBD.

Take-Home Messages

- Inflammatory polyps are commonplace in chronic IBD and rarely cause symptoms other than being a potential source of bleeding.
- Rarely, segmental mass-like agglomerations of inflammatory polyps form in IBD, both UC and CD. This condition, referred to as massive, giant, or filiform inflammatory polyposis, may cause luminal obstruction and elicit clinical suspicion of CD-associated stricture or carcinoma.
- The segments involved by polyposis may exhibit Crohn-like features, including chronic fissuring ulcers and transmural chronic inflammation, which are likely caused by fecal entrapment and stasis.
- The distinction between UC and CD should be based on the pathology of the rest of the colon in conjunction with preoperative clinical data.
- A pathological diagnosis of indeterminate colitis is recommended when the polyposis is extensive or if insufficient supportive clinical data are available.

Reference: [3]

Case 5

Case History

A 40-year-old woman with ulcerative pancolitis since age 13 underwent an endoscopic surveillance examination in which a 2-cm nodule was found in the proximal sigmoid colon. She was offered a choice of continued surveillance or colectomy and opted for the latter.

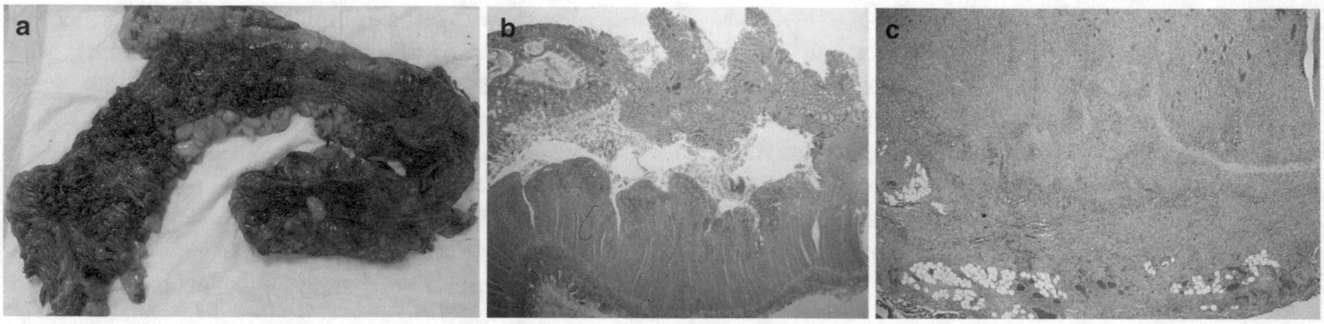

Fig. 6.44 (Case 4). (**a**) Subtotal colectomy specimen showing massive segmental inflammatory polyposis. (**b**) Ulcerated colonic mucosa covered by a canopy of partially detached mucosa. Note the fissuring ulcers and transmural chronic inflammation. (**c**) Ulcerative colitis with Crohn-like transmural chronic inflammation and subserosal fibrosis limited to the segment with massive inflammatory polyposis

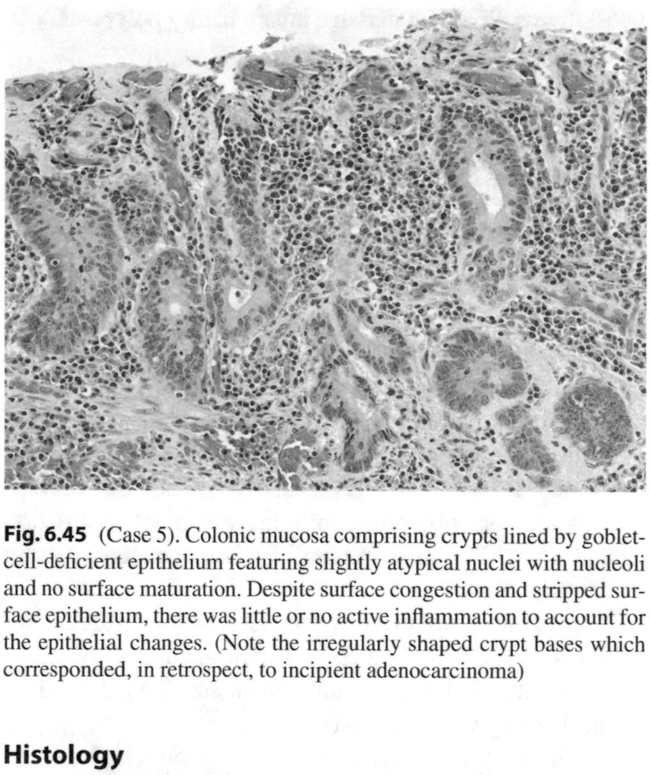

Fig. 6.45 (Case 5). Colonic mucosa comprising crypts lined by goblet-cell-deficient epithelium featuring slightly atypical nuclei with nucleoli and no surface maturation. Despite surface congestion and stripped surface epithelium, there was little or no active inflammation to account for the epithelial changes. (Note the irregularly shaped crypt bases which corresponded, in retrospect, to incipient adenocarcinoma)

Histology

A section from the nodular area revealed chronic inflammation with surface congestion and stripped surface epithelium but little or no active inflammation. The crypts were lined by columnar cells with basally polarized, mildly hyperchromatic, and pleomorphic nuclei and slightly eosinophilic cytoplasm. Goblet cells were absent. There was no evidence of maturation toward the surface. Several of the basal glands had irregular contours (Fig. 6.45).

Differential Diagnosis

- Indefinite for dysplasia
- Low-grade dysplasia
- High-grade dysplasia

The changes were interpreted as LGD, goblet-cell-deficient type, based on the lack of active inflammation, the extent and uniformity of the nuclear atypia, and the lack of surface maturation.

Follow-Up

A total colectomy was performed.

Histology

Lower magnification of the nodular area in the sigmoid colon revealed deep mural invasion by small glands with open lumens and irregular to elliptical profiles (Fig. 6.46a). The nuclei were relatively bland, and there was no surrounding desmoplasia (Fig. 6.46b); however, deeper regions of the tumor contained clusters of poorly differentiated glands with desmoplastic stroma (Fig. 6.46c and d).

Differential Diagnosis

- Superficial misplaced dysplastic glands with transition to poorly differentiated adenocarcinoma
- Conventional moderately to poorly differentiated adenocarcinoma
- Low-grade tubuloglandular adenocarcinoma with progression to poorly differentiated adenocarcinoma

Ancillary Studies

None.

Final Diagnosis

Low-grade tubuloglandular adenocarcinoma with progression to poorly differentiated adenocarcinoma.

Take-Home Messages

- Although inflammation can result in reactive epithelial changes that mimic dysplasia, the distinction can often be made based on the presence or absence of maturation.
- A diagnosis of LGD should lead to serious consideration of colectomy, especially when associated with a visible mass.
- LGD can progress directly to adenocarcinoma without an obligatory stage of HGD.

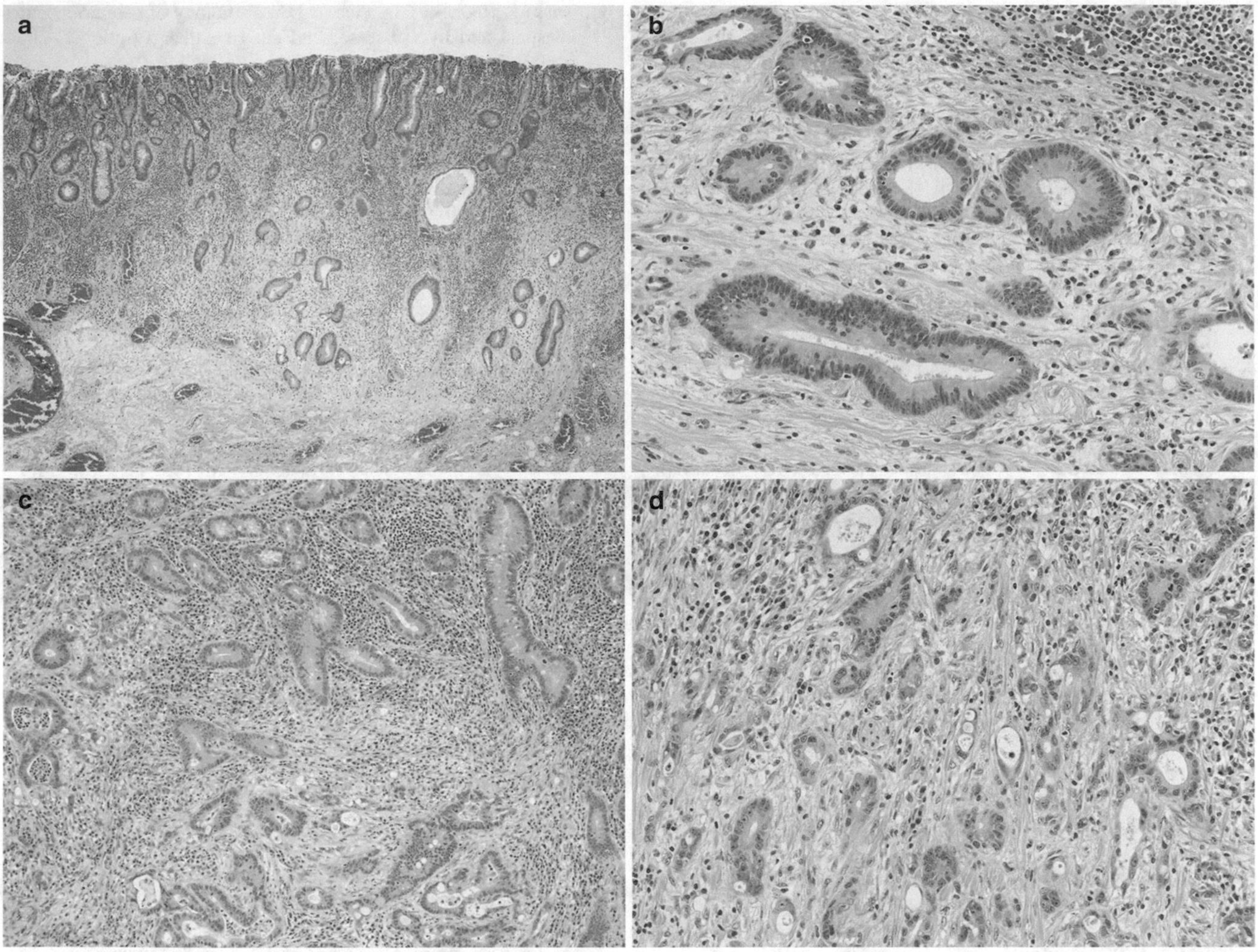

Fig. 6.46 (Case 5). (**a**) Low-grade tubuloglandular adenocarcinoma at low magnification consisted of deeply invasive elliptical glands with open lumens and little or no desmoplastic stromal reaction. (**b**) The invasive glands at higher magnification were round to elliptical. Cytologically, they closely resembled the overlying dysplastic mucosal crypts. (**c**) The deepest regions of the tumor consisted of conventional poorly differentiated adenocarcinoma. (**d**) Poorly differentiated adenocarcinoma with desmoplastic reaction

- Low-grade tubuloglandular adenocarcinoma is a distinctive cancer subtype that accounts for approximately 10% of IBD-related intestinal cancers.
- It usually originates from LGD or even indefinite dysplasia.
- It carries an excellent prognosis on its own but can progress to more aggressive histological subtypes.

Reference: [69]

References

1. Fenoglio-Preiser CM. Gastrointestinal pathology: an atlas and text, vol. xiii. 3rd ed. Philadelphia: Wolters Kluwer/Lippincott Williams & Wilkins; 2008. p. 1296.
2. Riddell RH, Jain D, Lewin KJ, Lewin KJ. Lewin, Weinstein, and Riddell's gastrointestinal pathology and its clinical implications. 2nd ed. Philadelphia: Wolters K`luwer/Lippincott Williams & Wilkins Health; 2014.
3. Naymagon S, Mikulasovich M, Gui X, Ullman TA, Harpaz N. Crohn's-like clinical and pathological manifestations of giant inflammatory polyposis in IBD: a potential diagnostic pitfall. J Crohns Colitis. 2014;8(7):635–40.
4. Yantiss RK, Odze RD. Diagnostic difficulties in inflammatory bowel disease pathology. Histopathology. 2006;48(2):116–32.
5. Guindi M, Riddell RH. Indeterminate colitis. J Clin Pathol. 2004;57(12):1233–44.
6. Jackson KL, Stocchi L, Duraes L, Rencuzogullari A, Bennett AE, Remzi FH. Long-term outcomes in indeterminate colitis patients undergoing Ileal pouch-anal anastomosis: function, quality of life, and complications. J Gastrointest Surg. 2017;21(1):56–61.
7. Martland GT, Shepherd NA. Indeterminate colitis: definition, diagnosis, implications and a plea for nosological sanity. Histopathology. 2007;50(1):83–96.
8. Netz U, Galbraith NJ, O'Brien S, Carter J, Manek S, Petras RE, et al. Long-term outcomes following ileal pouch-anal anastomosis in patients with indeterminate colitis. Surgery. 2018;163(3):535–41.
9. Odze RD. A contemporary and critical appraisal of 'indeterminate colitis'. Mod Pathol. 2015;28(Suppl 1):S30–46.
10. Feakins RM. British Society of G. inflammatory bowel disease biopsies: updated British Society of Gastroenterology reporting guidelines. J Clin Pathol. 2013;66(12):1005–26.

11. Goldenring JR. Pyloric metaplasia, pseudopyloric metaplasia, ulcer-associated cell lineage and spasmolytic polypeptide-expressing metaplasia: reparative lineages in the gastrointestinal mucosa. J Pathol. 2018;245(2):132–7.
12. Magro F, Langner C, Driessen A, Ensari A, Geboes K, Mantzaris GJ, et al. European consensus on the histopathology of inflammatory bowel disease. J Crohns Colitis. 2013;7(10):827–51.
13. Tanaka M, Riddell RH, Saito H, Soma Y, Hidaka H, Kudo H. Morphologic criteria applicable to biopsy specimens for effective distinction of inflammatory bowel disease from other forms of colitis and of Crohn's disease from ulcerative colitis. Scand J Gastroenterol. 1999;34(1):55–67.
14. Feakins RM. Ulcerative colitis or Crohn's disease? Pitfalls Probl Histopathol. 2014;64(3):317–35.
15. North American Society for Pediatric Gastroenterology H, Nutrition, Colitis Foundation of A, Bousvaros A, Antonioli DA, Colletti RB, et al. Differentiating ulcerative colitis from Crohn disease in children and young adults: report of a working group of the north American Society for Pediatric Gastroenterology, hepatology, and nutrition and the Crohn's and Colitis Foundation of America. J Pediatr Gastroenterol Nutr. 2007;44(5):653–74.
16. Cerilli LA, Greenson JK. The differential diagnosis of colitis in endoscopic biopsy specimens: a review article. Arch Pathol Lab Med. 2012;136(8):854–64.
17. Kaiser L, Surawicz CM. Infectious causes of chronic diarrhoea. Best Pract Res Clin Gastroenterol. 2012;26(5):563–71.
18. Lin WC, Chang CW, Chen MJ, Chu CH, Shih SC, Hsu TC, et al. Challenges in the diagnosis of ulcerative colitis with concomitant bacterial infections and chronic infectious colitis. PLoS One. 2017;12(12):e0189377.
19. Schumacher G, Sandstedt B, Mollby R, Kollberg B. Clinical and histologic features differentiating non-relapsing colitis from first attacks of inflammatory bowel disease. Scand J Gastroenterol. 1991;26(2):151–61.
20. Adler BL, Pezhouh MK, Kim A, Luan L, Zhu Q, Gani F, et al. Histopathological and immunophenotypic features of ipilimumab-associated colitis compared to ulcerative colitis. J Intern Med. 2018;283(6):568–77.
21. Bhalme M, Hayes S, Norton A, Lal S, Chinoy H, Paine P. Rituximab-associated colitis. Inflamm Bowel Dis. 2013;19(3):E41–3.
22. Calmet FH, Yarur AJ, Pukazhendhi G, Ahmad J, Bhamidimarri KR. Endoscopic and histological features of mycophenolate mofetil colitis in patients after solid organ transplantation. Ann Gastroenterol. 2015;28(3):366–73.
23. Chen JH, Pezhouh MK, Lauwers GY, Masia R. Histopathologic features of colitis due to immunotherapy with anti-PD-1 antibodies. Am J Surg Pathol. 2017;41(5):643–54.
24. Dubeau MF, Iacucci M, Beck PL, Moran GW, Kaplan GG, Ghosh S, et al. Drug-induced inflammatory bowel disease and IBD-like conditions. Inflamm Bowel Dis. 2013;19(2):445–56.
25. Riddell RH, Tanaka M, Mazzoleni G. Non-steroidal anti-inflammatory drugs as a possible cause of collagenous colitis: a case-control study. Gut. 1992;33(5):683–6.
26. Su Q, Zhang X, Shen X, Hou Y, Sun Z, Gao ZH. Risk of immune-related colitis with PD-1/PD-L1 inhibitors vs chemotherapy in solid tumors: systems assessment. J Cancer. 2018;9(9):1614–22.
27. Harpaz N. Pathology of inflammatory bowel disease in children. Pediat Inflamm Bowel Dis Perspect Conseq. 2009;14:51–66.
28. Levine A. Pediatric inflammatory bowel disease: is it different? Dig Dis. 2009;27(3):212–4.
29. Markowitz J, Kahn E, Grancher K, Hyams J, Treem W, Daum F. Atypical rectosigmoid histology in children with newly diagnosed ulcerative colitis. Am J Gastroenterol. 1993;88(12):2034–7.
30. Rubio CA, Orrego A, Nesi G, Finkel Y. Frequency of epithelioid granulomas in colonoscopic biopsy specimens from paediatric and adult patients with Crohn's colitis. J Clin Pathol. 2007;60(11):1268–72.
31. Russo P, Ruchelli ED, Piccoli DA. Pathology of pediatric gastrointestinal and liver disease. 2nd ed. Heidelberg: Springer; 2014. p. 699.
32. Gentile NM, Murray JA, Pardi DS. Autoimmune enteropathy: a review and update of clinical management. Curr Gastroenterol Rep. 2012;14(5):380–5.
33. Masia R, Peyton S, Lauwers GY, Brown I. Gastrointestinal biopsy findings of autoimmune enteropathy: a review of 25 cases. Am J Surg Pathol. 2014;38(10):1319–29.
34. Uzzan M, Ko HM, Mehandru S, Cunningham-Rundles C. Gastrointestinal disorders associated with common variable immune deficiency (CVID) and chronic granulomatous disease (CGD). Curr Gastroenterol Rep. 2016;18(4):17.
35. Abdullah BA, Gupta SK, Croffie JM, Pfefferkorn MD, Molleston JP, Corkins MR, et al. The role of esophagogastroduodenoscopy in the initial evaluation of childhood inflammatory bowel disease: a 7-year study. J Pediatr Gastroenterol Nutr. 2002;35(5):636–40.
36. Lenaerts C, Roy CC, Vaillancourt M, Weber AM, Morin CL, Seidman E. High incidence of upper gastrointestinal tract involvement in children with Crohn disease. Pediatrics. 1989;83(5):777–81.
37. Lin J, McKenna BJ, Appelman HD. Morphologic findings in upper gastrointestinal biopsies of patients with ulcerative colitis: a controlled study. Am J Surg Pathol. 2010;34(11):1672–7.
38. Tobin JM, Sinha B, Ramani P, Saleh AR, Murphy MS. Upper gastrointestinal mucosal disease in pediatric Crohn disease and ulcerative colitis: a blinded, controlled study. J Pediatr Gastroenterol Nutr. 2001;32(4):443–8.
39. Valdez R, Appelman HD, Bronner MP, Greenson JK. Diffuse duodenitis associated with ulcerative colitis. Am J Surg Pathol. 2000;24(10):1407–13.
40. Chang S, Shen B, Remzi F. When not to pouch: important considerations for patient selection for Ileal pouch-anal anastomosis. Gastroenterol Hepatol (N Y). 2017;13(8):466–75.
41. Lightner AL, Mathis KL, Dozois EJ, Hahnsloser D, Loftus EV Jr, Raffals LE, et al. Results at up to 30 years after Ileal pouch-anal anastomosis for chronic ulcerative colitis. Inflamm Bowel Dis. 2017;23(5):781–90.
42. Murrell ZA, Melmed GY, Ippoliti A, Vasiliauskas EA, Dubinsky M, Targan SR, et al. A prospective evaluation of the long-term outcome of ileal pouch-anal anastomosis in patients with inflammatory bowel disease-unclassified and indeterminate colitis. Dis Colon Rectum. 2009;52(5):872–8.
43. Sagar PM, Dozois RR, Wolff BG. Long-term results of ileal pouch-anal anastomosis in patients with Crohn's disease. Dis Colon Rectum. 1996;39(8):893–8.
44. Shen B, Remzi FH, Lavery IC, Lashner BA, Fazio VW. A proposed classification of ileal pouch disorders and associated complications after restorative proctocolectomy. Clin Gastroenterol Hepatol. 2008;6(2):145–58; quiz 24.
45. Sherman J, Greenstein AJ, Greenstein AJ. Ileal j pouch complications and surgical solutions: a review. Inflamm Bowel Dis. 2014;20(9):1678–85.
46. Wu H, Shen B. Crohn's disease of the pouch: diagnosis and management. Expert Rev Gastroenterol Hepatol. 2009;3(2):155–65.
47. Harpaz N, Ward SC, Mescoli C, Itzkowitz SH, Polydorides AD. Precancerous lesions in inflammatory bowel disease. Best Pract Res Clin Gastroenterol. 2013;27(2):257–67.
48. Riddell RH, Goldman H, Ransohoff DF, Appelman HD, Fenoglio CM, Haggitt RC, et al. Dysplasia in inflammatory bowel disease: standardized classification with provisional clinical applications. Hum Pathol. 1983;14(11):931–68.
49. Schlemper RJ, Riddell RH, Kato Y, Borchard F, Cooper HS, Dawsey SM, et al. The Vienna classification of gastrointestinal epithelial neoplasia. Gut. 2000;47(2):251–5.

50. Ko HM, Harpaz N, McBride RB, Cui M, Ye F, Zhang D, et al. Serrated colorectal polyps in inflammatory bowel disease. Mod Pathol. 2015;28(12):1584–93.
51. Harpaz N, Goldblum J, Shepherd N, Riddell R, Rubio C, Vieth M, et al. Novel classification of dysplasia in IBD. Mod Pathol. 2017;30:174A.
52. Harpaz N, Polydorides AD. Colorectal dysplasia in chronic inflammatory bowel disease: pathology, clinical implications, and pathogenesis. Arch Pathol Lab Med. 2010;134(6):876–95.
53. Mark-Christensen A, Laurberg S, Haboubi N. Dysplasia in inflammatory bowel disease: historical review, critical histopathological analysis, and clinical implications. Inflamm Bowel Dis. 2018.
54. Dorer R, Odze RD. AMACR immunostaining is useful in detecting dysplastic epithelium in Barrett's esophagus, ulcerative colitis, and Crohn's disease. Am J Surg Pathol. 2006;30(7):871–7.
55. Marx A, Wandrey T, Simon P, Wewer A, Grob T, Reichelt U, et al. Combined alpha-methylacyl coenzyme a racemase/p53 analysis to identify dysplasia in inflammatory bowel disease. Hum Pathol. 2009;40(2):166–73.
56. Nathanson JW, Yadron NE, Farnan J, Kinnear S, Hart J, Rubin DT. p53 mutations are associated with dysplasia and progression of dysplasia in patients with Crohn's disease. Dig Dis Sci. 2008;53(2):474–80.
57. Xie H, Xiao SY, Pai R, Jiang W, Shadrach B, Carver P, et al. Diagnostic utility of TP53 and cytokeratin 7 immunohistochemistry in idiopathic inflammatory bowel disease-associated neoplasia. Mod Pathol. 2014;27(2):303–13.
58. Laine L, Kaltenbach T, Barkun A, McQuaid KR, Subramanian V, Soetikno R, et al. SCENIC international consensus statement on surveillance and management of dysplasia in inflammatory bowel disease. Gastrointest Endosc. 2015;81(3):489–501 e26.
59. Watanabe T, Ajioka Y, Mitsuyama K, Watanabe K, Hanai H, Nakase H, et al. Comparison of targeted vs random biopsies for surveillance of ulcerative colitis-associated colorectal Cancer. Gastroenterology. 2016;151(6):1122–30.
60. Canavan C, Abrams KR, Mayberry J. Meta-analysis: colorectal and small bowel cancer risk in patients with Crohn's disease. Aliment Pharmacol Ther. 2006;23(8):1097–104.
61. Connell WR, Sheffield JP, Kamm MA, Ritchie JK, Hawley PR, Lennard-Jones JE. Lower gastrointestinal malignancy in Crohn's disease. Gut. 1994;35(3):347–52.
62. Connell WR, Talbot IC, Harpaz N, Britto N, Wilkinson KH, Kamm MA, et al. Clinicopathological characteristics of colorectal carcinoma complicating ulcerative colitis. Gut. 1994;35(10):1419–23.
63. Friedman S, Rubin PH, Bodian C, Goldstein E, Harpaz N, Present DH. Screening and surveillance colonoscopy in chronic Crohn's colitis. Gastroenterology. 2001;120(4):820–6.
64. Harpaz N, Talbot IC. Colorectal cancer in idiopathic inflammatory bowel disease. Semin Diagn Pathol. 1996;13(4):339–57.
65. Palascak-Juif V, Bouvier AM, Cosnes J, Flourie B, Bouche O, Cadiot G, et al. Small bowel adenocarcinoma in patients with Crohn's disease compared with small bowel adenocarcinoma de novo. Inflamm Bowel Dis. 2005;11(9):828–32.
66. Garcia Rodriguez LA, Ruigomez A, Panes J. Acute gastroenteritis is followed by an increased risk of inflammatory bowel disease. Gastroenterology. 2006;130(6):1588–94.
67. Surawicz CM, Haggitt RC, Husseman M, McFarland LV. Mucosal biopsy diagnosis of colitis: acute self-limited colitis and idiopathic inflammatory bowel disease. Gastroenterology. 1994;107(3):755–63.
68. Ma Y, Ko H, Sfreddo H, Harpaz N. Histological characteristics of IBD-associated dysplasia in non-targeted colorectal biopsies. Gastroenterol. 2017;152(5):S374–S5.
69. Levi GS, Harpaz N. Intestinal low-grade tubuloglandular adenocarcinoma in inflammatory bowel disease. Am J Surg Pathol. 2006;30(8):1022–9.

Non-IBD Noninfectious Colitis

7

Jingmei Lin and Henry D. Appelman

List of Frequently Asked Questions

1. Can I make the diagnosis of microscopic colitis if I do not know the patient's symptoms and endoscopic findings?
2. What are the typical histologic characteristics of microscopic colitis?
3. How is lymphocytic colitis distinguished from collagenous colitis?
4. Is it necessary to count intraepithelial lymphocytes or to apply immunohistochemistry to confirm the diagnosis of lymphocytic colitis?
5. Is microscopic colitis a patchy disease?
6. Does the presence of rare crypt abscesses and/or focal crypt architectural distortion exclude the diagnosis of microscopic colitis if all other features are present?
7. Should I do a Masson trichrome stain routinely when I suspect a microscopic colitis to see if it is collagenous colitis?
8. How can colon biopsies be signed out with slightly increased intraepithelial lymphocytes?
9. What if I see a nondistorted biopsy in which there is obvious epithelial injury and an increased number of lamina propria inflammatory cells but no increase in surface epithelial lymphocytes or subepithelial collagen band?
10. What if I see a nondistorted biopsy in which there is obvious epithelial injury, an increased number of lamina propria inflammatory cells, and a thickened subepithelial collagen band but no increase in surface epithelial lymphocytes?
11. Does a biopsy with a great increase in surface epithelial lymphocytes but with a normal-appearing lamina propria qualify as lymphocytic colitis?
12. From a clinical standpoint, does it make any difference if it is lymphocytic or collagenous?
13. What are the low power features that should make me suspect a microscopic colitis rather than ulcerative or Crohn colitis?
14. What is diverticular disease and what does diverticular-disease-associated colitis look like in a biopsy?
15. How is the diagnosis of diverticular-disease-associated colitis proven?
16. What are the key features to differentiate diverticular-disease-associated colitis from inflammatory bowel disease?
17. What are the histologic features in a biopsy or resection specimen that support the diagnosis of ischemic injury?
18. In addition to bone marrow or stem cell transplant, can solid organ transplants cause GVHD?
19. How is ischemic colitis distinguished from pseudomembranous colitis?
20. If a biopsy looks like acute ischemic injury but it comes from the right colon in a teenager, what is the most likely cause of the injury?
21. What are the typical histologic characteristics of fibromuscular dysplasia?
22. Is it possible purely on histologic grounds to make a diagnosis of chronic ischemic injury?
23. What histologic features should make me consider diversion colitis as a possibility?
24. What clinical data do I need to make the diagnosis of diversion colitis with confidence?
25. What are the key histologic features of pneumatosis intestinalis/coli?
26. Is radiation colitis a specific disease?
27. What changes in the mucosa should make me suspect radiation injury?
28. What are the potential etiologies or risk factors for necrotizing enterocolitis in pediatric population?
29. What are the pathologic features of necrotizing enterocolitis?

J. Lin (✉)
Indiana University, Indianapolis, IN, USA
e-mail: jinglin@iupui.edu

H. D. Appelman
University of Michigan, Ann Arbor, MI, USA

H. L. Wang, Z. E. Chen (eds.), *Practical Gastrointestinal Pathology*, Practical Anatomic Pathology,
https://doi.org/10.1007/978-3-030-51268-2_7

30. What are the key clinicopathologic features of Behçet disease?
31. What are the key features to differentiate intestinal Behçet disease from Crohn disease?
32. What are the typical histologic characteristics of irritable bowel syndrome?

Frequently Asked Questions

1. **Can I make the diagnosis of microscopic colitis if I do not know the patient's symptoms and endoscopic findings?**

   Microscopic colitis is a clinicopathological diagnosis. Therefore, patients' symptoms and endoscopic findings are important components in diagnosing microscopic colitis.

   The typical symptom is nonbloody or watery diarrhea that is defined as being persistent for over 4 weeks. When microscopic colitis is clinically suspected, a colonoscopy workup is considered.

   Normal endoscopy is a key element emphasized in the original definition of microscopic colitis. However, subtle endoscopic findings have been described in some patients, which include edema, patchy erythema, mucosal fragility, nodularity, and alterations of vascular pattern. Rare cases may show focal erosion or even ulceration.

   References: [1–7]

2. **What are the typical histologic characteristics of microscopic colitis?**

   Histologic evaluation is the gold standard to diagnose microscopic colitis, which is essential to differentiate between two major subtypes, and to exclude other causes of chronic diarrhea.

   Increased Intraepithelial Lymphocytes (IELs)

   The predominant histologic feature of microscopic colitis is IEL (Fig. 7.1a–d). IEL is more prominent in lymphocytic colitis than in collagenous colitis. The cutoff number to define IEL is not well established and accepted. Some authors recommend a cutoff value of 20 IELs per 100 surface epithelial cells, and others refer to at least 15 IELs per 100 surface enterocytes.

   Surface Epithelial Damage

   The surface epithelium often shows features of damage, including loss of mucin, vacuolization, flattening, and sloughing. Sloughing of surface epithelial cells is commonly seen in collagenous colitis (Fig. 7.2a–d).

   Inflammation in the Lamina Propria

   The cellularity in the lamina propria is usually diffusely increased, which appears bluish at low power examination (Figs. 7.1 and 7.2). The inflammatory infiltrates consist mainly of lymphocytes and plasma cells, with occasional eosinophils and neutrophils.

   Thickened Collagen Band Underneath the Surface Epithelium

   The pathognomonic feature of collagenous colitis is the thickened collagen band underneath the surface epithelium that might appear irregular, jagged, and patchy (Fig. 7.2a–d). It may contain entrapped capillaries and inflammatory cells. The thickness of collagen band is more than 10 μm on a well-oriented biopsy specimen (a small lymphocyte is 7–10 μm in diameter, which can be used as a reference). In most cases, routine H&E stain is sufficient to make the diagnosis. In borderline cases, Masson trichrome stain may be helpful to highlight the condensed subepithelial collagen band.

   References: [8–11]

3. **How is lymphocytic colitis distinguished from collagenous colitis?**

   Lymphocytic colitis and collagenous colitis are difficult to distinguish from each other based on clinical presentation and endoscopic findings. Histology is the gold standard to distinguish them (Figs. 7.1 and 7.2). The histologic features to differentiate these subtypes are summarized in Table 7.1. Generally speaking:

   - Lymphocytic colitis is characterized by IEL, surface epithelial damage, and inflammation in the lamina propria.
   - Collagenous colitis is characterized by IEL, surface epithelial damage, inflammation in the lamina propria, and thickened collagen band underneath the surface epithelium.
   - Although there may be subtle differences in the degree of IEL and surface epithelial damage between lymphocytic colitis and collagenous colitis, the key feature to distinguish them is the presence or absence of thickened subepithelial collagen band.

   References: [1, 9]

4. **Is it necessary to count intraepithelial lymphocytes or to apply immunohistochemistry to confirm the diagnosis of lymphocytic colitis?**

   In the vast majority of cases of lymphocytic colitis, IELs are prominent enough that it is not necessary to count on H&E slides. In cases where the presence of IELs is borderline, manual counting might be helpful. In counting such cases, only IELs between the cryptal spaces should be considered. The surface epithelium overlying lymphoid aggregates that likely contains more IELs should be avoided.

   IELs consist mainly of CD3+ T cells. In general, H&E itself is sufficient to make the diagnosis. Applying immunohistochemistry to highlight intraepithelial CD3+ T cells is not necessary but might be helpful for borderline cases (Fig. 7.3).

   References: [8, 9, 12]

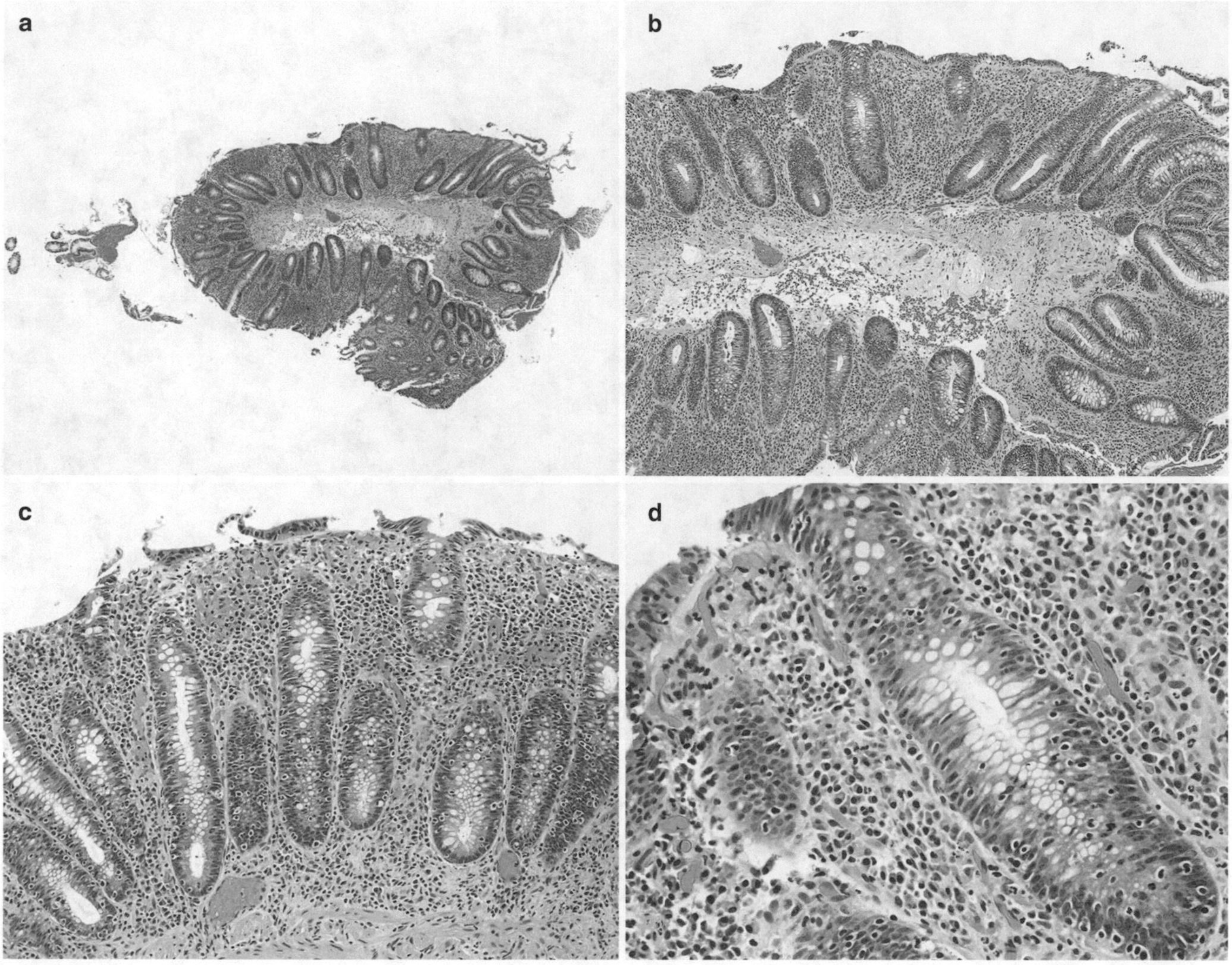

Fig. 7.1 Histologic features of lymphocytic colitis. Lymphocytic colitis is characterized by increased intraepithelial lymphocytes, surface epithelial damage, and inflammation in the lamina propria. The cellularity in the lamina propria is usually diffusely increased, which appears bluish at low power examination (**a** and **b**). The inflammatory infiltrate consists mainly of lymphocytes and plasma cells, with occasional eosinophils and neutrophils. The surface epithelium shows features of damage, including loss of mucin, flattening, and sloughing (**c**). The predominant histologic feature is increased numbers of intraepithelial lymphocytes (**d**)

5. Is microscopic colitis a patchy disease?

Yes, it is well known that pathologic findings of microscopic colitis can be patchy and discontinuous.

Studies have shown that microscopic colitis more commonly affects the right colon (cecum and ascending colon) with less frequent involvement in the sigmoid colon and rectum. Biopsies obtained only from the rectosigmoid colon might fail to detect 20–40% of cases of microscopic colitis.

As such, it is recommended to take multiple random biopsies throughout the entire colon, rather than just from a specific segment, in suspicious patients who present with chronic nonbloody watery diarrhea with normal or nearly normal colonoscopy. The biopsy specimens from different locations of the bowel are better to be submitted in separate containers.

References: [1, 9]

6. Does the presence of rare crypt abscesses and/or focal crypt architectural distortion exclude the diagnosis of microscopic colitis if all other features are present?

Foci of cryptitis and crypt abscesses have been reported to occur in 30–38% of patients with microscopic colitis. However, these should be focal and mild in nature rather than diffuse and predominant.

Preservation of the normal crypt architecture is expected for the diagnosis of microscopic colitis, which is a useful feature to distinguish it from inflammatory bowel disease (IBD). However, focal and mild crypt architectural distortion can be seen in the setting of microscopic colitis, which is not an unusual finding.

References: [1, 9]

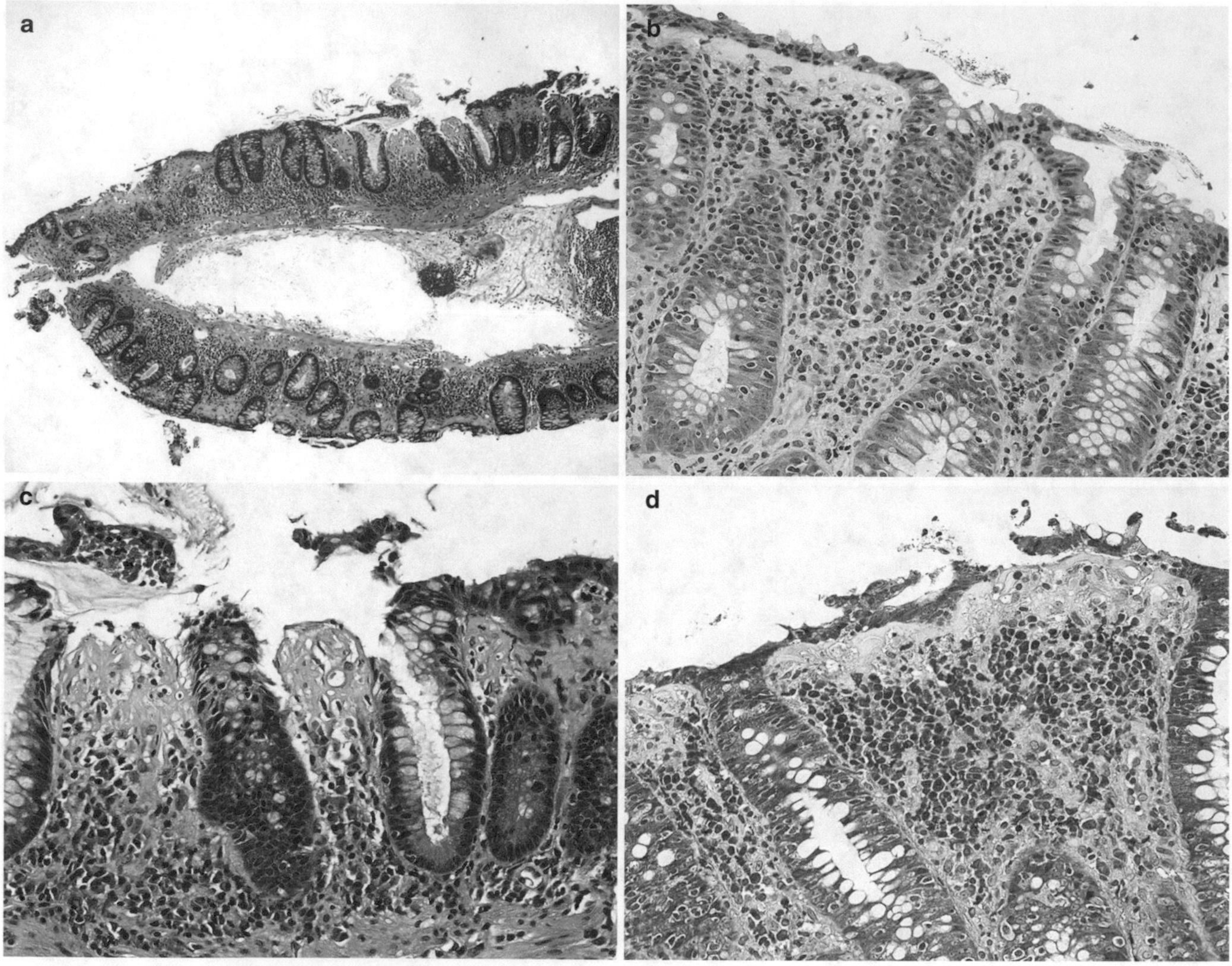

Fig. 7.2 Histologic features of collagenous colitis. Collagenous colitis is characterized by increased intraepithelial lymphocytes, surface epithelial damage, inflammation in the lamina propria, and thickened collagen band underneath the surface epithelium. Sloughing of surface epithelia is common (**a** and **c**). Increased intraepithelial lymphocytes can be prominent or less prominent than that seen in lymphocytic colitis (**b**). Thickened collagen band underneath the surface epithelium is pathognomonic, which can be highlighted by Masson trichrome stain (**d**)

7. **Should I do a Masson trichrome stain routinely when I suspect a microscopic colitis to see if it is collagenous colitis?**

In most cases, thickened subepithelial collagen band is easily visible on H&E sections, even at a low power view. It does not extend around the crypts and is appreciated between the crypts immediately beneath the surface epithelium. As mentioned previously, the distribution of thickened collagen band can be patchy in collagenous colitis. Routine Masson trichrome stain is thus unnecessary.

In cases in which the thickening of the subepithelial collagen band appears equivocal or suspicious or in specimens that are tangentially sectioned showing thickened basement membrane, applying Masson trichrome stain can be helpful (Fig. 7.2d).

References: [1, 9]

Table 7.1 Histologic comparison between lymphocytic colitis and collagenous colitis

	Lymphocytic colitis	Collagenous colitis
Increased intraepithelial lymphocytes	Present, more prominent, more diffuse	Present, less prominent, more patchy
Surface epithelial damage	Present	Present, more severe
Inflammation in the lamina propria	Present	Present
Thickened subepithelial collagen band	Absent	Present, can be patchy

8. **How can colon biopsies be signed out with slightly increased intraepithelial lymphocytes?**

There are cases where patients present with chronic watery diarrhea but the biopsies show only subtle epithelial

injury, minimally increased lymphoplasmacytic infiltrates in the lamina propria, and slightly increased IELs (<15 per 100 surface epithelial cells). In those cases, the diagnosis may be better to be as descriptive as "slightly increased intraepithelial lymphocytes" or as suggestive as "atypical or borderline for microscopic colitis." A comment that includes potential differentials such as microscopic colitis, celiac disease, infectious etiology, and medication-induced injury may be useful. These patients should be followed properly. Studies have shown that some of them may develop typical microscopic colitis subsequently.
Reference: [12]

9. **What if I see a nondistorted biopsy in which there is obvious epithelial injury and an increased number of lamina propria inflammatory cells but no increase in surface epithelial lymphocytes or subepithelial collagen band?**

In a patient who has typical symptoms and endoscopic findings of microscopic colitis, multiple biopsies taken throughout the entire colon may show obvious epithelial injury and increased numbers of lamina propria inflammatory cells, which raise the suspicion for microscopic colitis. However, the number of IELs is not increased, and the subepithelial collagen band is not thickened, which thus do not fulfill the diagnostic criteria. In such a case, a note in the pathology report to suggest clinical follow-up is appropriate.
Reference: [12]

10. **What if I see a nondistorted biopsy in which there is obvious epithelial injury, an increased number of lamina propria inflammatory cells, and a thickened subepithelial collagen band but no increase in surface epithelial lymphocytes?**

The increase of IELs in collagenous colitis is typically patchy and may not be as apparent as those seen in lymphocytic colitis. In the appropriate clinical setting, the finding of a thickened subepithelial collagen band, along with epithelial injury and increased numbers of lamina propria inflammatory cells, is sufficient for the diagnosis of collagenous colitis in the absence of increased IELs.
Reference: [12]

11. **Does a biopsy with a great increase in surface epithelial lymphocytes but with a normal-appearing lamina propria qualify as lymphocytic colitis?**

Isolated increase in IELs itself does not qualify as lymphocytic colitis if the lamina propria appears normal and epithelium exhibits no features of injury. This is debatable, however, because some patients with isolated IELs develop full-blown lymphocytic colitis subsequently. As such, lymphocytic colitis should be kept as a top differential diagnosis. Increased IELs in the colon is also known to be associated with various conditions, such as inflammatory bowel disease (usually accompanied by crypt architectural distortion or having a clinical history), celiac disease, autoimmune enteropathy (particularly in pediatric patients), food allergy, medications, infections, among others.
Reference: [13]

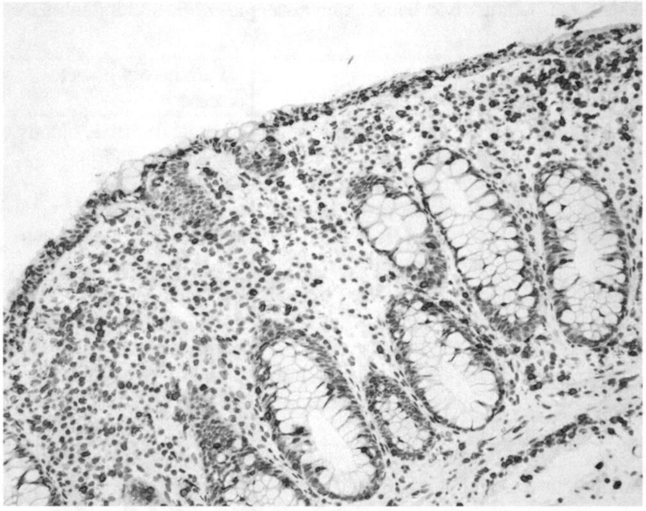

Fig. 7.3 CD3 immunostain highlights intraepithelial and lamina propria T lymphocytes, which can be helpful in borderline cases for lymphocytic colitis

12. **From a clinical standpoint, does it make any difference if it is lymphocytic or collagenous?**

From a clinical, especially management, standpoint, it does not really make much difference because the treatment is the same. For these patients, the first step is to stop potentially inciting medications, specifically nonsteroidal anti-inflammatory drugs (NSAIDs), proton pump inhibitors (PPIs), selective serotonin reuptake inhibitors (SSRIs), and statins, if possible. There are multiple approaches to treat microscopic colitis. Oral budesonide can effectively induce clinical remission and maintain remission for both types of microscopic colitis, although relapse frequently occurs after withdraw. Antidiarrheal agents and cholestyramine may be useful for symptom management. Biologics and immunomodulators (such as azathioprine, 6-mercaptopurine, methotrexate, and tumor necrosis factor (TNF) inhibitor) and even surgery (such as ileostomy for diversion of fecal stream) have been tried with clinical improvement in patients who have failed the initial therapy or present with refractory or steroid-dependent microscopic colitis.
References: [14–16]

13. **What are the low power features that should make me suspect a microscopic colitis rather than ulcerative or Crohn colitis?**

IBD-like histologic features, such as crypt architectural distortion, Paneth cell metaplasia (in the left colon and rectum), active inflammation (cryptitis and crypt

Table 7.2 Comparison between microscopic colitis and inflammatory bowel disease

	Microscopic colitis	Inflammatory bowel disease
Symptom	Chronic profound watery, nonbloody diarrhea, abdominal pain/cramping, weight loss, and fecal incontinence	Chronic diarrhea, bloody stool, fever, fatigue, abdominal pain/cramping, reduced appetite, and weight loss
Endoscopy	Normal or nearly normal (mild edema, patchy erythema, mucosal fragility, nodularity, and alterations of vascular pattern)	Erythema, edema, granularity and friability of the mucosa, pseudopolyp, erosion, ulcer, cobblestoning, and stricture
Crypt architecture	Well preserved, or focal mild distortion	Prominent, either diffuse or patchy
Active inflammation	None, or focal and mild	Prominent, diffuse or patchy, often ulcerated
Dysplasia	No	Maybe

abscess), and surface erosion can be seen in microscopic colitis, but these are usually focal and mild in nature. The overall crypt architecture is well preserved at low power examination. Assessment of multiple biopsies from the colon and/or small bowel, in combination with clinical presentation and endoscopic and radiographic findings, is useful to distinguish these two entities.

Evidently, microscopic colitis and IBD are not mutually exclusive. Studies have shown that the intermittent phases of microscopic colitis and IBD occur in rare patients. Microscopic colitis might be a part of the spectrum of IBD or an epiphenomenon that is superimposed on predisposed individuals. Useful features to distinguish microscopic colitis from IBD are summarized in Table 7.2.
References: [12, 17–23]

14. What is diverticular disease and what does diverticular-disease-associated colitis look like in a biopsy?

Diverticular disease in the colon is defined as small outpouchings (diverticula) lined by colonic mucosa that extend deep into or through the muscularis propria. It can occur anywhere in the colon but is most common in the sigmoid colon. The pure presence of one or more diverticula is termed diverticulosis (Fig. 7.4a). If one or more diverticula become inflamed, it is called diverticulitis (Fig. 7.4b), which may lead to a number of serious complications such as abscess formation, perforation, and stricturing.

Endoscopically, mucosal changes are limited to the affected segment (Fig. 7.4c). In a mucosal biopsy specimen, diverticular-disease-associated colitis (diverticulitis) may display similar histologic features as those of IBD, such as crypt architectural distortion, cryptitis, crypt abscess, and ulceration (Fig. 7.4d–f). Paneth cell metaplasia may be seen in the left colon.
Reference: [24]

15. How is the diagnosis of diverticular-disease-associated colitis proven?

The diagnosis of diverticular-disease-associated colitis is based on clinical, endoscopic, and histologic findings. It is common in males in the sixth decade of life, which most often involves the sigmoid colon.

In addition to the identification of diverticular orifices, endoscopy may show similar findings as those of IBD. These may include erythema, edema, granularity and friability of the mucosa, pseudopolyp, erosion, ulcer, and stricture. Sparing of the diverticular orifices from inflammation is commonly seen in diverticular-associated colitis, which may serve as a useful feature to distinguish it from IBD by endoscopists (Fig. 7.4f).
References: [24–26]

16. What are the key features to differentiate diverticular-disease-associated colitis from inflammatory bowel disease?

Given the overlapping features, diverticular-disease-associated colitis and IBD can be difficult to distinguish from each other based on histology alone. Clinical presentation and endoscopic findings are essential to the differential diagnosis.

In diverticular-disease-associated colitis, diverticulosis is recognized endoscopically and grossly. The histological findings of nongranulomatous inflammation and crypt architectural distortion are limited to the colon segment that is involved by diverticular disease.

As such, colonic biopsy should be obtained from the involved colon segments, as well as the parts that appear normal and are away from diverticular disease. For example, ileum and rectum are usually histologically unremarkable in patients who have diverticular-disease-associated colitis. This is in contrast to Crohn disease, which often involves the ileum, and ulcerative colitis, which often involves the rectum. Useful features to distinguish diverticular-disease-associated colitis from IBD are summarized in Table 7.3.

A good approach to examine resected specimens is to longitudinally slice the bowel at 0.5–1.0-cm interval after fixation, which provides a better view to identify diverticula (outpouchings) and areas of abscess and perforation within the bowel wall.
References: [24–26]

17. What are the histologic features in a biopsy or resection specimen that support the diagnosis of ischemic injury?

Microscopically, epithelial sloughing, necrosis of the superficial layer of the mucosa, and occasionally pseudomembrane-like materials on the mucosal surface are appreciated at low power magnification. In contrast, the crypt architecture in the deep portion of the mucosa is largely preserved, although the crypts

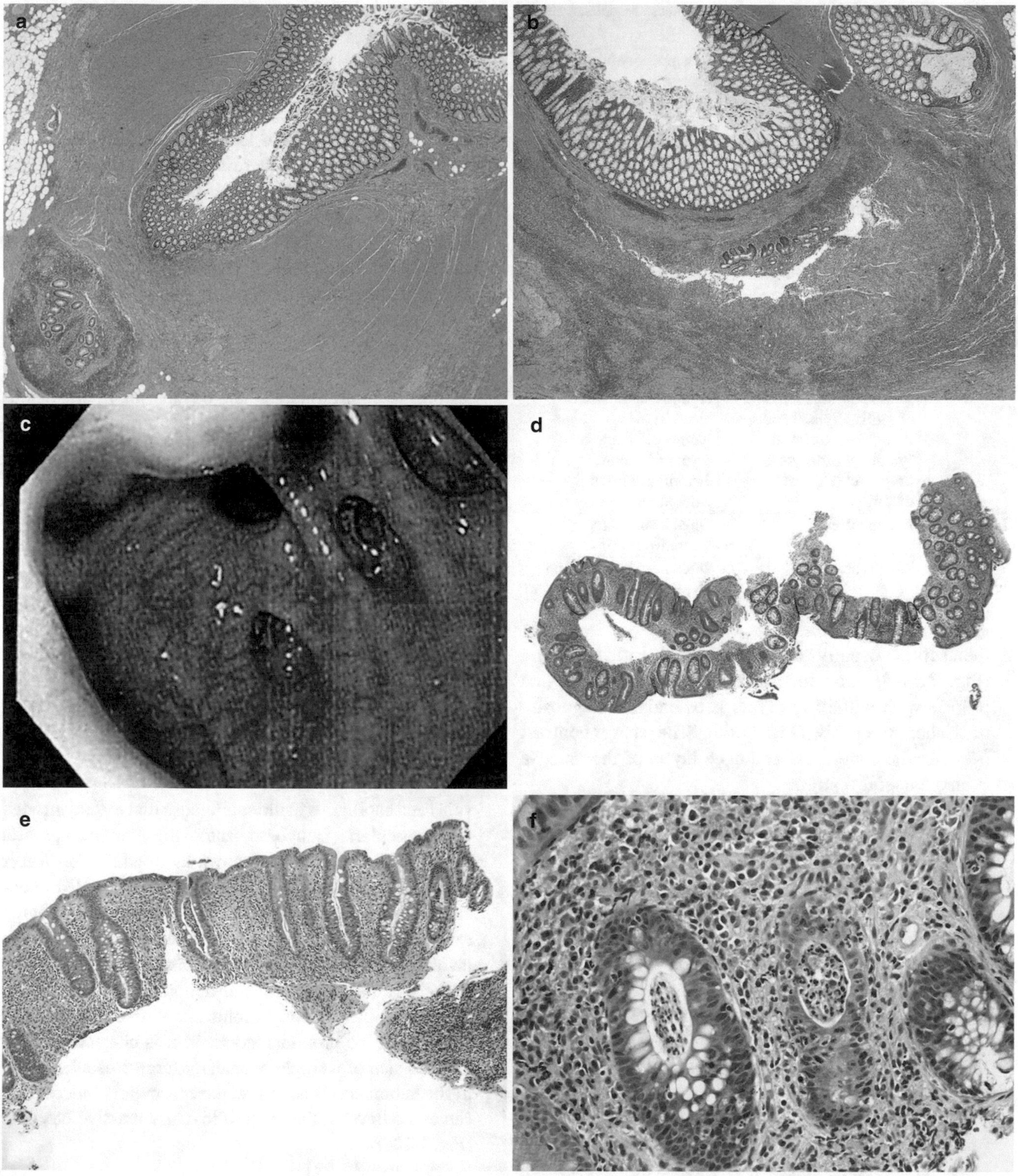

Fig. 7.4 Histologic and endoscopic features of diverticular disease. Diverticulosis features outpouching of the colonic mucosa into or through the muscularis propria without active inflammation (**a**). Diverticulitis shows associated active inflammation, which may lead to abscess formation (**b**) or perforation, resembling those seen in inflammatory bowel disease. Endoscopy can show erythema, granularity, friability, pseudopolyp, erosion, or ulcer that is limited to the segment with diverticulosis (**c**). Microscopically, diverticular-disease-associated colitis may display crypt architectural distortion (**d**), cryptitis, and crypt abscess (**e** and **f**)

Table 7.3 Comparison between diverticular-disease-associated colitis and inflammatory bowel disease

	Diverticular-disease-associated colitis	Inflammatory bowel disease
Symptom	Rectal bleeding, diarrhea, and/or abdominal pain	Chronic diarrhea, bloody stool, fever, fatigue, abdominal pain/cramping, reduced appetite, and weight loss
Endoscopy	Diverticulosis where the inflammation is detected within the interdiverticular mucosa and sparing the diverticular orifices	Diffuse or patchy erythema, edema, granularity and friability of the mucosa, pseudopolyp, erosion, ulcer, cobblestoning, and stricture
Pathology	Nonspecific nongranulomatous inflammation, including cryptitis, crypt abscess, ulcer, abscess, basal lymphoplasmacytosis, crypt architectural distortion	Chronic and active inflammation, including cryptitis, crypt abscess, ulcer, basal lymphoplasmacytosis, crypt architectural distortion, with or without granulomas
Rectum	Not involved	Often involved in ulcerative colitis
Terminal ileum	Not involved	Often involved in Crohn disease

themselves usually appear atrophic and withering (Fig. 7.5a–d). On mucosal biopsy, hyalinized lamina propria with withering crypts is essentially diagnostic of ischemic colitis (Fig. 7.6a). The sharp contrast between the superficial and deep layers of the mucosa is also a useful feature.

On resection specimens, ischemic colitis, enteritis, or enterocolitis may show congestion, hemorrhage, mucosal necrosis, submucosal edema, or full-thickness bowel necrosis (Fig. 7.6b). These findings may be diffuse or segmental. Lamina propria hyalinization with withering crypts may be seen at the transitional areas between necrosis and viable mucosa (Fig. 7.6c). Thrombi, emboli, features of vasculitis, or vascular abnormalities may be seen in mesenteric, subserosal, or submucosal blood vessels (see question 18 below).
References: [25–27]

18. What are the potential etiologies for ischemic bowel injury?

Ischemic colitis, enteritis, or enterocolitis occurs as a result of compromised intestinal blood flow, which can cause injury ranging from mild damage to the superficial layer of the mucosa, to mucosal necrosis, to full-thickness (transmural) necrosis of the intestinal wall. Congestion, edema, and hemorrhage are common in injured areas, as described in question 17.

Various conditions can cause ischemia, and patients with extensive comorbidities have an increased risk. Potential causes of ischemic bowel injury are listed in Table 7.4 (Figs. 7.7, 7.8 and 7.9).

For resected ischemic bowels, the mesenteric blood vessels should be grossly examined and representative sections of the mesenteric vessels should be submitted for histologic examination to look for thrombi, emboli, features of vasculitis, and other vascular anomalies. It should be cautioned, however, that the findings of thrombi and vasculitis in necrotic tissue do not necessarily indicate the underlying etiology as these likely represent secondary changes commonly seen in necrotic areas (Fig. 7.6d). On the other hand, their presence in nonnecrotic regions is more indicative of the underlying etiology.

In addition to ischemic injury, gastrointestinal bleeding is another clinical presentation caused by vascular lesions. Examples include angiodysplasia, arteriovenous malformation (AVM), Dieulafoy lesion, and hereditary hemorrhagic telangiectasia (HHT). AVM is a developmental disorder resulting from abnormal communication between arteries and veins and may present at any age. In the gastrointestinal tract, it is most commonly seen in the rectum and sigmoid colon and may present as a mass or polypoid lesion. Histologically, it is characterized by a cluster of tortuous and dilated arteries and arterialized veins (Fig. 7.10a). On the other hand, angiodysplasia is an acquired, aging-related lesion mainly seen in elderly patients. It can involve the entire gastrointestinal tract but is more commonly seen in the colon. Typical endoscopic findings are discrete, small (usually <1 cm), flat or slightly raised, often multiple red lesions (Fig. 7.10b). Histologically, the lesion comprises a cluster of dilated veins and capillaries in the submucosa that extend through the muscularis mucosae into the lamina propria (Fig. 7.10c). HHT is also known as Rendu-Osler-Weber disease. It may resemble angiodysplasia or AVM endoscopically and histologically, but it differs by having extragastrointestinal telangiectatic lesions such as those involving the skin and mucous membranes. Dieulafoy lesion is a distinctive vascular abnormality that can also be seen in the entire gastrointestinal tract but is more common in the proximal stomach. It is characterized by the presence of a single, unusually large muscular artery in the submucosa just below the muscularis mucosae. It can erode through the mucosa to cause massive bleeding (Fig. 7.10d).
References: [25–27]

19. How is ischemic colitis distinguished from pseudomembranous colitis?

Ischemic colitis and pseudomembranous colitis can be difficult to distinguish from each other based on clinical presentation and endoscopic findings. Endoscopic impression of pseudomembranes is often caused by *Clostridium difficile*, but it may involve an ischemic

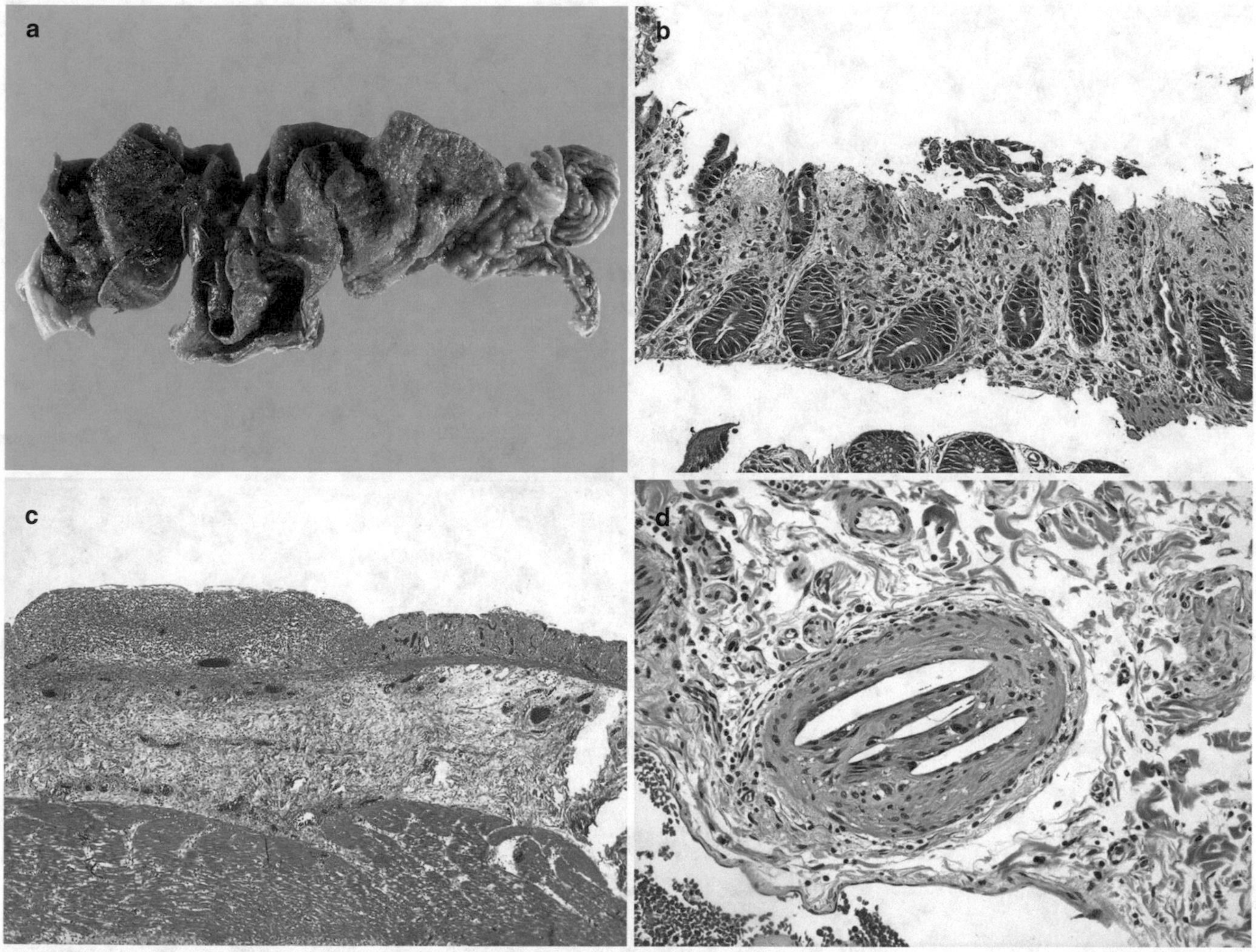

Fig. 7.5 Gross and histologic features of ischemic colitis. Gross examination reveals a segment of colon with dusky discoloration and thinning of the bowel wall. A sharp demarcation is noted between the ischemic segment and adjacent uninvolved colon (**a**). On mucosal biopsy, the superficial layer of the mucosa is injured with epithelial sloughing (**b**). Lamina propria fibrosis/hyalinization is noted. In contrast, the crypt architecture in the deep portion of the mucosa is preserved, although some of the crypts appear atrophic and withering. The sharp contrast between the superficial and deep portions of the mucosa is an important feature of ischemic colitis at low power examination. Histologic section of resected bowel shows complete mucosal necrosis due to ischemia (**c**). An atheroembolus is identified in a medium-size artery (**d**)

mechanism. When results of *C. difficile* toxin assay are negative and symptoms persist despite empiric treatment, colonic biopsies should be obtained as histology can offer helpful clues to the underlying diagnosis. Examples of ischemic colitis with pseudomembranes and *C. difficile* pseudomembranous colitis are shown in Fig. 7.11a and b. Useful features to distinguish these two types of colitis are summarized in Table 7.5.
References: [28, 29]

20. **If a biopsy looks like acute ischemic injury but it comes from the right colon in a teenager, what is the most likely cause of the injury?**

Acute ischemic colitis mostly occurs in old patients, particularly in debilitated elderly women. The left colon is more commonly affected, specifically in the watershed areas of the splenic flexure and rectosigmoid junction. When it occurs in older patients, cardiovascular disease is the most common etiology. It can also occur in young people, such as illicit drug abusers, long-distance runners, and women who take oral contraceptives. A retrospective study of 19 patients who had cocaine-associated colitis found that most of the injury affected the right colon.
References: [25–27, 30]

21. **What are the typical histologic characteristics of fibromuscular dysplasia?**

Fibromuscular dysplasia is a noninflammatory, nonatherosclerotic arterial disease of the medium-sized arteries throughout the body that causes arterial stenosis, occlusion, aneurysm, and dissection. The most common presenting symptoms are abdominal pain, hypertension,

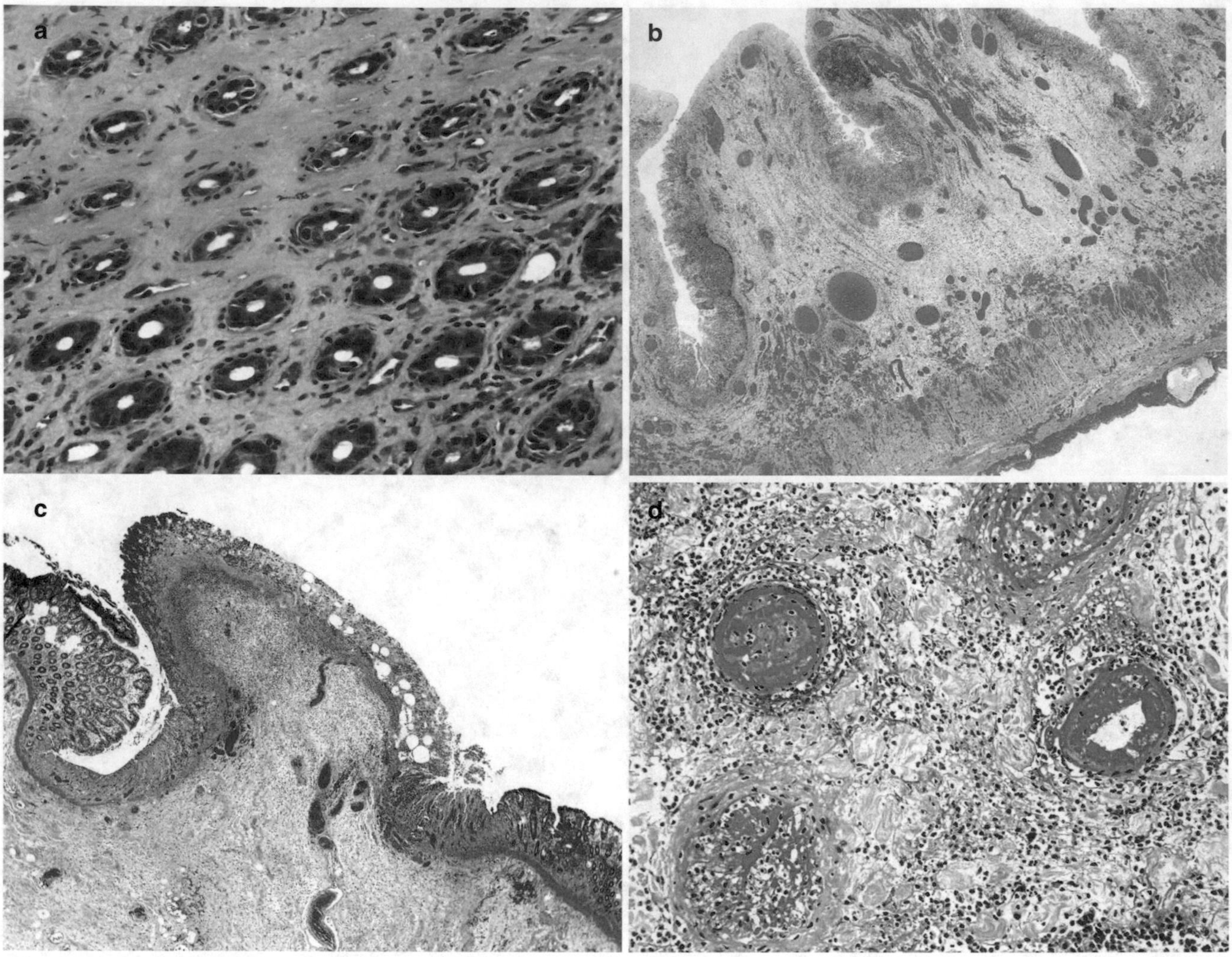

Fig. 7.6 On mucosal biopsy, lamina propria hyalinization with crypt withering is essentially diagnostic of ischemic colitis (**a**). On resection specimens, ischemic colitis, enteritis, or enterocolitis may show congestion, hemorrhage, mucosal necrosis, submucosal edema, and full-thickness bowel necrosis (**b**). Lamina propria hyalinization with withering crypts may be seen at the transitional areas between necrosis and viable mucosa (**c**). Vasculitis with fibrinoid necrosis and fibrin thrombi is seen in the background of necrosis in this case, which may or may not represent the underlying etiology for ischemia (**d**)

diarrhea, nausea, and vomiting. Death can occur when intestinal ischemia is severe.

Angiography, the gold standard, shows diagnostic features of narrowing of the vasculature with a beaded appearance. Histologically, the arterial muscle of intestinal artery is replaced by fibroplasia, which can involve different layers of intima, media, perimedia, and adventitia (Fig. 7.7).
References: [31–33]

22. Is it possible purely on histologic grounds to make a diagnosis of chronic ischemic injury?

The chronic phase of ischemic injury exhibits submucosal fibrosis and stricture formation, although the changes are not entirely specific. As such, if a biopsy deep enough or a resection specimen shows submucosal fibrosis and stricture formation from a patient who has recent ischemia, a diagnosis of chronic ischemic injury is appropriate.
References: [25–27]

23. What histologic features should make me consider diversion colitis as a possibility?

Grossly, the disused colon segment shows diffuse granularity, erythema, blurring of vascular pattern, and mucous plugs. Other findings include varying degrees of mucosal friability, edema, aphthous ulcer, and bleeding.

Microscopically, lymphoid follicular hyperplasia is pathognomonic for diversion colitis, which is easily appreciated at low power examination (Fig. 7.12a). Aphthous ulcer, mild cryptitis, and mild crypt distortion can also be appreciated (Fig. 7.12b).
References: [25, 34–37]

24. What clinical data do I need to make the diagnosis of diversion colitis with confidence?

Diversion colitis is a clinicopathological diagnosis. It occurs in a segment of large bowel that is diverted from the fecal stream, commonly in patients who have a blinded colon segment or rectum distal to an ileostomy or colostomy. It is thought to result from a deficiency of nutrients (mainly butyrate and short-chain fatty acids) derived from bacterial fermentation that is provided by the fecal stream.

Patients are often asymptomatic. Symptomatic patients present with rectal bleeding, tenesmus, mucous discharge, and abdominal pain.

References: [25, 34–37]

25. What are the key histologic features of pneumatosis intestinalis/coli?

Pneumatosis intestinalis or pneumatosis coli is characterized by the presence of gas cysts in the mucosa, submucosa, or subserosa of the intestine. It can be idiopathic

Table 7.4 Potential etiologies of ischemic bowel injury

Major vascular occlusion or obstruction
Trauma, thrombosis (arterial and venous), embolism (Fig. 7.5c), occupying mass lesion, adhesion, stricture, volvulus, intussusception, strangulated hernia, motility disorders (scleroderma, ileus, etc.), diverticular disease
Diseases of blood vessels
Fibromuscular dysplasia of mesenteric arteries (Fig. 7.7a–d), enterocolic lymphocytic phlebitis (Fig. 7.8) or idiopathic myointimal hyperplasia of mesenteric veins, idiopathic mesenteric phlebosclerosis, diabetes mellitus, rheumatoid arthritis, amyloidosis, radiation, systemic lupus erythematous, polyarteritis nodosa, scleroderma, Behçet disease, Takayasu arteritis, thromboangiitis obliterans, Buerger disease, allergic granulomatosis (Churg-Strauss syndrome), Henoch-Schönlein purpura, granulomatosis with polyangiitis (Wegener granulomatosis), microscopic polyangiitis, and other systemic vascular diseases
Surgery
Abdominal aortic aneurysm repair, cardiovascular surgery with cardiopulmonary bypass
Shock
Heart failure, hypovolemia, sepsis, neurogenic insult, anaphylaxis, blood loss, dehydration
Illicit drugs and other medications
Cocaine, methamphetamines, antihypertensives (calcium channel blockers), diuretics, estrogens/oral contraceptives, danazol, NSAIDs, digitalis, catecholamines, neuroleptics, Ma-huang (herbal supplements), interferons, TNFα inhibitors, antipsychotics, Kayexalate (Fig. 7.9a–d), cholestyramine (Fig. 7.9e–f), sevelamer, cold medicines
Hematologic disorders
Sickle cell disease, thrombophilia, protein C/S deficiency, antiphospholipid antibody, factor V Leiden mutation, antithrombin III deficiency, polycythemia vera, paroxysmal nocturnal hemoglobinuria, hypercoagulable state
Long-distance running

NSAIDs nonsteroidal anti-inflammatory drugs, *TNF* tumor necrosis factor

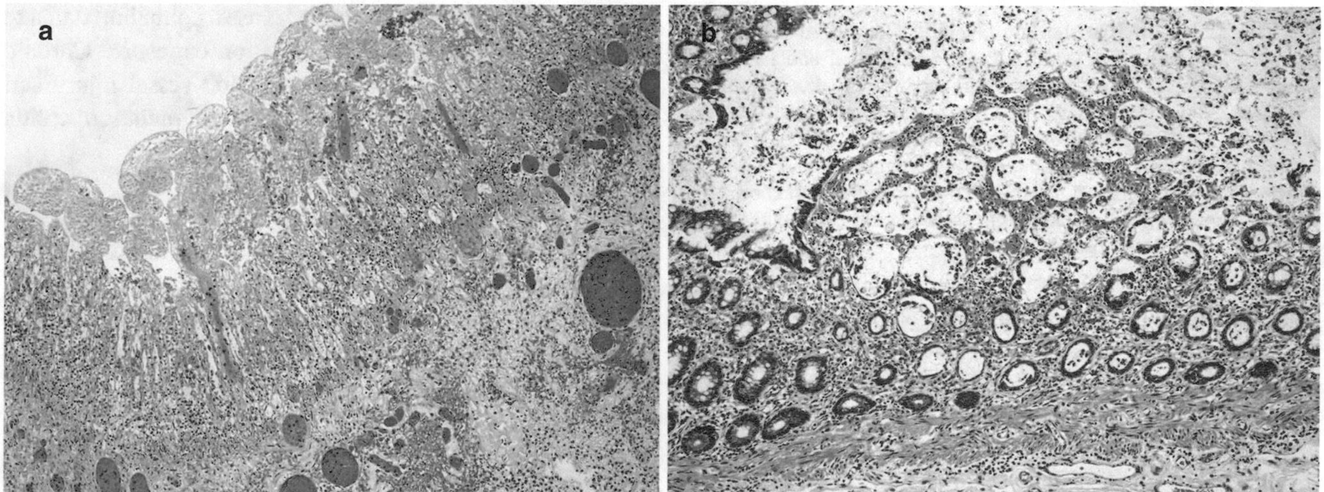

Fig. 7.7 Ischemic enterocolitis secondary to fibromuscular dysplasia. This patient was a 48-year-old female who underwent extensive resection of the entire small bowel and the transverse colon, which showed extensive transmural necrosis (**a**). Some viable areas showed ruptured crypts and pseudomembrane formation, resembling pseudomembranous colitis (**b**). Marked fibromuscular thickening involving the intima of the mesenteric arteries is noted, which caused nearly complete luminal obliteration (**c** and **d**)

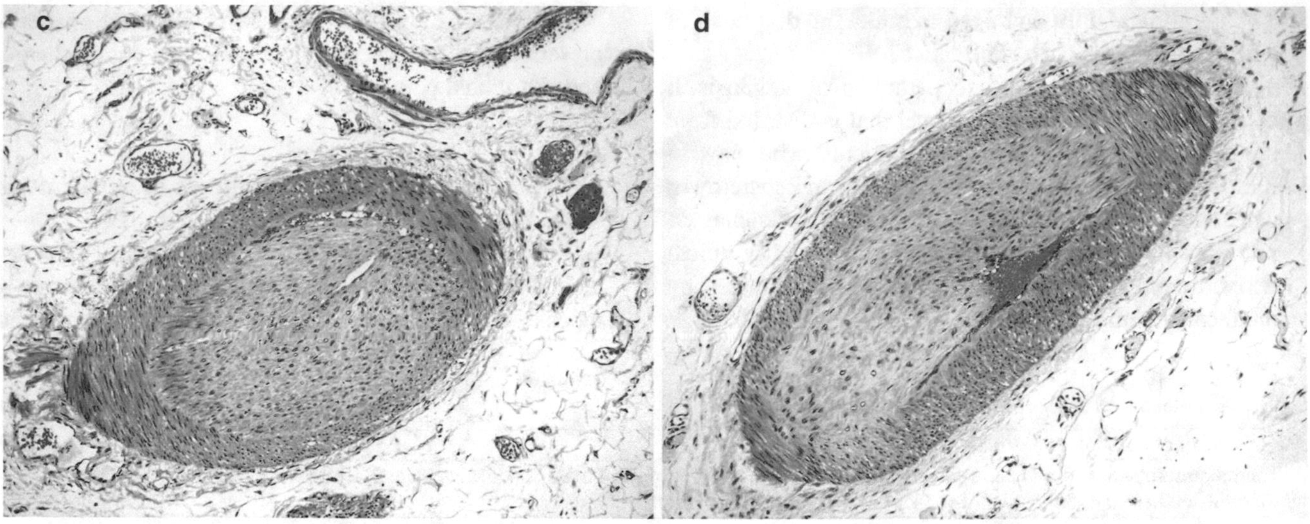

Fig. 7.7 (continued)

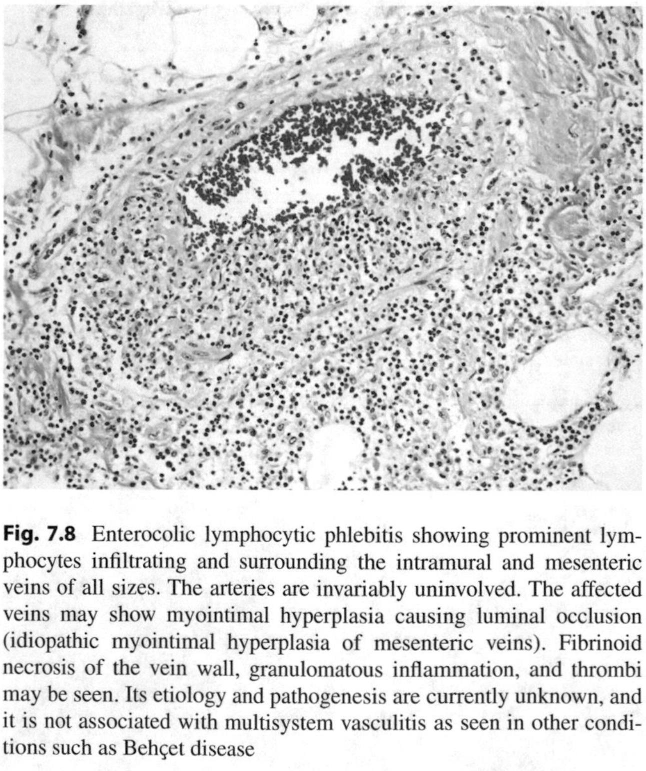

Fig. 7.8 Enterocolic lymphocytic phlebitis showing prominent lymphocytes infiltrating and surrounding the intramural and mesenteric veins of all sizes. The arteries are invariably uninvolved. The affected veins may show myointimal hyperplasia causing luminal occlusion (idiopathic myointimal hyperplasia of mesenteric veins). Fibrinoid necrosis of the vein wall, granulomatous inflammation, and thrombi may be seen. Its etiology and pathogenesis are currently unknown, and it is not associated with multisystem vasculitis as seen in other conditions such as Behçet disease

or secondary to a wide variety of gastrointestinal and nongastrointestinal illnesses. The pathogenesis is multifactorial, which includes mechanical, bacterial, and biochemical causes.

Grossly, submucosal cysts are often polypoid with the overlying mucosa demonstrating a bluish hue. Subserosal cysts are typically found near the mesentery as glistening and pale-bluish blebs (see case 5 in Case Presentation).

Microscopically, gas-filled cysts are confined to the mucosa, submucosa, or subserosa or involve all three layers. Among them, subserosal cysts are commonly seen. All cysts are essentially pseudocysts because of lack of an epithelial lining. However, they may be lined or surrounded by a rim of histiocytes, multinucleated giant cells, lymphocytes, neutrophils, eosinophils, granulomas, and fibrosis, especially when collapse happens (Fig. 7.13a and b). Bleeding and mucosal erosions may occur. Bowel necrosis occurs when the disease is severe.
Reference: [38]

26. **Is radiation colitis a specific disease?**

Radiation colitis is a specific entity that occurs within hours to years after regional radiotherapy in patients with gynecologic, urologic, and rectal cancers. The risk and the severity of the disease are directly related to radiation dose. Acute radiation colitis causes epithelial damage within hours to days after radiation exposure. Chronic radiation colitis is secondary to blood vessel injury and stricture formation. The diagnosis of radiation colitis requires clinicopathological correlation.
References: [25, 39, 40]

27. **What changes in the mucosa should make me suspect radiation injury?**

Microscopically, a wide range of histologic features, including cryptitis, crypt abscess, granulation tissue, and ulceration with profound epithelial damage, are often seen (Fig. 7.14a). However, these findings are not specific and are significantly overlapped with damages caused by other etiologies.

The hallmark of chronic radiation colitis is telangiectasia of the mucosal capillaries with lamina propria hyalinization (Fig. 7.14b and c). Enlarged fibroblasts with cytological atypia and submucosal fibrosis can be seen,

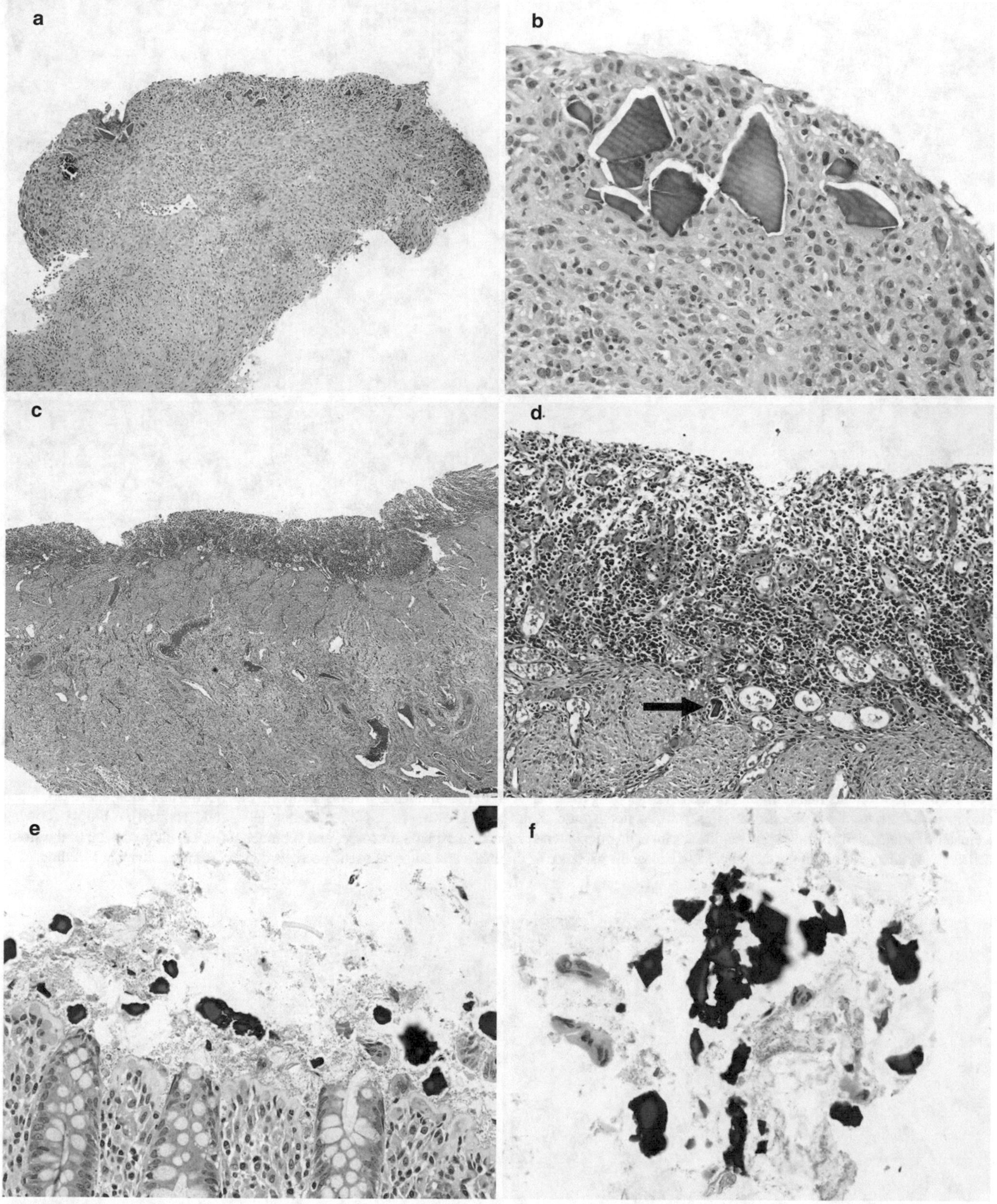

Fig. 7.9 Histologic features of ischemic colitis caused by Kayexalate and cholestyramine crystals. Sodium polystyrene sulfonate (Kayexalate), a medicine to treat hyperkaliemia, was given to a 53-year-old male who had renal failure. The patient presented with abdominal pain and diarrhea. A colon biopsy showed ulceration with multiple rhomboid and basophilic crystals in a fish scale-like pattern (**a** and **b**). The disease progressed, and segmental colectomy was performed that displayed extensive ulceration with granulation tissue (**c** and **d**). Kayexalate crystals embedded in ulcerated areas were noted (**d**, arrow). Cholestyramine is a nonabsorbable ion-exchange resin that is often used to treat hypercholesterolemia and bile-salt-induced diarrhea. Crystals of this medication have been found to be associated with erosion, ulceration, and active inflammation in the colon. Cholestyramine crystals display a uniform bright purple color with smooth glassy texture (**e** and **f**)

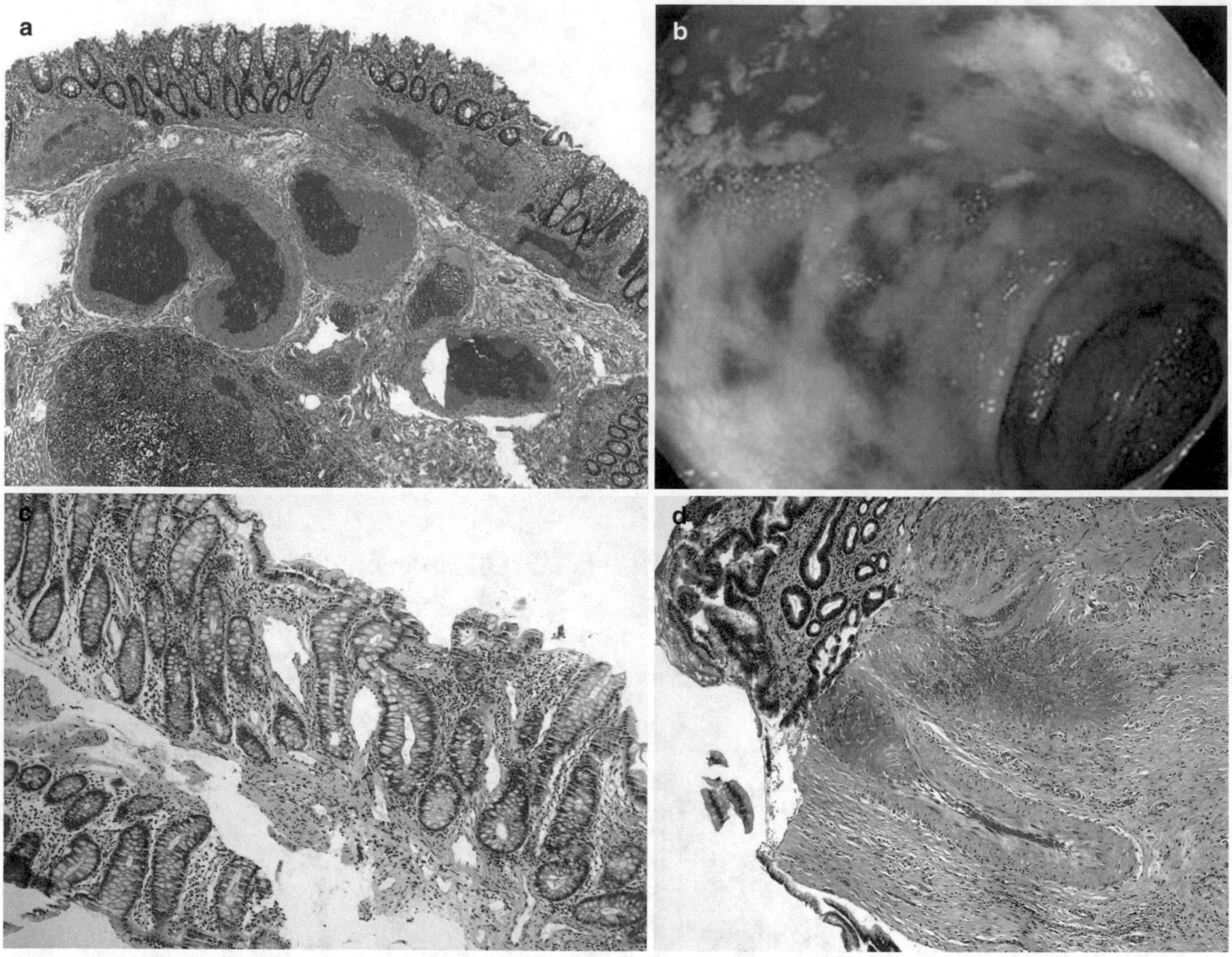

Fig. 7.10 Arteriovenous malformation of the colon showing a cluster of abnormal arteries and veins involving the mucosa and submucosa (**a**). It can also involve the muscularis propria and subserosa. Angiodysplasia of the colon showing multiple red lesions under endoscopy (**b**). A biopsy showing a cluster of dilated veins/venules and capillaries involving the lamina propria, muscularis mucosae, and submucosa (**c**). Dieulafoy lesion of the stomach showing a large artery in the submucosa (**d**). Note the presence of thrombus and adjacent tissue necrosis due to recent erosion and bleeding

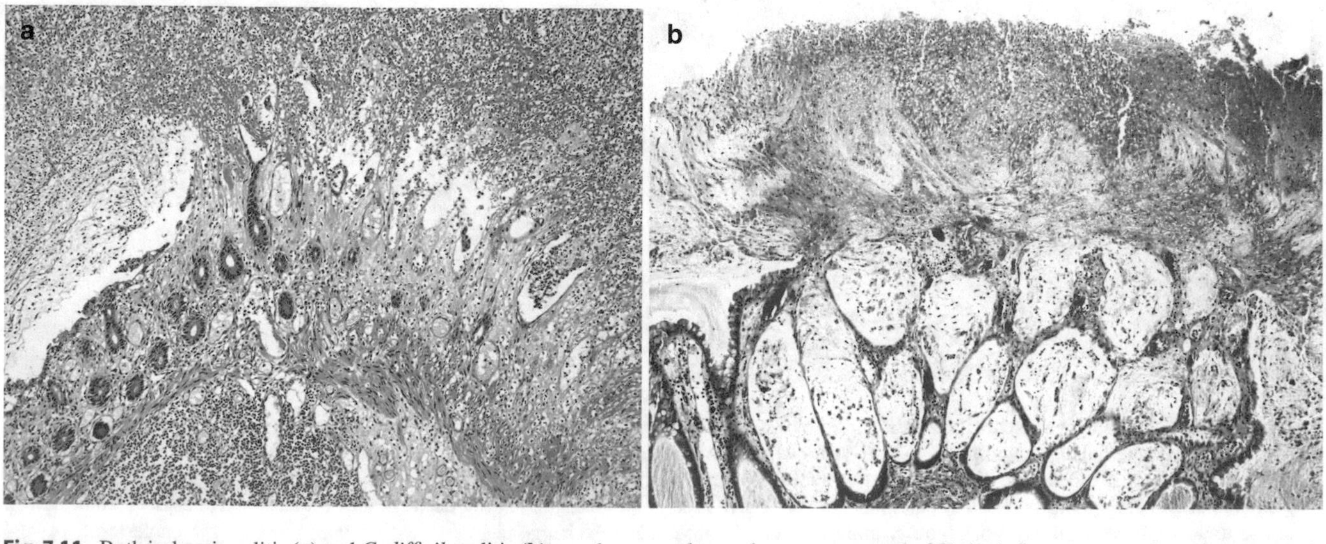

Fig. 7.11 Both ischemic colitis (**a**) and *C. difficile* colitis (**b**) can show pseudomembranes composed of fibrinoinflammatory and mucinous materials. Ruptured crypts (so-called volcano lesions) can also be seen in both conditions but may be more prominent in *C. difficile*-associated pseudomembranous colitis

which can be marked and profound and should not be misinterpreted as malignancy (Fig. 7.14d).
References: [25, 39, 40]

28. **What are the potential etiologies or risk factors for necrotizing enterocolitis in pediatric population?**

Necrotizing enterocolitis is the most common cause of intestinal perforation and short gut syndrome in neonatal intensive care units, which tends to affect premature infants. The pathogenesis of necrotizing enterocolitis is not completely understood. It often occurs at the beginning of enteral feeding. The clinical presentation varies, ranging from mild, self-limited gastrointestinal disturbance to a fulminant course with intestinal necrosis, perforation, sepsis, and death. Intestinal necrosis and perforation are indications for surgery. The possible underlying causes are summarized in Table 7.6.
References: [27, 41]

Table 7.5 Comparison between ischemic colitis and *C. difficile* pseudomembranous colitis

	Ischemic colitis	*C. difficile* pseudomembranous colitis
Endoscopy	Darkened or pale mucosa, petechial bleeding, mass- or polyp-like lesion, or a local process of pseudomembranes	pseudomembranes as yellow-white plaques
C. difficile toxin assay	Negative	Positive
Hyalinized lamina propria	Pathognomonic	No
Atrophic or withering crypts	Common	Less common
Lamina propria hemorrhage	Common	Less common
Full-thickness mucosal necrosis	Common	Less common

29. **What are the pathologic features of necrotizing enterocolitis?**

Necrotizing enterocolitis affects both small bowel and colon, especially the ileocecal region. The affected bowel appears distended, grayish, and purple, and the intestinal wall becomes thin and fragile. Grossly discernable gas bubbles that indicate pneumatosis occurs as a result of fermentation of intraluminal contents due to bacterial overgrowth. Histologically, ischemic enterocolitis with coagulative necrosis is the predominant feature that may affect mucosa or up to the full thickness of the bowel wall. Cryptitis and crypt abscess are not striking with few inflammatory cells in the lamina propria.
References: [41]

30. **What are the key clinicopathologic features of Behçet disease?**

Behçet disease is a rare chronic vasculitic disorder that involves multiple organs. Clinically, it is characterized by the triad of uveitis, aphthous stomatitis, and genital ulcer. It affects young adults and tends to be more severe in males. The gastrointestinal tract involvement is relatively uncommon. Endoscopically, well-demarcated ulcer occurs, especially at the ileocecal valve. Histologically, it is characterized by "punch out" or "flask-shaped" ulcers in contrast to the adjacent unremarkable mucosa.
Reference: [25]

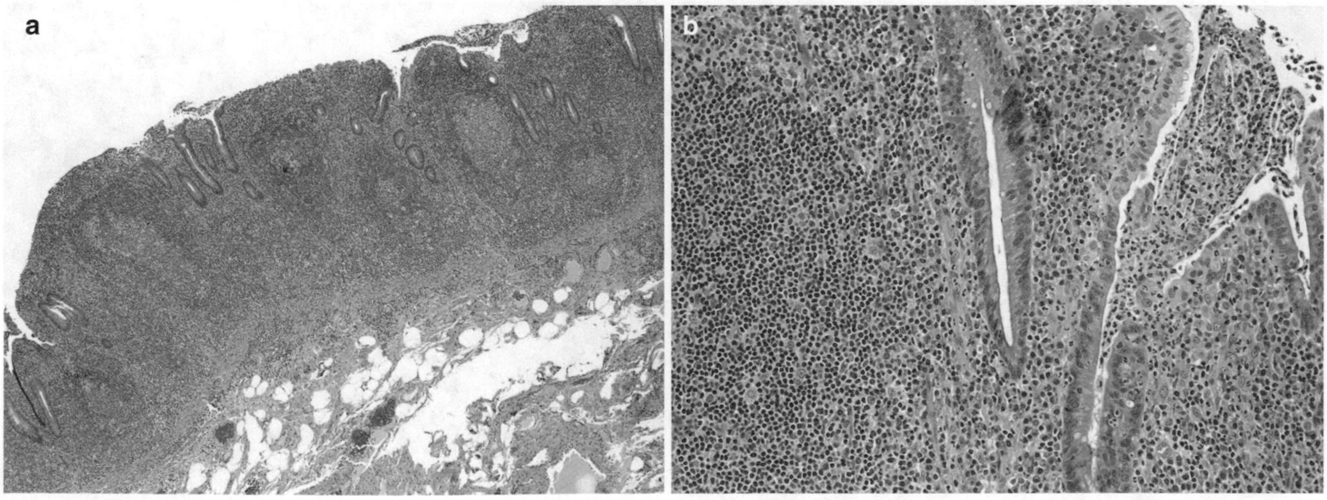

Fig. 7.12 Diversion colitis features lymphoid hyperplasia in the mucosa (**a**). Active inflammation, such as cryptitis, crypt abscess, and erosion/superficial ulceration, as well as mild crypt architectural distortion, can be seen (**b**)

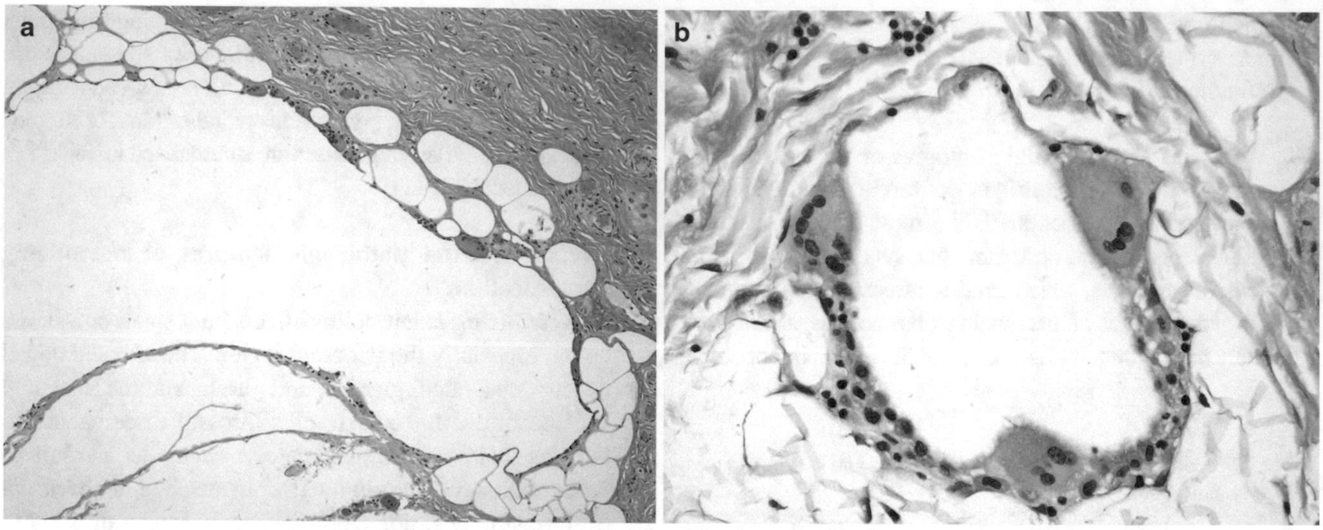

Fig. 7.13 Pneumatosis intestinalis/coli shows variably sized empty air spaces, which are frequently lined by a rim of histiocytes and/or multinucleated giant cells (**a** and **b**)

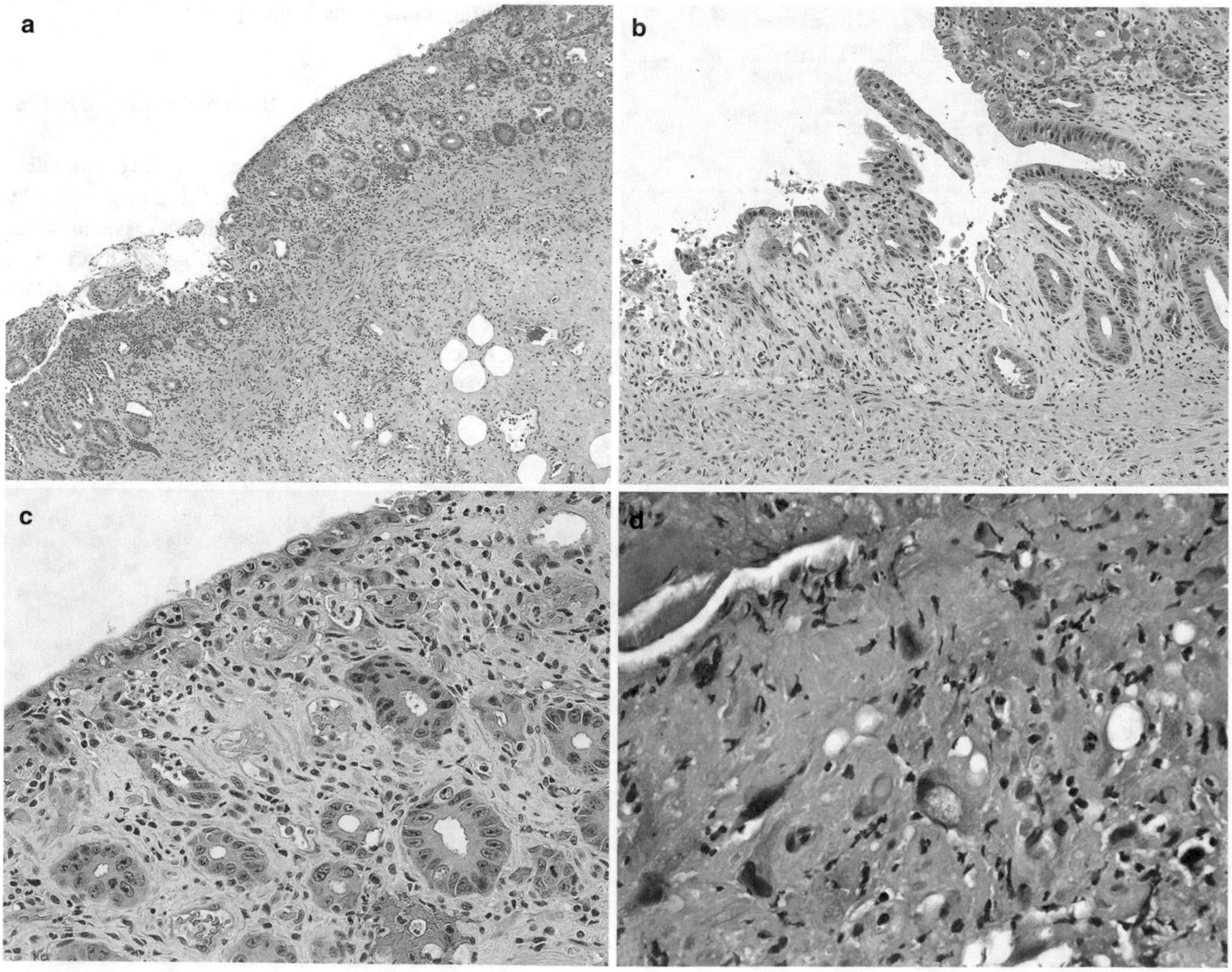

Fig. 7.14 Histologic features of radiation colitis. The patient was a 55-year-old female who had ovarian serous carcinoma status post chemoradiation presented with diarrhea. A rectal biopsy showed extensive necrosis. The disease progressed, and rectosigmoid resection was performed. Microscopically, ulceration with profound epithelial damage, cryptitis, and crypt abscess were appreciated (**a**). A prominent histologic feature was telangiectasia of the mucosal capillaries with predominantly perivascular hyalinization (**b** and **c**). Enlarged fibroblasts with cytological atypia were seen in ulcerated areas (**d**)

Table 7.6 Common conditions to cause necrotizing enterocolitis

Maternal and gestational conditions
Maternal diabetes, drug abuse, preeclampsia, anti-C Rhesus incompatibility, intrauterine growth retardation, premature rupture of the membranes
Organic conditions
Congenital cardiac anomalies, gastroschisis, myelomeningocele, Hirschsprung disease, anorectal malformation
Medical conditions
Hypoglycemia, polycythemia, cow's milk allergy, respiratory distress syndrome
Hyperosmolar feedings

Table 7.7 Comparison between Behçet disease and Crohn disease

	Behçet disease	Crohn disease
Population	Asian and Mediterranean	North European and American
Extraintestinal manifestations	Uveitis, arthritis, pyoderma gangrenosum, erythema nodosum, genital ulcers, joints and neurological involvement, vaso-occlusive disease, and thrombosis	Uveitis, arthritis, pyoderma gangrenosum, erythema nodosum, and anemia
Endoscopy	Large, discrete, round or oval-shaped ulcers that are single or few numbers (≤5) with focal distribution, discrete border, and deep penetration	Discontinuous distribution of longitudinal ulcer, cobblestone appearance, or small aphthous ulcers arranged in a longitudinal fashion
Histology	Mesenteric vasculitis affects small veins and venules, which leads to ischemia and necrosis of the intestine	Discontinuous crypt architectural distortion, cryptitis, crypt abscess, and epithelioid granulomas

31. What are the key features to differentiate intestinal Behçet disease from Crohn disease?

Behçet disease is an inflammatory disease with multisystemic involvement. There are no pathognomonic laboratory tests to define Behçet disease. Crohn disease primarily affects the gastrointestinal tract from mouth to anus with various extraintestinal involvements (skin rash, arthritis, and uveitis). The most frequently involved site in the gastrointestinal tract is the ileocecal valve region in both Behçet disease and Crohn disease. As such, when the gastrointestinal tract is involved by Behçet disease, the overlapping features make it difficult to distinguish from Crohn disease. Histologically, the presence of epithelioid granulomas in biopsy specimen suggests Crohn disease, while vasculitides (such as lymphocytic phlebitis) are more suggestive of Behçet disease. Management approaches are similar in various aspects. Useful features to distinguish Behçet disease from Crohn disease are summarized in Table 7.7.

References: [42–44]

32. What are the typical histologic characteristics of irritable bowel syndrome?

Irritable bowel syndrome (IBS) is the most common functional gastrointestinal disease with a prevalence of 5–20% worldwide. The presentation of symptom commonly includes diarrhea and constipation in a relapsing remitting manner. Because the symptoms of IBS often overlap with other gastrointestinal disease, in order to make an accurate diagnosis of IBS, colonoscopy and/or upper gastrointestinal endoscopy are required. Defined as a functional gastrointestinal disorder, no structure abnormality is emphasized in the diagnosis of IBS, although recently a density alteration of endocrine/paracrine cells has been described. Currently, a histologic finding within the normal range on H&E is expected in mucosal biopsies from IBS patients.

References: [45–48]

Case Presentation

Case 1

Learning Objectives

1. To become familiar with the endoscopic and histologic features of the disease
2. To generate the differential diagnosis

Case History

A 56-year-old male presented with chronic watery diarrhea. The patient is otherwise healthy.

Endoscopy

The endoscopy is nearly normal.

Histologic Findings

- Low power examination shows surface epithelial damage and increased numbers of lamina propria inflammatory cells (Fig. 7.15a and b).
- High power examination reveals increased IELs (Fig. 7.15c).

Differential Diagnosis

- Microscopic colitis
- Infectious colitis
- Inflammatory bowel disease

Final Diagnosis

Lymphocytic colitis.

Take-Home Messages

- Lymphocytic colitis is characterized by increased IELs, surface epithelial damage, and inflammation in the lamina propria.

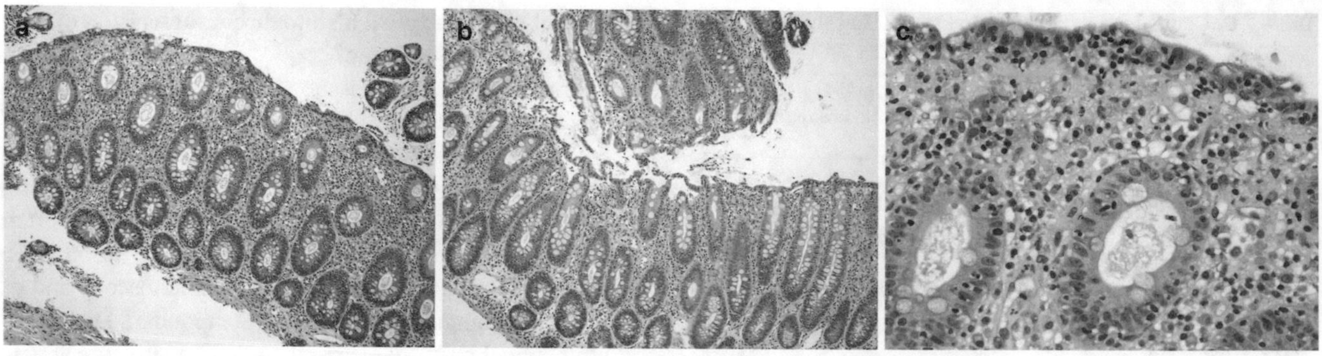

Fig. 7.15 (Case 1). Low power examination shows surface epithelial damage and increased numbers of lamina propria inflammatory cells (**a**) and (**b**). High power examination reveals increased numbers of intraepithelial lymphocytes (**c**)

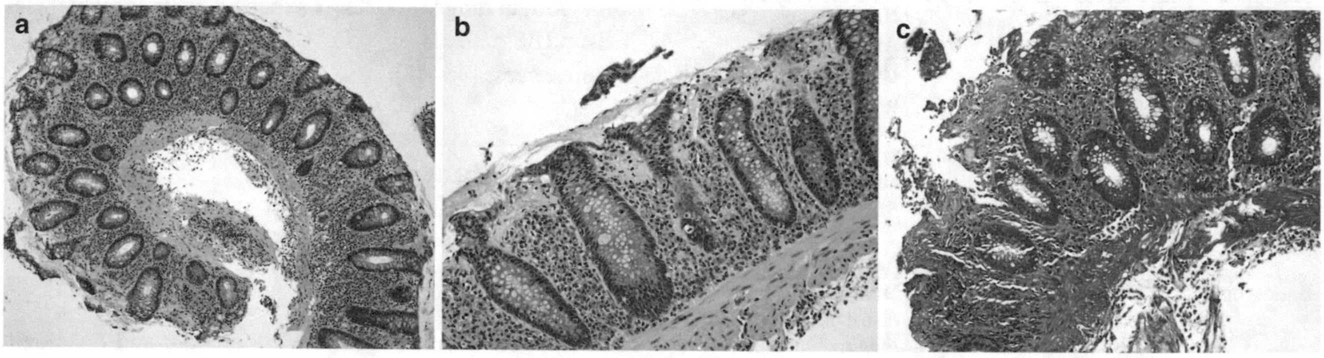

Fig. 7.16 (Case 2). Low power examination shows surface epithelial damage, increased numbers of lamina propria inflammatory cells, and thickened collagen band underneath the surface epithelium (**a** and **b**). Trichrome stain highlights the thickened subepithelial collagen band (**c**)

- Endoscopically, it is normal or nearly normal.
  References: [1–7, 9–11, 49]

Case 2

Learning Objectives

1. To become familiar with the endoscopic and histologic features of the disease
2. To generate the differential diagnosis

Case History

A 60-year-old female presented with chronic watery diarrhea. The patient is otherwise healthy.

Endoscopy

The endoscopy is nearly normal.

Histologic Findings

- Microscopic examination shows surface epithelial damage with patchy detachment, increased numbers of inflammatory cells in lamina propria, and a thickened collagen band underneath the surface epithelium with entrapped inflammatory cells and capillaries (Fig. 7.16a and b). There is a variable increase of IELs.

Differential Diagnosis

- Microscopic colitis
- Infectious colitis
- Inflammatory bowel disease

Ancillary Studies

- Trichrome stain highlights the thickened collagen band underneath the surface epithelium (Fig. 7.16c).

Final Diagnosis

Collagenous colitis.

Take-Home Messages

- Collagenous colitis is characterized by a thickened collagen band underneath the surface epithelium. Other features include increased IELs, surface epithelial damage, and inflammation in the lamina propria.
- Endoscopically, it is normal or nearly normal.
  References: [9–11, 49]

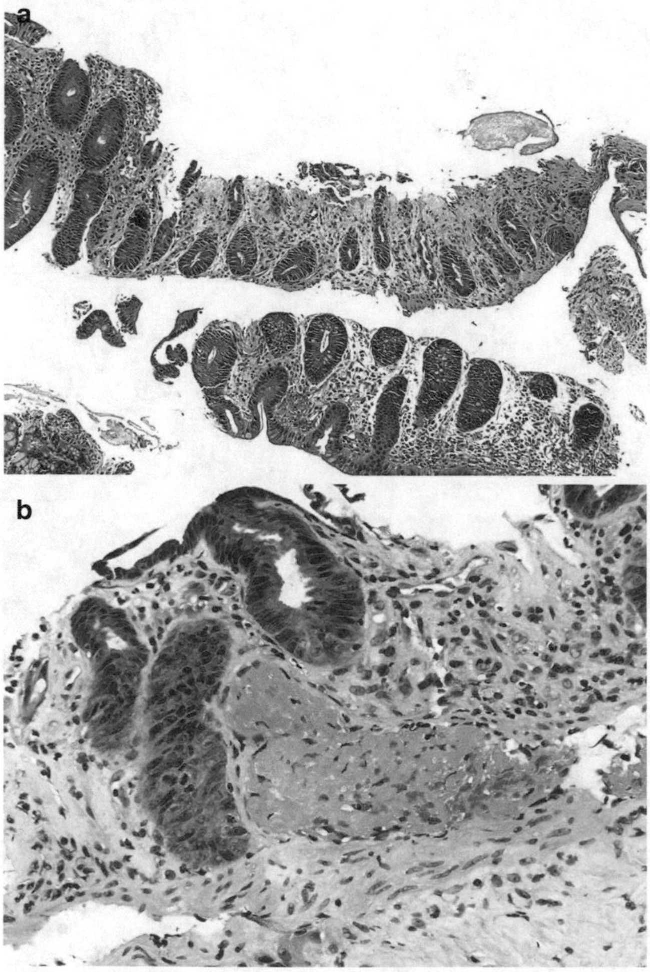

Fig. 7.17 (Case 3). Low power examination shows loss of the surface epithelium, withered deep crypts, and hyalinization of the lamina propria with minimal inflammation (**a**). High power examination reveals the presence of an organizing fibrin thrombus in a lamina propria blood vessel (**b**)

Case 3

Learning Objectives

1. To become familiar with the endoscopic and histologic features of the disease
2. To generate the differential diagnosis

Case History

A 70-year-old female presented with abdominal pain and bloody diarrhea. She has had cardiac arrhythmia for several years.

Endoscopy

Colonoscopy shows edema and petechial bleeding in the right colon.

Histologic Findings

- Low power examination shows focal loss of the surface epithelium, withered deep crypts, and hyalinization of the lamina propria with minimal inflammation (Fig. 7.17a).
- High power examination shows a fibrin thrombus in deeper mucosa (Fig. 7.17b).

Differential Diagnosis

- Infectious colitis
- Inflammatory bowel disease
- NSAID-induced colitis
- Radiation colitis
- Ischemic colitis

Final Diagnosis

Ischemic colitis.

Take-Home Messages

- Ischemic colitis is characterized by superficial mucosal necrosis, withered crypts in the deep layer of the mucosa, and hyalinized lamina propria with minimal inflammation.
- The sharp contrast between the superficial and deep layers of the mucosa is a useful feature for the diagnosis at low power examination.

References: [25, 26]

Case 4

Learning Objectives

1. To become familiar with the endoscopic or gross features of the disease
2. To become familiar with the histologic features of the disease
3. To generate the differential diagnosis

Case History

A 54-year-old male with a known history of Crohn disease had a total abdominal colectomy and end ileostomy for perforated colitis 2 years ago. He presented with lower abdominal discomfort, mucous discharge, and low-grade fever. His recent endoscopy demonstrated granularity and erythema of the rectum. Ileostomy takedown and incisional hernia repair were performed.

Gross

The disused rectum shows diffuse nodularity, granularity, and blurring of vascular pattern (Fig. 7.18a).

Histologic Findings

- Low (Fig. 7.18b) and medium (Fig. 7.18c) power examinations show profound lymphoid follicular hyperplasia.

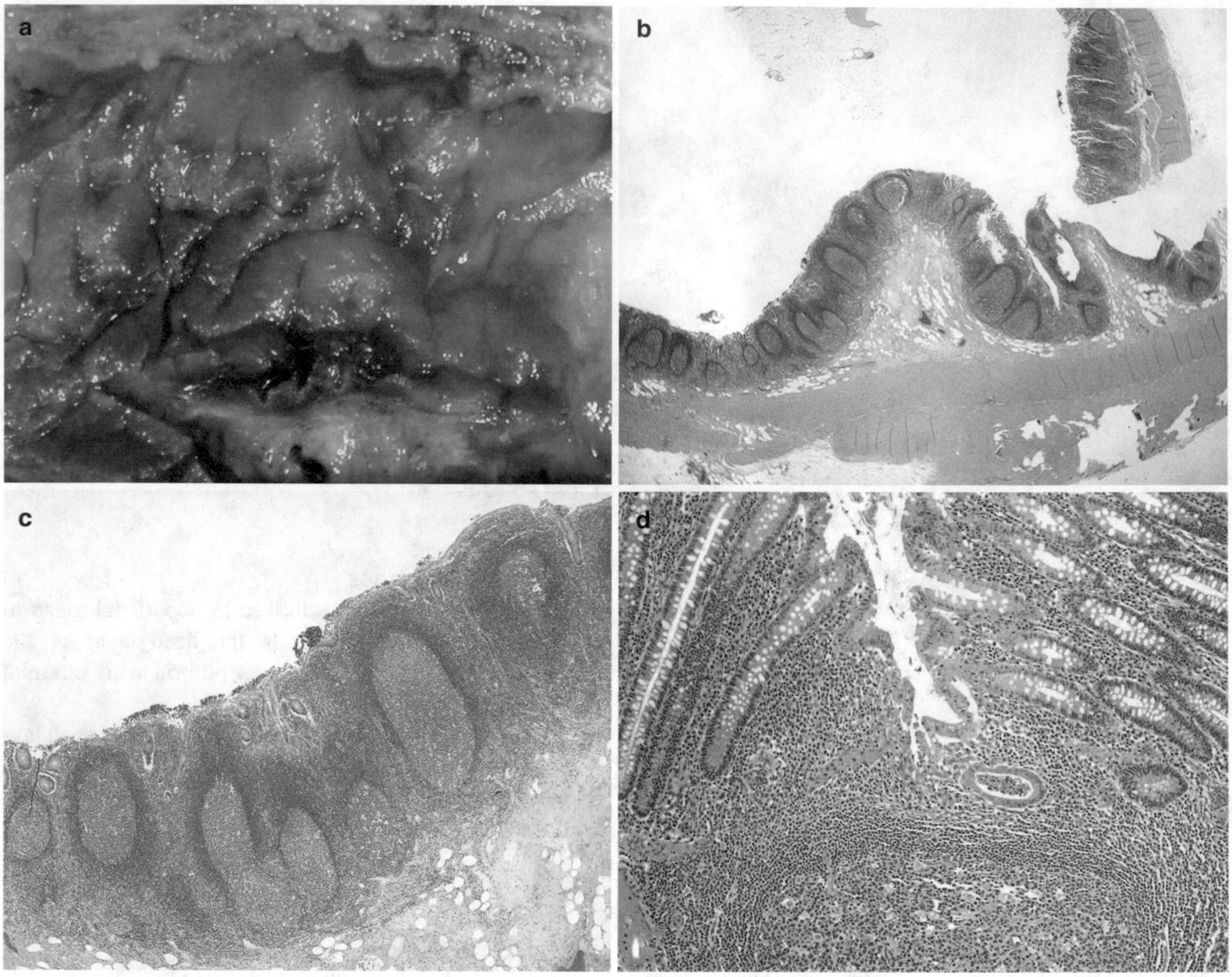

Fig. 7.18 (Case 4). Grossly, the disused colon segment shows diffuse nodularity, granularity, and blurring of vascular pattern (**a**). Low (**b**) and medium (**c**) power examinations show profound lymphoid hyperplasia. Focal aphthous ulcer with crypt abscess is seen (**d**)

- High power examination reveals focal aphthous ulcer with crypt abscess (Fig. 7.18d).

Differential Diagnosis

- Flare of Crohn disease
- Infectious disease
- Diversion colitis

Final Diagnosis

Diversion colitis.

Take-Home Messages

- Diversion colitis refers to the pathologic changes limited to the dysfunctioned segment of the colon due to lack of fecal stream.
- Lymphoid follicular hyperplasia is the pathognomonic finding.
  References: [25, 34–37]

Case 5

Learning Objectives

1. To become familiar with the gross features of the disease
2. To become familiar with the histologic features of the disease
3. To generate the differential diagnosis

Case History

A 71-year-old male presents with nausea, vomiting, abdominal distention, abdominal pain, and diarrhea. Physical examination showed signs of peritonitis (abdominal rigidity and rebound tenderness). Partial colectomy was performed.

Gross

The resected colon shows multiple glistening, pale-bluish, and gas-filled blebs (Fig. 7.19a).

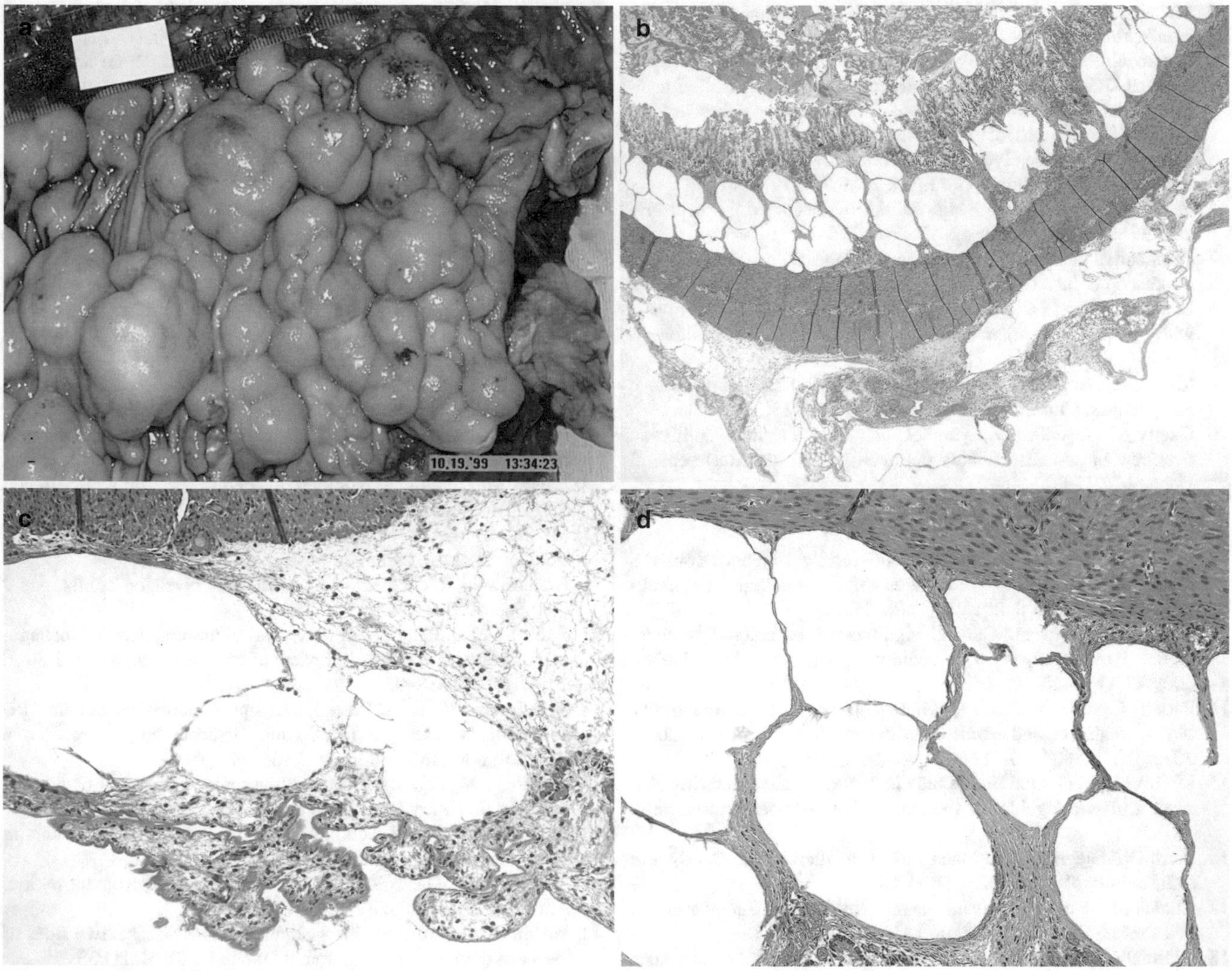

Fig. 7.19 (Case 5). Grossly, the resected segment of colon shows multiple glistening and pale bluish blebs (**a**). Microscopically, multiple gas-filled cysts are seen in the submucosa (**b**) and subserosa (**b** and **c**). The cysts are devoid of an epithelial lining in this case (**d**)

Histologic Findings

Microscopic examination reveals multiple gas-filled cysts in the submucosa (Fig. 7.19b) and subserosa (Fig. 7.19b and c) of the bowel wall. Superficial epithelial sloughing and mucosal necrosis are appreciated (Fig. 7.19b). The cysts are devoid of an epithelial lining (Fig. 7.19d).

Differential Diagnosis

- Pneumatosis coli
- Colon polyps
- Ischemia colitis
- Diverticulosis

Final Diagnosis

Pneumatosis coli.

Take-Home Messages

- Histologically, pneumatosis coli is characterized by multiple gas-filled cysts in the mucosa, submucosa, and subserosa of the intestinal wall. Multinucleated giant cells may be present, which line the air spaces and should not be misinterpreted as epithelial lining.
  Reference: [38]

References

1. Okamoto R, et al. Diagnosis and treatment of microscopic colitis. Clin J Gastroenterol. 2016;9(4):169–74.
2. Fernandez-Banares F, et al. Epidemiological risk factors in microscopic colitis: a prospective case-control study. Inflamm Bowel Dis. 2013;19(2):411–7.

3. Macaigne G, et al. Microscopic colitis or functional bowel disease with diarrhea: a French prospective multicenter study. Am J Gastroenterol. 2014;109(9):1461–70.
4. Nguyen GC, et al. American gastroenterological association institute guideline on the medical management of microscopic colitis. Gastroenterology. 2016;150(1):242–6; quiz e17–8.
5. Park HS, et al. Does lymphocytic colitis always present with normal endoscopic findings? Gut Liver. 2015;9(2):197–201.
6. Yung DE, et al. Microscopic colitis: a misnomer for a clearly defined entity? Endoscopy. 2015;47(8):754–7.
7. Bromberg DJ, Reed J, Gill JA. Microscopic colitis that is not so microscopic. Int J Color Dis. 2016;31(3):723–4.
8. Langner C, et al. Histology of microscopic colitis-review with a practical approach for pathologists. Histopathology. 2015;66(5):613–26.
9. Munch A, Langner C. Microscopic colitis: clinical and pathologic perspectives. Clin Gastroenterol Hepatol. 2015;13(2):228–36.
10. Chetty R, Govender D. Lymphocytic and collagenous colitis: an overview of so-called microscopic colitis. Nat Rev Gastroenterol Hepatol. 2012;9(4):209–18.
11. Yen EF, Pardi DS. Review of the microscopic colitides. Curr Gastroenterol Rep. 2011;13(5):458–64.
12. Mahajan D, et al. Lymphocytic colitis and collagenous colitis: a review of clinicopathologic features and immunologic abnormalities. Adv Anat Pathol. 2012;19(1):28–38.
13. Najarian RM, et al. Clinical significance of colonic intraepithelial lymphocytosis in a pediatric population. Mod Pathol. 2009;22(1):13–20.
14. Park T, Cave D, Marshall C. Microscopic colitis: a review of etiology, treatment and refractory disease. World J Gastroenterol. 2015;21(29):8804–10.
15. Miehlke S, et al. Oral budesonide in gastrointestinal and liver disease: a practical guide for the clinician. J Gastroenterol Hepatol. 2018.
16. Pardi DS. Diagnosis and Management of Microscopic Colitis. Am J Gastroenterol. 2017;112(1):78–85.
17. Chandratre S, et al. Simultaneous occurrence of collagenous colitis and Crohn's disease. Digestion. 1987;36(1):55–60.
18. Giardiello FM, Jackson FW, Lazenby AJ. Metachronous occurrence of collagenous colitis and ulcerative colitis. Gut. 1991;32(4):447–9.
19. Pokorny CS, Kneale KL, Henderson CJ. Progression of collagenous colitis to ulcerative colitis. J Clin Gastroenterol. 2001;32(5):435–8.
20. Freeman HJ, Berean KW, Nimmo M. Evolution of collagenous colitis into severe and extensive ulcerative colitis. Can J Gastroenterol. 2007;21(5):315–8.
21. Haque M, Florin T. Progression of ulcerative colitis to collagenous colitis: chance, evolution or association? Inflamm Bowel Dis. 2007;13(10):1321.
22. Osman H, et al. Intermittent inflammatory bowel disease and microscopic colitis: variant or epiphenomenon? Gastroenterol Hepatol. 2015;2(1):1–7.
23. Goldstein NS, Gyorfi T. Focal lymphocytic colitis and collagenous colitis: patterns of Crohn's colitis? Am J Surg Pathol. 1999;23(9):1075–81.
24. Schembri J, et al. Segmental colitis associated with diverticulosis: is it the coexistence of colonic diverticulosis and inflammatory bowel disease? Ann Gastroenterol. 2017;30(3):257–61.
25. Nielsen OH, Vainer B, Rask-Madsen J. Non-IBD and noninfectious colitis. Nat Clin Pract Gastroenterol Hepatol. 2008;5(1):28–39.
26. Villanacci V, et al. Non-IBD colitides: clinically useful histopathological clues. Rev Esp Enferm Dig. 2011;103(7):366–72.
27. Odze RD, Goldblum JR. Surgical pathology of the GI tract, liver, biliary tract, and pancreas. 3rd ed; 2015.
28. Dignan CR, Greenson JK. Can ischemic colitis be differentiated from C difficile colitis in biopsy specimens? Am J Surg Pathol. 1997;21(6):706–10.
29. Tang DM, et al. Pseudomembranous colitis: not always caused by Clostridium difficile. Case Rep Med. 2014;2014:812704.
30. Ellis CN, McAlexander WW. Enterocolitis associated with cocaine use. Dis Colon Rectum. 2005;48(12):2313–6.
31. Olin JW, et al. The United States registry for fibromuscular dysplasia: results in the first 447 patients. Circulation. 2012;125(25):3182–90.
32. Brinza EK, Gornik HL. Fibromuscular dysplasia: advances in understanding and management. Cleve Clin J Med. 2016;83(11 Suppl 2):S45–51.
33. Ko M, et al. Diagnosis and management of fibromuscular dysplasia and segmental arterial mediolysis in gastroenterology field: a mini-review. World J Gastroenterol. 2018;24(32):3637–49.
34. Bayasi M, Quiogue J. Noninfectious colitides. Clin Colon Rectal Surg. 2015;28(2):87–92.
35. Ma CK, Gottlieb C, Haas PA. Diversion colitis: a clinicopathologic study of 21 cases. Hum Pathol. 1990;21(4):429–36.
36. Komorowski RA. Histologic spectrum of diversion colitis. Am J Surg Pathol. 1990;14(6):548–54.
37. Kabir SI, et al. Pathophysiology, clinical presentation and management of diversion colitis: a review of current literature. Int J Surg. 2014;12(10):1088–92.
38. Higashizono K, et al. Postoperative pneumatosis intestinalis (PI) and portal venous gas (PVG) may indicate bowel necrosis: a 52-case study. BMC Surg. 2016;16(1):42.
39. Berthrong M, Fajardo LF. Radiation injury in surgical pathology. Part II. Alimentary tract. Am J Surg Pathol. 1981;5(2):153–78.
40. Hasleton PS, Carr N, Schofield PF. Vascular changes in radiation bowel disease. Histopathology. 1985;9(5):517–34.
41. Zamir O, et al. Gastrointestinal perforations in the neonatal-period. Am J Perinatol. 1988;5(2):131–3.
42. Valenti S, et al. Intestinal Behcet and Crohn's disease: two sides of the same coin. Pediatr Rheumatol Online J. 2017;15(1):33.
43. Yazisiz V. Similarities and differences between Behcet's disease and Crohn's disease. World J Gastrointest Pathophysiol. 2014;5(3):228–38.
44. Zhang T, et al. Comparison between intestinal Behcet's disease and Crohn's disease in characteristics of symptom, endoscopy, and radiology. Gastroenterol Res Pract. 2017;2017:3918746.
45. Canavan C, West J, Card T. The epidemiology of irritable bowel syndrome. Clin Epidemiol. 2014;6:71–80.
46. Ford AC, et al. Irritable bowel syndrome: a 10-yr natural history of symptoms and factors that influence consultation behavior. Am J Gastroenterol. 2008;103(5):1229–39. quiz 1240.
47. El-Salhy M, et al. Is irritable bowel syndrome an organic disorder? World J Gastroenterol. 2014;20(2):384–400.
48. Drossman DA. Functional gastrointestinal disorders: history, pathophysiology, clinical features and Rome IV. Gastroenterology. 2016
49. Magro F, et al. European consensus on the histopathology of inflammatory bowel disease. J Crohns Colitis. 2013;7(10):827–51.

Appendiceal Diseases

8

Yuna Gong, Hanlin L. Wang, and Sergei Tatishchev

List of Frequently Asked Questions

1. What are the histologic features of acute appendicitis?
2. What are the most common causes of acute appendicitis?
3. What is periappendicitis and what is the clinical significance of the diagnosis?
4. What is the clinical significance of granulomatous appendicitis?
5. What is the clinical significance of eosinophilic appendicitis?
6. What are the most common parasitic infections in the appendix?
7. What is appendiceal diverticulosis?
8. What is the current who classification of appendiceal neuroendocrine neoplasms?
9. What is tubular neuroendocrine tumor?
10. What is the current classification of appendiceal epithelial tumors?
11. What is goblet cell adenocarcinoma?
12. What are the clinical features of goblet cell adenocarcinoma?
13. What are the gross and histologic features of goblet cell adenocarcinoma?
14. How is goblet cell adenocarcinoma graded and what is the prognostic significance of grading?
15. What are the immunohistochemical features of goblet cell adenocarcinoma?
16. What molecular alterations have been found in goblet cell adenocarcinoma?
17. What is low-grade appendiceal mucinous neoplasm (LAMN)?
18. What is high-grade appendiceal mucinous neoplasm (HAMN)?
19. How are appendiceal mucinous neoplasms staged?
20. What is pseudomyxoma peritonei?
21. How can LAMN be distinguished from appendiceal adenoma, serrated lesions, retention cyst, ruptured diverticulum, endometriosis, and mucinous cystadenoma of the ovary?
22. What is mucinous adenocarcinoma of the appendix and how is it graded?

Y. Gong · S. Tatishchev (✉)
University of Southern California Keck School of Medicine, Los Angeles, CA, USA
e-mail: Sergei.Tatishchev@med.usc.edu

H. L. Wang
University of California at Los Angeles David Geffen School of Medicine, Los Angeles, CA, USA

Frequently Asked Questions

1. What are the histologic features of acute appendicitis?

- Histologic features of acute appendicitis vary by stage of inflammation. Early acute appendicitis may show neutrophilic infiltrates limited to the mucosa with cryptitis, crypt abscesses, and mucosal ulceration/erosion. With progression, transmural neutrophilic inflammation with involvement of the muscularis propria and serosa develops (suppurative appendicitis; Fig. 8.1a, b). Later stages may show transmural necrosis (gangrenous appendicitis; Fig. 8.1c) and eventually perforation in untreated cases. Thrombosis of the mural vessels may be seen. The presence of luminal neutrophils alone without involvement of the appendiceal wall is insufficient for the diagnosis of acute appendicitis.
- It should be noted that some question the usage of the term "acute appendicitis" to describe acute inflammation limited to the mucosa or submucosa, considering that these types of changes can be seen in incidental appendectomy specimens from patients without clinical symptoms of acute appendicitis. The term "acute appendicitis," it is argued, should thus be reserved for cases in which neutrophils extend into the muscularis propria. Others, however, consider mucosal or submucosal acute inflammation to be changes consistent with

H. L. Wang, Z. E. Chen (eds.), *Practical Gastrointestinal Pathology*, Practical Anatomic Pathology,
https://doi.org/10.1007/978-3-030-51268-2_8

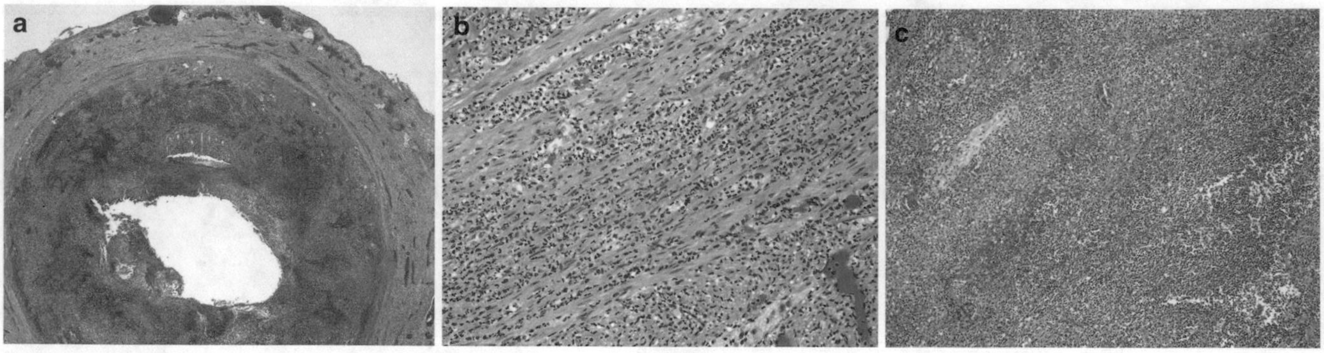

Fig. 8.1 A case of acute suppurative appendicitis showing transmural inflammation and extensive mucosal ulceration on low power view (**a**). Only residual crypts are recognized. Higher power view showing prominent neutrophils infiltrating the muscularis propria (**b**). Extensive transmural necrosis with abundant inflammatory infiltrates are seen in gangrenous appendicitis (**c**)

Table 8.1 Patterns of acute inflammation involving the appendix, suggested terminology, and clinical significance

Terminology or pattern	Microscopic description	Clinical significance
Acute intraluminal inflammation	Luminal accumulation of neutrophils only, no mucosal or transmural involvement	Probably none
Acute inflammation limited to mucosa or mucosa and submucosa (early or evolving acute appendicitis)	Neutrophils within mucosa, +/− ulceration/erosion, +/− involvement of submucosa	May not be responsible for patient's symptoms
Suppurative appendicitis	Transmural acute inflammation extending from mucosa to muscularis propria, +/− serosal involvement	An accepted cause of classic signs and symptoms associated with acute appendicitis (e.g., RLQ pain, fever, nausea/vomiting, abdominal distension)
Gangrenous appendicitis	Transmural acute inflammation with areas of tissue necrosis	Untreated gangrenous appendicitis can be complicated by perforation
Periappendicitis	Inflammation of serosa/subserosa, mesoappendix, or periappendiceal soft tissue	Usually seen as part of histologic findings in acute appendicitis; in the absence of mucosal or mucosal/submucosal involvement, an extraappendiceal cause may need to be considered, such as inflammatory pelvic disease in female patients (e.g., salpingitis)

RLQ right lower quadrant

early or evolving acute appendicitis. Table 8.1 describes different patterns of acute inflammation involving the appendix and the suggested terminology.

- When an appendectomy specimen is examined grossly, the presence or absence of perforation should be described. The shaved appendectomy margin should always be submitted either in a separate cassette, in a cassette with the longitudinal section of the tip, or marked with ink for easy recognition if submitted with other cross sections. This is for an easy margin evaluation in case a neoplasm is incidentally found. If appendectomy is for a clinical diagnosis of acute appendicitis but histologic features of appendicitis are not seen in submitted sections, the entire appendix should be submitted for histologic examination.

References*:* [1–3]

2. **What are the most common causes of acute appendicitis?**

- The most commonly quoted cause of acute appendicitis is luminal obstruction, which can result from a variety of sources such as lymphoid hyperplasia, fecalith, tumor, foreign body (such as undigested food), and even parasitic worm. It is theorized that luminal obstruction and subsequent distension lead to superimposed bacterial infection and/or ischemic injury.
- However, not all cases of acute appendicitis are associated with identifiable source of luminal obstruction. Infection without obstruction, inflammatory bowel disease, and diverticular disease have all been linked to an increased incidence of acute appendicitis. Genetics and environmental factors can also increase a person's susceptibility to acute appendicitis.
- Fibrous obliteration of the appendiceal lumen is a common incidental finding in appendectomy specimens. It is typically seen at the tip, but the entire appendix can be involved. Histologically, the appendiceal lumen is replaced by a mixture of Schwann cells, fibroblasts, collagen, and fat (Fig. 8.2). Scattered lymphocytes and mast cells may be present. It is generally regarded as a reactive process related to aging or prior mucosal injury.

References*:* [1, 4–8]

3. **What is periappendicitis and what is the clinical significance of the diagnosis?**
   - As described in Table 8.1, periappendicitis can be seen as part of the histologic findings in acute appendicitis (Fig. 8.3a). Isolated form of periappendicitis is inflammation limited to the appendiceal serosa, subserosa, and mesoappendix (Fig. 8.3b). The inflammation spares the mucosa and submucosa and only rarely or superficially extends into the muscularis propria from the external aspect. It occurs in 1–5% of appendices resected for clinically suspected acute appendicitis. Isolated periappendicitis usually occurs due to the spread of inflammation from a nearby source, most commonly from salpingitis or other inflammatory pelvic diseases. Other causes may include urologic disorders, inflammatory bowel disease, colonic or adnexal neoplasms, infectious enterocolitis, Meckel diverticulitis, and abdominal aortic aneurysm. Isolated periappendicitis should only be diagnosed when the entire appendix has been examined and acute appendicitis is excluded, and the diagnosis should prompt a search for extraappendiceal pathologies if not already clinically evident.

   References*:* [9–13]

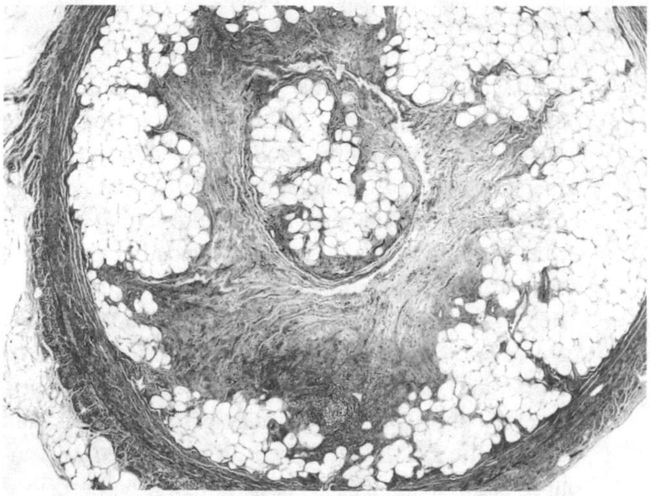

Fig. 8.2 Fibrous obliteration of the appendiceal lumen showing replacement by Schwann cells, fibroblasts, collagen, and fat

4. **What is the clinical significance of granulomatous appendicitis?**
   - Granulomatous appendicitis is a rare finding seen in <1% of all appendectomy specimens. It is divided into two categories based on etiology: primary (idiopathic) and secondary. Idiopathic granulomatous appendicitis is a diagnosis of exclusion that predominantly affects young adults and generally shows a benign clinical course after appendectomy. Historically it was thought to be primary Crohn disease of the appendix but is now recognized as a distinct entity. Secondary granulomatous appendicitis is associated with varied causes, both infectious and noninfectious. Infectious cases are more prevalent in tropical or subtropical regions and include bacterial (e.g., tuberculosis, *Yersinia*), fungal (e.g., *Candida*, *Histoplasma*), and parasitic agents. Noninfectious causes include but are not limited to Crohn disease, sarcoidosis, foreign body reaction, and interval appendectomy. Interval appendectomy describes the practice of nonoperative management and delayed surgery for patients with phlegmon or abscess formation. Allowing the acute inflammation to subside before attempting resection has been associated with a lower rate of complications. However, these patients are also at risk for recurrent or subacute

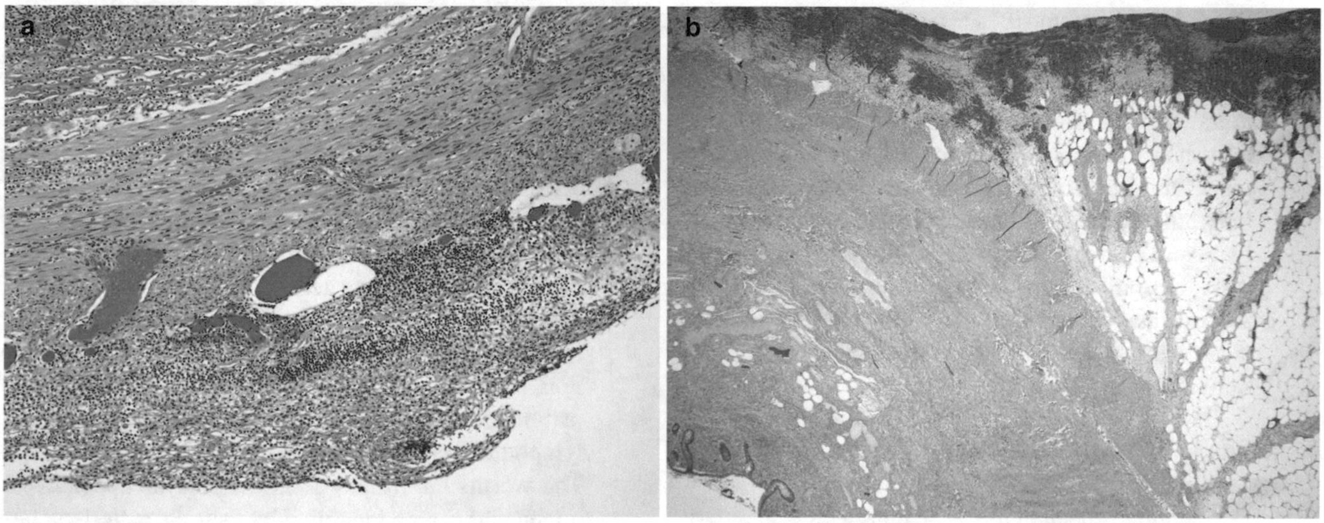

Fig. 8.3 Periappendicitis is characterized by inflammation involving the serosa and mesoappendix of the appendix, which can be part of the histologic spectrum of acute appendicitis (**a**) or isolated (**b**). The isolated form is usually associated with a nearby inflammatory process such as salpingitis

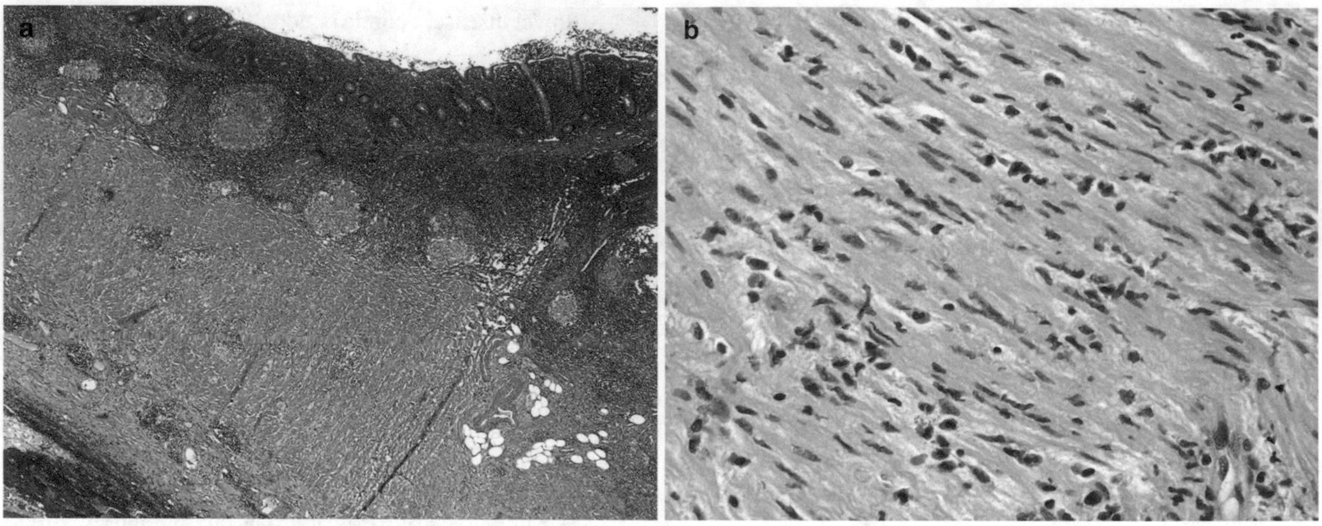

Fig. 8.4 Granulomatous appendicitis showing numerous noncaseating granulomas (**a**). Eosinophilic appendicitis features prominent eosinophils infiltrating the appendiceal wall (**b**). Neutrophils are inconspicuous in granulomatous and eosinophilic appendicitis

episodes of appendicitis, with some of those cases eventually developing into granulomatous appendicitis.

- Granulomatous appendicitis can present with symptoms similar to acute appendicitis, or symptoms associated with the underlying disease, or as an incidental finding. Histologic features vary by etiology. Idiopathic granulomatous appendicitis is typically characterized by numerous, nonnecrotizing granulomas (Fig. 8.4a). Chronic changes such as transmural lymphoid aggregates, fissures, and fibrosis can also be seen. Crohn disease can show similar findings but typically has more active inflammation and only occasional granulomas. Patients with idiopathic granulomatous appendicitis do not have Crohn disease elsewhere in the gastrointestinal tract.
- Secondary granulomatous appendicitis may show features of an underlying disease. Sarcoidosis usually shows numerous nonnecrotizing granulomas and mural fibrosis. Similarly, interval appendicitis generally shows nonnecrotizing granulomas but can have other microscopic findings such as xanthogranulomatous inflammation, eosinophilic infiltrate, transmural lymphoid aggregates, and mural fibrosis. On the other hand, appendicitis resulting from bacterial infections such as tuberculosis and *Yersinia* are characterized by necrotizing granulomas and active inflammation.

References*:* [14–18]

5. **What is the clinical significance of eosinophilic appendicitis?**
   - Eosinophilic appendicitis is a nonspecific diagnosis used to describe a variety of disease processes that show an increased eosinophilic infiltrate in the appendiceal wall (Fig. 8.4b). A significant neutrophilic component is absent by definition. However, acute eosinophilic appendicitis is usually seen in the setting of symptoms of acute appendicitis and grossly inflamed appendices, thus likely representing an early event in the progression of acute appendicitis and not necessarily a distinct entity in and of itself.
   - There are cases of eosinophilic appendicitis that involve parasitic infection, such as *Strongyloides stercoralis* and *Enterobius vermicularis.* These cases, however, usually involve a mix of neutrophilic and eosinophilic infiltrates, albeit with a prominent eosinophilic component. These cases may best be described as eosinophil-predominant acute appendicitis.
   - Lastly, some cases that have been described as "eosinophilic appendicitis" show a mix of eosinophils, lymphocytes, and histiocytes, which likely represent resolving, subacute, or interval appendicitis.

   References*:* [19–23]

6. **What are the most common parasitic infections in the appendix?**
   - The most common parasite found in the appendix is the *Enterobius vermicularis* (pinworm). The incidence of infection varies by region, ranging from 1.3% in Turkey to 8.7% in Czechoslovakia. In many cases, resident *E. vermicularis* do not cause acute inflammation, but they can be associated with a range of histopathologic changes, including acute appendicitis, lymphoid hyperplasia, eosinophilia, and peritonitis. The worms are usually found within the appendiceal lumen and can be identified by their characteristic lateral cuticular alae (Fig. 8.5). Eggs and internal organs can also be seen.

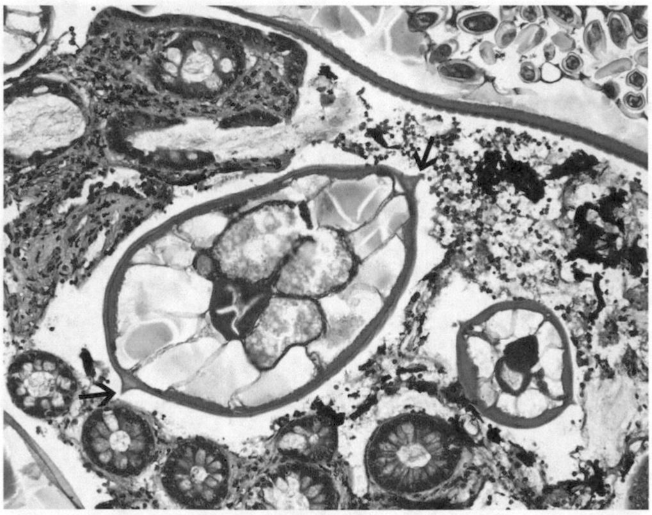

Fig. 8.5 *Enterobius vermicularis* in the appendiceal lumen. Note the characteristic lateral cuticular alae (arrows) and eggs

- Other less common parasites involving the appendix may include *Ascaris lumbricoides*, *Strongyloides stercoralis*, *Schistosoma japonicum*, and *Taenia* spp. Protozoans such as *Cryptosporidium*, and *Entamoeba histolytica* can also be seen.
  References*:* [24–29]

7. **What is appendiceal diverticulosis?**
   - There are two types of appendiceal diverticulosis: congenital (true) and acquired (false), with an incidence of 0.014% and 1.9%, respectively. Congenital diverticula retain all three appendiceal layers, whereas acquired diverticula (also known as pseudodiverticula) histologically show herniation of mucosa and submucosa through a defect of the muscular layer. Appendiceal diverticulosis is not associated with colonic diverticular disease.
   - Congenital diverticulosis is considered a developmental abnormality. The etiology and pathogenesis of acquired diverticulosis are poorly understood, but both inflammatory and noninflammatory mechanisms have been suggested. The noninflammatory factors include chronic luminal obstruction leading to mucosal herniation along the weak points of the appendiceal wall, such as the site of penetrating arteries. This might explain why acquired diverticula can be multiple, which give the appendix a beaded appearance, and are typically found in the distal portion of the appendix on the mesenteric edge. In contrast, congenital diverticula are located on the antimesenteric aspect of the appendix.
   - Appendiceal diverticulosis is usually asymptomatic. When a diverticulum becomes inflamed, the condition is described as diverticulitis and clinically it is commonly diagnosed as acute appendicitis. The incidence of appendiceal diverticulitis is estimated to range from 0.004% to 2.8%.
   - Appendiceal diverticulitis occurs in relatively older patients as compared to acute appendicitis (42.7 ± 15.4 vs. 29.1 ± 17.7 years, respectively) and has a male predominance. In contrast to acute appendicitis, clinical symptoms (i.e., abdominal pain) that develop in the setting of acute diverticulitis tend to be milder and intermittent.
   - Acquired appendiceal diverticula have a higher risk of perforation (particularly in the setting of diverticulitis) and increased mortality rates. According to Yamana et al., perforation of appendiceal diverticula is found in one third of all clinically detected cases versus ~10% of acute appendicitis cases unrelated to diverticulosis.
   - Microscopically, an appendiceal diverticulum may measure up to 5 mm in diameter and closely resembles its colonic counterpart (Fig. 8.6a). Mucosa can be markedly attenuated. Similar to colonic diverticulitis, the inflammatory process is localized to the diverticulum. Once the inflammation extends along the appendiceal wall, it turns into acute appendicitis. Periappendicitis and periappendiceal abscess formation are frequent findings, especially when there is perforation. Ruptured diverticulum often shows mucosal denudation and mucin extrusion into the appendiceal lumen, into the muscular wall, and onto the serosal surface (Fig. 8.6b), which should not be mistaken for low-grade mucinous neoplasm (see Question 21).
     References*:* [30–36]

8. **What is the current who classification of appendiceal neuroendocrine neoplasms?**
   - According to the fifth edition of WHO Classification of Digestive System Tumors, neuroendocrine neoplasms of the appendix are classified into well-differentiated neuroendocrine tumor (NET), poorly differentiated neuroendocrine carcinoma (NEC), and mixed neuroendocrine-nonneuroendocrine neoplasm (MiNEN) (Table 8.2). This classification is in line with those for the entire gastrointestinal tract, which are discussed in detail in Chap. 17. Goblet cell adenocarcinoma (GCA, previously termed "goblet cell carcinoid") is removed in this classification because it is no longer considered to be a unique subtype of appendiceal neuroendocrine neoplasms.
   - Well-differentiated NETs are graded based on Ki-67 proliferative index and mitotic count (see Chap. 17, Question 5). When there is a discordance, the grade is based on the highest of the two.
   - There are instances when tumors have a typical morphology of well-differentiated NET and a

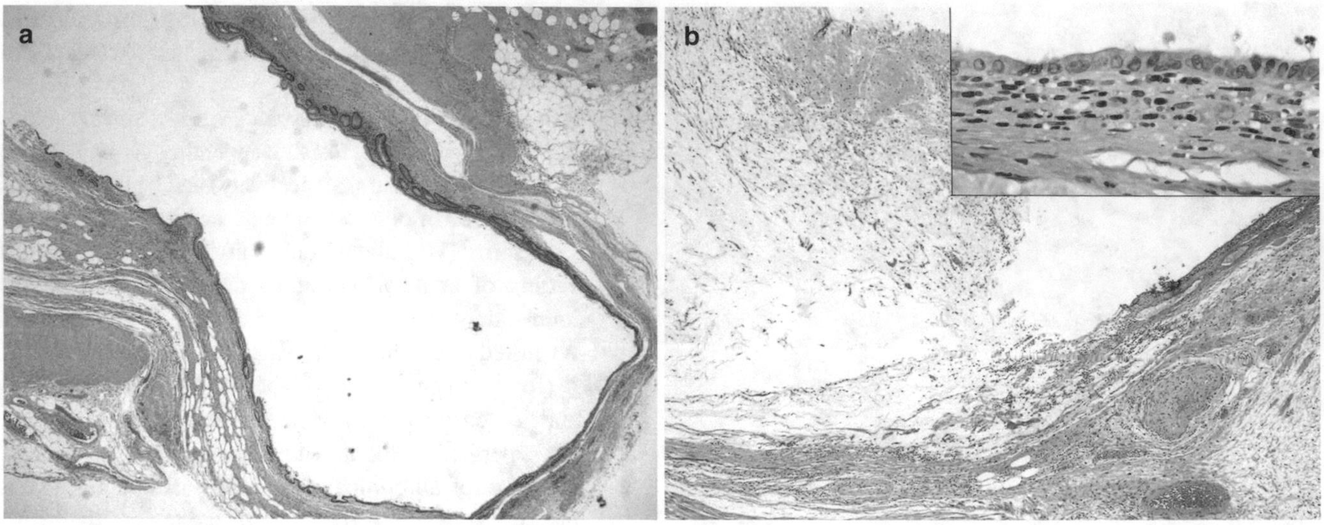

Fig. 8.6 An appendiceal diverticulum characterized by pouching out of the mucosa into the subserosa (**a**). Mucosal denudation and mucin extrusion into the lumen and the appendiceal wall are seen, particularly in ruptured diverticulum (**b**). The herniated mucosa can be markedly attenuated with minimal residual lamina propria and focal loss of crypts (**b**, inset)

Table 8.2 Classification of appendiceal neuroendocrine neoplasms

Neuroendocrine tumor (NET)
Neuroendocrine tumor, grade 1
Neuroendocrine tumor, grade 2
Neuroendocrine tumor, grade 3
L-cell tumor
Glucagon-like peptide-producing tumor
PP/PYY-producing tumor
Enterochromaffin-cell carcinoid
Serotonin-producing carcinoid
Neuroendocrine carcinoma (NEC)
Large cell neuroendocrine carcinoma
Small cell neuroendocrine carcinoma
Mixed neuroendocrine-nonneuroendocrine neoplasm (MiNEN)

mitotic count of <20 per 2 mm^2 but a Ki-67 index of >20%. These tumors are classified as grade 3 well-differentiated NETs rather than poorly differentiated NECs. These tumors have been shown to behave less aggressively than NECs but have a worse prognosis than grade 2 NETs. They do not have the genetic abnormalities seen in poorly differentiated NECs and are less responsive to platinum-based chemotherapy.

- Well-differentiated NETs of the appendix are commonly of enterochromaffin-cell or L-cell type. There is no need to specify the cell type in pathology report, however, because determination of cell type has no therapeutic or prognostic value.
- MiNEN is rare in the appendix. It consists of both epithelial (usually adenocarcinoma) and neuroendocrine (usually NEC) components, each constituting at least 30% of the tumor volume.

References*:* [37–40]

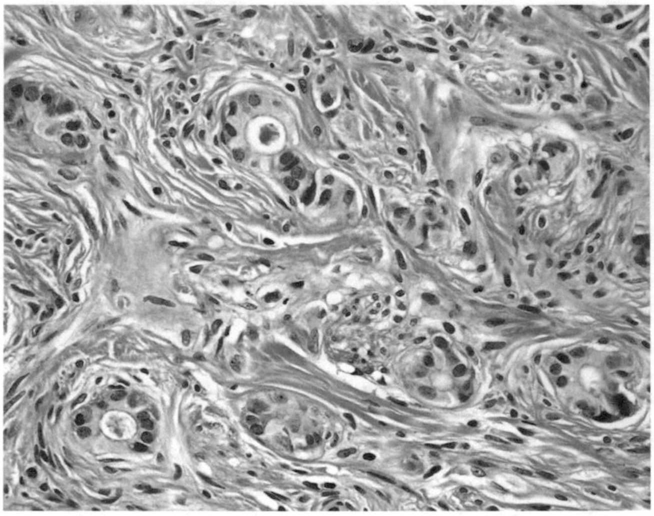

Fig. 8.7 Tubular neuroendocrine tumor showing small tubules dispersed in a fibrotic stroma. No cytologic atypia or mitotic activity is seen. A few tubules have pink mucinous materials in the lumens

9. What is tubular neuroendocrine tumor?

- Tubular NET (previously termed "tubular carcinoid") is a rare subtype of L-cell NET unique to the appendix. It is usually an incidental finding in the tip or distal half of the appendix.
- The age of patients in reported cases ranges from 16 to 85 years. It is seen in both male and female patients.
- The tumor size in reported cases ranges from 3 to 10 mm. It primarily involves the submucosa, but may extend into the muscularis propria and rarely the subserosa, and shows little contact with the overlying mucosa. It is composed of discrete small round tubules dispersed in a fibrotic stroma (Fig. 8.7). Some tubules

appear compressed to form short solid cords. Tumor cells are cuboidal to low columnar with no cytologic atypia or mitotic activity. Occasional Paneth cells may be present. Some of the tubules have inspissated mucin in their lumens.

- Tumor cells are at least focally positive for synaptophysin and/or chromogranin; variably positive for CEA, CK7, and CK20; and frequently positive for glucagon. Increased transcription of proglucagon mRNA has also been reported in tubular carcinoids. Ki-67 proliferative index is typically ≤2%.
- Tubular NETs are uniformly benign. They never recur or metastasize after appendectomy. The main clinical significance of establishing a correct diagnosis is not to confuse it with metastatic well-differentiated adenocarcinoma or GCA since the mucosa is typically spared by the tumor.

References*:* [41–46]

10. What is the current classification of appendiceal epithelial tumors?

- The current WHO classification of epithelial tumors of the appendix is shown in Table 8.3, and the classification by the Peritoneal Surface Oncology Group International (PSOGI) is shown in Table 8.4. The main difference is the inclusion of GCA in the WHO classification.

References*:* [47, 48]

11. What is goblet cell adenocarcinoma?

- GCA had been termed "goblet cell carcinoid" until 2019, when the name was changed by the new WHO tumor classification. Historically, this tumor has also been variably called adenocarcinoid, mucinous carcinoid, microglandular goblet cell carcinoid, amphicrine neoplasm, mucin-producing neuroendocrine tumor or carcinoma, crypt cell carcinoma or adenocarcinoma, mixed carcinoid-adenocarcinoma, mixed goblet cell carcinoid-adenocarcinoma, mixed adenoneuroendocrine carcinoma, and adenocarcinoma ex goblet cell carcinoid. These terms are not currently recommended, but goblet cell carcinoma is an acceptable alternative term for GCA per WHO.
- GCA is almost exclusively seen in the appendix. True extraappendiceal GCAs are exceedingly rare. Cases have been described in the stomach, ileum, and colorectum, but most of these reported cases did not have the entire appendix examined histologically. Therefore, GCAs found in locations other than the appendix are likely extraappendiceal presentations (metastasis) of an occult appendiceal primary.
- Despite the name change, GCA is an amphicrine neoplasm composed of goblet-like mucinous cells admixed with variable numbers of endocrine cells. Its histogenesis remains to be elucidated, and it has been hypothesized to derive from the pluripotent intestinal

Table 8.3 WHO classification of epithelial tumors of the appendix

Hyperplastic polyp
Sessile serrated lesion without dysplasia
Serrated dysplasia, low grade
Serrated dysplasia, high grade
Low-grade appendiceal mucinous neoplasm (LAMN)
High-grade appendiceal mucinous neoplasm (HAMN)
Adenocarcinoma NOS
Mucinous adenocarcinoma
Signet-ring cell adenocarcinoma
Carcinoma, undifferentiated, NOS
Goblet cell adenocarcinoma (GCA)

Table 8.4 PSOGI classification of noncarcinoid epithelial neoplasia of the appendix

Terminology	Description
Adenoma – Tubular, tubulovillous, or villous	Adenoma resembling traditional colorectal type, confined to mucosa with intact muscularis mucosae
Serrated polyp, with or without dysplasia	Lesion with serrated features, confined to the mucosa with intact muscularis mucosae
Low-grade appendiceal mucinous neoplasm (LAMN)	Mucinous neoplasm with low-grade cytologic atypia and any of: Loss of muscularis mucosae Fibrosis of submucosa "Pushing invasion" (expansile or diverticulum-like growth) Dissection of acellular mucin in wall Undulating or flattened epithelial growth Rupture of appendix Mucin and/or cells outside appendix
High-grade appendiceal mucinous neoplasm (HAMN)	Mucinous neoplasm with architectural features of LAMN and no infiltrative invasion but with high-grade cytologic atypia
Mucinous adenocarcinoma – Well, moderately, or poorly differentiated	Mucinous neoplasm with infiltrative invasion[a]
Poorly differentiated (mucinous) adenocarcinoma with signet-ring cells	Neoplasm with signet-ring cells (≤50% of cells)
(Mucinous) signet-ring cell carcinoma	Neoplasm with signet-ring cells (>50% of cells)
Adenocarcinoma – Well, moderately, or poorly differentiated	Nonmucinous adenocarcinoma resembling traditional colorectal type

PSOGI Peritoneal Surface Oncology Group International

[a]Features of infiltrative invasion include tumor budding (discohesive single cells or clusters of less than five cells) and/or small, irregular glands, typically within a desmoplastic stroma characterized by a proteoglycan-rich extracellular matrix with activated fibroblasts/myofibroblasts with vesicular nuclei

stem cells at the base of crypts that are capable of undergoing dual mucinous and neuroendocrine differentiation. Apparently, the new name "goblet cell adenocarcinoma" does not reflect the histogenesis of the tumor because it is clearly not derived from goblet cells. Furthermore, GCA is not the only type of carcinoma that has goblet-like cells. In fact, goblet-like cells can be variably present in other types of adenocarcinoma, such as conventional colorectal adenocarcinoma. Morphologically, the distinction between goblet-like cells and signet-ring cells is a known challenge.

- According to the National Organization for Rare Disorders, GCA has an estimated incidence of ~1 case per two million population. European epidemiologic studies showed an incidence of 0.01–0.05/100,000/year. It is found in 0.3 to 0.9% pf appendectomies but accounts for 35% to 58% of all appendiceal neoplasms and ~ 14% of all malignant neoplasms of the appendix.

  References*:* [47, 49–55]

12. **What are the clinical features of goblet cell adenocarcinoma?**

    GCA is only seen in adults, with a mean age of 50–60 years (ranging from 18 to 89 years). There is no sex predilection.

    - The most common presentation is acute appendicitis. In patients with disseminated disease, a palpable right lower quadrant abdominal mass or nonspecific abdominal pain may be the initial presentation. GCA tends to have peritoneal carcinomatosis rather than spreading to other parts of the body outside the abdomen, but bone and lymph node metastases have been reported. There is a high predilection for GCA to metastasize to the ovaries in female patients for reasons that are not well understood. GCA is an incidental finding in only 3% of cases.

      References*:* [49, 50, 54–58]

13. **What are the gross and histologic features of goblet cell adenocarcinoma?**

    - Most GCAs originate in the tip of the appendix, followed by the base. It is exceptionally rare for GCA to form a discrete mass lesion. The appendix may be grossly normal appearing or show ill-defined nodular or circumferential thickening of the wall, which can be overlooked on gross examination. The tumor size is thus difficult to measure for most cases. In a study by Tang et al., the estimated tumor size, which represents the longitudinal length of tumor extension, is >2 cm in the majority of their cases.
    - Histologically, GCA exhibits low-grade and high-grade growth patterns. The hallmark of low-grade pattern is circumferential infiltration of the appendiceal wall in a concentric fashion (Fig. 8.8a) by small tight round or oval clusters, tubules, nests, or short cords of tumor cells composed predominantly of goblet-like mucinous cells (Fig. 8.8b). Variable numbers of neuroendocrine cells and occasional Paneth cells are present. Luminal formation may be seen in some tumor clusters to form a tubular structure. The goblet-like cells are cytologically bland with compressed nuclei, minimal nuclear atypia, infrequent mitosis, and conspicuous cytoplasmic mucin. Some tumor clusters or tubules may not contain any goblet-like cells, which should still be included in the category of low-grade pattern as long as they maintain a simple clustered or tubular architecture (Fig. 8.8c). Mild architectural disarray or tubular fusion is allowed, however. Extracellular mucin is frequently present in low-grade GCAs (Fig. 8.8d), which can be abundant. The appendiceal mucosa is characteristically spared, which does not show adenomatous change. However, connection of tumor clusters to the base of crypts or focal extension into the lamina propria may be demonstrated in some cases (Fig. 8.8e). Despite its infiltrative growth, low-grade GCAs do not show desmoplastic reaction (Fig. 8.8b, c). Perineural invasion is common, but it does not appear to have prognostic significance.
    - High-grade pattern is seen in at least half of GCA cases. It includes any histologic feature that deviates from the simple clustered or tubular architecture and/or from low-grade cytology. Specifically, it includes single discohesive infiltrating mucinous (goblet-like or signet-ring-like) or nonmucinous cells (Fig. 8.9a, b), large solid sheets or large irregular aggregates of goblet-like or signet-ring-like cells (Fig. 8.9c, d), single file of nonmucinous cells (Fig. 8.9e), complex (anastomosing or cribriforming) structures, and high-grade cytologic features with obvious nuclear atypia (Fig. 8.9f), numerous mitoses, and atypical mitotic figures. A component of conventional gland-forming adenocarcinoma may be present in some cases. Desmoplasia with associated destruction of the muscularis propria is common (Fig. 8.9b, d). Necrosis may be seen. Lymphovascular invasion is more commonly seen in high-grade tumors.

      References*:* [49, 55, 59, 60]

14. **How is goblet cell adenocarcinoma graded and what is the prognostic significance of grading?**

    - While multiple grading systems have been proposed, the currently recommended system by the WHO

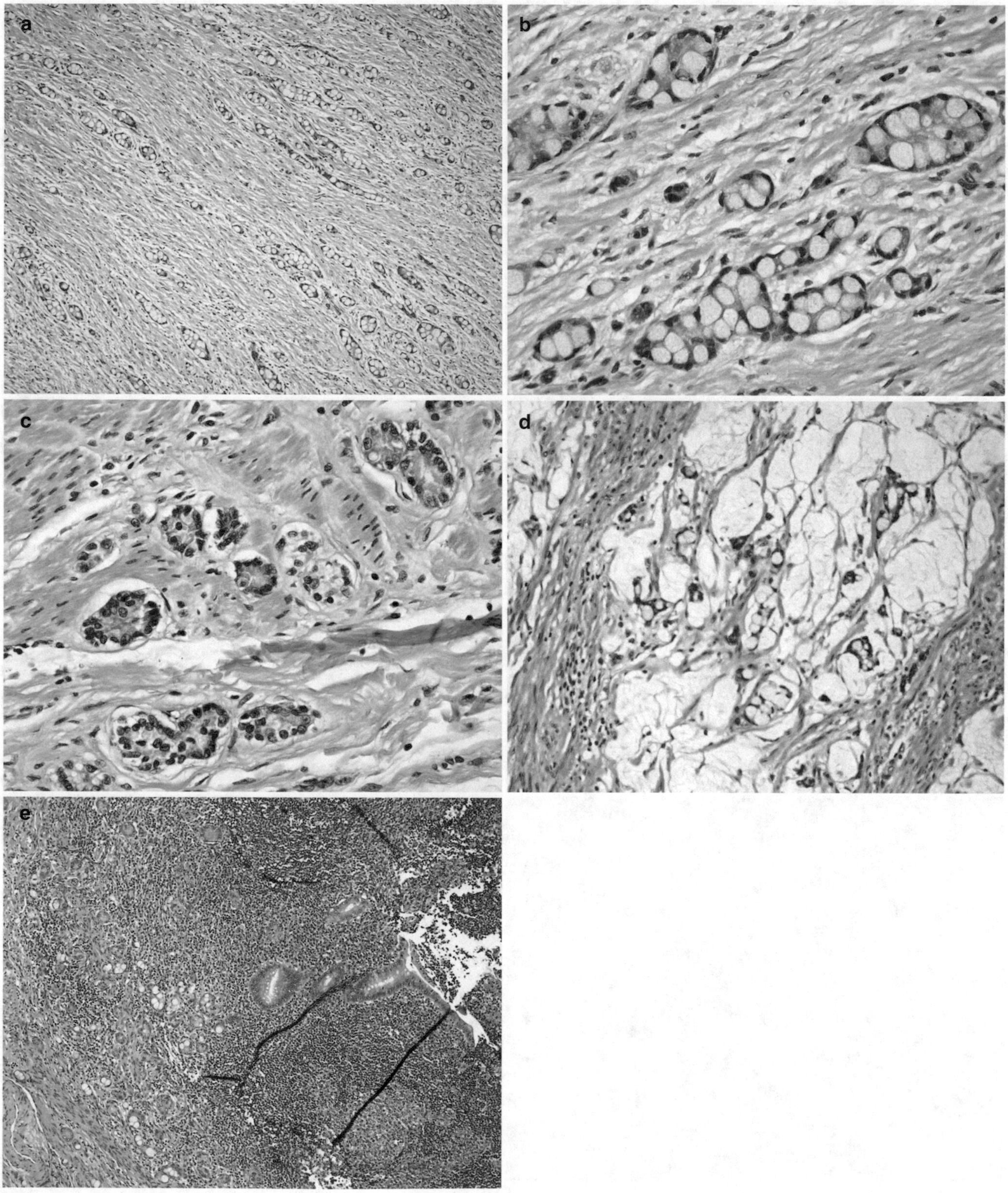

Fig. 8.8 Goblet cell adenocarcinoma showing low-grade histologic features. The tumor circumferentially involves the appendiceal wall in a concentric fashion (**a**). Tumor cells form small tight clusters, tubules, nests, or cords, composed predominantly of goblet-like mucinous cells (**b**). Clusters or tubules without a significant number of goblet-like cells may also be seen (**c**). Extracellular mucin is frequently present (**d**). There is no desmoplastic reaction. Nuclear atypia is minimal, and mitotic figures are infrequent. No adenomatous change is seen in the appendiceal mucosa (**e**)

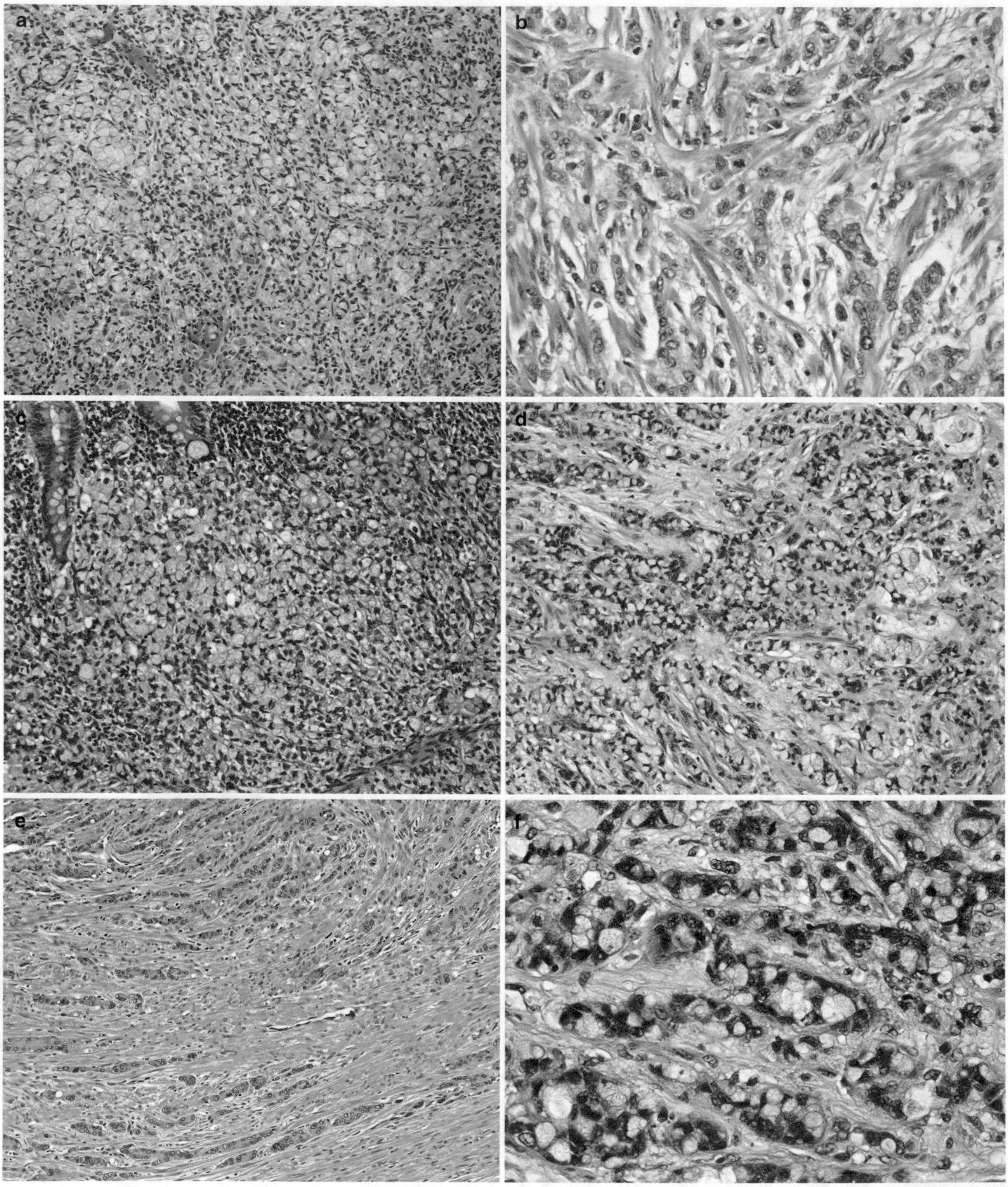

Fig. 8.9 Goblet cell adenocarcinoma showing high-grade histologic features. Examples include single discohesive infiltrating signet-ring-like cells (**a**) or nonmucinous cells (**b**), large solid sheets (**c**) or large irregular aggregates (**d**) of signet-ring-like cells, single file of nonmucinous cells (**e**), and high-grade cytology with obvious nuclear atypia (**f**). Desmoplasia is prominent. Note the presence of focal low-grade features in panels **a** (left) and **d** (right)

Table 8.5 Grading system for goblet cell adenocarcinoma

Grade	High-grade pattern	Low-grade pattern
1 (low grade)	<25%	>75%
2 (intermediate grade)	25–50%	50–75%
3 (high grade)	>50%	<50%

adopted the one proposed by Yozu et al. in 2018. This three-tiered grading system is based on the histologic assessment on the proportion of tumor cells that exhibit low-grade and high-grade growth patterns (Table 8.5). As discussed in Question 13, the main difference between low-grade and high-grade patterns is whether the clustered or tubular architecture is preserved or lost. Cytologic atypia is also a consideration. A tumor may show several intermixed high-grade features, which should be combined to constitute the total proportion. High-grade (grade 3) GCA is distinguished from conventional adenocarcinoma, such as signet-ring cell adenocarcinoma, by having at least focal recognizable classic low-grade GCA component (Fig. 8.9a, d).

- In the study by Yozu et al., patients with low-, intermediate-, and high-grade GCAs had median overall survivals of 204, 86, and 29 months, respectively. The 5- and 10-year survival rates were 82% and 78%, 55% and 33%, and 22% and 4% for low-, intermediate-, and high-grade tumors, respectively. Although tumor stage is also an important prognostic factor, this grading system seemed to be able to predict overall patient survival independently of stage.
- To achieve accurate grading, the entire appendix should be submitted for histologic examination. This also allows for more accurate pT staging and better margin evaluation, which further help decide whether right hemicolectomy is needed.

  References*:* [49, 60]

15. What are the immunohistochemical features of goblet cell adenocarcinoma?

- Low-grade GCAs consistently express CK20, CDX2, SATB2, and CEA and variably express CK7. A variable number of tumor cells also express neuroendocrine markers such as synaptophysin and chromogranin, which usually show a focal, patchy, or scattered staining pattern but a diffuse staining pattern can also be seen. However, staining for neuroendocrine markers is unnecessary for the diagnosis since it is no longer considered to be a neuroendocrine tumor.
- Ki-67 labeling index is around 10% in low-grade GCAs and can be markedly increased (up to 80%) in high-grade tumors. Studies have shown that Ki-67 labeling index by itself has no prognostic significance for GCA tumors and thus should not be used to help guide treatment strategies. Although high-grade tumors may show a higher Ki-67 labeling index than low-grade tumors, it is not recommended for grading GCAs.

  References*:* [49, 59, 61]

16. What molecular alterations have been found in goblet cell adenocarcinoma?

- The currently available molecular studies on GCAs have mainly focused on the comparison with conventional colorectal adenocarcinoma and intestinal neuroendocrine tumor. Briefly, mutations that are relatively common in colorectal adenocarcinoma, such as those involving the *KRAS*, *BRAF*, *APC*, and *TP53* genes, are only rarely detected in GCA cases. Loss of DNA mismatch repair protein expression or microsatellite instability-high is also a rare occurrence in these tumors. The available data indicate that GCA bears little molecular resemblance to colorectal adenocarcinoma.

  References*:* [49, 62–67]

17. What is low-grade appendiceal mucinous neoplasm (LAMN)?

- LAMN is most commonly seen in patients in their fifth to sixth decade of life (ranging from 20 to 89 years), with a female predilection. The most common presentation is a palpable abdominal or pelvic mass. It may also present with symptoms of acute appendicitis or be an incidental finding. Abdominal distension, umbilical hernia, and abdominal pain may develop in patients with peritoneal dissemination (pseudomyxoma peritonei). Ovarian metastasis is quite common in female patients, which may be the initial presentation of the disease.
- On gross examination, the appendix can appear unremarkable or may be enlarged with a mucin-distended lumen (Fig. 8.10a, b). Appendiceal wall may be thickened or attenuated with chronic changes such as fibrosis, hyalinization, or calcification. Rupture with serosal deposits of mucin can be seen. To ensure accurate staging (see Question 19), the entire appendix should be submitted for histologic examination.
- Histologically, LAMN is defined as a mucinous neoplasm with low-grade cytology. As described in Table 8.4, LAMN typically shows a loss of the lamina propria and muscularis mucosae, fibrosis of the submucosa, "pushing" invasion (expansile or diverticulum-like growth) into the muscular wall, dissection of acellular mucin in the wall, and cellular or acellular mucin outside the appendix. LAMN can involve part of the appendix or in its entirety and usually exhibits circumferential involvement of the mucosa (Fig. 8.11a). The neoplastic epithelial cells are typically columnar and hypermucinous. They have basally located, small, relatively uniform, pen-

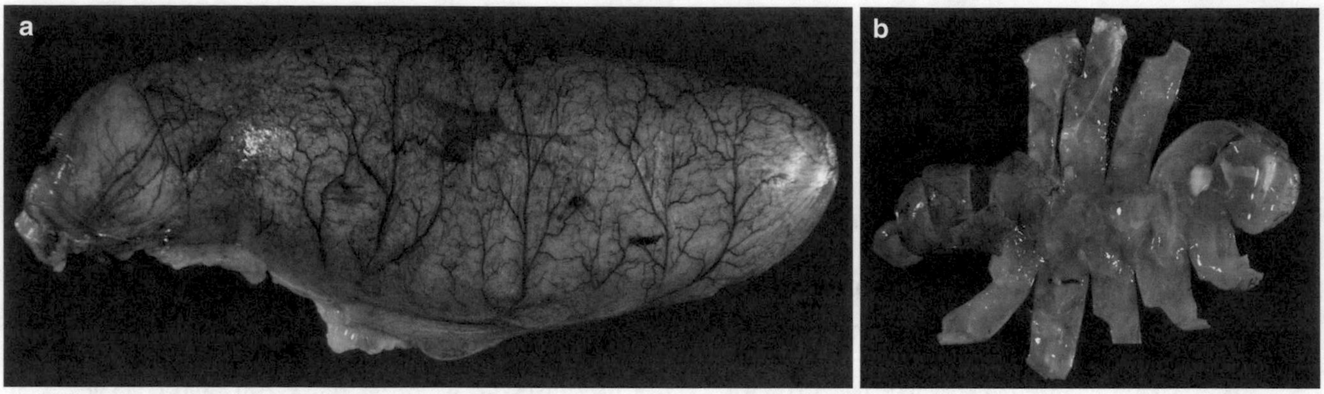

Fig. 8.10 An appendectomy specimen showing an enlarged appendix (**a**) distended by abundant mucin (**b**). The appendiceal wall appears attenuated grossly

cillate, and mildly pseudostratified nuclei; cytoplasmic mucin vacuoles; and no more than occasional mitosis (Fig. 8.11b). Architecturally, tumor cells can have a villous or undulating arrangement (Fig. 8.11c, d), resembling villous adenoma or low-grade dysplasia in the colon. Some cases may show a straight monolayer of mucinous epithelium, which can be partially flattened/attenuated and mucin depleted (Fig. 8.11e). Complex architectural arrangements such as cribriform or extensive papillary structures should not be seen. The neoplastic cells replace the appendiceal mucosa and sit directly on the fibrotic submucosal tissue. Lymphoid follicles, which are normally present in the appendix, are typically absent in LAMN. Some cases may show extensive surface denudation with only focal neoplastic cells remaining (Fig. 8.11f), further emphasizing the importance of submitting the entire appendix for histologic examination if a mucinous lesion is encountered.

- Biologically, LAMN has the potential for extraappendiceal dissemination and is considered as low-grade adenocarcinoma. Its prognosis is stage dependent (see Question 19). LAMNs limited to the appendix have a negligible risk of recurrent disease. Cases with acellular mucin involving the peritoneum have a small but measurable risk of intraperitoneal recurrence (~3%). The recurrence rate for cases with peritoneal cellular mucin deposits is much higher (~36%). The prognosis is also influenced by the grade of tumor cells involving the peritoneum, the extensiveness of peritoneal disease, and the possibility of complete cytoreduction.
- Molecularly, LAMNs frequently harbor *KRAS* and *GNAS* mutations. *BRAF* and *TP53* mutations and loss of DNA mismatch repair protein expression or microsatellite instability-high are uncommon in LAMNs.

References*:* [48, 68–71]

18. What is high-grade appendiceal mucinous neoplasm (HAMN)?

HAMN is a newly recognized appendiceal mucinous neoplasm that essentially shares the same histologic characteristics of LAMN but shows at least focal high-grade features (Fig. 8.12). The area of HAMN may exhibit a cribriforming or micropapillary architecture. Tumor cell nuclei are enlarged, hyperchromatic, round, or pleomorphic, which may be stratified or remain as a single layer. Mitotic figures can be frequent, and atypical mitosis can be seen. Single-cell necrosis and luminal necrotic debris may be present.

Clinical data on this extremely rare entity are limited, but the few cases reported in the literature described a highly aggressive clinical course. It is recommended that histologic evidence of invasive adenocarcinoma should be searched when a HAMN is diagnosed. Classification of HAMN lesions with cellular mucin on the visceral peritoneum is unclear. Some investigators believe that cases of HAMN-like mucinous neoplasm with serosal deposits of tumor cells with high-grade cytology likely represent undersampled invasive mucinous adenocarcinomas. These lesions are best considered as mucinous adenocarcinomas and should not be classified as HAMNs.

References*:* [48, 68, 70, 71]

19. How are appendiceal mucinous neoplasms staged?

- Considering the unique growth pattern, the American Joint Committee on Cancer (AJCC) eighth edition has created a pT staging protocol specifically for LAMN (Table 8.6), which differs from that used for conventional appendiceal carcinomas (see Chap. 18, Question 17). However, the same N and M staging criteria are applied to LAMN, although lymph node involvement is exceedingly rare.

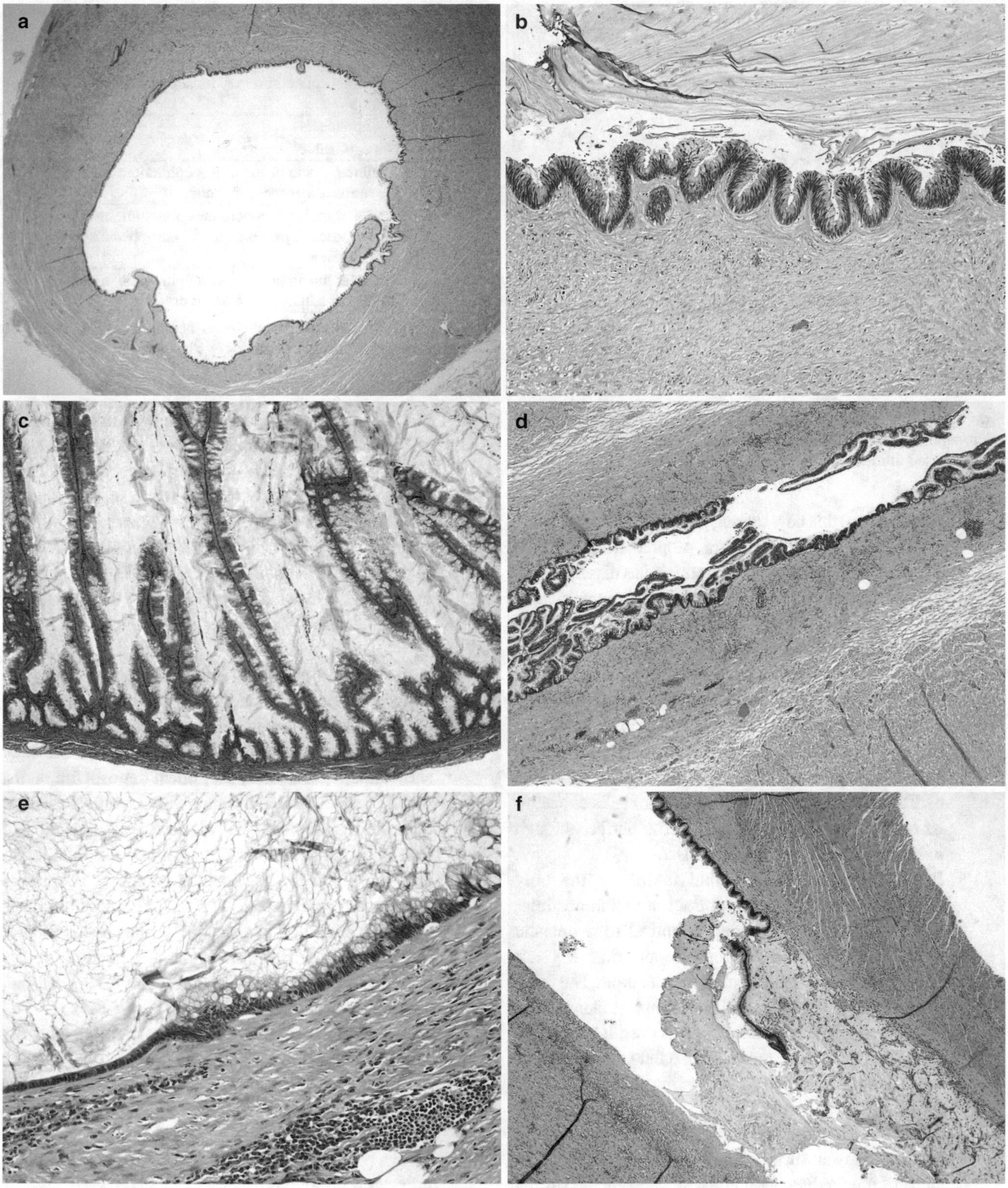

Fig. 8.11 Low-grade appendiceal mucinous neoplasm showing circumferential involvement of the mucosa (**a**). The neoplastic epithelial cells have basally located, pencillate, and mildly pseudostratified nuclei, as well as cytoplasmic mucin (**b**), with a villous (**c**), undulating (**d**), or straight linear (**e**) arrangement. Partial flattening with mucin depletion (**e**, left) or extensive denudation (**f**) can be seen. Neoplastic cells replace the appendiceal mucosa and sit directly on the fibrotic submucosal tissue. Lymphoid follicles are typically absent

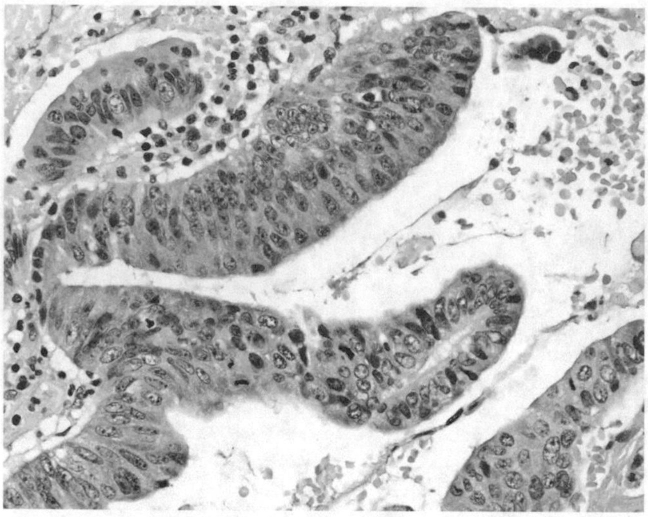

Fig. 8.12 High-grade appendiceal mucinous neoplasm showing micropapillary architecture, enlarged nuclei, loss of nuclear polarity, and increased mitotic activity

- According to this new staging protocol, all LAMNs that are confined by the muscularis propria are assigned as Tis, even if acellular or cellular mucin has dissected into the muscularis propria (Fig. 8.13a). Therefore, there is no T1 or T2 for LAMNs. The rationale for this is that the depth of appendiceal wall involvement is not a risk factor for recurrence as long as the tumor is confined to the appendix. However, if acellular mucin or mucinous epithelium extends beyond the muscularis propria into the subserosa, mesoappendix, or serosal surface, the tumor should be staged as T3 (Fig. 8.13b) or T4a (Fig. 8.13c, d). Tumor with perforation where tumor cells or acellular mucin is continuous with the serosal surface through inflammation is also considered T4a.
- It should be emphasized that LAMN is the only tumor in the gastrointestinal tract in which acellular mucin is used for T staging, identical to neoplastic cells. For other carcinomas, neoplastic cells are needed and acellular mucin does not count. The presence of acellular mucin within lymph nodes should not be considered nodal metastasis even for LAMN.
- Care should be exercised when handling the specimens to minimize knife "carry-over" of mucin and/or cells to the appendiceal surface. When evaluating the visceral peritoneum, avoid overinterpreting "carry-over" mucin for true serosal surface involvement by looking for signs of mucin dissection in the submesothelial stroma and signs of tissue reaction around the mucin, such as inflammatory response, mesothelial hyperplasia, and neovascularization (Figs. 8.13d and 8.14a, b).
- According to the AJCC eighth edition, the staging system for invasive adenocarcinomas should be used for HAMN because of its high risk of recurrence. However, how that staging system should be applied to HAMN is not specifically addressed. Since HAMN may show only focal high-grade features but is otherwise identical to LAMN, confusions exist on how to stage T1 and T2 lesions and whether acellular mucin should be used to stage T2, T3, and T4a. Presumably, the unique category of Tis for LAMN is not applicable to HAMN. Further clarification is needed for this rare new entity.

  References*:* [68–72]

Table 8.6 Unique T definition for LAMN, AJCC eighth edition

T category	Criteria
Tis	Confined by the muscularis propria; acellular mucin or mucinous epithelium may invade into the muscularis propria
T1	Not applicable
T2	Not applicable
T3	Acellular mucin or mucinous epithelium extends into the subserosa or mesoappendix
T4a	Acellular mucin or mucinous epithelium involves the serosa (visceral peritoneum) of the appendix or mesoappendix
T4b	Acellular mucin or mucinous epithelium directly invades or adheres to adjacent organs or structures

LAMN low-grade appendiceal mucinous neoplasm, *AJCC* American Joint Committee on Cancer, *Tis* tumor or carcinoma in situ

20. What is pseudomyxoma peritonei?

- Pseudomyxoma peritonei (PMP) is a malignant condition defined by the presence of intraperitoneal acellular mucin and/or mucinous epithelium. PMP may show mucinous ascites, peritoneal deposits/implants, omental cake, and ovarian involvement. It is most commonly associated with a perforated appendiceal mucinous neoplasm but can also be seen in association with other tumors such as mucinous neoplasms of the ovary, pancreas, colon, stomach, and gallbladder. The classification system proposed by PSOGI divides PMP into four categories, depending on the presence of epithelium, degree of cytologic atypia, and presence of signet-ring cells (Table 8.7).
- In general, the grades of peritoneal tumor and the appendiceal primary are concordant. Discordance may occur, however, which usually shows a higher grade in peritoneal disease. For those cases, the grades should be separately reported, and the grade of the peritoneal tumor is likely to have a greater impact on prognosis.

  References*:* [48, 73, 74]

21. How can LAMN be distinguished from appendiceal adenoma, serrated lesions, retention cyst, ruptured diverticulum, endometriosis, and mucinous cystadenoma of the ovary?

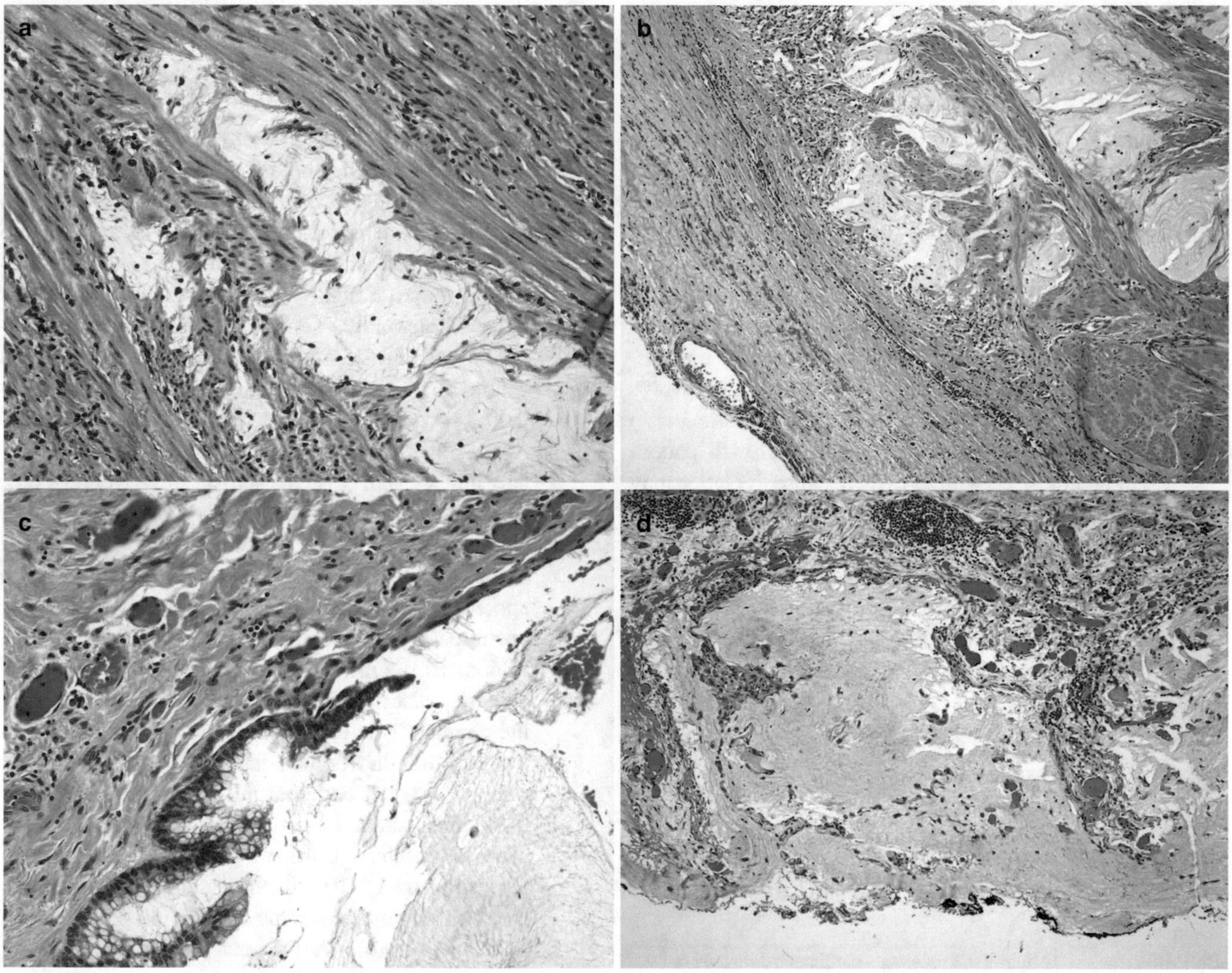

Fig. 8.13 Examples of various stages of low-grade appendiceal mucinous neoplasm. (**a**) Tis, acellular mucin involving the muscularis propria. (**b**) pT3, acellular mucin dissects through the muscularis propria into the subserosa. (**c** and **d**) pT4a, cellular and acellular mucin involving the serosal surface

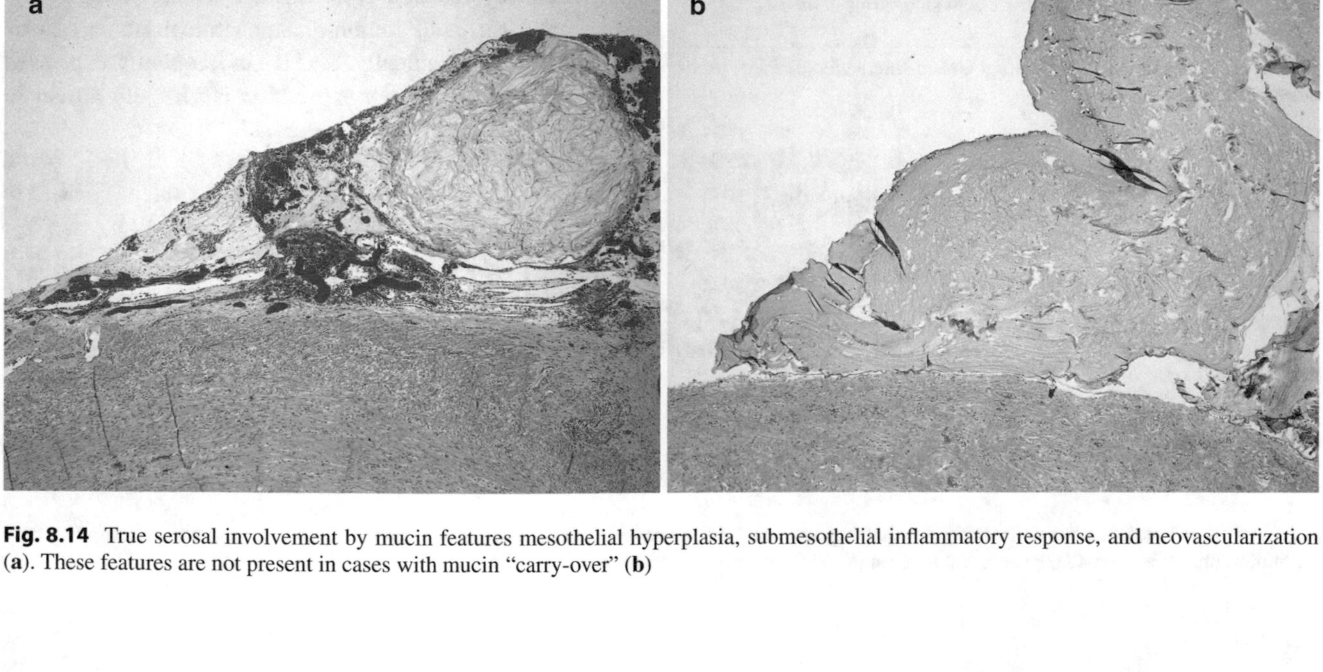

Fig. 8.14 True serosal involvement by mucin features mesothelial hyperplasia, submesothelial inflammatory response, and neovascularization (**a**). These features are not present in cases with mucin "carry-over" (**b**)

- Conventional appendiceal adenomas resemble their colorectal counterparts and can be classified as tubular, tubulovillous, or villous subtypes. Unlike LAMNs, adenomas lack the abundant cytologic mucin and have preserved mucosal architecture with intact lamina propria and muscularis mucosae (Fig. 8.15a). The entire appendix should be submitted to rule out the possibility of associated adenocarcinoma.
- Similarly, appendiceal serrated lesions (hyperplastic polyp, sessile serrated adenoma/polyp without or with cytologic dysplasia) also resemble their colorectal counterparts. They may circumferentially involve the appendiceal mucosa or form a discrete polyp (Fig. 8.15b, c). The circumferential growth pattern can be confused with LAMN because the latter may also show a villous or filiform architecture. However, prominent serration is not a feature of LAMN. Like conventional adenomas, appendiceal serrated lesions also maintain the normal mucosal architecture with preserved lamina propria and muscularis mucosae. Diagnosis of conventional adenomas and serrated lesions in specimens with perforation or peritoneal dissemination should be reconsidered as it is highly unlikely for these lesions to dissect through the appendiceal wall.
- Retention cyst is caused by luminal obstruction and may show marked mucosal atrophy with attenuated epithelial lining and diminished lamina propria, which can be confused with LAMN. However, there should be at least focal areas of attenuated but preserved mucosal architecture. If possible, the entire appendix should be submitted for histologic examination to rule out the possibility of LAMN. There should be no significant nuclear atypia or villous epithelial proliferation seen in retention cysts.
- Ruptured diverticulum can show mucin within the appendiceal wall or on the serosal surface (Fig. 8.6b), similar to LAMN. However, ruptured diverticulum should show intact, nonmucinous appendiceal mucosa at least focally. Submission of the entire appendix and step sections may be necessary to demonstrate the presence of diverticulum.
- Endometriosis may involve the appendix but should be easily distinguished from LAMN by recognizing the characteristic endometrial type glands, endometrial stroma, and hemosiderin. However, confusion may arise when endometrial glands develop mucinous metaplasia. In difficult cases, immunohistochemical stains (estrogen receptor, progesterone receptor, and CD10) to help identify endometrial-type epithelium and stroma are helpful.
- In women, LAMN has a tendency to spread to the ovaries. In fact, there is now a consensus that most mucinous tumors of the ovary are metastatic from the appendix. However, there are still cases where the distinction from an ovarian primary (such as mucinous cystadenoma) is needed. While morphologically difficult, immunohistochemical stains can be helpful. Specifically, SATB2 is frequently expressed in LAMNs, but its expression is virtually absent in

Table 8.7 PSOGI classification of pseudomyxoma peritonei

Category	PSOGI terminology
Mucin without epithelial cells	Acellular mucin
PMP with low-grade histologic features	Low-grade mucinous carcinoma peritonei or disseminated peritoneal adenomucinosis (DPAM)
PMP with high-grade histologic features	High-grade mucinous carcinoma peritonei or peritoneal mucinous carcinomatosis (PMCA)
PMP with signet-ring cells	High-grade mucinous carcinoma peritonei with signet-ring cells or peritoneal mucinous carcinomatosis with signet-ring cells (PMCA-S)

PSOGI Peritoneal Surface Oncology Group International, *PMP* pseudomyxoma peritonei

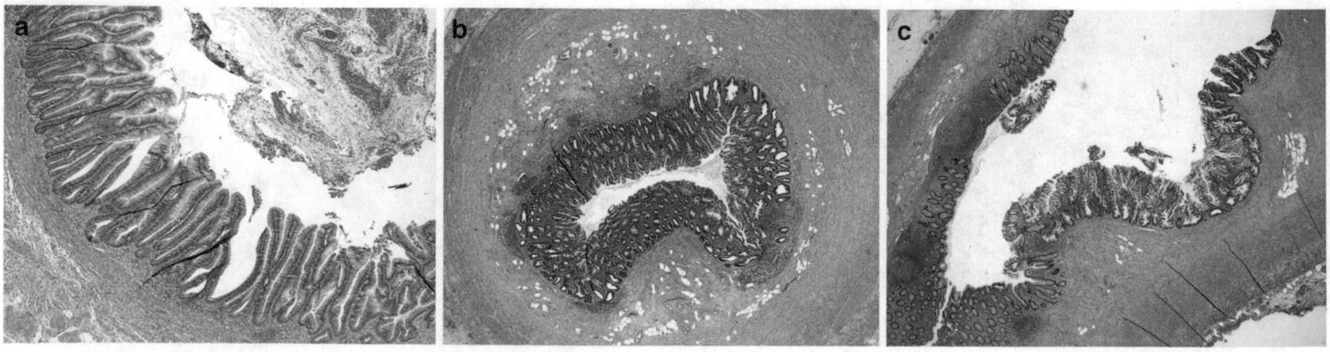

Fig. 8.15 A villous adenoma of the appendix showing preserved lamina propria and muscularis mucosae (**a**). Sessile serrated adenoma/polyp may circumferentially involve the appendiceal mucosa (**b**) or form a discrete polyp (**c**)

primary ovarian mucinous tumors. Ovarian mucinous tumors also show a CK7+/CK20+ or CK7+/CK20- pattern, whereas LAMNs tend to show a CK7-/CK20+ pattern. PAX8 is frequently expressed in ovarian tumors but negative in LAMNs.
References: [34, 48, 68, 75–78]

22. What is mucinous adenocarcinoma of the appendix and how is it graded?

- Mucinous adenocarcinoma differs from LAMN and HAMN by showing infiltrative invasion. Similar to those seen in other parts of the gastrointestinal tract, it is defined by abundant extracellular mucin composing >50% of the tumor volume. The mucin pools contain free-floating clusters or strips of neoplastic epithelium or individual tumor cells. Variable number of signet-ring cells may also be present. If the percentage of signet-ring cells is ≤50%, the tumor is designated as mucinous adenocarcinoma with signet-ring cells. If >50%, the tumor is classified as signet-ring cell carcinoma. Signet-ring cells may float in mucin pools or infiltrate stroma. It is believed that signet-ring cells floating in mucin pools may not have the same prognostic significance as those infiltrating tissue.
- Mucinous adenocarcinoma constitutes 40–50% of all appendiceal carcinomas, whereas they make up only 8–10% of all colorectal carcinomas. In the colon, mucinous adenocarcinomas are commonly associated with Lynch syndrome, microsatellite instability, right-sided tumors, and younger patients. In the appendix, however, studies so far have not shown a strong association with familial syndromes, microsatellite instability, or *BRAF* mutation. Instead, a high incidence of *KRAS* mutation is seen, involving 50–80% of well to moderately differentiated tumors and ~ 20% of poorly differentiated tumors. Another common mutation associated with appendiceal mucinous adenocarcinomas is *GNAS* mutation, seen in 30–70% of cases.
- Both the appendiceal mucinous adenocarcinoma and the peritoneal component (if present) can be graded using a three-tier system, as recommended by AJCC eighth edition. This grading system is based on the scheme proposed by Davidson et al., which stratifies tumors based on cytologic features, tumor cellularity, invasion, and signet-ring cells (Table 8.8, Fig. 8.16). As mentioned earlier, the grades of the appendiceal primary and peritoneal components are usually concordant. If not, the overall grade assigned should reflect the higher component.
- Significant survival differences are observed between the different grades of appendiceal mucinous adenocarcinomas. In a recent analysis of Surveillance, Epidemiology and End Results (SEER) data of 1375 mucinous adenocarcinomas, the adjusted hazard ratios for stage IV moderately and poorly differentiated histologic grades were 1.63 and 4.94, respectively. A recent study on 5971 mucinous neoplasms culled from the National Cancer Data Base (NCDB) showed a 5-year overall survival rate for patients with mucinous adenocarcinoma (stages I–III) of 74.9%, 63.2%, and 51.5% for well, moderate, and poor differentiation, respectively. For stage IV disease, the 5-year overall survival rates were 56.7%, 31.5%, and 11.3% for well, moderate, and poor differentiation, respectively.
Reference: [72, 79–88]

Case 1

Learning Objectives

1. To become familiar with the histologic features of the lesion
2. To become familiar with the clinical significance and differential diagnosis of the lesion

Table 8.8 Three-tier grading system for mucinous adenocarcinoma of the appendix

Grade	Histology
Well-differentiated (G1) (=LAMN) (Fig. 8.16a)	Low-grade cytologic atypia No signet-ring cells Lack of typical features of infiltrative invasion If peritoneum is involved: Acellular mucin or low cellularity (<20%) Lack of infiltrative invasion of the peritoneum or other organs Absence of lymphovascular or perineural invasion
Moderately differentiated (G2) (Fig. 8.16b)	Mixed low- and high-grade cytologic atypia or diffuse high grade No signet-ring cell component Most cases show features of invasion (at least focally), but rare cases may lack invasion (HAMN) If the peritoneum is involved: Often high cellularity (>20%) Infiltrative invasion into the peritoneum or other organs may be seen Lymphovascular and perineural invasion may be present
Poorly differentiated (G3) (Fig. 8.16c)	High-grade cytologic atypia Usually have signet-ring cell component If the peritoneum is involved: Often high cellularity (>20%) Infiltrative invasion into the peritoneum or other organs may be seen Lymphovascular and perineural invasion may be present

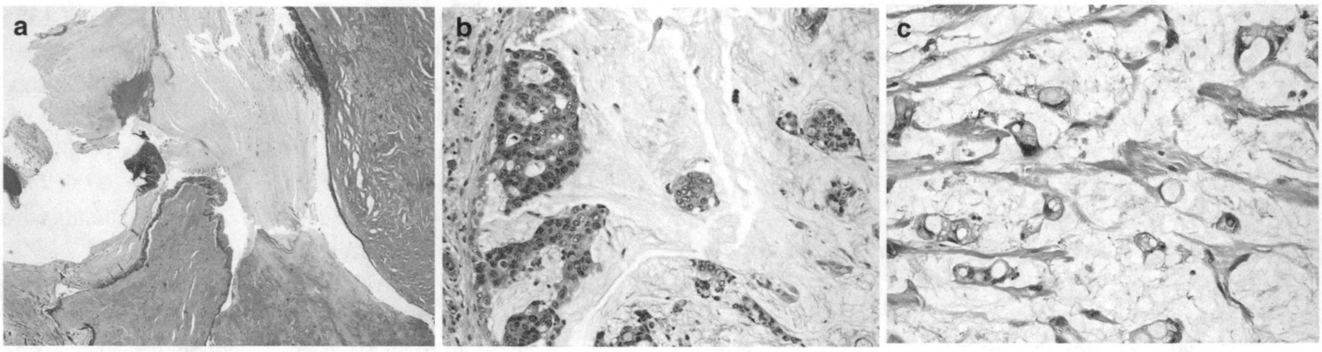

Fig. 8.16 Mucinous adenocarcinoma of the appendix. (**a**) Well-differentiated, resembling low-grade appendiceal mucinous neoplasm; (**b**) moderately differentiated, showing high-grade features, including complex architecture and prominent nuclear atypia; and (**c**) poorly differentiated, showing the presence of signet-ring cells

Case History

A 41-year-old male presented with symptoms and signs of acute appendicitis and underwent laparoscopic appendectomy.

Gross Findings

The resected appendix measured 7.2 cm in length and 1.1 cm in maximum diameter. Purulent exudate was noted on the serosal surface. A 0.7-cm fecalith was present in the lumen. No perforation or discrete lesion was identified. The proximal margin (shave), distal tip (longitudinal), and representative cross sections were submitted for histologic examination.

Histologic Findings

Histologic sections showed features of acute suppurative appendicitis with periappendicitis and luminal fecalith (Fig. 8.17a, b). In addition, multiple small tubular structures were noted in the appendiceal tip section, occupying an area of ~2 mm in the submucosa (Fig. 8.17c). The cells lining the tubules were cuboidal and exhibited no cytologic atypia (Fig. 8.17d). No mitotic figures were identified. Pink luminal secretions were seen in some of the tubules. No adenomatous change or dysplasia was appreciated in the appendiceal mucosa.

Differential Diagnosis

- Metastatic well-differentiated adenocarcinoma
- Tubular neuroendocrine tumor (tubular carcinoid)
- Conventional low-grade well-differentiated neuroendocrine tumor

IHC and Other Ancillary Studies

None.

Final Diagnosis

Tubular neuroendocrine tumor (tubular carcinoid).

Take-Home Messages

- Tubular NET or tubular carcinoid is a rare subtype of L-cell NET unique to the appendix.
- It is usually an incidental finding in the appendiceal tip.
- It is always benign and never recurs or metastasizes after appendectomy. The only clinical significance is not to mistake it for metastatic adenocarcinoma.
  References*:* [41, 42]

Case 2

Learning Objectives

1. To become familiar with the histologic features of the tumor
2. To become familiar with the immunohistochemical staining patterns of the tumor
3. To become familiar with the grading system for the tumor

Case History

A 66-year-old female presented with vague abdominal discomfort. Imaging studies showed a 5.5 x 3.7 x 3.1-cm mass involving the left adnexa. Left ovary was not identifiable. There was a suggestion of peritoneal nodularity in the right greater than left lower quadrants associated with

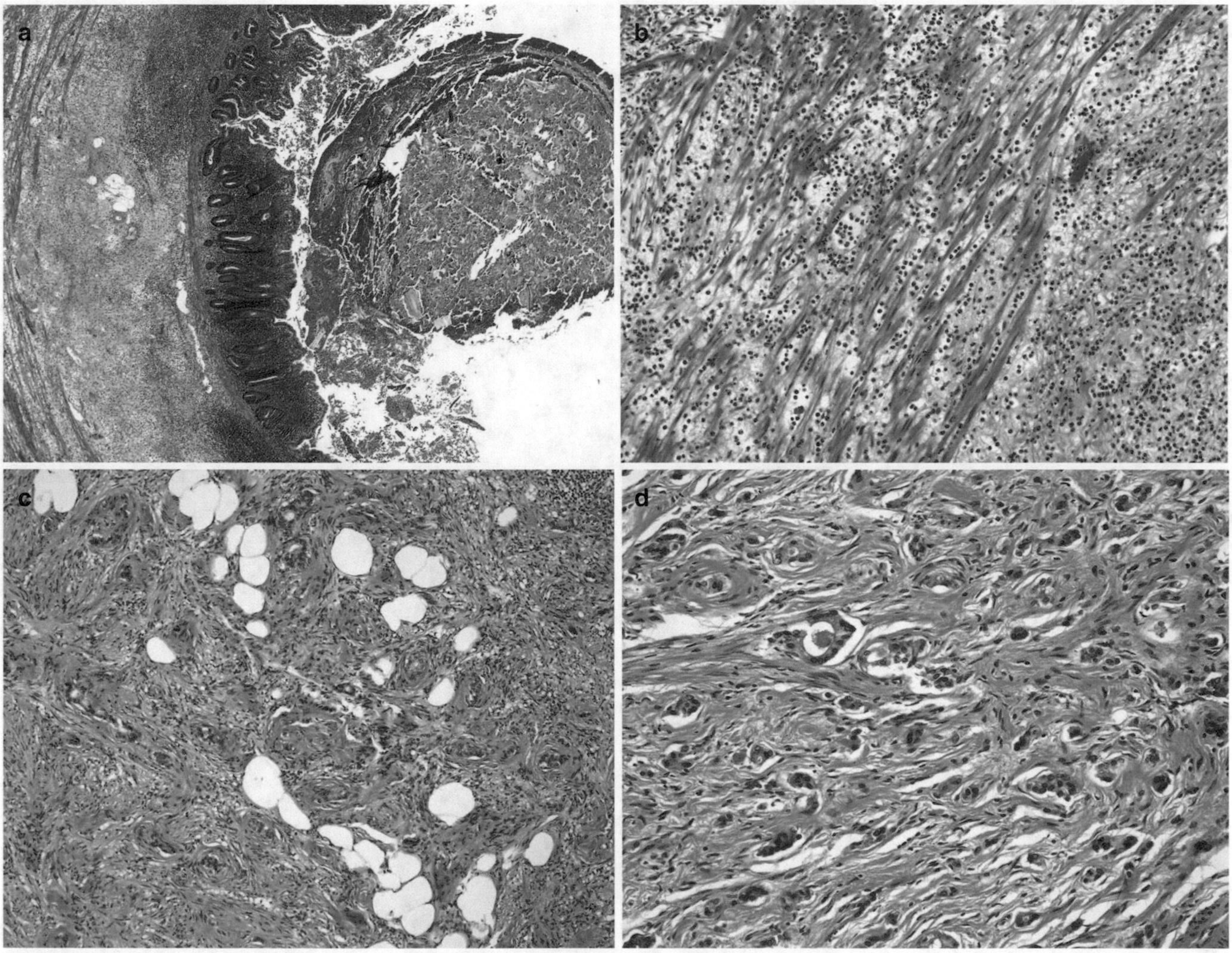

Fig. 8.17 (Case 1). Low power view showing features of acute appendicitis with luminal fecalith (**a**). High power view showing neutrophil infiltration of the appendiceal wall (**b**). Scattered small tubular structures noted in the appendiceal tip, involving the submucosa (**c**). Higher power view of the tubular structures (**d**)

minimal ascites, worrisome for peritoneal carcinomatosis. The bowel appeared unremarkable on imaging studies. The patient underwent diagnostic laparoscopy, followed by total abdominal hysterectomy with bilateral salpingo-oophorectomy, small bowel resection, appendectomy, and omentectomy. Intraoperatively, the presence of a right adnexal mass and peritoneal carcinomatosis was confirmed. Additionally, tumor was found in the appendix and ileum.

Gross Findings

The appendix measured 5.1 cm in length and 2.2 cm in maximum diameter. The appendiceal wall is diffusely thickened and firm. The tip was cystically distended, which appeared multilocular and mucin containing. The mesoappendix was studded with multiple small white nodules. The right ovary was distorted by numerous nodules and two dominant masses measuring 2.2 and 2.6 cm in maximum dimension. Tumor implants were noted in the right broad ligament, omentum, and small bowel serosal surface.

Histologic Findings

Histologic sections of the appendix showed an infiltrating neoplasm with areas of gland formation, clusters of goblet- or signet-ring-like cells, and areas of mucin production. Tumor cells invaded the lamina propria, but no adenomatous change or dysplasia was demonstrated in the mucosa (Fig. 8.18a, b). Some of the goblet- or signet-ring-like cells formed small clusters in mucin pools (Fig. 8.18c), while others formed irregular clusters or large sheets infiltrating

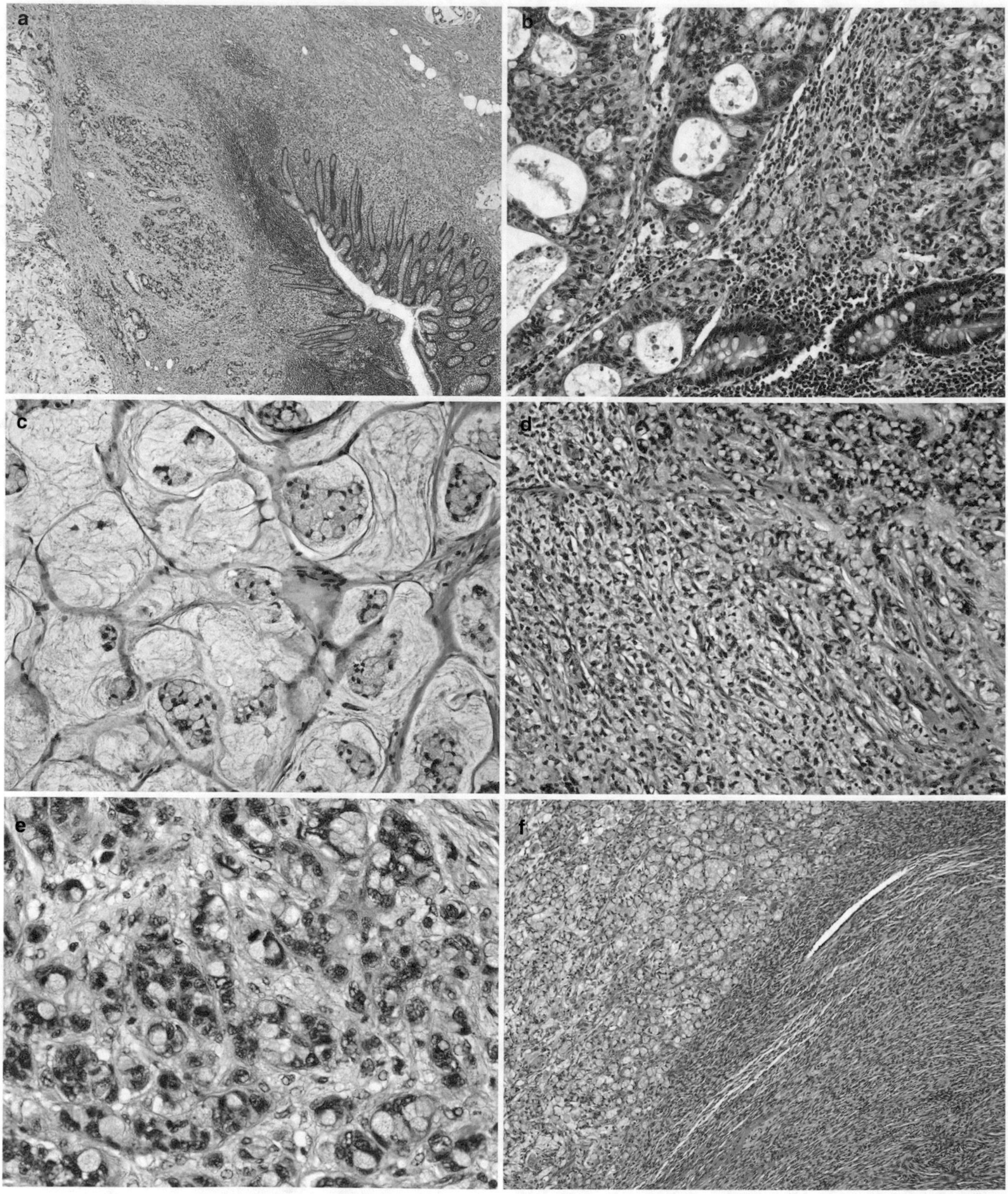

Fig. 8.18 (Case 2). (**a**) Low power examination of the appendix showing an infiltrating neoplasm with areas of gland formation, clustering, and mucin production. (**b**) High power view showing a mixture of gland-forming and goblet- or signet-ring-like components. (**c**) Small clusters of goblet- or signet-ring-like cells were seen in mucin pools in focal areas. (**d**) Sheets or irregular clusters of infiltrating goblet- or signet-ring-like cells were also seen. (**e**) Nuclear atypia and mitotic activity were evident. (**f**) Histologic examination of the right adnexal mass showing tumor involvement of the ovary with predominantly goblet- or signet-ring-like cells

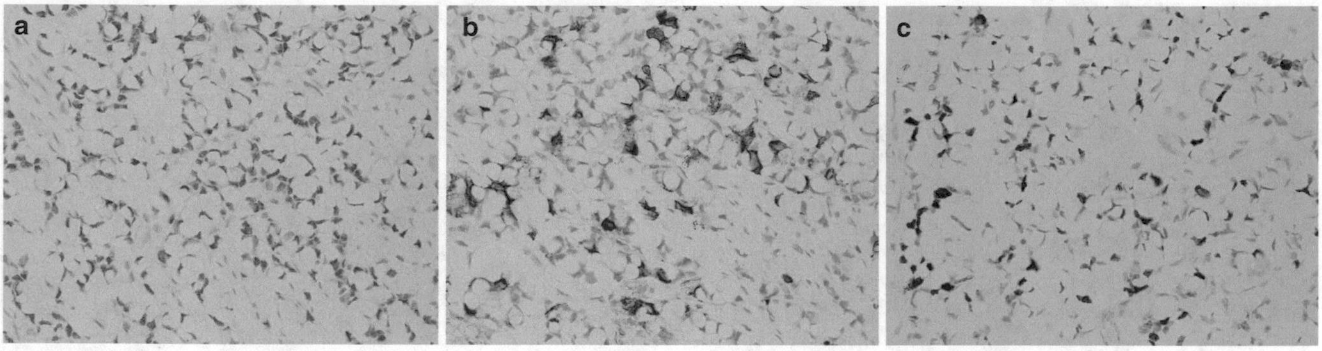

Fig. 8.19 (Case 2). Immunohistochemistry performed on a representative section of the appendix. (**a**) CDX2, (**b**) synaptophysin, and (**c**) Ki-67

the appendiceal wall (Fig. 8.18d). Single goblet- or signet-ring-like cells were also noted. Marked nuclear atypia was evident in most tumor cells (Fig. 8.18e). Histologic examination of the right adnexal mass showed tumor involvement of the ovary with predominantly signet-ring-like cells (Fig. 8.18f). Tumor cells also involved the left adnexa, omentum, and small bowel and were seen in a peritoneal wall biopsy.

Differential Diagnosis

- Goblet cell adenocarcinoma
- Signet-ring cell carcinoma
- Metastatic poorly differentiated adenocarcinoma

IHC and Other Ancillary Findings

A limited panel of immunostains were performed on a representative section of the appendix. Tumor cells were strongly and diffusely positive for CK20 and CDX2 (Fig. 8.19a), patchy positive for chromogranin and synaptophysin (Fig. 8.19b), and negative for CK7. Immunostain for Ki-67 showed a labeling index of >50% in many areas (Fig. 8.19c).

Final Diagnosis

Goblet cell adenocarcinoma, high-grade (grade 3), with intraperitoneal metastasis.

Take-Home Messages

- GCA seldom forms a discrete mass. It has a high tendency to spread by peritoneal carcinomatosis and to metastasize to ovaries in female patients.
- It is graded by the proportion of tumor cells that show low-grade and high-grade growth patterns (Table 8.5). This case showed several intermixed high-grade features such as irregular clusters and sheets of goblet- or signet-ring-like cells, complex glandular structures, and prominent nuclear atypia. Collectively, these high-grade components accounted for >80% of the tumor volume.
- The distinction between high-grade GCA and poorly differentiated adenocarcinoma (such as signet-ring cell carcinoma) relies on the presence (at least focal) or absence of low-grade GCA component in the tumor. In this example, focal low-grade GCA component was present, characterized by a clustered architecture and low-grade cytology (Fig. 8.18c).
- GCA cells variably express neuroendocrine markers. Ki-67 labeling index can be high in high-grade tumors.

References*:* [49, 60]

Case 3

Learning Objectives

1. To become familiar with the histologic features of the lesion
2. To become familiar with the differential diagnosis of the lesion

Case History

A 73-year-old male presented with rectal bleeding. The patient had a documented history of "adenocarcinoma ex goblet cell carcinoid" of the appendix, status post ileocecectomy 2 years ago. Histopathologic examination of the resection specimen at that time showed tumor cells invading through the visceral peritoneum of the appendix (pT4a), extending into the adjacent terminal ileum and cecum, and metastasizing to nine of nine lymph nodes (pN2). The appendectomy margin was negative for tumor involvement. Postoperatively, the patient received multiple cycles of adjuvant chemotherapy, which was complicated by sigmoid

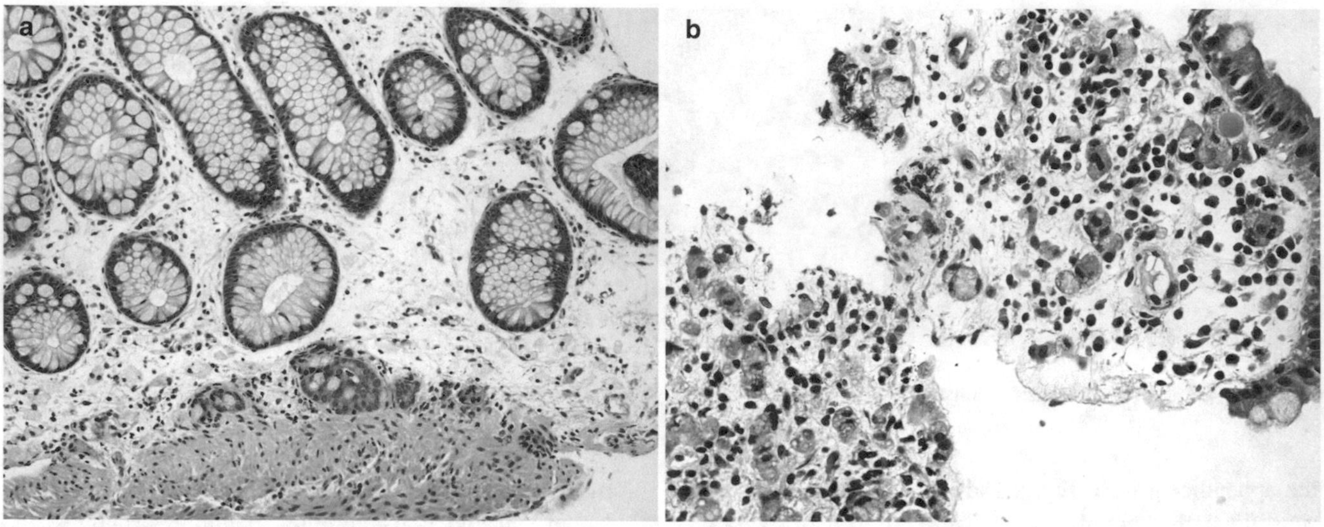

Fig. 8.20 (Case 3). The rectal biopsy showed a few small clusters of (**a**) or individual (**b**) neoplastic cells involving the lamina propria. Intracytoplasmic mucin was noted in some tumor cells

stricture. Sigmoidoscopy at this time identified an indwelling colonic stent embedded into the rectal wall, where mucosal friability was noted. The area with the stent was biopsied.

Histologic Findings

The biopsy consisted of multiple 0.1–0.4-cm pieces of rectal mucosa, a few of which showed small clusters of or individual neoplastic cells involving the lamina propria. Some of the neoplastic cells have intracytoplasmic mucin (Fig. 8.20a, b). No adenomatous change was seen in colonic epithelium.

Differential Diagnosis

- Signet-ring cell carcinoma of rectal primary
- Goblet cell adenocarcinoma of rectal primary
- Metastatic goblet cell adenocarcinoma of appendiceal origin

IHC and Other Ancillary Studies

None.

Final Diagnosis

Metastatic goblet cell adenocarcinoma of appendiceal origin.

Take-Home Messages

- True extraappendiceal GCAs are exceedingly rare. An appendiceal origin must be ruled out before an extraappendiceal primary is considered.

References*:* [49, 53]

Case 4

Learning Objectives

1. To become familiar with the histologic features of the lesion
2. To become familiar with the differential diagnosis of the lesion

Case History

A 70-year-old female presented with abdominal pain in the right lower quadrant. CT showed a fluid-filled dilated appendix with mild hyperemia, suspicious for early appendicitis. The patient underwent laparoscopic appendectomy.

Gross Findings

The appendix measured 7 cm in length and 0.7 cm in diameter. No peroration or discrete lesion was identified.

Histologic Findings

The entire appendix was submitted for histologic examination, which showed distorted serrated crypts with prominent basal dilatation that circumferentially involved the appendiceal mucosa (Fig. 8.21a). The appendectomy margin was not involved, however. There were several demarcated foci where the crypts assumed a villous architecture. Nuclear enlargement, stratification, and pleomorphism; partial mucin depletion; and lack of surface maturation were noted in these foci (Fig. 8.21b–d). Areas showing hyepermucinous changes were also noted, characterized by prominent villiform architecture lined by tall columnar epithelial cells with abundant cytoplasmic mucin and small, basally located nuclei with minimal nuclear atypia (Fig. 8.21e, f). Goblet cells were markedly reduced in number in these areas.

Differential Diagnosis

- Low-grade appendiceal mucinous neoplasm
- High-grade appendiceal mucinous neoplasm
- Appendiceal sessile serrated lesion with cytologic dysplasia
- Appendiceal villous or tubulovillous adenoma

IHC and Other Ancillary Studies

None.

Final Diagnosis

Appendiceal sessile serrated lesion with cytologic dysplasia.

Take-Home Messages

- Appendiceal serrated lesions resemble their colorectal counterparts histologically but may diffusely and circumferentially involve the appendiceal mucosa.
- Areas showing cytologic dysplasia are usually sharply demarcated from nondysplastic serrated lesions and can be multifocal.
- Different histologic subtypes of dysplasia have been recognized in serrated lesions. The most common is intestinal or adenomatous dysplasia, which resembles that seen in conventional adenomas of the colorectum. Serrated dysplasia maintains the serrated appearance but exhibits nuclear atypia, increased mitotic activity, and cytoplasmic mucin reduction. Serrated dysplasia may also show cytoplasmic eosinophilia, reminiscent of traditional serrated adenoma. Hypermucinous (or mucinous) dysplasia usually shows little cytologic atypia. More than one subtype can be present in a single lesion, as seen in this case.
- Serrated lesions with dysplasia are distinguished from LAMN by having preserved lamina propria and muscularis mucosae, including the presence of lymphoid follicles.
- No further therapy is needed for serrated lesions with or without cytologic dysplasia if no invasive adenocarcinoma is identified and the appendectomy margin is not involved. There is no risk for disseminated disease.

References*:* [48, 68, 76]

Case 5

Learning Objectives

1. To become familiar with the histologic features of the lesion
2. To become familiar with the differential diagnosis of the lesion
3. To become familiar with the staging system for the lesion

Case History

A 74-year-old male presented with increasing abdominal pain and waist size during the past 5 months. Imaging studies showed a large cystic lesion in the right lower abdomen extending into the pelvis and up toward the liver. He underwent exploratory laparotomy with excision of a 10-cm right pelvic mucinous lesion, omentectomy, splenectomy, cholecystectomy, right hemicolectomy, partial resection of the diaphragm, and abdominal/pelvic peritonectomies. Intraoperative frozen sections were performed on omental and right pelvic cyst biopsies.

Gross Findings

In the right hemicolectomy specimen, a ruptured and dilated appendix was identified, which had a diameter of 1.5 cm. No mass lesion was identified in this specimen. The mesentery and the serosal surface of the bowel were studded with numerous nodules ranging from 0.1 to 0.5 cm. The cut surface of the right pelvic lesion showed numerous cystic spaces with mucin.

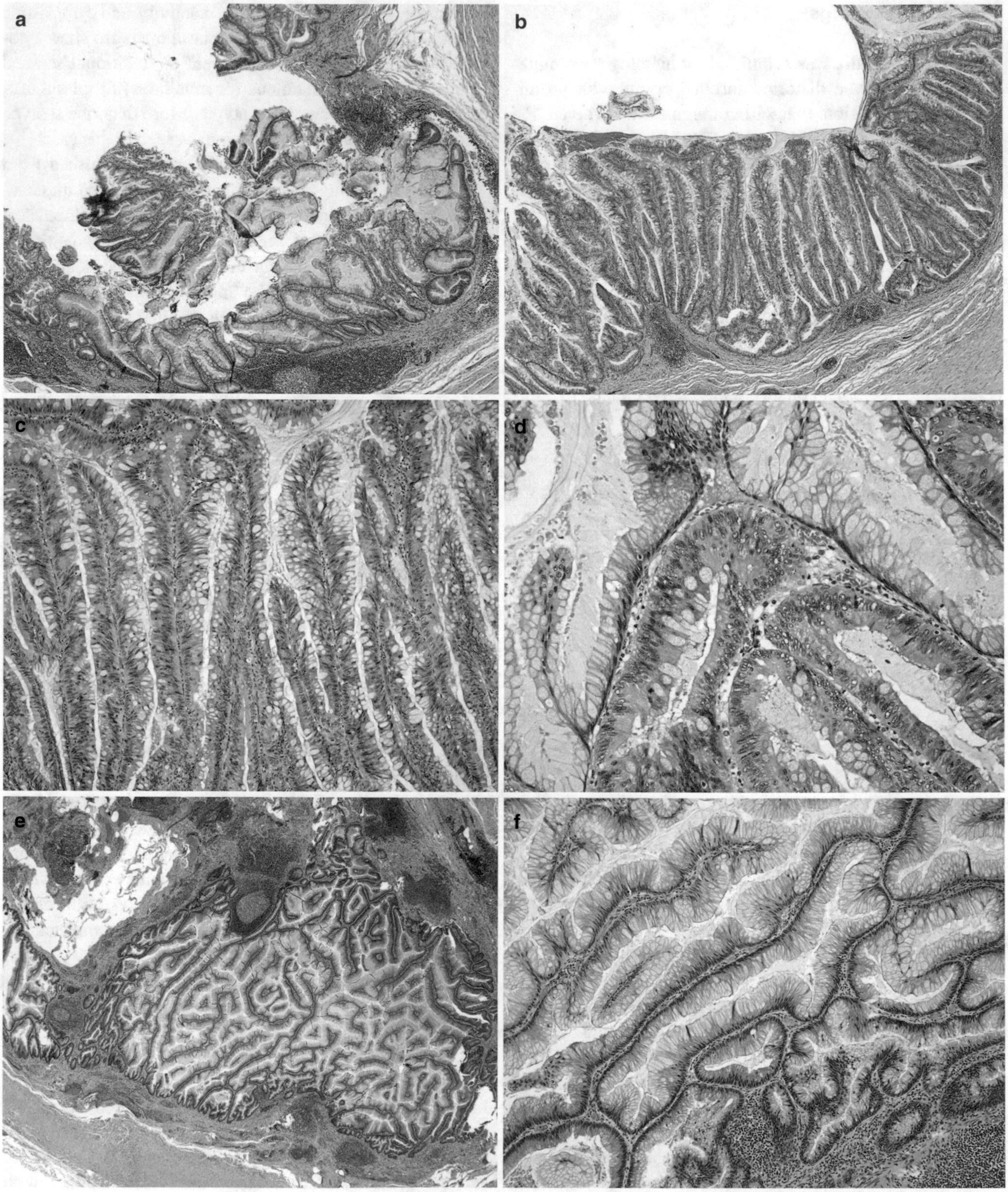

Fig. 8.21 (Case 4). (**a**) A cross section of the appendix showing distorted serrated crypts diffusely involving the mucosa. The lamina propria, muscularis mucosae, and lymphoid follicles were preserved. (**b**) In this area, the crypts showed a villous architecture, but basal dilatation was maintained in some of the crypts. (**c**) The epithelial cells in this area showed nuclear enlargement and stratification and lacked surface maturation. (**d**) These crypts were easily separated from adjacent crypts. (**e**) A different area showed hypermucinous changes with a villiform architecture. Note the presence of lymphoid follicles. (**f**) The epithelial cells with hypermucinous changes were tall columnar with abundant cytoplasmic mucin and small, basally located nuclei. There was minimal, if any, nuclear atypia

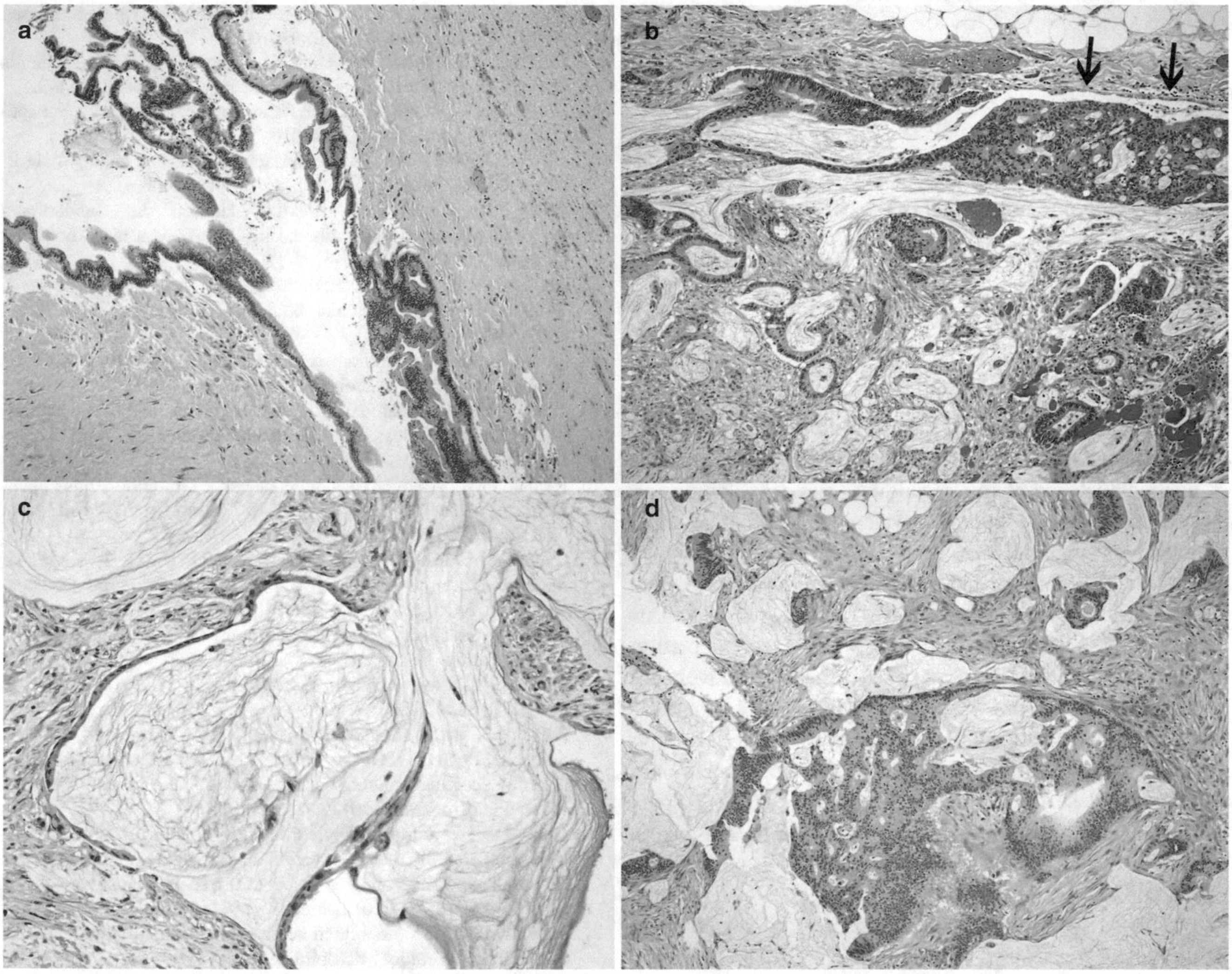

Fig. 8.22 (Case 5). (**a**) A section of the appendix showing a single layer of undulating mucinous epithelium sitting on fibrotic submucosa. Only mild cytologic atypia was noted. (**b**) A section including the appendiceal serosa and mesoappendix showed the presence of mucinous epithelial cells on the serosal surface. Note the partial preservation of mesothelial lining (arrows). Tumor cells formed glandular structures with focal cribriforming. (**c**, **d**) Representative sections of the right pelvic cystic lesion showed mucinous neoplasm with simple and complex structures. Desmoplasia was evident

Histologic Findings

Histologic examination of the appendix showed a single layer of undulating mucinous epithelium sitting on fibrotic submucosa, which exhibited features of low-grade cytologic atypia (Fig. 8.22a). Mucinous epithelial cells extended to the serosal surface of the appendix, where they formed glandular structures, some with a complex architecture (Fig. 8.22b). Tumor cells with histologic features similar to those seen on the appendiceal surface were also present on the serosal surface of the bowel and in the right pelvic cystic lesion, omentum, falciform ligament, gallbladder, porta hepatis, spleen, diaphragm, and peritoneum (Fig. 8.22c, d). Desmoplasia was evident. Signet-ring cells were not identified. Nineteen lymph nodes were retrieved from the right hemicolectomy specimen, which were all negative for metastasis.

Differential Diagnosis

- Appendiceal adenoma with high-grade dysplasia
- Low-grade appendiceal mucinous neoplasm with high-grade mucinous carcinoma peritonei
- High-grade appendiceal mucinous neoplasm with high-grade mucinous carcinoma peritonei
- Mucinous adenocarcinoma, moderately differentiated

IHC and Other Ancillary Studies

None.

Final Diagnosis

Low-grade appendiceal mucinous neoplasm with high-grade mucinous carcinoma peritonei (pT4a, pN0, pM1b).

Take-Home Messages

- LAMN and HAMN are distinguished from mucinous adenocarcinoma by showing "pushing" invasion, instead of infiltrative invasion, of the appendiceal wall. However, the current definition of well-differentiated mucinous adenocarcinoma of the appendix is somewhat confusing because it is essentially equivalent to LAMN and lacks infiltrative-type invasion.
- HAMN also lacks features of infiltrative invasion. A neoplasm with the architecture of LAMN but showing any focus of unequivocal high-grade histology should be diagnosed as HAMN. HAMN may be more likely to harbor invasive carcinoma when the entire appendix is histologically examined.
- LAMNs that show cellular or acellular mucin dissecting through the muscularis propria into the subserosa or onto the serosal surface are staged as pT3 or pT4a, respectively. Lesions limited to the submucosa or muscularis propria are all considered Tis, and thus pT1 and pT2 are not applicable to LAMNs.
- For LAMNs, high-grade features may be observed in peritoneal metastasis, as seen in this case. The grades of appendiceal primary and peritoneal disease should be separately reported for those cases because the higher grade of the peritoneal metastasis is likely to have a more significant impact on prognosis.

  References*:* [48, 68, 72]

References

1. Carr NJ. The pathology of acute appendicitis. Ann Diagn Pathol. 2000;4(1):46–58.
2. Herd ME, Cross PA, Dutt S. Histological audit of acute appendicitis. J Clin Pathol. 1992;45(5):456–8.
3. Ahmed MJ. Incidental acute focal appendicitis in incidentally removed vermiform appendices. W V Med J. 1966;62(6):151–4.
4. Warren S. The etiology of acute appendicitis. Am J Pathol. 1925;1(2):241–6.
5. Hiraiwa H, Umemoto M, Take H. Prevalence of appendectomy in Japanese families. Acta Paediatr Jpn. 1995;37(6):691–3.
6. Ergul E. Heredity and familial tendency of acute appendicitis. Scand J Surg. 2007;96(4):290–2.
7. Bhangu A, Søreide K, Di Saverio S, Assarsson JH, Drake FT. Acute appendicitis: modern understanding of pathogenesis, diagnosis, and management. Lancet. 2015;386(10000):1278–87.
8. Wei PL, Chen CS, Keller JJ, Lin HC. Monthly variation in acute appendicitis incidence: a 10-year nationwide population-based study. J Surg Res. 2012;178(2):670–6.
9. Fink AS, Kosakowski CA, Hiatt JR, Cochran AJ. Periappendicitis is a significant clinical finding. Am J Surg. 1990;159(6):564–8.
10. Chaudhary P, Nabi I, Arora MP. Periappendicitis: our 13 year experience. Int J Surg. 2014;12(9):1010–3.
11. Mårdh PA, Wølner-Hanssen P. Periappendicitis and chlamydial salpingitis. Surg Gynecol Obstet. 1985;160(4):304–6.
12. Bloch AV, Kock KF, Saxtoft Hansen L, Sandermann J. Periappendicitis and diagnostic consequences. Ann Chir Gynaecol. 1988;77(4):151–4.
13. Mukherjee A, Schlenker E, LaMasters T, Johnson M, Brunz J, Thomas E. Periappendicitis: is it a clinical entity? Am Surg. 2002;68(10):913–6.
14. AbdullGaffar B. Granulomatous diseases and granulomas of the appendix. Int J Surg Pathol. 2010;18(1):14–20.
15. Dudley TH Jr, Dean PJ. Idiopathic granulomatous appendicitis, or Crohn's disease of the appendix revisited. Hum Pathol. 1993;24(6):595–601.
16. Richards ML, Aberger FJ, Landercasper J. Granulomatous appendicitis: Crohn's disease, atypical Crohn's or not Crohn's at all? J Am Coll Surg. 1997;185(1):13–7.
17. Oliak D, Yamini D, Udani VM, Lewis RJ, Arnell T, Vargas H, Stamos MJ. Initial nonoperative management for periappendiceal abscess. Dis Colon Rectum. 2001;44(7):936–41.
18. Guo G, Greenson JK. Histopathology of interval (delayed) appendectomy specimens: strong association with granulomatous and xanthogranulomatous appendicitis. Am J Surg Pathol. 2003;27(8):1147–51.
19. Akbulut S, Tas M, Sogutcu N, Arikanoglu Z, Basbug M, Ulku A, Semur H, Yagmur Y. Unusual histopathological findings in appendectomy specimens: a retrospective analysis and literature review. World J Gastroenterol. 2011;17(15):1961–70.
20. Cruz DB, Friedrisch BK, Fontanive Junior V, da Rocha VW. Eosinophilic acute appendicitis caused by Strongyloides stercoralis and Enterobius vermicularis in an HIV-positive patient. BMJ Case Rep. 2012;2012.
21. Aravindan KP. Eosinophils in acute appendicitis: possible significance. Indian J Pathol Microbiol. 1997;40(4):491–8.
22. Aravindan KP, Vijayaraghavan D, Manipadam MT. Acute eosinophilic appendicitis and the significance of eosinophil - edema lesion. Indian J Pathol Microbiol. 2010;53(2):258–61.
23. Ciani S, Chuaqui B. Histological features of resolving acute, non-complicated phlegmonous appendicitis. Pathol Res Pract. 2000;196(2):89–93.
24. Yildirim S, Nursal TZ, Tarim A, Kayaselcuk F, Noyan T. A rare cause of acute appendicitis: parasitic infection. Scand J Infect Dis. 2005;37(10):757–9.
25. Yabanoğlu H, Aytaç HÖ, Türk E, Karagülle E, Calışkan K, Belli S, Kayaselçuk F, Tarım MA. Parasitic infections of the appendix as a cause of appendectomy in adult patients. Turkiye Parazitol Derg. 2014;38(1):12–6.
26. Aydin O. Incidental parasitic infestations in surgically removed appendices: a retrospective analysis. Diagn Pathol. 2007;2:16.
27. da Silva DF, da Silva RJ, da Silva MG, Sartorelli AC, Rodrigues MA. Parasitic infection of the appendix as a cause of acute appendicitis. Parasitol Res. 2007;102(1):99–102.
28. Cerva L, Schrottenbaum M, Kliment V. Intestinal parasites: a study of human appendices. Folia Parasitol (Praha). 1991;38(1):5–9.
29. Kanoksil W, Larbcharoensub N, Soontrapa P, Phongkitkarun S, Sriphojanart S, Nitiyanant P. Eosinophilic appendicitis caused by Schistosoma japonicum: a case report and review of the literature. Southeast Asian J Trop Med Public Health. 2010;41(5):1065–70.
30. Altieri ML, Piozzi GN, Salvatori P, Mirra M, Piccolo G, Olivari N. Appendiceal diverticulitis, a rare relevant pathology: presenta-

tion of a case report and review of the literature. Int J Surg Case Rep. 2017;33:31–4.
31. Sohn TJ, Chang YS, Kang JH, Kim DH, Lee TS, Han JK, Kim SH, Hong YO. Clinical characteristics of acute appendiceal diverticulitis. J Korean Surg Soc. 2013;84(1):33–7.
32. Dupre MP, Jadavji I, Matshes E, Urbanski SJ. Diverticular disease of the vermiform appendix: a diagnostic clue to underlying appendiceal neoplasm. Hum Pathol. 2008;39(12):1823–6.
33. Yardimci AH, Bektas CT, Pasaoglu E, Kinaci E, Ozer C, Sevinc MM, Mahmutoglu AS, Kilickesmez O. Retrospective study of 24 cases of acute appendiceal diverticulitis: CT findings and pathological correlations. Jpn J Radiol. 2017;35(5):225–32.
34. Abdullgaffar B. Diverticulosis and diverticulitis of the appendix. Int J Surg Pathol. 2009;17(3):231–7.
35. Yamana I, Kawamoto S, Inada K, Nagao S, Yoshida T, Yamashita Y. Clinical characteristics of 12 cases of appendiceal diverticulitis: a comparison with 378 cases of acute appendicitis. Surg Today. 2012;42(4):363–7.
36. Phillips BJ, Perry CW. Appendiceal diverticulitis. Mayo Clin Proc. 1999;74(9):890–2.
37. Alexandraki KI, Kaltsas GA, Grozinsky-Glasberg S, Chatzellis E, Grossman AB. Appendiceal neuroendocrine neoplasms: diagnosis and management. Endocr Relat Cancer. 2016;23(1):R27–41.
38. Moris D, Tsilimigras DI, Vagios S, Ntanasis-Stathopoulos I, Karachaliou GS, Papalampros A, Alexandrou A, Blazer DG. 3RD, Felekouras E. neuroendocrine neoplasms of the appendix: a review of the literature. Anticancer Res. 2018;38(2):601–11.
39. Yachida S, Vakiani E, White CM, Zhong Y, Saunders T, Morgan R, de Wilde RF, Maitra A, Hicks J, Demarzo AM, Shi C, Sharma R, Laheru D, Edil BH, Wolfgang CL, Schulick RD, Hruban RH, Tang LH, Klimstra DS, Iacobuzio-Donahue CA. Small cell and large cell neuroendocrine carcinomas of the pancreas are genetically similar and distinct from well-differentiated pancreatic neuroendocrine tumors. Am J Surg Pathol. 2012;36(2):173–84.
40. Sorbye H, Strosberg J, Baudin E, Klimstra DS, Yao JC. Gastroenteropancreatic high-grade neuroendocrine carcinoma. Cancer. 2014;120(18):2814–23.
41. Emre A, Akbulut S, Bozdag Z, Yilmaz M, Kanlioz M, Emre R, Sahin N. Routine histopathologic examination of appendectomy specimens: retrospective analysis of 1255 patients. Int Surg. 2013;98(4):354–62.
42. Matsukuma KE, Montgomery EA. Tubular carcinoids of the appendix: the CK7/CK20 immunophenotype can be a diagnostic pitfall. J Clin Pathol. 2012;65(7):666–8.
43. Burke AP, Sobin LH, Federspiel BH, Shekitka KM. Appendiceal carcinoids: correlation of histology and immunohistochemistry. Mod Pathol. 1989;2(6):630–7.
44. Burke AP, Sobin LH, Federspiel BH, Shekitka KM, Helwig EB. Goblet cell carcinoids and related tumors of the vermiform appendix. Am J Clin Pathol. 1990;94(1):27–35.
45. Carr NJ, Sobin LH. Neuroendocrine tumors of the appendix. Semin Diagn Pathol. 2004;21(2):108–19.
46. Shaw PA, Pringle JH. The demonstration of a subset of carcinoid tumours of the appendix by in situ hybridization using synthetic probes to proglucagon mRNA. J Pathol. 1992;167(4):375–80.
47. WHO Classification of Tumours Editorial Board. Digestive system tumours. 5th ed. Lyon: IARC; 2019. p. 136.
48. Carr NJ, Cecil TD, Mohamed F, Sobin LH, Sugarbaker PH, González-Moreno S, Taflampas P, Chapman S, Moran BJ, Peritoneal Surface Oncology Group International. A consensus for classification and pathologic reporting of pseudomyxoma peritonei and associated appendiceal neoplasia: the results of the Peritoneal Surface Oncology Group International (PSOGI) Modified Delphi Process. Am J Surg Pathol. 2016;40(1):14–26.
49. Zhang K, Meyerson C, Kassardjian A, Westbrook LM, Zheng W, Wang HL. Goblet cell carcinoid/carcinoma: an update. Adv Anat Pathol. 2019;26(2):75–83.
50. Roy P, Chetty R. Goblet cell carcinoid tumors of the appendix: an overview. World J Gastrointest Oncol. 2010;2(6):251–8.
51. Lambert LA. Goblet cell carcinoid. National Organization for Rare Disorders (NORD). Available from https://rarediseases.org/rare-diseases/goblet-cell-carcinoid/. Accessed 29 Nov 2019.
52. Pape UF, Perren A, Niederle B, Gross D, Gress T, Costa F, Arnold R, Denecke T, Plöckinger U, Salazar R, Grossman A, Barcelona Consensus Conference Participants. ENETS consensus guidelines for the management of patients with neuroendocrine neoplasms from the jejuno-ileum and the appendix including goblet cell carcinomas. Neuroendocrinology. 2012;95(2):135–56.
53. Gui X, Qin L, Gao ZH, Falck V, Harpaz N. Goblet cell carcinoids at extraappendiceal locations of gastrointestinal tract: an underrecognized diagnostic pitfall. J Surg Oncol. 2011;103(8):790–5.
54. McGory ML, Maggard MA, Kang H, O'Connell JB, Ko CY. Malignancies of the appendix: beyond case series reports. Dis Colon Rectum. 2005;48(12):2264–71.
55. Wang HL, Dhall D. Goblet or signet ring cells: that is the question. Adv Anat Pathol. 2009;16(4):247–54.
56. O'Donnell ME, Carson J, Garstin WI. Surgical treatment of malignant carcinoid tumours of the appendix. Int J Clin Pract. 2007;61(3):431–7.
57. Pham TH, Wolff B, Abraham SC, Drelichman E. Surgical and chemotherapy treatment outcomes of goblet cell carcinoid: a tertiary cancer center experience. Ann Surg Oncol. 2006;13(3):370–6.
58. Varisco B, McAlvin B, Dias J, Franga D. Adenocarcinoid of the appendix: is right hemicolectomy necessary? A meta-analysis of retrospective chart reviews. Am Surg. 2004;70(7):593–9.
59. Tang LH, Shia J, Soslow RA, Dhall D, Wong WD, O'Reilly E, Qin J, Paty P, Weiser MR, Guillem J, Temple L, Sobin LH, Klimstra DS. Pathologic classification and clinical behavior of the spectrum of goblet cell carcinoid tumors of the appendix. Am J Surg Pathol. 2008;32(10):1429–43.
60. Yozu M, Johncilla ME, Srivastava A, Ryan DP, Cusack JC, Doyle L, Setia N, Yang M, Lauwers GY, Odze RD, Misdraji J. Histologic and outcome study supports reclassifying appendiceal goblet cell carcinoids as goblet cell adenocarcinomas, and grading and staging similarly to colonic adenocarcinomas. Am J Surg Pathol. 2018;42(7):898–910.
61. Liu E, Telem DA, Warner RR, Dikman A, Divino CM. The role of Ki-67 in predicting biological behavior of goblet cell carcinoid tumor in appendix. Am J Surg. 2011;202(4):400–3.
62. Stancu M, Wu TT, Wallace C, Houlihan PS, Hamilton SR, Rashid A. Genetic alterations in goblet cell carcinoids of the vermiform appendix and comparison with gastrointestinal carcinoid tumors. Mod Pathol. 2003;16(12):1189–98.
63. Zhang Y, Zulfiqar M, Bluth MH, Bhalla A, Beydoun R. Molecular diagnostics in the neoplasms of small intestine and appendix: 2018 update. Clin Lab Med. 2018;38(2):343–55.
64. Dimmler A, Geddert H, Faller G. EGFR, KRAS, BRAF-mutations and microsatellite instability are absent in goblet cell carcinoids of the appendix. Pathol Res Pract. 2014;210(5):274–8.
65. Kidd M, Modlin IM, Mane SM, Camp RL, Eick G, Latich I. The role of genetic markers-NAP1L1, MAGE-D2, and MTA1-in defining small-intestinal carcinoid neoplasia. Ann Surg Oncol. 2006;13(2):253–62.
66. Modlin IM, Kidd M, Latich I, Zikusoka MN, Eick GN, Mane SM, Camp RL. Genetic differentiation of appendiceal tumor malignancy: a guide for the perplexed. Ann Surg. 2006;244(1):52–60.
67. Jesinghaus M, Konukiewitz B, Foersch S, Stenzinger A, Steiger K, Muckenhuber A, Groß C, Mollenhauer M, Roth W, Detlefsen S, Weichert W, Klöppel G, Pfarr N, Schlitter AM. Appendiceal goblet cell carcinoids and adenocarcinomas ex-goblet cell carcinoid are genetically distinct from primary colorectal-type adenocarcinoma of the appendix. Mod Pathol. 2018;31(5):829–39.

68. Valasek MA, Pai RK. An update on the diagnosis, grading, and staging of appendiceal mucinous neoplasms. Adv Anat Pathol. 2018;25(1):38–60.
69. Yantiss RK, Shia J, Klimstra DS, Hahn HP, Odze RD, Misdraji J. Prognostic significance of localized extra-appendiceal mucin deposition in appendiceal mucinous neoplasms. Am J Surg Pathol. 2009;33(2):248–55.
70. Pai RK, Beck AH, Norton JA, Longacre TA. Appendiceal mucinous neoplasms: clinicopathologic study of 116 cases with analysis of factors predicting recurrence. Am J Surg Pathol. 2009;33(10):1425–39.
71. Misdraji J, Yantiss RK, Graeme-Cook FM, Balis UJ, Young RH. Appendiceal mucinous neoplasms: a clinicopathologic analysis of 107 cases. Am J Surg Pathol. 2003;27(8):1089–103.
72. Amin MB, Greene FL, Edge SB, Compton CC, Gershenwald JE, Brookland RK, Meyer L, Gress DM, Byrd DR, Winchester DP. The eighth edition AJCC cancer staging manual: continuing to build a bridge from a population-based to a more "personalized" approach to cancer staging. CA Cancer J Clin. 2017;67(2):93–9.
73. Rosenberger LH, Stein LH, Witkiewicz AK, Kennedy EP, Yeo CJ. Intraductal papillary mucinous neoplasm (IPMN) with extra-pancreatic mucin: a case series and review of the literature. J Gastrointest Surg. 2012;16(4):762–70.
74. McKenney JK, Soslow RA, Longacre TA. Ovarian mature teratomas with mucinous epithelial neoplasms: morphologic heterogeneity and association with pseudomyxoma peritonei. Am J Surg Pathol. 2008;32(5):645–55.
75. Carr NJ, Bibeau F, Bradley RF, Dartigues P, Feakins RM, Geisinger KR, Gui X, Isaac S, Milione M, Misdraji J, Pai RK, Rodriguez-Justo M, Sobin LH, van Velthuysen MF, Yantiss RK. The histopathological classification, diagnosis and differential diagnosis of mucinous appendiceal neoplasms, appendiceal adenocarcinomas and pseudomyxoma peritonei. Histopathology. 2017;71(6):847–58.
76. Rubio CA. Serrated adenomas of the appendix. J Clin Pathol. 2004;57(9):946–9.
77. Wang HL, Kim CJ, Koo J, Zhou W, Choi EK, Arcega R, Chen ZE, Wang H, Zhang L, Lin F. Practical immunohistochemistry in neoplastic pathology of the gastrointestinal tract, liver, biliary tract, and pancreas. Arch Pathol Lab Med. 2017;141(9):1155–80.
78. Schmoeckel E, Kirchner T, Mayr D. SATB2 is a supportive marker for the differentiation of a primary mucinous tumor of the ovary and an ovarian metastasis of a low-grade appendiceal mucinous neoplasm (LAMN): a series of seven cases. Pathol Res Pract. 2018;214(3):426–30.
79. Asare EA, Compton CC, Hanna NN, Kosinski LA, Washington MK, Kakar S, Weiser MR, Overman MJ. The impact of stage, grade, and mucinous histology on the efficacy of systemic chemotherapy in adenocarcinomas of the appendix: analysis of the National Cancer Data Base. Cancer. 2016;122(2):213–21.
80. Symonds DA, Vickery AL. Mucinous carcinoma of the colon and rectum. Cancer. 1976;37(4):1891–900.
81. Verhulst J, Ferdinande L, Demetter P, Ceelen W. Mucinous subtype as prognostic factor in colorectal cancer: a systematic review and meta-analysis. J Clin Pathol. 2012;65(5):381–8.
82. Kabbani W, Houlihan PS, Luthra R, Hamilton SR, Rashid A. Mucinous and nonmucinous appendiceal adenocarcinomas: different clinicopathological features but similar genetic alterations. Mod Pathol. 2002;15(6):599–605.
83. Zauber P, Berman E, Marotta S, Sabbath-Solitare M, Bishop T. Ki-ras gene mutations are invariably present in low-grade mucinous tumors of the vermiform appendix. Scand J Gastroenterol. 2011;46(7–8):869–74.
84. Cerame MA. A 25-year review of adenocarcinoma of the appendix. A frequently perforating carcinoma. Dis Colon Rectum. 1988;31(2):145–50.
85. Singhi AD, Davison JM, Choudry HA, Pingpank JF, Ahrendt SA, Holtzman MP, Zureikat AH, Zeh HJ, Ramalingam L, Mantha G, Nikiforova M, Bartlett DL, Pai RK. GNAS is frequently mutated in both low-grade and high-grade disseminated appendiceal mucinous neoplasms but does not affect survival. Hum Pathol. 2014;45(8):1737–43.
86. Noguchi R, Yano H, Gohda Y, Suda R, Igari T, Ohta Y, Yamashita N, Yamaguchi K, Terakado Y, Ikenoue T, Furukawa Y. Molecular profiles of high-grade and low-grade pseudomyxoma peritonei. Cancer Med. 2015;4(12):1809–16.
87. Davison JM, Choudry HA, Pingpank JF, Ahrendt SA, Holtzman MP, Zureikat AH, Zeh HJ, Ramalingam L, Zhu B, Nikiforova M, Bartlett DL, Pai RK. Clinicopathologic and molecular analysis of disseminated appendiceal mucinous neoplasms: identification of factors predicting survival and proposed criteria for a three-tiered assessment of tumor grade. Mod Pathol. 2014;27(11):1521–39.
88. Overman MJ, Fournier K, Hu CY, Eng C, Taggart M, Royal R, Mansfield P, Chang GJ. Improving the AJCC/TNM staging for adenocarcinomas of the appendix: the prognostic impact of histological grade. Ann Surg. 2013;257(6):1072–8.

Anal Diseases

9

Upasana Joneja and Jinru Shia

List of Frequently Asked Questions

1. What does the term "anus" mean?
2. What are the common benign medical conditions that affect the anus?
3. Does inflammatory bowel disease (IBD) affect the anus, and are there characteristic pathological features?
4. What tumors occur in the anus, and how are they classified?
5. Are there unique features of skin adnexal tumors that involve the perianal skin?
6. How does the american joint committee on cancer (AJCC) define the anus and stage anal tumors?
7. What is Bowen disease?
8. Are there differences between verrucous carcinoma and giant condyloma of Buschke–Lowenstein?
9. What is the difference between "cloacogenic carcinoma" and squamous cell carcinoma?
10. What types of adenocarcinoma occur in the anus?
11. What comes under the differential diagnosis of high-grade or high-grade-appearing cellular neoplasms in the anus?

Frequently Asked Questions

1. What does the term "anus" mean?

- The term "anus" refers to the terminal portion of the large bowel, including its opening at the lower end (Fig. 9.1). It encompasses (1) the anal canal, which can be defined surgically, histologically, or anatomically, and (2) the perianal skin (also known as the anal margin.

References: [1–4]

U. Joneja
Cooper University Hospital, Camden, NJ, USA

J. Shia (✉)
Memorial Sloan Kettering Cancer Center, New York, NY, USA

Surgical Anal Canal

- Superior border: the anorectal ring or the junction of the puborectalis portion of the levator ani muscle with the external anal sphincter.
- Inferior border: the anal verge (where the anal squamous mucosa meets the anal margin skin).
- It corresponds to the segment that is invested by the internal anal sphincter, about 4.0 cm in length; the dentate (pectinate) line is located roughly at the midpoint.

Histologic Anal Canal

- Superior portion is lined by colorectal-type glandular mucosa.
- Anal transition zone (ATZ) is lined by a mucosal epithelium that may exhibit varying appearances, often composed of multiple cell layers (Fig. 9.2a) containing mucin, endocrine cells, and melanocytes. Scattered foci of colorectal crypts or small areas of mature squamous epithelium may also be seen (Fig. 9.2b). In some individuals, this histologic transitional zone may be absent altogether.
- Distal portion is lined by squamous mucosa.
- The "dentate line" corresponds to the ATZ.
- The "anal verge" corresponds to the junction between squamous mucosa (lacks skin adnexa) and anal margin skin (has skin adnexa and is hair bearing).
- Anal glands exist in the wall of the anal canal. Their ducts open into the anal canal. The openings are typically in the ATZ (Fig. 9.3a).
- The anal duct epithelium and the ATZ epithelium share morphological and immunohistochemical characteristics: both tend to be positive for CK7 and negative for CK20 (Fig. 9.3b).
- The various epithelial elements in the anal canal account for the different types of neoplasms occurring in this region.

Reference: [5]

H. L. Wang, Z. E. Chen (eds.), *Practical Gastrointestinal Pathology*, Practical Anatomic Pathology,
https://doi.org/10.1007/978-3-030-51268-2_9

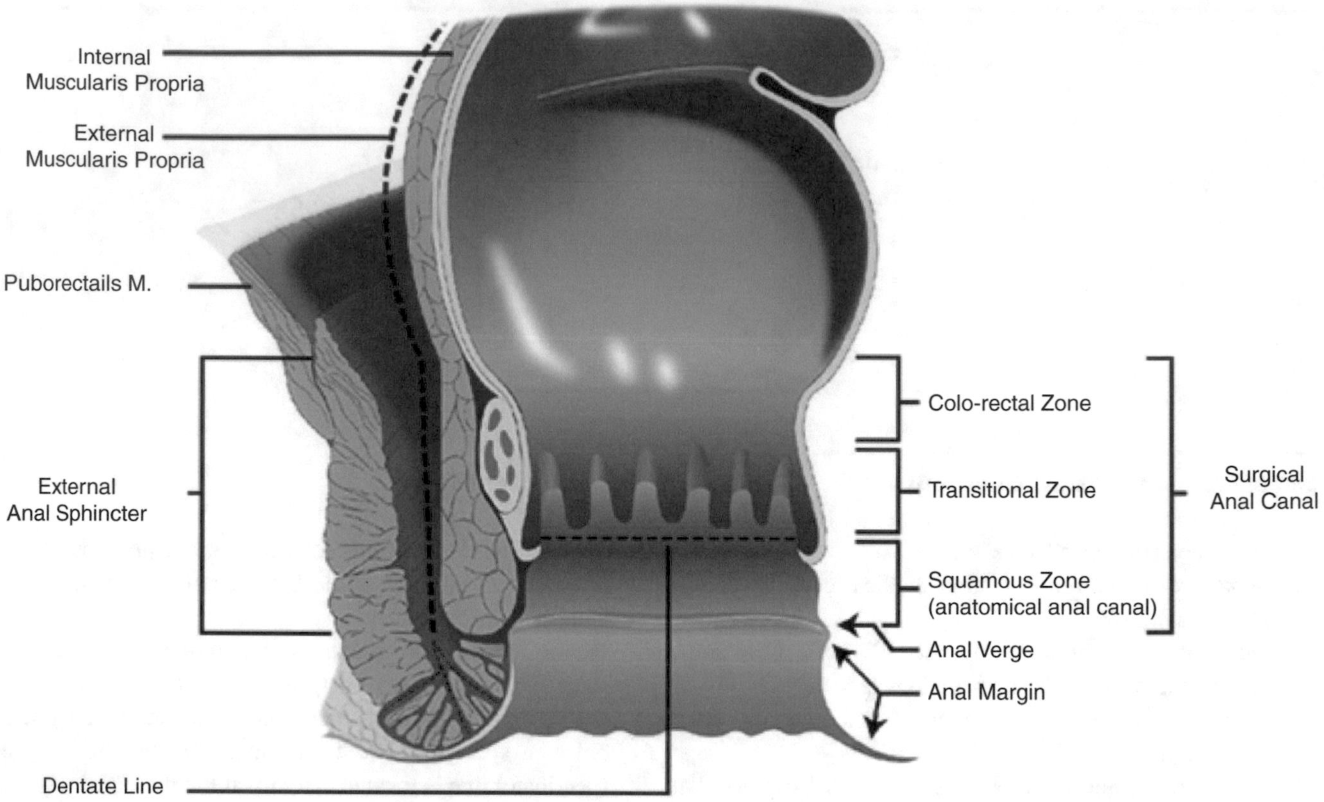

Fig. 9.1 Schematic drawing of the anus (Shia [3])

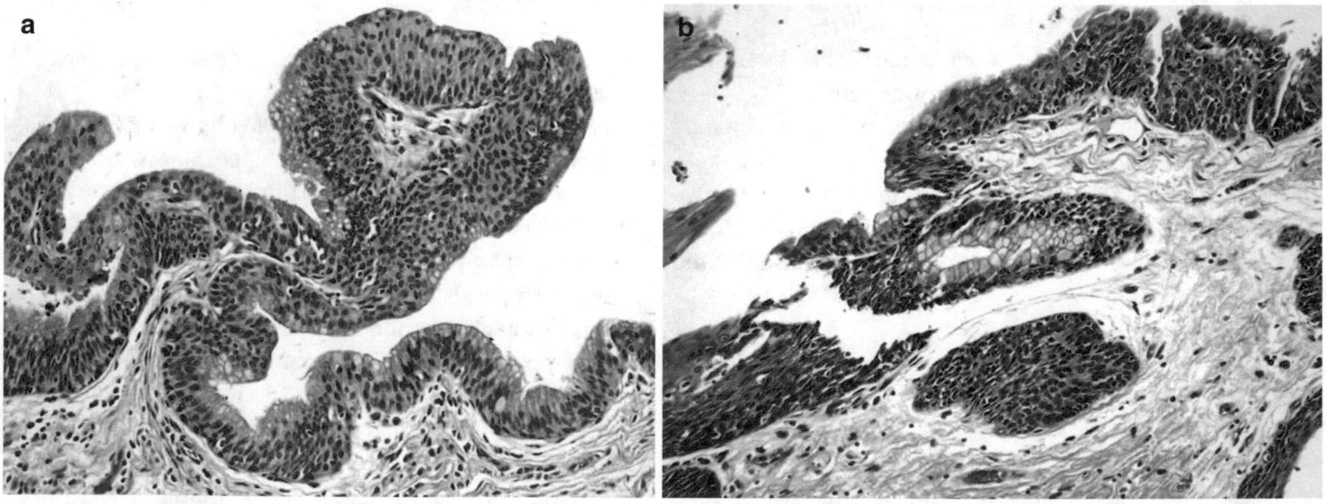

Fig. 9.2 Histologic appearance of the anal transition zone mucosa. Rather frequently, the transition zone mucosa is composed of multiple cell layers with some containing cytoplasmic mucin (**a**). In some cases, scattered rectal crypts are seen intermixed with squamous or transitional-type epithelium (**b**)

Anatomical Anal Canal

- Superior border: dentate line/ATZ
- Inferior border: anal verge (squamous mucocutaneous junction)

Perianal Skin

- Also known as "anal margin," the current AJCC staging manual refers to it as "perianus." It is the skin around the anal verge for a radius of 5 cm. The significance lies in its

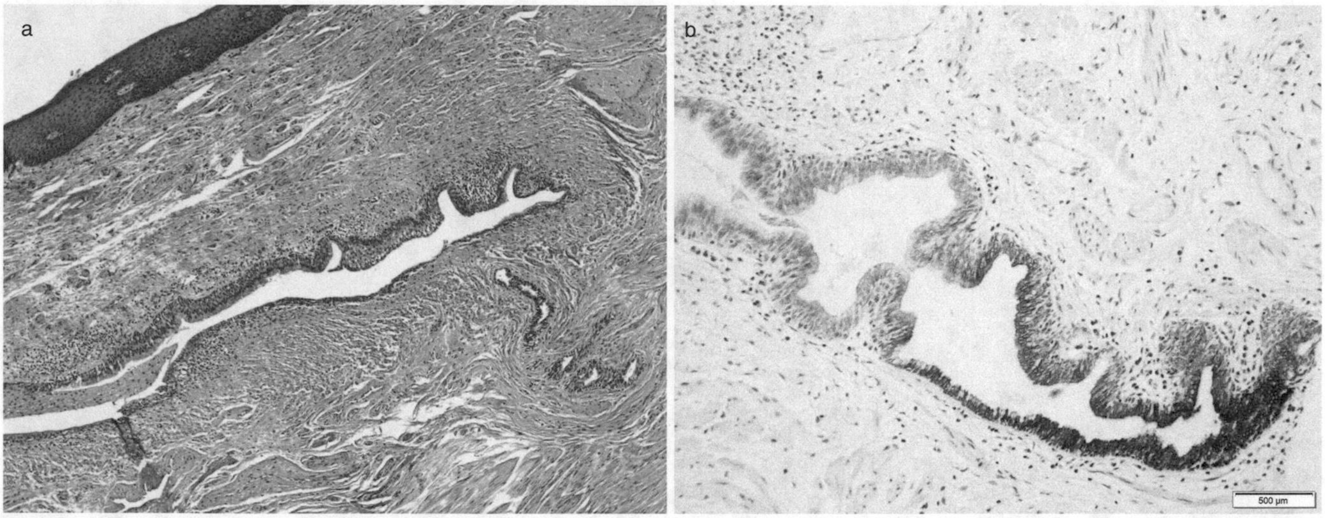

Fig. 9.3 Photomicrograph showing a long profile of an anal duct next to a group of smaller anal glands situated in the wall of the anal canal (**a**). The anal duct epithelial cells show variable degrees of immunoreactivity to CK7 (**b**)

proclivity to surface erosion or injury and consequently susceptibility to human papillomavirus (HPV) infection.

Reference: [6]

2. **What are the common benign medical conditions that affect the anus?**
   - A wide variety of medical conditions can affect the anal region, including but not limited to anal fissure, anal ulcer, anal fistula, "polyps" (including the so-called fibroepithelial polyp/hypertrophied anal papillae and "inflammatory cloacogenic polyp"), "solitary rectal ulcer," hemorrhoids, rectal varices, and the so-called Dieulafoy lesion.

Anal Fistula

- It is often a result of an intersphincteric abscess originating in an anal duct or a complication of other conditions such as inflammatory bowel disease (particularly Crohn disease), tuberculosis, and actinomycosis.
- It typically has an internal opening within the anal canal, usually at the dentate line/ATZ. The fistulous tract may lead to the skin or end blindly in the perianal soft tissue.
- It is important that tissue obtained from an anal fistula be examined microscopically. It may help establish the etiology and is necessary to rule out neoplasia. Cancer risk in Crohn-disease-associated fistula is well established. Such cancers are often mucinous.
- Microscopically, most have a lining that is made of granulation tissue, although epithelium may eventually grow at either end of the tract. The diagnosis of Crohn-disease-associated fistula may be suggested by the presence of non-caseating granulomas, but it is important not to confuse them with foreign-body-type giant cell reaction, sometimes seen in nonspecific fistulas (see also question 3).

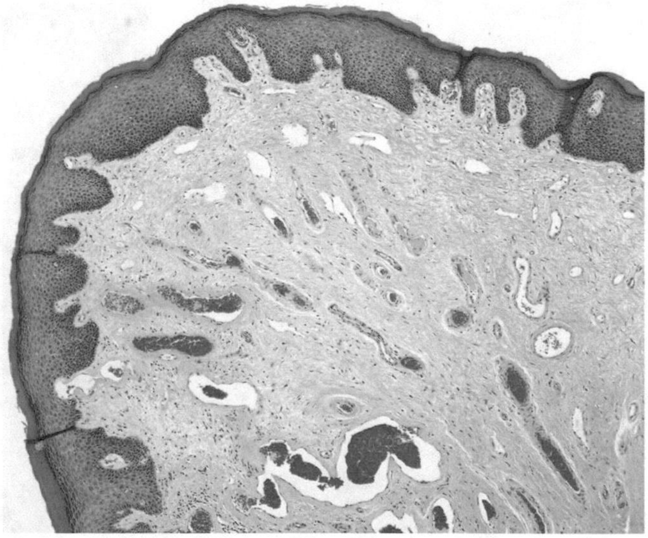

Fig. 9.4 A fibroepithelial polyp composed of polypoid tissue with squamous epithelium encompassing a fibrotic stroma that contains prominent congested vessels. (Image courtesy of Meredith Pittman, MD)

Hypertrophied Papillae

- Synonyms: fibroepithelial polyp, fibrous polyp, "anal tag."
- It is a hyperplastic process secondary to chronic injury.
- Microscopic appearance: polypoid tissue with squamous epithelium encompassing a loose or sometimes fibrotic stroma (Fig. 9.4). Atypical or "bizarre" stromal cells with large and/or multiple nuclei and stellate cytoplasmic outlines may be seen. These cells may be immunoreactive for CD34. Prominent vessels, often hyalinized, are a frequent finding.

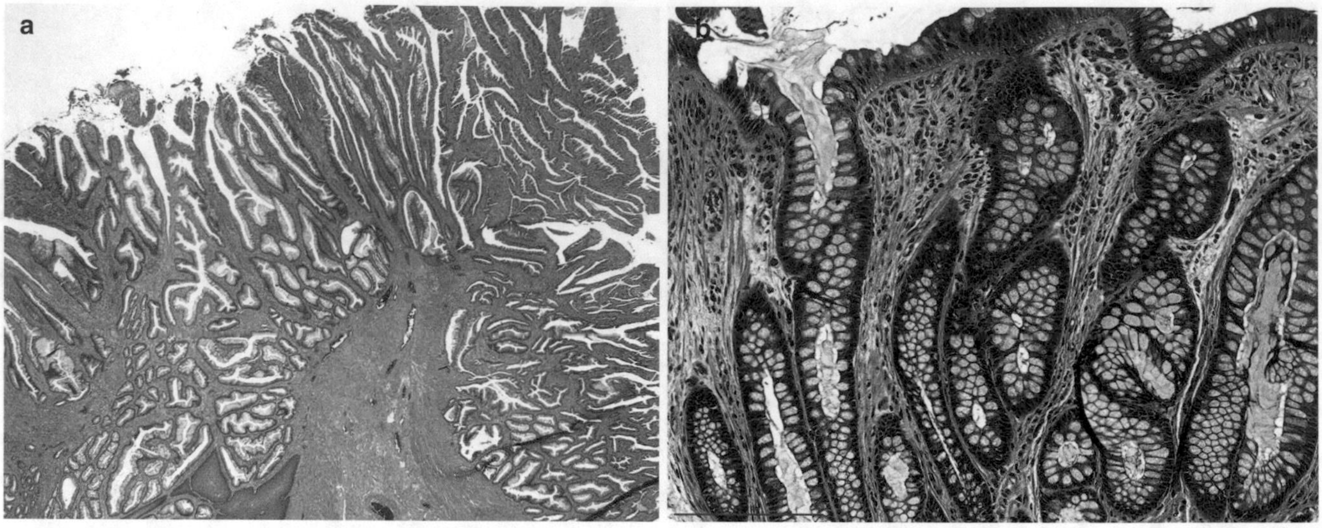

Fig. 9.5 A so-called inflammatory cloacogenic polyp showing a villous architecture at low power view, resembling a villous or tubulovillous adenoma (**a**). High power view demonstrating vertically oriented smooth-muscle fibers coursing in-between elongated and tortuous crypts (**b**)

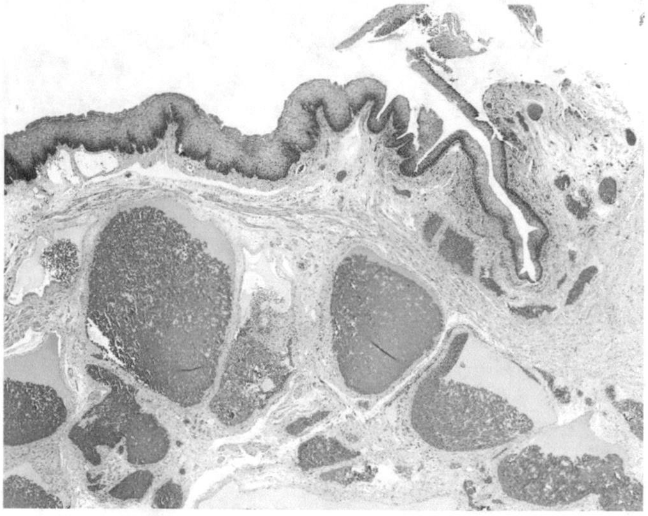

Fig. 9.6 External hemorrhoidal tissue showing ectatic vessels with congestion underneath anal squamous epithelium. (Image courtesy of Meredith Pittman, MD). Organizing thrombus is a common finding

- Some authors prefer to reserve the diagnosis of "hypertrophied anal papillae" for cases in which the stroma is composed of loose fibrovascular tissue and use "anal fibroepithelial polyp" when the stroma shows predominantly fibrous changes.

Inflammatory Cloacogenic Polyp

- It falls under the umbrella of mucosal-prolapse-induced lesions such as colitis cystica profunda, solitary rectal ulcer syndrome, and diverticular disease. It is sometimes related to hemorrhoids and is located in the ATZ.
- Microscopic appearance: (1) hyperplastic mucosa containing ATZ-type and squamous-type epithelia, with surface erosion, stroma edema, vascular ectasia, inflammatory cells, and granulation tissue, and (2) vertically oriented smooth-muscle fibers coursing in-between elongated and tortuous crypts (Fig. 9.5a, b).
- Differential diagnosis may include prolapsed rectal adenoma, hamartomatous polyp, and hyperplastic polyp.

Hemorrhoids, Varices, and Dieulafoy Lesion

- "Internal hemorrhoids" originate above the dentate line and are covered by columnar epithelium.
- "External hemorrhoids" occur below the dentate line and are covered by squamous epithelium (Fig. 9.6).
- Many disease conditions can resemble hemorrhoids clinically: granulomatous disease, tuberculosis, lymphoma, dysplasia/condyloma, carcinoma, melanoma.
- Anorectal varices typically occur in the setting of portal hypertension and can exhibit histologic changes mimicking hemorrhoids, including subepithelial dilated vessels with a thickened wall and associated hemorrhage. Diagnosis of varices is usually made via endoscopic findings and clinical history, not through biopsy, due to the risk of bleeding.
- Dieulafoy lesion, a condition more commonly seen in the stomach, can rarely be a cause of heavy bleeding from the anorectal region. It is characterized by a dilated, aberrant, submucosal artery (~3 mm) that injures the overlying mucosa in the absence of an underlying ulcer, aneurysm, or intrinsic abnormality. As with varices, the diagnosis of Dieulafoy lesion is rarely a pathological one; rather, it is achieved based on endoscopic findings.

References: [7, 8]

3. **Does inflammatory bowel disease (IBD) affect the anus, and are there characteristic pathological features?**
   - IBD can affect the anal canal and perianal skin. The clinical findings are typically nonspecific and may simulate infectious conditions (important examples include syphilis and lymphogranuloma venereum) or neoplastic conditions. As such, increased awareness and careful pathological examination of all tissue samples are important.

   Reference: [9]

Ulcerative Colitis

- The inflammatory changes in the anus are typically nonspecific and often indistinguishable from the appearance in patients without colitis, both clinically and pathologically.

Crohn Disease

- Anal manifestations may include fissures, fistulas, ulcers, strictures, fibroepithelial polyps/skin tags, and hemorrhoids.
- Increased risk of anal squamous and glandular neoplasia is observed. The higher risk may be related to an increased rate of high-risk HPV (mostly HPV16) infection. Anal fistula has been associated with fistula-associated squamous cell carcinoma and adenocarcinoma; the latter is typically of mucinous type. A long-standing fistula with a change of draining contents from purulent to mucinous should particularly raise the suspicion of carcinoma and warrant tissue diagnosis (also see question 10).
- As is the case with ulcerative colitis, pathological findings are nonspecific. But noncaseating granulomas (not associated with infection), when present, favor Crohn disease, especially in a young patient with no other alternative explanation.

References: [10, 11]

Syphilis and Lymphogranuloma Venereum (LGV) Are Among the Differential Diagnoses for Anal IBD

- *Treponema pallidum* is the bacterium responsible for syphilis, and the causative agent for LGV is *Chlamydia trachomatis* serovar L1, L2, or L3. Both are sexually transmitted infectious conditions; HIV+ men who have sex with men are at increased risk of contracting the infections.
- Both can show inflammatory changes in the anus that may raise concern of IBD (Fig. 9.7a). A recent study by Arnold et al. suggests the following histologic features as more supportive of syphilis or LGV than IBD: minimal active chronic crypt-centric damage, lack of mucosal eosinophilia, submucosal plasma cells, endothelial swelling, and perivascular plasma cells.
- Final diagnosis requires close clinical and pathological correlation and testing of pathogenic infectious agents. Immunohistochemistry for *Treponema pallidum* is available and can be helpful (Fig. 9.7b).

References: [9, 12]

4. **What tumors occur in the anus, and how are they classified?**

   See tumors enlisted by the fourth and fifth editions of the World Health Organization (WHO) classification of digestive system tumors (Tables 9.1 and 9.2).
   - Overall, carcinomas of the anus and anal canal account for 2.7% of all gastrointestinal malignancies [13]. In 2018, an estimated 8580 new cases (2960 men and 5620 women) of anal cancers occurred in the United States. About 80% of the carcinomas are squamous cell carcinomas; the rest are adenocarcinomas.
   - Mesenchymal tumors are rare, and it is often difficult to determine their exact point of origin.

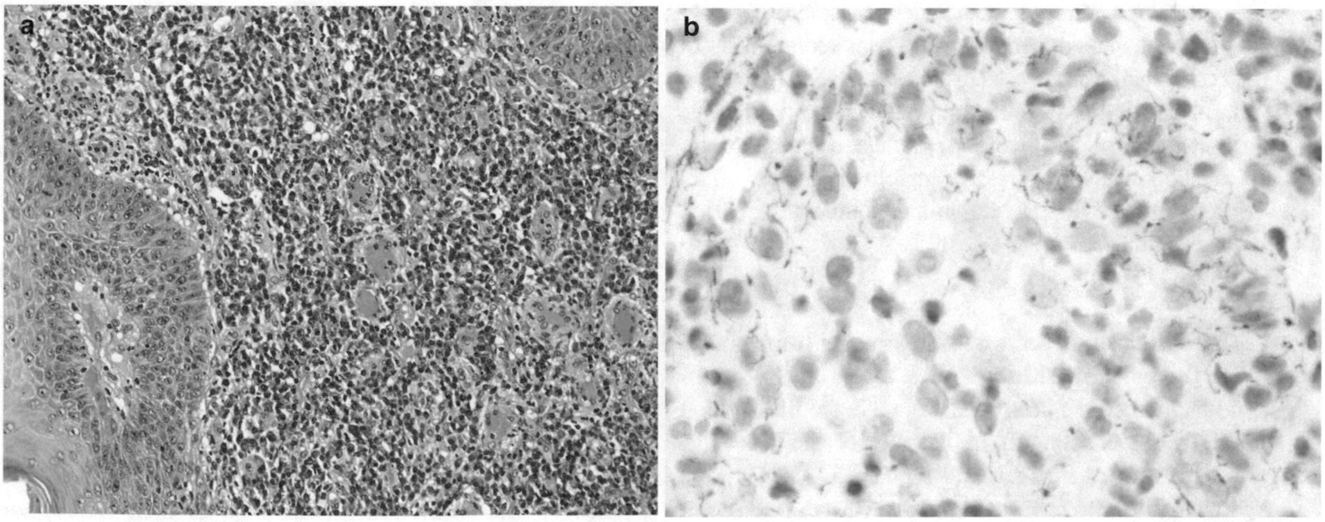

Fig. 9.7 A case of anal syphilis showing dense plasma-cell-rich infiltrates on biopsy (**a**). Surface erosion/superficial ulceration is noted in other areas. Immunostaining for spirochetes demonstrates the presence of numerous organisms (**b**)

Table 9.1 Fourth Edition WHO classification of anal tumors [20]

Epithelial tumors
Premalignant lesions (of anal canal epithelium)
Anal intraepithelial neoplasia (dysplasia), low grade
Anal intraepithelial neoplasia (dysplasia), high grade
Bowen disease
Perianal squamous intraepithelial neoplasia
Paget disease
Carcinoma (of anal canal epithelium)
Squamous cell carcinoma
Verrucous carcinoma
Undifferentiated carcinoma
Adenocarcinoma
Mucinous adenocarcinoma
Neuroendocrine neoplasms (of anal canal epithelium)
Neuroendocrine tumor (NET)
Neuroendocrine carcinoma (NEC), large-cell or small-cell type
Mixed adenoneuroendocrine carcinoma
Mesenchymal tumors
Lymphoma
Secondary tumors

Table 9.2 Fifth edition WHO classification of anal tumors [21]

Benign epithelial tumors and precursors
Squamous intraepithelial neoplasia, low grade
Squamous intraepithelial neoplasia, high grade
Malignant epithelial tumors
Squamous cell carcinoma NOS
Verrucous squamous cell carcinoma
Adenocarcinoma NOS
Neuroendocrine tumor NOS
Neuroendocrine tumor, grade 1
Neuroendocrine tumor, grade 2
Neuroendocrine tumor, grade 3
Neuroendocrine carcinoma NOS
Large cell neuroendocrine carcinoma
Small cell neuroendocrine carcinoma
Mixed neuroendocrine-nonneuroendocrine neoplasm (MiNEN)

- Mesenchymal entities may include hemangioma, lymphangioma, hemangiopericytoma, angiosarcoma, Kaposi sarcoma, malignant fibrous histiocytoma, leiomyoma and leiomyosarcoma, rhabdomyoma and rhabdomyosarcoma, peripheral nerve sheath tumors, granular cell tumor, spindle cell lipoma, and aggressive angiomyxoma.
- Other tumors include lymphoma, follicular dendritic cell sarcoma, and metastases.

Reference: [13]

5. **Are there unique features of skin adnexal tumors that involve the perianal skin?**
   - Although not specifically mentioned in the fifth edition WHO classification of the Tumors of the Digestive System, various skin adnexal tumors may involve the perianal skin, and some have unique features when compared to their counterparts in other skin regions.

   References: [14, 15]

Hidradenoma Papilliferum

- It is a benign tumor unique to the anogenital region. The most common site is the labia, followed by the vulva and perianal skin, although "ectopic" lesions involving the eyelid and external auditory canal are on record. It occurs almost exclusively in females and is thought to have its origin in apocrine glands or "mammary-like" glands. It typically presents as a solitary asymptomatic nodule or cyst-like lesion, usually <2 cm in size.
- Microscopic appearance (Fig. 9.8a–c): typically in the form of branching and anastomosing tubules with intervening fibrous tissue bands, resulting in a complex papillary configuration, and there is presence of a luminal layer (cuboidal to columnar, positive for AE1/AE3, CK5/6, GCDFP, and ER) and a myoepithelial layer (positive for S100, calponin, and smooth muscle actin (SMA)). Tumor cells may have some stratification and mild pleomorphism.

Reference: [14]

Trichoepithelioma

- It occurs in both sexes. The clinical and pathological features are similar to its counterpart in other skin regions, except that perianal tumors may reach a larger size to several centimeters at presentation.

Other Tumors

- Tumors such as fibroadenoma, apocrine mixed tumor, "lactating adenoma," and phyllodes tumor have been described to occur in the anogenital region. They are more affinitive to the genital part than to the anal region.
- Anal Paget disease and basal cell carcinoma are discussed in questions 10 and 11.

6. **How does the american joint committee on cancer (AJCC) define the anus and stage anal tumors?**
   - According to the eighth edition AJCC Cancer Staging Manual, carcinomas of the anal canal and "perianus" (formally "anal margin") are staged the same, and the classification system applies to both squamous cell carcinoma and adenocarcinoma.

   Reference: [6]

Clinical Definition

- Anal cancer: cancers that develop from the anal canal mucosa (glandular, transitional, or squamous) that cannot be visualized in their entirety while gentle traction is placed on the buttocks

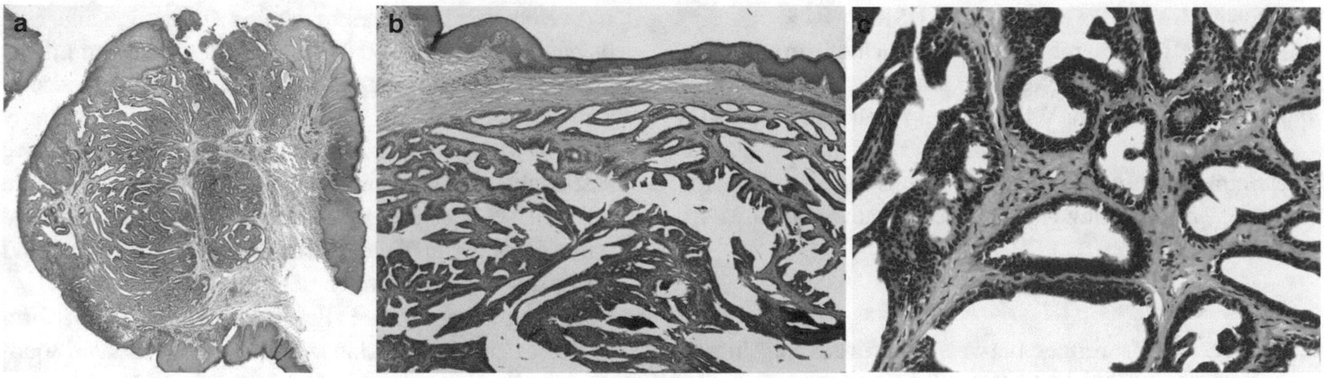

Fig. 9.8 An anal hidradenoma papilliferum exhibiting branching tubules with intervening fibrous tissue bands, resulting in a complex papillary configuration (**a**, **b**). Higher power view showing the lining epithelium to be composed of two layers of cells (**c**)

- Perianal cancer: cancers that arise within the skin at or distal to the squamous mucocutaneous junction, can be seen in their entirety with gentle traction placed on the buttocks, and are within 5 cm of the anus

AJCC Definition

- For pathological staging purposes, the AJCC staging manual arbitrarily defines the anal canal as beginning at 1–2 cm above the dentate line and recommends that tumors with an epicenter that is located 2 cm or less above the dentate line be staged as anal canal cancer.

References: [16, 17]

AJCC Staging Schema (Table 9.3)

- pT staging is based on tumor size.
- pN staging differs from staging for colon and rectum; most notably, inguinal lymph nodes are regarded as regional for anal malignancies.

7. **What is Bowen disease?**
    - Bowen disease is adopted from cutaneous terminology and refers to squamous cell carcinoma in situ of the perianal skin. More recently, the term "anal intraepithelial neoplasia (AIN)" has been proposed to embrace the entire range of precancerous squamous lesions. HPV infection is a common etiology.

The Lower Anogenital Squamous Terminology (LAST) Proposal

- It is being used in current practice.
- It is a unified terminology for lower ano- and genital tracts.
- It applies to both cytology and histology.

Reference: [18]

- It encompasses all HPV-associated precancerous squamous proliferations.
- Two-tiered terminology:
    - LSIL/AIN1 (low-grade squamous intraepithelial lesion/anal intraepithelial neoplasia).
    - HSIL/AIN2-AIN3 (high-grade squamous intraepithelial lesion/anal intraepithelial neoplasia).
- AIN refers to anal canal intraepithelial neoplasia; for perianal skin (anal margin), perianal intraepithelial neoplasia (PAIN) is recommended.
- LSIL includes lesions presenting cytopathic effects of HPV (condyloma and koilocytosis) that may or may not have associated features of intraepithelial neoplasia.

Table 9.3 Tumor–node–metastasis (TNM) classification of carcinoma of the anus

T category	T criteria
TX	Primary tumor not assessed
T0	No evidence of primary tumor
Tis	High-grade squamous intraepithelial lesion (previously termed carcinoma in situ, Bowen disease, anal intraepithelial neoplasias II–III, high-grade anal intraepithelial neoplasia)
T1	Tumor ≤2 cm
T2	Tumor >2 cm but ≤5 cm
T3	Tumor >5 cm
T4	Tumor of any size invading adjacent organ(s), such as the vagina, urethra, or bladder
N category	N criteria
NX	Regional lymph nodes cannot be assessed
N0	No regional lymph node metastasis
N1	Metastasis in inguinal, mesorectal, internal iliac, or external iliac nodes
N1a	Metastasis in inguinal, mesorectal, or internal iliac nodes
N1b	Metastasis in external iliac nodes
N1c	Metastasis in external iliac with any N1a nodes
M category	M criteria
M0	No distant metastasis
M1	Distant metastasis

Eighth edition AJCC staging manual

- "Bowen disease" is equivalent to HSIL/PAIN 3.
- Positive p16 immunohistochemistry in the form of diffuse and strong nuclear or nuclear plus cytoplasmic staining involving at least one third of the epithelial thickness supports the diagnosis of HSIL. Focal or patchy nuclear staining can be seen in reactive lesions and LSIL. Isolated cytoplasmic staining is considered negative (Fig. 9.9a–d).

Reference: [18]

8. **Are there differences between verrucous carcinoma and giant condyloma of Buschke–Lowenstein?**
   - Most literature reports and textbooks, including the fourth edition WHO Classification of Tumors of the Digestive System, state that the two terms are regarded as synonymous. However, recent data seem to suggest that they may be distinct diseases.

   Reference: [19]

Verrucous Carcinoma (VC)

- It can occur in the skin and squamous mucosa of various sites, including the head and neck, urinary bladder, and anogenital region. It is commonly regarded as a variant of well-differentiated squamous cell carcinoma.
- It develops slowly, typically assuming a coarse irregular exophytic growth (Fig. 9.10a), but can cause downward tissue destruction if left untreated. Pure VC does not metastasize.
- The etiology of VC remains controversial. Initially thought to be HPV driven, recently emerged data have cast doubt on this belief. Using multiple polymerase chain reaction (PCR)-based assays covering at least 89 HPV types, Zidar et al. failed to detect alpha-, gamma-, and mu-papillomaviruses in ten of ten VC cases.
- Microscopic appearance (Fig. 9.11a–c): it is in the form of thick club-shaped islands of well-differentiated squamous epithelium with marked keratosis and parakeratosis, lack of the usual cytological criteria of malignancy, and invasion with a well-defined pushing border at its base. The cells are typically large and "spinous" and lack koilocytosis. Mitoses are rare and basally located if present.

Reference: [19]

Giant Condyloma of Buschke–Lowenstein (GCBL)

- This tumor was originally described in the penis, but it can occur in the anus and other sites. It is associated with HPV infection, typically HPV6 and HPV11.

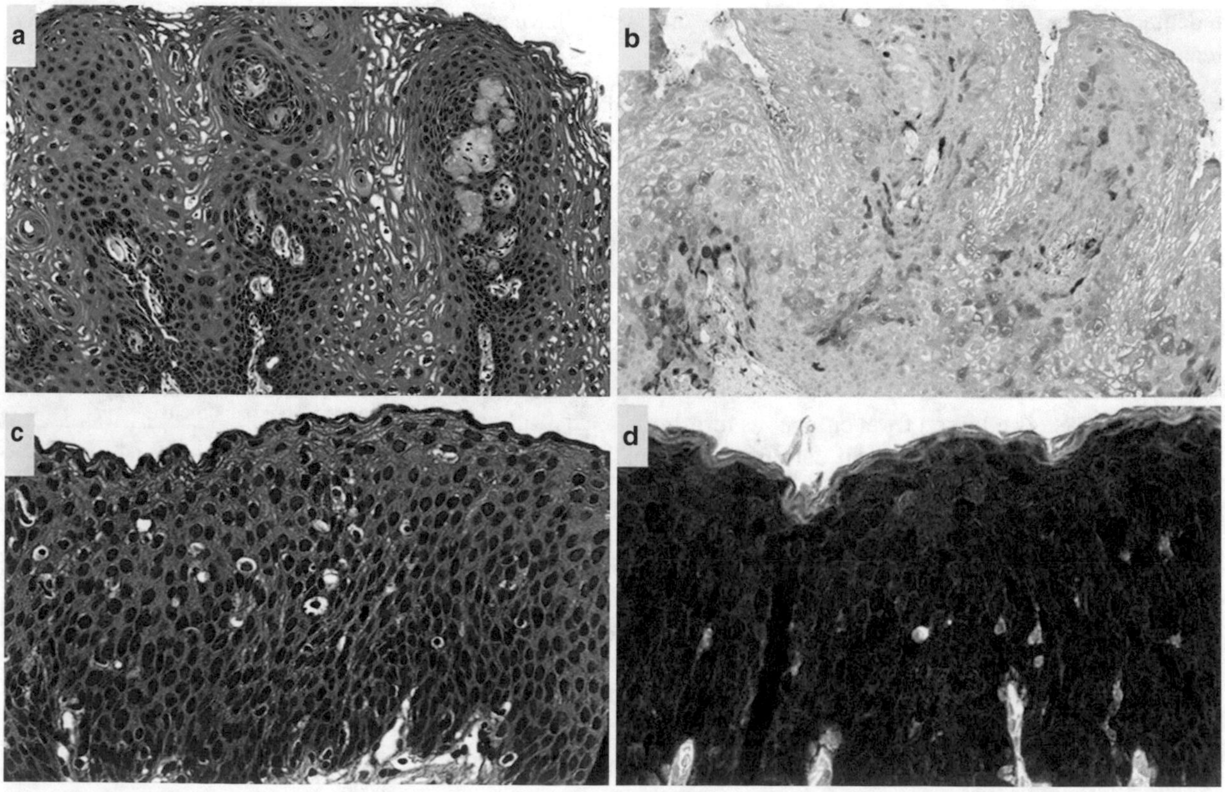

Fig. 9.9 p16 immunohistochemistry can help detect high-grade versus low-grade squamous intraepithelial lesion. A low-grade squamous lesion with koilocytic changes (**a**) shows only patchy nuclear labeling for p16 (**b**), whereas a high-grade squamous lesion with full-thickness cytologic atypia (**c**) exhibits diffuse and strong nuclear (plus cytoplasmic) labeling for p16 (**d**)

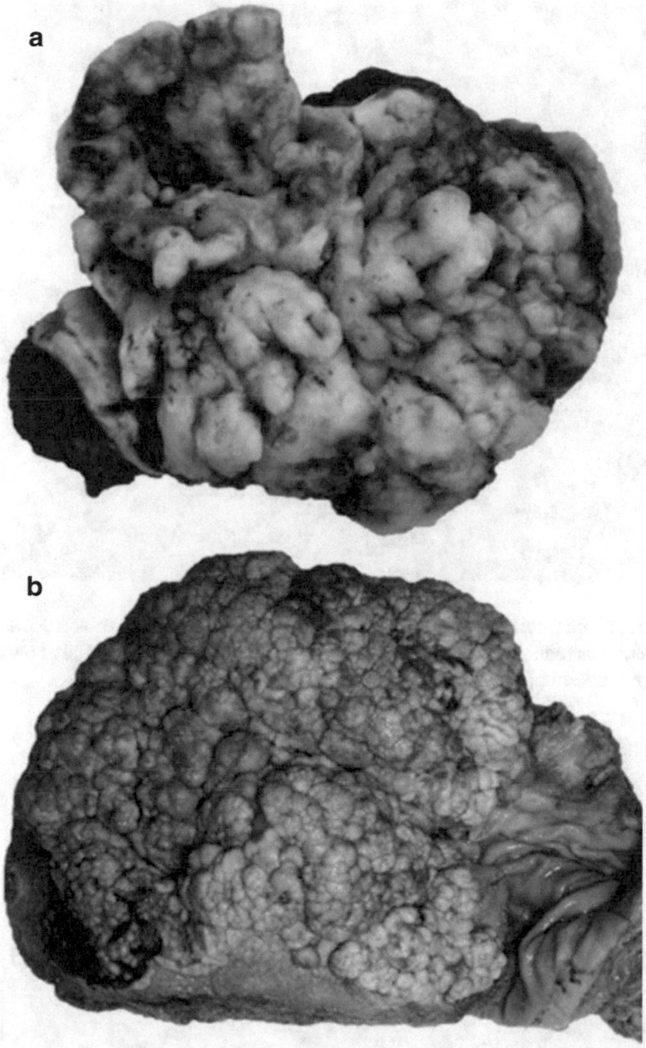

Fig. 9.10 Gross appearance of verrucous carcinoma and giant condyloma of Buschke–Lowenstein. Panel **a** illustrates a verrucous carcinoma with exophytic growth and a coarse, irregular warty surface. Panel **b** illustrates a giant condyloma that also has an exophytic growth but with a more regular, fine warty surface. (From [19], with permission)

- The biology of the tumor remains an area of controversy: some believe that GCBL can result in tissue destruction and is malignant, while others regard it as a benign condition and suspect that the cases reported as having destructive growth may actually be examples of VC.
- Typical lesion grows exophytically and exceeds 10 cm in greatest dimension (Fig. 9.10b).
- Microscopic appearance (Fig. 9.12a–c): acanthosis and papillomatosis of orderly arranged epithelial layers, an intact but maybe irregular base, and having koilocytosis.

Recommendations for Diagnosis

- Acknowledge controversy and uncertainty in terminology.
- Describe the presence or absence of "pushing" pattern of invasion (infiltrative invasion should place the tumor in the category of invasive squamous cell carcinoma, which can metastasize).
- Describe the presence or absence of appreciable HPV viral cytopathic changes.
- Test HPV.

Main differences between VC and GCBL: VC is not HPV associated and thus lacks viral cytopathic effect and it is locally destructive with both exophytic and endophytic growth patterns; On the other hand, GCBL is associated with low-risk HPV and thus exhibits viral cytopathic effect and shows an exophytic growth pattern only. Since invasive squamous cell carcinoma with the potential of metastasis can develop from VC, a definitive diagnosis of VC should not be made on a small superficial biopsy.

9. **What is the difference between "cloacogenic carcinoma" and squamous cell carcinoma?**
   - Once regarded as separate subgroups, the current WHO classification enlists both cloacogenic carcinoma and squamous cell carcinoma, along with other related variants (including mucoepidermoid and adenoid cystic), under one common terminology: squamous cell carcinoma.

   Reference: [21]

"Cloacogenic Carcinoma"

- The term stems from the assumption that these tumors originate from the embryonic remnant of the cloacal membrane in the ATZ.
- Synonyms include transitional carcinoma and basaloid carcinoma. Similar tumors may also be termed mucoepidermoid carcinoma or adenoid cystic carcinoma.
- Morphological patterns (Fig. 9.13a–d) vary and may include the following:
  - Nested and trabecular growth of small cells without intercellular bridges.
  - Peripheral palisading similar to cutaneous basal cell carcinoma.
  - Small cystic foci lined by mucin-producing cells (the reason for the former designation of mucoepidermoid carcinoma).
  - Lobular growth containing prominent eosinophilic, hyaline, paucicellular basement membrane-like material around and within tumor nests, resulting in an appearance simulating that of an adenoid cystic carcinoma.
  - Central necrosis and mitotic figures may be prominent, but cellular pleomorphism is not typical.
  - Components with conventional squamous cell carcinoma are common.
- The term "cloacogenic carcinoma" is now abandoned by WHO, and "squamous cell carcinoma" is used to encompass

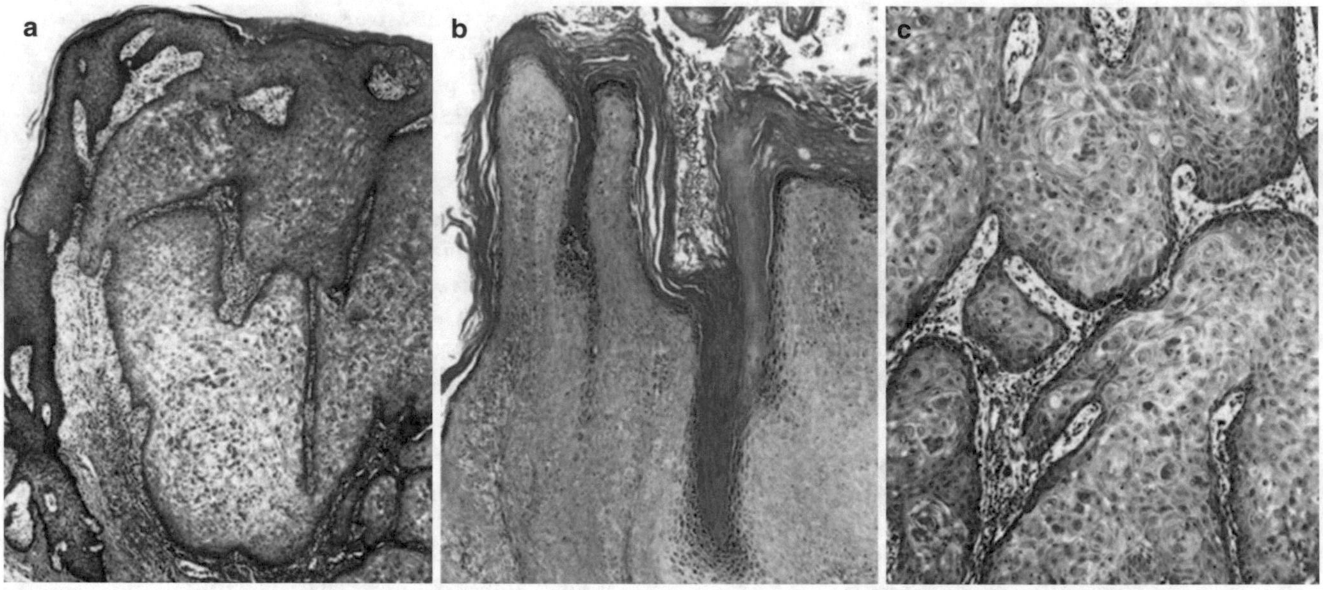

Fig. 9.11 Microscopic appearance of verrucous carcinoma. Panel **a** illustrates the transition from the normal squamous epithelium to verrucous carcinoma. Panel **b** illustrates elongated projections with marked surface keratosis (church spire keratosis). Panel **c** illustrates that the invasive part of the tumor is composed of thick islands of well-differentiated squamous epithelium. (From [19], with permission)

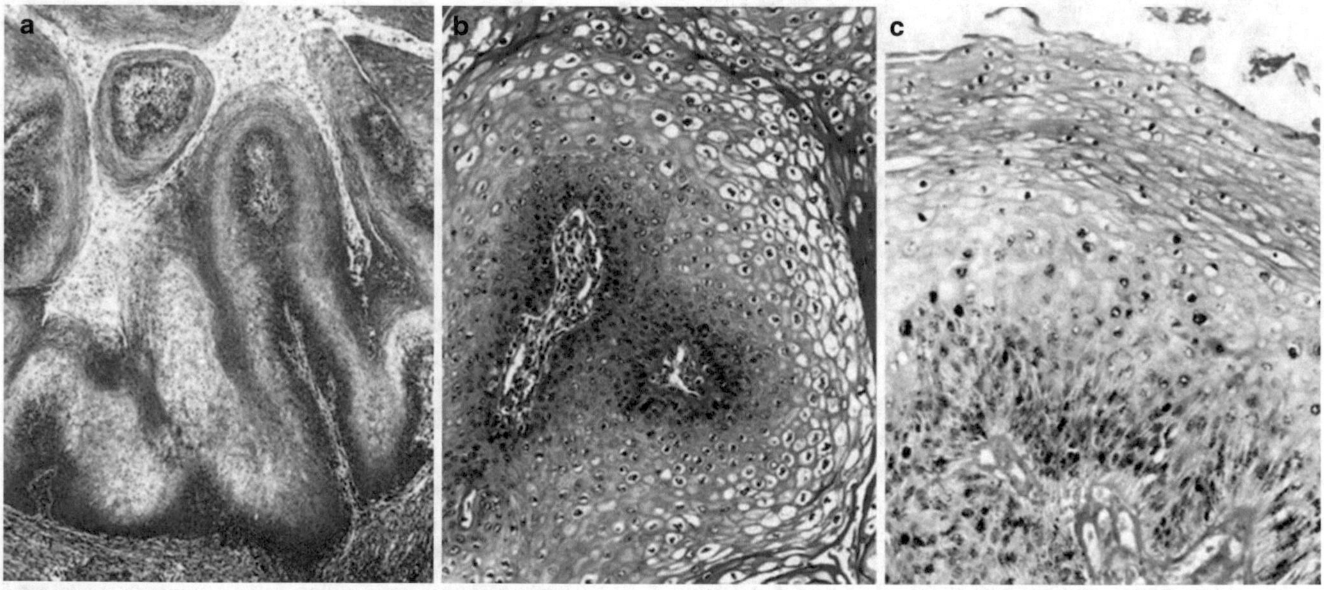

Fig. 9.12 Microscopic appearance of giant condyloma of Buschke–Lowenstein. Panel **a** illustrates well-formed papillae with parakeratosis. Panel **b** illustrates koilocytosis with enlarged, dark nuclei surrounded by a clear cytoplasmic area, present mainly in the upper half of the epithelium. Panel **c** illustrates that in situ hybridization for human papillomavirus 6 (HPV6) is positive in many epithelial cells. (From [19], with permission)

all squamous cell carcinomas and variants. Other terms, such as "mucoepidermoid carcinoma," are also discouraged in order to avoid clinical confusion. However, for tumors with striking basaloid appearance, the description "squamous cell carcinoma with basaloid features" may still be used.

- Basis for the recommendation: many tumors show more than one subtype, the diagnostic reproducibility of the subtypes is low, and there is no proven prognostic influence (Fig. 9.14a–c).
- However, some patterns with prognostic implication or reflecting different etiology are still worth mentioning:
  - Squamous cell carcinoma with mucinous microcysts (areas with well-formed acinar or cystic spaces containing mucin that are Alcian blue and Periodic acid–Schiff-Diastase (PASD) positive).
  - Small cell (anaplastic) carcinoma: the word "anaplastic" is used to distinguish it from small cell neuroendocrine carcinoma. Typical morphology includes a

uniform pattern of small tumor cells with nuclear molding, high mitotic rate, extensive apoptosis, and diffuse infiltration in the surrounding stroma.
- Poor keratinization, prominent basaloid features, and small tumor cell size are related to infection with high-risk HPV.

References: [21–26]

10. What types of adenocarcinoma occur in the anus?

- Most adenocarcinomas detected in the anal canal are downward extension of distal rectal adenocarcinomas. Adenocarcinomas primary to the anal canal can occur and include two major subtypes: mucosal and extramucosal. The former is believed to originate from the glandular epithelium of the anal canal (primarily from the colorectal epithelium in the upper zone), and the latter may be associated with anal gland or anal fistula. Additionally, primary Paget disease of the perianal skin may evolve into invasive adenocarcinoma and extend to the anal canal.

Mucosal Type Adenocarcinoma

- It originates from glandular cells lining the surface of the anal canal and is histologically indistinguishable from upper rectal adenocarcinoma.
- It tends to have a "CK7 positive/CK20 positive" staining pattern (this is true with rectal adenocarcinoma as well, whereas colonic adenocarcinomas typically have a "CK7 negative/CK20 positive" phenotype).
- Their anal canal location implies different tumor–node–metastasis (TNM) staging than rectal adenocarcinoma: tumors with their epicenter located within 2 cm above the dentate line are to be staged according to TNM classification for anal carcinomas (Fig. 9.15a–c).

Reference: [6]

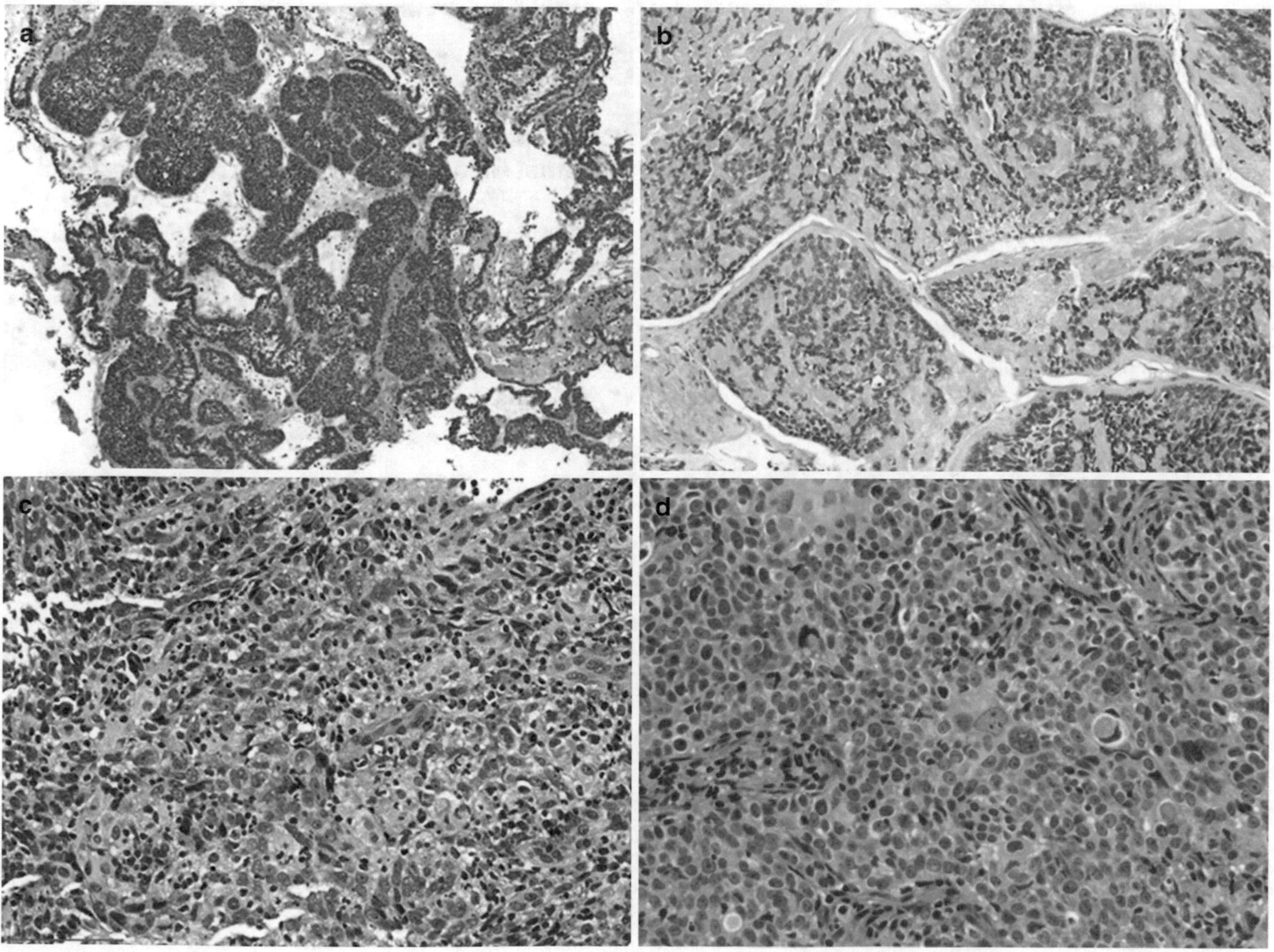

Fig. 9.13 Squamous cell carcinomas arising in ATZ may show varied morphological patterns, including basaloid (**a**), adenoid cystic-like (**b**), or simply poorly differentiated (**c, d**). In case **c**, the tumor is associated with prominent lymphoid infiltrates simulating lymphoepithelioma morphology

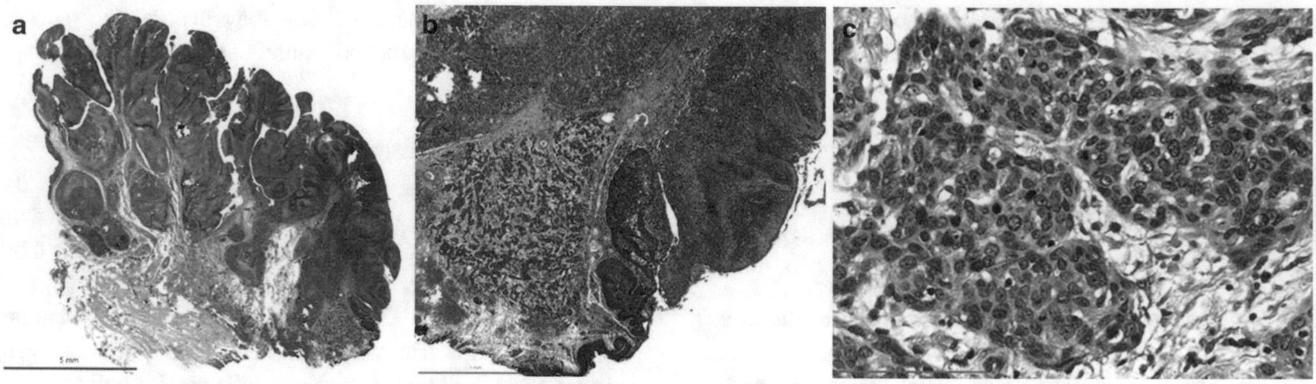

Fig. 9.14 An anal squamous cell carcinoma showing apparent intratumoral variation in H&E morphology. Low power view illustrating an overall "verrucoid" growth pattern with broad fronds pushing downward (**a**). Higher power view (**b**, of right lower corner of **a**) reveals variations: some grow in larger groups (left upper panel of **b**), while others show small nests with more intervening stroma (left lower panel of **b**). The latter component is further magnified (**c**) to show high-grade small hyperchromatic cells with frequent apoptosis and mitosis. Immunostains for neuroendocrine markers chromogranin and synaptophysin are negative (not shown)

Anal Gland Adenocarcinoma

- It originates from the epithelium of the anal gland or anal duct.
- Histologic spectrum remains to be defined. While typical cases have haphazardly dispersed glands with cuboidal cells and scant mucin (Fig. 9.16a), atypical forms may show tumor cell stratification, solid growth, or prominent mucin production. It lacks a luminal in situ component—an important histologic feature in establishing the diagnosis (Fig. 9.16b).
- By immunohistochemistry, tumor cells typically express CK7 and MUC5AC and do not express CK20 or CDX2. Tumor cells are also negative for CK5/6 and p63, even though these markers are positive in benign anal glands.
- Major differential diagnoses include metastases from sites such as the gynaecologic tract and breast.

Fistula-Associated Adenocarcinoma

- It is associated with a preexisting, usually long-standing, anal fistula. The fistula may be idiopathic or as a manifestation of Crohn disease (also see question 3). The speculated histogenesis is variable, which may be related to anal gland epithelium, transitional epithelium, or rectal epithelium.
- The majority of cases are mucinous. An adenoma or adenoma-like component can be seen lining the fistula tract (Fig. 9.17a, b).
- Available immunohistochemical studies support the presumed variability in histogenesis: some show intestinal phenotype (positive for CK20 and MUC2); others show anal-gland-like mucin composition (no immunoreactivity to O-acetyl sialic acid groups).
- Diagnosis hinges on the presence of a preexisting fistula and the exclusion of secondary involvement by a carcinoma from elsewhere, particularly the rectum or upper colon.

Extramucosal Anal Canal Adenocarcinoma, Nonanal Gland Type and Nonfistula Associated

- This type of adenocarcinoma is newly recognized in our practice and described in a recent publication. The reported cases had an intestinal phenotype. Histogenetically, it may be related to nonfistulating intramural glandular structures such as embryological remnants.

Reference: [27]

Anal Paget Disease

- Primary anal Paget disease originates from the perianal (anal margin) skin. It is commonly believed to be an intraepidermal adenocarcinoma with skin appendage differentiation. It can become invasive to involve the perianal and ischiorectal region, mimicking primary anal canal adenocarcinoma.
- Secondary Paget disease represents pagetoid extension of tumor cells from an anorectal carcinoma (rarely, adenoma) into the squamous epithelium of the anal canal or perianus. It may be contiguous or discontiguous with the underlying tumor. It may occur concurrently with the underlying tumor or months to years before or after the underlying tumor becomes detectable.
- Histologically, Paget cells (primary or secondary) are typically large, with abundant pale cytoplasm, and may

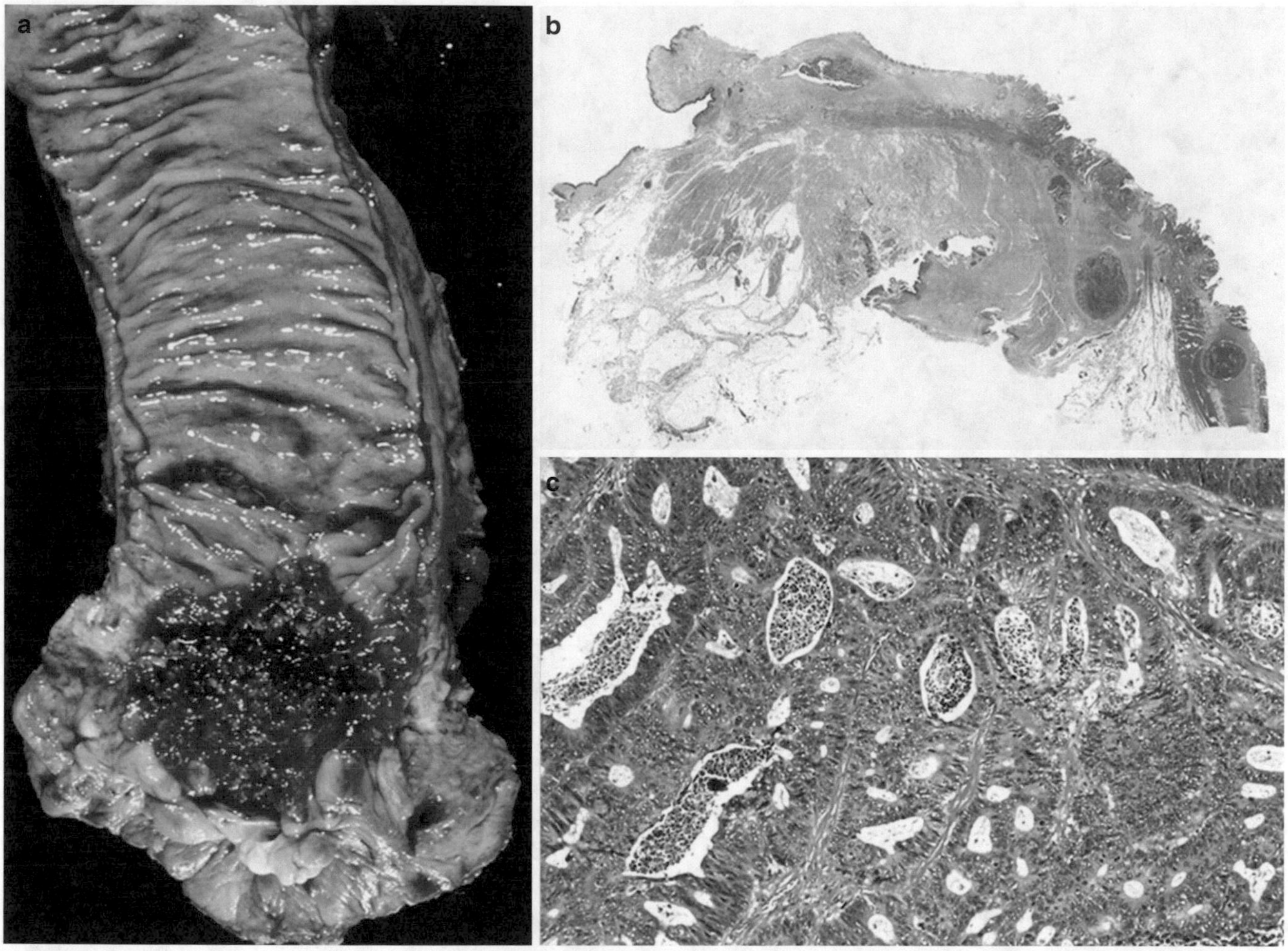

Fig. 9.15 An intestinal-type adenocarcinoma with its epicenter at 1.9 cm above the dentate line, as seen on an opened abdominoperineal resection specimen with a thin rim of perianal skin (**a**). The tumor was treated with neoadjuvant chemoradiation but achieved only partial response. Scanning power view (**b**) of one representative tumor section showing some fibrosis toward the distal portion of the tumor, but overt residual tumor foci are seen more proximally. High power view (**c**) showing typical gland forming colorectal-type adenocarcinoma

contain intracellular mucin with signet ring cell morphology (Fig. 9.18a). The cells are mostly arranged individually but can occasionally form nests and gland-like structures. The affected squamous epithelium may show prominent hyperplasia with elongated and sometimes "anastomosing" rete ridges and associated atypia, mimicking squamous dysplasia.

- Immunohistochemistry for primary Paget cells:
  - Typically coexpress CK7 and gross cystic disease fluid protein (GCDFP).
  - Typically do not express CK20 or CDX2.
- Immunohistochemistry for secondary Paget cells associated with rectal-type adenocarcinoma:
  - Tend to express not only CK20 but also CK7 in both the Paget cells and the associated adenocarcinoma (Fig. 9.18b).

11. **What comes under the differential diagnosis of high-grade or high-grade-appearing cellular neoplasms in the anus?**
    - A wide variety of anal tumors can assume a high-grade or high-grade-appearing cellular morphology, typically with a diffuse growth pattern. They include squamous cell carcinoma with basaloid or small cell (anaplastic) features, basal cell carcinoma of the perianal skin, adenocarcinoma, neuroendocrine neoplasms (particularly poorly differentiated neuroendocrine carcinoma, small cell or nonsmall cell type), malignant melanoma, lymphoma, epithelioid sarcoma (such as epithelioid angiosarcoma and epithelioid gastrointestinal stromal tumor). Tables 9.4 and 9.5 summarize the diagnostic features and common pitfalls for these neoplasms. Figure 9.19a–d illustrates a few typical examples.

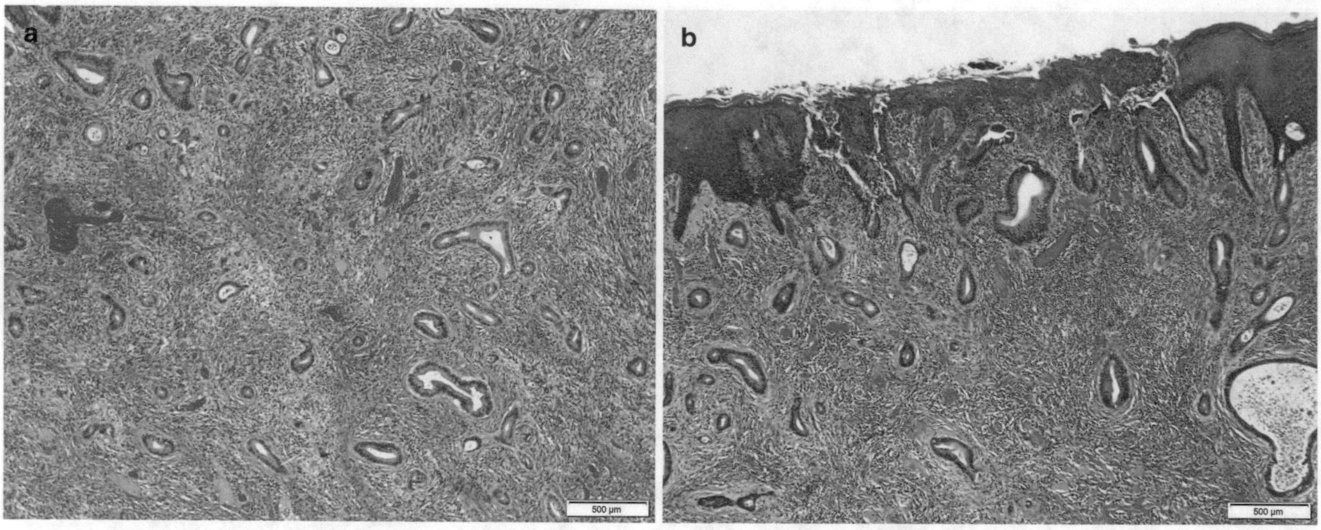

Fig. 9.16 An anal gland adenocarcinoma showing haphazardly dispersed glands with cuboidal cells and only inconspicuous intracellular mucin (**a**). The tumor undermines the squamous epithelium (and may colonize it), but a mucosal precursor lesion is lacking (**b**)

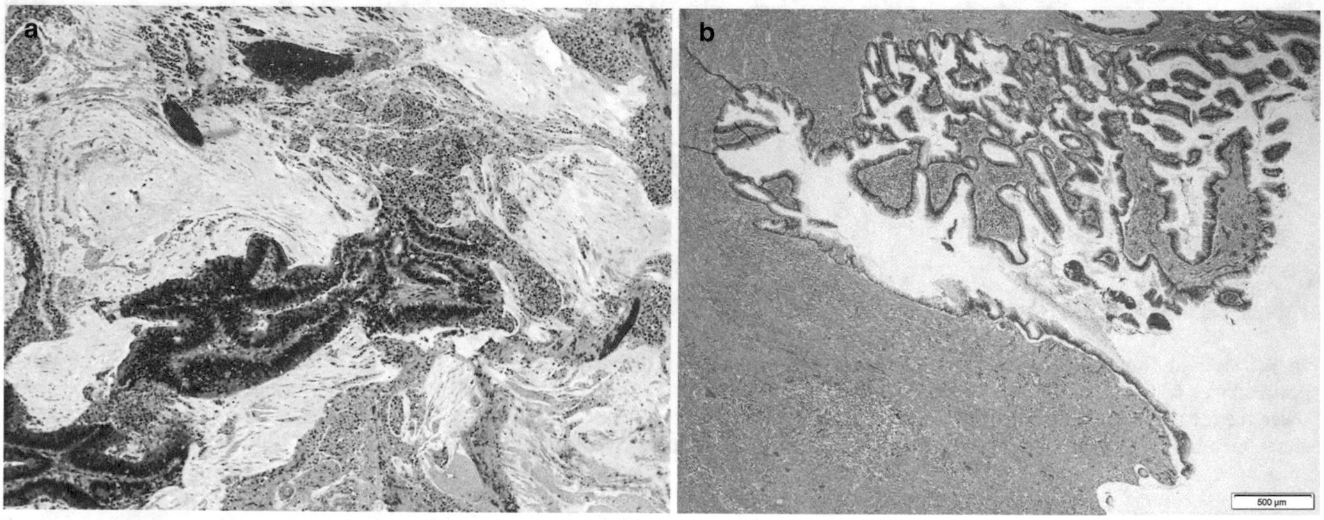

Fig. 9.17 An anal-fistula-associated adenocarcinoma exhibiting mucinous morphology (**a**). Note the prominent inflammatory component in the background. Another fistula-associated adenocarcinoma showing a region with an adenoma-like component involving the fistula tract (**b**)

Poorly Differentiated Squamous Cell Carcinoma (Also See Question 9)

- A thorough examination typically reveals areas that have discernible evidence of squamous differentiation.
- Beware that poorly differentiated neuroendocrine carcinomas, particularly small cell carcinoma, can have areas with squamous differentiation. Usually, in this setting, the squamous differentiation is abrupt and forms squamous pearls.
- Immunohistochemical stains often show positivity for keratin 34BE12 and CK 5/6, and p63/4A4.

Basal Cell Carcinoma from Anal Margin Skin

- Although it is a skin disease typically associated with sun exposure, it can occur in the anal margin skin, which may then extend to involve the anal canal. Etiology is unknown for the anal location.
- It shares histologic features with basal cell carcinoma in other sites of the body, commonly with solid and adenoid patterns (Fig. 9.20a, b).
- Major differential diagnosis: squamous cell carcinoma with basaloid features. Helpful clues:

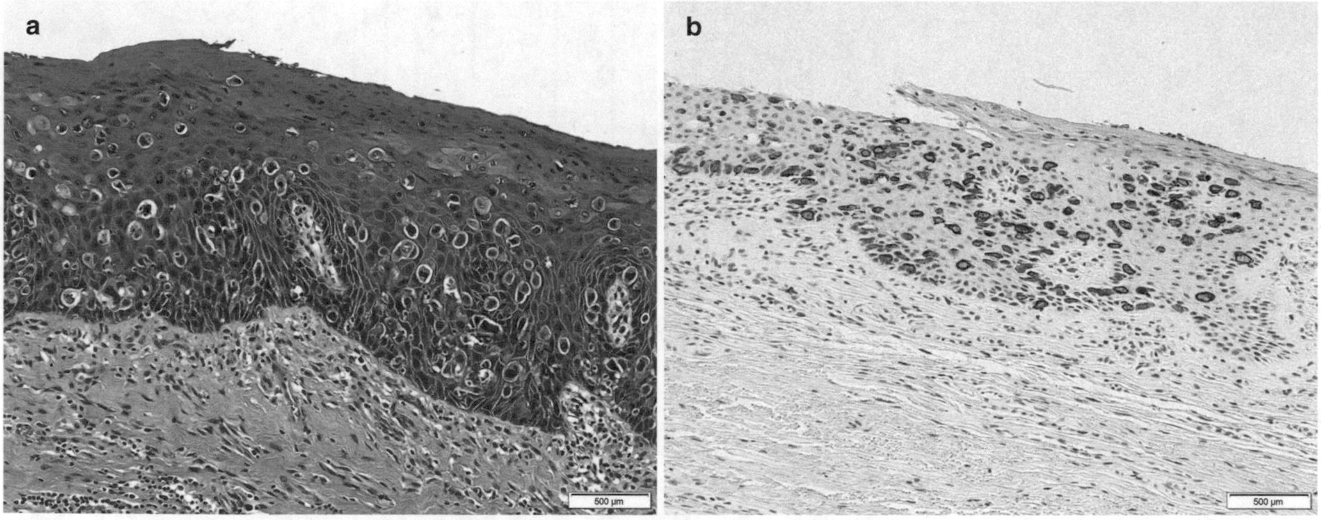

Fig. 9.18 Secondary anal Paget disease. Panel A illustrates the histologic appearance of Paget cells. Panel B shows that the Paget cells are positive for CK20 by immunohistochemistry

- – Basal cell carcinoma is centered in the perianal skin (tumors with its epicenter in the anal canal are unlikely to be basal cell carcinoma).
- – Basal cell carcinoma tends to have conspicuous peripheral palisading and less cellular pleomorphism.
- – Basal cell carcinoma is not associated with precursor squamous dysplasia.

- Immunohistochemical stains typical of basal cell carcinoma:
  - – Positive Ber-EP4 (Fig. 9.20c) and BCL2.
  - – Negative keratins AE1, 13, 19, and 22.
  - – Negative EMA.
  - – Squamous cell carcinomas characteristically show the opposite staining patterns for the above markers, although a minor subset may show positivity for Ber-EP4 or BCL2 as well.

  Reference: [28]

Neuroendocrine Neoplasms

- Well-differentiated neuroendocrine tumors (carcinoid tumors) can occasionally be mitotically active (falling into WHO grade 3 category) and pose challenges in the distinction from poorly differentiated neuroendocrine carcinoma.
- Poorly differentiated neuroendocrine carcinomas may coexist with either an adenocarcinoma or a squamous cell carcinoma component.
- Poorly differentiated neuroendocrine carcinomas, particularly small cell carcinoma, can exhibit abrupt squamous differentiation and may show squamous pearls (Fig. 9.21a, b).
- Poorly differentiated neuroendocrine carcinomas may be positive for TTF1. They may also show loss of RB and abnormal staining for p53 (diffusely positive or totally negative). However, lack of these patterns does not exclude the diagnosis.

Malignant Melanoma

- It may be cutaneous or mucosal depending on the location in the perianal skin versus the anal canal.
- It is often pigmented, with histologic and immunophenotypical features similar to melanoma in other sites.

Lymphoma

- It has histologic and immunophenotypical features similar to lymphomas in other sites.
- It is more common in patients with AIDS, particularly homosexual men.

Epithelioid Sarcomas

- Many mesenchymal and neurogenic neoplasms may occur in the anus. Major entities that come to the differential diagnosis of anal cellular neoplasms include epithelioid angiosarcoma and epithelioid gastrointestinal stromal tumor.
- These tumors share histologic and immunophenotypical features with their counterparts in other sites of the body.

Table 9.4 Morphological and immunophenotypical features of anal malignancies [3]

Tumor types		Morphology	Immunohistochemical staining						
			HMW keratin	4A4/p63	Ber-EP4	Ki-67	NE markers	Melanoma markers	Lymphoma markers
Squamous cell carcinoma		Squamous differentiation	++	++	–	Not relevant	–	–	–
Basal cell carcinoma		Peripheral palisading, not associated with squamous dysplasia	+	+	+	Not relevant	–	–	–
Adenocarcinoma		Mucin, gland formation	–/+	–	+/–	Not relevant	–	–	–
NE neoplasm	Well-differentiated NET	Trabecular, organoid, or nested. Typically with low mitotic activity	–	–		<20%, usually <10%	++	–	–
	Small cell carcinoma	Can have foci of squamous differentiation	– (Squamous foci +)	– (Squamous foci +)		Usually >50%	+	–	–
	Large cell neuroendocrine carcinoma	May simulate carcinoid, but with high mitotic activity and often foci of necrosis	–	–		Usually >30-50%	+	–	–
Melanoma		In situ component, melanin pigment	–	–		Not relevant	–	++	–
Sarcoma		Lacks cohesiveness	–	–		Not relevant	–	–	–
Lymphoma		Lacks cohesiveness	–	–		Variable	–	–	++

NE neuroendocrine; *NET*, neuroendocrine tumor.

Case Presentations

Case 1

Learning Objectives

1. To be familiar with the terminology for anal squamous lesions
2. To know the utility of Ki-67 and p16 immunohistochemistry in diagnosing squamous neoplasia
3. To be aware of the common pitfalls in diagnosing invasiveness in squamous cell carcinoma

Table 9.5 Potential pitfalls in immunohistochemistry of anal tumors [3]

Melanoma versus GIST	A103 (melan A) may stain some epithelioid GISTs [33]
	C-kit stains not only GIST but also melanoma
Poorly differentiated carcinoma versus sarcoma	CK18 may be positive in GISTs and smooth muscle tumors
Neuroendocrine tumors versus others	Neuroendocrine tumors can be positive for CK7 and/or CK20
	Small cell carcinoma primary to the anal canal may be positive for TTF-1

Case History

A 48-year-old male patient presented with "a possible anal hemorrhoid," which was excised.

Gross Findings

One irregular fragment of pink-tan rubbery tissue, polypoid appearing, measuring 0.8 × 0.5 × 0.3 cm. The specimen is sectioned and entirely submitted.

Histologic Findings

Histologic features are illustrated in Figs. 9.22, 9.23, and 9.24.

Differential Diagnosis

- Condyloma acuminatum with high-grade dysplasia
- Squamous cell carcinoma in situ
- Bowen disease
- In situ and invasive squamous cell carcinoma

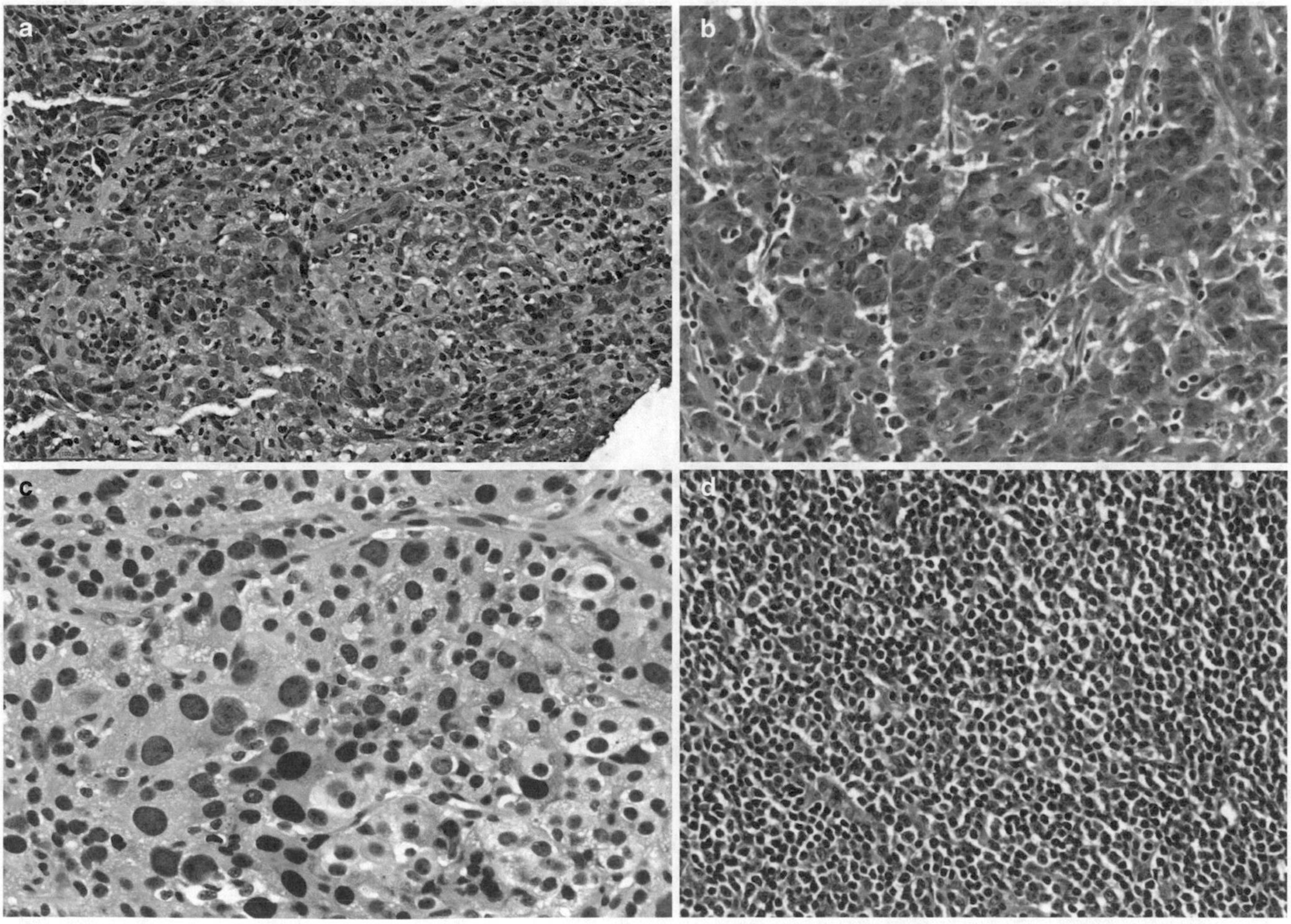

Fig. 9.19 Examples of anal malignant neoplasms that exhibit high cellularity and solid growth: a poorly differentiated squamous cell carcinoma (**a**), a poorly differentiated adenocarcinoma (**b**), a malignant melanoma (**c**), and a lymphoma (**d**)

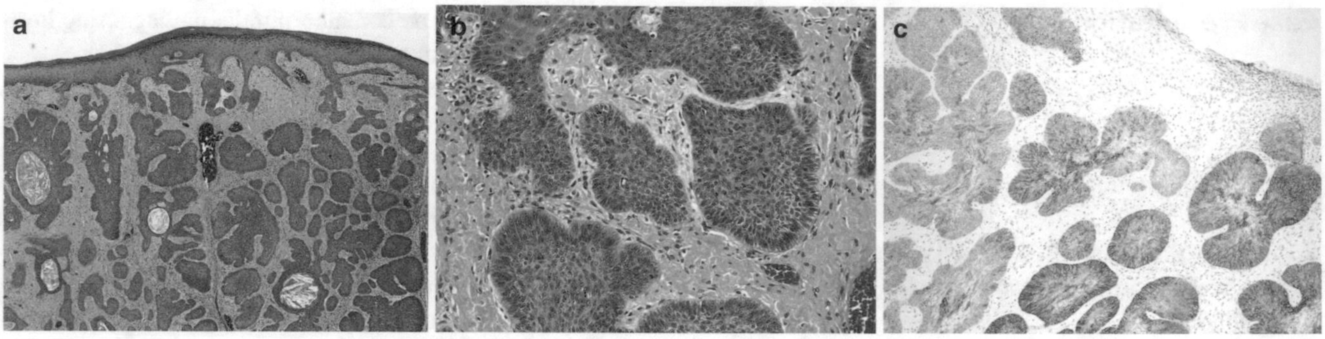

Fig. 9.20 Basal cell carcinoma of the anal margin skin showing irregular nests of squamoid cells arising from the basal layers of the overlying squamous epithelium (**a**). Peripheral palisading is evident (**b**). Tumor cells are positive for Ber-EP4 (**c**)

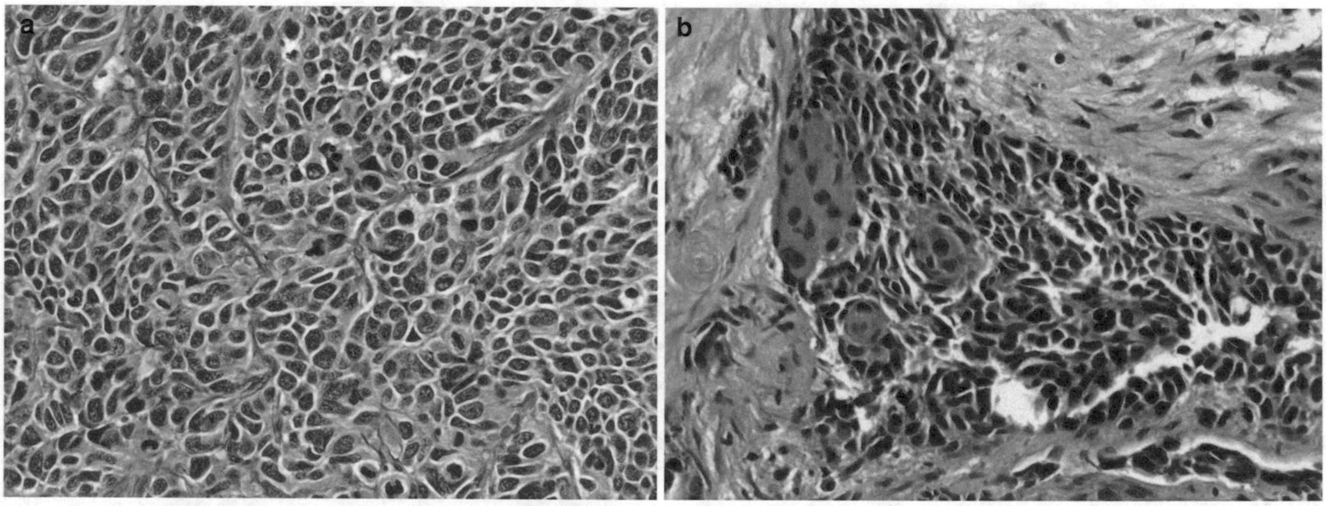

Fig. 9.21 A poorly differentiated neuroendocrine carcinoma with a morphology that is more closely related to small cell carcinoma than large cell neuroendocrine carcinoma (**a**) showing an area with abrupt squamous differentiation (**b**)

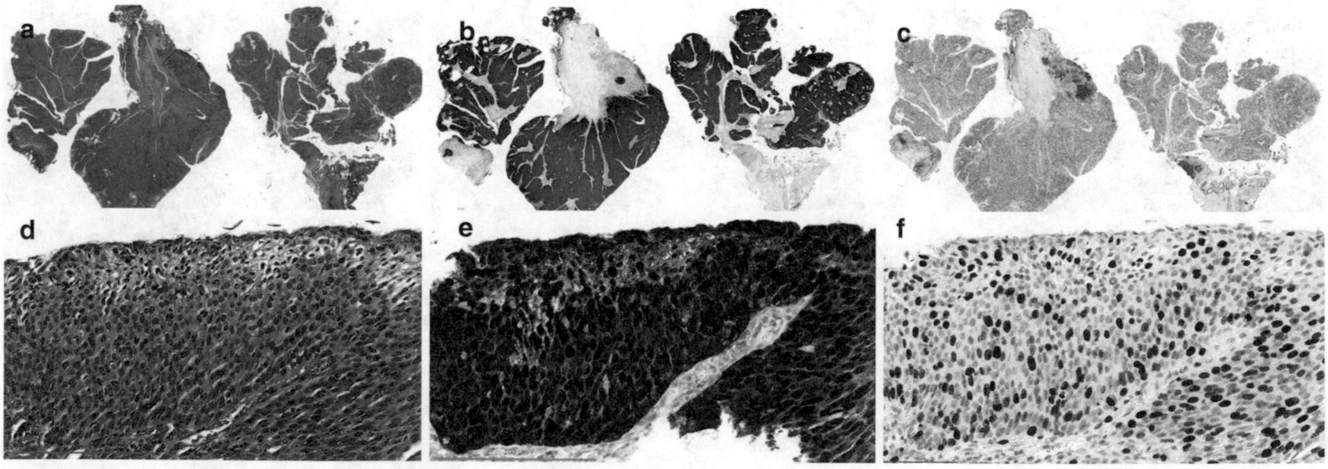

Fig. 9.22 (Case 1). Photomicrographs of an anal squamous cell carcinoma. Panels **a–c** illustrate the scanning power view of all three sections of this case (**a**, H&E; **b**, immunohistochemistry for p16; and **c**, immunohistochemistry for KI-67). Panels **d–f** illustrate squamous dysplasia of severe degree (**d**, H&E; **e**, immunohistochemistry for p16; and **f**, immunohistochemistry for KI-67)

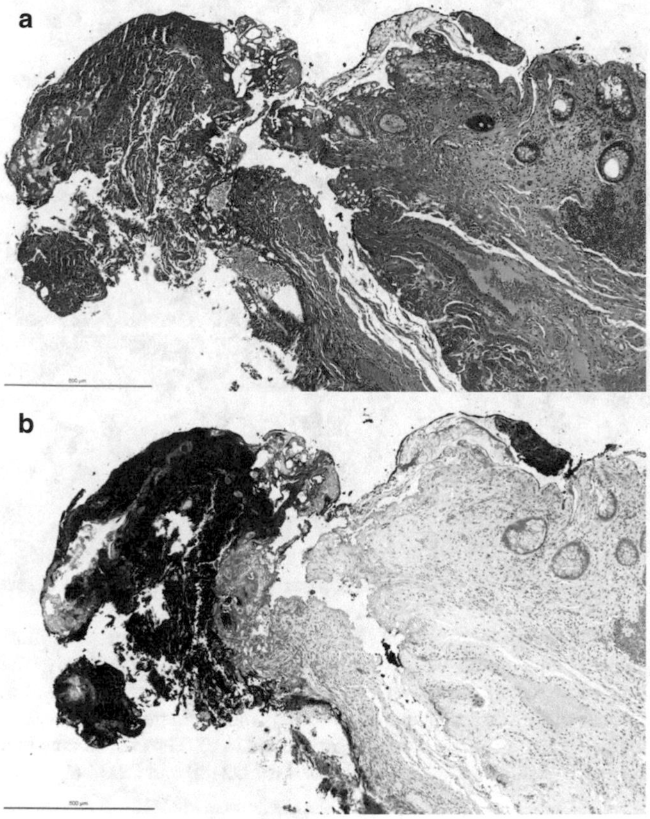

Fig. 9.23 (Case 1). Photomicrograph of the same case illustrated in Fig. 9.22. A cauterized tissue margin (**a**) revealing high-grade squamous dysplasia by showing diffuse and strong immunohistochemical staining for p16 (**b**)

Immunohistochemistry and Other Ancillary Studies

- Ki-67
- P16

Final Diagnosis

In situ and invasive squamous cell carcinoma.

Discussion and Take-Home Messages

This case represents a common scenario whereby malignant anal lesions come as unexpected findings in minor surgical specimens (e.g., hemorrhoidectomies). Histologic evaluation of all anal tissue samples is essential.

The malignant lesion depicted here is a squamous cell carcinoma arising in a background of high-grade squamous dysplasia (see case 4 for further discussion on squamous dysplasia). Condyloma with high-grade dysplasia, squamous cell carcinoma in situ, and Bowen disease are all terms referring to high-grade squamous precursor lesions that are typically associated with high-risk HPV infection, mostly HPV 16.

Condylomas typically have papillary excrescences lined by hyperkeratotic squamous epithelium with variable degrees of koilocytic changes. High-grade dysplasia can occur but only infrequently. Squamous cell carcinoma in situ and Bowen disease are synonymous in terms of the degree of dysplasia: both with high-grade dysplasia, but Bowen disease has traditionally been used more for perianal skin lesions.

As discussed in question 7, current recommendation lumps all precursor lesions with dysplasia into a two-tiered system: LSIL/AIN 1 (low-grade squamous intraepithelial lesion/anal intraepithelial neoplasia) or HSIL/AIN2-AIN3 (high-grade squamous intraepithelial lesion/anal intraepithelial neoplasia).

The microscopic images of the case indicate that there is apparent H&E evidence of HSIL/AIN3 (Fig. 9.22a, d). Further in support of this, immunostain for p16 shows strong and diffuse "block-positive" nuclear and cytoplasmic labeling, and Ki-67 shows proliferative activity in full thickness of the epithelium. These two immunomarkers have been shown to be particularly useful in dealing with squamous lesions where the dysplastic changes on H&E fall into the gray zone between low- and high-grade lesions (particularly in small biopsy samples). In this particular case, the stains also helped identify AIN at cauterized margins which was not easily discernible on H&E due to cautery artifact (Fig. 9.23a). Concordant with the p16 positivity (Fig. 9.23b), in situ hybridization for high-risk HPV showed conspicuous positive signals in the lesional cells.

As the dysplastic epithelium appears confluent with prominent downward expansion, a difficult diagnostic question in this case is whether some of the downward nodular-appearing proliferations represent true invasion. This is a diagnostic dilemma commonly encountered in superficial squamous cell carcinomas. Helpful features in detecting true invasion in borderline cases include the following:

- Presence of at least focal "endophytic" growth (Fig. 9.24a, double arrow indicated area). In general, LSIL lesions tend to be exophytic with koilocytes, HSIL lesions tend to be flat, and invasive carcinomas are endophytic.
- Confluence of endophytic or downward proliferating nodules. Tangential cutting may also result in confluence of nodules in some tissue fragments, but this should not be seen in all fragments.
- Proliferating nodules are irregular (Fig. 9.24a, b), while confluent nodules from tangential cutting often have less irregularity.
- Proliferating nodules lack a good basal palisading layer (Fig. 9.24a, b).
- Paradoxical maturation of the leading edge of proliferating nodules (Fig. 9.24a, c).
- Presence of lymphovascular invasion, which can masquerade as proliferating nodules (Fig. 9.24a, d–f).

The presence of all these features in this case led to the final diagnosis of invasive squamous cell carcinoma. The staging of this tumor will be based on tumor size. The term "superficially invasive squamous cell carcinoma" is recom-

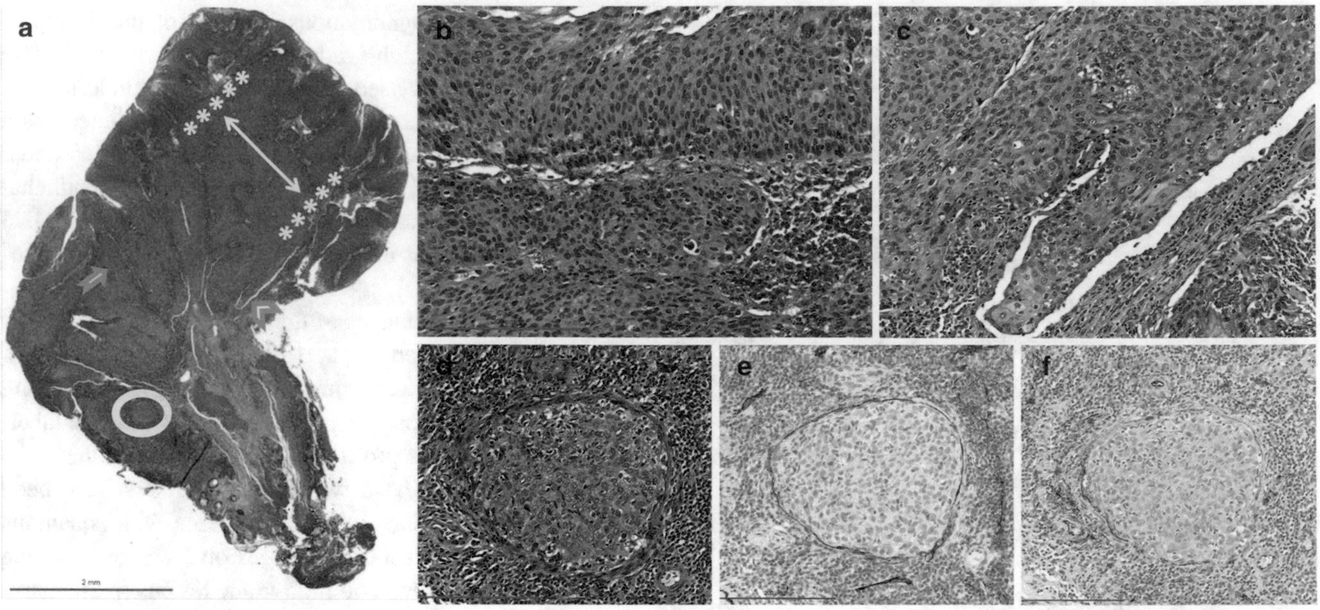

Fig. 9.24 (Case 1). Photomicrograph of the same case illustrated in Fig. 9.22. In one tissue fragment (**a**), various diagnostic features are illustrated. The double-arrow-indicated area (upper right of **a**) illustrates an example of endophytic growth, which involves this section diffusely. The endophytic growth shows irregularity and lacks a well-defined peripheral palisading layer (an example area is marked by a single arrow in **a**, magnified in **b**, which presents as irregular groups underneath an evaginated focus of surface squamous dysplasia). Paradoxical maturation is seen at the periphery of the downward proliferating nodules (an example area is indicated by an arrow head in **a**, magnified in **c**). The circled area in **a** is magnified in **d**, which shows a focus of lymphovascular invasion (**d**) confirmed by immunohistochemical stains for D2–40 and CD34 (**f**)

mended for minimally invasive lesions (microinvasion) that are completely excised. These cases are potentially amenable to conservative surgical treatment. The criteria used for superficially invasive carcinoma in the anal region are identical to those for cervical lesions: an invasive depth of ≤3 mm from the basement membrane of the point of origin, and a horizontal spread of ≤7 mm in maximum extent. It should be emphasized that these criteria should apply only to completely excised lesions with negative surgical margins. The histologic measurements can be challenging in fragmented, cauterized or poorly oriented specimens. The presence or absence of lymphovascular invasion should be reported. If multiple independent foci of superficially invasive carcinoma are present, the number and size range should also be reported.
References: [29, 30]

Case 2

Learning Objectives

1. To be familiar with the differential between reactive atypia versus neoplasia for anal glandular lesions
2. To know the types of adenocarcinoma that can affect the anus
3. To understand the current views on the varied histogenesis of anal adenocarcinomas

Case History

A 57-year-old otherwise healthy female with no history of IBD or malignancy presented with "knots near the anus." The initial clinical impression was "thrombosed external hemorrhoids." Four months later, after failing to respond to "high fiber diet, stool softeners and topical hydrocortisone," the lesion was reexamined and appeared like a mass, about 2 cm in size, in the left posterior quadrant of the soft tissue under the anal margin skin, with no luminal component in the anal canal or rectum. This was excised.

Gross Findings

One tissue fragment labeled as "lesion" is unoriented and irregular, measuring 2.0 × 1.0 × 1.0 cm. A second fragment from the "deep margin of the lesion" is also irregular, measuring 1.0 × 0.5 × 0.5 cm. Both fragments are sectioned and entirely submitted.

Histologic Findings

Histologic features are illustrated in Fig. 9.25a–d.

Differential Diagnosis

- "Inverted" inflammatory/cloacogenic polyp
- Ectopic rectal tissue
- Ectopic rectal tissue with adenoma
- Anal adenocarcinoma, mucinous type, extramucosal in location

Immunohistochemistry and Other Ancillary Studies

- CK7 negative
- CK20 positive

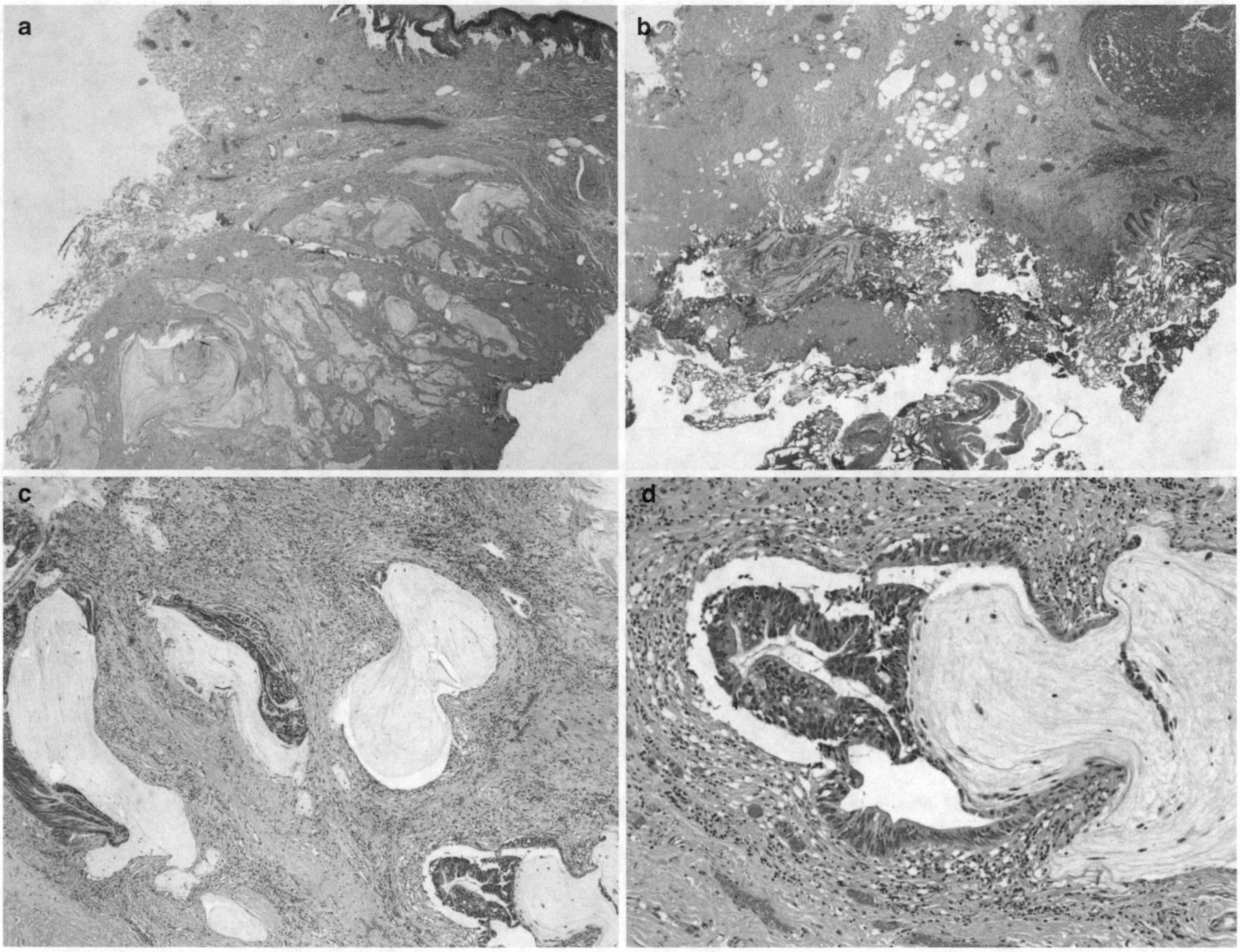

Fig. 9.25 (Case 2). An anal canal extramucosal lesion showing abundant stroma-dissecting mucin (**a**), background rectal-type mucosa embedded in soft tissue (**b**), and neoplastic glands lining or floating in mucin pools (**c**, **d**)

Final Diagnosis

Anal adenocarcinoma, mucinous type, extramucosal in location.

Discussion and Take-Home Messages

This case exemplifies the nonspecificity of the clinical symptoms of anal adenocarcinoma, which often results in delay in diagnosis.

The diagnosis of adenocarcinoma in this case is based on the histologic features illustrated in Fig. 9.25, including:

- Irregular distribution of the neoplastic glands
- Dissecting quality of the mucin pools
- Foci where neoplastic glands are in or at the periphery of the mucin pools

The tumor is of intestinal type, both morphologically and immunophenotypically. The interpretational challenge of this case mainly relates to the histogenesis. The presence of rectal-type glandular mucosa in the lesion (Fig. 9.25b) coupled with the lack of a luminal component in the anal canal or rectum (as determined by the tumor location and the clinical impression) raises the concern whether this could represent a form of "inverted inflammatory/cloacogenic" polyp with associated reactive atypia (Fig. 9.26a, b, an example case from a different patient). However, the atypia is too severe to be explained by a reactive process. Alternative explanations are:

- A fistula-associated adenocarcinoma: we regard it as unlikely due to (1) its association with rectal-type mucosa and its intestinal phenotype (fistular lesions are commonly thought to be of anal gland origin, although some may be intestinal as well) and (2) the negative clinical history of fistula (typical fistula-associated cancer patients have a history of long-standing anal fistula prior to cancer diagnosis).
- An adenocarcinoma associated with nonfistulating intramural glandular structures: this is our favored interpretation for the case. The rectal type mucosa (Fig. 9.25b) likely represents acquired (or congenital) mucosal herniation/malformation (or alternatively embryological remnants).

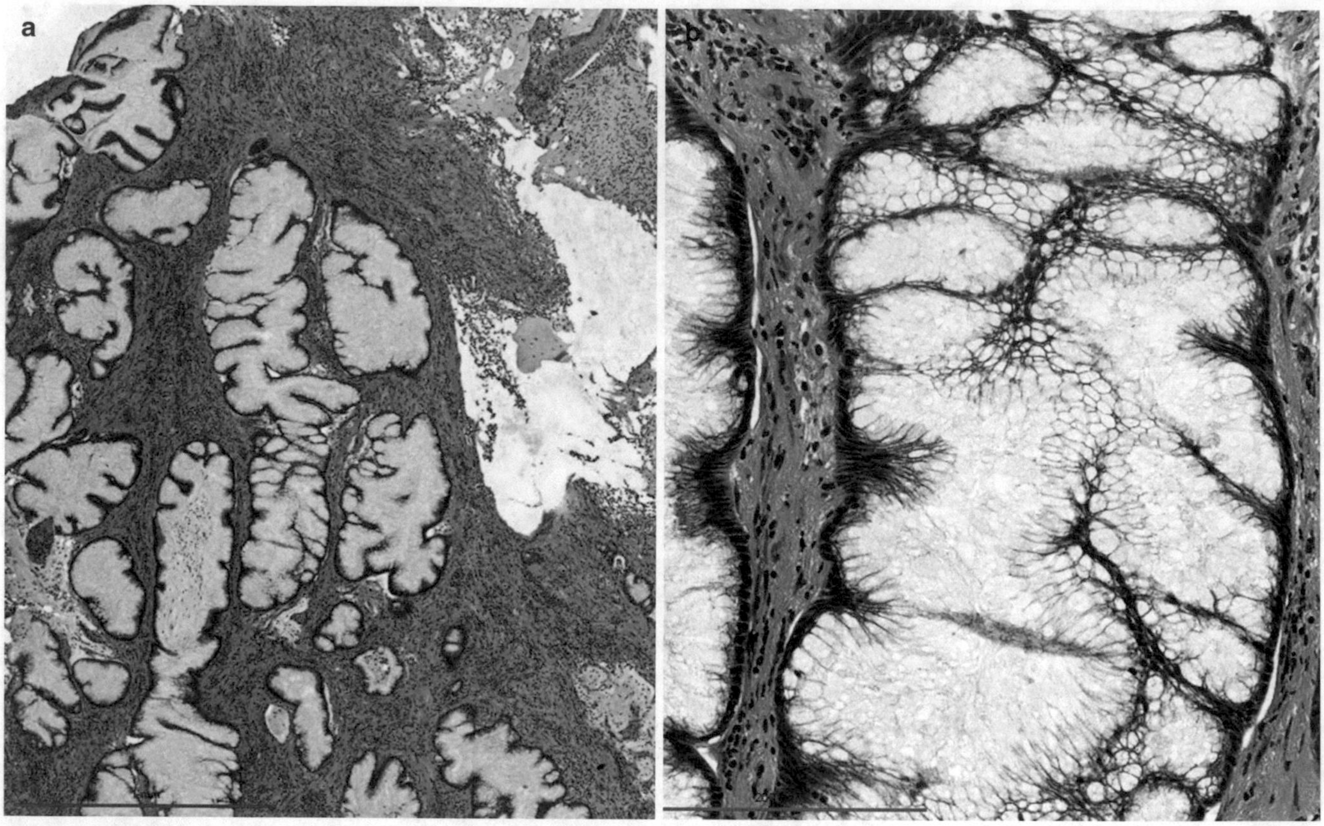

Fig. 9.26 (Case 2). An "inverted" inflammatory polyp (from a different patient) showing hyperplastic (cytologically bland) glandular mucosa with an inflamed stroma (**a**, **b**)

Similar cases of extramural intestinal-type anal adenocarcinoma have indeed been reported in the literature.

As discussed in question 10, three subtypes of extramucosal adenocarcinomas are currently recognized: anal gland adenocarcinoma; fistula-associated carcinoma; and extramucosal anal canal adenocarcinoma, nonanal gland type and nonfistula associated. Diagnosis of the third subtype requires exclusion of alternative primaries (i.e., anal gland type or fistula associated) and exclusion of direct extension from a tumor nearby (particularly that arising from the luminal mucosa of the anal canal or rectum) or a metastasis.

It is to be noted that in both fistula and nonfistulating scenarios, extramucosal anal glandular neoplasia may contain adenoma or adenoma-like component. This is present in the current case.
Reference: [27]

Case 3

Learning Objectives

1. To become familiar with the morphological patterns of anal Paget cells
2. To understand the histogenesis of the two types of anal Paget disease
3. To know the clinical implication of a diagnosis of anal Paget disease

Case History

A female patient, at age 50, presented with a long-standing history of anal pruritus and was found to have anal Paget disease upon biopsy. She was treated with wide local excision at our institution, followed by observation and topical treatment with her local physician. At age 59, she returned with a complaint of rectal bleeding. A lesion was detected in the anal canal, and an abdominoperineal resection (APR) was performed.

Gross Findings

Initial local excision shows eczematous patches of the perianal skin. The APR specimen 9 years later reveals a mucosa-based mass lesion immediately above the dentate line.

Histologic Findings

Sections from the initial local excision exhibit florid Paget cells involving the perianal skin (Fig. 9.27). The APR specimen 9 years later shows a 2.2-cm (pT2) node-negative adenocarcinoma (Fig. 9.28a–c), with prominent secondary Paget disease that involves anal canal squamous mucosa (Fig. 9.28d, e) and the perianal skin and extends close to the distal anal margin.

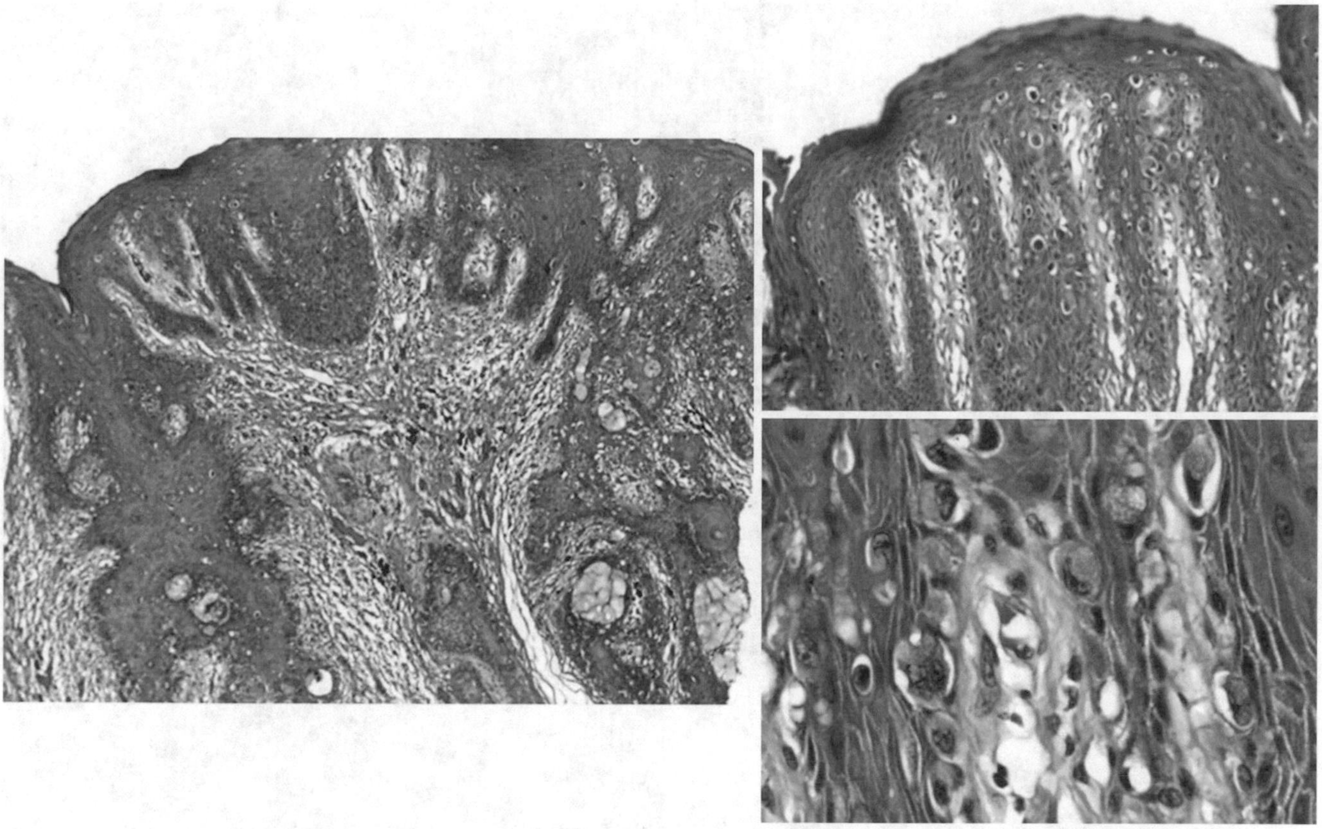

Fig. 9.27 (Case 3). Photomicrographs illustrating anal Paget disease involving the perianal skin. Low power view (left panel) demonstrating epidermal hyperplasia in diseased skin. Medium and high power view (right upper and lower panels, respectively) highlighting the intraepithelial adenocarcinoma cells

Differential Diagnosis
Paget disease, primary versus secondary

Immunohistochemistry and Other Ancillary Studies
- CAM5.2 positive
- GCDFP-15/BRST 2 negative
- CK7 positive
- CK20 positive
- CDX2 positive

Final Diagnosis
Secondary anal Paget disease associated with a pT2N0 mucosal-type anal adenocarcinoma, with first manifestation of Paget disease occurring 9 years prior to the detection of the associated carcinoma.

Discussion and Take-Home Messages
Interesting points in this case are as follows:

- Secondary anal Paget disease can occur metachronously with the associated underlying malignancy, which may be months to years before or after the associated malignancy becomes detectable.
- Immunohistochemical stains can be helpful in distinguishing primary versus secondary Paget disease (see also question 10).
- Paget cells can be large and pale, resembling melanocytes, or signet ring like with intracellular mucin.
- Both primary and secondary Paget cells can have mucin production. Thus, signet ring cell morphology alone is not a reliable criterion to distinguish the two types of Paget disease.
- A diagnosis of primary Paget disease should prompt surveillance for recurrence or progression to invasive disease. Secondary Paget disease should prompt investigation of an internal malignancy. On rare occasions, the underlying tumor associated with secondary anal Paget disease has been found to be adenoma only.

Reference: [31, 32]

Case 4

Learning Objectives
1. To become familiar with the terminology for anal squamous intraepithelial lesion
2. To know the utility of Ki-67 and p16 immunohistochemistry and HPV in situ hybridization in diagnosing anal squamous intraepithelial lesion

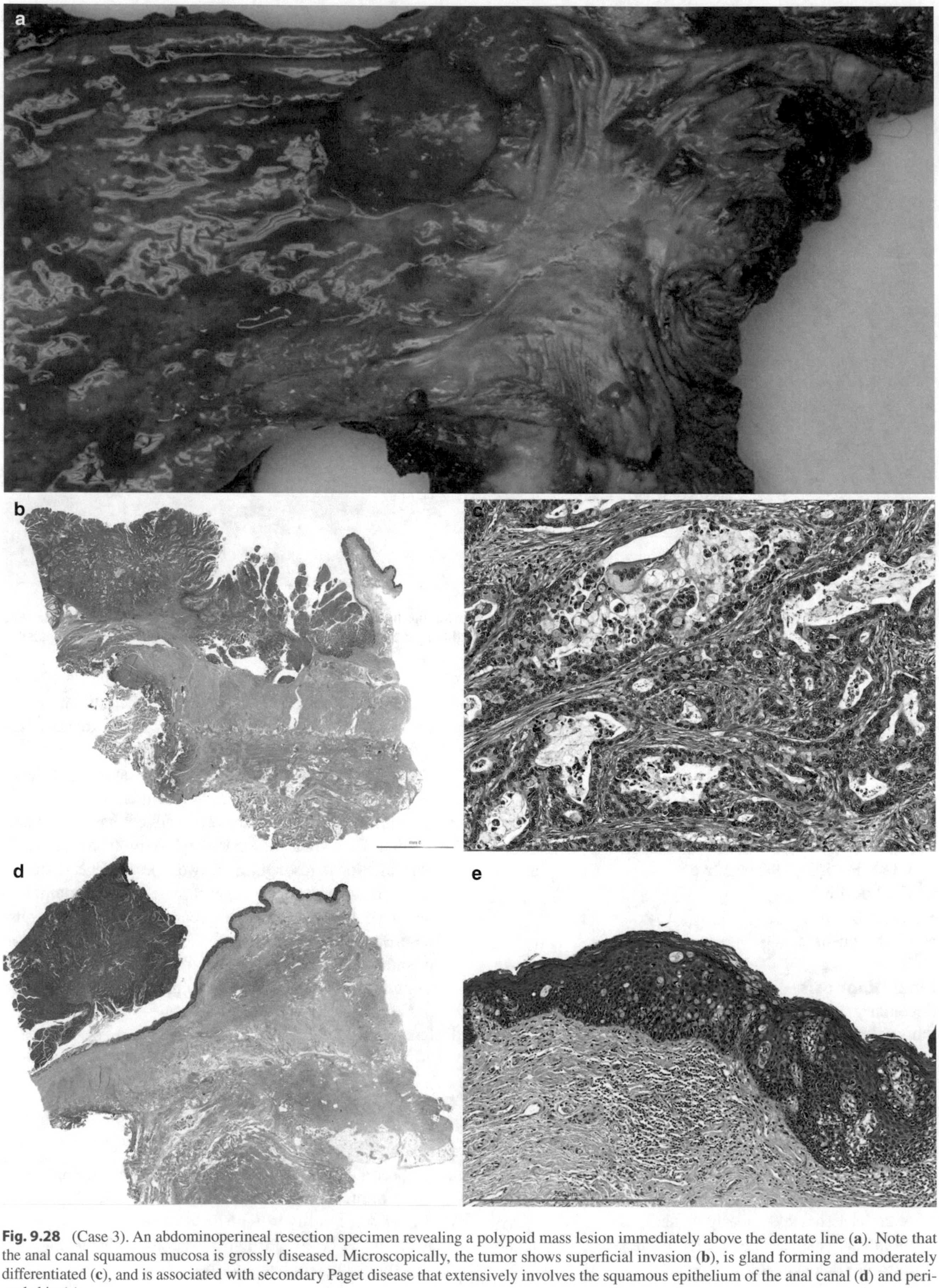

Fig. 9.28 (Case 3). An abdominoperineal resection specimen revealing a polypoid mass lesion immediately above the dentate line (**a**). Note that the anal canal squamous mucosa is grossly diseased. Microscopically, the tumor shows superficial invasion (**b**), is gland forming and moderately differentiated (**c**), and is associated with secondary Paget disease that extensively involves the squamous epithelium of the anal canal (**d**) and perianal skin (**e**)

3. To know the clinical implication of a diagnosis of anal squamous intraepithelial lesion

Case History

A 30-year-old man with an anal Pap smear showing atypical squamous cells of undetermined significance (ASC-US). Anal examination showed a nodular lesion, which was excised.

Gross Findings

The specimen was designated as "anal condyloma" and consisted of two tan-pink, wrinkled, and mucosal-lined tissue fragments measuring 0.8 and 0.6 cm in maximum dimension.

Histologic Findings

Sections show papillary squamous proliferation with broad fronds (Fig. 9.29a). Cells in the superficial layers show perinuclear halos consistent with viral cytopathic effect (koilocytes). Occasional binucleated cells and dyskeratotic cells are seen. A few neutrophils are also seen in the superficial layers (Fig. 9.29b). A few mitotic figures are noted in the basal layers (Fig. 9.29c).

Differential Diagnosis

Condyloma acuminatum, no other differentials

Immunohistochemistry and Other Ancillary Studies

No immunostains or other ancillary studies needed

Final Diagnosis

Condyloma acuminatum.

Discussion and Take-Home Messages

- The terms anal squamous intraepithelial neoplasia (AIN) and anal squamous intraepithelial lesion (SIL) are used interchangeably in practice based on personal preference. AIN is stratified into low grade and high grade categories. In some centers, AIN1, AIN2, and AIN3 are also used, where AIN1 is low grade and both AIN2 and AIN3 are considered high grade. As discussed in question 7, current recommendation lumps all precursor lesions into a two-tiered system: LSIL/AIN1 or HSIL/AIN2-AIN3. It has been recommended that p16 immunohistochemistry be performed if a morphologic diagnosis of AIN2 is to be specifically entertained. A strong and diffuse block-like staining pattern supports a diagnosis of high-grade precancerous lesion, whereas negative or non-block positive staining favors an interpretation of low-grade disease or a non-HPV-associated process.
- Low-grade AIN (AIN1) is characterized by dysplastic cells involving the lower third of the squamous epithelium. The dysplastic cells typically exhibit enlarged and hyperchromatic nuclei with irregular nuclear contours and increased mitoses. It is frequently associated with low-risk HPV, and viral cytopathic effects (koilocytosis) are frequently seen, usually in the superficial layers. HPV cytopathic effects feature enlarged or raisinoid nuclei with perinuclear halos. Binucleated or multinucleated cells may be seen.
- Pure HPV cytopathic effects in the absence of classical dysplastic features should still be diagnosed as AIN1. There is no need to separate it from conventional AIN1.
- Condyloma acuminatum of the anus belongs to the low grade category. Whether it should be called AIN1, condyloma/AIN1, or just condyloma may be of academic interest but will not have any impact on patient care. In our practice, we call a warty or nodular anal lesion condyloma but AIN1 if the biopsy is random or from abnormal-appearing anal mucosa revealed by acetic acid or Lugol staining.
- For cases where AIN1 is suspected but histologic findings are insufficient, in situ hybridization for low-risk HPV can be helpful. Positive staining will help confirm the diagnosis of AIN1, whereas negative staining will help rule out the possibility with more confidence (Fig. 9.30a–c).

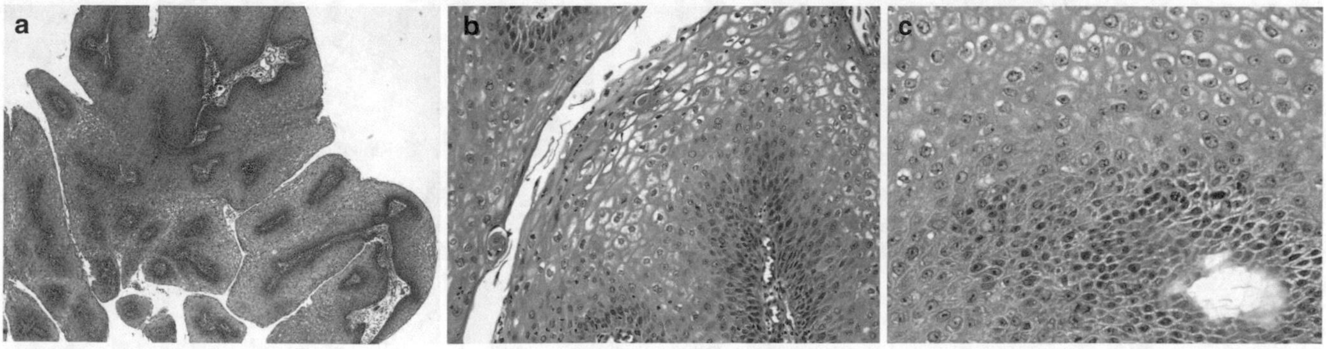

Fig. 9.29 (Case 4). Excision of an anal nodular lesion showing papillary squamous proliferation with broad fronds (**a**). Cells in the superficial layers show perinuclear halos. A few binucleated cells and dyskeratotic cells are seen. A few neutrophils are also seen in the superficial layers (**b**). A few mitotic figures are noted in the basal layers (**c**)

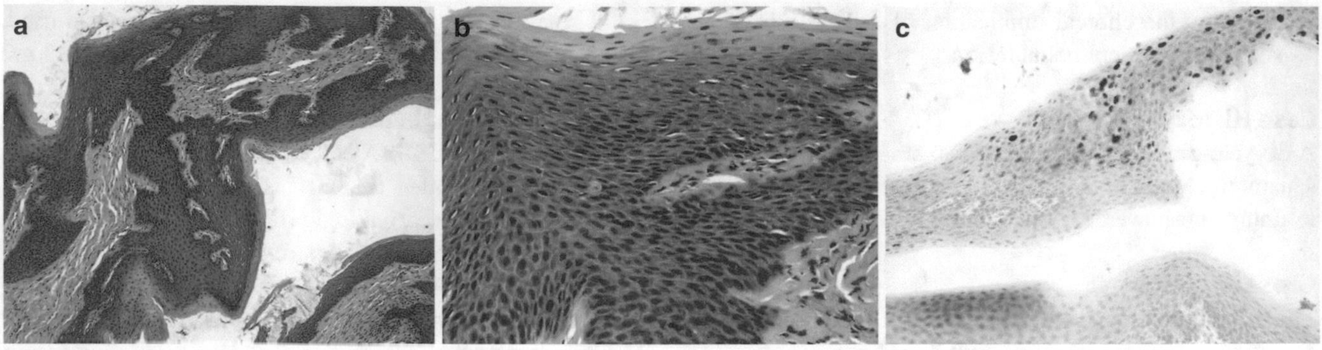

Fig. 9.30 (Discussed in case 4). Random anal biopsy from a patient with an anal condyloma status post fulguration showing squamous mucosa with parakeratosis (**a**). A few slightly atypical squamous cells are noted, but no HPV cytopathic effects are seen. No mitoses are identified (**b**). However, in situ hybridization for low-risk HPV is positive, consistent with a diagnosis of AIN1

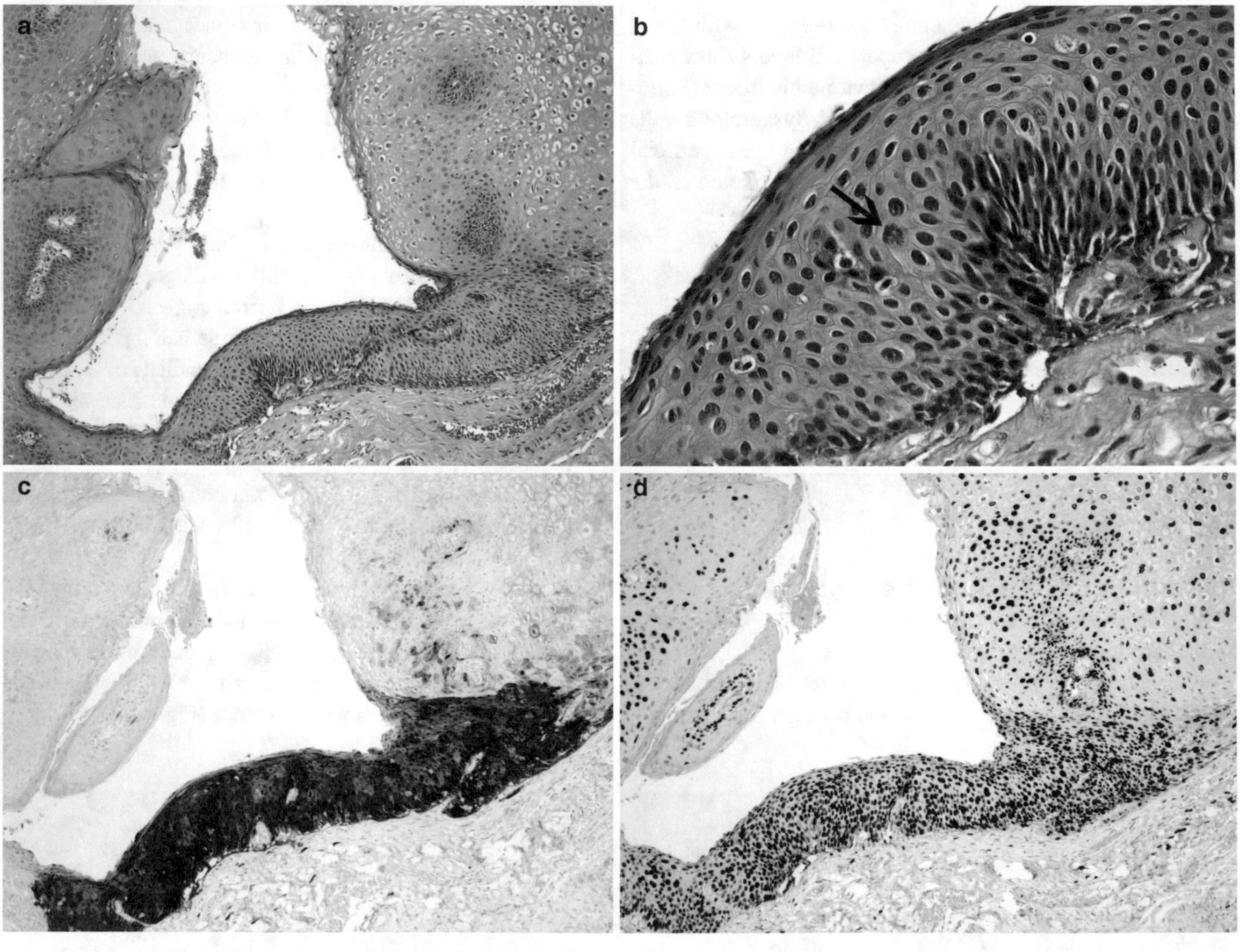

Fig. 9.31 (Discussed in case 4). A case of condyloma showing a focal area with increased nuclear density (**a**). Higher power view showing nuclear enlargement and hyperchromasia extending beyond the lower third. A mitotic figure is seen in the middle third (arrow) (**b**). Immunostain for p16 shows a strong, diffuse, and band-like pattern in this area (**c**). Diffuse Ki-67 positive cells are also demonstrated in this area, extending to the surface (**d**)

- High-grade AIN is characterized by dysplastic cells extending into the middle (AIN2) or upper (AIN3) third of the squamous epithelium. Some use AIN3 and squamous cell carcinoma in situ interchangeably, but others would split them based on whether the full thickness of the squamous epithelium is involved (i.e., if the bottom and top look the same). In our practice, we routinely call it AIN3, except when a superficial biopsy is from a mass lesion and the possibility of invasive squamous cell carcinoma cannot be assessed in the biopsy. For cases where AIN2 and AIN3 are difficult to separate, a diagnosis of AIN2–3 is appropriate, which would not change patient management.

- High-grade AIN is typically associated with high-risk HPV.
- Focal or multifocal high-grade AIN can be seen in condylomas. Mitoses may be seen in the middle or upper third. In cases where low grade and high grade are difficult to separate or when high-grade AIN is difficult to separate from immature-appearing anal transitional epithelium, immunostains for p16 and Ki-67 can be extremely helpful. A strong, diffuse, and block-like p16 staining pattern and diffuse Ki-67 positivity seen in the middle and upper thirds are essentially diagnostic of high-grade AIN (Fig. 9.31a–d). AIN1 and anal transitional epithelium either are negative for p16 or show focal/patchy weak positivity. Ki-67 positive cells are limited to the lower third for AIN1 or sparse in the bottom layers for anal transitional epithelium.

References

1. Fetissof F, Dubois MP, Assan R, et al. Endocrine cells in the anal canal. Virchows Arch A Pathol Anat Histopathol. 1984;404:39–47.
2. Clemmensen OJ, Fenger C. Melanocytes in the anal canal epithelium. Histopathology. 1991;18:237–41.
3. Shia J. An update on tumors of the anal canal. Arch Pathol Lab Med. 2010;134:1601–11.
4. Ramalingam P, Hart WR, Goldblum JR. Cytokeratin subset immunostaining in rectal adenocarcinoma and normal anal glands. Arch Pathol Lab Med. 2001;125:1074–7.
5. Fenger C. The anal transitional zone. Acta Pathol Microbiol Immunol Scand Suppl. 1987;289:1–42.
6. Welton ML, Steel SR, Goodman KA, et al. Chapter 21: Anus. In: Amin MB, et al., editors. AJCC cancer staging manual. 8th ed. New York: Springer; 2017. p. 275–84.
7. Nojkov B, Cappell MS. Gastrointestinal bleeding from Dieulafoy's lesion: clinical presentation, endoscopic findings, and endoscopic therapy. World J Gastrointest Endosc. 2015;7:295–307.
8. Dogan U, Gomceli I, Koc U, Habibi M, Bulbuller N. Rectal dieulafoy lesions: a rare etiology of chronic lower gastrointestinal bleeding. Case Rep Med. 2014;2014:180230.
9. Arnold CA, Roth R, Arsenescu R, et al. Sexually transmitted infectious colitis vs inflammatory bowel disease: distinguishing features from a case-controlled study. Am J Clin Pathol. 2015;144:771–81.
10. Beaugerie L, Carrat F, Nahon S, et al. High risk of anal and rectal cancer in patients with anal and/or perianal Crohn's disease. Clin Gastroenterol Hepatol. 2018;16:892–9. e2
11. Vuitton L, Jacquin E, Parmentier AL, et al. High prevalence of anal canal high-risk human papillomavirus infection in patients with Crohn's disease. Clin Gastroenterol Hepatol. 2018;16:1768–1776.e5.
12. Grillova L, Bawa T, Mikalova L, et al. Molecular characterization of Treponema pallidum subsp. pallidum in Switzerland and France with a new multilocus sequence typing scheme. PLoS One. 2018;13:e0200773.
13. Siegel RL, Miller KD, Jemal A. Cancer statistics, 2018. CA Cancer J Clin. 2018;68:7–30.
14. Kazakov DV, Spagnolo DV, Kacerovska D, Michal M. Lesions of anogenital mammary-like glands: an update. Adv Anat Pathol. 2011;18:1–28.
15. Parks A, Branch KD, Metcalf J, Underwood P, Young J. Hidradenoma papilliferum with mixed histopathologic features of syringocystadenoma papilliferum and anogenital mammary-like glands: report of a case and review of the literature. Am J Dermatopathol. 2012;34:104–9.
16. Compton CC. Colorectal carcinoma: diagnostic, prognostic, and molecular features. Mod Pathol. 2003;16:376–88.
17. American Joint Committe on Cancer. Vagina. In: Greene F, Page DL, Fleming ID, Fritz AG, Balch CM, Haller DG, Morrow M, editors. AJCC cancer staging manual. New York: Springer; 2002.
18. Darragh TM, Colgan TJ, Cox JT, et al. The lower Anogenital squamous terminology standardization project for HPV-associated lesions: background and consensus recommendations from the College of American Pathologists and the American Society for Colposcopy and Cervical Pathology. Arch Pathol Lab Med. 2012;136:1266–97.
19. Zidar N, Langner C, Odar K, et al. Anal verrucous carcinoma is not related to infection with human papillomaviruses and should be distinguished from giant condyloma (Buschke-Lowenstein tumour). Histopathology. 2017;70:938–45.
20. Bosman FT, Carneiro F, Hruban RH, et al., editors. WHO classificaiton of tumours of the digestive system. Lyon: IARC Press; 2010. p. 184.
21. WHO Classification of Tumours Editorial Board. WHO classificaiton of tumours of the digestive system. Lyon: IARC Press; 2019. p. 194.
22. Sink JD, Kramer SA, Copeland DD, Seigler HF. Cloacogenic carcinoma. Ann Surg. 1978;188:53–9.
23. Chetty R, Serra S, Hsieh E. Basaloid squamous carcinoma of the anal canal with an adenoid cystic pattern: histologic and immunohistochemical reappraisal of an unusual variant. Am J Surg Pathol. 2005;29:1668–72.
24. Williams GR, Talbot IC. Anal carcinoma--a histological review. Histopathology. 1994;25:507–16.
25. Shepherd NA, Scholefield JH, Love SB, England J, Northover JM. Prognostic factors in anal squamous carcinoma: a multivariate analysis of clinical, pathological and flow cytometric parameters in 235 cases. Histopathology. 1990;16:545–55.
26. Frisch M, Fenger C, van den Brule AJ, et al. Variants of squamous cell carcinoma of the anal canal and perianal skin and their relation to human papillomaviruses. Cancer Res. 1999;59:753–7.
27. Gill PS, Wong N. Primary peri-anal adenocarcinoma of intestinal type - a new proposed entity. Histopathology. 2018;73:157–61.
28. Patil DT, Goldblum JR, Billings SD. Clinicopathological analysis of basal cell carcinoma of the anal region and its distinction from basaloid squamous cell carcinoma. Mod Pathol. 2013;26:1382–9.
29. Bala R, Pinsky BA, Beck AH, et al. p16 is superior to ProEx C in identifying high-grade squamous intraepithelial lesions (HSIL) of the anal canal. Am J Surg Pathol. 2013;37:659–68.
30. Fiedler U, Christian S, Koidl S, et al. The sialomucin CD34 is a marker of lymphatic endothelial cells in human tumors. Am J Pathol. 2006;168:1045–53.
31. Minicozzi A, Borzellino G, Momo R, et al. Perianal Paget's disease: presentation of six cases and literature review. Int J Color Dis. 2010;25:1–7.
32. Chumbalkar V, Jennings TA, Ainechi S, Lee EC, Lee H. Extramammary Paget's disease of anal canal associated with rectal adenoma without invasive carcinoma. Gastroenterology Res. 2016;9:99–102.
33. Guler ML, Daniels JA, Abraham SC, Montgomery EA. Expression of melanoma antigens in epithelioid gastrointestinal stromal tumors: a potential diagnostic pitfall. Arch Pathol Lab Med. 2008;132:1302–6.

Infections of the Gastrointestinal Tract

10

Michael Bachman and Laura W. Lamps

List of Frequently Asked Questions

1. How reliable is a PCR result obtained from formalin-fixed, paraffin-embedded tissue blocks for the diagnosis of infections?
2. What GI infections are most likely to mimic other commonly encountered GI diseases, such as chronic idiopathic IBD, celiac disease, and ischemia?
3. What are the most common pathogens that are superimposed on chronic idiopathic IBD, and what is the clinical significance?
4. How well are plasma CMV PCR results, tissue CMV PCR results, and CMV inclusions identified in tissue correlated?
5. What are the best ways to differentiate between the different viruses commonly encountered in surgical pathology?
6. What are the most common infectious manifestations of AIDS in the GI tract?
7. What are the best ways to confirm high-risk HPV infection in the anus, and what are the clinical implications?
8. What are the best ways to differentiate between the different fungi that are commonly encountered in surgical pathology?
9. What are the best methodologies for diagnosing Helicobacter pylori infection, and how are drug-resistant organisms detected and managed?
10. What are the best ways to diagnose Whipple disease?
11. What are the best ways to diagnose mycobacterial infection in the GI tract and to distinguish tubercular from non-tubercular mycobacteria?
12. What is the best way to distinguish chronic idiopathic IBD from sexually transmitted infectious mimics?
13. What are the best ways to diagnose intestinal spirochetosis, and what is the clinical significance?
14. What is the clinical significance of a positive result with a stool PCR assay, and how does that correlate with biopsy findings?
15. What are the most commonly encountered causes of antibiotic-associated injury other than C. difficile, and what are the best ways to diagnose them?
16. How do the different laboratory methodologies for the diagnosis of C. difficile correlate with clinical scenario and biopsy findings?
17. What are the best morphologic and laboratory methods for distinguishing between commonly encountered protozoa in the GI tract?
18. What are clinically significant helminths, and how are they distinguished?

Frequently Asked Questions

1. How reliable is a PCR result obtained from formalin-fixed, paraffin-embedded tissue blocks for the diagnosis of infections?

The use of polymerase chain reaction (PCR)-based assays to detect pathogens in formalin-fixed, routinely processed, paraffin-embedded (FFPE) tissue specimens poses many challenges. Formalin fixation itself enhances DNA degradation and inhibits DNA amplification. It has been reported that fixation times of less than 24 h are optimal, a goal that may not be possible to meet in routine laboratories. Degradation of DNA also appears to increase if the specimen is fixed at room temperature (which most are) and with length of time of block storage. Fixatives other than formalin (such as mercuric or picric acid-based fixatives) may even further limit DNA yield.

There are no generally accepted recommendations that guide laboratories regarding fixation, processing, and

M. Bachman · L. W. Lamps (✉)
University of Michigan, Ann Arbor, MI, USA
e-mail: lwlamps@med.umich.edu

H. L. Wang, Z. E. Chen (eds.), *Practical Gastrointestinal Pathology*, Practical Anatomic Pathology,
https://doi.org/10.1007/978-3-030-51268-2_10

extraction techniques for FFPE tissue. Commercial extraction kits are usually designed for use on fresh or frozen specimens and may not be able to adequately handle the tiny quantities of DNA present in many mucosal biopsy specimens. The lesional tissue in small specimens may also be exhausted by the time they are subjected to molecular analysis (particularly if many stains are performed), and thus, sampling error may cause a negative result even when the patient truly has an infection. Conversely, specimen contamination with bacteria, yeasts, and molds that exist widely in nature may also pose a problem with false-positive results.

The success of PCR-based assays in FFPE tissue samples also appears to vary with the target and the specific assay used. Variation in the assay used, as well as the extremely wide range of sample types and study sizes in the literature, makes accurate assessment of sensitivity and specificity for any individual pathogen difficult.

In terms of the use of PCR to detect viruses in FFPE specimens, attempts to detect high-risk human papillomavirus (HPV) in head and neck squamous cell carcinomas have been quite successful using commercial assays, with a reported 100% sensitivity and 91% specificity. Similarly, attempts to detect cytomegalovirus (CMV) in FFPE gastrointestinal (GI) biopsies have also been successful, with a reported sensitivity of 96% and specificity of 98%.

Detection of fungi in FFPE tissue using pan-fungal assays with sequencing has been more challenging, with one recent study reporting a sensitivity of 53% and specificity of 65%; interestingly, the sensitivity was higher when yeasts were the target and lower when attempting to detect filamentous fungi. The sensitivity and specificity using various PCR assays in detecting tubercular and non-tubercular mycobacteria have varied, with reported sensitivities of 70–87% and specificities of 95–100% for *Mycobacterium tuberculosis* and 35–50% and 96–100% for non-tubercular mycobacteria, respectively. Sensitivity improved when organisms were seen on special stains, as one would expect.

Application of molecular technology, while often invaluable, must be done with the knowledge (by both pathologists and clinicians) of the limitations of the test. As with all ancillary testing, the result of a PCR assay must be correlated with the histologic findings, as well as the available clinical and laboratory data. Although technology continues to improve, the use of PCR-based assays in FFPE specimens remains challenging, and when possible, it is always a good idea to attempt to preserve fresh or frozen tissue for both molecular studies and microbial culture techniques.

References: [1–6]

2. **What GI infections are most likely to mimic other commonly encountered GI diseases, such as chronic idiopathic IBD, celiac disease, and ischemia?**

Surgical pathologists should be aware of GI infections that mimic other commonly encountered GI diseases, such as chronic idiopathic inflammatory bowel disease (IBD), ischemic colitis, and celiac disease. These infections and the diseases that they mimic are summarized in Table 10.1.

Patients who undergo endoscopic evaluation and biopsy generally have unusual clinical features such as chronic or debilitating diarrhea, evidence of systemic disease, or a history of immunocompromise. One of the most valuable (and least expensive) diagnostic aids for the pathologist is review of the medical record and/or a discussion with the gastroenterologist regarding duration of symptoms, colonoscopic findings, travel history, food intake history (such as sushi or poorly cooked meat), sexual practices, and immune status.

- *Infections that mimic chronic idiopathic inflammatory bowel disease.*

The infections that are most likely to mimic IBD include those caused by food-borne and waterborne pathogens *Salmonella*, *Shigella*, *Yersinia*, *Campylobacter*, and *Aeromonas* species (Table 10.2) and the sexually acquired pathogens of syphilis and lymphogranuloma venereum (LGV) (see later section). In general, these pathogens mimic IBD histologically because they cause architectural distortion, basal plasmacytosis, or granulomas and endoscopically because of the distribution and appearance of the mucosa.

Table 10.1 Infections that can mimic chronic idiopathic inflammatory bowel disease, celiac disease, and ischemic colitis

Mimics of Crohn disease	Mimics of ulcerative colitis	Mimics of ischemic colitis	Mimics of celiac disease
Salmonella typhimurium	*Shigella* species	Enterohemorrhagic *Escherichia coli*	HIV-associated enteritis
Shigella species	Non-typhoid *Salmonella* species	*Clostridium difficile* (pseudomembranous colitis)	Coccidians
Yersinia	*Aeromonas* species	*Clostridium perfringens*	Viral gastroenteritis
Mycobacterium tuberculosis	*Campylobacter* (rarely)		
Aeromonas species	Lymphogranuloma venereum		
Campylobacter (rarely)	Syphilis		

Table 10.2 Infections most likely to mimic chronic idiopathic inflammatory bowel disease

	Aeromonas	*Campylobacter*	*Salmonella* (typhoid)	*Salmonella* (non-typhoid)	*Shigella*	*Yersinia*
Acquisition	Food and water, particularly pond water	Food and water, particularly undercooked meat	Food and water, particularly where sanitation is poor	Food and water, particularly where sanitation is poor	Food and water, particularly where sanitation is poor	Meat, especially undercooked pork; dairy products; water
Macroscopic findings that mimic IBD	Segmental disease; mucosal ulceration	Erythema, ulcers, friability, hemorrhage	Ileocecal involvement; thickened wall, aphthous ulcers	Mucosal friability, erythema	Pancolitis initially; patchier distribution as it resolves. Variably present with pseudomembranes and ulcers	Thick, edematous wall with aphthous ulcers centered on Peyer patches. Ileum and right colon most often involved
Pertinent histologic features	Usually AITC; focal architectural distortion	Usually AITC; architectural distortion rare	Architectural distortion, mononuclear infiltrate	Usually AITC; occasionally architectural distortion	Most severe in rectum. Early AITC; marked architectural distortion with resolution. Pseudomembranes may be seen	Transmural inflammation, granulomas, ulcers, mural fibrosis

IBD inflammatory bowel disease, *AITC* acute infectious type colitis

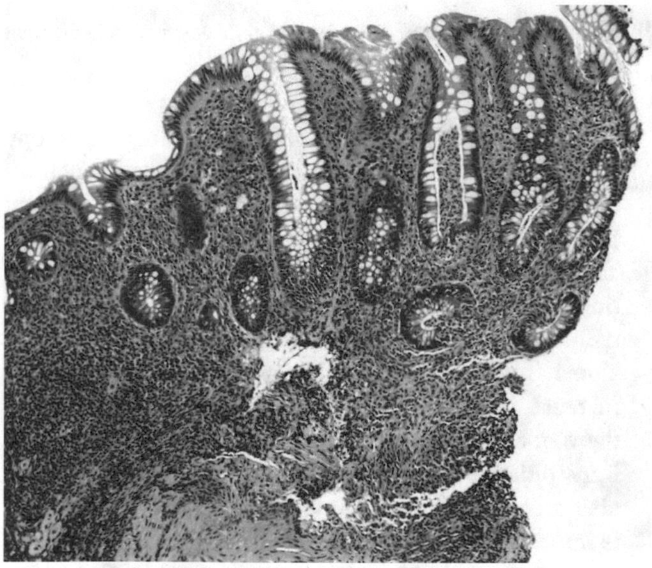

Fig. 10.1 *Aeromonas* colitis. Ileocecal valve biopsy shows active colitis in a background of mild architectural distortion and basal plasmacytosis. The right colon segmental distribution mimicked Crohn disease macroscopically

- *Aeromonas* (Fig. 10.1) species are increasingly recognized as causes of gastroenteritis in humans. Children are most commonly affected, and most frequently present in the late spring, summer, and early fall. A mild self-limited diarrheal illness is most common, but a more severe, dysentery-like illness occurs in 15–25% of patients, which is most likely to mimic IBD endoscopically.

Campylobacter species are a major cause of diarrhea worldwide and remain the most common stool isolate in the United States. *Campylobacter jejuni* is most commonly associated with food-borne gastroenteritis; *C. fetus* and the other less common species are more often seen in immunosuppressed patients and homosexual men. The incidence of this infection in HIV-positive patients is higher than that in the general population, and severe, chronic, recurrent, or disseminated infections are more common in this group. Symptoms generally resolve within 1–2 weeks, but relapse is common.

The majority of clinically important *Salmonella* (Fig. 10.2a, b) are in the species *S. enterica,* and are differentiated by serotyping. They are an important cause of both food poisoning and traveler's diarrhea. The discussion of *Salmonella* infection is generally divided into typhoid and non-typhoid serovars. Enteric (typhoid) fever is usually caused by *S.* Typhi, but may also be associated with *S.* Paratyphi. Non-typhoid serovars that are likely to cause infection include *S.* Enteritidis, *S.* Typhimurium, and *S.* Muenchen, among others. Historically, enteric fever was considered to be a much more severe disease than non-typhoid salmonellosis, but more recent literature suggests a greater degree of overlap both clinically and pathologically.

Shigella are virulent, invasive Gram-negative bacilli that are a major cause of infectious diarrhea worldwide. Shigellosis is most common in developing countries where sanitation is poor. Children under the age of 6 years are commonly affected, as are homosexual males and debilitated patients. Constitutional symptoms are the earliest manifestation, including abdominal pain, malaise, and fever, accompanied by diarrhea.

Yersinia (Fig. 10.3) is one of the most common causes of bacterial enteritis in Western and Northern Europe, and numerous cases have been documented in

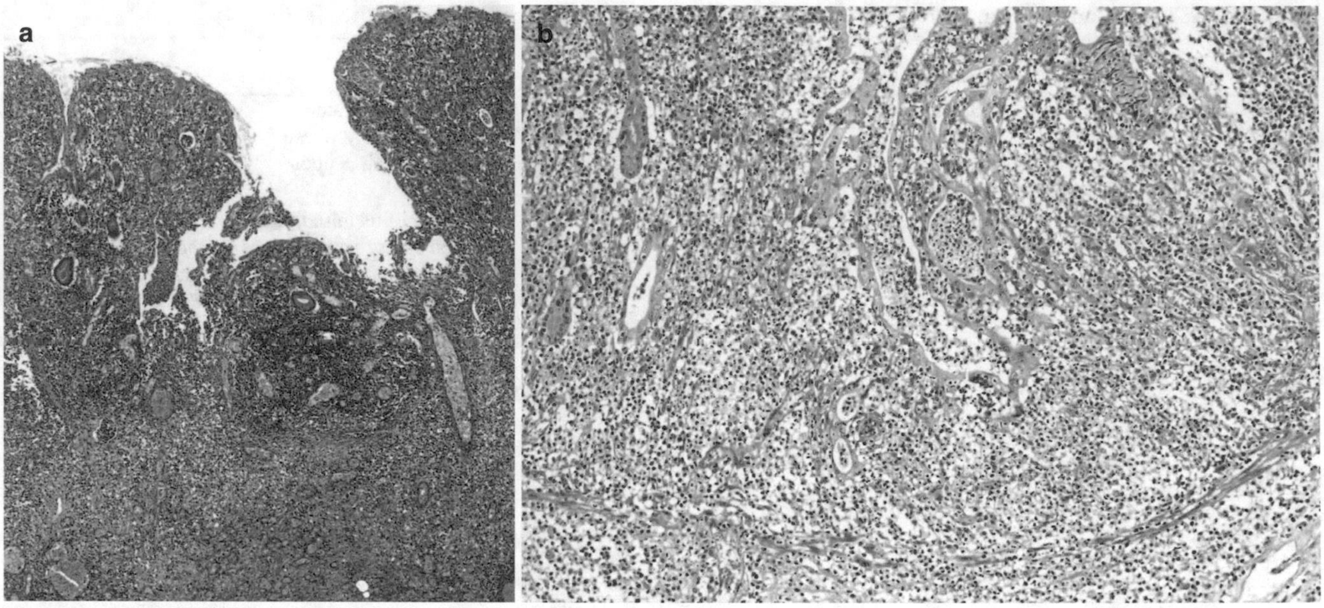

Fig. 10.2 *Salmonella* enterocolitis. Aphthous ulcer in the ileocecal valve (**a**) and marked architectural distortion and crypt destruction in the right colon (**b**) can mimic chronic idiopathic inflammatory bowel disease

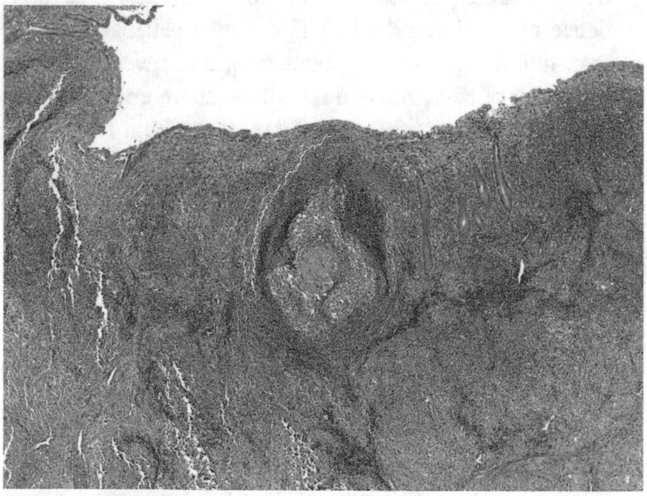

Fig. 10.3 *Yersinia* colitis. Features such as marked thickening of the wall, mucosal ulceration, granulomas, and prominent lymphoid follicles can mimic Crohn disease

North America and Australia. *Yersinia enterocolitica* and *Y. pseudotuberculosis* are the two species that cause human GI disease. Immunocompromised and debilitated patients, as well as patients on deferoxamine or with iron overload due to other causes, are at particular risk of serious disease. Crohn disease and yersiniosis may be very difficult, if not impossible, to distinguish from one another histologically. Features that may favor Crohn disease include cobblestoning of mucosa and creeping fat grossly, and changes of chronicity microscopically including crypt distortion, thickening of the muscularis mucosae, and prominent neural hyperplasia.

Since most patients do not present for endoscopy until several weeks after the onset of symptoms, pathologists are less and less frequently exposed to the typical histologic features of acute infectious enterocolitis. This is important, because the resolving phase of infection is more challenging to diagnose. At this stage, mononuclear cells often predominate, with only occasional foci of neutrophilic cryptitis and a patchy increase in lamina propria inflammation; in addition, there may be abundant plasma cells and increased intraepithelial lymphocytes. Since these features are also seen in Crohn disease and in lymphocytic colitis, it is important to be aware of the duration of the patient's symptoms, and, ideally, the culture or PCR results, because a specific diagnosis may be difficult to determine on histologic grounds alone.

- *Infections that mimic ischemia.* The enterohemorrhagic or Shiga-toxin-producing Escherichia coli (EHEC or STEC) are the bacteria that most frequently cause infections that mimic ischemia (Fig. 10.4a, b). The most common strain of enterohemorrhagic *E. coli* is 0157:H7. The bacteria adhere to intestinal epithelial cells and produce a cytotoxin similar to that produced by *Shigella dysenteriae*; however, unlike *S. dysenteriae*, there is no tissue invasion. Although contaminated meat is the most frequent mode of transmission, infection may also occur through contaminated water, milk, produce, and person-to-person contact. Characteristic symptoms include bloody diarrhea and severe abdominal cramps. The fact that fever is mild or absent and that only one-third of patients have fecal

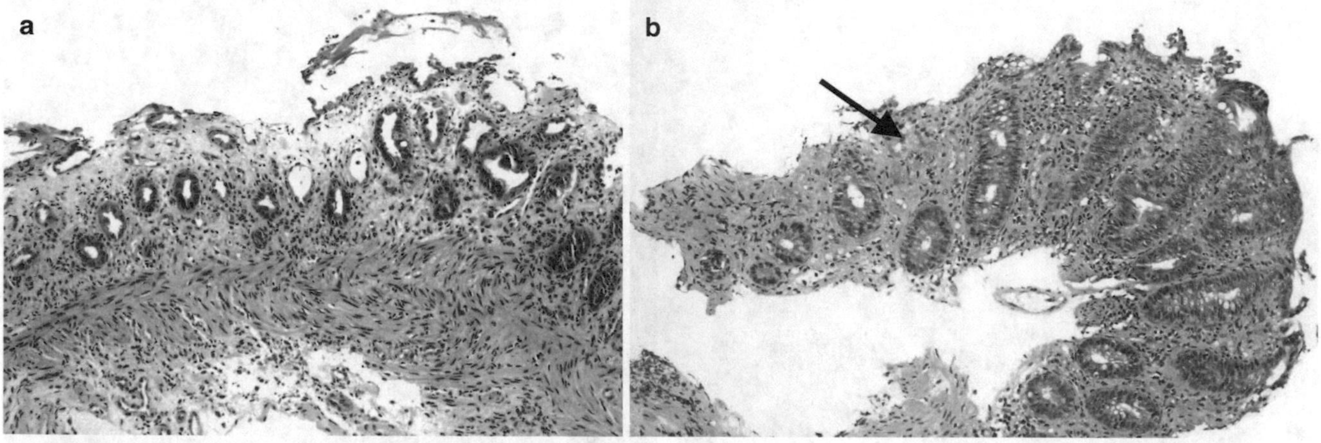

Fig. 10.4 Enterohemorrhagic *E. coli*-associated colitis. Lamina propria hyalinization and crypt withering mimic ischemic colitis in this biopsy from the right colon (**a**). Fibrin thrombi (arrow) may be prominent (**b**)

leukocytes may cause a confusing clinical picture. Infected patients are at risk for the hemolytic–uremic syndrome or thrombotic thrombocytopenic purpura, particularly children and the elderly.

Endoscopically, the right side of the colon is typically more severely affected, which is unusual for ischemic colitis. Edema is common, which may be so severe as to cause obstruction; erosions, ulcers, and hemorrhage are also commonly seen. The histologic features are typical of ischemic colitis, as the cytotoxin is postulated to induce an ischemic insult. Findings include marked edema and hemorrhage in the lamina propria and submucosa, with associated mucosal neutrophils, crypt withering, and necrosis. Microthrombi may be seen within small vessels, and pseudomembranes are rarely present.

Clostridium difficile may also produce histologic changes that mimic ischemia. A hyalinized lamina propria favors the diagnosis of ischemia, and dilated crypts with an "exploding" or "volcanic" exudate, as well as intercrypt necrosis, favors *C. difficile*. Endoscopically, pseudomembrane formation is more common in *C. difficile* infection, whereas the presence of a polypoid or mass lesion is more indicative of ischemia.

- *Infections that mimic celiac disease*. Many different infections can cause villous blunting and increased intraepithelial lymphocytes, including viral gastroenteritis, HIV-associated enteropathy, and infection by coccidians. Clinical history and laboratory studies are often the most useful in distinguishing these from celiac disease. HIV-associated enteropathy and viral infection are more likely to have increased apoptotic enterocytes, and organisms can often be found in coccidial infection after a dedicated search and/or the use of special stains.

The detection of pathogens that can mimic other commonly encountered GI diseases has become easier with the development of multiplex PCR assays. A number of Food and Drug Administration (FDA)-cleared assays are available (e.g., xTAG Gastrointestinal Pathogen Panel and VERIGENE Enteric Pathogens Test, Luminex, Austin, Texas; BioFire FilmArray Gastrointestinal Panel, Biofire, Salt Lake City, Utah) that can detect a combination of bacteria, viruses, and parasites (as many as 22 pathogens) in as little as an hour. These assays target epidemiologically common causes of acute gastroenteritis, such as *Salmonella*, *Shigella*, *Campylobacter*, *Giardia*, *Cryptosporidum*, and Norovirus. Some assays target the virulence genes of these pathogens, such as the stx1/stx2 genes produced by *E. coli* O157:H7 and other EHEC strains, whereas others target genes conserved at the species level. The required specimen is typically stool in Cary–Blair preservative. As these tests are used to diagnose gastroenteritis, the laboratory will expect a liquid specimen and may routinely reject formed stools as inappropriate for testing.

Multiplex molecular assays are expensive, however, and targets vary by manufacturer and are not exhaustive. For these reasons, traditional culture methods remain appropriate in some cases. Routine stool cultures on selective and differential media can be used to detect *Salmonella* and *Shigella*. *Campylobacter* can be cultured on selective media at 42 °C in microaerophilic conditions (5% O_2, 10% CO_2, 85% N_2), which can be achieved either by single-use gas pack bags or specialized incubators. *Yersinia* can be grown on routine or selective Cefsulodin-Irgasan-Novobiocin (CIN) agar, but requires incubation at 25 °C for optimal recovery. *Aeromonas* can also be recovered on routine agar from stool cultures or recovered on CIN agar at 25 °C along with *Yersinia*.

Selective Sorbital-MacConkey agar can be used to detect *E. coli* 0157:H7 but will not detect other EHEC serotypes. Other serotypes can, however, be detected by

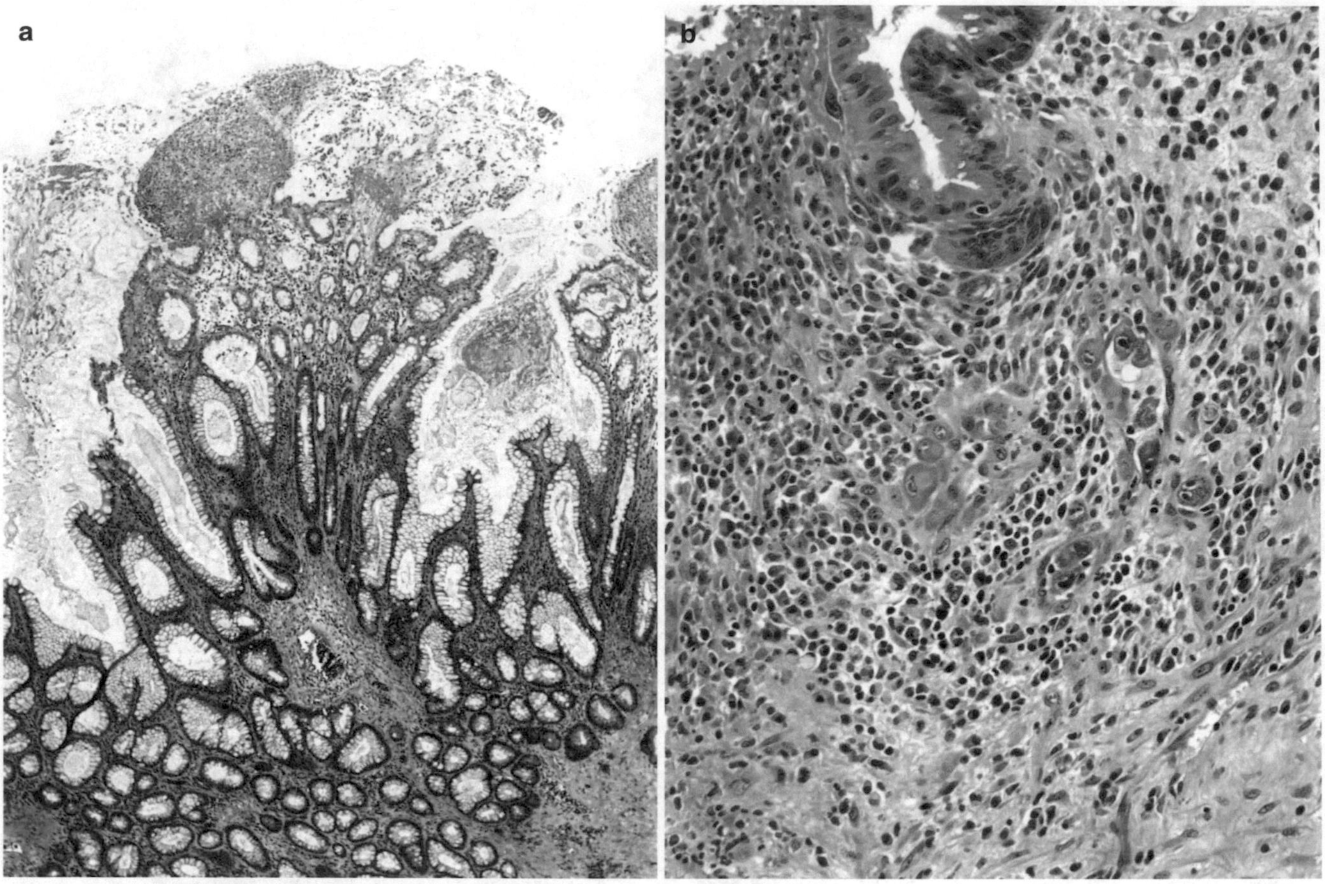

Fig. 10.5 This patient with ulcerative colitis has superimposed *C. difficile* infection (**a**) as well as CMV (**b**). Note the crypt architectural distortion characteristic of ulcerative colitis, and the overlying pseudomembrane typical of *C. difficile*. The CMV inclusions are present within endothelial cells

immunoassays for the shigatoxins or by some of the multiplex molecular assays above. An immunohistochemical stain for this organism has also been described, but is not widely available and opinions vary on its usefulness.

Stool culture for *M. tuberculosis* may be available in laboratories with biosafety protections in place for this pathogen. Diagnosis of *C. difficile* infection presents numerous challenges since approaches vary in terms of sensitivity and specificity for disease. The Infectious Diseases Society of America recommend a combination of antigen testing for toxin and detection of *C. difficile* by antigen or nucleic acid amplification test (NAAT), where having both positive are consistent with infection (see section below).

References: [7–15]

3. **What are the most common pathogens that are superimposed on chronic idiopathic IBD, and what is the clinical significance?**

A number of pathogens can superinfect patients with ulcerative colitis and Crohn disease, often with significant clinical implications. In IBD patients who are experiencing flares, the prevalence of *C. difficile* infection is much higher than that in patients with inactive IBD or without IBD. The use of steroids and immunomodulators is independently associated with the development of *C. difficile* infection as well. Recurrent *C. difficile* infection is common in this population, and hospitalization is not infrequent. Interestingly, biopsies may not show the classic findings of pseudomembranous colitis typically seen in non-IBD patients.

The association between CMV and IBD has been recognized for decades, although the clinical significance remains a subject of debate. CMV infection is associated with steroids and immunomodulators, but not tumor necrosis factor agonists. CMV infection has also been associated with a more severe course of disease, although this remains somewhat controversial. Crohn disease patients seem to be less affected by CMV superinfection. Interestingly, *C. difficile* is more common in IBD patients with CMV infection, and the combination is associated with poor outcomes (Fig. 10.5a, b).

Other infections that have been described in the context of IBD patients, especially those on long-term immunosuppression, include tuberculosis, *C. jejuni*, and

Epstein–Barr virus. Of note, primary EBV infection is considered to be a risk factor for the development of lymphoproliferative disorders in patients treated with thiopurines.
References: [16–25]

4. **How well are plasma CMV PCR results, tissue CMV PCR results, and CMV inclusions identified in tissue correlated?**

In patients infected with CMV, the GI tract can be a site of both asymptomatic shedding and tissue-invasive disease. The risk of invasive disease is greatest in immunocompromised patients, including solid organ and hematopoietic stem cell recipients, HIV-positive patients, and those on immunomodulatory drugs. Immunosuppression can increase asymptomatic shedding as well as the risk of invasive disease; therefore, the goal of diagnostic testing is to distinguish between these two viral processes.

In the setting of suspected invasive disease in the GI tract, there are two types of samples with diagnostic value: plasma and GI biopsy tissue. PCR can be performed on both types of samples, whereas viral culture, histology, and immunohistochemistry (IHC) can be performed only on biopsy tissue. However, the two approaches differ in their ability to detect tissue-invasive disease with the necessary sensitivity and specificity.

Quantitative plasma CMV PCR is used to detect viremia and to measure the viral load in the blood of infected patients. There are now multiple FDA-approved assays and an international standard against which these assays can be calibrated. These assays are most useful in detecting changes in viral load over time because an increase may indicate CMV infection with an associated viral syndrome or invasive disease. Currently, there are no established thresholds that are diagnostic of invasive CMV infection, and patients with latent infections may have baseline viral loads that vary over time.

For HIV-positive patients, the correlation between plasma PCR and invasive GI disease is poor, with both a low positive predictive value and insufficient negative predictive value. In solid organ transplant recipients, the correlation is better, but depends on the serologic status of the donor and recipient; although overall, the assay is 85% sensitive and 95% specific, it is only 72% sensitive in CMV donor-positive/recipient-positive patients. Therefore, plasma PCR is a useful adjunctive test, but it cannot completely exclude or confirm GI CMV infection. An important caveat is that most of these data are based on older generations of PCR assays; as analytical sensitivities improve with newer assays, it may be valuable to reassess the corresponding clinical sensitivity.

Histology and detection of the characteristic inclusions remain the gold standard for diagnosing GI tissue-invasive disease. However, the number of inclusions that indicate clinically significant disease remains controversial, and the presence of CMV inclusions in a tissue biopsy does not necessarily correlate with plasma PCR results or viral culture. Culture and PCR from biopsy tissue both have high sensitivity but low specificity, as they can detect both shedding virus and true disease. This is especially true in HIV-positive patients, where cultures can be positive without any clinical evidence of disease in patients with low CD4 counts.

In immunocompromised patients, even isolated CMV inclusions can indicate clinically significant disease, and the lack of plasma PCR positivity does not diminish the significance of rare inclusions. It is also important to note that the higher the number of biopsies obtained, the greater the likelihood of finding inclusions. In one study, 11 biopsies in ulcerative colitis and 16 in Crohn disease were required to achieve an 80% probability of a CMV positive biopsy. This number of biopsies is rarely achieved in routine clinical practice.

The need for CMV IHC in these cases also remains a subject of debate. Recent studies have supported the use of IHC in a supporting role, when no inclusions are found, or when suspicious cells that need confirmation by IHC are found. These studies have argued against clinician-initiated or “up-front” ordering. In a review of cases that were positive for CMV IHC, the relative sensitivity of finding inclusions without IHC was 75%, and specificity was 98%. Although IHC may be useful in cases with only rare inclusions, or no definite inclusions, this study indicated that there was no change in clinical management based on this low-level detection of CMV. In summary, the diagnosis of clinically significant CMV infection remains dependent upon careful correlation between clinical, histologic, and laboratory information.
References: [26–32]

5. **What are the best ways to differentiate between the different viruses commonly encountered in surgical pathology?**

The viruses that are most commonly encountered in GI pathology are CMV, herpes simplex virus (HSV), adenovirus, and varicella zoster (Table 10.3). The histologic spectrum of CMV infection is extremely variable, ranging from minimal inflammation to deep ulcers with prominent granulation tissue and necrosis. Histologic features may include a mixed inflammatory infiltrate typically with numerous neutrophils, cryptitis of glandular epithelium, crypt abscesses, crypt atrophy and loss, and numerous apoptotic enterocytes. Prominent aggregates of macrophages may surround viral inclusions within the inflammatory infiltrate and sometimes in a perivascular distribution within granulation tissue.

Table 10.3 Histologic comparison of commonly encountered viral infections

	CMV	Adenovirus	HSV/VZV
Cell involved	Stromal and endothelial cells; macrophages; rarely epithelial cells	Epithelial only Predominantly surface Predominantly goblet cells in the colon	Epithelial cells, usually squamous
Location of inclusion	Nucleus and cytoplasm	Exclusively intranuclear	Intranuclear
Characteristics of inclusion	"Owl's eye" morphology in nucleus; basophilic and granular in cytoplasm	Basophilic "smudge cell" filling entire nucleus most common; rarely acidophilic inclusions with halos	Homogeneous with "ground glass" appearance or acidophilic with clear halo and peripheral chromatin margination
Associated changes	Cellular enlargement Apoptosis Mixed inflammatory infiltrate Vasculitis	Surface cell disorder, loss of orientation, degeneration; cells not enlarged	Sloughing of epithelial cells, neutrophilic infiltrate; multinucleated cells common

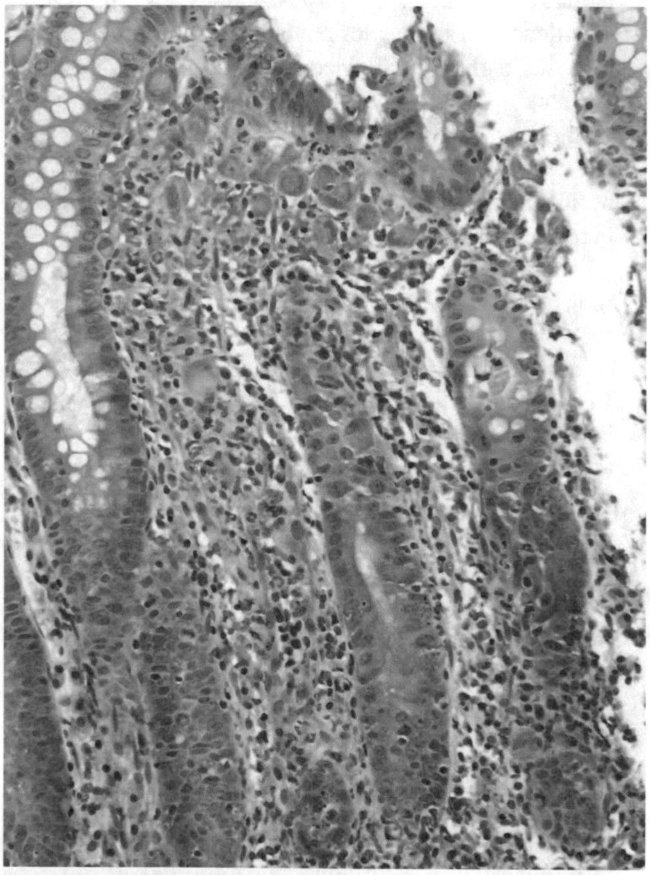

Fig. 10.6 CMV colitis. Numerous CMV inclusions, both "owl's eye" and granular, are present, primarily within stromal cells and endothelial cells

Inclusions with virtually no associated inflammatory reaction may occur in severely immunocompromised patients.

Infected cells show both nuclear and cytoplasmic enlargement (Fig. 10.6), hence the name "cytomegalovirus." Intranuclear inclusions have the characteristic "owl's eye" appearance, whereas cytoplasmic inclusions are basophilic and granular. Inclusions are usually found in endothelial cells, stromal cells, and macrophages, and rarely in epithelial cells. In addition, unlike adenovirus and herpes, CMV inclusions are often found deep within ulcer bases rather than at the edges of ulcers or in the superficial mucosa. An exception to this rule is the fact that prominent CMV inclusions with minimal inflammatory response may be seen in the glandular cells of the stomach.

The histologic features of HSV-1 and HSV-2 infections are indistinguishable. Histologic findings, regardless of site, include ulceration; acantholytic, sloughed epithelial cells; and a neutrophilic infiltrate (Fig. 10.7a–d). Similar to CMV, prominent aggregates of macrophages may be seen within the inflammatory exudate as well. The best place to search for HSV inclusions is within the squamous epithelium at the edges of ulcers and in sloughed epithelial cells within the exudate. There are two types of nuclear inclusions: the characteristic homogenous "ground glass" inclusion and the much rarer acidophilic Cowdry type A inclusion with a surrounding clear halo and peripheral chromatin margination. Inclusions may be single or multinucleate. Herpes zoster/varicella, which may rarely infect the GI tract, produces lesions and inclusions identical to HSV, but patients more often present with rashes.

Adenovirus infection of the tubal gut (Fig. 10.8a, b) is often associated with degenerative changes of the surface epithelium, such as epithelial cell disorder, loss of cell orientation (especially goblet cells), apoptosis, and sloughing of epithelial cells. Mild villous blunting may be seen in the small bowel. Adenovirus inclusions, known as "smudge cells," are exclusively intranuclear and fill the entire nucleus, but the cell itself is not enlarged. They have enlarged, basophilic nuclei without a clear nuclear membrane. Inclusions are usually present within surface epithelial cells, particularly goblet cells, in which they are often crescent-shaped; they are only rarely seen within crypts.

IHC, which is widely commercially available, is very useful in distinguishing between these viruses. PCR assays are also available, although it may be difficult to distinguish active disease from viral shedding based on PCR results alone. As described in the section above on

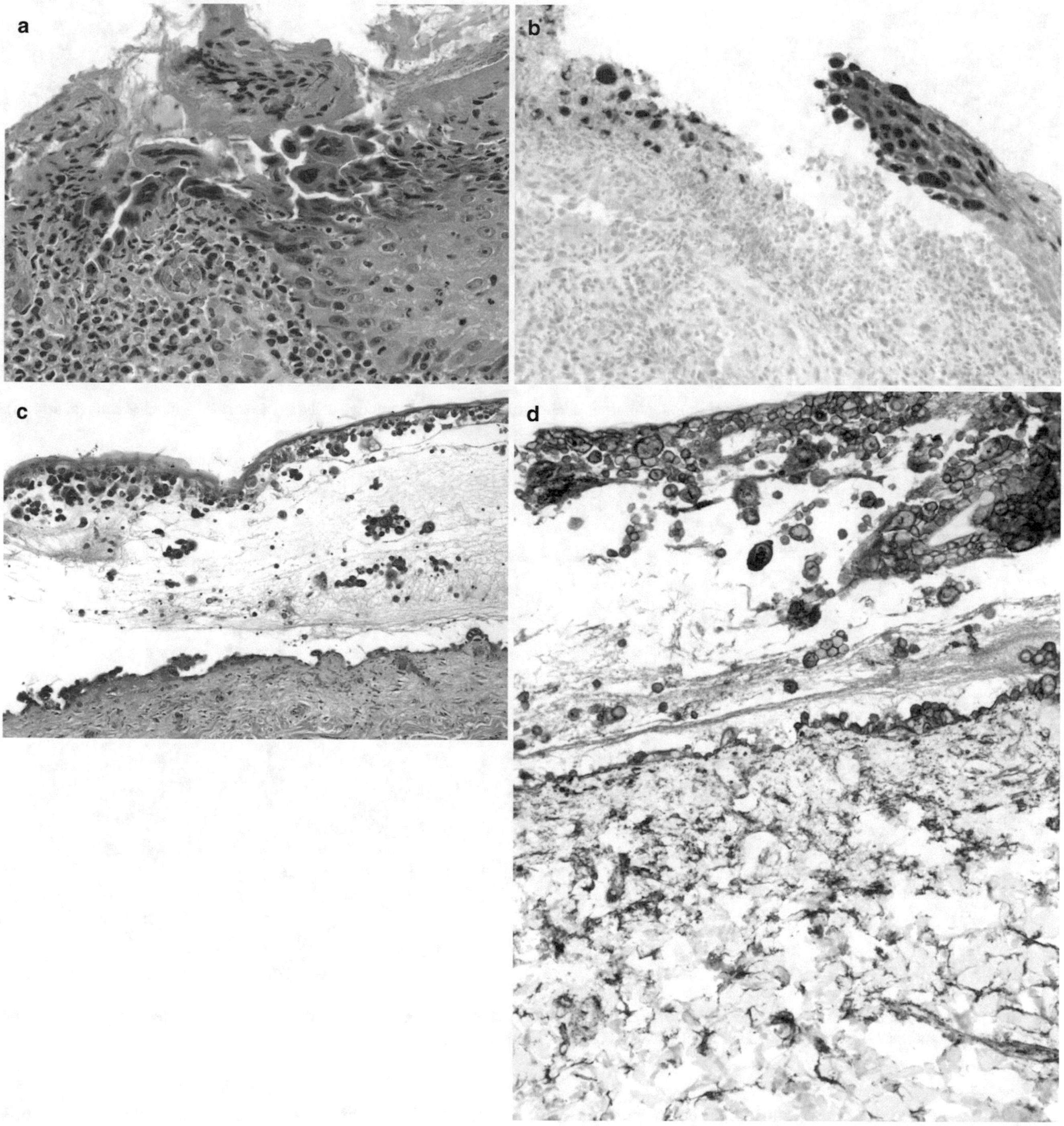

Fig. 10.7 Anal herpes simplex virus. Typical "ground glass" herpetic inclusions have associated acute inflammation and acantholytic squamous epithelial cells (**a**). IHC for HSV highlights the inclusions (**b**). The VZV inclusions are virtually indistinguishable from HSV on H&E (**c**), and IHC for VZV is required for differentiation (**d**)

CMV, the detection of characteristic inclusions in tissue is the most specific way to diagnose tissue-invasive disease.

For HSV, there are a number of PCR assays available that detect and differentiate between HSV-1 and -2, and some laboratories have validated these assays on tissue biopsies in addition to swabs from mucocutaneous tissue. Viral culture for HSV is also still widely available. Serology has little value in diagnosing the cause of a lesion suspected of HSV or CMV infection, as it will be positive in patients latently infected with the virus as well as in those with active infection. For adenovirus, the types most commonly associated with gastroenteritis are 40 and 41, although other types have been associated with diarrhea in case control studies. Most commercial PCR

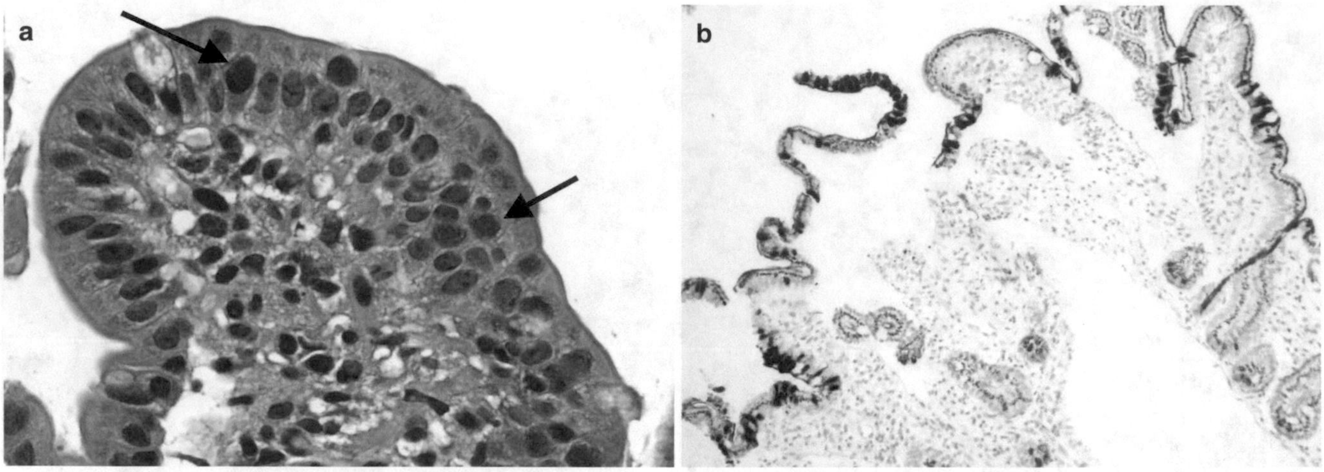

Fig. 10.8 Adenovirus. This small bowel biopsy shows numerous adenovirus inclusions, or smudge cells, in the surface epithelial cells (**a**, arrows). IHC helps to confirm the diagnosis (**b**, courtesy Dr. Maria Westerhoff)

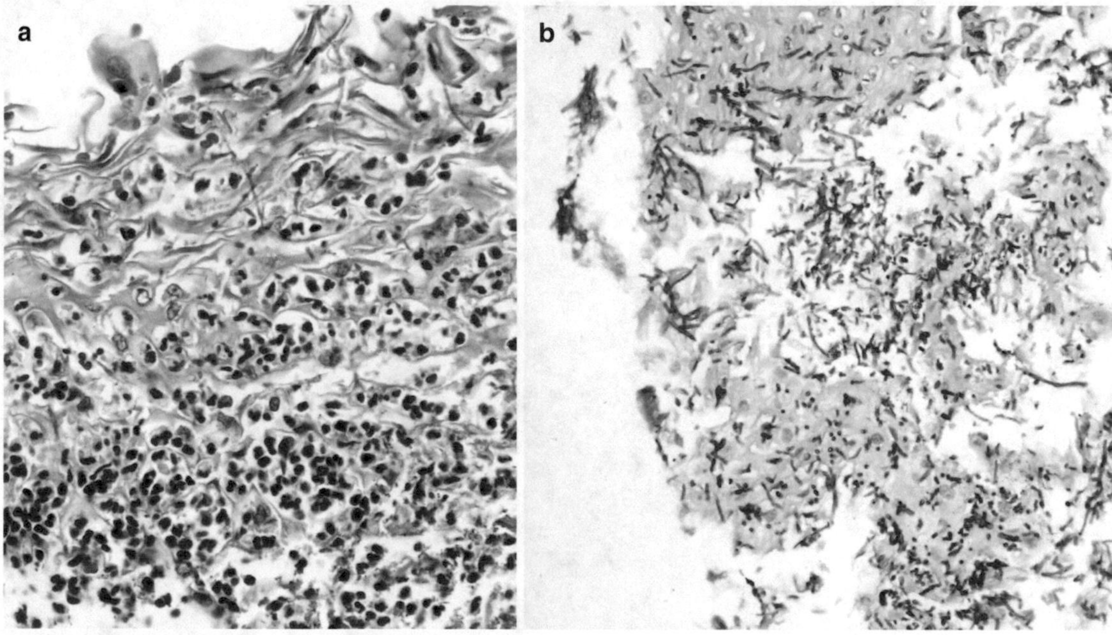

Fig. 10.9 *Candida* esophagitis. Invasive *Candida* are seen in the surface epithelium of an esophageal biopsy, with associated acute inflammation and sloughing squamous debris (**a**). PAS stain highlights the buds and pseudohyphae (**b**)

assays designed to detect causes of gastroenteritis are specific to 40/41, as are antigen-based assays. Adenovirus PCR assays with broad inclusivity of different types are also available and may be helpful if adenovirus other than 40/41 is suspected. Adenovirus serology is helpful in epidemiology studies but not in diagnosis (Table 10.3). References: [33–41]

6. What are the most common infectious manifestations of AIDS in the GI tract?

Although the incidence and prevalence of GI infections in HIV-positive patients have changed dramatically with the introduction of highly active anti-retroviral therapy (HAART), infections remain an important problem in this patient population.

Candida esophagitis (Fig. 10.9a, b) remains the most common cause of infectious esophagitis in AIDS paitents, particularly in HIV-positive patients with a high viral load and/or a CD4 count of less than 200 cells/μL. Infection with *Talaromyces* (formerly *Penicillium*) *marneffei* (Fig. 10.10a–c) is also increasing in both endemic and nonendemic areas. Disseminated histoplasmosis remains common as well, particularly in Brazil and parts of Africa such as French Guiana.

CMV is one of the most common GI pathogens in HIV-positive patients overall, and CMV and HSV are

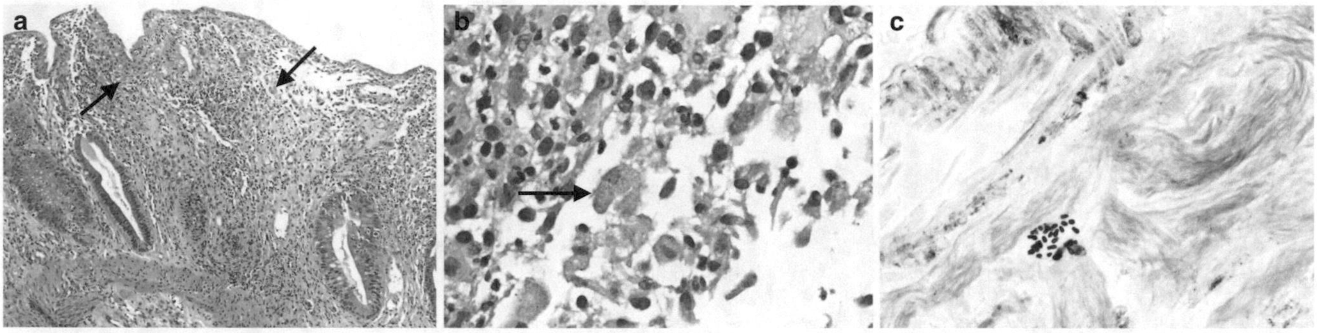

Fig. 10.10 *Penicillium marneffei* colitis. Macrophages filled with organisms (arrows) are difficult to detect in a background of marked colitis with mucosal destruction (**a**). Higher power view shows macrophages filled with tiny yeasts (**b**, arrow). GMS stain highlights the small non-budding yeasts (**c**)

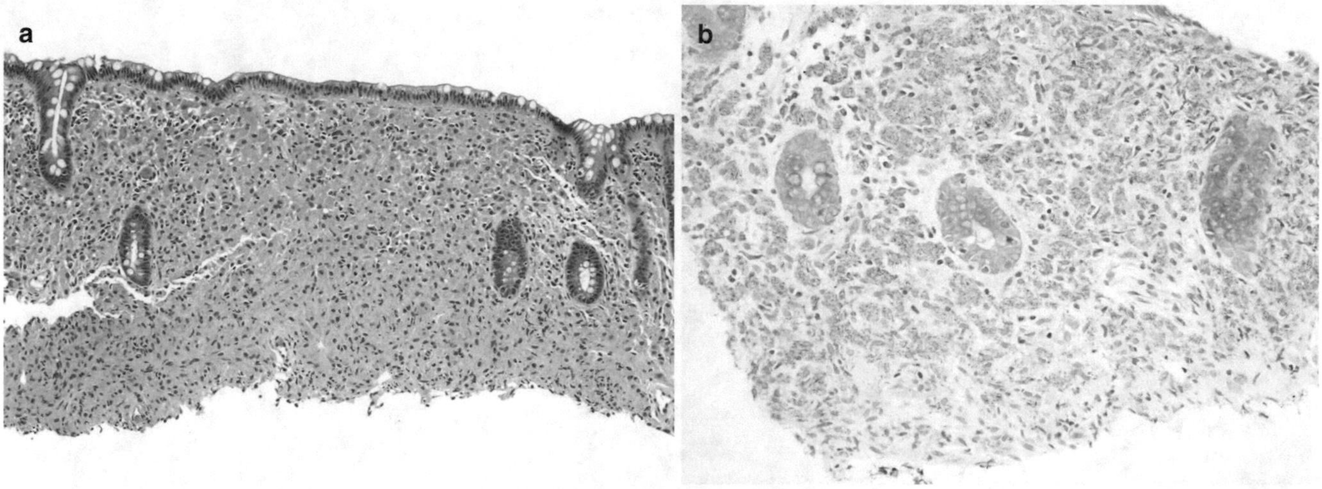

Fig. 10.11 *Mycobacterium avium-intracellulare* colitis. The mucosa is filled with an infiltrate composed almost exclusively of histiocytes (**a**). Ziehl-Neelsen stain highlights numerous mycobacteria in this patient with AIDS (**b**)

frequent causes of esophageal ulcers. Lesions secondary to anorectal HPV infection are frequently seen and do not appear to be affected by HAART.

Mycobacterium avium-intracellulare is still a common intestinal pathogen (Fig. 10.11a, b), and the sexually transmitted bacterial proctocolitides are increasing in men who have sex with men (MSM) (see below).

Parasitic infections remain a significant problem in this population, including *Giarda* spp., *Entamoeba histolytica*, *Toxoplasmosis*, *Cryptosporidium*, *Cyclospora*, *Cystoisospora*, and *Microsporidia*, and these pathogens also are seen more commonly in patients with low CD4 counts.

References: [42–47]

7. **What are the best ways to confirm high-risk HPV infection in the anus, and what are the clinical implications?**

Anal squamous intraepithelial neoplasia (AIN) is relatively uncommon compared to the incidence of cervical intraepithelial neoplasia in the female genital tract. However, the incidence is rising, particularly in HIV-positive men and homosexual men who practice receptive anal intercourse. An overall slight female predominance still persists though because patients with genital HPV-related disease are at high risk of anal neoplasia.

Low-grade squamous intraepithelial neoplasia (LSIL) is usually associated with low-risk HPV genotypes such as 6 and 11; these have a lower risk of progression to malignancy than high-risk genotypes. Similarly, high-grade squamous intraepithelial neoplasia (HSIL) and invasive squamous carcinoma are typically associated with high-risk HPV genotypes such as 16 and 18. Although these genotype associations are typical, some LSIL are associated with high-risk HPV genotypes, and conversely, HSIL may harbor low-risk genotypes. Furthermore, some patients (particularly HIV-positive patients) are infected by multiple genotypes.

Approximately 80–90% of anal squamous cell carcinomas are associated with HPV infection; HPV 16 is present in the majority of cases, followed by HPV 18. Similar to AIN, there is a strong association between anal squamous cell carcinoma and receptive anal intercourse, as well as multiple lifetime sexual partners.

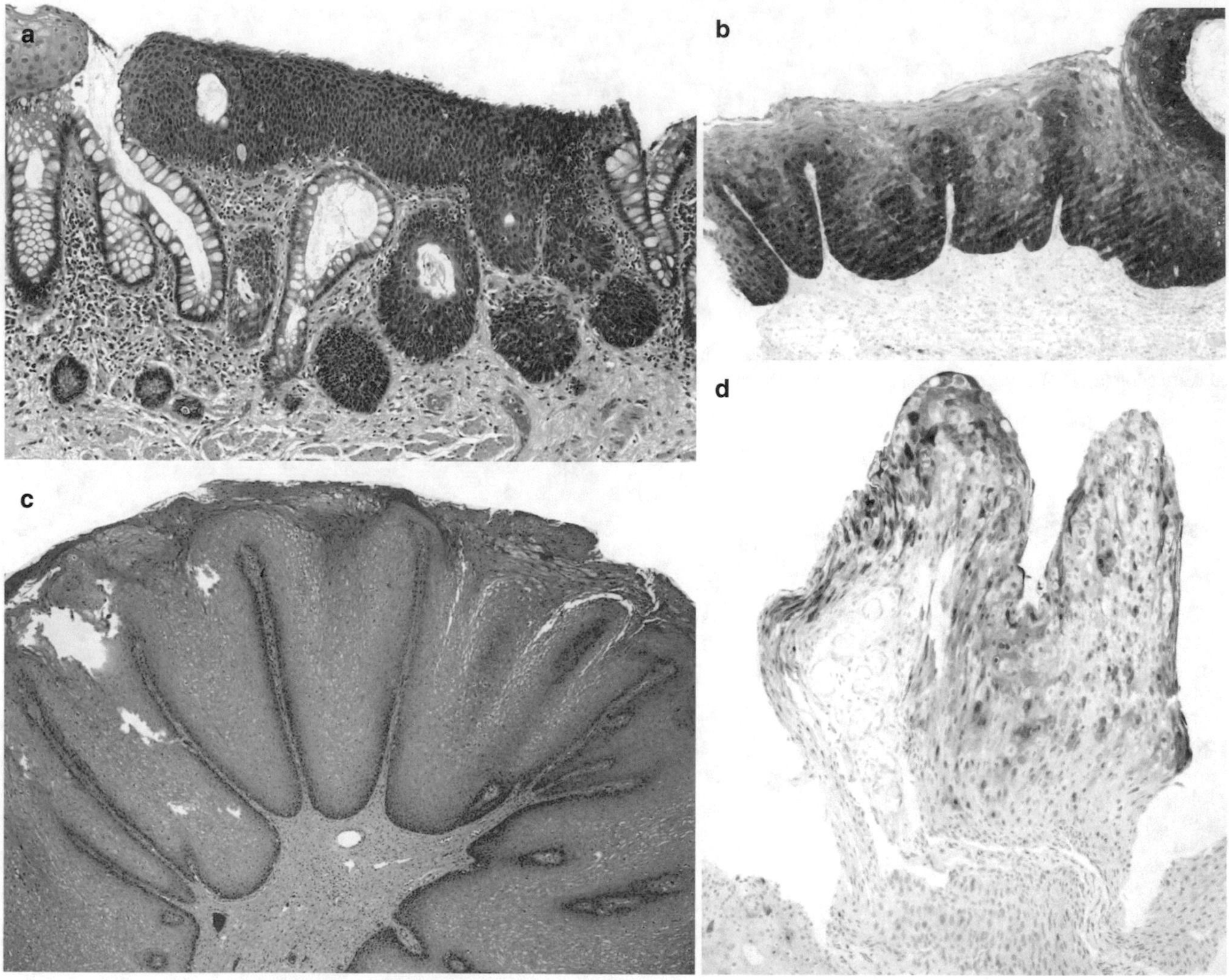

Fig. 10.12 Anal intraepithleial neoplasia. An anal biopsy shows AIN3, with full-thickness involvement of the mucosa by enlarged, hyperchromatic nuclei with no surface maturation (**a**). p16 IHC shows diffuse strong block-like staining (**b**). AIN1/condyloma acuminatum of the anus (**c**). p16 IHC is typically patchy and weak in low-grade squamous intraepithelial lesions (**d**)

Infection with high-risk HPV genotypes upregulates p16, a tumor suppressor gene product that is a surrogate marker of HPV infection, and is associated with increased cellular proliferation. HSIL typically shows diffuse, block-like overexpression of p16 on IHC, whereas LGSIL and reactive processes usually show absent or weak, patchy staining (Fig. 10.12a–d). Both LGSIL and HGSIL typically show abnormal Ki-67 staining, defined as nuclear positivity in the upper two-thirds of the epithelium. HPV CISH (chromogenic in situ hybridization) may also be used to detect both low- and high-risk HPV, and this assay correlates well with p16 expression by IHC.

The strong link between HPV and progression to anal squamous cell carcinoma has some parallels to the paradigm of cervical cancer and suggests that screening programs may help prevent cancer in patients at risk. Like the cervix, the anus has a transformation zone from squamous to columnar epithelium that is susceptible to HPV infection. The infected cells progress in a stepwise manner toward neoplasia and, like cervical cancer, these changes can be detected by cytology. Since multiple FDA-approved assays have been developed to detect HPV 16, 18, and other high-risk types, they can be readily modified to test anal cytology specimens. In fact, the sensitivity of a DNA-based assay for cervical HPV detection approaches 100% for AIN2/3. Similar to colposcopy to follow-up abnormal screening, high-resolution anoscopy can be used to visualize and biopsy suspicious lesions.

Unlike cervical cancer, anal cancer prevalence is too low to justify population-based screening, but the prevalence of HPV in patients at risk of anal cancer is so high that screening may not be informative. In a survey of HPV testing of HIV-positive men, 79% were positive for

Table 10.4 Morphologic features of fungi that may be encountered in the gastrointestinal tract

Organism	Primary geographic distribution	Morphologic features	Host reaction	Major differential diagnoses
Aspergillus species	Worldwide	Hyphae-Septate Uniform width Branching-Regular Acute angles	Ischemic necrosis with angioinvasion Acute inflammation Occasionally granulomatous	Mucormycosis *Fusarium* Dematiaceous fungi
Mucormycosis	Worldwide, associated with diabetics more than any other mycosis	Hyphae-Pauciseptate Ribbon-like Thin walls Branching-Haphazard	Similar to *Aspergillus*	Similar to *Aspergillus*; *Basidiobolus ranarum*
Candida albicans and similar species	Worldwide	Mixture of budding yeasts and pseudohyphae or hyphae; occasional septate hyphae	Usually suppurative, with variable necrosis and ulceration Occasionally granulomatous Occasional angioinvasion	*Aspergillus*
Cryptococcus spp.	Worldwide	Highly pleomorphic (4–7 μm) Uninucleate Narrow-based buds Variably mucicarmine-positive; Fontana-Masson-positive	Usually suppurative; may have extensive necrosis Sometimes granulomatous "Soap bubble" sign	Histoplasmosis
Histoplasma capsulatum var. capsulatum	Worldwide, but endemic to Ohio, the Mississippi river basins; parts of Central and South America; St. Lawrence river basin in Canada	Uniform small (2–5 μm), uninucleate ovoid yeasts Narrow-based buds Intracellular "Halo" effect around organism on H&E	Lymphohistiocytic infiltrate with parasitized histiocytes Occasional granulomas	*Cryptococcus* *P. marneffei* *C. glabrata* *P. carinii* Intracellular parasites
Pneumocystis carinii	Worldwide	Ovoid Cup- or crescent-shaped if collapsed No buds Internal enhancing detail	Characteristic foamy casts May have suppurative or granulomatous inflammation as well	Histoplasmosis Small parasites *P. marneffei*

a carcinogenic HPV type on anal cytology, 31% had HPV 16, and 20% had AIN2/3. This translates to a poor specificity for AIN2/3 (26%) and few patients who will have a negative test and be reassured of low risk of anal cancer. This is supported more broadly by a meta-analysis showing pooled sensitivity of 91% but specificity of 31%. The combination of HPV 16/18 detection and high-grade cytology appears to improve both sensitivity and specificity. Furthermore, baseline detection of HPV 16/18 in LSIL has been associated with increased risk of progression to HSIL. On the other hand, resection of anal lesions has a greater risk of significant side effects than cervical treatments, including anal sphincter dysfunction, pain, stenosis, and incontinence. Currently, there are no large randomized controlled trials to help provide practice guidelines for anal cancer screening.

References: [48–55]

8. **What are the best ways to differentiate between the different fungi that are commonly encountered in surgical pathology?**

Tissue biopsy is a very important tool in the diagnosis of fungal infections, as fungal cultures may require days to weeks for adequate growth and analysis, and molecular studies may also take a week or more. In addition, material for culture is often not obtained. Accurate speciation of fungal infections is critical because it significantly affects antifungal therapy. Fungal infections of the GI tract (with the exception of *Candida* esophagitis) are often part of a disseminated disease process, but GI symptoms and signs may be the presenting manifestations. Inflammatory reaction to fungi in immunosuppressed patients may be markedly blunted, and thus, seemingly normal tissue at low power may actually contain fungi; therefore, vigilance is required in immunosuppressed patients who are at risk for these infections.

The incidence of invasive fungal infections, including fungal infections of the GI tract, has increased significantly over the past 30 years as the number of patients with organ transplants, AIDS, and other immunodeficiency states and on long-term immunosuppression has risen. It is important to note that although GI fungal infections occur most commonly in immunocompromised patients, they are certainly not limited to that population, and virtually, all fungi have been reported to cause infection in immunocompetent persons as well.

For the purposes of this discussion, it is helpful to divide fungi morphologically into filamentous fungi and budding yeasts. The most important of these are summarized in Table 10.4.

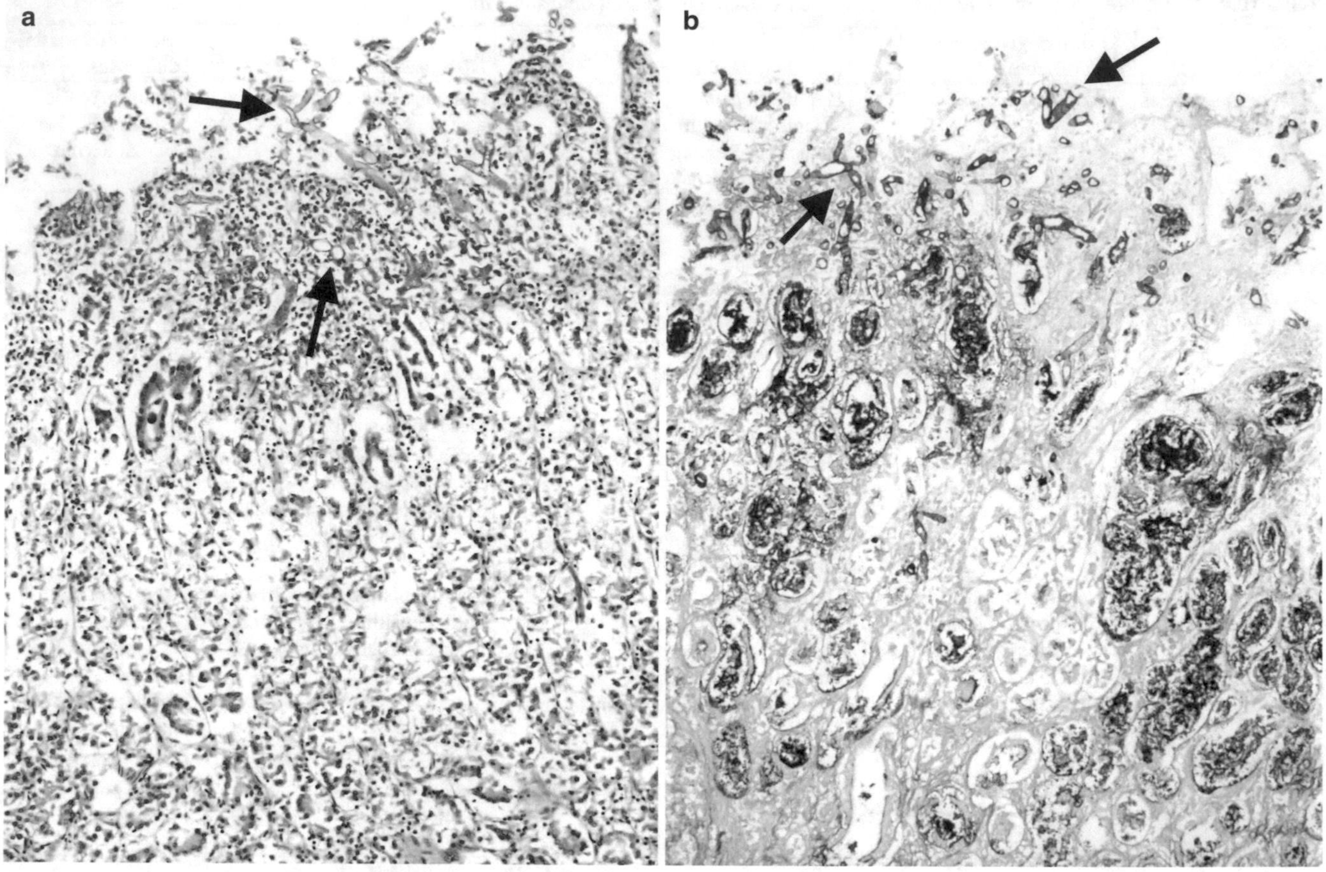

Fig. 10.13 *Mucor*. A gastric biopsy from a diabetic patient shows broad, ribbon-like, pauciseptate fungi within the inflammatory infiltrate (**a**, arrows). GMS stain highlights the Mucor, including their optically clear centers on cut section (**b**, arrows)

Organisms are often identifiable on H&E sections in heavy infections, but GMS and PAS stains remain invaluable diagnostic aids. Fungi often can be correctly classified in tissue sections based on morphology; however, fungi exposed to antifungal therapy or ambient air may produce bizarre and unusual forms.

The filamentous fungi most often encountered in tissue sections include *Aspergillus* spp. and the *Aspergillus*-like fungi such as *Fusarium*, *Mucor*, and *Candida* spp. *Mucor* produces broad, ribbon-like pauciseptate hyphae with irregular walls, which branch randomly at various angles (Fig. 10.13a, b). When cut at cross section, they have optically clear centers. They are angioinvasive and frequently associated with extensive necrosis. In contrast to *Mucor*, *Aspergillus* has septate hyphae of uniform width that branch at acute angles (Fig. 10.14a, b). *Fusarium*, an emerging filamentous fungal pathogen that is also associated with neutropenia, is indistinguishable from *Aspergillus* on morphologic grounds alone. *Basidiobolus ranarum* is a more recently described GI fungal pathogen that is related to *Mucor*. Basidiobolomycosis has an almost pathognomonic tissue reaction, featuring numerous eosinophils, necrosis, granulomas, and a Splendore-Hoeppli protein reaction to the fungi (Fig. 10.15a, b). The fungi are generally fewer than what is seen in mucormycosis, with fewer branches and a "crinkled cellophane ball" appearance in tissue sections. *Candida* species are often a mixture of budding yeasts and hyphae or pseudohyphae (see section above) and are Gram-positive. The dematiaceous, or naturally pigmented, fungi are rarely seen in the GI tract, but cases have been reported in immunocompromised patients. Their natural pigment can be seen on H&E stains, but speciation requires culture or molecular studies.

Budding yeasts more likely to be seen in the GI tract include *Histoplasma* spp. and *Cryptococcus* spp. *Histoplasma* are uniformly small and ovoid and produce narrow-based buds at the pointed end (Fig. 10.16a–c). They also have a "halo" around the organisms on H&E. *Cryptococcus* are much more pleomorphic in size and also have narrow-based buds and may produce a "soap bubble" effect in tissue due to the dense capsule (Fig. 10.17a–c). Historically, *Cryptococcus* species were usually mucicarmine-positive, but capsule-deficient organisms are increasingly common. Fontana-Masson

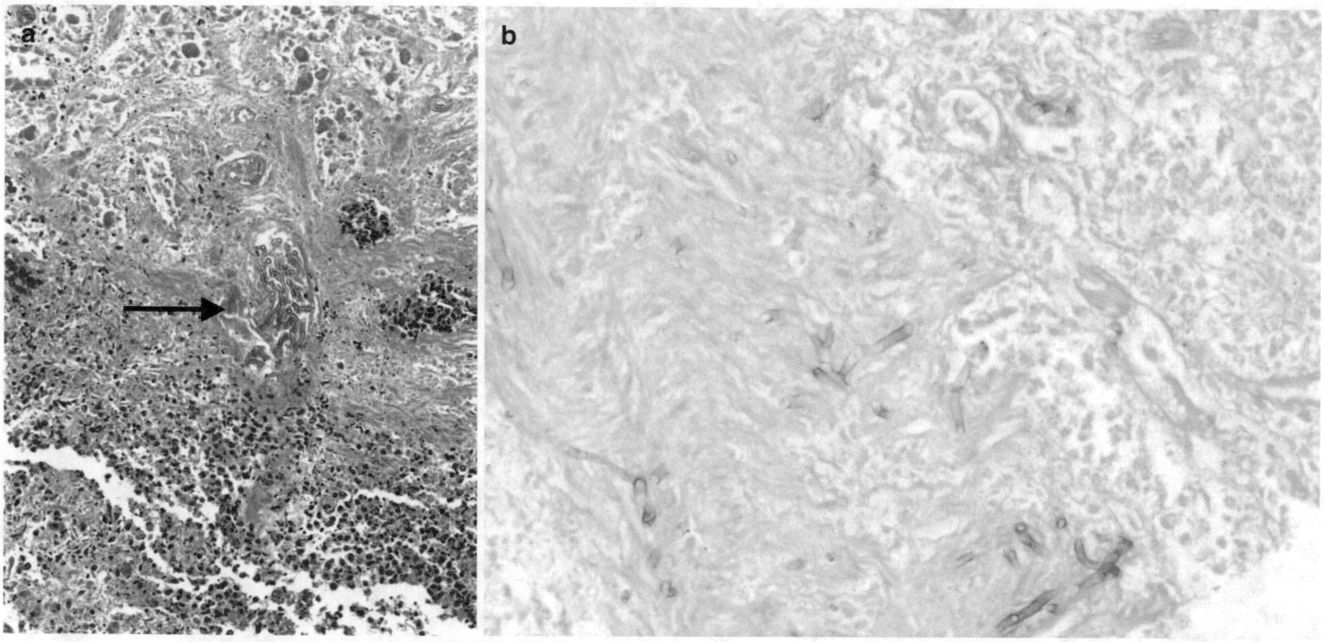

Fig. 10.14 *Aspergillus*. Aspergillus fills the vessels in the wall of the stomach of a bone marrow transplant patient, with associated tissue necrosis (**a**, arrow). GMS stain shows septate hyphae of uniform width that branch at acute angles (**b**)

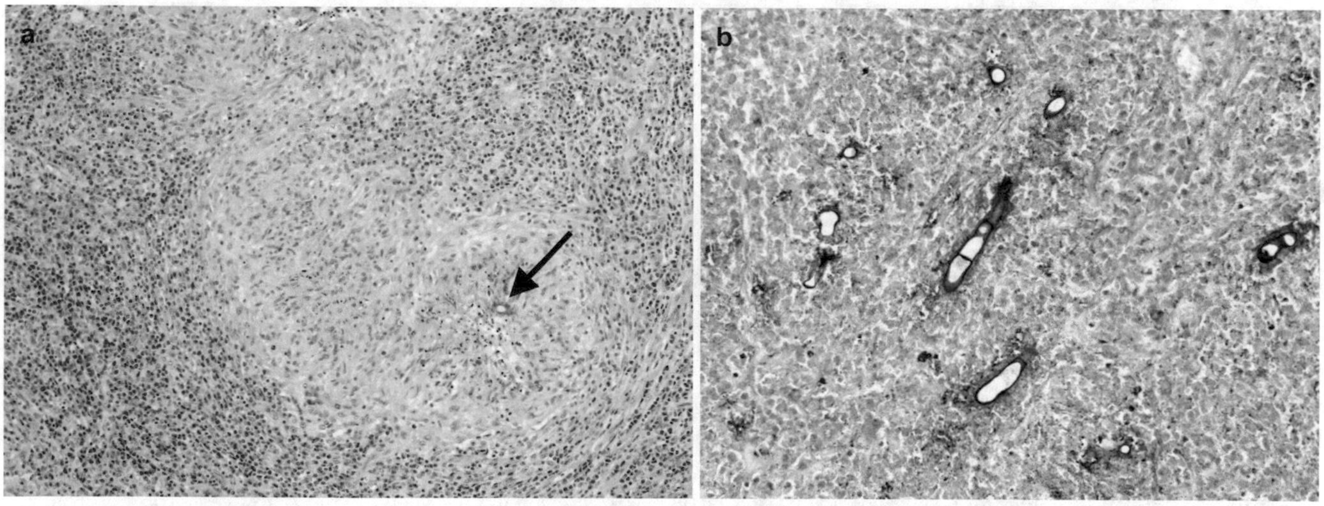

Fig. 10.15 *Basidiobolus ranarum*. The classic histologic features include granulomas with a striking eosinophilic infiltrate. A fungal organism is surrounded by Splendore-Hoeppli protein (**a**, arrow). GMS stain highlights the fungi, which are pauciseptate (**b**)

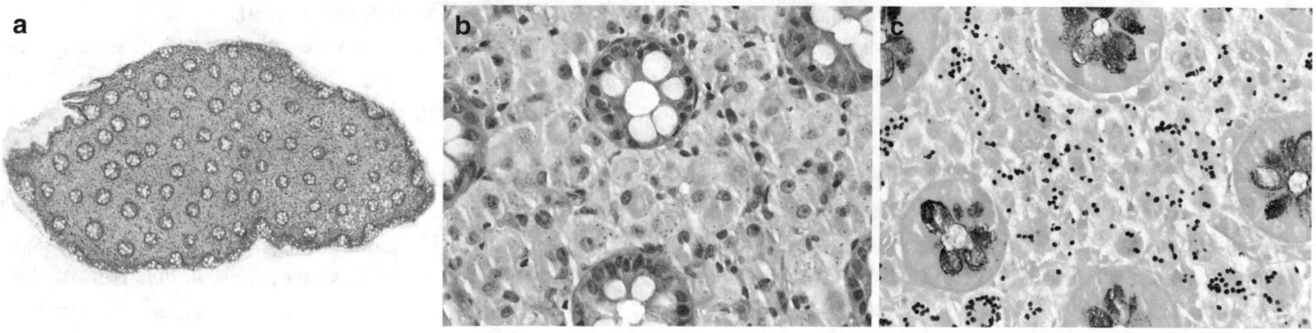

Fig. 10.16 Histoplasmosis. This colon biopsy shows a diffuse macrophage infiltrate in the lamina propria (**a**). Higher power view shows the intracellular organisms, which have a tiny "halo" around each yeast (**b**). GMS shows uniform small yeasts with a narrow-based bud at the pointed pole (**c**)

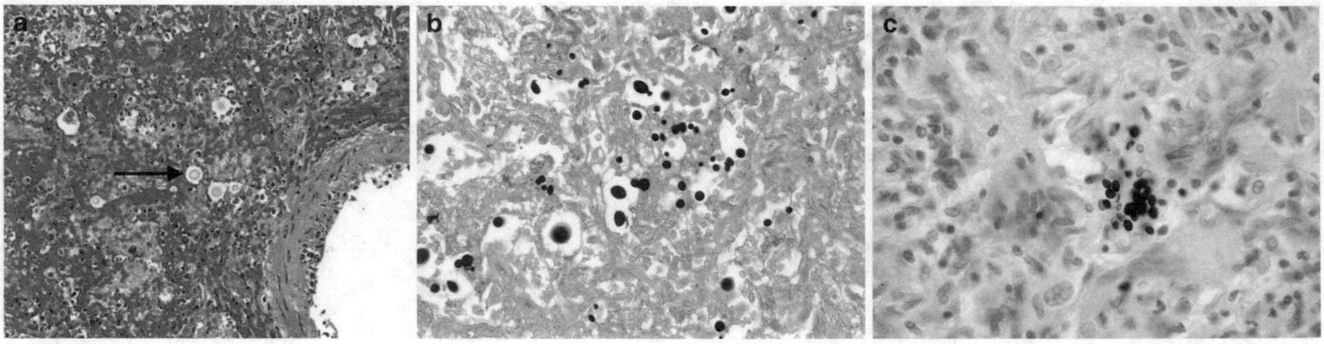

Fig. 10.17 *Cryptococcus*. This abscess containing *Cryptococcus* highlights the prominent capsule and the "soap bubble" around the yeast (**a**, arrow). GMS stain shows the pleomorphic size of the fungi and the narrow-based budding (**b**). Fontana-Masson stain is positive, even in capsule-deficient strains (**c**)

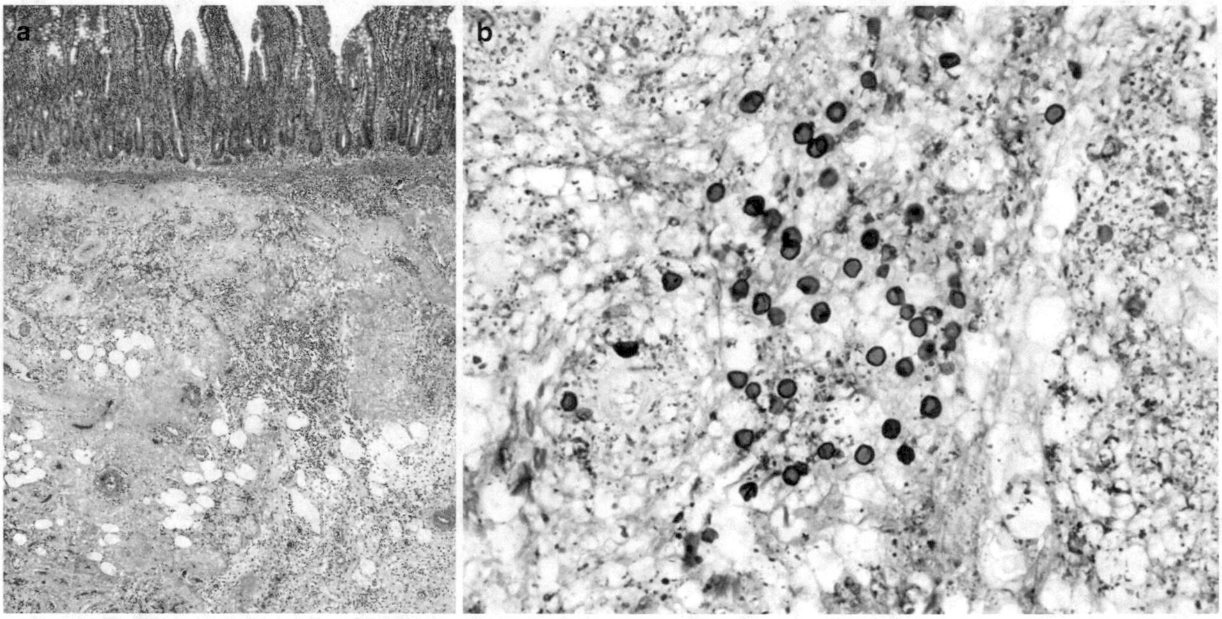

Fig. 10.18 Small bowel with *Pneumocystis carinii*. The foamy-cast infiltrate is identical to that seen in the lung (**a**). GMS shows cup-shaped organisms with focally visible internal structure, and no budding (**b**)

stains are helpful in detecting *Cryptococcus*, particularly if capsule-deficient. *Penicillium marneffei* is rarely seen in the GI tract, but infection does occur (see section above). It is small, like *Histoplasma*, but does not bud, and large forms may have a central septation. *Pneumocystis carinii* (Fig. 10.18a, b) is also similar in size to *Histoplasma*, but has a more cup-shaped morphology with a distinct internal structure and lacks buds. It is also extracellular, with a foamy-cast tissue reaction.

When fungal infection is in the differential diagnosis prior to biopsy, a separate specimen should be submitted for fungal stain and culture. Primary stains such as calcofluor white are fluorescent, enabling high sensitivity while screening large areas of the slide. Culture also enables definitive identification of fungi that have morphologic mimics, particularly the dimorphic fungi for which DNA hybridization or conversion between the mold and yeast form is required. Culture also provides the ability to perform antifungal susceptibility testing, results of which can vary significantly for *Candida* species and which have growing importance in the treatment of mold infections as well.

If a fungal infection was an unexpected finding and fresh tissue is not available, PCR from formalin-fixed, paraffin-embedded tissue can be used for identification. These assays are either species-specific for common pathogens such as *Histoplasma* and *Pneumocystis* or broad-range assays that use primers that anneal to conserved DNA regions and sequencing to identify the genus and species. The analytical sensitivity of these assays is limited by the degradation of nucleic acids by formalin. These tests are often expensive, require extended amounts of time for results, and are only available in special labs; thus, judicious use and thorough evaluation using the above tools is warranted. IHC may also play a role in diagnosis from paraffin-embedded tissue, although it may suffer from cross-reactivity between fungal species.

Non-invasive fungal diagnostics that can complement a histologic diagnosis include serology and antigen tests. These assays are based on detecting fungal cell wall elements and their antibodies in host tissue and body fluids. Urine antigen testing is particularly useful for endemic fungi such as *Histoplasma* and the combination of antigen testing with antibody testing through enzyme immunoassay (EIA), immunodiffusion and/or complement fixation increases the overall diagnostic yield of testing. Knowledge of the patient's geographic and/or travel history also may be very helpful in test selection and diagnosis, particularly when endemic fungi are suspected. Galactomannan is a component of the *Aspergillus* cell wall released during growth, and the galactomannan assay is a serologic test that is helpful in diagnosing invasive aspergillosis. The beta (1.3) D glucan assay is an antigen test that is positive in many disseminated fungal infections, with important exceptions including *Zygomycetes*, *Cryptococcus*, and *Blastomyces*.

References: [56–65]

9. **What are the best methodologies for diagnosing Helicobacter pylori infection, and how are drug-resistant organisms detected and managed?**

Helicobacter pylori, originally named *Campylobacter pyloridis*, is a spirillar Gram-negative bacterium that infects the stomach. It remains one of the most common bacterial infections worldwide and reportedly infects over half of the entire human race. The incidence is decreasing, but the specific reasons for this are unknown.

Although the exact mechanisms by which *H. pylori* causes disease remain unclear, *H. pylori* infection is associated with many GI diseases, including chronic and atrophic gastritis, peptic ulcers, gastric adenocarcinoma, and lymphomas of the mucosa-associated lymphoid tissue type. Many infected patients are asymptomatic.

The bacteria are tiny (2–5 μm), slightly basophilic, spirillar, and "comma" or "seagull" shaped (Fig. 10.19). They are usually present in the mucus layer at the surface of the epithelium, both at the luminal surface and within the pits. Invasive organisms are only rarely seen. The distribution of bacteria may be very focal and patchy. In addition, under suboptimal conditions, the typically spirillar bacteria may undergo transformation to coccoid forms (Fig. 10.20) that closely resemble mucus droplets, other bacteria, or other organisms such as fungal spores or coccidians. Coccoid forms are usually admixed with at least some spirillar forms, and the diagnosis of infection when only coccoid forms are present should be considered with caution.

The need for special stains in the diagnosis of HP remains controversial, although most agree that some form of stain is very helpful (if not absolutely necessary), particularly if the patient has been treated previously. Useful stains include Giemsa, Diff-quick, and silver impregnation stains such as the Warthin-Starry or Steiner. The latter may be combined with H&E and Alcian blue (pH 2.5) to produce the "triple" or "Genta" stain that also allows for evaluation of gastric morphology. Silver impregnation stains are expensive and technically more difficult, but the bacteria are easy to identify using this method as they stain dark black and appear fatter. Gram stain and the fluorescent acridine orange stain also will detect *H. pylori*, although these are not routinely used. The more recently introduced immunostain (Fig. 10.21) has gained increasing popularity due to the ease of use,

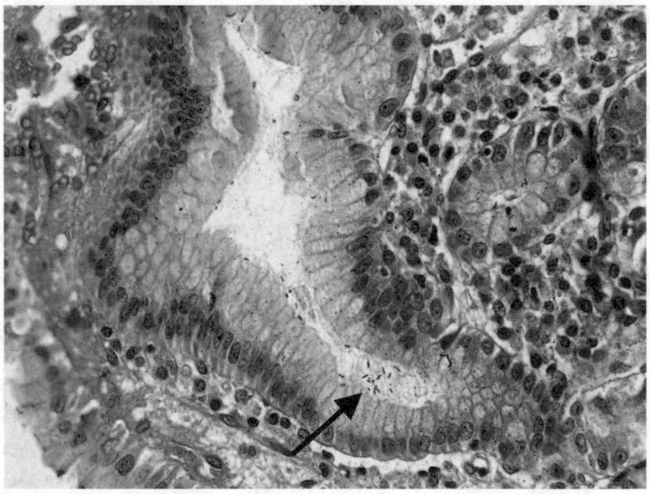

Fig. 10.19 *H. pylori* are seen as small, seagull-shaped bacteria that stain black (arrow) on this triple stain

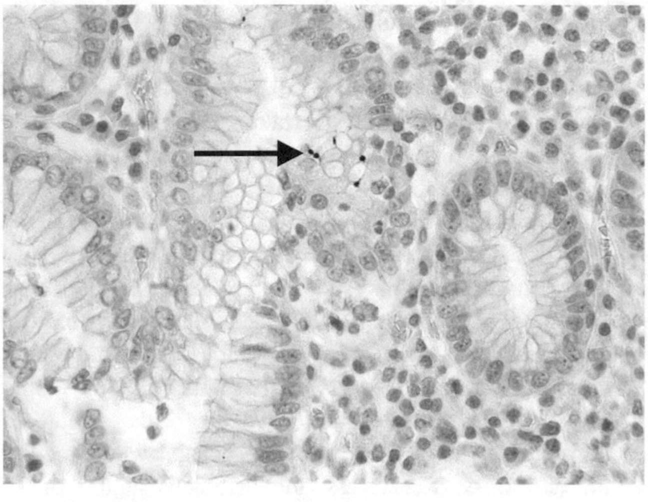

Fig. 10.20 Following treatment, *H. pylori* may assume a coccoid morphology (*H. pylori* IHC, arrow)

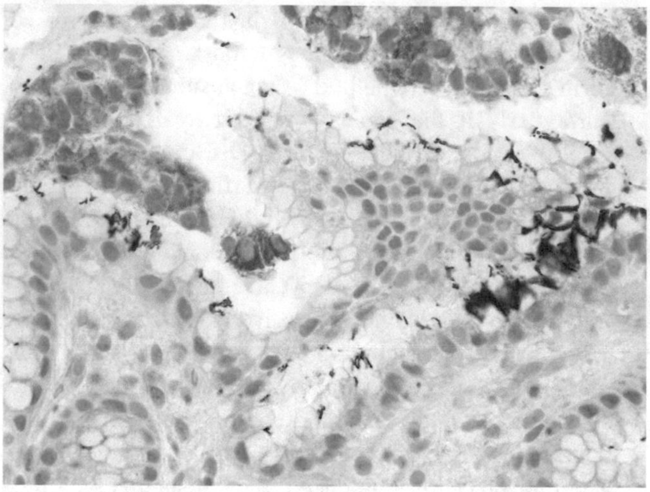

Fig. 10.21 IHC for *H. pylori* reveals numerous seagull-shaped organisms at the surface of the epithelium

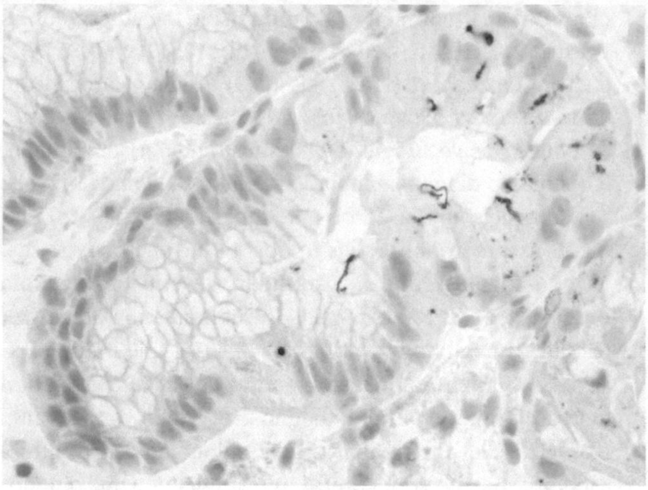

Fig. 10.22 *Helicobacter heilmannii* is larger and more tightly spiraled than *H. pylori*, but is detectable with the same immunohistochemical stain

ease of identification of the organism, and the sensitivity and specificity.

Based on the American College of Gastroenterology guidelines, the overall approach to diagnosis of *H. pylori* differs by clinical features and whether endoscopy is indicated. If endoscopy is performed, biopsy should also be performed and diagnosis can be made by rapid urea test on the tissue with equivalent sensitivity and specificity to histology. If endoscopy is not required, there are several non-invasive test modalities available with excellent test performance. The urea breath test relies on ingestion of ^{13}C-labeled urea and subsequent detection of labeled CO_2 after breakdown of the urea by *H. pylori*. Overall accuracy is excellent. Alternatively, stool antigen testing that has nearly the same accuracy as urea breath test but at lower cost can be performed. For both the urea breath test and stool antigen test, the patient should discontinue proton pump inhibitors (PPIs) 2 weeks before testing. Serology has limited utility since it cannot distinguish past from current infection. It may be helpful in cases where the patient cannot stop taking PPIs.

Antibiotic resistance in *H. pylori* can complicate therapy, and susceptibility testing is technically challenging. Surveys in the United States over the past 20 years found rates of resistance at 20–21% for metronidazole, 13–16% for clarithromycin, and 31% for levofloxacin. Therefore, empiric therapy may fail and susceptibility testing may be needed to develop a successful antibiotic regimen. There is currently controversy over whether initial therapy should rely on susceptibility results or whether testing should be done after an initial failure, an approach that would require repeat biopsy. Regardless, the fastidious nature of *H. pylori* makes culture and subsequent susceptibility testing challenging. Culture requires microaerobic conditions (4% O_2, 5% CO_2, 5% H_2, 86% N_2) and the organisms can rapidly lose viability during transport. Even if a laboratory is equipped to culture the organism, they may not be able to perform susceptibility testing, leading to another transport stage and risk of viability loss. Because of these challenges, molecular assays that detect common mutations are emerging, leading to antibiotic resistance.

Helicobacter heilmannii is a less commonly encountered *Helicobacter* species formerly known as *Gastrospirillum hominis*. It causes symptoms similar to *H. pylori* infection, and co-infection with *H. pylori* has been well-documented. It is longer (4–10 μm in length) and more tightly spiraled than *H. pylori* (Fig. 10.22), but it is detectable with all of the same histochemical stains used for *H. pylori* detection and also reacts with the anti-*H. pylori* immunohistochemical stains.

Please see Chap. 4, questions 6–15, for additional discussion on *H. pylori* gastritis.

References: [65–72]

10. What are the best ways to diagnose Whipple disease?

Eighty-four years after Dr. George H. Whipple initially reported the disease, the actinobacterium *Tropheryma whippelii*, also known as the Whipple's bacillus, was identified. Whipple disease can affect virtually any organ system, and thus, the clinical presentation is very variable. Polyarthritis is often the first manifestation, and it may precede GI symptoms by years. Other characteristic symptoms include low-grade fever, weight loss, malabsorption, and lymphadenopathy, as well as significant neuropsychiatric manifestations.

The diagnosis of Whipple disease usually starts with a mucosal biopsy from the small bowel. The characteristic histologic lesion is a striking macrophage infiltrate in the lamina propria and submucosa, which blunts and distends the villi. Involvement may be diffuse or patchy.

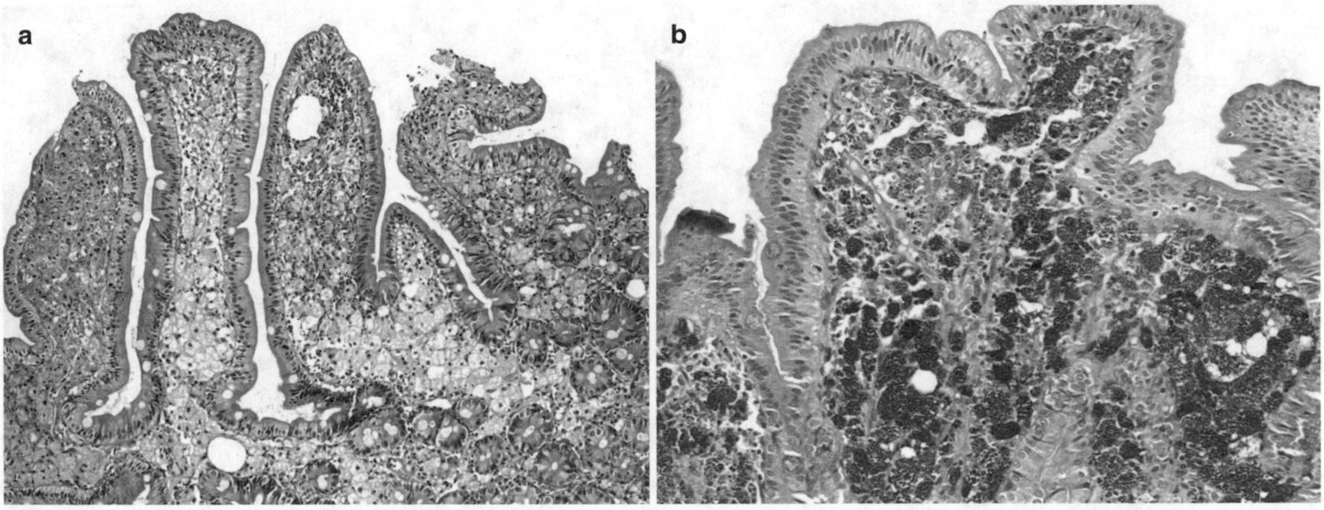

Fig. 10.23 Whipple disease. The small bowel mucosa contains an infiltrate of macrophages that distend the villi (**a**). Fat droplets are also visible. PAS stain highlights the macrophage infiltrate (**b**)

The macrophages are packed with bacilli, which are strongly PAS-positive (Fig. 10.23a, b). Neutrophils are often present, but there is usually no associated mononuclear inflammatory infiltrate. The lamina propria often contains small foci of fat, and overlying vacuolization of surface enterocytes may also occur. Epithelioid granulomas are present in a minority of cases. It is important to note that PAS-positive macrophages may persist in biopsies for years, even in patients who have been treated with long-term antibiotic therapy.

IHC has been used to identify the bacillus, but is not widely available, and it can also be identified by electron microscopy. Although PAS-positive macrophages are consistent with Whipple disease, they may also be seen in other bacterial and fungal infections. PCR is a more specific and perhaps more sensitive method and should be performed along with histologic examination and PAS staining. As the prevalence is exceedingly low, estimated to be 3 per 1,000,000 people with ~12 new cases diagnosed per year worldwide, the chance of a false-positive is high. Therefore, if PCR is positive, confirmation with a second assay that targets a different genomic region is recommended. PCR can be performed on a paraffin block, although as discussed above, the yield from PCR from fresh tissue is superior to paraffin-embedded tissue.

References: [72–75]

11. **What are the best ways to diagnose mycobacterial infection in the GI tract and to distinguish tubercular from non-tubercular mycobacteria?**

- *Mycobacterium tuberculosis*

Tuberculosis remains common in developing countries, but there has also been a resurgence in industrialized countries. In large measure, this is secondary to AIDS, but immigration and institutional overcrowding are also contributing factors. GI tuberculosis can be acquired through swallowing infected sputum in cases of pulmonary tuberculosis; ingestion of contaminated milk; as part of hematogenous spread from pulmonary or military disease; and through direct extension from adjacent organs.

It is important to note that GI symptoms may be the initial manifestation of disease and that primary GI tuberculosis in the absence of pulmonary infection has been well-documented. Extrapulmonary manifestations are also more common in AIDS patients. Tuberculosis has recently been associated with the use of infliximab, a tumor necrosis factor alpha-neutralizing agent used in the treatment of Crohn disease and autoimmune diseases. The emergence of infection is often associated with initiation of treatment, and a majority of patients have extrapulmonary manifestations.

The ileocecal and jejuno-ileal segments are most commonly involved. Strictures and ulcers (often seen together) are the most common endoscopic findings. The ulcers are often circumferential and transverse; multiple and segmental lesions with skip areas are common, which can easily mimic Crohn disease. Thickened mucosal folds and inflammatory nodules are also frequent findings. When the ileum is involved, the ileocecal valve is often deformed and gaping. Large inflammatory masses known as tuberculoma are another manifestation, which also most frequently involves the ileocecum. Mesenteric lymphadenopathy is very common.

The characteristic histologic lesion consists of granulomas, which are caseating and often confluent and present at any level of the gut wall but most commonly in the submucosa (Fig. 10.24a, b). Giant cells are often present, and a

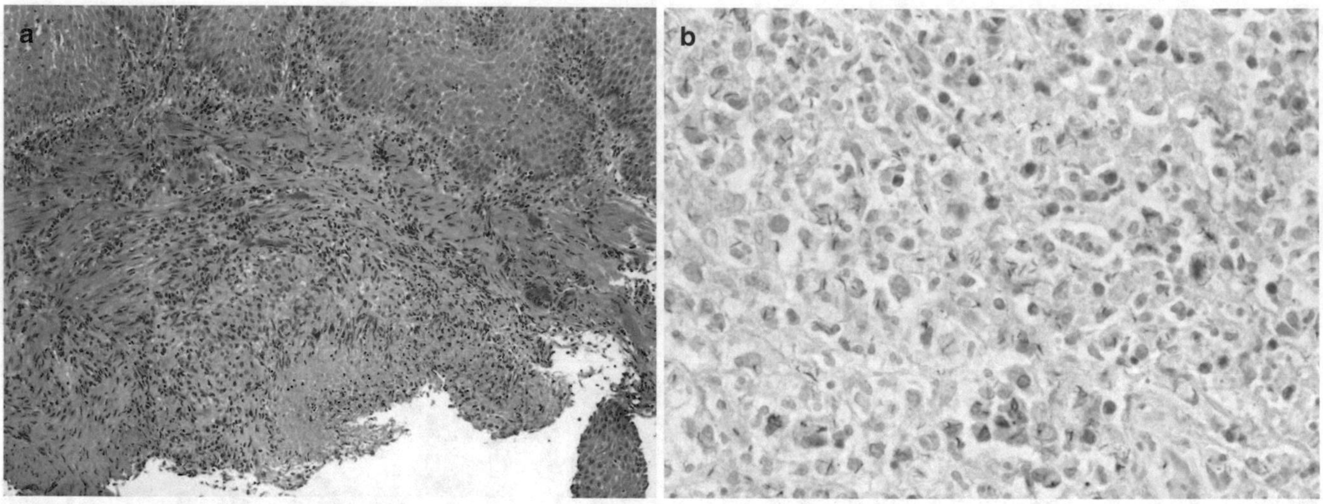

Fig. 10.24 Tuberculosis. A caseating granuloma is present in the submucosa of the esophagus (**a**). Ziehl-Neelsen stain shows numerous mycobacteria (**b**)

rim of lymphocytes can be seen at the periphery of the granulomas. Architectural distortion that mimics IBD can be seen overlying areas of granulomatous inflammation. The wall of the bowel is thickened and edematous, with transmural inflammation, lymphoid hyperplasia, and fibrosis in later stages of disease. Ulcers are common and may be superficial or deep; they can overlie hyperplastic Peyer patches, producing aphthoid ulcers that also mimic Crohn disease. Some atypical mycobacteria, such as *M. kansasii* and *M. bovis*, may cause similar pathologic findings.

Acid-fast stains may demonstrate organisms, often within necrotic areas or macrophages. The acid-fast bacilli of *M. tuberculosis* are typically rod-shaped and have a "beaded" morphology. Organisms may be abundant in immunocompromised patients, yet rare and hard to find in immunocompetent persons. The number of organisms also varies with the age of the lesion and previous antitubercular therapy.

- *Mycobacterium avium-intracellulare complex (MAI)*

MAI is the most common mycobacterium isolated from the GI tract. It is usually found in patients with AIDS and other immune-compromising conditions, and disseminated MAI infection remains the most common systemic bacterial infection among AIDS patients, but it is also found in immunocompetent patients. GI involvement is usually a feature of disseminated infection.

The small bowel is preferentially involved, but colonic and gastroesophageal involvement can occur. Endoscopy is often normal, but when macroscopic findings are present, they usually consist of tiny granular white mucosal nodules with surrounding erythema. Small ulcers and mucosal hemorrhage have been noted as well. Histologic manifestations vary with the immune status of the patient. Immunocompetent patients may have well-formed, epithelioid granulomas, either with or without necrosis. Small bowel biopsies from immunocompromised patients show villi distended by a diffuse infiltration of histiocytes containing bacilli (see section above), with little inflammatory response.

Bacilli stain with acid-fast stains, as well as PAS and GMS (as any rapidly dividing bacteria may stain positively on GMS stain), and this should not dissuade the pathologist from an erroneous diagnosis of fungal infection. Organisms are generally abundant in the immunocompromised host, but harder to detect in immunocompetent patients.

It is very important to distinguish atypical mycobacterial infection from *M. tuberculosis*, because the antitubercular drug regimen varies. MAI is more likely to produce diffuse histiocytic infiltrates and poorly formed granulomas with abundant organisms, as opposed to the well-formed granulomas typical of tuberculosis. Rarely, other atypical mycobacteria (e.g. *M. fortuitum*, *M. chelonei*, or *M. sulgai*) infect the GI tract and cause histologic findings similar to MAI infection.

Biopsy tissue is the appropriate culture source in most cases where mycobacterial infection of the GI tract is being considered. Stool culture is only recommended when MAI is suspected in an immunocompromised patient. Mycobacterial culture first requires decontamination of the specimen to prevent overgrowth of the culture by more rapidly growing bacteria. This decontamination process is a fine balance, as rigorous methods can also reduce recovery of *Mycobacteria* itself. Once decontaminated, the sample can be used to inoculate automated broth culture systems, slants, or plates. The automated system has an advantage in that it facilitates the rapid growth of organisms. Once the instrument signals that a broth is positive, an acid-fast stain is used to confirm the growth of *Mycobacteria* as opposed to a co-inoculated contaminant. Then the broth must be inoculated to agar slants or plates to isolate the organism.

Identification of *Mycobacteria* is increasingly performed by nucleic acid hybridization or MALDI-TOF mass spectrometry, replacing slower traditional identification biochemical methods. In some laboratories, nucleic acid hybridization is performed on broth cultures, providing rapid identification of *M. tuberculosis*, *M. kansasii*, and MAI. Cultures identified at the broth stage are still cultured on agar for isolation and susceptibility testing. If this preliminary testing is negative, identification is performed once colonies are isolated. MALDI-TOF is a rapid and reliable identification method, although differentiation of closely related species such as *M. intracellulare* and *M. chimera* can be challenging. In these cases, either more sophisticated analysis of the MALDI-TOF spectrum, or gene sequencing, is required.

Direct detection and identification can also be performed by PCR, either from fresh tissue or paraffin-embedded tissue. The latter can be helpful when acid-fast organisms are seen on histopathology but culture was not ordered. Targeted identification can be performed using real-time PCR, or broad-range PCR can be performed followed by sequencing of the amplicon for identification purposes.

References: [76–80]

12. **What is the best way to distinguish chronic idiopathic IBD from sexually transmitted infectious mimics?**

The two sexually transmitted infections most likely to mimic IBD are syphilis, or infection with *Treponema pallidum*, and LGV, or infection with *Chlamydia trachomatis*.

The incidence of syphilis is increasing, especially among men who practice anal-receptive intercourse and/or are HIV-positive. It is likely that anorectal syphilis is underdiagnosed, due to its variable clinical findings as well as low index of clinical suspicion. When GI syphilis presents as proctitis, symptoms typically include pain that is exacerbated with defecation, tenesmus, constipation, bleeding, and anal discharge, which may be mucoid or bloody. Some patients remain asymptomatic or have only minimal complaints.

Endoscopic findings are nonspecific and include ulcers, fissures, and inflammatory polypoid lesions, which may mimic IBD macroscopically. Histologically, the most common feature is a dense lymphohistiocytic infiltrate, often with admixed plasma cells and prominent lymphoid aggregates (Fig. 10.25a–c). Neutrophilic cryptitis and crypt abscesses may be present and may be associated with gland destruction, but neutrophilic inflammation and crypt architectural distortion are usually less prominent than the mononuclear cell infiltrate. Granulomas have been reported in rare cases, and small vessels with prominent endothelial cells may be noted. Occasional cases of syphilitic proctitis have the acute self-limited colitis pattern, without substantially increased plasma cells. Silver impregnation stains (Warthin-Starry, Steiner, and Dieterle) may be helpful in highlighting *T. pallidum* organisms, but these have poor sensitivity. IHC directed against the pathogen is significantly more sensitive than the silver stains.

In the last 20 years, outbreaks of LGV proctitis have appeared in North America, Europe, and Australia, most often among the MSM population. The primary stage of infection is characterized by rectal pain, bleeding, mucopurulent discharge, tenesmus, and constipation. Lymphadenopathy develops during the second stage, and the tertiary stage involves complications of longstanding chronic proctitis, including fistulae and strictures. Although some patients with anorectal LGV also have evidence of urethral infection, many do not.

The endoscopic appearance of *Chlamydia* proctitis ranges from unremarkable to mucosal hyperemia, friability, ulcers, purulent exudate, and strictures that mimic IBD. The inflammatory infiltrate of LGV

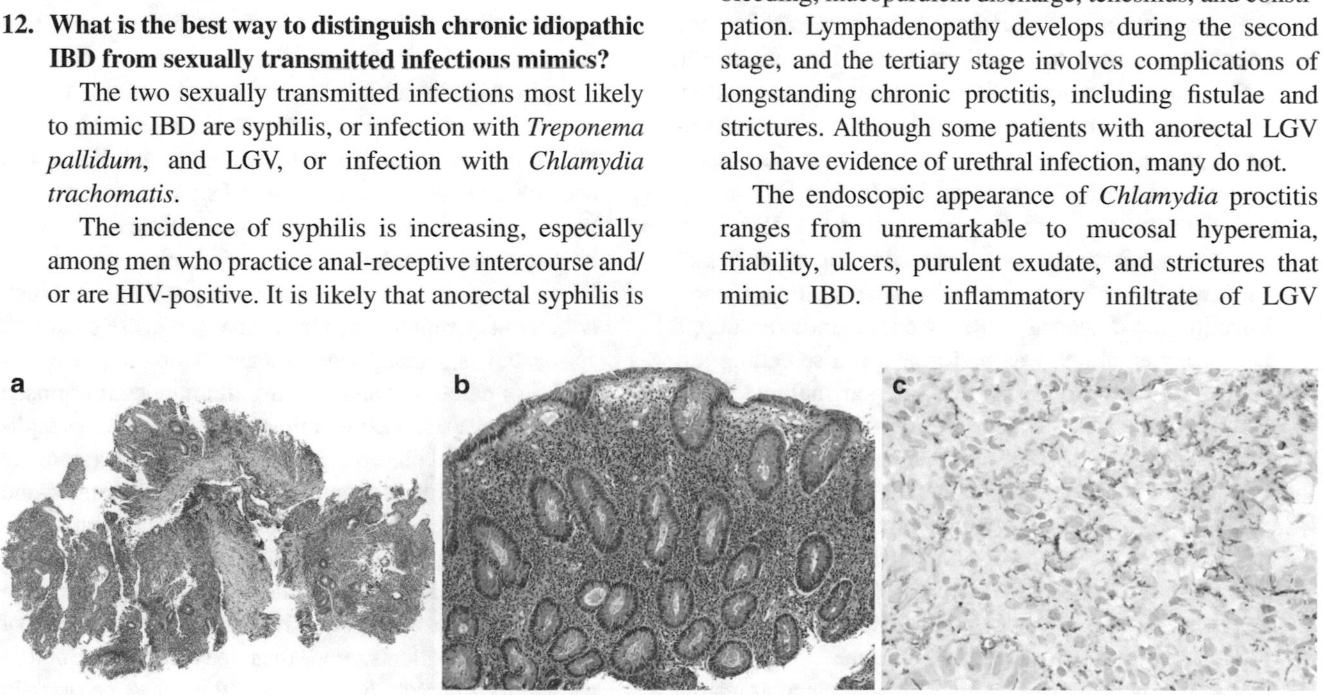

Fig. 10.25 Syphilitic proctitis. A low power view shows a lymphoplasmacytic infiltrate with architectural distortion (**a**). Another case shows expansion of the lamina propria by a mononuclear cell infiltrate, but minimal active inflammation (**b**). IHC highlights numerous organisms (**c**)

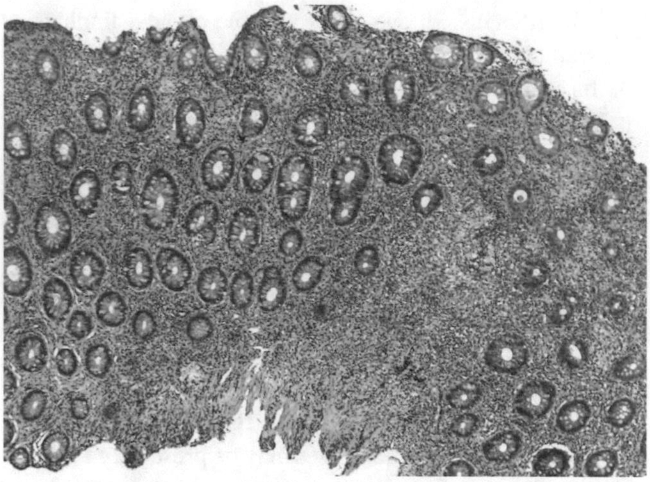

Fig. 10.26 LGV proctitis. The lamina propria is expanded by a lymphohistiocytic infiltrate, and there are several loose granulomas

proctitis, similar to syphilitic proctitis, consists of a lymphoplasmacytic infiltrate that may contain abundant neutrophils (Fig. 10.26). Granulomatous inflammation is occasionally present. A prominent follicular proctitis with associated architectural distortion has also been described.

Both syphilis and LGV may mimic IBD histologically and endoscopically, and laboratory testing may be required to make the distinction. A presumptive diagnosis of syphilis is made through serologic testing with both non-treponemal and treponemal tests. Non-treoponemal tests detect antibodies against lipoidal antigens and can be used to track serologic responses to therapy, but have limitations in both sensitivity and specificity. These tests include Rapid Plasma Reagin (RPR) and Venereal Disease Research Laboratory (VDRL) tests. Treponemal tests detect antibodies developed against the pathogen, and include fluorescent treponemal antibody absorbed test (FTA-ABS) and *T. pallidum* passive particle agglutination (TP-PA) tests. Treponemal tests are highly sensitive for all stages of infection but can remain positive after treatment, complicating the diagnosis of re-infection. Until recently, a non-treponemal test was performed as a screening test followed by confirmation with a treponemal test. Now, some laboratories are screening with treponemal EIA tests, due to the ease of automating these assays, and confirming with a non-treponemal test. In this algorithm, a negative non-treponemal test should be followed up by a second treponemal test to distinguish a false-positive from a past infection. In managing syphilis, it is important to be familiar with the laboratory algorithm where testing will be performed.

LGV may be supported by positive molecular testing for *C. trachomatis*, using an assay that detects genotypes L1–3 associated with the disease. Most commercial assays detect these genotypes but do not distinguish them from others. NAATs have become the diagnostic method of choice for *C. trachomatis* due to their sensitivity, specificity, and speed. Although these tests do not have FDA approval for rectal specimens, many laboratories have performed the necessary validation to show good performance with this specimen type. Bacterial culture may be a useful supplement by providing information of antibiotic sensitivity. Serologic testing for *C. trachomatis*-specific antibodies may also be used to establish a diagnosis, but is not as quick or sensitive, particularly in early infection where antibodies have not been formed, as nucleic acid testing-based modalities

References: [81–88]

13. **What are the best ways to diagnose intestinal spirochetosis, and what is the clinical significance?**

Intestinal spirochetosis is characterized by the presence of bacteria with spiral morphology on the luminal surface of the large bowel mucosa. A heterogeneous group of related organisms are involved, most importantly *Brachyspira aalborgi* and *Brachyspira pilosicoli*, which are genetically unrelated to *T. pallidum,* the causative agent of syphilis. Patients with spirochetosis may harbor one or both of these species.

The prevalence of spirochetosis ranges from 2% to 16% in industrialized nations, but is significantly higher in developing countries and homosexual and HIV-positive patients, where prevalence has been reported to be as high as 50% based on tissue biopsy and stool culture.

Spirochetosis has been associated with a wide variety of conditions including diverticular disease, IBD, hyperplastic polyps, and adenomatous polyps, and it also has been found in children. The clinical significance remains controversial, however. Patients with spirochetosis may have symptoms such as diarrhea, abdominal pain, lower GI bleeding, and anorectal pain and discharge, but they are often asymptomatic. Furthermore, it is not clear that spirochetosis actually causes these symptoms in symptomatic patients, and many immunocompromised patients have other concomitant infections that complicate the clinical picture. Conversely, many symptomatic patients appear to respond to antimicrobial therapy, and ultrastructural studies have suggested that the spirochetes cause epithelial damage at that level despite the typical lack of associated inflammation and tissue damage. *B. pilosicoli* has been isolated from the blood of seriously ill patients, and thus may represent a true pathogen, whereas *B. aalborgi* (the more commonly detected species) has not, and thus, some authorities

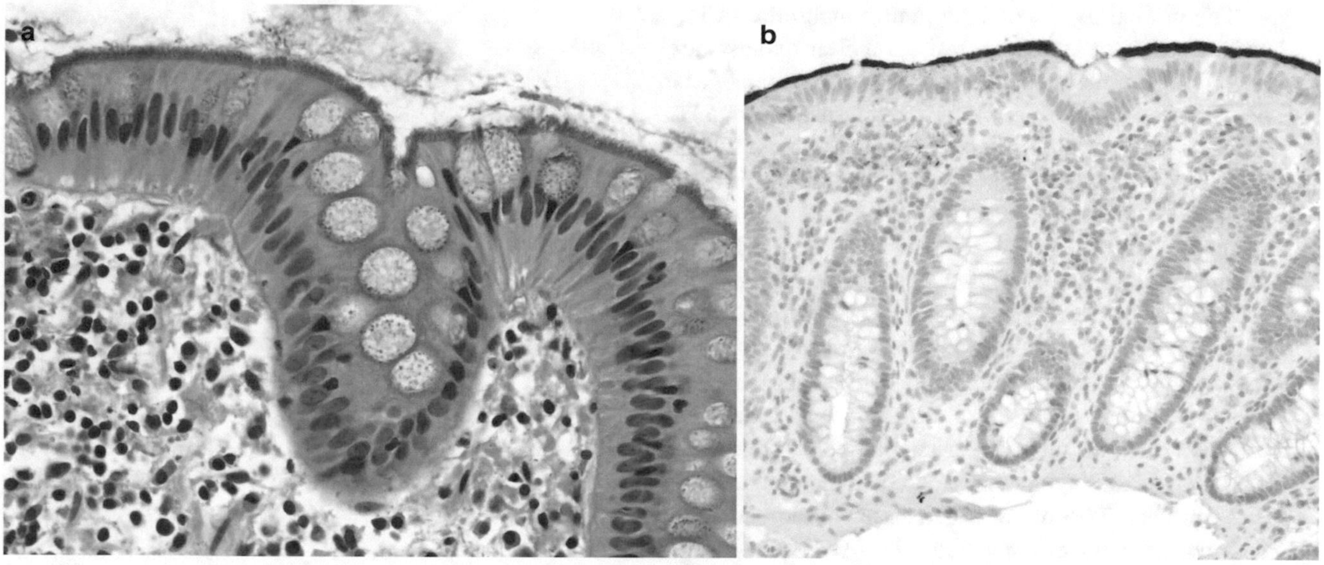

Fig. 10.27 Spirochetosis. On H&E, organisms appear as a thick, fuzzy, "fringed" border at the luminal surface (**a**). Treponeme IHC highlights the organisms (**b**)

believe it is merely a commensal, but the status of both organisms as true pathogens remains controversial. Given the controversy regarding clinical significance, some reserve antimicrobial therapy for patients who have severe or persistent symptoms.

Spirochetosis affects the large bowel, and any segment may be involved, including the appendix. Endoscopic abnormalities are typically mild (mucosal edema or erythema) or completely absent. Histologically, spirochetosis produces a fuzzy, "fringed," 2–3-μm-thick blue-purple line at the luminal border of the mucosa that can be seen on routine H&E sections (Fig. 10.27a, b). The distribution of organisms can be patchy and focal. It is believed that the bacteria do not invade, although there are rare reports of alleged minimal invasion when many organisms are present. Inflammation is usually absent, although neutrophilic cryptitis is rarely seen. The spirochetes stain intensely with Warthin-Starry or similar silver impregnation stains, which highlight their spirillar morphology. They may also stain with alcian blue (pH 2.5) and PAS stains, but they do not stain distinctly with tissue Gram stain. The treponeme immunostain used for syphilis will also stain cases of spirochetosis and is regarded by many as superior, as the quality of silver impregnation stains varies widely. PCR and in situ hybridization assays also exist for identification of the specific organisms, but this is not widely available.

It is important to distinguish spirochetosis from a prominent glycocalyx, which does not stain with silver impregnation stains or IHC directed against the bacteria. Some type of special stain or immunostain is recommended in the evaluation of cases where spirochetosis is suspected, both to avoid underdiagnosis and to avoid mistaking a prominent glycocalyx for organisms. Occasionally, enteroadherent *E. coli* have a similar histologic appearance, but *E. coli* are Gram-negative and lack spirillar morphology.

References: [89–95]

14. **What is the clinical significance of a positive result with a stool PCR assay, and how does that correlate with biopsy findings?**

Recently, multiplex PCR assays have received FDA approval for pathogen detection and identification of agents that cause gastroenteritis and infectious colitis from stool specimens. These assays use nucleic acid amplification, typically PCR, followed by detection through fluorescent dyes, array hybridization, or bead-based hybridization to specific probes. They can detect as many as 22 bacteria, viruses, and parasites combined, often within 1–5 h of specimen receipt. These assays hold promise in that they are highly sensitive and rapid. In addition, they allow consolidation of multiple laboratory work flows, because without these PCR-based assays, a combination of cultures, immmunoassays, microscopic examination, and targeted PCR would be needed to test for all of the possible causes of infectious diarrhea. However, the breadth of multiplex PCR testing is also a challenge, in that these assays detect pathogens that can differ widely in their epidemiology, virulence, and incidence of co-infection, making the interpretation of positive results challenging. The clinical significance of a positive result is often unclear, and there are currently few studies that have correlated biopsy findings with positive stool PCR assays.

The critical aspect of interpreting multiplex PCRs, and indeed most laboratory tests, is a clear understanding of the pre-test probability for the various pathogens being tested. For some enteric pathogens, the rate of detection in asymptomatic controls is equivalent to that in patients with GI complaints, making the significance of a positive stool PCR assay dubious. GI complaints are strongly associated with pathogens such as *Campylobacter* and *Salmonella* spp., but strength of association between symptoms and the presence of a pathogen is much less for other organisms and is also less in young children compared with adults. Another example is that of traveler's diarrhea. It is clear that travelers often acquire pathogens, but the pathogens do not always cause symptoms. For example, in a study of 382 travelers, 75% of patients had an enteric pathogen detected after travel compared with 4% before travel. Pathogen detection was strongly associated with traveler's diarrhea (odds ratios >3), but this association was not absolute: 61% of asymptomatic travelers had also acquired a pathogen compared with 83% of patients with active or resolved traveler's diarrhea.

In one large study correlating stool PCR assays with colon biopsies obtained within a week of the positive stool PCR test, 75% of patients had histologic abnormalities on biopsy. Many of these patients had morphologic evidence of pseudomembranous colitis, and a PCR result positive for *C. difficile*. Of the remainder of patients with a positive stool PCR assay, many had IBD, and the significance of a PCR assay positive for pathogens such as enteropathogenic *E. coli* or Norovirus in this population remains unclear, although the potential causative role of these organisms in a IBD flare is worthy of further consideration.

In cases where the differential diagnosis is between infectious and non-infectious etiologies, interpretation of PCR assays remains challenging, and by performing these multiplex assays, we are essentially learning the epidemiology of these pathogens in real time.

References: [96–99]

15. What are the most commonly encountered causes of antibiotic-associated injury other than C. difficile, and what are the best ways to diagnose them?

The vast majority of cases of antibiotic-associated diarrhea are due to *C. difficile* infection (see below), but other pathogens have been implicated as well. *Clostridium perfringens* and *Staphyloccus aureus* (including MRSA) have also been suggested as causes of antibiotic-associated diarrhea based on stool studies, but pathologic features have not been well-described.

Klebsiella oxytoca is a recently recognized pathogen that has been experimentally and epidemiologically linked to antibiotic-associated hemorrhagic colitis. Associated drugs include penicillins, cephalosporins, and pristinamycin, and symptoms and lesions typically resolve quickly after withdrawal of the antibiotic. Endoscopic findings include a segmental hemorrhagic colitis, without pseudomembranes. Histologic findings have not been well-characterized, but case reports describe an active hemorrhagic colitis with neutrophilic infiltrates and crypt abscesses, but no architectural distortion or other features of chronicity (Fig. 10.28). The *K. oxytoca* toxin has been identified as tilavalline, a peptide produced by nonribosomal peptide synthetases. Toxin-producing strains of *K. oxytoca* are found in feces from both hemorrhagic colitis and asymptomatic patients, suggesting that *K. oxytoca* can cause opportunistic infections when a colonizing strain is able to expand in density after antibiotic treatment. They are also phylogenetically distinguishable from respiratory infection isolates, suggesting that mutually exclusive subsets of *K. oxytoca* cause colitis and pneumonia. Unlike *Salmonella* and *Shigella*, there are no standardized approaches for isolating *K. oxytoca* from stool samples using selective and differential agar. This makes isolating *K. oxytoca* from stool samples challenging with routinely available media. Once isolated, *K. oxytoca* can be preliminarily distinguished from *K. pneumoniae* by a rapid indole test and definitively identified by MALDI-TOF mass spectrometry.

References: [100–104]

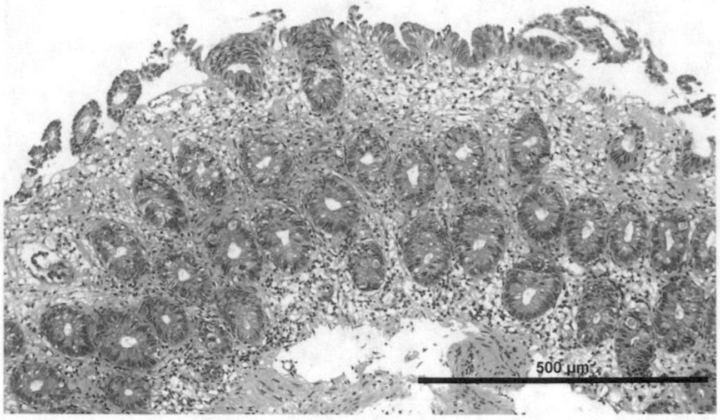

Fig. 10.28 *Klebsiella oxytoca* antibiotic-associated hemorrhagic colitis. Colon biopsy shows a hemorrhagic colitis with marked reactive epithelial changes, and no features of chronicity or pseudomembranes. (Courtesy Dr. Gregor Gorkiewicz)

16. How do the different laboratory methodologies for the diagnosis of C. difficile correlate with clinical scenario and biopsy findings?

The association between *C. difficile* and antibiotic-associated diarrhea was initially described in the 1970s, and the incidence has dramatically increased since then.

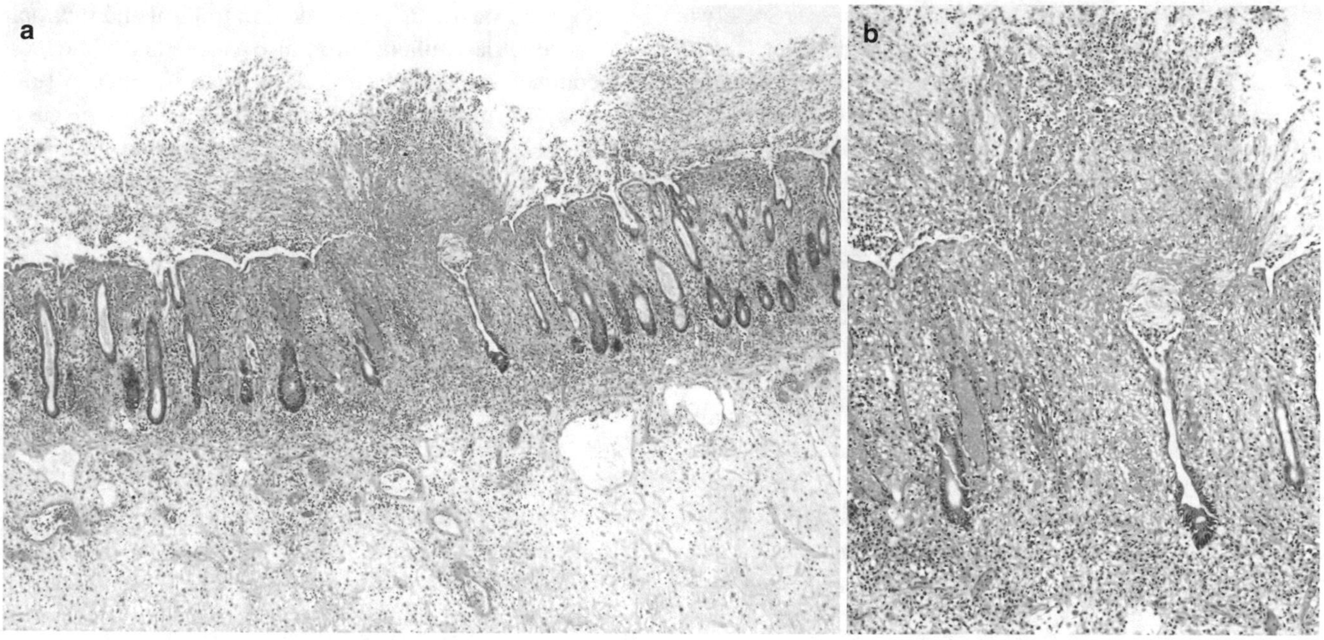

Fig. 10.29 *C difficile* colitis. Low power view shows the classic exploding crypts with volcano-shaped pseudomembranes (**a**). Higher power shows the intercrypt necrosis and admixed fibrin and inflammatory cells in the pseudomembrane (**b**)

C. difficile is the most common nosocomial GI pathogen. Infection is usually related to prior antibiotic exposure, particularly orally administered antibiotics, because the bacteria cannot infect in the presence of normal colonic flora. The majority of patients are elderly, although infection is certainly not limited to this group. In addition to prior antibiotic use, other risk factors for infection include severe co-morbid conditions, indwelling nasogastric tubes, GI procedures, antacids, admission to an intensive care unit, and length of hospitalization. Since 2010, rates have declined in Europe but stabilized at high levels in the United States. Similarly, the epidemic ribosome 027 strain, associated with both increased rates and severity of infection, has decreased in Europe but remains a significant subset of infections in the United States.

Endoscopically, classic *C. difficile*-associated pseudomembranous colitis features yellow-white pseudomembranes that bleed when scraped off the mucosa. Any segment of the bowel can be affected, including the small bowel and the appendix, but pseudomembranes are most common in the distal left colon. Histologically, the classic lesion is a volcano- or mushroom-shaped exudate, with intercrypt necrosis and ballooned crypts that give rise to the laminated pseudomembranes composed of fibrin, mucin, and neutrophils (Fig. 10.29a, b). More severe and prolonged pseudomembranous colitis may lead to full-thickness mucosal necrosis. Nonspecific, less characteristic lesions, usually focal active colitis with occasional crypt abscesses but lacking pseudomembranous features, have been well-described in association with a positive *C. difficile* toxin assay. Endoscopy is not routinely recommended in patients with typical symptoms of *C. difficile* infection who have positive laboratory testing. However, it can be valuable in patients with persistent or recurrent symptoms and negative laboratory testing or patients who fail conventional therapy.

Diagnosis of *C. difficile* infection is both a success of translational research and an ongoing challenge in optimizing clinical sensitivity and specificity. The success in *C. difficile* diagnosis was in establishing that the pathophysiology of the disease is directly attributable to two toxins encoded by the *tcdA* and *tcdB* genes. As not all strains of *C. difficile* carry these toxins, diagnostic testing is focused on detecting either toxin in the stool sample or their genes within the bacteria. However, the challenge is that patients may have toxigenic *C. difficile* detected in their stool without any evidence of infection. For purposes of test interpretation, this is considered to be asymptomatic colonization, although the true physiologic state of *C. difficile* in these patients is unclear. Detectable *C. difficile* in an asymptomatic patient is difficult to interpret. The risk of infection in the patient is unclear and likely declines over time, but evidence is emerging that these patients may spread *C. difficile* within healthcare facilities. However, current evidence is not strong enough to support any interventions or contact precautions in asymptomatic patients with positive test results.

The 2017 update of the Infectious Diseases Society of America (IDSA) clinical practice guidelines for *C. difficile* defines infection as "the presence of symptoms (usually diarrhea) and either a stool test positive for *C. difficile* toxins or detection of toxigenic *C. difficile*, or colonoscopic or histopathologic findings revealing pseudomembranous colitis." For accurate diagnosis, these guidelines recommend testing patients who have had an acute onset of diarrhea with three or more unformed stools within 24 h, and best practice is to have institutional guidelines for sample submission that includes only non-formed stools and not testing patients on laxatives.

There are a number of testing modalities that can be used separately or in combination to optimize diagnostic accuracy. Antigen testing for glutamate dehydrogenase (GDH) is highly sensitive as it is expressed in all strains, but has low specificity since it may be expressed in non-toxigenic strains as well. Conversely, antigen tests for toxins have low analytical sensitivity but high specificity for disease since a positive result means the toxins are being produced within the GI tract. Finally, NAAT for toxin genes is highly sensitive for toxigenic *C. difficile*, but the specificity of this test is controversial. If institutional guidelines for specimen submission are established, NAAT testing alone is acceptable, and some investigators consider this approach optimal for both clinical care and infection prevention. With or without institutional guidelines for specimen submission, algorithms that combine modalities are appropriate for diagnosis. One common algorithm is testing with highly sensitive GDH antigen with follow-up toxin antigen testing. Discrepancies between the two tests may be due to low toxin antigen sensitivity and can be arbitrated by NAAT. Alternatively, NAAT can be performed and followed up by toxin testing. As with many tests, the critical step in *C. difficile* diagnosis occurs before the sample reaches the laboratory: selecting patients with an appropriate pre-test probability of having the disease in question.

References: [14, 105–108]

17. What are the best morphologic and laboratory methods for distinguishing between commonly encountered protozoa in the GI tract?

Protozoa are most prevalent in tropical and subtropical countries, although they also cause some of the most common intestinal infections in North America. A summary of protozoa affecting the GI tract is given in Table 10.5. Protozoa are often diagnosed in stool samples, but may also be encountered in tissue sections; those encountered in tissue sections are the focus of this discussion.

- *Balantidium coli* is the largest protozoan and also the only ciliate capable of causing disease in humans. It is common in the tropics, especially the Philippines, where it is most often a parasite infecting pigs and other domestic and wild animals. Because of this, human infections are commonly linked to close contact with pigs, water contaminated with pig excreta, and butchering. Although most human infections are asymptomatic, infection may produce a spectrum of clinical and pathologic changes similar to that of *E. histolytica*. *B. coli* typically infects the terminal ileum and colon, particularly the rectosigmoid, causing mucosal ulceration, edema, hemorrhage, and necrosis. The inflammatory infiltrate is often predominantly mononuclear, and inflammation and necrosis may be transmural. Rare manifestations include appendicitis and superinfection of patients with IBD.

B. coli are distinguished from amoebae by their large size (50–200 µm in length by 40–70 µm in diameter), prominent kidney bean-shaped macronuclei, smaller round micronuclei, and the presence of hundreds of cilia that beat in coordinated rhythm (Fig. 10.30a, b). Because of this distinctive appearance and their size, they are easily identified in tissue sections.

- *Entamoeba histolytica* infects approximately 10% of the world's population, predominantly in tropical and subtropical regions. In the United States, it is most often seen in immigrants, overseas travelers, male homosexuals, and institutionalized persons. Infection is usually acquired through contaminated water or food and can be spread by the fecal–oral route; sexual transmission has been rarely reported. Risk factors for symptomatic

Table 10.5 Selected protozoa affecting the gastrointestinal tract

Amoebae	Flagellates	Coccidians	Ciliates	Uncertain
Entamoeba histolytica	*Trypanosoma cruzi*	Microsporidia	*Balantidium coli*	*Blastocystis hominis*
Entamoeba coli *Entamoeba hartmani* *Entamoeba polecki*	*Leishmania donovanii* and related species	Cyclospora		
Endolimax nana	*Giardia lamblia*	Cryptosporidium		
Iodamoeba butschlii	*Dientamoeba fragilis*	*Isospora belli*		
		Toxoplasma gondii		

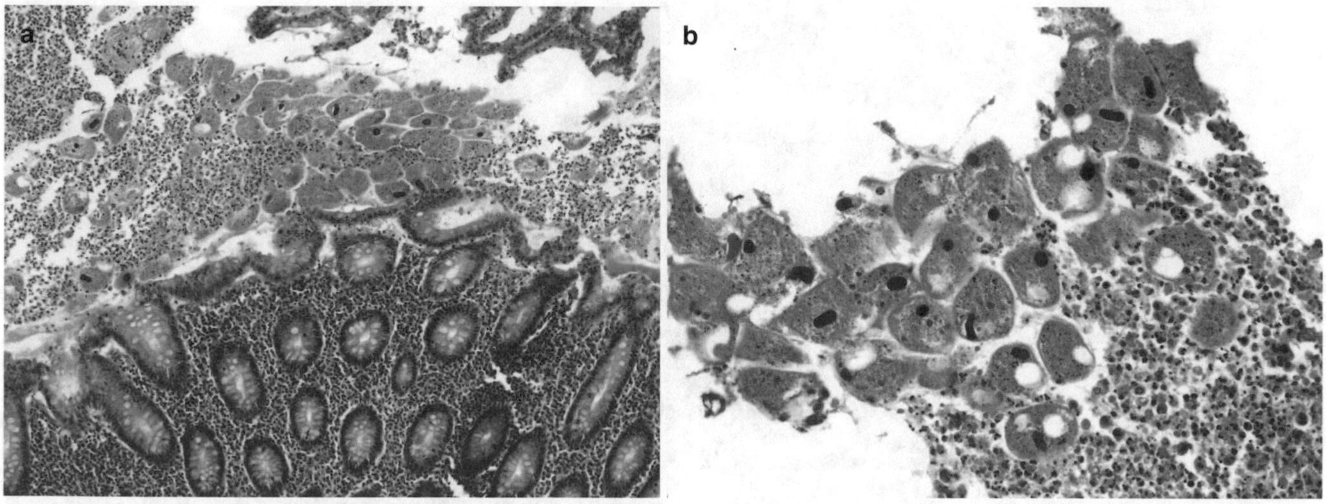

Fig. 10.30 *Balantidium coli*. Appendiceal infection with a large number of organisms admixed with neutrophilic inflammation (**a**). The parasites are very large, with large kidney-bean-shaped nuclei and peripheral cilia (**b**)

infection include pediatric age group, malnutrition, pregnancy, immunosuppression, and steroid use.

The spectrum of infection is extremely broad. Many infected patients are asymptomatic or have only vague, nonspecific GI complaints. Symptomatic patients most commonly have diarrhea, abdominal cramps, and variable right lower quadrant tenderness; this has been referred to as "nondysenteric" amebiasis. Invasive disease, most often manifested as amoebic dysentery or liver abscess, reportedly occurs in less than 10% of infected persons. Amebic dysentery presents suddenly, approximately 1–3 weeks after exposure to the motile protozoan, with severe abdominal cramps, tenesmus, fever, and diarrhea. *E. histolytica* is occasionally found in the appendix, generally in association with heavy infection of the right colon.

The cecum is the most common site of involvement, followed by the right colon, rectum, sigmoid, then appendix. Colonoscopy may be normal in asymptomatic patients or those with mild disease. When patients do have colonoscopic findings, they typically include small ulcers, which may coalesce to form large, irregular geographic or serpiginous lesions. The ulcers may undermine adjacent mucosa to produce the classic "flask-shaped" ulceration. The intervening mucosa is often grossly normal. Unusual findings include fulminant colitis resembling ulcerative colitis; pseudomembrane formation mimicking *C. difficile*-related pseudomembranous colitis; and large inflammatory masses consisting of organisms and granulation tissue (amoebomas).

In asymptomatic patients or those with only mild symptoms, histologic findings may range from normal to a heavy mixed inflammatory infiltrate. Organisms may be particularly difficult (if not impossible) to detect in these patients. In symptomatic patients, early lesions may show a mild neutrophilic infiltrate. However, a common feature is abundant amorphous eosinophilic necrotic material at the luminal surface, containing nuclear debris and organisms, but few intact neutrophils (Fig. 10.31a–e). In more advanced disease, ulcers are often deep, extending into the submucosa and undermining adjacent mucosa, which can show gland distortion that can mimic IBD. In early lesions, the organisms are concentrated at the luminal surface and in ulcers, usually within the necrotic material. Invasive amoebae may occasionally be detected within the bowel wall.

Amoebic trophozoites have distinct cell membranes with foamy cytoplasm, and round, eccentrically located nuclei with peripheral margination of chromatin and a central karyosome. The presence of ingested red blood cells is essentially pathognomonic of *E. histolytica* and helps to distinguish it from nonpathogenic amoebae. Distinction of trophozoites from macrophages within inflammatory exudates may be difficult, particularly in poorly fixed tissue sections. Amoebae are trichrome and PAS-positive; in addition, their nuclei are usually smaller, more rounded, and pale and have a more open nuclear chromatin pattern than macrophage nuclei. In addition, macrophages stain with CD68, CD163, and alpha-1-antitrypsin, whereas amoebae do not. In stool samples, in the absence of ingested red blood cells, *E. histolytica* cannot be distinguished morphologically from the nonpathogenic *E. dispar*. However, multiplex PCR assays are available that are specific for the detection of *E. histolytica*.

B. coli may mimic *E. histolytica* histologically, but it is much larger, has a kidney-bean-shaped macronucleus, and is ciliated. *E. histolytica* may be distinguished from most other amoebae by the presence of ingested red blood cells.

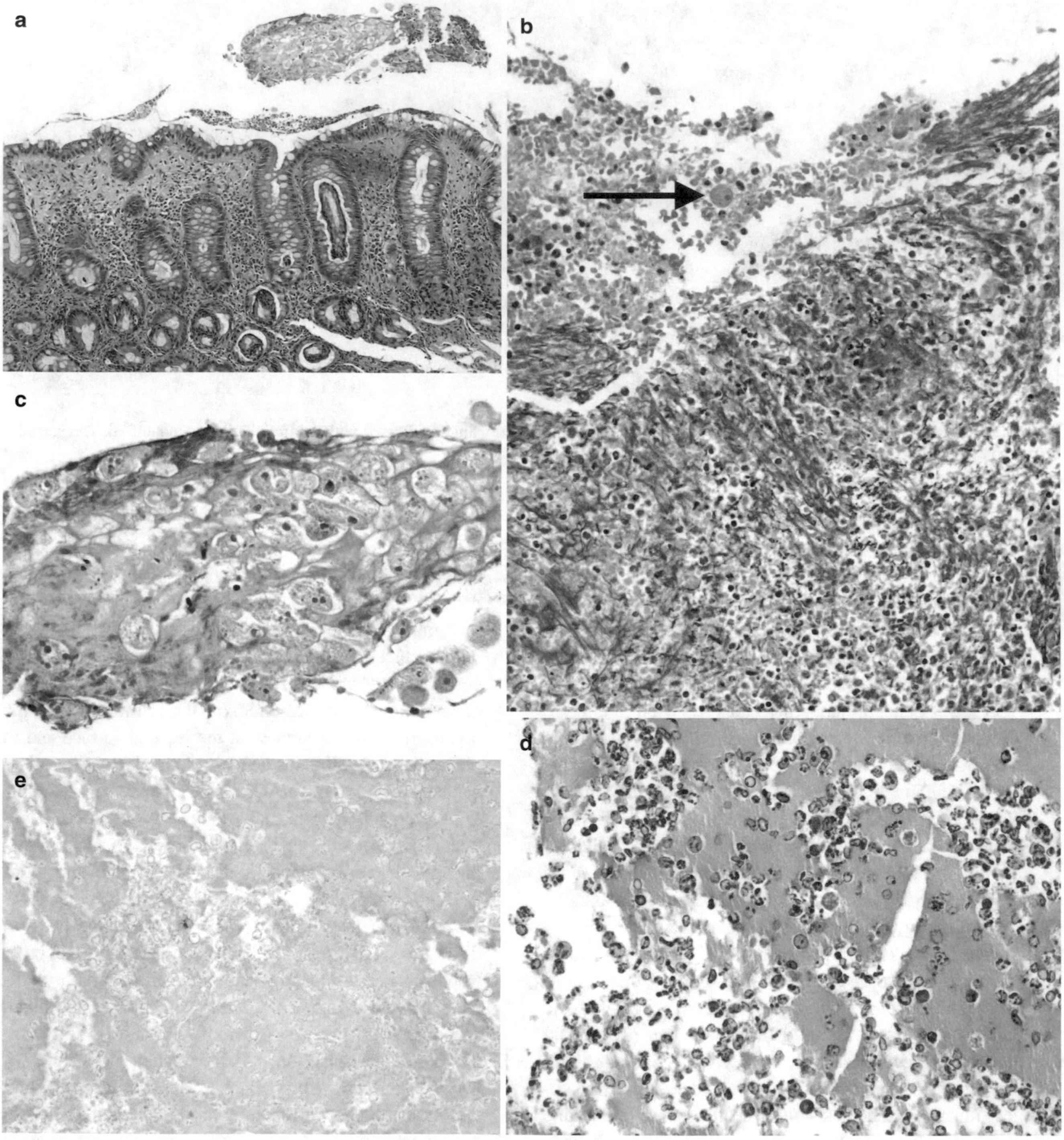

Fig. 10.31 Amebiasis. Colon biopsy shows minimal inflammation, with a few amoeba admixed with neutrophils overlying the epithelium (**a**). A single amoeba (arrow) is present amidst abundant amorphous debris with few intact neutrophils (**b**). At high power, *E. histolytica* have foamy cytoplasm, round nuclei with open chromatin, and contain ingested red blood cells (**c**). Amoeba stain positively with trichrome (**d**) and are negative for macrophage markers such as CD163 (**e**)

The differential diagnosis of amebiasis also includes other GI diseases such as Crohn disease, ulcerative colitis, *C. difficile*-related pseudomembranous colitis, and other infections. Although amebiasis can cause architectural distortion, other features of IBD are absent in amebiasis, such as marked basal lymphoplasmacytosis, transmural lymphoid aggregates, mural fibrosis, granulomas, and neural hyperplasia. A careful search for trophozoites in unusual cases of IBD or in specimens from patients from endemic regions is war-

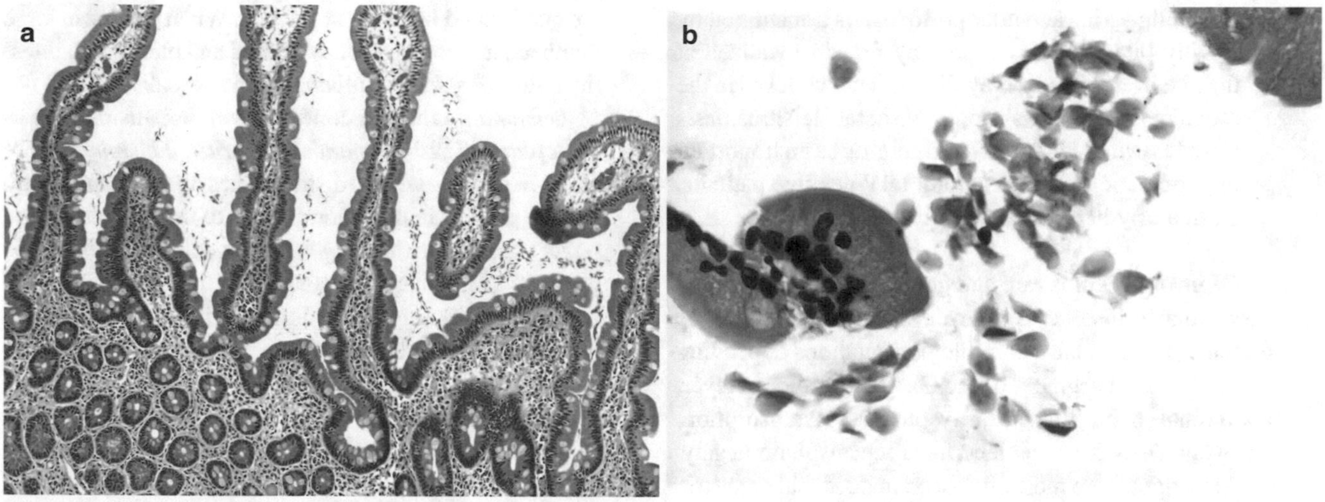

Fig. 10.32 Giardiasis. At low power, *Giardia* at the surface of the duodenum have a "falling leaves" appearance (**a**). There is minimal attendant inflammation. At high power, the pear shape and ovoid nuclei can be better appreciated (**b**)

ranted, however, as immunosuppression can cause life-threatening complications.

- *Giardia lamblia* infection occurs throughout temperate and tropical regions worldwide. It is one of the most common human protozoal enteric pathogens, and it is the most clinically significant protozoan pathogen in the United States. Risk factors for infection include pediatric age group, travel to foreign countries, use of drinking and recreational water from untreated sources, institutional settings (including daycare centers), living with an infected child, and immune compromise, particularly common variable immunodeficiency.

Transmission is through contaminated water or food, and person-to-person transmission via the fecal–oral route is quite common. Transmission via oral–anal sexual practices has also been well-documented. The cyst is the infective form, and it is extremely hardy and chlorine-resistant; *Giardia* can survive in water for several months. The mechanism by which *Giardia* causes illness remains poorly understood.

Many infections are asymptomatic. Patients with acute giardiasis present with diarrhea and weight loss, variably accompanied by abdominal pain and distension, nausea, vomiting, flatulence, evidence of malabsorption, and fatigue. Infection may resolve spontaneously, but often persists for weeks or months if untreated. Many patients go on to develop chronic giardiasis, featuring diarrhea accompanied by marked weight loss, signs of malabsorption, and anemia. Complications include dehydration, especially in children, and failure to thrive among infants and small children.

Giardia is found primarily in the proximal small bowel, although they may be found rarely in the stomach and colon. Endoscopic examination is generally unremarkable, and small bowel biopsies usually show no tissue reaction to the organism at all. A minority of cases show mild to moderate villous blunting, crypt hyperplasia, and increased lamina propria inflammation. Trophozoites are found at the luminal surface, and tissue invasion is not a feature of giardiasis (Fig. 10.32a, b). The flagellated trophozoites resemble pears cut lengthwise and contain two ovoid nuclei with a central karyosome. The somewhat scattered distribution of the parasite at the luminal surface has been referred to as "falling leaves." Absence or a marked decrease of plasma cells in the lamina propria in a patient with giardiasis should alert the pathologist to the possibility of an underlying immunodeficiency disorder such as common variable immunodeficiency.

Giardia do not closely resemble other intestinal protozoa, but they can be hard to find, and examination of multiple levels is often necessary to establish the diagnosis. Touch cytology (imprint from endoscopic biopsy specimens performed before the tissue is placed in formalin) may significantly increase diagnostic yield, since many of the luminal trophozoites may be washed away during tissue processing. CD117 will also highlight the organism.

From stool samples of symptomatic patients, *Giardia* can be identified by their distinctive morphology. However, EIAs have better test performance and are more cost-effective than stool ova and parasite (O&P) examination. Multiplex PCR tests also include assays for this parasite.

- Leishmaniasis, caused by *Leishmania donovani* and related species, is endemic in over 80 countries in Africa, Asia, South and Central America, and Europe.

The obligate intracellular protozoan is transmitted by sandfly bites; the infection may remain localized at the site of the bite or may disseminate widely via the reticuloendothelial system. Visceral leishmaniasis (also known as kala-azar) is emerging as an important opportunistic infection among HIV-positive patients, particularly in Southwestern Europe.

GI involvement is rare and generally part of a widely disseminated disease. Any level of the GI tract may be affected. Patients have variable presentations depending on the involved segment of the GI tract, including fever, abdominal pain, diarrhea, dysphagia, malabsorption, and weight loss. Many patients have hepatosplenomegaly.

Amastigotes are most often seen in duodenal or gastric biopsies, but are also found in the colon. Amastigote-containing macrophages are seen within the lamina propria (Fig. 10.33). The amastigotes are rounded, 2–4 μm basophilic organisms with a round to oval central nucleus and a thin external membrane. The kinetoplast lies tangentially or at right angles to the nucleus, producing the characteristic "double-knot" configuration. Organisms are highlighted by Giemsa staining. When present in large numbers, macrophages may distend and blunt small intestinal villi. Associated inflammation is usually absent.

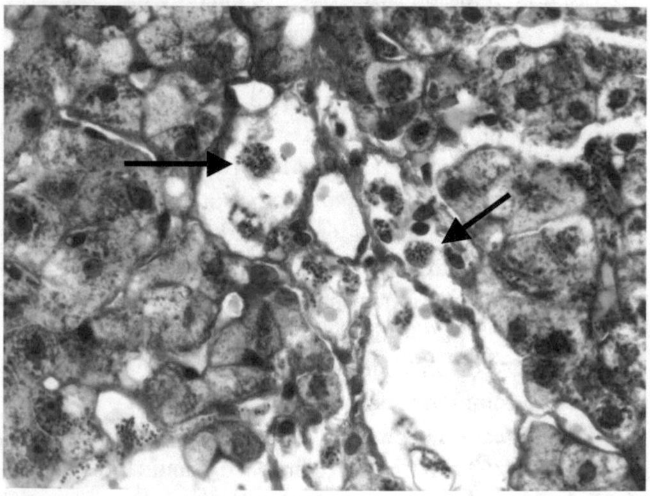

Fig. 10.33 Leishmaniasis. Giemsa stain highlights organisms within macrophages (arrows). The kinetoplast is barely visible as a more purple-staining dot

Leishmania may be confused with organisms such as *Histoplasma* and *Trypanosoma cruzi*. *Leishmania* are GMS-negative, which distinguishes them from fungi, and are present in the macrophages of the lamina propria rather than surrounding the myenteric plexus (as opposed to Chagas disease). The kinetoplast of *Leishmania* distinguishes it from *Toxoplasma*, which may also stain with Giemsa.

- Coccidial infection is particularly important when considering the differential diagnosis of diarrhea in patients with AIDS. However, all are capable of causing diarrhea (often prolonged) in otherwise healthy patients. Although all four of these organisms are still typically grouped as coccidians for purposes of discussion, Microsporidia are now classified as fungi, and Cryptosporidia have been placed in a separate parasite category known as the Gregorines.

Transmission is normally via the fecal–oral route, either directly or through contaminated food and water. Many infections are asymptomatic; symptomatic patients generally present with diarrhea, variably accompanied by fever, weight loss, abdominal pain, and malaise. In immunocompetent persons, infection is usually self-limited, but immunocompromised patients are at risk for chronic severe diarrhea with associated malabsorption, dehydration, and eventual death.

Endoscopic findings are usually absent or mild. A comparison of the morphologic features in biopsy specimens of the most important GI coccidians is given in Table 10.6 and discussed below. Although typical staining properties are listed, they may vary with the form of the organism and tissue fixation. Almost all other intracellular organisms that could be confused with coccidians are present within macrophages and do not occur within epithelial cells at the luminal surface (e.g. *Leishmania*, *Toxoplasma*, or *Histoplasma*).

Table 10.6 A Comparison of the morphologic features of enteric coccidians in tissue sections

Feature	Microsporidia	Cryptosporidia	Cyclospora	Cystoisospora
Size	2–3 μm spores (smallest coccidian)	2–5 μm	2–3 μm schizonts 5–6 μm merozoites	15–20 μm (largest coccidian)
Location	Epithelial cells; rarely macrophages	Apical surface	Upper-third of epithelial cell	Epithelial cells and macrophages
Staining properties	Modified trichrome-, Giemsa-, Gram-, and Warthin-Starry-positive	Giemsa- and Gram stain-positive	Acid-fast-, auramine-positive; GMS-, PAS-, Giemsa-negative	Giemsa-, Gram-, and PAS-positive
Other	May be birefringent under polarized light	Organism bulges out of the luminal surface of enterocyte apex	Parasitophorous vacuole	Parasitophorous vacuole; eosinophilic infiltrate

Cryptosporidium is most common in the small bowel, but may infect any segment of the GI tract. It rarely infects the pancreaticobiliary tree, causing sclerosing cholangitis, pancreatitis, or acalculous cholecystitis. The characteristic appearance is that of a 2–5 μm, basophilic spherical body that protrudes or bulges from the apex of the enterocyte at the luminal surface, giving a "blue beads" appearance in H&E sections (Fig. 10.34). They may be found in crypts or in surface epithelium. Associated mucosal changes include villous atrophy (occasionally severe), crypt hyperplasia, mixed lamina propria inflammation, and rarely cryptitis. Surface epithelial cells may show degenerative changes and nuclear disarray. *Cryptosporidium* may be distinguished from most other coccidians by their size and unique apical location. In stool specimens, *Cryptospordium* are 2–4-μm-diameter acid-fast spherical oocysts that are positive by modified acid-fast stain. EIAs have superior performance to microscopy and can be bundled with *Giardia* immunoassays as a cost-effective approach to diagnosing two of the most common intestinal parasites. Alternatively, multiplex PCR assays can be used to detect *Cryptosporidium*.

Cyclospora cayetanensis most commonly infects the small bowel as well. Histologic changes in mucosal biopsies are similar to other coccidians, including mild villous blunting, patchy lamina propria inflammation, and surface epithelial disarray. Intracellular forms of *Cyclospora* include 2–3 μm schizonts and 5–6 μm banana-shaped merozoites located within enterocytes (Fig. 10.35), often within the upper-third of the enterocyte, within a parasitophorous vacuole. In stool specimens, *Cyclospora* are 7–8-μm-diameter round oocysts best visualized with a modified acid-fast stain and larger than *Cryptosporidium*. Sporulated oocysts contain two 6 × 4 μm sporocysts, each with two sporozoites. Some multiplex PCR assays also include *Cyclospora*.

Cystoisospora sp. (formerly *Isospora*) is the largest coccidian (15–20 μm in tissue sections). The small bowel is most commonly involved, although the colon and biliary tree may also be affected. Histologic changes include villous blunting, which may be severe; villous fusion; surface epithelial disarray; mixed inflammation in the lamina propria, often with prominent eosinophils; and fibrosis of the lamina propria (Fig. 10.36a, b). Tissue reaction may be minimal, however. When crescent-shaped, *Cyclospora* may be confused with *Cystoisospora*, which are larger. In stool specimens, *Cystoisospora* are identified as oblong acid-fast oocysts averaging 32 × 14 μm in size usually containing one or two round sporoblasts that mature into infectious sporocysts.

Microsporidia spp. affect all levels of the GI tract, including the biliary tree, but the small bowel is the most common. Histologic findings include focal mild villous blunting, a patchy lamina propria lymphoplasmacytic infiltrate, variably increased surface intraepithelial lymphocytes, vacuolization of the surface epithelium, and surface epithelial cell disarray (Fig. 10.37a, b). There may be minimal to no tissue reaction, however. The organisms are present as small 2–3 μm spores, as well as large plasmodia that are located within the supranuclear cytoplasm of epithelial cells or occasionally lamina propria macrophages. Associated vacuoles may cup or flatten the enterocyte nucleus. In stool samples, the small spores (0.8–4 μm depending on species) can be detected by specialized chromotrope stains or fungal stains such as the calcofluor white fluorescent stain.

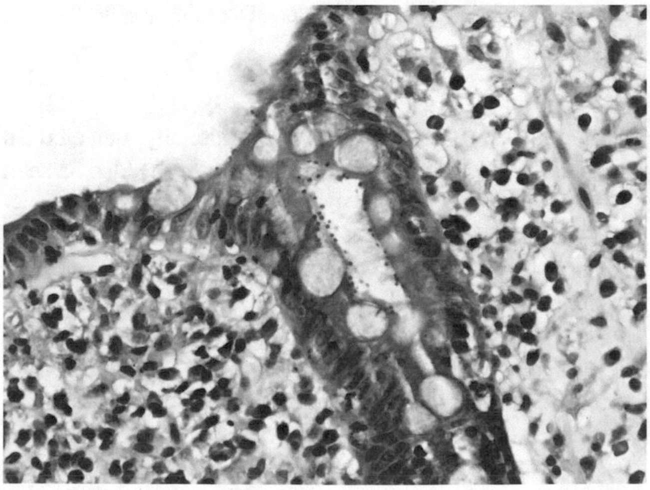

Fig. 10.34 *Cryptosporidium. Cryptosporidium* appear as blue beads at the luminal surface and within the crypts of the colonic epithelium. Associated inflammation is mild, but there are increased intraepithelial lymphocytes and surface epithelial disarray

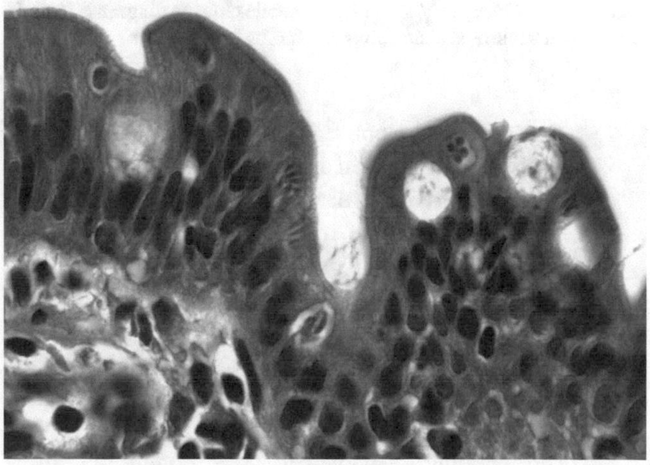

Fig. 10.35 *Cyclospora*. Both the round schizonts and crescent-shaped merozoites are present, within clear parasitophorous vacuoles

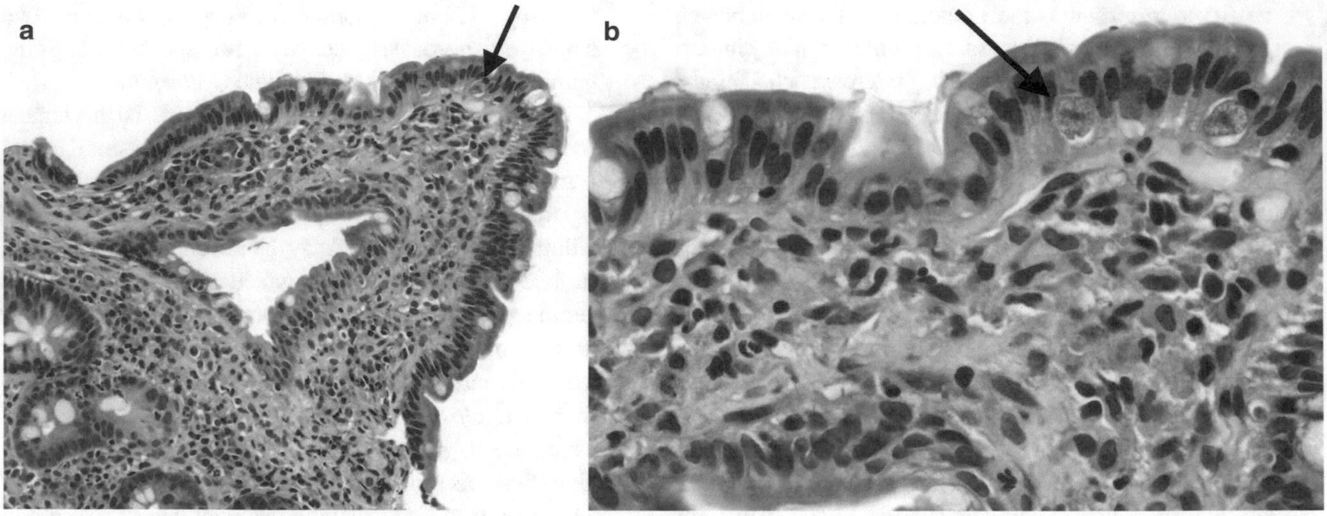

Fig. 10.36 *Cystoisospora*. A duodenal biopsy shows organisms in the surface epithelium, with a neutrophilc and eosinophilic infiltrate in the lamina propria (**a**, arrow). A higher power view of the organism demonstrates their large size and surrounding parasitophorous vacuole (**b**, arrow)

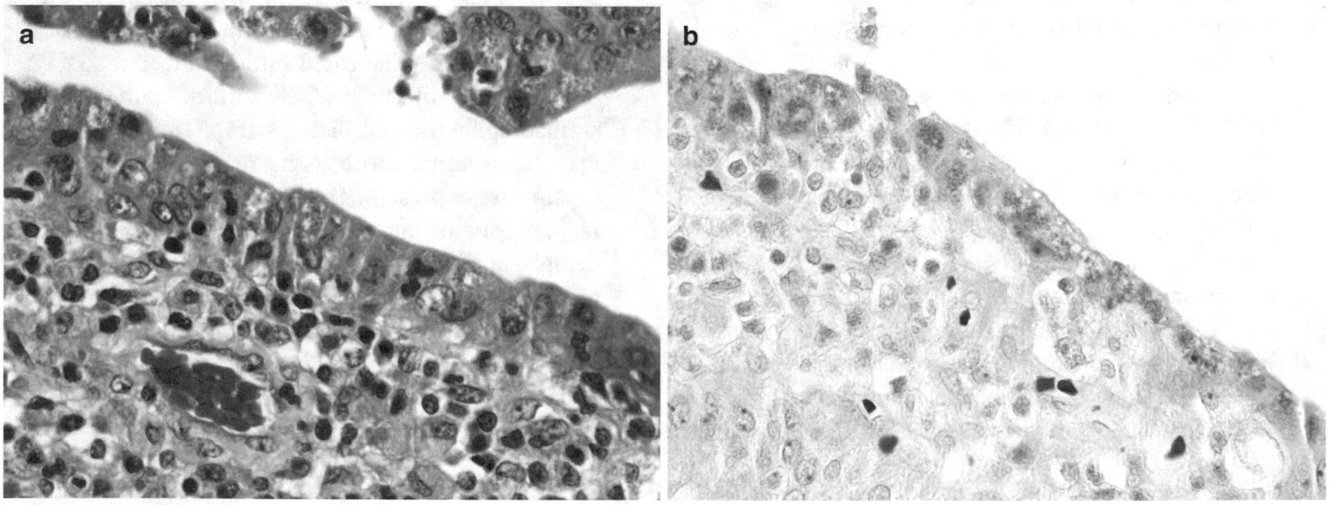

Fig. 10.37 *Microsporidia*. On H&E, subtle clues to diagnosis include surface epithelial disarray and vacuolization of the luminal epithelium (**a**). A modified trichrome stain stains the spores bright red (**b**)

- *T. gondii*. GI toxoplasmosis is primarily a disease of immunocompromised hosts and usually presents in patients with disseminated disease. Gastric and colonic involvement are the most common. Both crescent-shaped tachyzoites as well as tissue cysts containing bradyzoites may be present within tissue sections.

References: [109–124]

18. What are clinically significant helminths, and how are they distinguished?

The helminths, or worms, that commonly affect humans include the trematodes (flukes), cestodes (tapeworms), and nematodes (roundworms) (Table 10.7). Although the most common method of diagnosing GI helminthic infections is examination of stool for O&P (see below), helminths are occasionally detected in biopsy or resection specimens. Worms may also be seen endoscopically.

GI helminths have a worldwide distribution, but the clinical significance varies with geography, in that they are more often a cause of serious disease in nations with deficient sanitation, excessive poverty, and hot, humid climates. Helminths can cause severe, life-threatening nutritional problems, particularly in children. Infection can also be encountered in immigrants and patients who have traveled to endemic areas and may be an important problem in immunocompromised hosts.

The most common site of infection is the small bowel, although the stomach and large bowel may occasionally be involved. Hookworms, roundworms (both *Ascaris* and *Enterobius*), and whipworms are the most common helminths found in humans.

- Fluke infection, which is food-borne, remains a worldwide public health problem, particularly in Asia and the Pacific. Most clinically significant infections are due to *Fasciolopsis buski, Echinostoma* spp., and *Heterophyes* spp. Flukes are ovoid to flat, fleshy worms ranging in size from 1.0 mm (*Heterophyes*) to 7.5 cm (*Fasciolopsis*) that can be seen endoscopically. They are ingested along with aquatic plants, fish, shellfish, or amphibians, and symptoms usually occur as a result of heavy infection. Mild anemia and eosinophilia are common, and GI symptoms include diarrhea, which may alternate with constipation, abdominal pain, anorexia, nausea, vomiting, and malabsorption. Obstruction and GI bleeding have also been described. *Heterophyes* species can actually penetrate the wall of the intestine, with associated ulceration and inflammation.

Schistosomiasis is one of the most common diseases in the world. All species of *Schistosoma* that infect humans can cause significant GI disease. These trematodes are endemic to Africa, Asia, and parts of the Americas. In the United States, infected patients are often immigrants or travelers. Humans become infected by exposure to contaminated water. The histologic findings in schistosomiasis result from inflammation and fibrosis in reaction to the eggs deposited in tissue; the worms themselves cause little damage. On H&E, the calcified eggs are generally dark blue or black and somewhat amorphous. There is variably present associated granulomatous inflammation or fibrosis (Fig. 10.38a, b).

- Tapeworms occasionally cause GI disease in humans. They are flat and segmented, consisting of a head (scolex) and multiple segments (proglottids), but no true body cavity. They range in size from 2.5 mm (*Hymenolepsis*) to 30 m (*Taenia saginata*). The latter can live for up to 20 years.

Table 10.7 General classification of clinically significant helminths

	Trematodes (flukes)	Cestodes (tapeworms)	Nematodes (roundworms)
Examples	*Fasciola* (liver fluke) *Fasciolopsis* (giant intestinal fluke) *Echinostoma* (intestinal fluke) *Schistosoma* *Clonorchis*, *Opisthorchis* (Asian liver fluke, biliary fluke) *Heterophyes* *Paragonimus*	*Diphyllobothrium* (fish tapeworm) *Taenia* (pork and beef tapeworm) *Echinococcus* *Hymenolepsis* (dwarf tapeworm)	*Trichuris* (whipworm) *Capillaria* *Trichinella* *Strongyloides* *Ancylostoma* (hookworm) *Ascaris* (roundworm) *Toxocara* (visceral larva migrans) *Anisakis* *Angiostrongylus* *Oesophagostoma* *Enterobius* (pinworm, threadworm)
Important characteristics	Fish are principal hosts Flat, sometimes leaf-shaped bodies with oral and ventral suckers	Have scolex and proglottids	One of the largest and most widespread groups of multicellular animals Affect virtually all plants and animals Elongated, cylindrical bodies

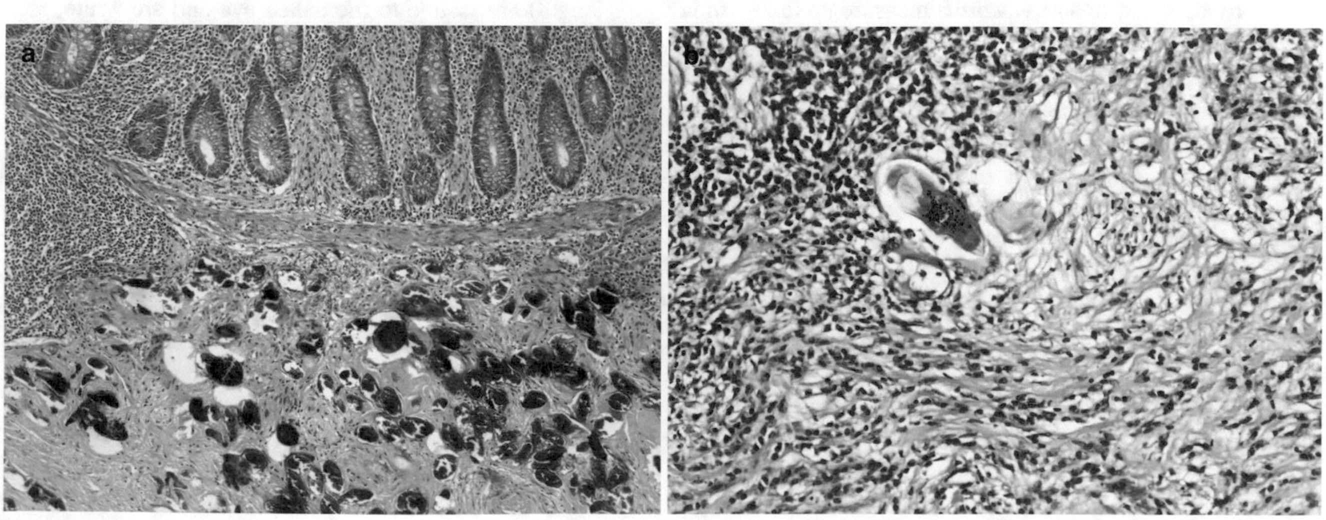

Fig. 10.38 Schistosomiasis. The Schistosome eggs are often calcified, as seen in this appendix, and often have associated fibrosis and giant cells (**a**). Embryonated eggs are occasionally seen (**b**)

T. saginata is endemic in Latin America and Africa, with moderate prevalence in Europe, Japan, and South Asia, reflecting cattle farming in areas with poor sanitation. Infection is acquired through eating undercooked beef. *T. solium* has a worldwide distribution that similarly correlates with pig farming, ingestion of raw and undercooked pork, and poor sanitation; it is endemic to Southeast Asia, Central and South America, Mexico, the Philippines, Africa, India, Eastern Europe, and Micronesia. Most patients with tapeworms are asymptomatic, although some patients have GI symptoms. Patients may pass proglottids, however.

Diphyllobothrium (fish tapeworm) is common in Northern Europe and Scandinavia, as well as the Great Lakes region in Michigan, and Alaska. Infection is acquired through eating raw fish, and most infections are asymptomatic, even though the worm can achieve a length of over 20 m. Symptoms including diarrhea, fatigue, dizziness, paresthesias, and increased appetite, and fish tapeworm is a rare cause of B12 deficiency.

Hymenolepsis nana (dwarf tapeworm) is the most common cestode infection in humans. It has a worldwide distribution and is more common in warm climates and areas of poor sanitation. It is the smallest adult tapeworm, measuring only 2.5–5 mm by 1.0 mm. Most infections are asymptomatic, although heavy infection may cause GI symptoms. Immunocompromised patients may be susceptible to very heavy worm burdens.

- A variety of nematodes cause human GI disease. *Ascaris lumbricoides* (roundworm) is the largest helminth of all, and one of the most common human parasites. It has a worldwide distribution, but is most common in Asia, Africa, and Latin America, in areas of poor sanitation; it most often affects children. The worms are ingested from exposure to contaminated food, water, or soil. *Ascarids* measure up to 30 cm in length and 6 mm in diameter, with a cylindrical, unsegmented body. Infection is usually asymptomatic, but heavy infection or worm migration can cause abdominal pain and distension, nausea, vomiting, and diarrhea. Patients may pass worms in either stool or vomit. Serious complications, including obstruction and volvulus, usually arise when enough worms are present to form a mass. Heavy worm burdens can also cause malnutrition and growth retardation, often complicated by the fact that children in endemic areas often have a poor diet in addition to parasitic infection. The worms may be seen with the naked eye endoscopically or in resection specimens.

Hookworms are common in all tropical and subtropical countries. Infection occurs either through penetration of the skin or direct ingestion. The worms attach to the small intestinal wall and ingest blood from mucosal capillaries, resulting in anemia, and thus, children and women of reproductive age are particularly susceptible. Other manifestations include abdominal pain, diarrhea, malnutrition, and childhood growth retardation. Endoscopically, the worms (measuring about 1 cm in length) are visible to the naked eye and are white, red-brown, or gray, depending on the amount of ingested blood or hemosiderin deposition. Pieces of worm may occasionally be detected in biopsy specimens.

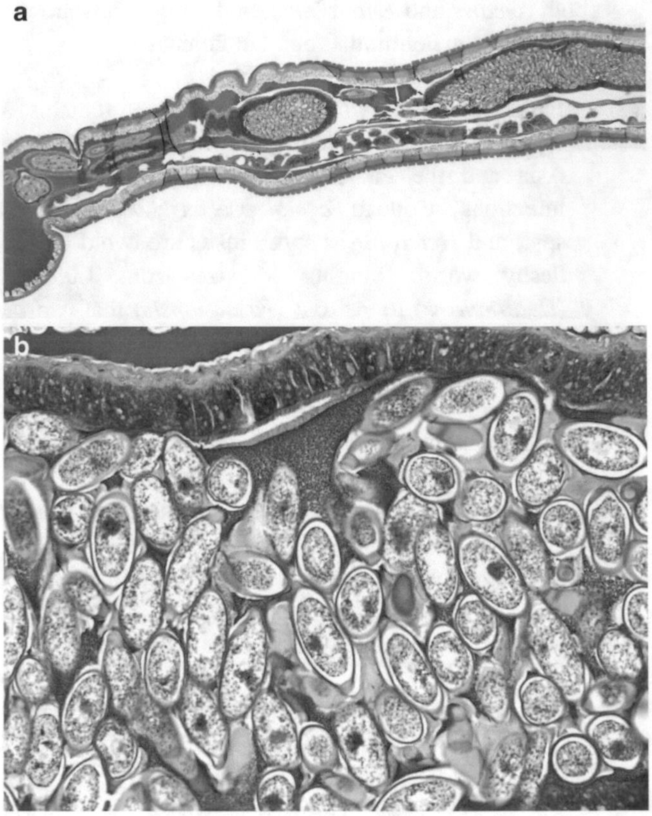

Fig. 10.39 Whipworm. The prominent somewhat irregular cuticle can be seen in this longitudinal microscopic section (**a**). At high power, the eggs within this female worm show the characteristic opercula at each end (**b**)

Whipworm is a soil helminth with a worldwide distribution, which is also most common in tropical climates. In the United States, it is most often seen in immigrants and in the rural Southeast. Infection is acquired by ingesting contaminated water or food. The worms measure 3–5 mm in length and may be seen endoscopically (Fig. 10.39a, b); only the male worms have the characteristic coiled, whip-like tail. Most infections are asymptomatic. Patients with heavier worm burdens may develop symptoms. Unusual clinical manifestations include an ulcerative inflammatory process similar to Crohn disease and rectal prolapse.

Pinworms are one of the most common human parasites, and it has been reported that pinworm infections

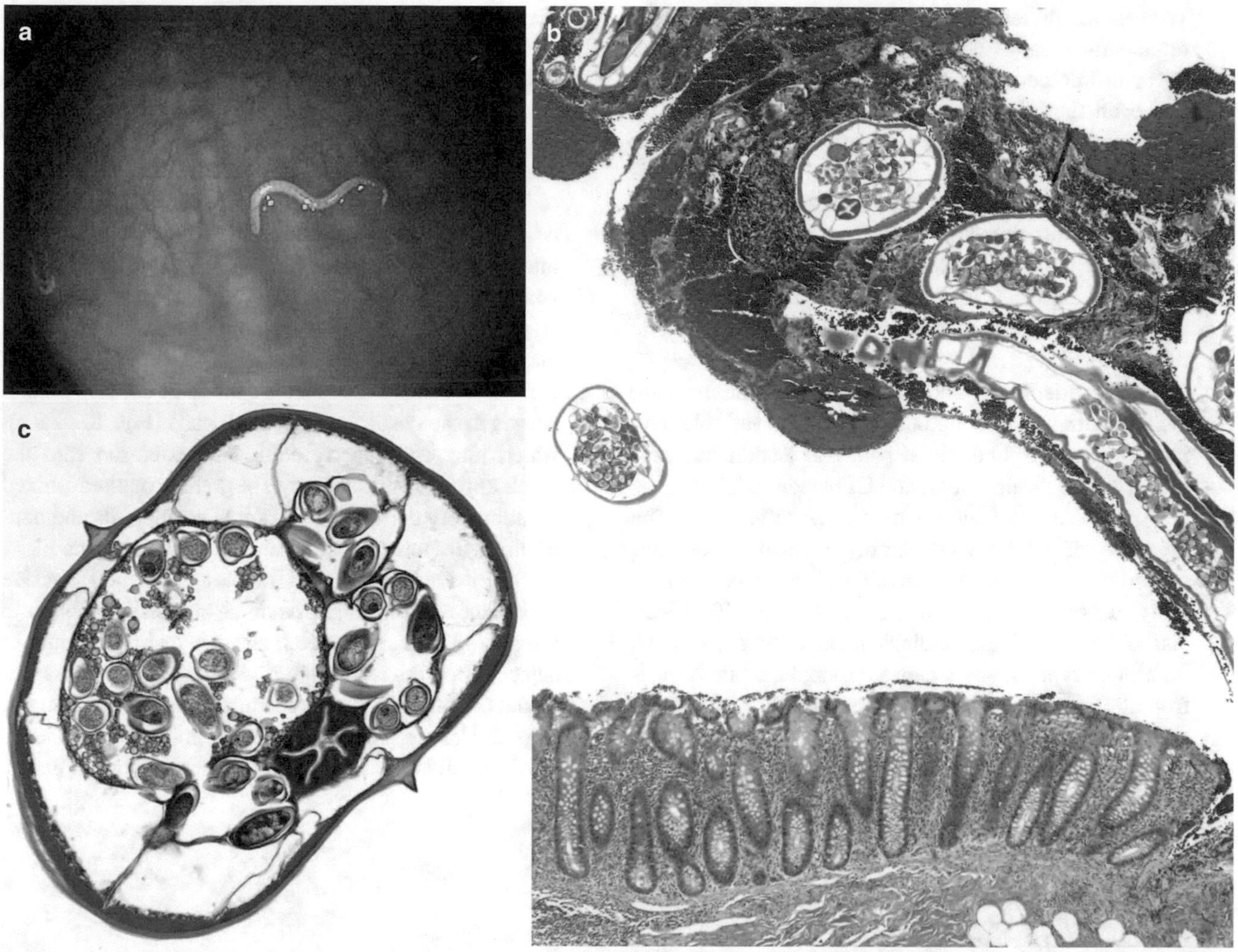

Fig. 10.40 Enterobiasis. Endoscopic view of a pinworm in the colon (**a**). The organisms are typically present in the lumen of the bowel or appendix, with no associated inflammation (**b**). At high power, the prominent eosinophilic cuticle and lateral ala can be seen (**c**). The ovoid eggs are flatter on one side

affect 4–28% of children worldwide. They have a worldwide distribution, but are more common in cold or temperate climates and in industrialized countries. They are very common in the United States and Northwestern Europe. The infective egg resides in dust and soil, and transmission is believed to be via the fecal–oral route. The worms live in the ileum, cecum, proximal colon, and appendix, and the female migrates to the anus to deposit eggs and die. The perianal eggs and worms produce the characteristic symptoms of pruritis ani. Heavy infections may cause abdominal pain, nausea, and vomiting.

In the colon the mucosa is usually normal, although rare cases of severe eosinophilic colitis associated with heavy pinworm infections have been reported. Granulomas, sometimes with necrosis, may develop as a reaction to degenerating worms or eggs.

The worms are 2–5 mm in length, white or ivory, and pointed at both ends; the posterior end is curved. They may be seen with the naked eye or endoscopically (Fig. 10.40a–c).

Strongyloides stercoralis has a worldwide distribution. It is endemic to tropical regions; in the United States, it is endemic to the Southeast. Strongyloidiasis occurs primarily in adults, many of whom are hospitalized, suffer from chronic illnesses, or are immunocompromised. Infection is contracted from soil containing the organism, which penetrates the skin, enters the venous system, travels to the lungs, and then migrates up the respiratory tree and down the esophagus to reach the small intestine. The female lives in the small intestine and lays eggs that hatch into rhabditiform larvae, which are excreted. An extremely important feature of the *Strongyloides* life cycle is that rhabditiform larvae can mature into infective filariform larvae within the host, via molting. This autoinfective (also known as hyperinfective) capability allows the organism to infect the host for long periods of time, sometimes upwards of 30 years.

Widespread dissemination (defined as migration of the organism to organs beyond the lung and GI tract) may occur in immunocompromised patients, causing severe and even fatal illness. Interestingly, AIDS patients do not appear to be unusually susceptible to strongyloidiasis. Corticosteroids appear to be responsible for the conversion of chronic, low-grade strongyloidiasis into fulminant disseminated infection in many cases. Fulminant strongyloidiasis is also associated with disseminated bacterial infections, apparently because the worms carry enteric bacteria with them as they invade the intestinal wall and migrate to other sites.

Many patients are asymptomatic. When patients are symptomatic, the symptoms are quite variable and include diarrhea, abdominal pain and tenderness, nausea, vomiting, weight loss, and GI bleeding.

Any segment of the GI tract may be affected. The presence of larvae with sharply pointed, sometimes curved tails within the glands of the GI mucosa, is essentially diagnostic of strongyloidiasis (Fig. 10.41a–c). Associated histologic findings include edema, villous blunting, cryptitis, and a dense eosinophilic and/or neutrophilic infiltrate in the lamina propria. In some cases, the parasites invade the lamina propria, which may result in nodular collections of eosinophils. Granulomas are occasionally present. In severe infections, larvae may be seen transmurally, and in lymphatics, small vessels, and rarely mesenteric lymph nodes.

Gastrointestinal anisakiasis is caused by ingesting raw or poorly cooked fresh fish that are parasitized by *Anisakis* species. The stomach is the most common site of involvement but the small bowel and colon can also be affected. The *Anisakis* larvae penetrate the gastric and intestinal walls, causing abdominal pain, nausea, and vomiting within 12 h after larval ingestion. Hypersensitivity symptoms and peripheral eosinophilia may develop in some patients. Histologically, large areas of necrosis with abscess formation develop around worms in the gastric or intestinal walls (Fig. 10.42a–c), which may cause perforation and extension into the omentum and mesentery. There are marked mixed inflammatory cell infiltrates rich in eosinophils and neutrophils. Granulomas and giant cells may be seen.

O&P examination and serology are non-invasive approaches for the diagnosis of gastrointestinal helminth infection. From stool specimens, the main procedure to detect helminths is through direct and concentrated wet mounts. Concentration procedures enrich for helminth eggs and larvae. The majority of helminths can be identified and distinguished from one another based on the

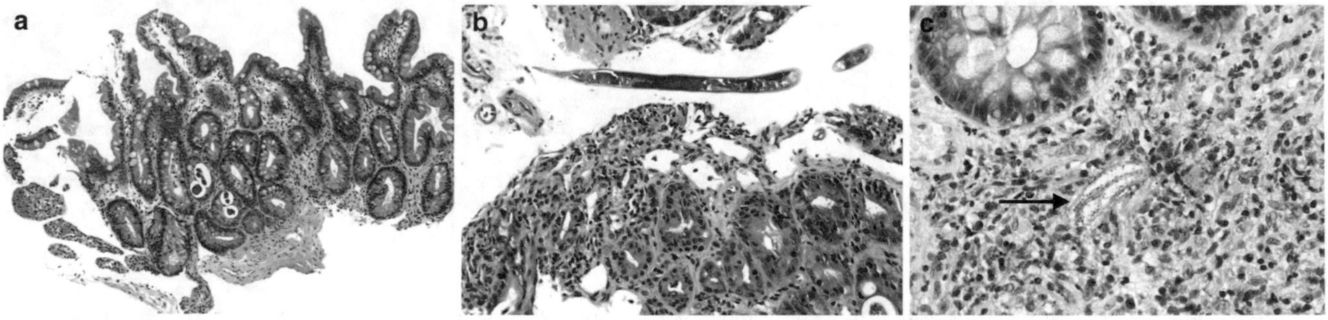

Fig. 10.41 Strongyloidiasis. *Strongyloides* within the epithelial cells of a small bowel biopsy (**a**). There is minimal inflammation. A worm with the characteristic sharply pointed tail is present in another field (**b**). Invasive worms may be difficult to detect in the lamina propria when cut in cross section (arrow) and are often surrounded by a dense eosinophilic infiltrate (**c**)

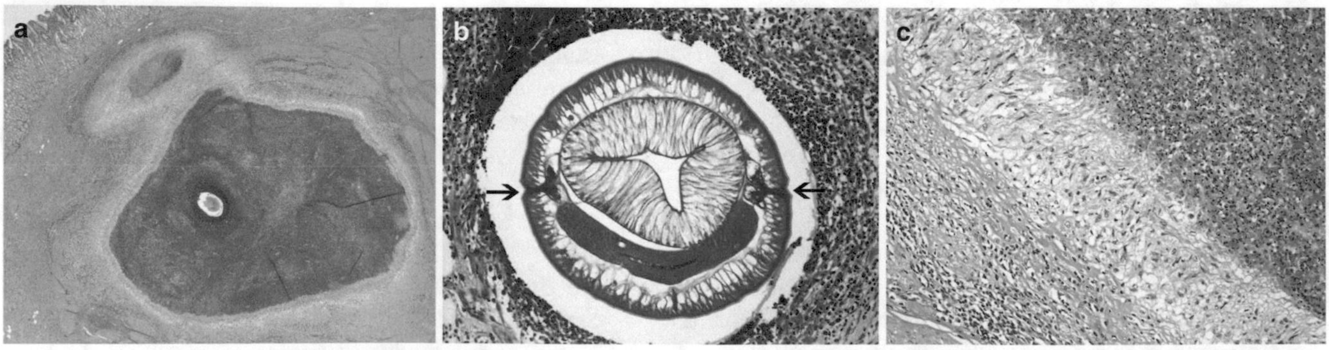

Fig. 10.42 Gastric anisakiasis. Large areas of necrosis and abscess formation surrounding *Anisakis* larvae (**a**). The worms penetrate through the full-thickness of the gastric wall and are seen in the omental tissue (**b**). Note the characteristic Y-shaped lateral cords (arrows) and the presence of numerous eosinophils and neutrophils around the worm. Granulomatous inflammation is evident at the periphery of abscesses in this case, with prominent palisading histiocytes (**c**)

size and morphology of their eggs in stool samples. This requires a well-trained parasitologist and a microscope with a micrometer for accurate egg measurement. The best sample for pinworm (*Enterobius*) diagnosis is a cellulose tape preparation, where the tape is applied to the anal folds and then applied to a glass slide for microscopy. Diagnosis of *S. stercoralis* can be challenging since O&P examination has low sensitivity. Instead serology can be used for initial testing, with follow-up testing to attempt to make a microbiological diagnosis. A concomitant eosinophilia may occur during acute infection although the correlation is imperfect. The preferred method of detection is agar culture using stool samples, where feces is inoculated and worms are detected as trails of bacteria after incubation that have been dragged along by the worms. These worms can then be recovered and identified by microscopic examination.

References: [124–138]

Case Presentation

Case 1

Learning Objectives

1. To become familiar with the infectious mimics of chronic idiopathic IBD
2. To become familiar with the common sexually transmitted proctocolitides
3. To understand the laboratory diagnosis of sexually transmitted proctocolitides

Case History

A 35-year-old man presented with rectal bleeding of 2 weeks' duration.

Colonoscopy

Diffuse friable mucosa from anus to sigmoid colon.

Histologic Findings

- Figure 10.43a: Sigmoid biopsy shows a dense lymphohistiocytic infiltrate with large lymphoid aggregates.
- Figure 10.43b: Other areas show ulceration with numerous plasma cells and loose granulomas.

Differential Diagnosis

- Chronic idiopathic IBD
- Lymphogranuloma venereum
- Anorectal syphilis

IHC and Other Ancillary Studies

- Positive spirochete immunostain (Fig. 10.43c).
- Positive RPR, VDRL, and treponeme serologies.
- Positive HIV serologies.

Final Diagnosis

Anorectal syphilis.

Take-Home Messages

1. Immunocompromised/immunosuppressed patients rarely get de novo chronic idiopathic IBD.
2. Syphilis mimics ulcerative colitis both macroscopically and histologically and should be considered in the differential diagnosis.
3. The anorectum and stomach are the sites most commonly affected in GI syphilis.

References: [81, 87]

Case 2

Learning Objectives

1. To become familiar with features of filamentous fungi in tissue sections
2. To become familiar with the risk factors for invasive GI fungal infections
3. To understand the laboratory diagnosis of medically important fungi

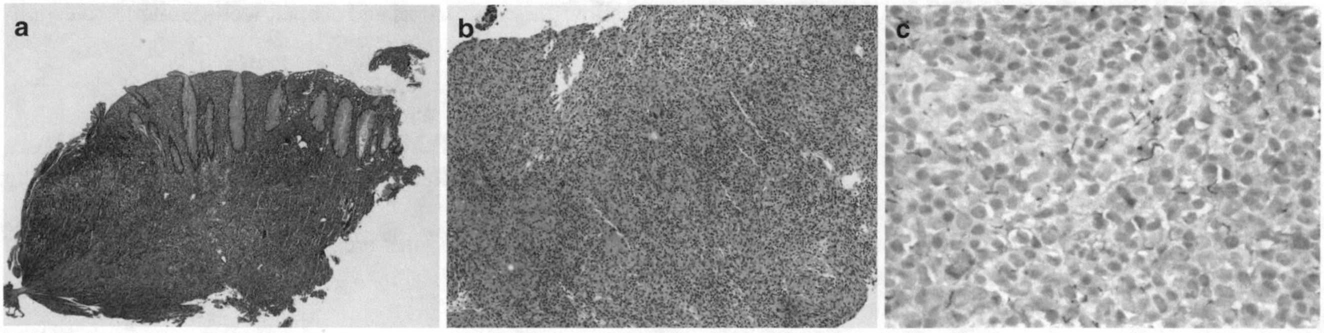

Fig. 10.43 (Case 1). A dense lymphohistiocytic infiltrate with large lymphoid aggregates is seen (**a**). Ulceration with numerous plasma cells and loose granulomas are also present (**b**). Positive immunostaining for spirochetes (**c**)

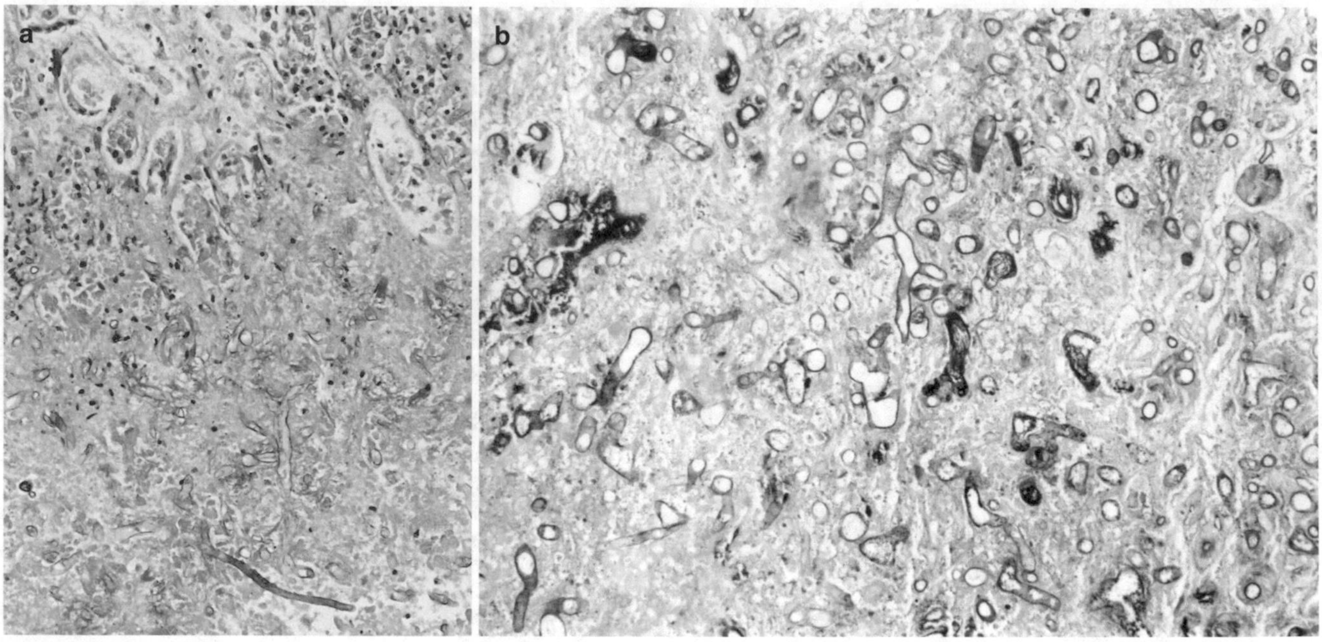

Fig. 10.44 (Case 2). Necrotic debris with ribbon-like, broad fungal hyphae (**a**). GMS stain highlights fungal organisms (**b**)

Case History
A 75-year-old severely debilitated woman with diabetes presented with upper GI bleeding.

Endoscopy
Large gastric ulcer with prominent, "heaped-up" edges that was macroscopically worrisome for carcinoma.

Histologic Findings
- Figure 10.44a: Necrotic ulcer debris contains large fungi with ribbon-like, broad hyphae.

Differential Diagnosis
- *Aspergillus* and similar fungi
- Mucormycosis
- *Candida* spp.
- *Basidiobolus ranarum*

IHC and Other Ancillary Studies
- GMS stain (Fig. 10.44b).
- Negative galactomannan and beta (1,3) glucan assays.
- No tissue preserved for culture.

Final Diagnosis
Mucormycosis.

Take-Home Messages
1. Mucor is an important fungal pathogen in diabetic, immunosuppressed, and malnourished patients.
2. GI mucormycosis most often involves the stomach or colon.
3. Preservation of tissue for fungal culture is ideal, although PCR can often be done from the paraffin block.

References: [56, 58, 62]

Case 3

Learning Objectives
1. To understand the morphologic differential diagnosis of commonly encountered GI viruses
2. To understand the available ancillary tests such as IHC and PCR

Case History
A 60-year-old man receiving chemotherapy for lung adenocarcinoma. He presented with odynophagia and epigastric pain.

Endoscopy
Shallow gastric erosions and deeper, well-demarcated esophageal ulcers.

Histologic Findings
- Figure 10.45a: Gastric epithelial cells contain odd basophilic inclusions with minimal surrounding inflammation.
- Figure 10.45b: Other areas show larger inclusions with prominent granules.

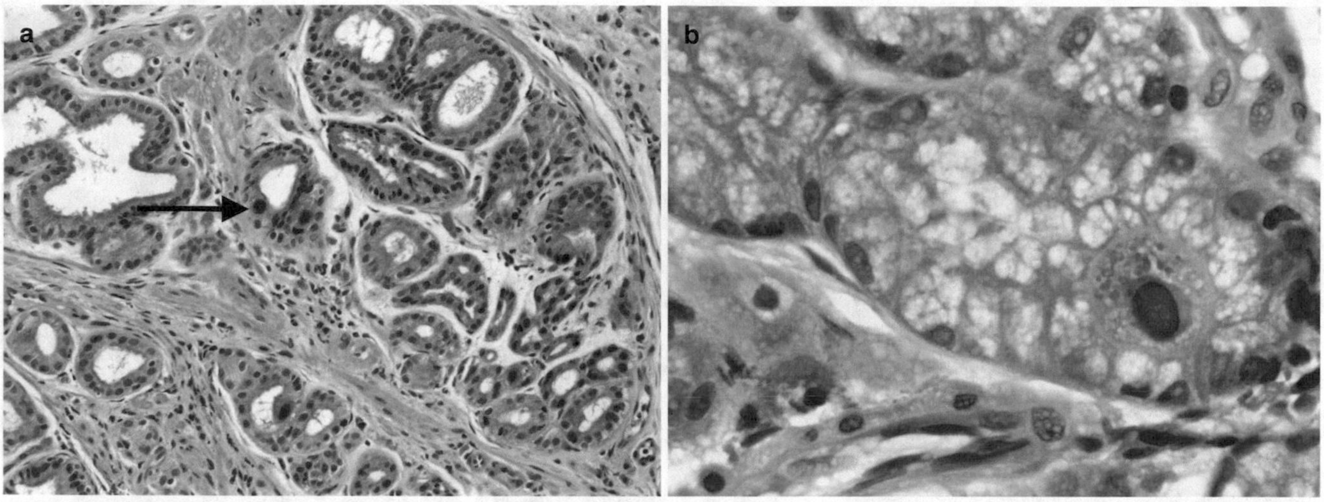

Fig. 10.45 (Case 3). A basophilic inclusion is noted in an epithelial cell of the gastric mucosa (**a**, arrow). There is only minimal surrounding inflammation. High power view shows intranuclear and cytoplasmic inclusions (**b**)

Differential Diagnosis

- CMV infection
- HSV infection
- Adenovirus infection
- Idiopathic giant esophageal ulcer

IHC and Other Ancillary Studies

- CMV IHC was positive.
- Weakly positive plasma CMV PCR.

Final Diagnosis

CMV esophagitis and gastritis.

Take-Home Messages

1. CMV most often affects stromal cells, endothelial cells, and macrophages, but occasionally infects epithelial cells. The appearance of the inclusions may be atypical in these circumstances.
2. IHC is a widely available and very helpful tool for distinguishing between the viruses that affect the GI tract.
3. Severely immunocompromised patients often have a very minimal inflammatory reaction.

References: [26, 33, 139]

Case 4

Learning Objectives

1. To understand the diagnostic features of invasive strongyloidiasis
2. To become familiar with the risk factors for strongyloidiasis

Case History

A 51-year-old female with a history of Crohn disease, on steroids for flare.

Right Hemicolectomy

Chronic, active colitis with perforation.

Histologic Findings

- Figure 10.46a: Chronic, active colitis with architectural distortion and basal plasmacytosis.
- Figure 10.46b: Occasional worms are seen within the colonic crypts.
- Figure 10.46c: Other areas show more numerous organisms.
- Figure 10.46d: Lymph nodes also contained characteristic organisms.

Differential Diagnosis

- Crohn disease
- Strongyloides infection

Final Diagnosis

Invasive strongyloidiasis.

Take-Home Messages

1. Fulminant strongyloides infection, often triggered by steroid use, can mimic chronic idiopathic IBD.
2. Finding larvae or worms with sharply pointed tails, within crypt epithelium, is essentially pathognomonic.

References: [140, 141]

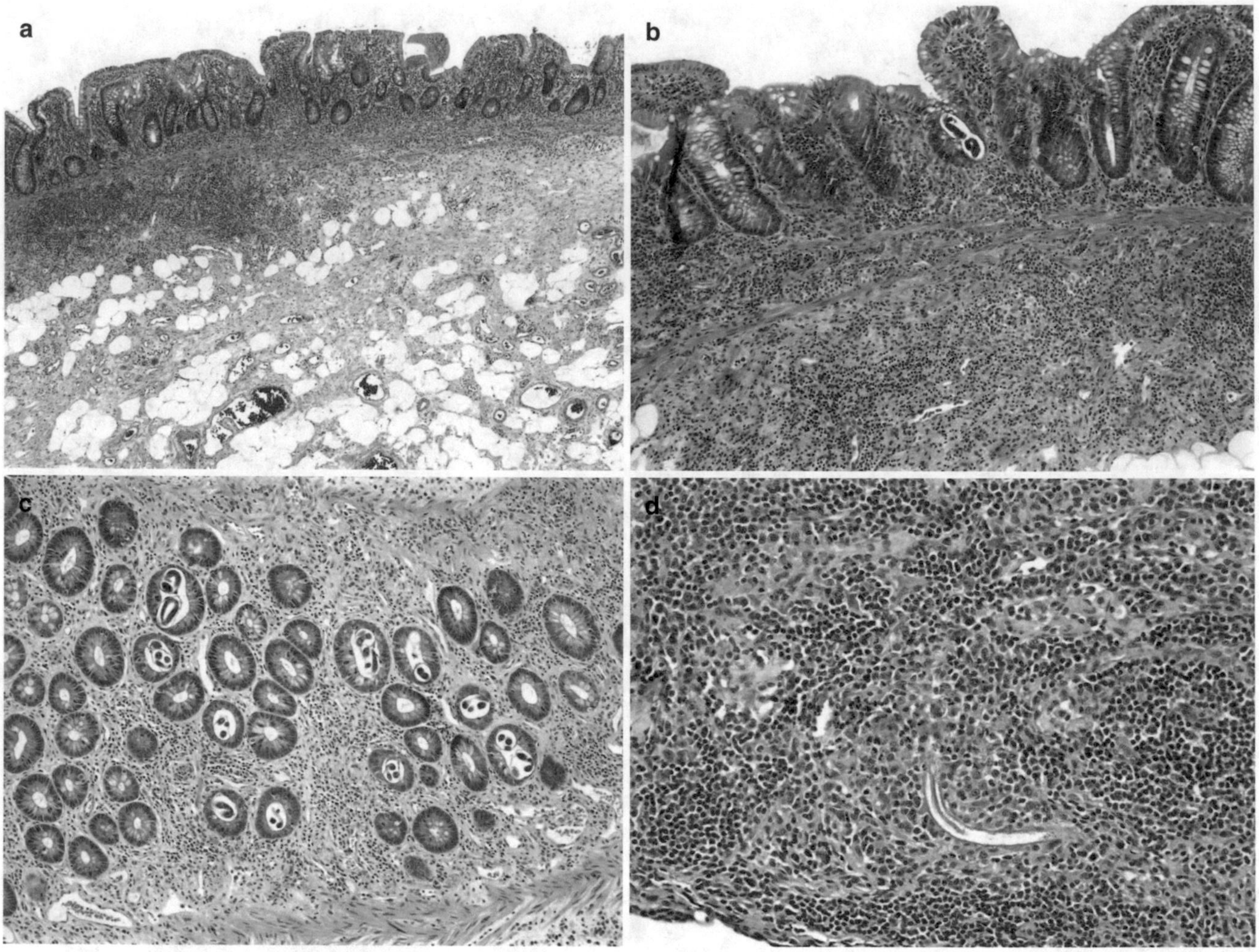

Fig. 10.46 (Case 4). Endoscopic biopsy shows chronic active colitis with crypt architectural distortion and areas of basal plasmacytosis (**a**). A worm is seen within the lumen of a crypt (**b**), but more organisms are seen in another area (**c**). An organism is present in a lymph node (**d**)

References

1. Babouee Flury B, Weisser M, Prince SS, et al. Performances of two different panfungal PCRs to detect mould DNA in formalin-fixed paraffin-embedded tissue: what are the limiting factors? BMC Infect Dis. 2014;14:692.
2. Kerr DA, Sweeney B, Arpin RN 3rd, et al. Automated extraction of formalin-fixed, paraffin-embedded tissue for high-risk human papillomavirus testing of head and neck squamous cell caricnomas using the Roche Cobas 4800 system. Arch Pathol Lab Med. 2016;140:844–8.
3. Kim YN, Kim KM, Choi HN, et al. Clinical usefulness of PCR for differential diagnosis of tuberculosis and nontuberculous mycobacterial infection in paraffin-embedded lung tissues. J Mol Diagn. 2015;17:597–604.
4. McCoy MH, Post K, Sen JD, et al. qPCR increased sensitivity to detect cytomegalovirus in formalin-fixed, paraffin-embedded tissue of gastrointestinal biopsies. Hum Pathol. 2014;45:48–53.
5. Seo AN, Park HJ, Lee HS, et al. Performance characteristics of nested polymerase chain reaction vs real-time PCR polymerase chain reaction methods for detecting mycobacterium tuberculosis complex in paraffin-embedded human tissues. Am J Clin Pathol. 2014;142:384–90.
6. Turashvili G, Yang W, McKinney S, et al. Nucleic acid quantity and quality from paraffin blocks: defining optimal fixation, processing and DNA/RNA extraction techniques. Exp Mol Pathol. 2012;92:33–43.
7. Dignan CR, Greenson JK. Can ischemic colitis be differentiated from *C. difficile* colitis in biopsy specimens? Am J Surg Path. 1997;21:706–10.
8. Fields PI, Swerdlow DL. Campylobacter jejuni. Clin Lab Med. 1999;9:489–503.
9. Gleason TH, Patterson SD. The pathology of *Yersinia enterocolitica* ileocolitis. Am J Surg Pathol. 1982;6:347–55.
10. Griffin PM, Olmstead LC, Petras RE. *Escherichia coli* 0157:H7-associated colitis: a clinical and histological study of 11 cases. Gastroenterol. 1990;99:142–9.
11. Lamps LW. Update on infectious enterocolitides and the diseases that they mimic. Histopathol. 2015;66:3–14.
12. Mathan MM, Mathan VI. Morphology of rectal mucosa of patients with shigellosis. Rev Inf Dis. 1991;13 Suppl 4:S314–8.
13. Merino S, Rubires X, Knochel S, Tomas JM. Emerging pathogens: Aeromonas spp. Int J Food Microbiol. 1995;28:157–68.
14. McDonald LC, Gerding DN, Johnson S, et al. Clinical practice guidelines for *Clostridium difficile* infection in adults and children: 2017 update by the Infectious Diseases Society of America (IDSA) and Society for Healthcare Epidemiology of America (SHEA). Clin Infect Dis. 2018;66(7):e1–e48.

15. Zhang H, Morrison S, Tang YW. Multiplex polymerase chain reaction tests for detection of pathogens associated with gastroenteritis. Clin Lab Med. 2015;35:461–86.
16. Garcia PG, Chebli LA, da Rocha Ribeiro TC, et al. Impact of superimposed Clostridium difficile infection in Crohn's or ulcerative colitis flares in the outpatient setting. Int J Color Dis. 2018; https://doi.org/10.1007/s00384-018-3105-8.
17. Garrido E, Carrera E, Manzano R, Lopez-Sanroman A. Clinical significance of cytomegalovirus infection in patients with inflammatory bowel disease. World J Gastroenterol. 2013;19:17–25.
18. Gordon J, Ramaswami A, Beuttler M, et al. EBV status and thiopurine use in pediatric IBD. J Pediatri Gastroenterol Nutr. 2016;62:711–4.
19. Kambham N, Vij R, Cartwright CA, Longacre T. Cytomegalovirus infection in steroid-refractory ulcerative colitis: a case-control study. Am J Surg Pathol. 2004;28:365–73.
20. Landsman MJ, Sultan M, Stevens M, et al. Diagnosis and management of common gastrointestinal tract infectious diseases in ulcerative colitis and Crohn's disease patients. Inflamm Bowel Dis. 2014;20:2503–10.
21. Maharshak N, Barzilay I, Zinger H, et al. Clostridum difficile infection in hospitalized patients with inflammatory bowel disease: prevalence, risk factors, and prognosis. Medicine (Baltimore). 2018;97(5):e9772.
22. McCurdy JD, Jones A, Enders FT, et al. A model for identifying cytomegalovirus in patient with inflammatory bowel disease. Clin Gastroenterol Hepatol. 2015;13:131–7.
23. McCurdy JD, Enders FT, Khanna S, et al. Increased rates of Clostridium difficile infection and poor outcomes in patients with IBD and cytomegalovirus. Inflamm Bowel Dis. 2016;22:2688–93.
24. Pillet S, Pozzetto B, Jarlot C, et al. Management of cytomegalovirus infection in inflammatory bowel disease. Dig Liver Dis. 2012;44:541–8.
25. Wang T, Matukas L, Streutker CJ. Histologic findings and clinical characteristics in acutely symptomatic ulcerative colitis patients with superimposed Clostridium difficile infection. Am J Clin Pathol. 2013;140:831–7.
26. Durand CM, Marr KA, Arnold CA, et al. Detection of cytomegalovirus DNA in plasma as an adjunct diagnostic for gastrointestinal tract disease in kidney and liver rransplant recipients. Clin Inf Dis. 2013;57(11):1550–9.
27. Guidelines for prevention and treatment of opportunistic infections in HIV-infected adults and adolescents; 2018, p. 1–433.
28. https://www.uptodate.com/contents/approach-to-the-diagnosis-of-cytomegalovirus-infection?topicRef=8291&source=see_link
29. Juric-Sekhar G, Upton MP, Swanson PE, Westerhoff M. Cytomegalovirus (CMV) in gastrointestinal mucosal biopsies: should a pathologist perform CMV immunohistochemistry if the clinician requests it? Hum Pathol. 2017;60:11–5.
30. McCurdy JD, Enders FT, Jones A, et al. Detection of cytomegalovirus in patients with inflammatory bowel disease: where to biopsy and how many biopsies? Inflamm Bowel Dis. 2015;21:2833–8.
31. Solomon IH, Hornick JL, Laga AC. Immunohistochemistry is rarely justified for the diagnosis of viral infections. Am J Clin Pathol. 2017;147:96–104.
32. Yan Z, Wang L, Dennis J, et al. Clinical significance of isolated cytomegalovirus-infected gastrointestinal cells. Int J Surgical Pathol. 2014;22:492–8.
33. Chetty R, Roskell DE. Cytomegalovirus infection in the gastrointestinal tract. J Clin Pathol. 1994;47:968–72.
34. Fica A, Cervera C, Perez N, et al. Immunohistochemically proven cytomegalovirus end-organ disease in solid organ transplant patients: clinical features and usefulness of conventional diagnostic tests. Transpl Inf Dis. 2007;9:203–10.
35. Goodell SE, Quinn TC, Mkrtichian E, et al. Herpes simplex virus proctitis in homosexual men: clinical, sigmoidoscopic, and histopathological features. New Eng J Med. 1983;308:868–71.
36. Kraus MD, Feran-Doza M, Garcia-Moliner ML, et al. Cytomegalovirus infection in the colon of bone marrow transplant patients. Mod Pathol. 1998;11:29–36.
37. Mallet E, Maitre M, Mouterde O. Complications of the digestive tract in varicella infection including two cases of erosive gastritis. Eur J Pediatr. 2006;165:64–5.
38. Shayan K, Saunders F, Roberts E, Cutz E. Adenovirus enterocolitis in pediatric patients following bone marrow transplantation: report of 2 cases and review of the literature. Arch Pathol Lab Med. 2003;127:1615–8.
39. Yan Z, Nguyen S, Poles M, et al. Adenovirus colitis in human immunodeficiency virus infection: an underdiagnosed entity. Am J Surg Pathol. 1998;22:1101–6.
40. Qiu FZ, Shen XX, Li GX, et al. Adenovirus associated with acute diarrhea: a case-control study. BMC Infect Dis. 2018;18:450.
41. Lion T. Adenovirus infections in immunocompetent and immunocompromised patients. Clin Microbiol Rev. 2014;27(3): 441–62.
42. Chen J, Zhang R, Shen Y, et al. Clinical characteristics and prognosis of penicilliosis among human immunodeficiency virus-infected patients in Eastern China. Am J Trop Med Hyg. 2017;96:1350–4.
43. Gronborg HL, Jespersen S, Honge BL, et al. Review of cytomegalovirus infection in HIV-infected individuals in Africa. Rev Med Virol 2017;27(1). https://doi.org/10.1002/rmv.1907.
44. Huppmann AR, Orenstein JM. Opportunistic disorders of the gastrointestinal tract in the age of highly active antiretroviral therapy. Hum Pathol. 2010;41:1777–87.
45. Nishimura S, Nagata N, Shimbo T, et al. Factors associated with esophageal candidiasis and its endoscopic severity in the era of antiretroviral therapy. PLoS One. 2013;8(3):e58217.
46. Nsagha DS, Njunda AL, Assob NJC, et al. Intestinal parasite infections in relation to CD4(+) T cell counts and diarrhea in HIV/AIDS patients with or without antiretroviral therapy in Cameroon. BMC Infect Dis. 2016;16:9.
47. Putot A, Perrin S, Jolivet A, Vantilcke V. HIV-associated disseminated histoplasmosis in western French Guiana, 2002-2012. Mycoses. 2015;58:160–6.
48. Alemany L, Saunier M, Alvarado-Cabrero I, et al. Human papillomavirus DNA prevalence and type distribution in anal carcinomas worldwide. Int J Cancer. 2015;136:98–107.
49. Bean SM, Eltoum I, Horton DK, et al. Immunohistochemical expression of p16 and Ki-67 correlates with degree of anal intraepithelial neoplasia. Am J Surg Pathol. 2007;31(4):555–61.
50. Clarke MA, Wentzensen N. Strategies for screening and early detection of anal cancers: a narrative and systematic review and meta-analysis of cytology, HPV testing, and other biomarkers. Cancer Cytopathol. 2018;126(7):447–60.
51. Liu Y, Sigel K, Gaisa MM. Human papillomavirus genotypes predict progression of anal low-grade squamous intraepithelial lesions. J Infect Dis. 2018;13:487.
52. Maniar KP, Nayar R. HPV-related squamous neoplasia of the lower anogenital tract: an update and review of recent guidelines. Adv Anat Pathol. 2014;21(5):341–58.
53. Pirog EC, Quint KD, Yantiss RY. p16.CDKN2A and Ki-67 enhance the detection of anal intraepithelial neoplasia and condyloma and correlate with human papillomavirus detection by polymerase chain reaction. Am J Surg Pathol. 2010;34:1449–55.
54. Roldan Urgoiti GB, Gustafson K, Klimowicz AC, et al. The prognostic value of HPV status and p16 expression in patients with carcinoma of the anal canal. PLoS One. 2014;9(10):e108790.
55. Wentzensen N, Follansbee S, Borgonovo S, et al. Analytic and clinical performance of cobas HPV testing in anal specimens

from HIV-positive men who have sex with men. J Clin Microbiol. 2014;52(8):2892–7.
56. Dictar MO, Maiolo E, Alexander B, et al. Mycoses in the transplanted patient. Med Mycol. 2000;38 Suppl 1:251–8.
57. Fleming RV, Walsh TJ, Anaissie EJ. Emerging and less common fungal pathogens. Infect Dis Clin N Am. 2002;16:915–33.
58. Gonzalez CE, Rinaldi MG, Sugar AM. Zygomycosis. Inf Dis Clin N Am. 2002;16:895–914.
59. Lamps LW, Lai KK, Milner DA Jr. Fungal infections of the gastrointestinal tract in the immunocompromised host: an update. Adv Anat Pathol. 2014;21:217–27.
60. Lyon DT, Schubert TT, Mantia AG. Phycomycosis of the gastrointestinal tract. Am J Gastroenterol. 1979;72:379–94.
61. Pilmis B, Puel A, Lortholary O, Lanternier F. New clinical phenotypes of fungal infections in special hosts. Clin Microbiol Infect. 2016;22:681–7.
62. Roden MM, Zaoutis TE, Buchanan WL, et al. Epidemiology and outcome of zygomycosis: a review of 929 reported cases. Clin Infect Dis. 2005;41:634–53.
63. Smilack JD. Gastrointestinal basidiobolomycosis. Clin Infect Dis. 1998;27:663–4.
64. Richer SM, Smedema ML, Durkin MM, et al. Improved diagnosis of acute pulmonary histoplasmosis by combining antigen and antibody detection. Clin Infect Dis. 2016;62(7):896–902.
65. Brown KE, Peura DA. Diagnosis of *Helicobacter pylori* infection. Gastroenterol Clin N Amer. 1993;22(1):105–15.
66. Laine L, Lewin DN, Naritoku W, Cohen H. Prospective comparison of H&E, Giemsa, and Genta stains for the diagnosis of *Helicobacter pylori*. Gastrointest Endosc. 1997;45:463–7.
67. Lash RH, Genta RM. Routine anti-Helicobacter immunohistochemical staining is significantly superior to reflex staining protocols for the detection of Helicobacter in gastric biopsy specimens. Helicobacter. 2016;21:581–5.
68. Solnick JV. Clinical significance of *Helicobacter* species other than *Helicobacter pylori*. Clin Inf DIs. 2003;36:349–54.
69. Stolte M, Kroher G, Meining A, et al. A comparison of *Helicobacter pylori* and *H. heilmannii* gastritis. A matched control study involving 404 patients. Scand J Gastroenterol. 1997;32:28–33.
70. Chey WD, Leontiadis GI, Howden CW, Moss SF. ACG clinical guideline: treatment of Helicobacter pylori infection. Am J Gastroenterol. 2017;112(2):212–39.
71. Fashner J, Gitu AC. Diagnosis and treatment of peptic ulcer disease and H. pylori infection. Am Fam Physician. 2015;91:236–42.
72. Bai JC, Mazure RM, Vazquez H, et al. Whipple's disease. Clin Gastroenterol Hepatol. 2004;2:849–60.
73. Dutly F, Altwegg M. Whipple's disease and "Tropheryma whippelii". Clin Microbiol Rev. 2001;14:561–83.
74. El-Abassi R, Soliman MY, Williams F, England JD. Whipple's disease. J Neurol Sci. 2017;377:197–206.
75. Dolmans RAV, Boel CHE, Lacle MM, Kusters JG. Clinical manifestations, treatment, and diagnosis of tropheryma whipplei infections. Clin Microbiol Rev. 2017;30(2):529–55.
76. Cenci E, Luciano E, Bucaioni M, et al. Evaluation of IVD 3.0 vitek MS matrix-assisted laser desorption ionization-time of flight mass spectrometry for identification of Mycobacterium tuberculsosi and nontuberculous mycobacteria and its use in routine diagnostics. Eur J Clin Microbiol Infect Dis. 2018; https://doi.org/10.1007/s10096-018-3326-3.
77. Farhi DC, Mason UG, Horsburgh CR. Pathologic findings in disseminated *Mycobacterium avium-intracellulare* infection: a report of 11 cases. Am J Clin Pathol. 1986;85:67–72.
78. Horvath KD, Whelan RL. Intestinal tuberculosis: return of an old disease. Am J Gastroenterol. 1998;93:692–6.
79. Marshall JB. Tuberculosis of the gastrointestinal tract and peritoneum. Am J Gastroenterol. 1993;88:989–99.
80. Pulimood AB, Peter S, Ramakrishna BS, et al. Segmental colonoscopic biopsies in the differentiation of ileocolonic tuberculosis from Crohn's disease. J Gastroenterol Hepatol. 2005;20:688–96.
81. Arnold CA, Limketkai BN, Illei PB, et al. Syphilitic and lymphogranuloma venereum (LGV) proctocolitis. Am J Surg Pathol. 2013;37:38–46.
82. Cunha CB, Friedman RK, de Boni RB, et al. Chlamydia trachomatis, Neisseria gonorrhoeae and syphilis among men who have sex with men in Brazil. BMC Public Health. 2015;15:686.
83. De Vrieze NH, de Vries HJ. Lymphogranuloma venereum among men who have sex with men. An epidemiological and clinical review. Expert Rev Anti-Infect Ther. 2014;12:697–704.
84. Foschi C, Marangoni A, D'Antuono A, et al. Prevalence and predictors of lymphogranuloma venereum in a high risk population attending a STD outpatients clinic in Italy. BMC Res Notes. 2014;7:225.
85. Hoentjen F, Rubin DT. Infectious proctitis: when to suspect it is not inflammatory bowel disease. Dig Dis Sci. 2012;57:269–73.
86. Hoie S, Knudson LS, Gerstoft J. Lymphogranuloma venereum proctitis: a differential diagnosis to inflammatory bowel disease. Scand J Gastroenterol. 2011;46:503–10.
87. Jawale R, Lai KK, Lamps LW. Sexually transmitted infections of the lower gastrointestinal tract. Virchows Arch. 2018;472:149–58.
88. Workowski KA, Bolan GA. Sexually transmitted diseases treatment guidelines, 2015. MMRW Recommend Rep. 2015;64(RR-03):1–137.
89. Esteve M, Salas A, Fernandez-Banares F, et al. Intestinal spirochetosis and chronic watery diarrhea: clinical and histological response to treatment and long term follow up. J Gastroenterol Hepatol. 2006;21:1326–33.
90. Korner M, Gebbers J-O. Clinical significance of human intestinal spirochetosis-a morphological approach. Infection. 2003;31:341–9.
91. Koteish A, Kannangai R, Abraham S, Torbenson M. Colonic spirochetosis in children and adults. Am J Clin Pathol. 2003;120:828–32.
92. O'Donnell S, Swan N, Crotty P, et al. Assessment of the clinical significance of intestinal spirochetosis. J Clin Pathol. 2008;61:1029–33.
93. Surawicz CM. Intestinal spirochetosis in homosexual men. Am J Med. 1988;82:587–92.
94. Uhlemann ER, Fenoglio-Preiser C. Intestinal spirochetosis (letter). Am J Surg Pathol. 2005;29:982.
95. Weisheit B, Bethke B, Stolte M. Human intestinal spirochetosis: analysis of the symptoms of 209 patients. Scand J Gastroenterol. 2007;42:1422–7.
96. Lääveri T, Antikainen J, Pakkanen SH, et al. Prospective study of pathogens in asymptomatic travellers and those with diarrhoea: aetiological agents revisited. Clin Microbiol Infect. 2016;22:1–7.
97. Mowers J, Lamps LW, Greenson J, et al. Clinical and histologic correlates of the FilmArray BioFire Gastrointestinal Panel. Mod Pathol. 2018;31:811A.
98. Mowers J, Lamps LW, Greenson J, et al. The clinical significance of enteropathogenic E. coli detected in stool multiplex PCR assays. Mod Pathol. 2018;31:813A.
99. van Coppenraet LESB, Boer MD-D, Ruijs GJHM, et al. Case–control comparison of bacterial and protozoan microorganisms associated with gastroenteritis: application of molecular detection. Clin Microbiol Infect. 2015;21(6):592.e9–592.e19.
100. Asha JN, Tompkins D, Wilcox MH. Comparative analysis of prevalence, risk factors, and molecular epidemiology of antibiotic associated diarrhea due to Clostridium difficile, Clostridium perfringens, and Staphylococcus aureus. J Clin Micrbiol. 2006;44:2785–91.
101. Cheng VCC, Yam WC, Tsang LL, et al. Epidemiology of Klebsiella oxytoca-associated diarrhea detected by Simmons

citrate agar supplemented with inositol, tryptophan, and bile salts. J Clin Microbiol. 2012;50(5):1571–9.
102. Herzog KAT, Schneditz G, Leitner E, et al. Genotypes of Klebsiella oxytoca isolates from patients with nosocomial pneumonia are distinct from those of isolates from patients with antibiotic-associated hemorrhagic colitis. J Clin Microbiol. 2014;52(5):1607–16.
103. Hogenauer C, Langner C, Beubler E, et al. Klebsiella oxytoca as a causative organism of antibiotic-associated hemorrhagic colitis. N Engl J Med. 2006;355:2418–26.
104. Lo TS, Borchardt SM. Antibiotic-associated diarrhea due to methicillin-resistant Staphyloccus aureus. Diagn Microbiol Infect Dis. 2009;63:388–9.
105. Burnham CAD, Carroll KC. Diagnosis of Clostridium difficile infection: an ongoing conundrum for clinicians and for clinical laboratories. Clin Microbiol Rev. 2013;26:604–30.
106. Farooq PD, Urrunaga NH, Tang DM, et al. Pseudomembranous colitis. Dis Mon. 2015;61:181–206.
107. Nash SV, Bourgeault R, Sands M. Colonic disease associated with a positive assay for *Clostridium difficile* toxin: a retrospective study. J Clin Gastro. 1997;25:476–9.
108. Surawicz CM, McFarland LV. Pseudomembranous colitis: causes and cures. Digestion. 1999;60:91–100.
109. Bertoli F, Espino M, Arosemena JR, et al. A spectrum in the pathology of toxoplasmosis in patients with acquired immunodeficiency syndrome. Arch Path Lab Med. 1995;19: 214–24.
110. Brandt H, Tamayo P. Pathology of human amebiasis. Hum Pathol. 1970;1:351–85.
111. Connor BA, Reidy J, Soave R. Cyclosporiasis: clinical and histopathologic correlates. Clin Inf Dis. 1999;28:1216–21.
112. Cooper CJ, Fleming R, Boman DA, Zuckerman MJ. Varied clinical manifestations of amebic colitis. South Med J. 2015;108:676–81.
113. Field AS, Milner DA Jr. Intestinal microsporidiosis. Clin Lab Med. 2015;35:445–59.
114. Goodgame R. Understanding intestinal spore-forming protozoa: *Cryptosporidia, Microsporidia, Isospora*, and *Cyclospora*. Ann Int Med. 1996;124:429–41.
115. Legua P, Seas C. Cystoisospora and cyclospora. Curr Opin Infect Dis. 2013;26:479–83.
116. Lewthwaite P, Gill GV, Hart CA, Beeching NJ. Gastrointestinal parasites in the immunocompromised. Curr Opin Infect Dis. 2005;18:427–35.
117. Minetti C, Chalmers RM, Beeching NJ, et al. Giardiasis. BMJ. 2016;355:i5369.
118. Oberhuber G, Kaster N, Stolte M. Giardiasis: a histologic analysis of 567 cases. Scand J Gastroenterol. 1997;32:48–51.
119. Schuster FL, Ramirez-Avila L. Current world status of Balantidium coli. Clin Microbiol Rev. 2008;21:626–38.
120. Sinelnikov I, Sion-Vardy N, Shaco-Levy R. C-kit (CD117) immunostain is useful fort he diagnosis of Giardia lamblia in duodenal biopsies. Hum Pathol. 2009;40:323–5.
121. Stanley SL Jr. Amoebiasis. Lancet. 2003;361(9362):1025–34.
122. Variyam EP, Gogate P, Hassan M, et al. Nondysenteric intestinal amebiasis: colonic morphology and search for *Entamoeba histolytica* adherence and invasion. Dig Dis Sci. 1989;34:732–40.
123. Wilson ME, Streit JA. Visceral leishmaniasis. Gastroenterol Clin N Amer. 1996;25(3):535.
124. Strickland GT. Gastrointestinal manifestations of schistosomiasis. Gut. 1994;35:1334–7.
125. Bruckner DA. Helminthic food-borne infections. Clin Lab Med. 1999;19(3):639–60.
126. Concha R, Harrington W Jr, Rogers AI. Intestinal strongyloidiasis: recognition, management, and determinants of outcome. J Clin Gastroenterol. 2005;39:203–11.
127. Cook GC. The clinical significance of gastrointestinal helminths – a review. Trans Roy Soc Trop Med Hyg. 1986;80:675–85.
128. Elsayed S, Yilmaz A, Hershfield N. *Trichuris trichiura* worm infection. Gastro Endosc. 2004;60:990–1.
129. Fried B, Gracyk T, Tamang L. Food-borne intestinal trematodiases in humans. Parasitol Res. 2004;93:159–70.
130. Kishimoto K, Hokama A, Hirata T, et al. Endoscopic and histopathological study on the duodenum of *Strongyloides stercoralis* hyperinfection. World J Gastroenterol. 2008;14: 1768–73.
131. Liu LX, Harinasuta KT. Liver and intestinal flukes. Gastroenterol Clin North Amer. 1996;25:627–36.
132. Ochoa B. Surgical complications of ascarisis. World J Surg. 1991;15:222–7.
133. Rivasi F, Pampiglione S, Boldorini R, Cardinale L. Histopathology of gastric and duodenal *Strongyloides stercoralis* locations in fifteen immunocompromised subjects. Arch Pathol Lab Med. 2006;130:1792–8.
134. Sinniah B, Leopairut RC, Connor DH, Voge M. Enterobiasis: a histopathological study of 259 patients. Ann Trop Med Parasitol. 1991;85:625–35.
135. Thompson BF, Fry LC, Wells CD, et al. The spectrum of GI strongyloidiasis: an endoscopic-pathologic study. Gastro Endosc. 2004;59:906–10.
136. Weight SC, Barrie WW. Colonic strongyloides infection masquerading as ulcerative colitis. J R Coll Surg Edinb. 1997;42:202–3.
137. https://www.cdc.gov/dpdx/diagnosticprocedures/stool/microexam.html
138. https://www.cdc.gov/dpdx/strongyloidiasis/index.html
139. Baehr PH, McDonald GB. Esophageal infections: risk factors, presentation, diagnosis, and treatment. Gastroenterology. 1994;106:509–32.
140. Nutman TB. Human infection with strongyloides stercoralis and other related Strongyloides species. Parasitology. 2017;144:263–73.
141. Qu Z, Kundu UR, Abadeer RA, Wanger A. Strongyloides colitis is a lethal mimic of ulcerative colitis: the key morphologic differential diagnosis. Hum Pathol. 2009;40:572–7.

Drug-Induced Gastrointestinal Tract Injury

11

Rifat Mannan, Kevin M. Waters, and Elizabeth Montgomery

List of Frequently Asked Questions

1. What are the commonly encountered medication-induced injury patterns in the GI tract?
2. What are the different non-specific drug-induced GI tract injury patterns?
3. What are the histologic changes associated with nonsteroidal anti-inflammatory drug (NSAID)-related GI tract mucosal injury?
4. What are the mucosal changes associated with iron therapy?
5. What is gastric mucosal calcinosis?
6. What are the histologic changes induced by proton pump inhibitors? Are they limited to the stomach?
7. Do radiation microspheres such as Yttrium-90 impart any specific GI tract mucosal injury pattern?
8. Which medications are associated with "mitotic arrest"-related changes in GI tract mucosa? Is it important to differentiate, and how can they be differentiated?
9. What are the injurious effects associated with angiotensin II receptor antagonists on GI tract mucosa?
10. What are the histologic changes associated with mycophenolate (CellCept) in GI tract mucosa? What is the closest histologic mimic and how can these be differentiated?
11. What are the different medication resins that are associated with GI tract injury? How can these be morphologically recognized?
12. What is melanosis coli? How is it different from pseudomelanosis enteri?
13. What are the GI tract injuries induced by different immunotherapy agents?

Esophagitis can be a frustrating diagnostic challenge as the esophagus has a limited number of mechanisms to deal with injury and many causes of esophageal damage create overlapping histologic pictures. While a pathology report may not be able to always offer a specific diagnosis, it is important to both exclude specific treatable conditions and recognize different patterns of injury that can produce a more precise differential diagnosis that, along with clinical history, endoscopic findings, and medication history, can lead a clinician to the proper treatment plan.

Frequently Asked Questions

Drug-induced injury to the gastrointestinal (GI) tract is fairly common, often with important clinical consequences. An aging population, coupled with an ever-expanding drug industry, and availability of a bewildering array of both prescription and over-the-counter medications offer increasing opportunities to encounter unwarranted side effects from different medications. Several factors such as dose, mechanism of action, drug interactions, and the individual's underlying health status can influence the type and severity of medication effects. Mucosal damage may occur due to direct physical injury or by altering mucosal immunity and local environmental milieu. Pathologic changes induced by the medications are varied, often non-specific, and can mimic various diseases, including neoplasms. An awareness of the spectrum of pathologic changes induced by various drugs is important in establishing a temporal relationship and avoiding misdiagnosis.

1. What are the commonly encountered medication-induced injury patterns in the GI tract?

R. Mannan (✉)
University of Pennsylvania Perelman School of Medicine, Philadelphia, PA, USA
e-mail: rifat.mannan@pennmedicine.upenn.edu

K. M. Waters
Cedars-Sinai Medical Center, Los Angeles, CA, USA

E. Montgomery
University of Miami Leonard M. Miller School of Medicine, Miami, FL, USA

H. L. Wang, Z. E. Chen (eds.), *Practical Gastrointestinal Pathology*, Practical Anatomic Pathology,
https://doi.org/10.1007/978-3-030-51268-2_11

Table 11.1 Common mucosal injury patterns and associated offending agents

Histologic pattern	Medications
Mucosal erosions, ulcerations, and strictures	NSAIDs KCl Iron Alendronate Kayexalate Sevelamer
Increased crypt apoptosis	NSAIDs Mycophenolate Ipilimumab Idelalisib Nivolumab Pembrolizumab Taxanes Colchicine
Ischemic colitis	NSAIDs Digitalis Estrogen Cocaine Ergotamine Sumatriptan Sodium polysterene sulfonate (Kayexalate)
Microscopic colitis (lymphocytic and/or collagenous colitis)	NSAIDs PPI (lansoprazole) Nivolumab Pembrolizumab Idelalisib H_2 antagonist SSRI Ticlopidine Simvastatin Flutamide Penicillin
Focal active colitis	NSAIDs Oral sodium phosphate
Mitotic arrest	Colchicine Taxanes
Pseudomembranous colitis	NSAIDs Antibiotics PPI

NSAIDs nonsteroidal anti-inflammatory drugs, *KCl* potassium chloride, *PPI* proton pump inhibitor, *SSRI* slow serotonin reuptake inhibitor

Different medications can lead to a variety of injury patterns in the GI tract, which can either be organ-specific or non-organ-specific. These injury patterns can be either non-specific (shared by various agents/diseases) or specific to certain medications.

- The majority of the medications cause non-specific injury patterns, which are shared among various agents (Table 11.1). Such changes also display overlap with those produced by infections and immune-mediated diseases. Clinical correlation is important to establish a temporal relationship with the offending agent.
- On the other hand, there exist a few medications that produce characteristic histologic changes, which can then be attributed to the particular agent (Table 11.2).

Table 11.2 Commonly used medications and their mucosal injury patterns

Medication	Histologic pattern
NSAIDs	Mucosal erosions, ulcerations, strictures Increased crypt apoptosis Ischemic colitis Focal active colitis Microscopic colitis
Mycophenolate	Increased crypt apoptosis Ischemic colitis Focal active colitis
Kayexalate Sevelemar	Mucosal ulcerations, erosions and strictures Ischemic colitis
Immunotherapy agents Idelalisib Ipilimumab Nivolumab Pembrolizumab	Increased crypt apoptosis Focal active colitis Lymphocytic colitis

NSAIDs nonsteroidal anti-inflammatory drugs

- In both instances, a knowledge of clinical features, endoscopic findings and underlying illnesses is helpful in ascertaining the offending agent.

Reference: [1]

2. **What are the different non-specific drug-induced GI tract injury patterns?**

The GI tract has only limited ways to respond to various injurious assaults imparted by different medications. Similar histologic changes can be seen in association with a variety of medications. Moreover, many non-specific injury patterns such as mucosal erosion, ulceration, stricture, focal inflammation, and apoptosis of epithelial cells can be due to infections, malformations, vascular insufficiency and immune-mediated injury. Hence, histology alone is not sufficient to implicate a specific drug as a cause of the observed injury. Pertinent clinical details including medication history, endoscopic findings and knowledge of predisposing conditions can alert the pathologist to consider drug-induced injury as an important differential diagnosis.

- *Pill esophagitis*
Pill esophagitis refers to caustic injury arising from direct contact between ingested pills and (usually) the esophageal mucosa. Local injury usually occurs due to stasis of the pill in areas of esophageal narrowing. The mid esophagus is a common location. Other sites of impaction include those affected by external compression, such as where the esophagus rests against the left main stem bronchus, the gastroesophageal junction, and the left atrium. Pills can also lodge in areas of prior injury. Elderly individuals are at particularly risk, as they are more likely to ingest medication without adequate amounts of water or consume medications in a

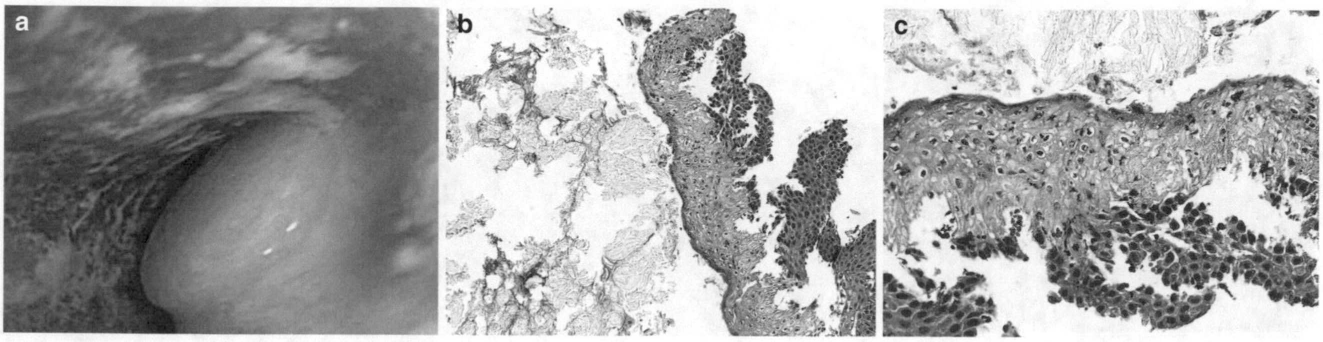

Fig. 11.1 Pill esophagitis. (**a**) A pill is embedded in the mucosa and the patient also has candidiasis, as evidenced by the whitish material. (Photograph courtesy of Dr. Christina Arnold). (**b**) Pill fragments appear as clear, colorless, refractile crystalline material associated with squamous epithelium surface necrosis and reactive epithelial changes. (**c**) A higher power view of the epithelium with overlying refractile pill fragments. This "mummified" surface can impart an esophagitis dissecans pattern

supine position shortly before bedtime. Endoscopic findings include erosions, ulcers, erythema, mucosal denudations, or strictures (mimicking malignancy) (Fig. 11.1a).

Common offending agents include nonsteroidal anti-inflammatory drugs (NSAIDs), antibiotics (doxycycline, tetracycline, and clindamycin are common), potassium chloride, iron supplements, and bisphosphonates. NSAIDs are likely the most common culprit, accounting for 41% of all cases of medication-induced pill esophagitis in one study.

Histologic changes are usually non-specific. Acute inflammation, granulation tissue, erosions, and ulcers are common. Polarizable crystalline material, when present, can be an important diagnostic clue (Fig. 11.1b, c). Pill esophagitis is well-described in association with bisphosphonates, especially alendronate, although injury associated with bisphosphonates has become far less common than in the past based on improved package labeling and patient instructions to take the pills with abundant liquid and not before sleeping. Abraham and colleagues described a series of ten patients who experienced erosive/ulcerative esophagitis while on alendronate therapy. The biopsies from all patients showed inflammatory exudates and inflamed granulation tissue, with or without polarizable crystalline material. Multinucleated giant cells may be seen. Adjacent squamous epithelium usually shows active inflammation and reactive changes with enlarged hyperchromatic nuclei. Regardless of histology, finding foreign material in association with esophageal injury should prompt consideration of pill-induced esophagitis. Fungal organisms and viral cytopathic effects should always be excluded. Patients are typically managed conservatively with proton pump inhibitors, withdrawal of the offending agent, or behavioral modifications such as tablet ingestion with adequate fluids while maintaining an upright posture.

Please also see Chap. 2, question 10, for additional discussion on this topic.

- *Sloughing esophagitis*
Also known as "esophagitis dissecans superficialis," this condition refers to a characteristic pattern of mucosal injury, with a dramatic endoscopic image and a blister-like appearance on microscopy. The patients are typically older, debilitated individuals, who are on "polypharmacy". In one study, association with psychoactive drugs was reported in 73% of the patients. Other disease associations include pemphigus vulgaris, heavy smoking, physical trauma (such as ingestion of hot liquid), immunosuppression, and impaired mobility. The endoscopic picture is characterized by whitish streaks or strips of peeling esophageal mucosa, predominantly involving the mid and distal esophagus (Fig. 11.2a). On histology, the esophageal epithelium has a 2-toned appearance, with a superficial eosinophilic zone of necrosis and an underlying deeper squamous epithelium that is either normal or appears more basophilic. There is often some degree of intraepithelial splitting, sometimes forming a distinct bulla but the cleft is in the middle of the epithelium rather than at the basal zone, in contrast to that in many skin diseases (Fig. 11.2b, c).

Please see Chap. 2, question 12, for additional discussion on this topic.

- *Chemical gastritis/Reactive gastropathy*
Initially described in association with bile reflux into the stomach (also known as "reflux gastritis") and usually encountered in the gastric antrum, chemical gastritis or reactive gastropathy refers to a non-specific response to a variety of gastric irritants. NSAIDs and alcohol are among the common offenders. Characteristic histology includes foveolar hyperplasia

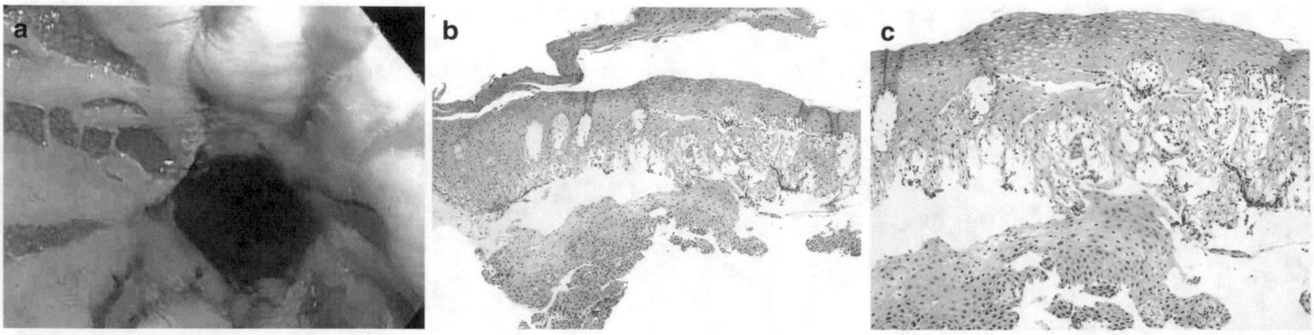

Fig. 11.2 Esophagitis dissecans superficialis. (**a**) Prominent streaks of white plaques are characteristic. (**b**) Squamous mucosa with a detached peeled off layer of superficial epithelium with parakeratosis. (**c**) High-power view of squamous epithelium with necrosis and superficial layer of parakeratosis. There is minimal inflammation

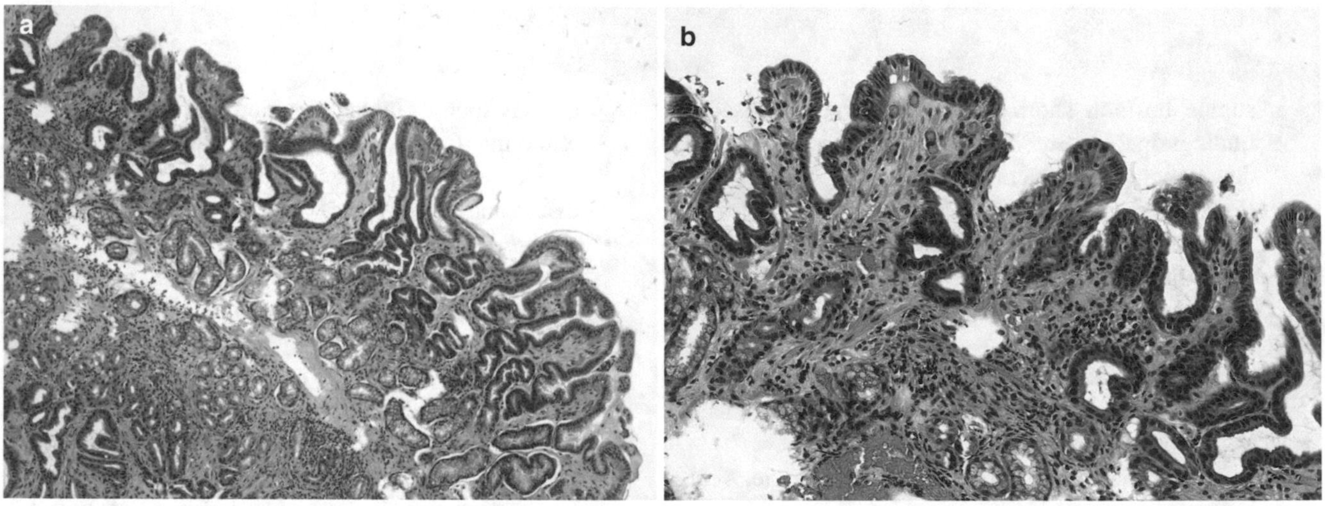

Fig. 11.3 Chemical gastritis/reactive gastropathy. (**a**) There is surface mucin loss, a corkscrew appearance of gastric pits and reactive epithelial changes, with minimal lamina propria inflammation. (**b**) High-power view highlighting loss of surface mucin, reactive epithelial changes, and splayed smooth muscle fibers in the lamina propria

with a "corkscrew" appearance to the pits, mucin-depleted epithelium, splaying of smooth muscle fibers in the lamina propria, edema, vascular congestion, and paucity of inflammatory cells in the lamina propria (Fig. 11.3a, b). Surface erosion can be seen, which is usually accompanied by a neutrophilic infiltrate.

Please see Chap. 5, questions 16–19, for additional discussion on this topic.

- *Microscopic colitis*
  Several drugs are implicated in the development of microscopic colitis, either lymphocytic or collagenous colitis. Proton pump inhibitors (especially lansoprazole) are common offenders. Other less frequently associated drugs include NSAIDs, ticlopidine, H_2 receptor antagonists (ranitidine, cimetidine), simvastatin, flutamide, carbamazepine, sertraline, penicillin, angiotensin II receptor antagonists, and immunotherapy agents (nivolumab, pembrolizumab, ipilimumab, etc.).

  Please see Chap. 7, questions 1–13, for additional discussion on this topic.
- *Ischemic colitis*
  An ischemic colitis pattern of injury is characterized by surface injury, mucin loss in crypts, "atrophic microcrypts," and hyalinization of the lamina propria (Fig. 11.4a, b). In younger patients, such changes should always raise the possibility of drug involvement. Commonly implicated agents include cocaine, decongestant medications, oral contraceptives, NSAIDs, and the migraine headache medication sumatriptan, among others. In the past, sodium polystyrene sulfonate (Kayexalate given for hyperkalemia in patients with renal failure) was associated with ischemic mucosal disease, but formulary changes to

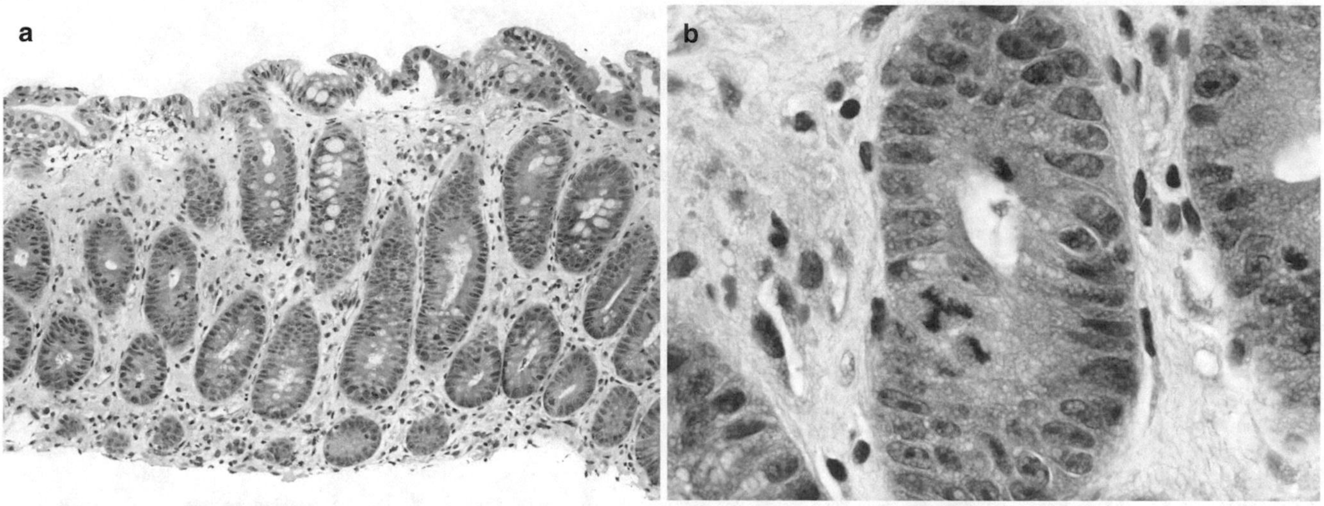

Fig. 11.4 Ischemic colitis. (**a**) This example shows focal surface damage, hyalinization of the lamina propria, mucin loss in the crypts, and reactive cytologic atypia. (**b**) High power showing presence of an atypical "tripolar" mitosis, which can mimic dysplasia

administration of this medication have vastly reduced ischemic complications.

Please see Chap. 7, questions 17–22, for additional discussion on this topic.

- *Focal active colitis*
  Focal active colitis is defined as cryptitis that involves one or only a few crypts, without evidence of chronic mucosal injury changes such as crypt architectural distortion (Fig. 11.5). Once common causes are ruled out (acute infections, ischemia, or Crohn disease), drugs should be considered as a potential offender. Two often reported drugs that are associated with focal active colitis include sodium phosphate bowel preparations and NSAIDs.
- *Increased epithelial apoptosis*
  Apoptotic cells are rare in the normal intestinal mucosa. The presence of substantially increased apoptotic bodies in the surface epithelium, or crypts in an otherwise normal looking mucosa (greater than 3 per 10 consecutive crypts), warrants correlation with clinical findings. Medications among the potential culprits include laxatives, oral sodium phosphate used for bowel preparation, NSAIDs, mycophenolic acid (MFA), angiotensin II receptor antagonists, and chemotherapeutic agents (especially 5-fluorouracil). Recently, immunotherapy agents (ipilimumab, idelalisib, nivolumab, pembrolizumab, etc.) have emerged as an important cause of increased epithelial apoptosis. However, non-drug-related causes of increased apoptosis, including graft-versus host disease (GVHD), common variable immunodeficiency, cytomegalovirus/adenovirus, and human immunodeficiency virus (HIV) enteropathy should always be ruled out before considering drugs.
  References: [1–33]

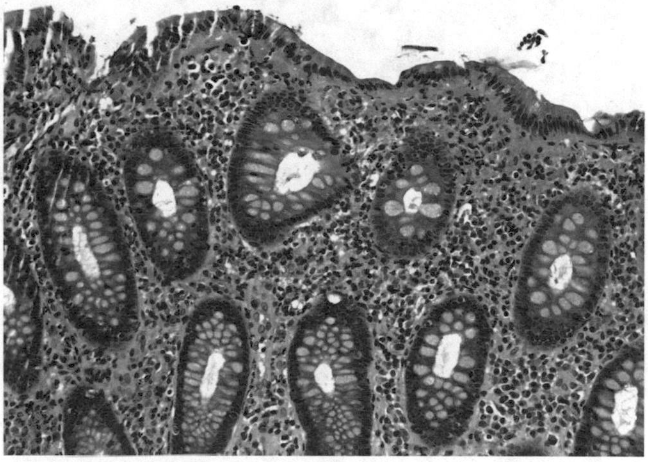

Fig. 11.5 Focal active colitis. Neutrophilic infiltration involving very few crypts

3. **What are the histologic changes associated with nonsteroidal anti-inflammatory drug (NSAID)-related GI tract mucosal injury?**

NSAIDs exert their analgesic and anti-inflammatory activity by inhibiting cyclooxygenase-1 (COX-1) and cyclooxygenase-2 (COX-2) activity, resulting in decreased prostaglandin synthesis. Common GI tract injuries include erosions and ulcers in the gastric mucosa. Classical NSAID-associated lesions show mucosal necrosis, resulting in erosions and ulcerations with sparse inflammatory infiltration, consisting mostly of neutrophils. Associated lesions can be found in the proximal duodenum, terminal ileum, and proximal large bowel. Gastric lesions are characterized by the so-called reactive gastropathy or chemical gastritis (described in question 2).

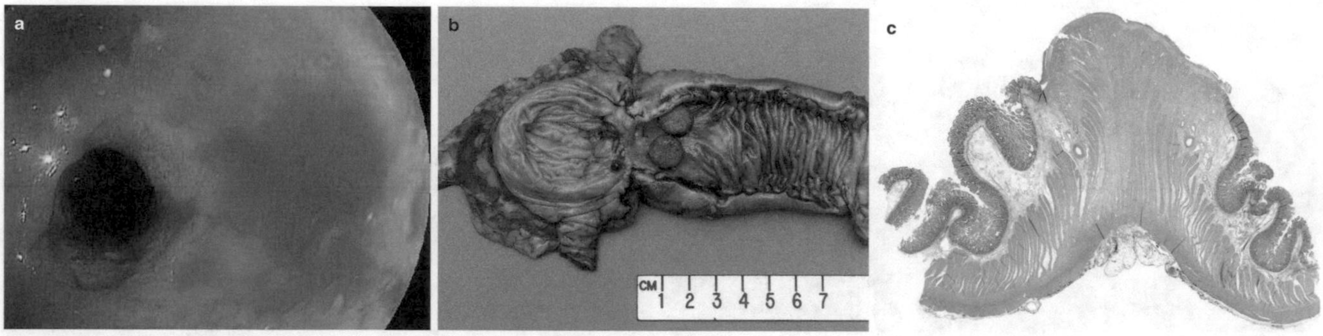

Fig. 11.6 Diaphragm disease. (**a**) Such mucosal ledges narrow the lumen and impede passage of the endoscope. (Photograph courtesy of Dr. Dora Lam-Himlin). (**b**) A small bowel resection necessitated due to intestinal obstruction. Some tablets can be seen that failed to pass through the mucosal diaphragm (photograph courtesy of Dr. Dora Lam-Himlin). (**c**) The submucosa is replaced by columns of fibromuscular tissue with an erosion at the top

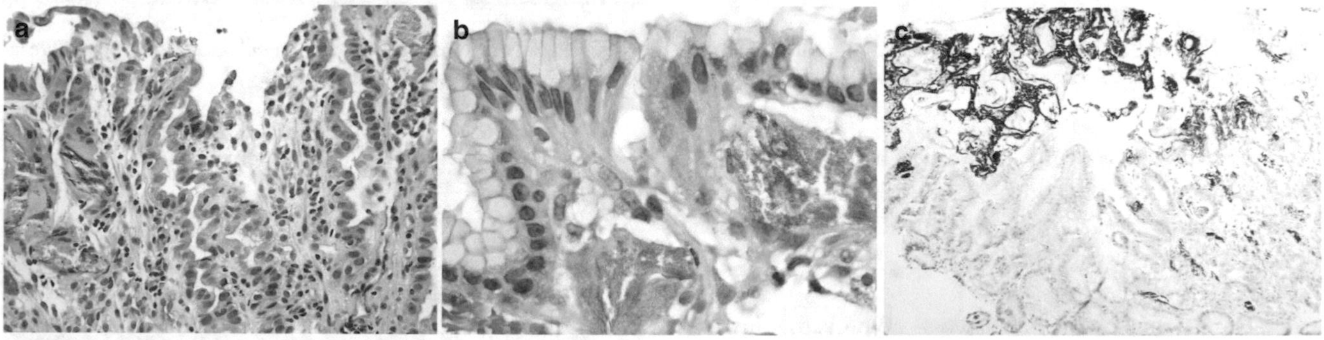

Fig. 11.7 Iron pill gastritis. (**a**) There is surface erosion, mucin loss, reactive epithelial changes, and golden brown iron deposits. (**b**) A higher magnification image better demonstrates the golden brown appearance of the ferrous sulfate crystals. (**c**) A Prussian blue stain highlights the iron crystals

- Diaphragm disease is a long-term adverse event of chronic NSAID use, which usually involves the small bowel. As a result of repetitive cycles of damage and repair, submucosal fibrosis arises in the form of concentric ridges that macroscopically appear as web-like luminal protrusions (Fig. 11.6a). These can cause small bowel obstruction, requiring surgical resection (Fig. 11.6b). Histology shows columns of perpendicularly oriented collagen fibers, extending from the mucosa into deeper regions of the submucosa, often with erosion at the apices (Fig. 11.6c).

References: [34–40]

4. **What are the mucosal changes associated with iron therapy?**

Oral iron supplements for anemia and other hematologic conditions are usually in the form of ferrous sulfate. These exert direct corrosive effects on mucosal surfaces of the upper GI tract, which is usually dose-dependent. Mucosal damage also results from local ischemia due to formation of microthrombi. Therapeutic doses elicit mild mucosal injury, which is most common in the stomach (iron pill gastritis), less frequent in the esophagus, and sometimes in the duodenum.

- On gastric biopsies, iron deposits appear in the tissue as extracellular clumps of non-polarizing golden brown crystalline material concentrated in the superficial lamina propria, around vessels and within vascular thrombi (Fig. 11.7a, b). These can be highlighted by an iron stain (Perl's Prussian blue) (Fig. 11.7c). The background mucosa usually shows erosions and ulcers. Sometimes reactive gastropathy/chemical gastritis type changes may also be encountered.
- Gastric siderosis refers to iron deposits in the form of hemosiderin in patients with systemic iron overload, such as from hereditary hemochromatosis, or other causes of secondary hemosiderosis. These appear as tiny golden brown granules, often observed within gastric glandular cells (Fig. 11.8a–c).
- Psedomelanosis intestinalis refers to spotty-brown-to-black pigmentation of the small intestinal mucosa that may be observed in association with oral iron therapy. These appear on the biopsy as iron deposits within the cytoplasm of macrophages located in small bowel

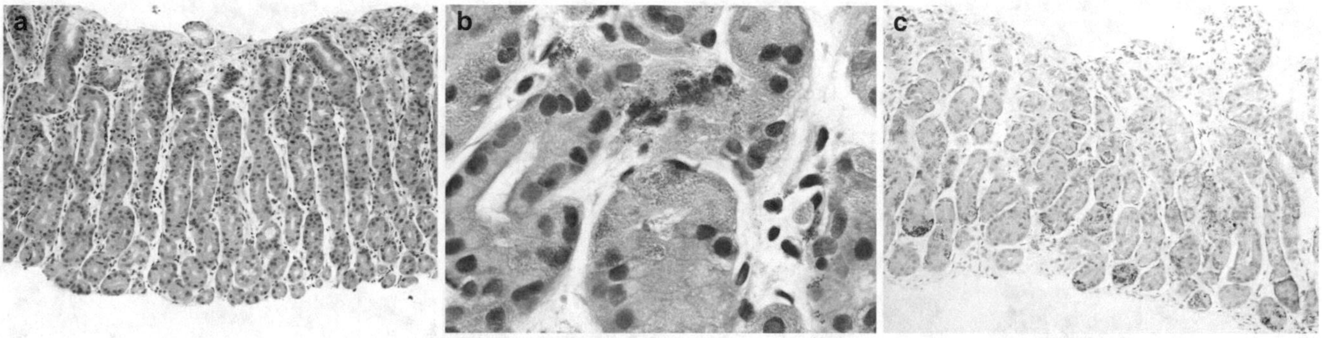

Fig. 11.8 Gastric siderosis. (**a**) Low power view of gastric oxyntic type mucosa with faint brownish tinge to the deep gastric glands. The superficial glands are mostly unremarkable. (**b**) Higher magnification highlights the brown-colored iron deposits in the cytoplasm of the deep gastric glands. (**c**) A Prussian blue stain highlights the intracytoplasmic iron

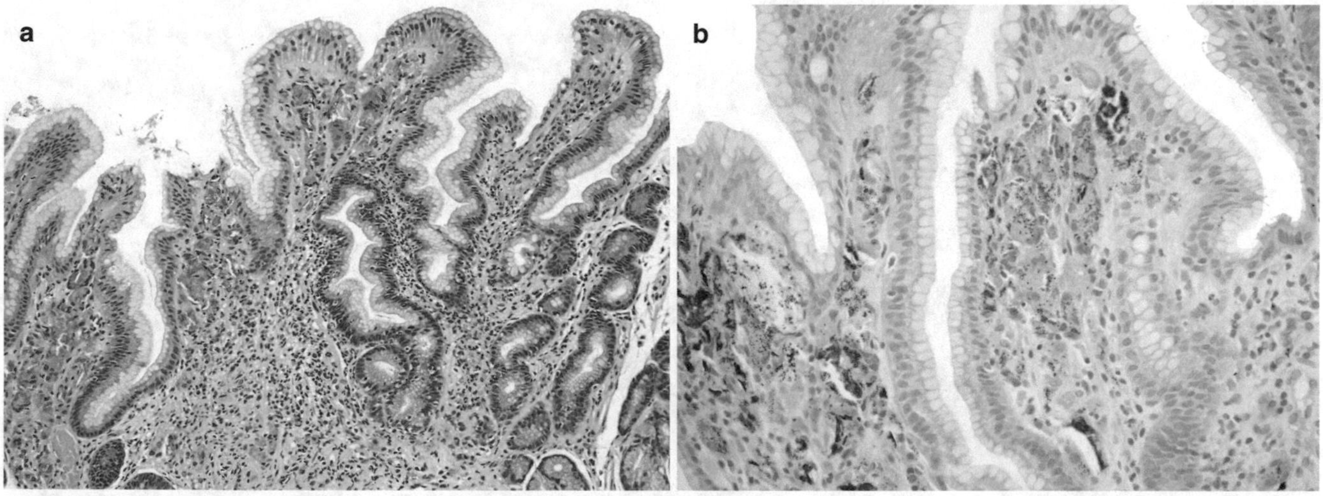

Fig. 11.9 Gastric mucosal calcinosis. (**a**) Calcium deposits are seen within the superficial lamina propria. (**b**) The calcium deposits are highlighted on a von Kossa stain

lamina propria. Such changes are also observed in patients with systemic iron overload and can also be associated with antihypertensive medications, such as hydralazine, propranolol, and thiazides.

References: [41–46]

5. **What is gastric mucosal calcinosis?**

Gastric mucosal calcinosis represents mucosal calcium deposits, usually in the antrum or in the body, typically located beneath the surface epithelium. This is an example of "metastatic calcification" (as opposed to "dystrophic calcification"), often observed in patients with disturbance in calcium and phosphate homeostasis. Patients with renal failure are a classical example, although mucosal calcinosis is also encountered in association with atrophic gastritis, hypervitaminosis A, organ transplantation, gastric neoplasias, and various clinical situations that can cause hypercalcemia/hyperphosphatemia. Among medications, calcium-containing antacids such as sucralfate are common offenders. Citrate-containing blood products and isotrenion are also implicated with mucosal calcinosis.

- On biopsy, the coarse black-purple pigment is usually extracellular and is present just beneath the surface epithelium at the tips of the foveolae (Fig. 11.9a). A von Kossa stain can be helpful, which imparts a black color to calcium (Fig. 11.9b). In one study, elemental microanalysis showed that these deposits contained aluminum, phosphate, calcium, and chlorine.
- A differential diagnosis is lanthanum carbonate deposition in the GI tract mucosa. Lanthanum carbonate is a phosphate binder that is administered orally to reduce phosphate absorption in patients with end-stage renal diseases. Deposition is most commonly seen in the stomach, but small bowel and colon can also be involved. The lamina propria is filled with abundant brown-purple, amorphous, mineral-like materials,

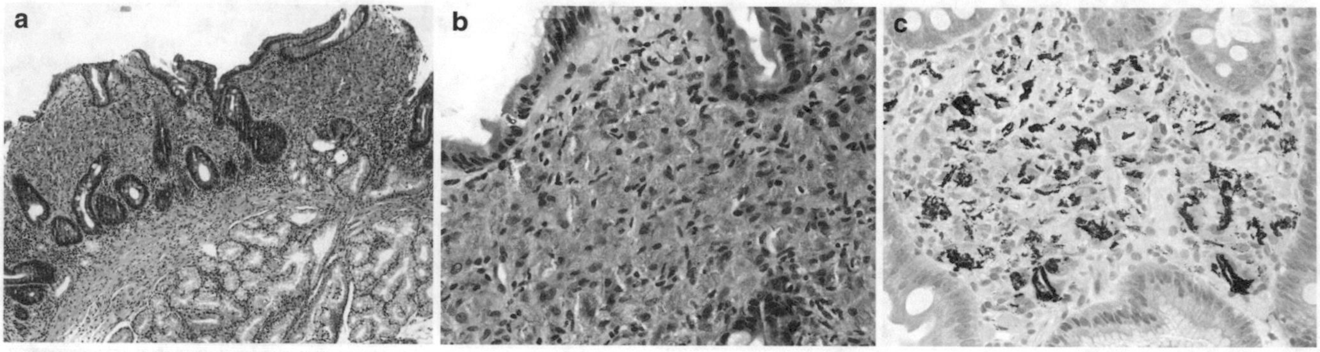

Fig. 11.10 Lanthanum deposition in duodenal mucosa. (**a**) Low power view of a duodenal biopsy showing histiocytic accumulation in the lamina propria, accompanied by villous blunting. (**b**) Higher power view showing brown-purple mineral-like materials in histiocytes, which stain black on von Kossa stain (**c**). The duodenal mucosa is nodular under endoscopy in this case

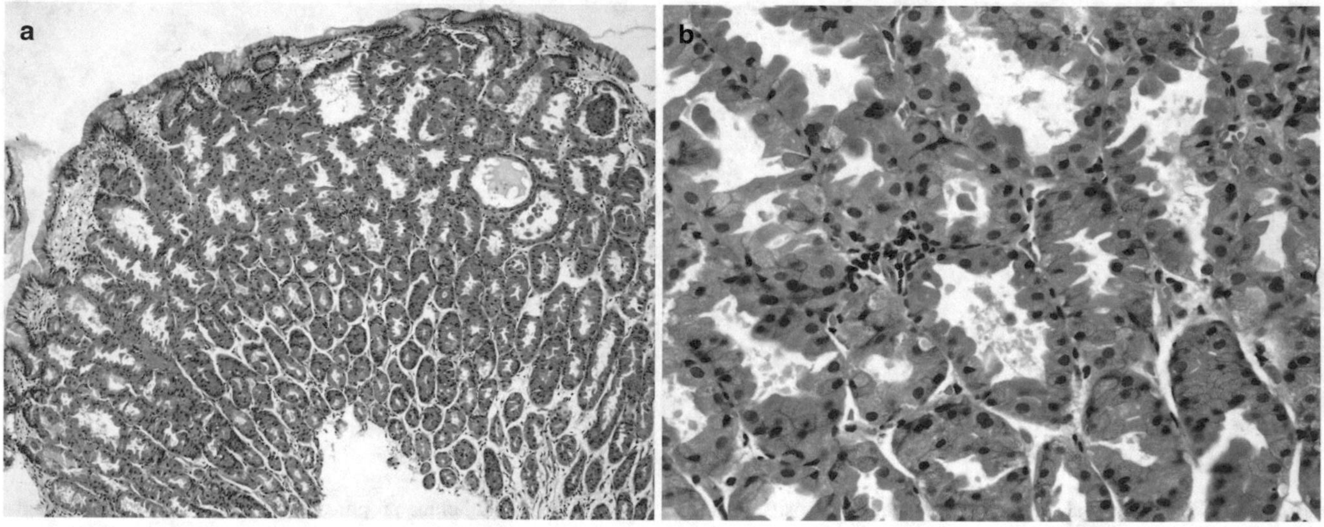

Fig. 11.11 Proton pump inhibitor effect. (**a**) Low power view with dilated oxyntic glands lined by plump appearing parietal cells. (**b**) High magnification shows the swollen "apocrine-like" parietal cell cytoplasm

which are mostly engulfed by histiocytes. A von Kossa stain can also be helpful, which reveals a black coloration (Fig. 11.10a–c).

References: [47–52]

6. **What are the histologic changes induced by proton pump inhibitors? Are they limited to the stomach?**

Proton pump inhibitors (PPIs) are commonly prescribed medications for various upper GI tract ailments, such as gastroesophageal reflux disease and eosinophilic esophagitis, and as a component of *Helicobacter pylori* eradication therapy and in patients with Zollinger-Ellison syndrome.

- PPI effect is classically observed in gastric parietal cells, which become hypertrophied, and take on the appearance of an apocrine-like cytoplasmic swelling (Fig. 11.11a, b). The oxyntic glands are typically dilated. Cytoplasmic protrusions and vacuolation are seen. In *H. pylori*-infected patients who are treated with PPI, the oxyntic mucosa shows parietal cell hypertrophy and persistent inflammation, while the antral mucosa tends to normalize. Sometimes *H. pylori* may be found within the canaliculi of the parietal cells. Gastritis predominantly involving the gastric corpus is an indication for long- term users of PPI to undergo *H. pylori* eradication.
- PPI-induced changes are not exclusive to the stomach. Recently, several PPIs, particularly lansoprazole, esomeprazole, and omeprazole, have been associated with a microscopic colitis pattern of injury. Though both lymphocytic colitis and collagenous colitis can occur, PPI injury is more strongly linked to the latter pattern of changes. The histologic appearance of PPI-related microscopic colitis is identical to that of idiopathic microscopic colitis. Though there is limited literature related to PPI-

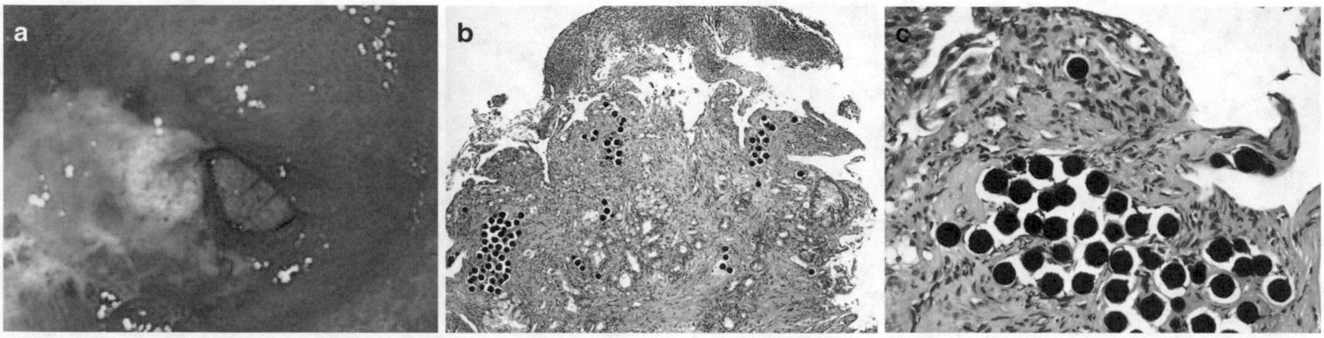

Fig. 11.12 Yttrium microspheres. (**a**) Endoscopic picture of gastric injury induced by Yttrium (photograph courtesy of Dr. Christina Arnold). (**b**) Low power view shows discrete, round blackish to purple spheres embedded in eroded gastric mucosa (**c**). High power of the distinctive appearing Yttrium microspheres embedded within the granulation tissue

associated microscopic colitis, it is important to consider it in the differential diagnosis of a microscopic colitis pattern, since withdrawal of PPI can be curative.

References: [20, 53–56]

7. **Do radiation microspheres such as Yttrium-90 impart any specific GI tract mucosal injury pattern?**

Yttrium-90 microspheres (under the trade names of TheraSphere, Sirtex, and SIR-Spheres) are used for "selective internal radiation therapy" for targeted therapy of unresectable primary and metastatic hepatic malignancies. Yttrium-90 is incorporated into microspheres and injected into the hepatic artery to preferentially target the neoplastic cells. Inadvertently, these radioactive beads can enter the arteries supplying the esophagus, stomach, duodenum, gallbladder, or stomach and impart ischemic and radiation type injury. On microscopy, these microspheres appear as uniform basophilic globules measuring 30–40 μm in diameter within mucosal/submucosal vessels, lamina propria, or glands (Fig. 11.12a–c).

References: [57, 58]

8. **Which medications are associated with "mitotic arrest"-related changes in GI tract mucosa? Is it important to differentiate, and how can they be differentiated?**

Two important types of medications, namely taxanes and colchicine, impart changes associated with "mitotic arrest" in GI epithelial cells.

- Taxanes (paclitaxel, docetaxel, and cabazitaxel) are chemotherapeutic agents used in the treatment of breast, ovarian, lung, prostate, and other carcinomas. Their mechanism of action involves stabilization of microtubule polymerization in proliferating cells, mitotic arrest, and apoptotic cell death. In contrast, colchicine is an alkaloid with anti-mitotic activity, predominantly used to treat gout and familial Mediterranean fever. It prevents tubulin protein polymerization, which is necessary for mitotic spindle formation, thereby causing mitotic arrest during metaphase.
- Colchicine and taxane effects are histologically indistinguishable, characterized by arrested mitotic figures, ring mitoses, and prominent apoptotic cell damage (Fig. 11.13a, b). Taxane-related lesions can occur anywhere in the GI tract, including the gallbladder, and predominantly affect the proliferative compartment of the epithelium. Colchicine effects are most prominent in the duodenum, but may also be encountered in the gastric antrum; changes are minimal in the colon.
- While histologic changes are identical between the two groups of drugs, there is a significant clinical difference. Taxane-related changes can be seen in the mucosa of any patient undergoing chemotherapy with this agent, indicating medication "effect." The characteristic findings are only seen within the first few days following intravenous administration of the agent (as well in patients who have toxicity from these medications). On the other hand, such histologic changes related to colchicine indicate toxicity, and the patient usually has underlying renal insufficiency. This requires immediate notification to the treating physician. Clinical correlation, with attention to the medication list, becomes very crucial in determining the offending agent.

References: [25, 36, 59–62]

9. **What are the injurious effects associated with angiotensin II receptor antagonists on GI tract mucosa?**

The angiotensin II receptor antagonist olmesartan (trade name Benicar) is one of several related compounds used for management of hypertension. Although it is essentially considered a safe medication, less than 1% of patients develop a severe diarrheal illness, often after taking the medication for many years. Olmesartan-associated sprue-like enteropathy was first described by Rubio-Tapia

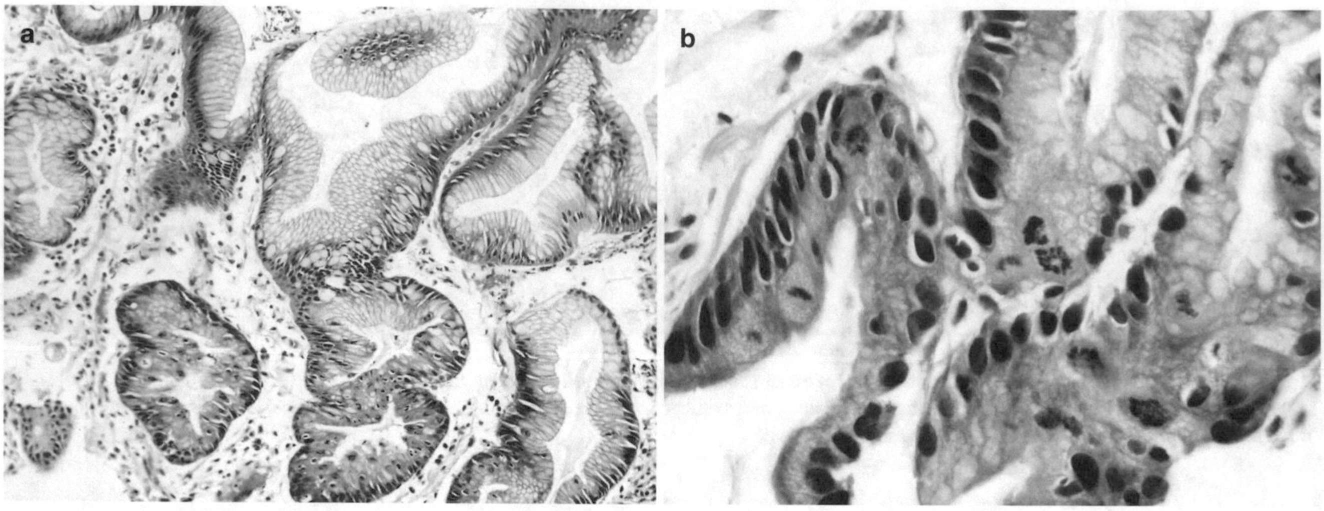

Fig. 11.13 Taxane effect. (**a**) The changes are visible in the proliferative component of gastric antrum, with prominent apoptosis, arrested mitotic figures, and ring mitoses. (**b**) Higher magnification highlights ring mitoses and prominent apoptosis

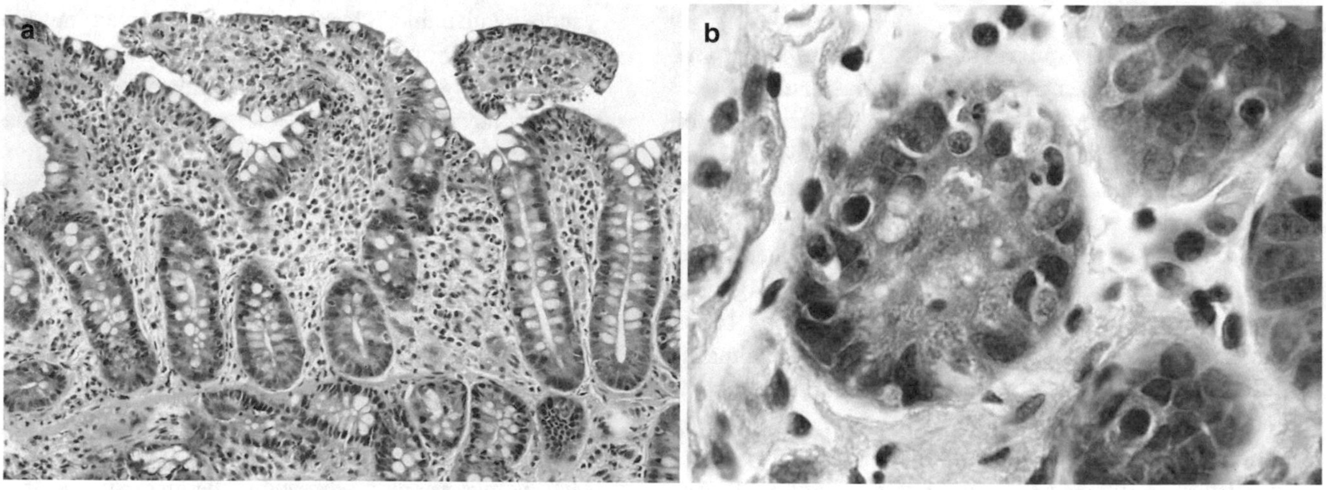

Fig. 11.14 Olmesartan-associated enteropathy. (**a**) This small bowel mucosa shows mild villous blunting with crypt hyperplasia and increased intraepithelial lymphocytes. (**b**) High magnification shows prominent crypt apoptosis

and his colleagues. Subsequently, about 150 additional cases have been published and the effects appear to be a class effect associated with all "sartan" compounds. Patients present with sudden onset of severe diarrhea, sometimes following a dose increase. Lesions have been reported primarily in the small bowel and stomach, although the colon can be involved.

- Histologic changes in the duodenum bear a striking resemblance to those of collagenous sprue or celiac disease, with intraepithelial lymphocytosis, increased lymphocytes and plasma cells in the lamina propria, and partial or total villous blunting (Fig. 11.14a). These may be accompanied by subepithelial collagen deposition, active inflammation, including eosinophils, and sometimes striking crypt cell apoptosis (Fig. 11.14b). Lymphocytic gastritis, collagenous gastritis, lymphocytic colitis, and collagenous colitis have also been described. While biopsy changes somewhat mimic celiac disease, patients lack serologic evidence, with negative anti-tissue transglutaminase and anti-endomysial antibody titers.

References: [1, 63–67]

10. What are the histologic changes associated with mycophenolate (CellCept) in GI tract mucosa? What is the closest histologic mimic and how can these be differentiated?

Mycophenolate mofetil (MMF) and its variants CellCept and Myfortic are agents used to prevent allograft rejection in solid organs, bone marrow, and stem cell transplant recipients. MMF is a prodrug that is

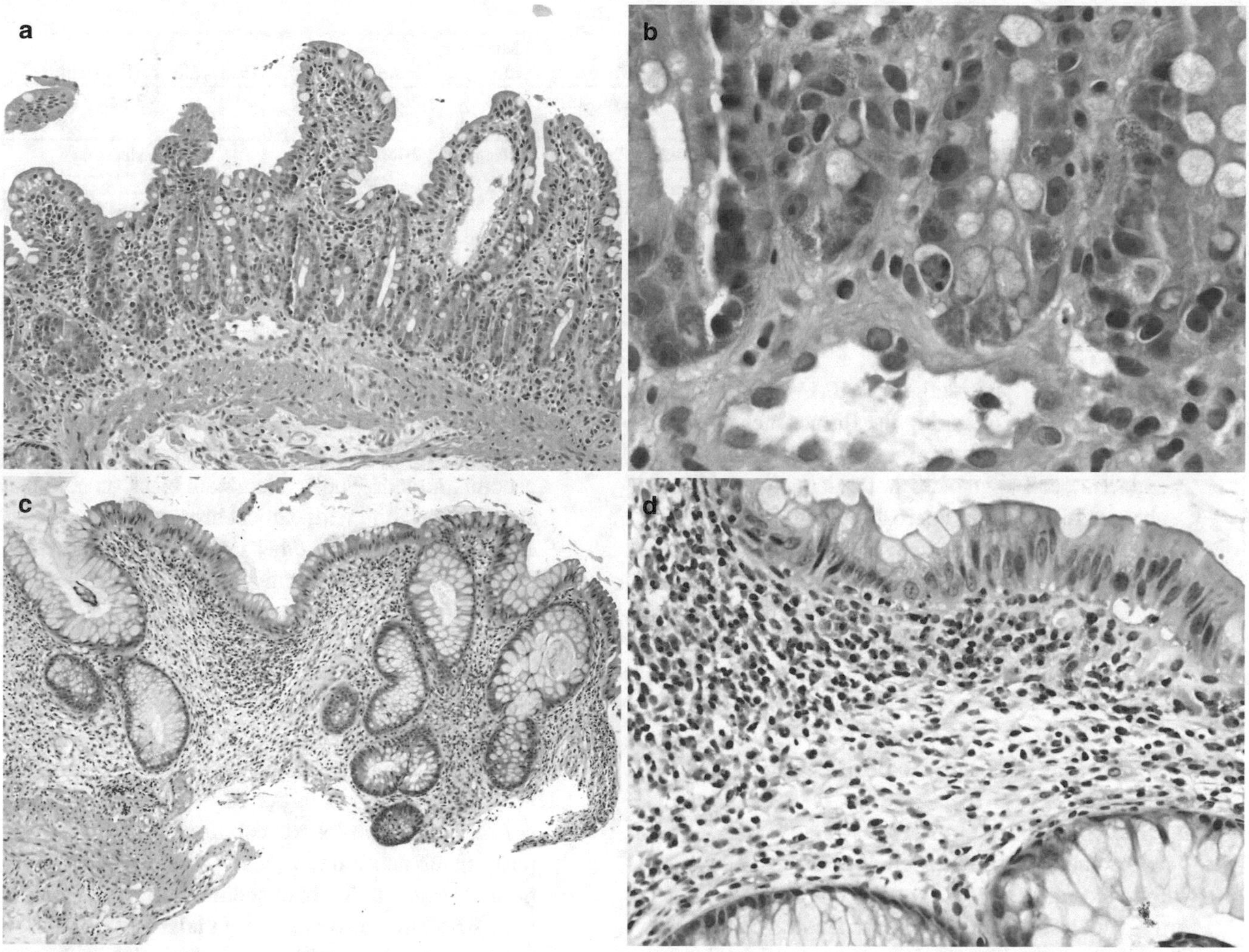

Fig. 11.15 Mycophenolate-associated injury. (**a**) The findings are essentially identical to those of GVHD, requiring knowledge of clinical history to separate the two. Crypt apoptosis is the key feature. (**b**) This small bowel biopsy shows prominent crypt apoptotic bodies. (**c**) Colonic mucosa with chronic mycophenolate-associated injury shows crypt architectural distortion with crypt loss and an edematous lamina propria; eosinophils are often prominent. (**d**) High-power view showing eosinophil-rich inflammation in colonic lamina propria

converted to metabolically active mycophenolic acid, which non-competitively inhibits inosine 5′-monophosphate dehydrogenase in the de novo purine synthesis pathway. Enterocytes are partly dependent on this pathway, and GI toxicity is one of the main limitations of the drug. Reported GI symptoms include diarrhea, nausea, vomiting, abdominal pain, malabsorption, and bleeding. MMF-associated damage may result in enterocolitis, but the upper GI tract can also be affected. Endoscopically, it manifests as ulcers and erosions.

- The key histologic finding is prominent apoptosis of intestinal crypts or gastric pits (Fig. 11.15a, b). In the stomach, finding greater than 3 apoptotic bodies per 10 glands can be considered in keeping with MFA injury. The esophagus is often spared since the squamous epithelium is less dependent on the de novo pathway of purine synthesis. Other less characteristic changes include mild distortion of crypt architecture, focal loss of crypts, and edema of lamina propria with sparse inflammatory cells (Fig. 11.15c, d). Dilated crypts lined by attenuated epithelial cells and crypt abscesses can also be seen.
- The closest differential diagnosis of MMF-associated injury is acute GVHD. Increased crypt apoptosis is also observed in GVHD. This distinction poses a major diagnostic challenge for pathologists and clinicians, particularly in patients who have had bone marrow transplants. While MMF-associated injury is cured with medication cessation, GVHD is treated with immunosuppressants. Clinical correlation is extremely important; if the patient has had bone marrow transplant rather than solid organ transplant, increased apoptosis may be a feature of either MFA

Table 11.3 Classical features of the medication resins

Generic name	Brand name	Clinical associations	Target	Mucosal injury	H&E	Fish scale	AFB stain
Sodium polystyrene sulfonate	Kayexalate	Hyperkalemia (renal failure)	Potassium	Yes	Purple	+	Black
Sevelamer	Renvela Renagel	Hyperphosphatemia (renal failure)	Phosphate	Possible	2-toned	+	Magenta
Bile acid Sequestrants	Cholestyramine Colestipol Colesevelam	Dyslipidemia	Bile acids	–	Bright orange	–	Dull yellow

AFB acid fast bacillus

injury, GVHD, or both. Star et al. reported on useful criteria to differentiate MFA colitis from GVHD. Features favoring the former include a triad of eosinophils >15 per high-power field, absence of endocrine cell aggregates in the lamina propria, and absence of apoptotic microabscesses. One important differential diagnostic consideration always worth keeping in mind is possible cytomegalovirus infection (and other viral infections) in such patients, which can manifest with prominent apoptosis. An immunostain can be helpful in excluding viral inclusions.

References: [68–71]

11. **What are the different medication resins that are associated with GI tract injury? How can these be morphologically recognized?**

Ion-exchange resins are non-absorbable medications, which are commonly orally ingested and their crystal forms can be seen anywhere along the luminal GI tract. The three most commonly encountered resins are sodium polystyrene sulfonate, sevelamer, and bile acid sequestrants (BAS). These have distinctive morphologic appearances on H&E. However, morphologic overlap is possible and helpful adjuncts include special stains (such as acid fast bacillus stain), review of the medication chart, and an awareness of relevant clinical details (Table 11.3).

- *Sodium polystyrene sulfonate*

  Known by the trade name Kayexalate, this is a cation exchange resin used to treat hyperkalemia in patients with renal failure. Initially, it was administered in an aqueous solution, which resulted in bezoar formation, which led to dispersion of the drug in hypertonic sorbitol solution in the past. As such, the resin itself was unassociated with injury, whereas the formulation in hypertonic sorbitol was. The latter form has been associated with severe osmotic injury to the mucosa but more recent formulations have mitigated these issues. However, this injury is still occasionally encountered, sometimes unassociated with hypertonic sorbitol. Kayexlate-associated injury can occur throughout the GI tract. On histology, the crystals appear as deeply basophilic rhomboid or triangular crystals that display a characteristic lamellated rectangular cracks ("fish-scale" pattern) (Fig. 11.16). An ischemic injury to the adjoining mucosa is a common accompaniment. The crystals stain black on acid fast stain. Correlation with clinical history is important to avoid confusion with other crystals, pill fragments, and even dystrophic calcification.

- *Sevelamer*

  Also known as renvela, sevelamer is an anion exchange resin used to treat hyperphosphatemia in patients with chronic kidney disease. This is a relatively new medication, and associated GI mucosal injury was first described in 2013, although there are no experimental data as per Kayexalate (above). The crystal has a "two-toned" color on H&E with bright pink linear accentuation and a rusty yellow background (Fig. 11.17). Like sodium polystyrene sulfonate, sevelamer also displays an internal "fish-scale" pattern, with "scales" that are typically wide and irregularly distributed. Sevelamer turns magenta on acid fast bacillus (AFB) stain. Though associated with mucosal injury, it is not clear whether it causes the injury or is an innocent bystander.

- *Bile acid sequestrants*

  Cholestyramine, colestipol, and colesevelam are the common BAS, which are used to treat hypercholesterolemia and hyperlipidemia. They are not known to cause direct mucosal injury. However, the crystals are often mistaken for sevelamer or sodium polysterene sulfonate. On H&E, they are polygonal, homogeneously eosinophilic and lack the internal "fish-scale" pattern (Fig. 11.16). They appear dull yellow on AFB stain. The various BAS resins are indistinguishable from each other, and classifying them requires correlation with the medication list.

  References: [25, 72–78]

12. **What is melanosis coli? How is it different from pseudomelanosis enteri?**

Melanosis coli is characterized by dark pigmentation of the colonic mucosa, often associated with use of laxatives, especially those containing anthraquinone.

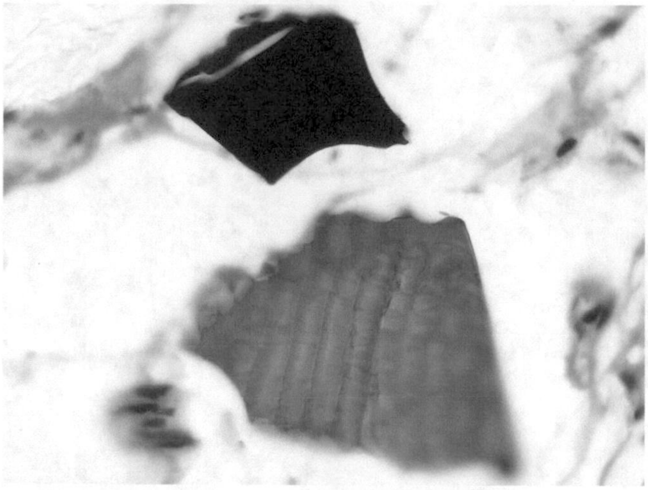

Fig. 11.16 Sodium polystyrene sulfonate (Kayexalate) and bile acid sequestrants. The Kayexalate crystal (below) is purple with evenly distributed rectangular cracks that resemble fish scales. The bile acid sequestrant crystal (above) is smooth, glassy, and eosinophilic, without "fish-scale" pattern

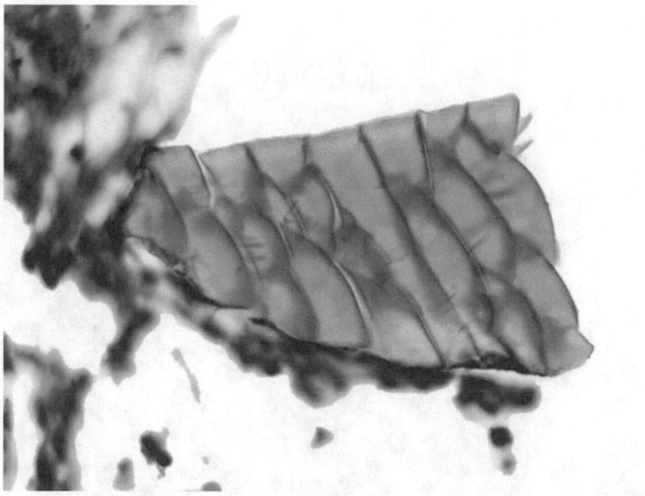

Fig. 11.17 Sevelamer. The crystal has a two-toned appearance, with rusty yellow structures interspersed by bright pink broad, irregularly spaced "fish scales"

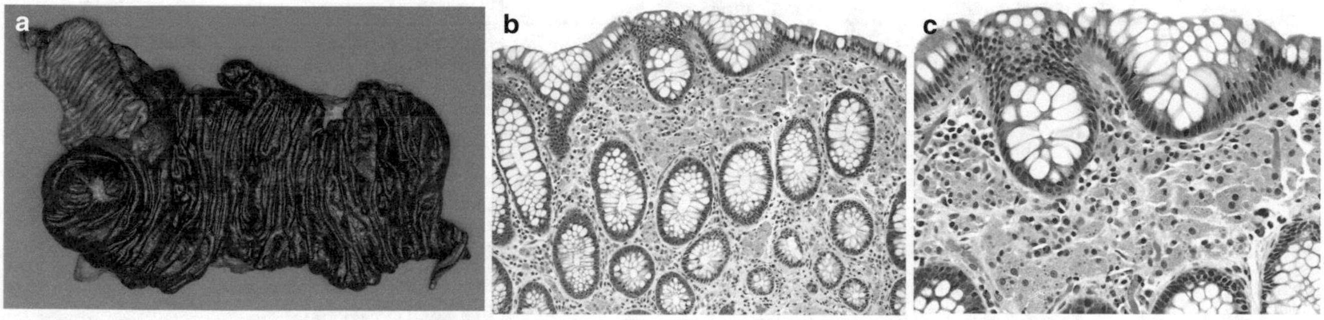

Fig. 11.18 Melanosis coli. (**a**) This colonic resection specimen is characterized by a large patch of dark-colored mucosa. (Photograph courtesy of Dr. Christina Arnold). (**b**) Pigment-laden macrophages in an otherwise unremarkable colonic mucosa. (**c**) The brown pigment in the macrophages is lipofuscin, not melanin

Unfortunately, the term "melanosis" is a misnomer, as the brown pigment is actually lipofuscin, not melanin. Apoptosis of colonic epithelial cells generates lipofuscin, which is phagocytosed by macrophages and imparts dark discoloration. Though commonly encountered in the cecum and rectum, melanosis coli can be found throughout the colorectum, appendix, and terminal ileum. Variable numbers of pigment-laden macrophages are found in the mucosa and, less frequently, submucosa (Fig. 11.18a–c).

- Pseudomelanosis, yet another misnomer, refers to the accumulation of pigmented macrophages in the lamina propria of the small bowel and less commonly of the stomach. Again, the pigment is not melanin, instead composed of varying amounts of iron, calcium, and sulfur. Common associations include hypertension, GI bleeding, renal failure, diabetes, oral iron supplementation, systemic iron overload, and antihypertensive medications, including hydralazine, propranolol, and thiazides. Biopsy shows macrophages filled with granular black or brown pigment, resembling melanin, which may be found at the villous tips (Fig. 11.19a, b), and stain variably with trichrome and iron stains.

References: [44–46, 79–82]

13. **What are the GI tract injuries induced by different immunotherapy agents?**

Immune checkpoint inhibitors have emerged as the latest armamentarium in the treatment of various advanced-stage malignancies. These agents block the co-inhibitory receptors on T cells to activate their cytotoxic immune function, which in turn exert anti-tumor activity. Commonly used agents are inhibitors against immunologically significant checkpoint molecules, such as cytotoxic T lymphocyte antigen 4 (CTLA-4) inhibitors ipilimumab and tremelimumab, programmed cell death

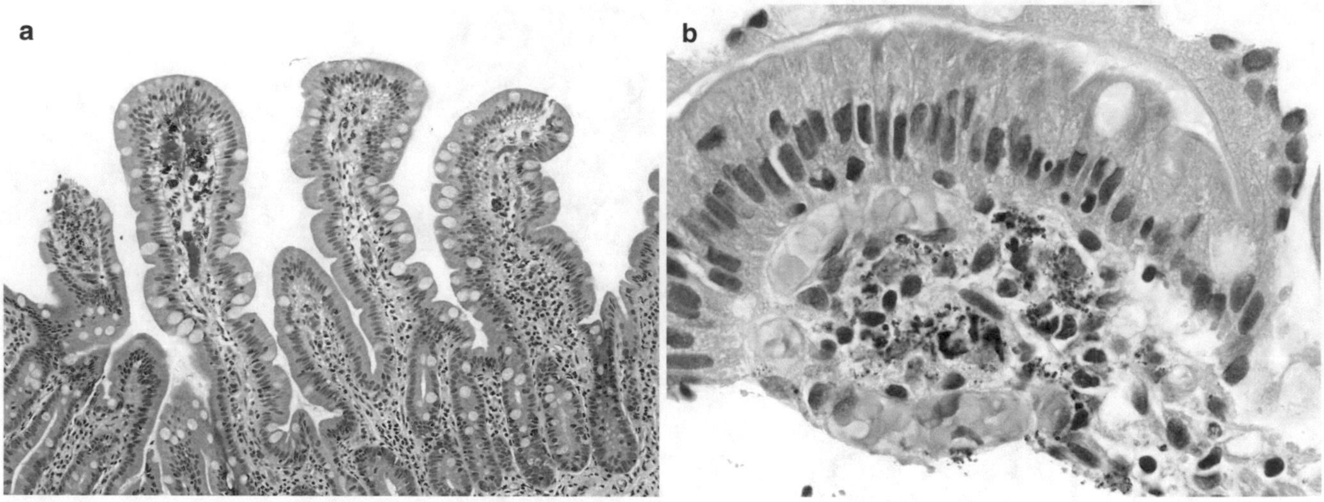

Fig. 11.19 Pseudomelanosis enteri. (**a**) Small bowel mucosa with lamina propria macrophages filled with granular black or brown pigment, mimicking melanin. (**b**) High-power view of the pigmented macrophages at the tip of a villus

Table 11.4 Summary of key immunotherapy agents and histologic changes associated with injury

Target molecule	Brand name	Indication	Histologic features
CTLA-4	Ipilimumab	Melanoma	Lamina propria expansion by lymphoplasmacytic infiltrate Increased crypt apoptosis Intraepithelial lymphocytosis
PD-1	Pembrolizumab Nivolumab	NSCLC, melanoma, RCC, MSI-H colon cancer	Active colitis pattern with increased crypt apoptosis and neutrophilic crypt abscesses Lymphocytic colitis pattern Features of chronicity in recurrent cases Ruptured crypt granuloma
PI3Kδ	Idelalisib	CLL, NHL	Intraepithelial lymphocytosis Increased crypt apoptosis Neutrophilic cryptitis

CLL chronic lymphocytic leukemia, *CTLA-4* cytotoxic T lymphocyte antigen-4, *MSI-H* microsatellite instability-high, *NHL* non-Hodgkin lymphoma, *NSCLC* non-small cell lung cancer, *PD-1* programmed death 1, *PI3Kδ* phosphoinositide-3 kinase delta, *RCC* renal cell carcinoma

protein 1 (PD-1) inhibitors nivolumab and pembrolizumab, and a phosphoinositide-3 kinase δ (PI3Kδ) inhibitor idelalisib (Table 11.4). Despite successful therapeutic responses, immune-related adverse events have been reported with the use of these agents. GI tract side effects, particularly diarrhea, are among the most commonly reported. The histologic features of immune checkpoint inhibitor-associated colitis consist of a spectrum of injury patterns, with significant overlap among individual agents as well as colitides due to various other etiologies.

- *Ipilimumab*
  Ipilimumab (Yervoy) is a monoclonal antibody directed against CTLA-4 that is used to treat various malignancies, of which melanoma is the prototype. Common GI side effects include diarrhea, abdominal pain, nausea, and vomiting. Histologic findings include active chronic injury with intraepithelial lymphocytosis, prominent crypt cell apoptosis (Fig. 11.20a, b), villous blunting (in the small bowel), and scattered neutrophil infiltrates.
- *PD-1 inhibitors*
  Pembrolizumab (Keytruda) and nivolumab (Opdivo) are commonly used PD-1 inhibitors administered against a host of malignancies including melanomas and mismatch-repair-deficient colorectal carcinomas. These inhibitors act on the PD-1/PD-L1 axis, releasing cytotoxic T cells to exert anti-tumor effects. These drugs essentially create iatrogenic autoimmunity to enhance destruction of tumor cells. Though the medications are overall well-tolerated, diarrhea is a common GI side effect. Endoscopic findings range from normal to varying degrees of colitis, including exudates, erythema, and ulcerations. The most commonly reported histologic pattern of injury is an

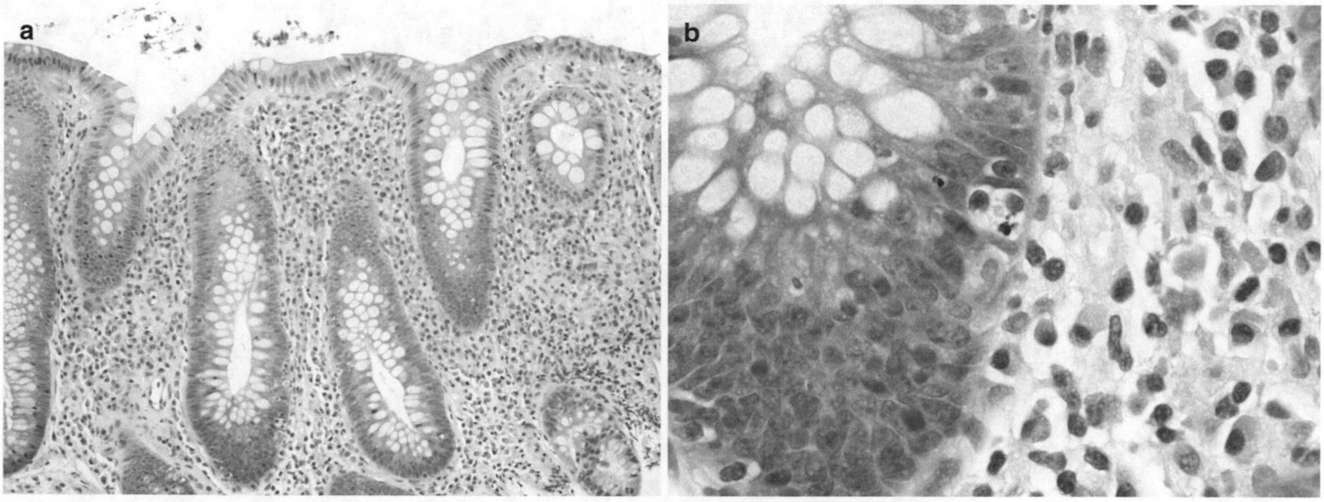

Fig. 11.20 Ipilimumab-associated injury. (**a**) Colonic mucosa with an expanded lamina propria, intraepithelial lymphocytosis, and crypt apoptosis. (**b**) Higher magnification showing an apoptotic body at the center of the image

active colitis with increased apoptosis and crypt atrophy/dropout (Fig. 11.21a, b), very similar to that observed with CTLA-4 inhibitor colitis. A lymphocytic colitis pattern of injury with intraepithelial lymphocytosis, along with surface epithelial injury and lymphoplasmacytic expansion of the lamina propria is also commonly encountered. There are rare reports of anti-PD-1-associated collagenous colitis.

- *Idelalisib*

  Idelalisib is a PI3Kδ inhibitor used to treat hematologic malignancies such as chronic lymphocytic leukemia/small lymphocytic lymphoma. Diarrhea is a commonly observed complication, occurring in about 45% of patients. Endoscopic changes range from focal mucosal erythema to severe pancolitis. Histologic changes are characterized by intraepithelial lymphocytosis, crypt epithelial cell apoptosis, loss of goblet cells, mild architectural distortion, and neutrophilic cryptitis (Fig. 11.22). In the small bowel, villous blunting along with intraepithelial lymphocytosis and crypt apoptosis has been reported.

  References: [22–25, 36, 83–92]

Case Presentation

Case 1

Learning Objectives

1. To learn the differential diagnosis of medication resins on GI biopsy specimens
2. To understand the role of ancillary aides and clinical correlation in identifying the agent

Case History

A 45-year-old woman on hemodialysis for renal failure presents with bloody diarrhea.

Endoscopic Finding

Area of mucosal necrosis involving the ascending colon.

Differential Diagnosis Prior to Slide Review

- Ischemic colitis
- Infectious colitis
- Malignancy
- Medication effect

Histologic Findings

- Colonic mucosa with ulceration, mucin loss in crypts, and hyalinization of lamina propria (Fig. 11.23).
- Detached purple colored polygonal crystals with regular lamellated fish-scale pattern.
- No evidence of dysplasia, granuloma, or viral cytopathic effects.

Differential Diagnosis after Slide Review

- Medication resins
  - Sodium polystyrene sulfonate (Kayexalate)
  - Sevelamer
  - BAS
  - Others
- Infectious colitis

IHC and Other Ancillary Studies

- Crystals appear black on AFB stain.
- Immunostaining for cytomegalovirus and adenovirus is negative.

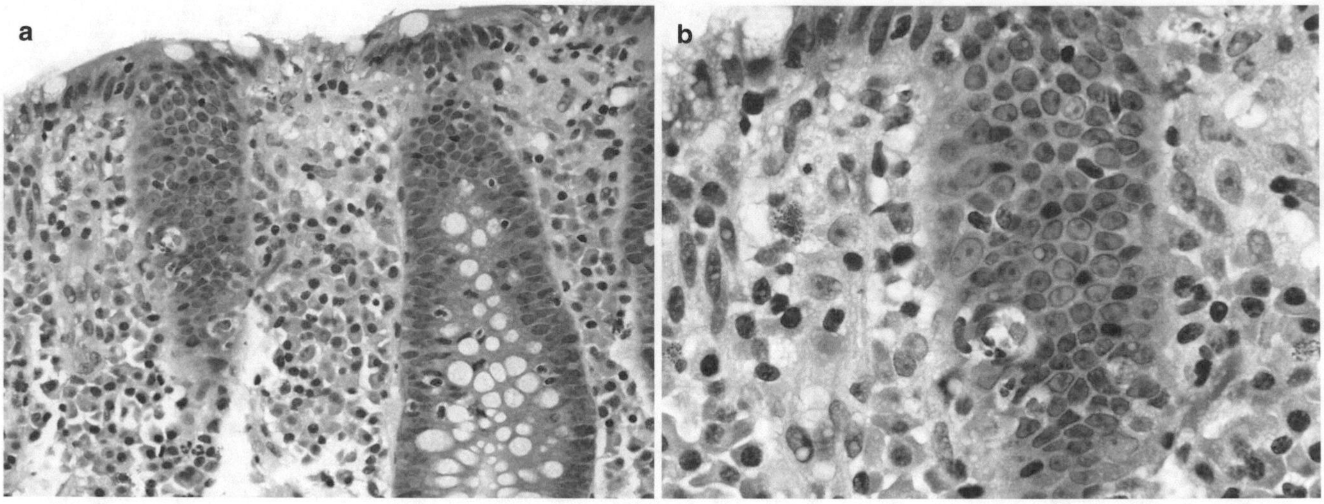

Fig. 11.21 Nivolumab-associated injury. The changes are similar to those observed with ipilimumab. (**a**) This example shows intraepithelial lymphocytosis, crypt apoptosis, and focal cryptitis. (**b**) An apoptotic body is present at the center of the image

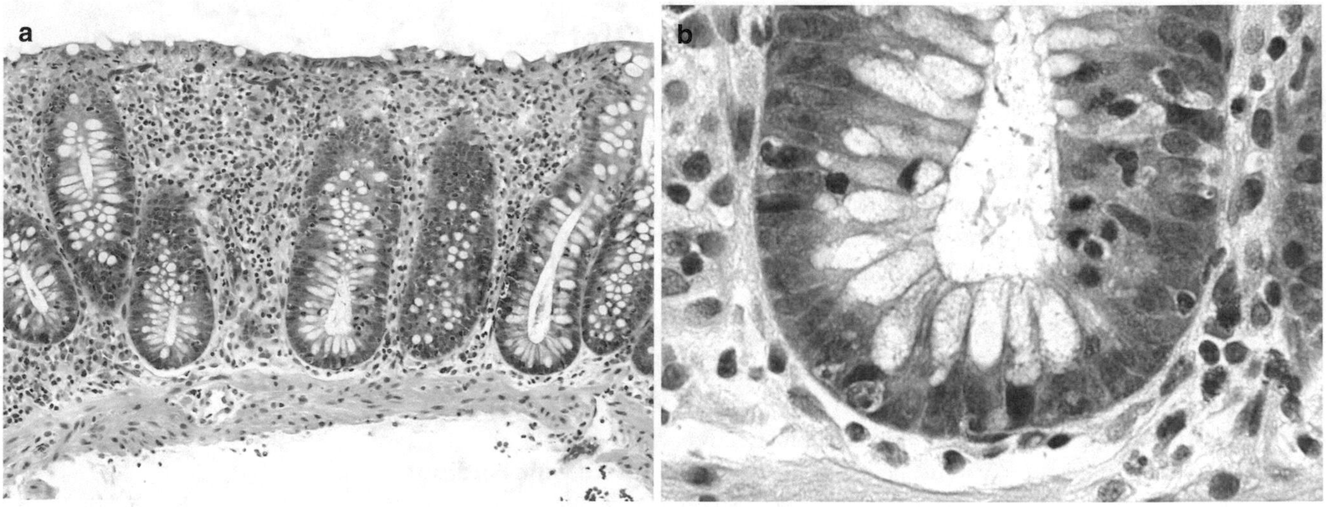

Fig. 11.22 Idelalisib-associated injury. (**a**) This colonic biopsy shows intraepithelial lymphocytosis, scattered cryptitis, and prominent crypt apoptosis. (**b**) This high-power image shows a few intraepithelial lymphocytes and an apoptotic body (lower left)

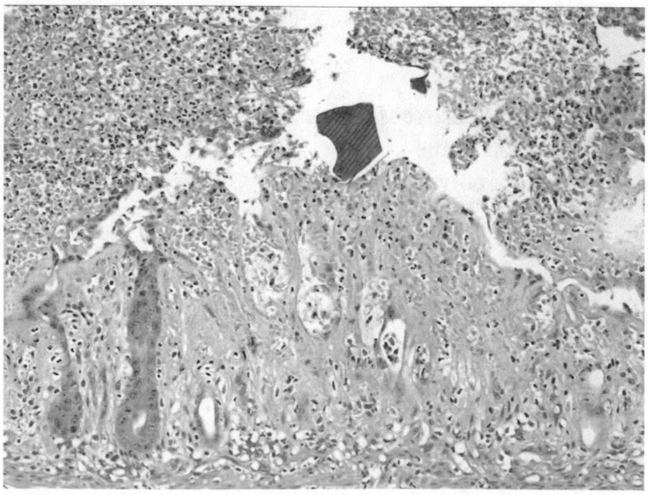

Fig. 11.23 (Case 1). Severe ischemic injury to the colonic mucosa. The purple Kayexalate crystal can be seen with regularly spaced rectangular cracks

Final Diagnosis

Ischemic colitis associated with Kayexalate crystals (confirmed after checking medication list).

Take-Home Messages

1. Kayexalate crystals can be associated with an ischemic colitis pattern of injury.
2. Noting the morphologic appearance of the crystals (purple color with fish-scale pattern for Kayexalate) is helpful in recognizing the type of resin.
3. Ancillary aids (such as AFB stain) and attention to the patient's clinical condition and associated medication history are important in identifying the offending agent.
4. Infectious agents, including viruses, should be excluded.

Case 2

Learning Objectives
1. Melanosis coli is not associated with melanin deposition
2. Medications are often an important association

Case History
A 65-year-old man underwent screening colonoscopy.

Endoscopic Finding
A patch of dark pigmentation in the ascending colon.

Differential Diagnosis Prior to Slide Review
- Tattoo mark
- Melanosis coli
- Malignant melanoma
- Old hemorrhage

Histologic Findings
- Colonic mucosa with pigment-laden macrophages in the lamina propria (Fig. 11.24a, b).
- Overlying normal colonic mucosa.

Differential Diagnosis after Slide Review
- Melanosis coli
- Old hemorrhage

IHC and Other Ancillary Studies
- Iron stain is negative.

Final Diagnosis
Melanosis coli (chart review revealed use of laxatives).

Take-Home Messages
1. Melanosis coli is an incidental benign finding, characterized by the presence of pigment-laden macrophages in the colonic lamina propria.
2. The deposited pigment is lipofuscin (not melanin), resulting from the apoptosis of colonic epithelial cells.
3. The condition is commonly associated with the use of laxatives, especially those containing anthraquinone.
4. An awareness of this common incidental finding is important to avoid unnecessary immunostaining for melanoma diagnosis.

Case 3

Learning Objectives
1. The presence of mitotic arrest and ring mitoses in gastric biopsies is associated with certain medications
2. Clinical correlation is required to ascertain the correct diagnosis

Case History
A 45-year-old man with a long standing history of gout presented with sudden-onset watery diarrhea.

Endoscopic Finding
A small area of ulceration in the gastric antrum.

Differential Diagnosis Prior to Slide Review
- *H. pylori* gastritis
- Chemical gastritis/reactive gastropathy
- Medication-associated injury
- Gastric malignancy

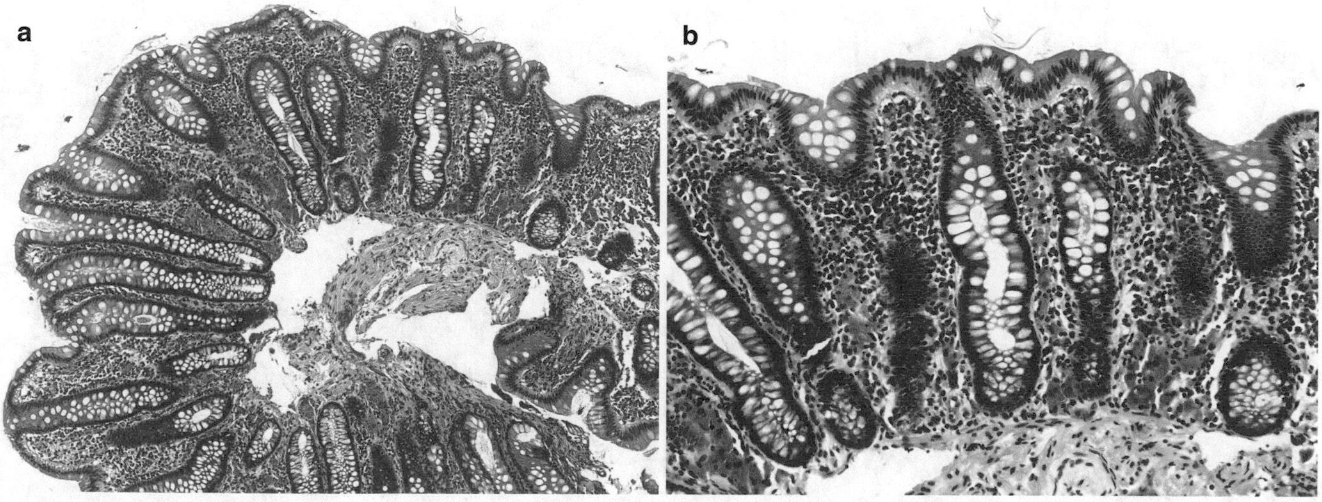

Fig. 11.24 (Case 2). (**a**) Colonic mucosa with pigment-laden macrophages in the lamina propria. (**b**). Higher magnification shows the brown pigment in the macrophages, which is lipofuscin, not melanin

Histologic Findings

- Gastric antral type mucosa with epithelial pseudostratification, prominent pit apoptosis, and ring mitoses. Minimal lamina propria inflammation (Fig. 11.25a, b).
- Absence of *H. pylori* organism on H&E; negative for epithelial dysplasia.

Differential Diagnosis after Slide Review

- Colchicine toxicity
- Taxane effect
- Other medications

IHC and Other Ancillary Studies

- None.

Final Diagnosis

Colchicine toxicity (chart review revealed acute renal failure and long-term use of colchicine for chronic gout).

Take-Home Messages

1. Ring mitoses on a biopsy specimen (usually small intestine and stomach), along with prominent crypt apoptosis, can be observed in association with both colchicine and taxane use.
2. It is extremely important to correlate with clinical details and medication list, since with taxanes, the findings are often incidental ("taxane effect"), whereas if the patient is taking colchicine, the findings likely reflect colchicine toxicity, necessitating immediate notification to the treating physician.

Case 4

Learning Objectives

1. Lymphocytic colitis is a pattern of injury with a wide range of associations
2. Knowledge of medication as an offending agent is important

Case History

A 68-year-old man with advanced-stage lung cancer presented with sudden-onset diarrhea.

Endoscopic Finding

Normal colonoscopy with an unremarkable terminal ileum.

Differential Diagnosis Prior to Slide Review

- Microscopic colitis
- Medication injury
- Infectious colitis

Histologic Findings

- Colonic mucosa with prominent intraepithelial lymphocytosis, focal surface epithelial injury, and expansion of superficial lamina propria by lymphoplasmacytic inflammation (Fig. 11.26a, b). Increased crypt apoptosis was also observed.
- There was no thickening of subepithelial collagen table; granulomas were absent.

Differential Diagnosis after Slide Review

- Idiopathic lymphocytic colitis
- Medication injury
- Viral infection

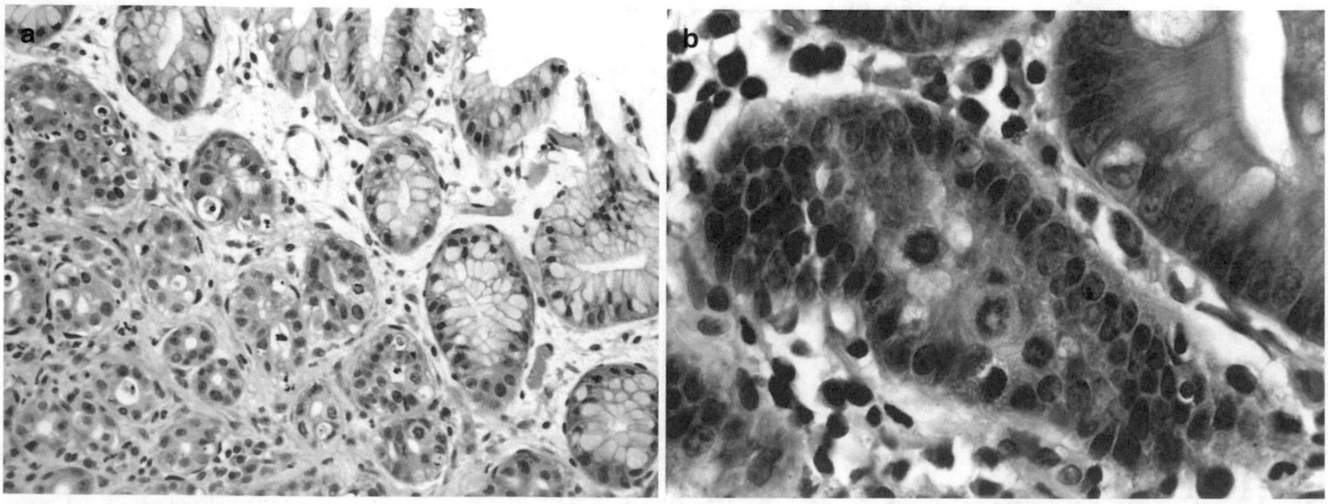

Fig. 11.25 (Case 3). (**a**) The changes are identical to those seen in taxane effect, with prominent apoptosis and arrested mitotic figures, including ring mitoses. (**b**) High-power view shows prominent ring mitoses, which is essentially the same as the findings observed in taxane effect

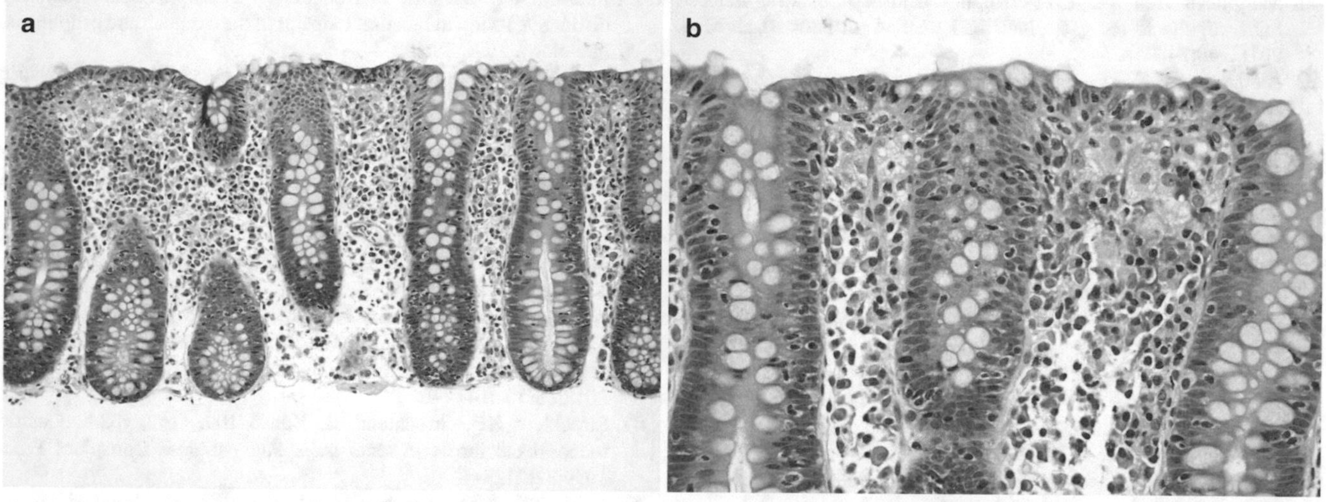

Fig. 11.26 (Case 4). (**a**) Low-power view showing intraepithelial lymphocytosis and surface epithelial injury. (**b**) Higher magnification shows surface epithelial injury and increased intraepithelial lymphocytes

IHC and Other Ancillary Studies

- Immunostains for cytomegalovirus and adenovirus were both negative.

Final Diagnosis

Nivolumab-associated colitis (chart review revealed that the patient was being treated with an anti-PD-1 agent nivolumab).

Take-Home Messages

1. A lymphocytic colitis pattern of injury can be associated with various medications or be idiopathic.
2. Though less common, use of immune checkpoint inhibitors (nivolumab, pembrolizumab, Ipilimumab) can also result in a lymphocytic colitis pattern (the most common finding with such agent is prominent crypt apoptosis with neutrophilic crypt micro abscesses).
3. Awareness of the clinical scenario and knowledge of medications that can be associated with a lymphocytic colitis pattern of injury is helpful in accurately pinpointing the offending agent.

References

1. Panarelli NC. Drug-induced injury in the gastrointestinal tract. Semin Diagn Pathol. 2014;31(2):165–75.
2. De Petris G, Gatius Caldero S, Chen L, Xiao SY, Dhungel BM, Wendel Spizcka AJ, Lam-Himlin D. Histopathological changes in the gastrointestinal tract due to drugs: an update for the surgical pathologist (part I of II). Int J Surg Pathol. 2014;22(2):120–8.
3. Abid S, Mumtaz K, Jafri W, Hamid S, Abbas Z, Shah HA, Khan AH. Pill-induced esophageal injury: endoscopic features and clinical outcomes. Endoscopy. 2005;37(8):740–4.
4. Eng J, Sabanathan S. Drug-induced esophagitis. Am J Gastroenterol. 1991;86:1127–33.
5. Kadayifci A, Gulsen MT, Koruk M, Savas MC. Doxycycline-induced pill esophagitis. Dis Esophagus. 2004;17(2):168–71.
6. Abbarah TR, Fredell JE, Ellenz GB. Ulceration by oral ferrous sulfate. J Am Med Assoc. 1976;236:2320.
7. Zografos GN, Georgiadou D, Thomas D, Kaltsas G, Digalakis M. Drug-induced esophagitis. Dis Esophagus. 2009;22(8):633–7.
8. Pemberton J. Oesophageal obstruction and ulceration caused by oral potassium therapy. Br Heart J. 1970;32:267–8.
9. Abraham SC, Cruz-Correa M, Lee LA, Yardley JH, Wu TT. Alendronate-associated esophageal injury: pathologic and endoscopic features. Mod Pathol. 1999;12(12):1152–7.
10. Carmack SW, Vemulapalli R, Spechler SJ, Genta RM. Esophagitis dissecans superficialis ("sloughing esophagitis"): a clinicopathologic study of 12 cases. Am J Surg Pathol. 2009;33(12):1789–94.
11. Coppola D, Lu L, Boyce HW Jr. Chronic esophagitis dissecans presenting with esophageal strictures: a case report. Hum Pathol. 2000;31(10):1313–7.
12. Moawad FJ, Appleman HD. Sloughing esophagitis: a spectacular histologic and endoscopic disease without a uniform clinical correlation. Ann N Y Acad Sci. 2016;1380:178–82.
13. Purdy JK, Appleman HD, McKenna BJ. Sloughing esophagitis is associated with chronic debilitation and medications that injure the esophageal mucosa. Mod Pathol. 2012;25:767–75.
14. Ponsot P, Molas G, Scoazec JY, Ruszniewski P, Hénin D, Bernades P. Chronic esophagitis dissecans: an unrecognized clinicopathologic entity? Gastrointest Endosc. 1997;45(1):38–45.
15. Hart PA, Romano RC, Moreira RK, Ravi K, Sweetser S. Esophagitis Dissecans Superficialis: clinical, endoscopic, and histologic features. Dig Dis Sci. 2015;60(7):2049–57.
16. Haber MM, Lopez I. Reflux gastritis in gastroesophageal reflux disease: a histopathological study. Ann Diagn Pathol. 1999;3:281–6.
17. Sobala GM, King RF, Axon AT, Dixon MF. Reflux gastritis in the intact stomach. J Clin Pathol. 1990;43(4):303–6.
18. Haber MM, Lopez I. Gastric histologic findings in patients with non-steroidal anti-inflammatory drug-associated gastric ulcer. Mod Pathol. 1999;12:592–8.
19. Pashankar DS, Bishop WP, Mitros FA. Chemical gastropathy: a distinct histopathologic entity in children. J Pediatr Gastroenterol Nutr. 2002;35:653–7.
20. Thomson RD, Lestina LS, Bensen SP, Toor A, Maheshwari Y, Ratcliffe NR. Lansoprazole-associated microscopic colitis: a case series. Am J Gastroenterol. 2002;97(11):2908–13.

21. Marginean EC. The ever-changing landscape of drug-induced injury of the lower gastrointestinal tract. Arch Pathol Lab Med. 2016;140:748–58.
22. Assarzadegan N, Montgomery E, Anders RA. Immune checkpoint inhibitor colitis: the flip side of the wonder drugs. Virchows Arch. 2018;472:125–33.
23. Chen JH, Pezhouh MK, Lauwers GY, Masia R. Histopathologic features of colitis due to immunotherapy with anti-PD-1 antibodies. Am J Surg Pathol. 2017;41:643–54.
24. Karamchandani DM, Chetty R. Immune checkpoint inhibitor-induced gastrointestinal and hepatic injury: pathologists' perspective. J Clin Pathol. 2018;71:665–71.
25. Voltaggio L, Lam-Himlin D, Limketkai BN, Singhi AD, Arnold CA. Message in a bottle: decoding medication injury patterns in the gastrointestinal tract. J Clin Pathol. 2014;67:903–12.
26. Niazi M, Kondru A, Levy J, Bloom AA. Spectrum of ischemic colitis in cocaine users. Dig Dis Sci. 1997;42:1537–41.
27. Elramah M, Einstein M, Mori N, Vakil N. High mortality of cocaine-related ischemic colitis: a hybrid cohort/case-control study. Gastrointest Endosc. 2012;75:1226–32.
28. Deana DG, Dean PJ. Reversible ischemic colitis in young women. Association with oral contraceptive use. Am J Surg Pathol. 1995;19:454–62.
29. Ghahremani GG, Meyers MA, Farman J, Port RB. Ischemic disease of the small bowel and colon associated with oral contraceptives. Gastrointest Radiol. 1977;2:221–8.
30. Puspok A, Kiener HP, Oberhuber G. Clinical, endoscopic and histologic spectrum of nonsteroidal anti-inflammatory drug-induced lesions in the colon. Dis Colon Rectum. 2000;43:685–91.
31. Volk EE, Shapiro BD, Easley KA, Goldblum JR. The clinical significance of a biopsy-based diagnosis of focal active colitis: a clinicopathologic study of 31 cases. Mod Pathol. 1998;11:789–94.
32. Goldstein NS, Cinenza AN. The histopathology of nonsteroidal anti-inflammatory drug-associated colitis. Am J Clin Pathol. 1998;110:622–8.
33. Driman DK, Preiksaitis HG. Colorectal inflammation and increased cell proliferation associated with oral sodium phosphate bowel preparation solution. Hum Pathol. 1998;29:972–8.
34. Lewis JD, Kimmel SE, Localio AR, Metz DC, Farrar JT, Nessel L, Brensinger C, McGibney K, Strom BL. Risk of serious upper gastrointestinal toxicity with over-the-counter nonaspirin nonsteroidal anti-inflammatory drugs. Gastroenterology. 2005;129(6):1865–74.
35. Langman MJ. Epidemiologic evidence on the association between peptic ulceration and anti-inflammatory drug use. Gastroenterology. 1989;96(2 Pt 2 Suppl):640–6.
36. Vieth M, Montgomery E. Medication-associated gastrointestinal tract injury. Virchows Arch. 2017;470:245–66.
37. Cortina G, Wren S, Armstrong B, Lewin K, Fajardo L. Clinical and pathologic overlap in nonsteroidal anti-inflammatory drug-related small bowel diaphragm disease and the neuromuscular and vascular hamartoma of the small bowel. Am J Surg Pathol. 1999;23:1414–7.
38. Lang J, Price AB, Levi AJ, Burke M, Gumpel JM, Bjarnason I. Diaphragm disease: pathology of disease of the small intestine induced by non-steroidal anti-inflammatory drugs. J Clin Pathol. 1988;41(5):516–26.
39. Zhao B, Sanati S, Eltorky M. Diaphragm disease: complete small bowel obstruction after long-term nonsteroidal anti-inflammatory drugs use. Ann Diagn Pathol. 2005;9:169–73.
40. Kelly ME, McMahon LE, Jaroszewski DE, Yousfi MM, De Petris G, Swain JM. Small-bowel diaphragm disease: seven surgical cases. Arch Surg. 2005;140(12):1162–6.
41. Abraham SC, Yardley JH, Wu TT. Erosive injury to the upper gastrointestinal tract in patients receiving iron medication: an underrecognized entity. Am J Surg Pathol. 1999;23:1241–7.
42. Eckstein RP, Symons P. Iron tablets cause histopathologically distinctive lesion in mucosal biopsies of the stomach and esophagus. Pathology. 1996;28:142–5.
43. Marginean EC, Bennick M, Cyczk J, Robert ME, Jain D. Gastric siderosis: patterns and significance. Am J Surg Pathol. 2006;30:514–20.
44. Kim SY, Choung RS, Kwon BS, Hyun JJ, Jung SW, Koo JS, Yim HJ, Lee SW, Choi JH. Small bowel pseudomelanosis associated with oral iron therapy. J Korean Med Sci. 2013;28(7):1103–6.
45. Lee HH, O'Donnell DB, Keren DF. Characteristics of melanosis duodeni: incorporation of endoscopy, pathology, and etiology. Endoscopy. 1987;19:107–9.
46. de Magalhães Costa MH, Fernandes Pegado Mda G, Vargas C, Castro ME, Madi K, Nunes T, Zaltman C. Pseudomelanosis duodeni associated with chronic renal failure. World J Gastroenterol. 2012;18(12):1414–6.
47. Strochlein KB, Strochlein JR, Kahan BD, Gruber SA. Gastric mucosal calcinosis in renal transplant patients. Transplant Proc. 1999;31:2124–6.
48. Hsieh TH, McCullough A, Aqel B. Gastric mucosal calcinosis. Gastrointest Endosc. 2011;73:1282–3.
49. Gorospe M, Fadare O. Gastric mucosal calcinosis: clinicopathologic considerations. Adv Anat Pathol. 2007;14:224–8.
50. Greenson JK, Trinidad SB, Pfeil SA, Brainard JA, McBride PT, Colijn HO, Tesi RJ, Lucas JG. Gastric mucosal calcinosis. Calcified aluminum phosphate deposits secondary to aluminum-containing antacids or sucralfate therapy in organ transplant patients. Am J Surg Pathol. 1993;17(1):45–50.
51. Haratake J, Yasunaga C, Ootani A, Shimajiri S, Matsuyama A, Hisaoka M. Peculiar histiocytic lesions with massive lanthanum deposition in dialysis patients treated with lanthanum carbonate. Am J Surg Pathol. 2015;39(6):767–71.
52. Ban S, Suzuki S, Kubota K, Ohshima S, Satoh H, Imada H, Ueda Y. Gastric mucosal status susceptible to lanthanum deposition in patients treated with dialysis and lanthanum carbonate. Ann Diagn Pathol. 2017;26:6–9.
53. Logan RP. The chemotherapeutic effects of H+/K+ inhibitors on helicobacter pylori infection. Pharmacol Ther. 1996;69:79–83.
54. Logan RP, Walker MM, Misiewicz JJ, Gummett PA, Karim QN, Baron JH. Changes in the intragastric distribution of helicobacter pylori during treatment with omeprazole. Gut. 1995;36:12–6.
55. Lundell L, Attwood S, Ell C, Fiocca R, Galmiche JP, Hatlebakk J, Lind T, Junghard O; LOTUS trial collaborators. Comparing laparoscopic antireflux surgery with esomeprazole in the management of patients with chronic gastro-oesophagealreflux disease: a 3-year interim analysis of the LOTUS trial. Gut. 2008;57(9):1207–13.
56. Simsek Z, Alagozlu H, Tuncer C, Dursun A. Lymphocytic colitis associated with lansoprazole treatment. Curr Ther Res Clin Exp. 2007;68(5):360–6.
57. Crowder CD, Grabowski C, Inampudi S, Sielaff T, Sherman CA, Batts KP. Selective internal radiation therapy-induced extrahepatic injury: an emerging cause of iatrogenic organ damage. Am J Surg Pathol. 2009;33(7):963–75.
58. Kennedy AS, Nutting C, Coldwell D, Gaiser J, Drachenberg C. Pathologic response and microdosimetry of (90) Y microspheres in man: review of four explanted whole livers. Int J Radiat Oncol Biol Phys. 2004;60(5):1552–63.
59. Joerger M. Treatment regimens of classical and newer taxanes. Cancer Chemother Pharmacol. 2016;77(2):221–33.
60. Iacobuzio-Donahue CA, Lee EL, Abraham SC, Yardley JH, Wu TT. Colchicine toxicity: distinct morphologic findings in gastrointestinal biopsies. Am J Surg Pathol. 2001;25(8):1067–73.
61. Daniels JA, Gibson MK, Xu L, Sun S, Canto MI, Heath E, Wang J, Brock M, Montgomery E. Gastrointestinal tract epithelial changes

associated with taxanes: marker of drug toxicity versus effect. Am J Surg Pathol. 2008;32(3):473–7.
62. Hruban RH, Yardley JH, Donehower RC, Boitnott JK. Taxol toxicity. Epithelial necrosis in the gastrointestinal tract associated with polymerized microtubule accumulation and mitotic arrest. Cancer. 1989;63(10):1944–50.
63. Rubio-Tapia A, Herman ML, Ludvigsson JF, Kelly DG, Mangan TF, Wu TT, Murray JA. Severe spruelike enteropathy associated with olmesartan. Mayo Clin Proc. 2012;87(8):732–8.
64. Burbure N, Lebwohl B, Arguelles-Grande C, Green PH, Bhagat G, Lagana S. Olmesartan-associated sprue-like enteropathy: a systematic review with emphasis on histopathology. Hum Pathol. 2016;50:127–34.
65. Lagana SM, Braunstein ED, Arguelles-Grande C, Bhagat G, Green PH, Lebwohl B. Sprue-like histology in patients with abdominal pain taking olmesartan compared with other angiotensin receptor blockers. J Clin Pathol. 2015;68(1):29–32.
66. Choi EY, McKenna BJ. Olmesartan-associated Enteropathy: a review of clinical and histologic findings. Arch Pathol Lab Med. 2015;139(10):1242–7.
67. Nielsen JA, Steephen A, Lewin M. Angiotensin-II inhibitor (olmesartan)-induced collagenous sprue with resolution following discontinuation of drug. World J Gastroenterol. 2013;19(40):6928–30.
68. Sievers TM, Rossi SJ, Ghobrial RM, Arriola E, Nishimura P, Kawano M, Holt CD. Mycophenolate mofetil. Pharmacotherapy. 1997;17(6):1178–97.
69. Papadimitriou JC, Cangro CB, Lustberg A, Khaled A, Nogueira J, Wiland A, Ramos E, Klassen DK, Drachenberg CB. Histologic features of mycophenolate mofetil-related colitis: a graft-versus-host disease-like pattern. Int J Surg Pathol. 2003;11(4):295–302.
70. Nguyen T, Park JY, Scudiere JR, Montgomery E. Mycophenolic acid (cellcept and myofortic) induced injury of the upper GI tract. Am J Surg Pathol. 2009;33(9):1355–63.
71. Star KV, Ho VT, Wang HH, Odze RD. Histologic features in colon biopsies can discriminate mycophenolate from GVHD-induced colitis. Am J Surg Pathol. 2013;37(9):1319–28.
72. Gonzalez RS, Lagana SM, Szeto O, Arnold CA. Challenges in diagnosing medication resins in surgical pathology specimens: a crystal-clear review guide. Arch Pathol Lab Med. 2017;141(9): 1276–82.
73. Abraham SC, Bhagavan BS, Lee LA, Rashid A, Wu TT. Upper gastrointestinal tract injury in patients receiving kayexalate (sodium polystyrene sulfonate) in sorbitol: clinical, endoscopic, and histopathologic findings. Am J Surg Pathol. 2001;25(5):637–44.
74. Harel Z, Harel S, Shah PS, Wald R, Perl J, Bell CM. Gastrointestinal adverse events with sodium polystyrene sulfonate (Kayexalate) use: a systematic review. Am J Med. 2013;126(3):264.e9–24.
75. Lillemoe KD, Romolo JL, Hamilton SR, Pennington LR, Burdick JF, Williams GM. Intestinal necrosis due to sodium polystyrene (Kayexalate) in sorbitol enemas: clinical and experimental support for the hypothesis. Surgery. 1987;101(3):267–72.
76. Rashid A, Hamilton SR. Necrosis of the gastrointestinal tract in uremic patients as a result of sodium polystyrene sulfonate (Kayexalate) in sorbitol: an underrecognized condition. Am J Surg Pathol. 1997;21(1):60–9.
77. Swanson BJ, Limketkai BN, Liu TC, Montgomery E, Nazari K, Park JY, Santangelo WC, Torbenson MS, Voltaggio L, Yearsley MM, Arnold CA. Sevelamer crystals in the gastrointestinal tract (GIT): a new entity associated with mucosal injury. Am J Surg Pathol. 2013;37(11):1686–93.
78. Arnold MA, Swanson BJ, Crowder CD, Frankel WL, Lam-Himlin D, Singhi AD, Stanich PP, Arnold CA. Colesevelam and colestipol: novel medication resins in the gastrointestinal tract. Am J Surg Pathol. 2014;38(11):1530–7.
79. Walker NI, Bennett RE, Axelsen RA. Melanosis coli. A consequence of anthraquinone-induced apoptosis of colonic epithelial cells. Am J Pathol. 1988;131(3):465–76.
80. Benavides SH, Morgante PE, Monserrat AJ, Zárate J, Porta EA. The pigment of melanosis coli: a lectin histochemical study. Gastrointest Endosc. 1997;46(2):131–8.
81. eL-Newihi HM, Lynch CA, Mihas AA. Case reports: pseudomelanosis duodeni: association with systemic hypertension. Am J Med Sci. 1995;310(3):111–4.
82. Kim SY, Koo JS, Hynun JJ, Jung SW, Choung RS, Yim HJ, Lee SW, Choi JH. Charcoal-induced pseudomelanosis ilei. Endoscopy. 2011;43 Suppl 2 UCTN:E380.
83. Kyi C, Postow MA. Checkpoint blocking antibodies in cancer immunotherapy. FEBS Lett. 2014;588(2):368–76.
84. Dolan DE, Gupta S. PD-1 pathway inhibitors: changing the landscape of cancer immunotherapy. Cancer Control. 2014;21(3):231–7.
85. Khoja L, Atenafu EG, Ye Q, Gedye C, Chappell M, Hogg D, Butler MO, Joshua AM. Real-world efficacy, toxicity and clinical management of ipilimumab treatment in metastatic melanoma. Oncol Lett. 2016;11(2):1581–5.
86. Garon EB, Rizvi NA, Hui R, Leighl N, Balmanoukian AS, Eder JP, Patnaik A, Aggarwal C, Gubens M, Horn L, Carcereny E, Ahn MJ, Felip E, Lee JS, Hellmann MD, Hamid O, Goldman JW, Soria JC, Dolled-Filhart M, Rutledge RZ, Zhang J, Lunceford JK, Rangwala R, Lubiniecki GM, Roach C, Emancipator K. Gandhi L; KEYNOTE-001 investigators. Pembrolizumab for the treatment of non-small-cell lung cancer. N Engl J Med. 2015;372(21):2018–28.
87. Wilkinson E. Nivolumab success in untreated metastatic melanoma. Lancet Oncol. 2015;16(1):e9.
88. Gonzalez RS, Salaria SN, Bohannon CD, Huber AR, Feely MM, Shi C. PD-1 inhibitor gastroenterocolitis: case series and appraisal of 'immunomodulatory gastroenterocolitis'. Histopathology. 2017;70(4):558–67.
89. Bavi P, Butler M, Serra S, Chetty R. Immune modulator-induced changes in the gastrointestinal tract. Histopathology. 2017;71(3):494–6.
90. Baroudjian B, Lourenco N, Pagès C, Chami I, Maillet M, Bertheau P, Bagot M, Gornet JM, Lebbé C, Allez M. Anti-PD1-induced collagenous colitis in a melanoma patient. Melanoma Res. 2016;26(3):308–11.
91. Barrientos JC. Idelalisib for the treatment of indolent non-Hodgkin lymphoma: a review of its clinical potential. Onco Targets Ther. 2016;9:2945–53.
92. Weidner AS, Panarelli NC, Geyer JT, Bhavsar EB, Furman RR, Leonard JP, Jessurun J, Yantiss RK. Idelalisib-associated colitis: histologic findings in 14 patients. Am J Surg Pathol. 2015;39(12):1661–7.

Eosinophilic, Mastocytic, and Histiocytic Diseases of the Gastrointestinal Tract

12

Michael G. Drage and Amitabh Srivastava

List of Frequently Asked Questions

1. What functions do eosinophils, mast cells, and basophils have in mucosal immunity?
2. What is the normal eosinophil count in the luminal GI tract?
3. What is the differential diagnosis of increased eosinophils in the esophagus?
4. What are the criteria for the diagnosis of eosinophilic esophagitis?
5. What is the current understanding of the pathogenesis of eosinophilic esophagitis?
6. What is the differential diagnosis of increased tissue eosinophils in the stomach and intestines?
7. What prognostic significance do eosinophils have in colonic biopsies of patients with inflammatory bowel disease?
8. How should tissue eosinophilia be reported?
9. What are normal mast cell counts in the GI tract?
10. What role do mast cells play in irritable bowel syndrome?
11. What is mastocytosis? How is it diagnosed?
12. How is mastocytosis classified?
13. What endoscopic and histologic features suggest systemic mastocytosis in the luminal GI tract?
14. What is the differential diagnosis for a histiocytic infiltrate in the luminal GI tract?
15. What is the differential diagnosis for granulomas in the GI tract?
16. What primary histiocytic disorders involve the GI tract?

M. G. Drage (✉)
University of Rochester, Rochester, NY, USA
e-mail: Michael_Drage@urmc.rochester.edu

A. Srivastava
Harvard Medical School and Brigham and Women's Hospital, Boston, MA, USA

Frequently Asked Questions

1. What functions do eosinophils, mast cells, and basophils have in mucosal immunity?

Mast cells, eosinophils, and basophils are granulocytes derived from myeloid progenitors that are crucial players in Th2 inflammatory response, the principal goal of which is to rapidly expel metazoan parasites that would otherwise elicit extensive collateral damage if destroyed within the body. Since they are the sentinel inflammatory cells designed to detect metazoan parasites, they contain abundant preformed granules that contain products to increase gastrointestinal (GI) secretions and motility, and potent vasodilators to recruit other inflammatory cells. Upon activation, they produce cytokines and lipid mediators that further guide the immune response.

Eosinophils are the most abundant of the three cell types, mast cells the second most abundant, and basophils are scarce and found only in the blood and bone marrow. Only eosinophils are constitutively present in significant quantities in the peripheral blood while mast cells are unique in their frequency in the submucosa, skin, and interstitial connective tissues of the body.

Interestingly, mast cells appear to have functionally distinct subpopulations. When found in the skin and intestinal submucosa, they have abundant heparin, histamine, and neutral proteases in their granules, and their survival shows little dependence on T cells. In mucosal sites such as the pulmonary alveoli and GI tract, their granules contain abundant chondroitin sulfate relative to histamine, and their survival is dependent upon IL-3 provided by local T cells.

Basophils are scarcest granulocytes in mammals (<1% of peripheral blood leukocytes). Like mast cells, they can capture antigen via FcεRI, but are distinct in their ability to rapidly generate and secrete IL-4 and IL-13. Activated mast cells recruit basophils via prostaglandin D2; thus, basophils may function as a potent amplifier of Th2

H. L. Wang, Z. E. Chen (eds.), *Practical Gastrointestinal Pathology*, Practical Anatomic Pathology,
https://doi.org/10.1007/978-3-030-51268-2_12

inflammation. Both mast cells and basophils are primary effectors of Th2-mediated disease; and therapies that target the effectors of mast cells and basophils are the mainstays of therapy for atopy.

2. **What is the normal eosinophil count in the luminal GI tract?**

Esophagus While most normal esophageal biopsies will not have any intraepithelial eosinophils, the finding of rare eosinophils in the absence of any epithelial injury is not considered diagnostic of esophagitis, and can be still considered "within normal limits." As is true elsewhere in the GI tract, epithelial injury is important in establishing a diagnosis of esophagitis, regardless of etiology.

Stomach Normal eosinophil counts in the stomach have been systematically evaluated recently. A retrospective review found a mean eosinophil count of 15.5 + 16.8 SD eosinophils/mm^2 (range 0–110) in controls (range 0–26 eosinophils/400× field with an ocular FN of 22), with the vast majority of control patients showing a peak density of around 50 eosinophils/mm^2 (12 eosinophils/400× high power field (HPF) with an ocular FN of 22), which is similar to what was reported in previous studies. There were no differences between antral and corpus biopsies and no differences based on patient age or geographic location.

Small intestine In the normal small intestine, eosinophils number up to 20 eosinophils/HPF in the duodenum, and up to 30 eosinophils/HPF in the ileum. The usual gradient is basal predominant with decreasing numbers toward the superficial lamina propria.

Colon Eosinophils are at their greatest density in the proximal colon, where the normal mucosa may harbor 20–50 eosinophils/HPF. The numbers of intramucosal eosinophils decrease progressively distally, with the lowest density in the rectum. Occasional eosinophils may be seen hugging the base of the colonic crypts and occasionally infiltrate the epithelium without evidence of epithelial injury. This finding alone is not sufficient to render a diagnosis of eosinophilic or active colitis (Fig. 12.1). Interestingly, some evidence suggests that the density of eosinophils in normal colonic mucosa varies by the season with increased numbers during seasons of greater allergens and also by location (reported normal densities greater in New Orleans compared to the northeastern United States).

In summary, while the normal number of lamina propria eosinophils depends on anatomic location of the biopsy, a common theme throughout the GI tract is that eosinophils are usually evenly dispersed throughout the biopsy with basal predominance in the lamina propria and are not associated with any epithelial damage. A greater density of eosinophils in the superficial lamina propria, with large clusters or aggregates, and/or significant infiltration into the epithelium should prompt a careful evaluation of the biopsies for a primary disorder with eosinophil-predominant mucosal injury.

References: [1–8]

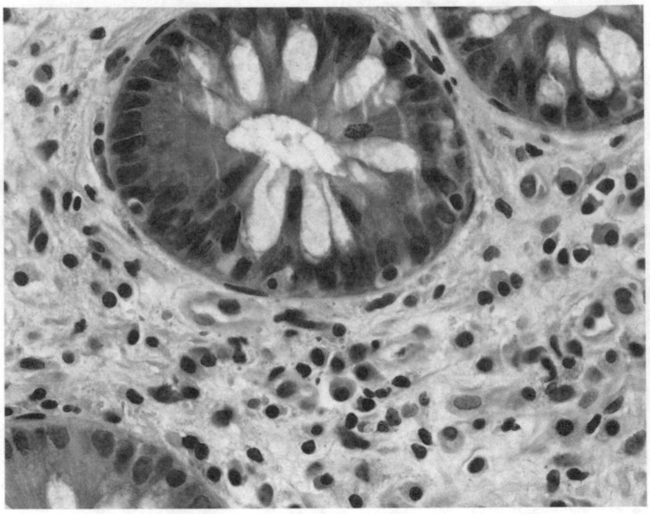

Fig. 12.1 Intraepithelial eosinophils can be occasionally seen in normal colonic mucosa, a finding more frequently seen in the right colon. The lack of epithelial injury, clustering, or increased density in the superficial lamina propria all argue against any pathology

3. **What is the differential diagnosis of increased eosinophils in the esophagus?**

Esophageal eosinophilia can arise in numerous settings. In the United States, gastroesophageal reflux disease (GERD) comprises the most common etiology for esophageal eosinophilia. Other etiologic considerations include eosinophilic esophagitis (EoE), pill esophagitis, radiation esophagitis, post-radiofrequency ablation, infections, esophageal involvement in eosinophilic gastroenteritis, and rare disorders such as hypereosinophilic syndrome involving the esophagus. GERD typically shows greater injury and abundance of eosinophils in the distal esophagus than the mid/proximal esophagus. Pill esophagitis (Fig. 12.2a–c) is typically characterized by a remarkably well-circumscribed focal erosion, usually at sites of esophageal narrowing at the upper sphincter, the aortic arch, the left main bronchus, and the lower esophageal sphincter. Patients with esophageal motility disorders, those with congestive heart failure and enlarged right atrium, and those with Schatzki rings in the distal esophagus are predisposed to developing pill esophagitis. Radiation esophagitis is accompanied by characteristic nuclear and cytoplasmic alterations in epithelial and stromal cells (Fig. 12.3a–c). Eosinophil-predominant esophagitis can also be seen sometimes in infections such as

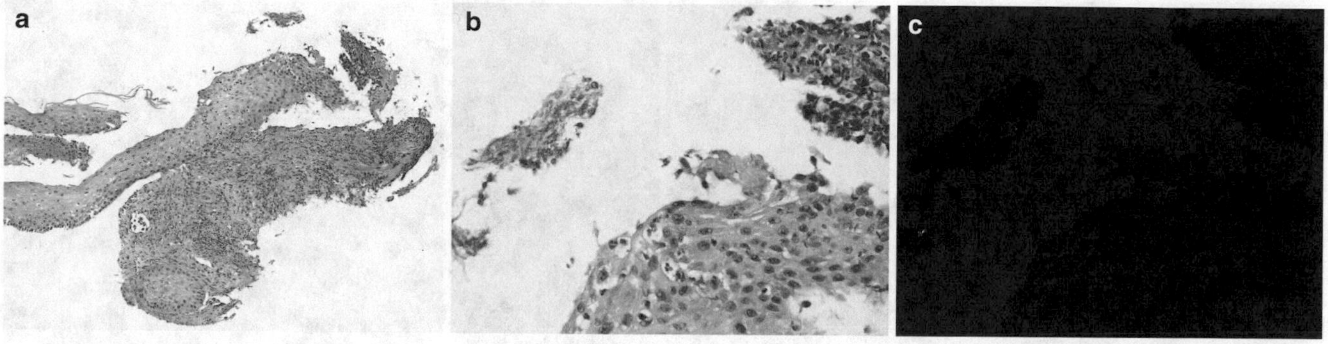

Fig. 12.2 Pill esophagitis showing a sharply circumscribed ulcer with minimal adjacent inflammation at low-power magnification (**a**). The mucosa immediately adjacent to the ulcer shows a relatively sparse infiltrate of eosinophils and neutrophils (**b**). The presence of polarizable foreign material (**c**; same field of view as **b**) permits a definitive diagnosis

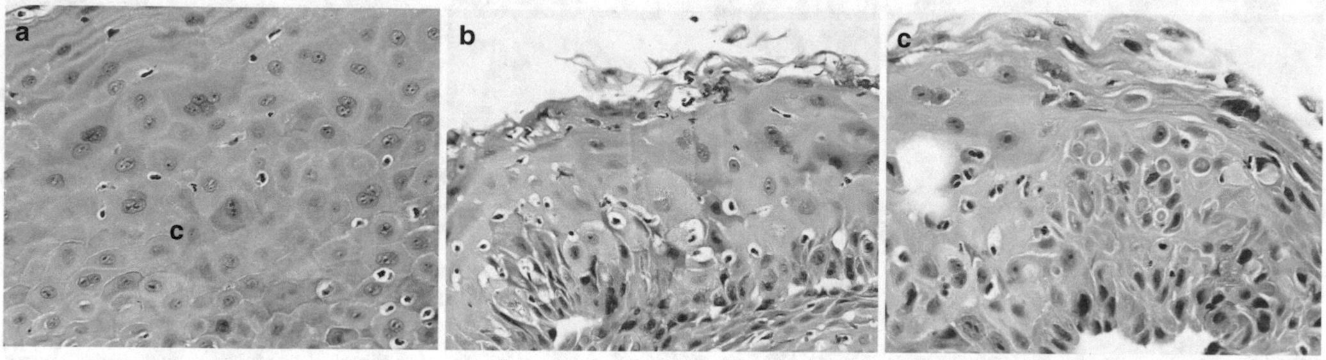

Fig. 12.3 Radiation esophagitis showing mild spongiosis and numerous intraepithelial eosinophils (**a**), including superficial microabscesses (**b**). The lack of basal cell hyperplasia and the presence of radiation-induced atypia, such as enlarged nuclei with irregular nucleoli, occasional cells with exaggerated atypia (**c**), scattered multinucleated cells and consistently preserved nuclear-to-cytoplasmic ratio indicate radiation effect as the etiology rather than primary eosinophilic esophagitis

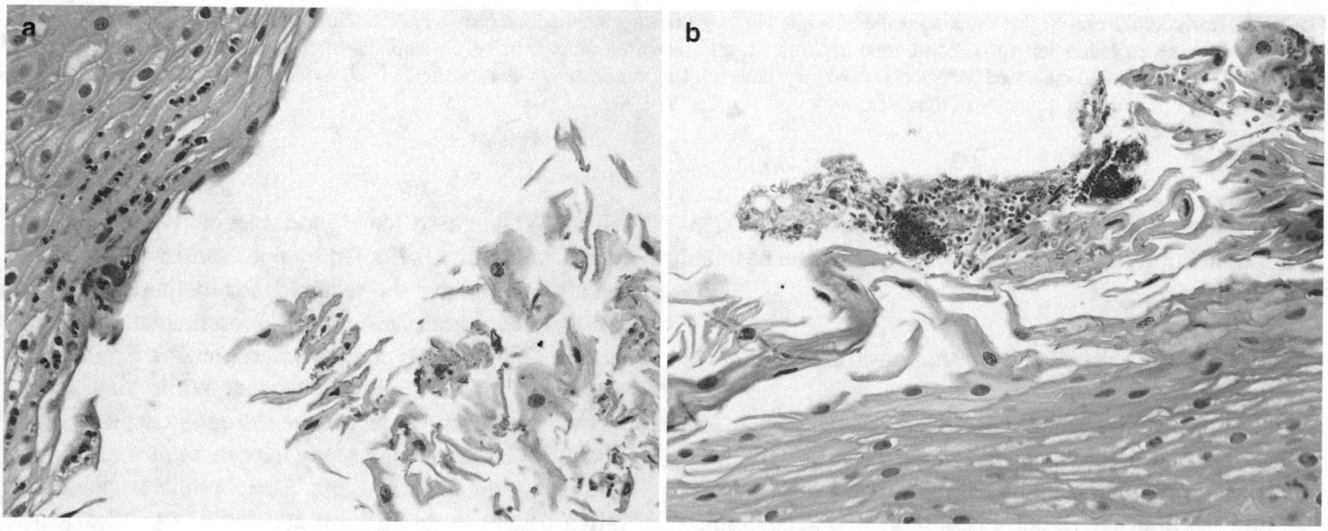

Fig. 12.4 Esophageal candidiasis showing spongiosis of the squamous epithelium and superficial eosinophilia (**a**). In an adjacent field, both yeast forms (center) and pseudohyphae (left) consistent with Candida species are easily appreciated (**b**). Even when eosinophils predominate, neutrophils are also seen in most cases of candidiasis

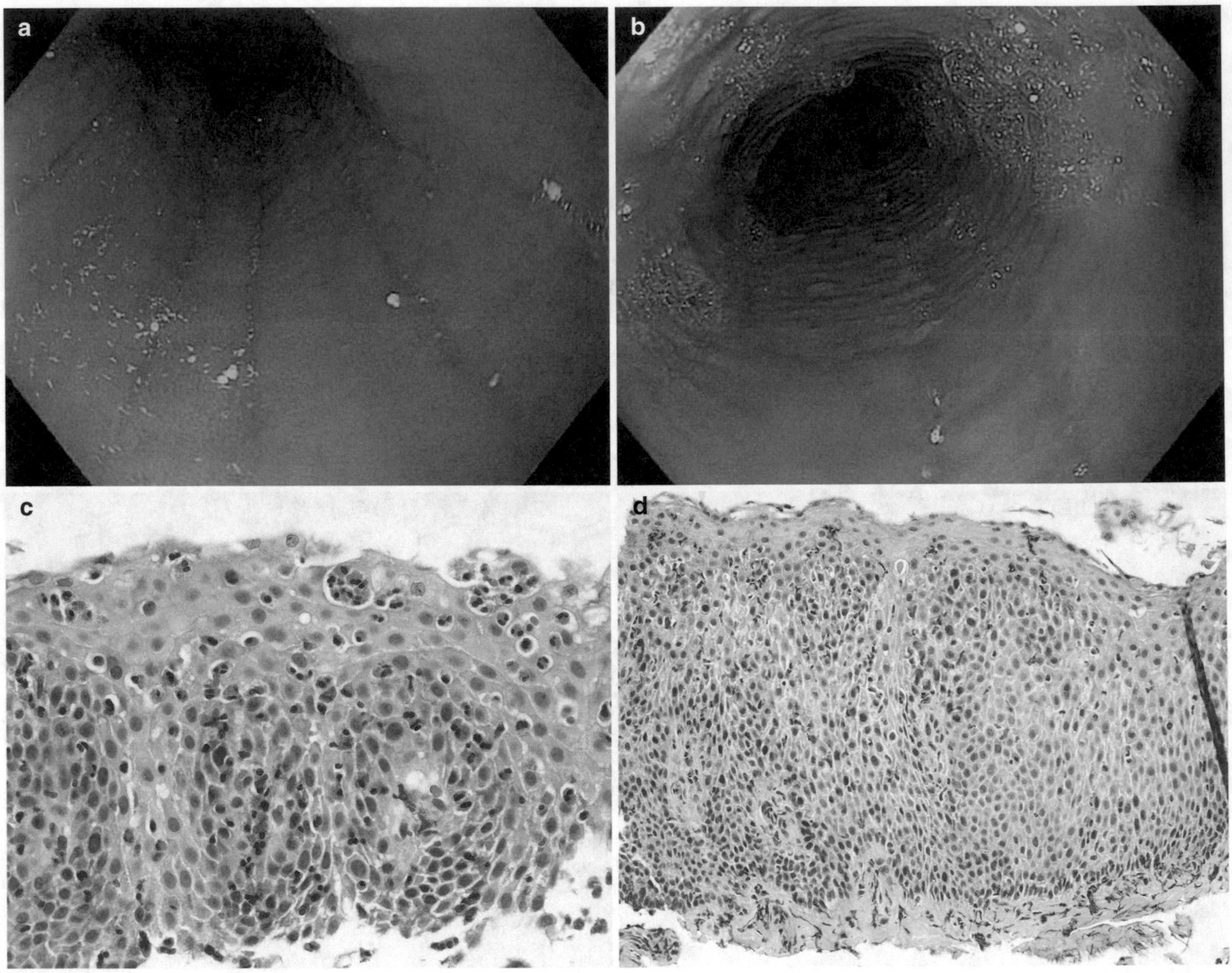

Fig. 12.5 Eosinophilic esophagitis showing scattered white plaques, stricture, longitudinal furrows (**a**) and rings (**b**) on endoscopy. Characteristic histologic features include spongiosis, basal zone hyperplasia, and increased intraepithelial eosinophils, often including superficial microabscesses, in a background of increased lymphocytes and mast cells (**c**). Chronic eosinophilic esophagitis leads to lamina propria fibrosis (**d**), representing the most problematic sequelae of the disease

candidiasis (Fig. 12.4a, b), although some degree of neutrophilic infiltrate and surface hyperkeratosis can be found even in these cases.

4. **What are the criteria for the diagnosis of eosinophilic esophagitis?**

   EoE is a clinicopathologic diagnosis and no single feature in isolation is diagnostic of the disorder. The most common presenting symptom is dysphagia (occasionally with food impaction), but it is important to keep in mind that some patients may be asymptomatic at the time of tissue biopsy. Characteristic abnormalities noted on endoscopy include mucosal edema, white exudates, rings ("feline esophagus"), longitudinal furrows, and strictures (Fig. 12.5a, b). The endoscopic findings can be scored using the EREFS criteria and the esophageal biopsy "pull sign." While these have good specificity (~90%) their diagnostic utility is limited by poor sensitivity (15–50%) and tissue biopsy is required for definite diagnosis. Furthermore, both the clinical presentation and endoscopic features of lymphocytic esophagitis overlap with those of eosinophilic esophagitis. While this further necessitates tissue biopsy, there are early data suggesting that distinction via endoscopy may be improved with the use of narrow band imaging. Eosinophilic esophagitis is often patchy in distribution and there is good evidence that 6–8 biopsies from the distal, and an additional 6–8 biopsies from the mid/proximal esophagus, are needed for adequate sensitivity to diagnose EoE. For the same reason, the pathologist must carefully examine each available tissue fragment or diagnostic findings may be easily missed.

Histologic features associated with EoE include spongiosis (intercellular edema), basal zone hyperplasia, increased eosinophils with clusters, aggregates, degranulating forms, and often superficial layering with eosinophilic microabscesses (Fig. 12.5c). Mast cells and lymphocytes may also be present in increased numbers. A numerical cutoff of a peak density of 15 eosinophils/HPF, in any part of the biopsy, is currently used for initial diagnosis. A more comprehensive scoring system utilizing a combination of the above histologic criteria has been reported but is not in widespread use. Lamina propria fibrosis (Fig. 12.5d) is a characteristic feature relevant to pathophysiology and explains the dysphagia symptoms present in most patients, but is of limited diagnostic utility because the majority of esophageal biopsies lack lamina propria for evaluation.

Proton pump inhibitor (PPI)-responsive EoE (PPI-REE) is now considered a subtype of EoE based on overlapping transcriptional signatures that are clearly distinct from those in patients with GERD. Laboratory tests to support the diagnosis of EoE are in development, of which creatinine-normalized levels of urine 3-bromotyrosine, a marker of eosinophil degranulation, appears to have the most potential. Importantly, the histologic endpoints for therapy and predictors of recurrence are not defined and are areas of active investigation. Peak eosinophil count <5/HPF after therapy is considered as a sign of histologic remission in most studies.

References: [3, 9–19]

5. **What is the current understanding of the pathogenesis of eosinophilic esophagitis?**

While the pathophysiology of EoE is not entirely understood, it is now established that EoE is driven by an ingested allergen combined with some other predisposing factor, such as altered epithelial permeability, either intrinsic or secondary to reflux, dysmotility, and/or predisposition for fibrosis. Its prevalence, currently 1:2000, with 3:1 male–female ratio, has increased in parallel to that of food allergy. Other manifestations of atopy, such as asthma and airway hyperresponsiveness, are frequent comorbidities in patients with EoE. As mentioned above, EoE and the related entity of PPI-REE, have a distinct transcriptional profile compared to GERD.

There is strong evidence for both heritable and environmental/epigenetic factors in the pathogenesis of EoE. Concordance for EoE amongst monozygotic twins is 58%, for dizygotic twins 36%, and non-twin siblings 2.4%. Treatment with elemental diet induces complete remission in nearly all pediatric patients and approximately 80–90% of adults. Less aggressive empiric elimination of the six most common food allergens results in remission rates of approximately 75% of patients, and reintroduction of allergens leads to recurrent tissue eosinophilia. While peak tissue eosinophil counts have been useful for diagnosis and correlate well with functional measures such as mucosal impedance and food impaction, emerging data suggest that tissue/blood eosinophilia are not required for symptoms. For instance, treatment with monoclonal antibody against IL-5 reduced tissue and blood eosinophils by 90%, whilst having no effect on symptoms. Furthermore, a case series reported an EoE-like syndrome in members of EoE families who lacked tissue and peripheral eosinophilia, but demonstrated similarly increased tissue T and mast cells, and a gene expression pattern remarkably similar to EoE.

Genome-wide association studies and candidate gene studies have identified multiple compelling candidates, most prominently thymic stromal lymphopoietin (TSLP) and calpain 14 (CAPN14), among others. TSLP is ubiquitously expressed by epithelial cells and induces local dendritic cells to polarize incoming lymphocytes to a Th2 inflammatory response; the type of inflammation driven by IL-4 and IL-13 and prototypically seen in allergy or metazoan parasite infection. Given its ubiquitous expression in epithelial cells, TSLP is involved in many atopic disorders. In contrast, expression of CAPN14 is limited to the esophagus and encodes a proteolytic enzyme, induced by IL-13, that directly increases epithelial barrier permeability. TGF-beta, a major fibrogenic signal produced by mast cells, plays a critical role in the fibrosis of chronic EoE, which leads to fibrostenotic disease and represents the most important unmet therapeutic need in these patients. Interestingly, some studies have demonstrated an increase in IgG4-positive plasma cells in EoE, raising the intriguing possibility of a relationship with systemic IgG4-related disease. A recent meta-analysis found that *Helicobacter pylori* gastritis is inversely associated with EoE.

In summary, EoE is an esophageal allergic hypersensitivity disorder likely due to factor(s) predisposing to increased permeability of the squamous epithelium. Surgical pathologists play an important role in evaluation of biopsies obtained from patients suspected of having EoE and in confirming histologic resolution posttreatment.

References: [14, 19–42]

6. **What is the differential diagnosis of increased tissue eosinophils in the stomach and intestines?**

The differential diagnosis of increased eosinophils in the stomach, small intestine, and colon is quite broad, and includes drug-induced mucosal injury, bacterial, fungal, and parasitic infections, inflammatory bowel disease (IBD), lymphocytic enteritides, celiac disease, connective tissue disease, vasculitides, Hodgkin lymphoma, myeloid neoplasms, infiltrative disorders such as systemic mastocytosis and Langerhans cell histiocytosis, a subset of mucosal inflammatory polyps, and the late phase of a healing ulcer from any etiology. This differential diagnosis varies somewhat by organ and location, and will thus be discussed by organ below.

Stomach and/or small intestine Tissue eosinophilia in the stomach is usually encountered in reactive/chemical gastropathy, healing erosion sites, drug hypersensitivity reaction, parasitic infections such as Anisakis or strongyloides (Fig. 12.6), less commonly as a manifestation of *H. pylori* gastritis, and rarely due to an idiopathic primary eosinophilic gastritis/gastroenteritis. In the small intestine, increased tissue eosinophils is frequently seen in IBD, parasitic infections, drug hypersensitivity reaction, and eosinophilic gastroenteritis. Primary idiopathic eosinophilic gastroenteritis may present with nonspecific upper GI symptoms such as vomiting and/or diarrhea, obstruction, or occasionally with ileus and pseudo-obstruction. Some patients with serosal involvement may develop an eosinophilic ascites.

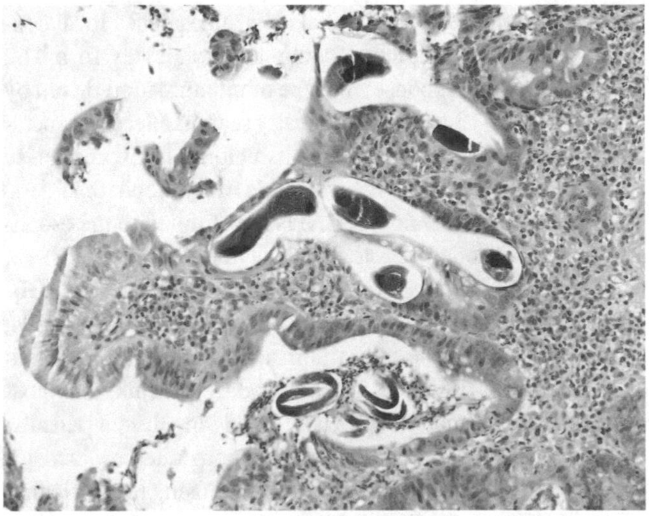

Fig. 12.6 Strongyloides stercolaris tends to reside within the crypts of the small intestine, stomach, and colon, occasionally with a prominent eosinophilic reaction

Colon In the colorectum, tissue eosinophilia is most often associated with IBD, lymphocytic or collagenous colitis, drug reaction commonly associated with NSAIDs, carbamazepine, clozapine, tacrolimus, mycophenolate, and rifampicin. Tissue eosinophilia can also be seen in parasitic and fungal infections, allergic reaction in pediatric patients, healing erosion/ulcers, pneumatosis coli, and as an infiltrate secondary to systemic mastocytosis or Langerhans cell histiocytosis.
References: [43–59]

7. **What prognostic significance do eosinophils have in colonic biopsies of patients with inflammatory bowel disease?**

Tissue eosinophilia and stool markers of eosinophil degranulation correlate with disease activity in IBD, and IL-5 levels predict recurrence of Crohn disease after resection. However, eosinophils may be prominent in posttreatment biopsies in asymptomatic IBD patients who have responded well to therapy. Data from murine models of colitis show conflicting evidence regarding the role of eosinophils in IBD: some models suggest the possibility that eosinophils may be protective in IBD rather than pathogenic, while others suggest a crucial pathogenetic role in the development of colitis. While eosinophilia is an intriguing and inconsistent finding in IBD (Fig. 12.7a, b), there are no definitive guidelines for interpretation.
References: [60–67]

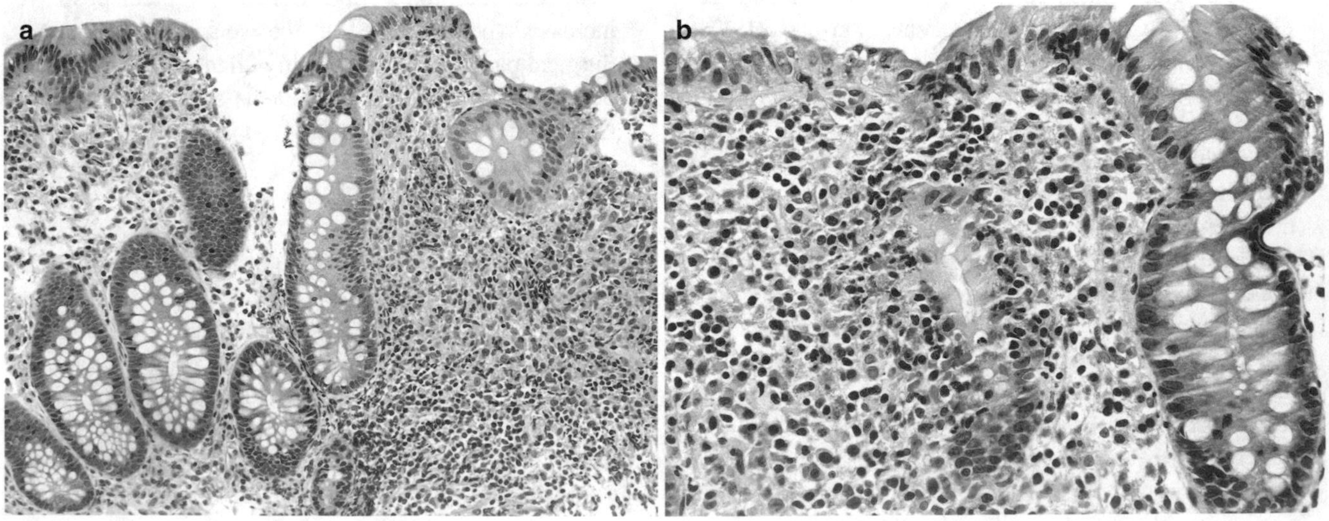

Fig. 12.7 Colonic biopsies from a patient with inflammatory bowel disease showing clustering of eosinophils (**a**) and injurious infiltration of a crypt (**b**)

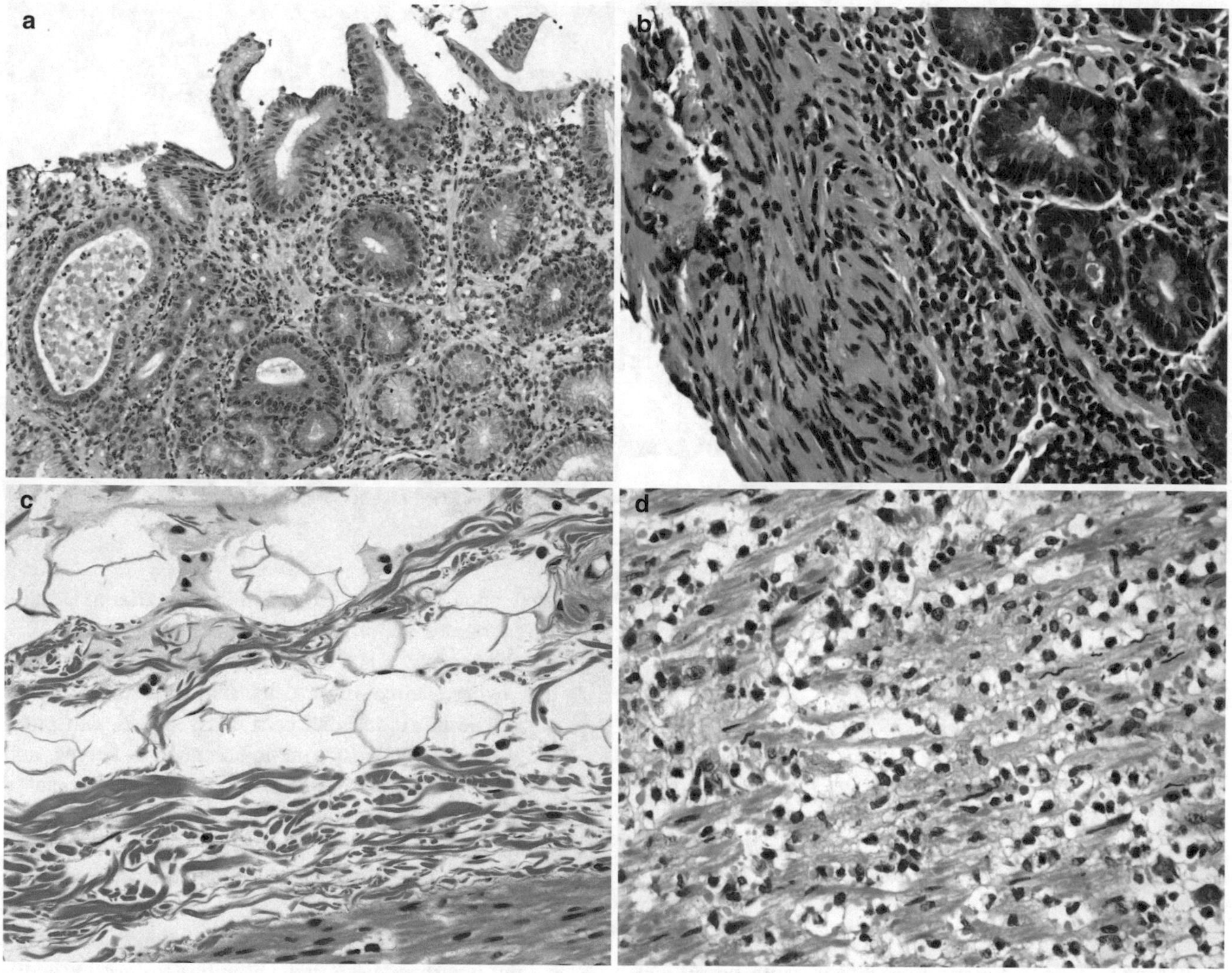

Fig. 12.8 Eosinophilic gastritis showing numerous eosinophils in the lamina propria with reactive epithelial changes (**a**). Eosinophilic infiltration of the muscularis mucosae is a useful diagnostic feature of eosinophilic gastroenteritis (**b**). Infiltration of the submucosa may also be present, which can be subtle (**c**). Infiltration of the muscularis propria is a diagnostic feature of mural form of eosinophilic gastroenteritis (**d**). Note the presence of patchy destruction of the muscle fibers with replacement fibrosis in this case

8. How should tissue eosinophilia be reported?

No clear consensus recommendations exist on how to report tissue eosinophilia in GI biopsies but a mild increase in lamina propria eosinophils without epithelial injury is usually reported either as "within normal limits" or as "mild prominence of lamina propria eosinophils, nonspecific." The designation of "eosinophilic gastritis/enteritis/colitis" is best reserved for samples in which tissue eosinophilia is marked with significant clusters/aggregates and is associated with intraepithelial infiltration and epithelial injury (Fig. 12.8a), or the infiltration extends deep into the muscularis mucosae or submucosa (Fig. 12.8b, c). Mural and serosal forms of eosinophilic gastroenteritis are diagnosed on resection specimens, where prominent eosinophils are seen to infiltrate the muscularis propria and subserosal tissue (Fig. 12.8d). Ulceration, edema, and wall thickening can be seen.

Importantly, depending on the clinical setting, the pathologist should make every effort to establish the etiology, such as consideration of autoimmune or *H. pylori* gastritis, mastocytosis or Langerhans cell infiltrate, and level deeper into the block to evaluate for an adjacent erosion and/or pill fragments/parasites. In the absence of a definite etiology on biopsies, a diagnosis of eosinophilic gastritis/enteritis/colitis or gastroenteritis will typically lead to additional testing based on the clinical history, such as presence of peripheral blood eosinophilia, stool exam for parasites, allergy testing, and/or TTG serologies.

9. What are normal mast cell counts in the GI tract?

Several studies have reported mast cell counts in the normal GI tract (Table 12.1). The mean highest mast cell count in a single high-power field (0.25 mm^2) is reported

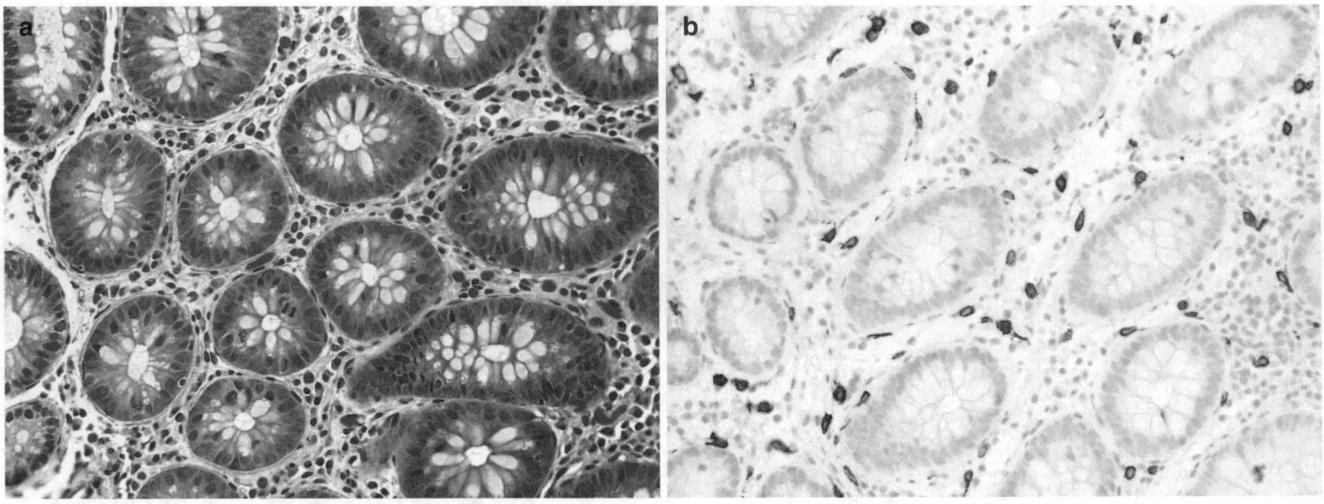

Fig. 12.9 The so-called mastocytic enterocolitis showing normal histology (**a**) but an increased number of lamina propria mast cells as demonstrated by Kit immunostaining (**b**)

Table 12.1 Mast cell counts in gastrointestinal mucosae

	Hahn and Hornick (2007) Mean (range)/HPF (0.25 mm^2)		Sokol et al. (2013) Mean ± SEM of 5 HPF (field area not reported)	
	Normal	Mastocytosis	Normal	Mastocytosis
Stomach	12 (5–21)	57 (24–90)	17.9 ± 1.8	20.5 ± 5.1
Duodenum	27 (4–51)	175 (74–339)	24.1 ± 2.7	40.3 ± 6.1
Ileum	32 (21–40)		28.4 ± 2.7	45.7 ± 3.5
Colon	21 (10–31)	209 (110–301)	14.4 ± 3.1	45.1 ± 8.8

HPF high power field, *SEM* standard error of the mean

to be around 26 (range 11–55) for asymptomatic patients, 30 (range 13–59) for patients with irritable bowel syndrome with diarrhea (IBS-D), and 28 (range 14–48) for patients with mast cell activation syndrome (59). Thus, nonneoplastic mast cell disorders are derangements of function but not number and counting mast cells in mucosal biopsies appears to have little clinical relevance.

In the normal colorectum, there appears to be a physiological variation in the distribution of intramucosal mast cells. Similar to eosinophils and other lamina propria inflammatory cells, mast cells have a higher density in the right colon and a lower density in the left colon and rectum.

References: [68, 69]

10. What role do mast cells play in irritable bowel syndrome?

IBS is a poorly defined, multifactorial entity characterized by abdominal distension, cramping, diarrhea or constipation or alternating bouts of both, relief of abdominal pain by bowel movement, with or without associated fatigue and sleep disturbances. Various clinical criteria exist to diagnose patients, the most widely used being the Rome III and Manning criteria. Despite the numerous abnormalities and comorbidities of IBS, which suggest a range of factors, there is some evidence that hyperreactive mast cells may contribute to the pathogenesis. Abdominal pain is associated with proximity of mast cells to colonic submucosal nerves, and mast cell granules have been shown to excite nociceptive receptors in the intestine. There is also symptomatic improvement after treatment with histamine receptor antagonists and cromolyn, an inhibitor of mast cell mediator release.

The terms "mastocytic enterocolitis" and "mastocytic colitis" have been used in the literature to describe endoscopic biopsies that exhibit normal histology but show an increased number of intramucosal mast cells as demonstrated by mast cell stains (Fig. 12.9a, b). The patients usually have a history of chronic diarrhea with no identifiable underlying etiology, unremarkable endoscopic findings and normal serum tryptase levels. A cutoff of >20 mast cells/HPF has been proposed for this diagnosis (only intact mast cells with visible nuclei and darkly stained cytoplasm should be counted). In this condition, mast cells are relatively evenly distributed in the lamina propria, with occasional cells infiltrating crypts, and do not form aggregates. It remains controversial, however, whether this entity truly exists because other studies have failed to demonstrate an increase in the number of intramucosal mast cells in IBS patients. As discussed above, functional derangements rather than increased numbers of mast cells appear to serve a role in IBS pathogenesis. Nevertheless, mast cell staining on endoscopic biopsies may still be requested occasionally by gastroenterologists.

References: [68, 70–75]

11. What is mastocytosis? How is it diagnosed?

The diagnosis of mastocytosis is a challenging problem in which surgical pathologists play a critical role. The symptoms of mastocytosis are the manifestations of systemic release of mast cell mediators and lead to a broad array of presenting symptoms. Histamine causes rapid vasodilation, bronchoconstriction, GI hypermotility, increased gastric acid production with consequent duodenal ulcers, headache, hypotension, pruritis, urticaria, angioedema, cramping, diarrhea, and/or anaphylaxis. Chymase can cause arrhythmias, myocardial ischemia, and hypotension. Occasionally, tissue eosinophilia results from excess IL-5 production and extensive mast cell burden in the marrow can result in osteoporosis.

If clinical suspicion for mastocytosis exists, the first diagnostic test is a bone marrow biopsy, which allows for definitive assessment of mastocytosis and evaluation of the presence or absence of any associated clonal non-mast-cell hematopoietic disorder. Mucosal GI biopsies can be used to establish the diagnosis and confirm classification as systemic mastocytosis. However, given the rarity of the disease and the variable clinical presentation, typically driven by GI symptoms present in 70% of mastocytosis patients, the first approach to determine the etiology of the patient's symptoms is often endoscopy of the luminal GI tract with biopsies. Furthermore, since a significant proportion of patients lack cutaneous manifestations, surgical pathologists will often diagnose mastocytosis in a GI biopsy where the diagnosis is not suspected by the gastroenterologist. Pathologists must, therefore, be always alert to this possibility when evaluating GI biopsies because in some cases the findings can be quite subtle and easily missed.

The objective clinicopathologic criteria used to diagnose systemic mastocytosis are classified as "Major Criterion" and "Minor Criteria"; with the diagnosis requiring either the presence of the major criterion and one minor criterion or the presence of ≥3 minor criteria (Table 12.2). The critical role of the surgical pathologist is evident by the fact that the sole major criterion is purely histologic: multifocal dense infiltrates of mast cells (≥15 mast cells in aggregates) detected in sections of bone marrow and/or other extracutaneous organs. Several of the minor criteria are also determined by the surgical pathologist, including abnormal morphology (spindled/ovoid shape) and aberrant expression of CD25. In suspected cases, the flow cytometry and molecular pathology laboratories can establish the presence of minor criteria such as aberrant expression of CD25 and/or CD2, and the presence of the *KIT* D816V mutation, respectively.

Interestingly, a recent case series reported incidental enterocolic mast cell aggregates that fulfilled the diagnostic criteria for systemic mastocytosis (tight clusters of ≥15 mast cells and coexpression of CD25) in 16 patients without clinical suspicion. Spontaneous resolution of symptoms occurred in all patients (mean follow-up: 54 months) and asymptomatic patients remained symptom-free (mean follow-up: 17 months). These observations suggest that incidental finding of mast cell aggregates in GI biopsies may not have apparent clinical significance because it is unlikely to reflect a systemic disease. However, in another study of 24 cases of systemic mastocytosis involving the GI tract, 16 (67%) had the first diagnosis made on GI biopsies. In this series, 18 patients had an indolent disease, but 6 had an aggressive clinical course.

References: [59, 68, 69, 76–80]

Table 12.2 Diagnostic criteria of systemic mastocytosis

Major criterion	
	Multifocal, dense infiltrates of mast cells (≥15 mast cells in aggregates) detected in sections of bone marrow and/or other extracutaneous organs
Minor criteria	
(a)	In biopsy sections of bone marrow or other extracutaneous organs, >25% of the mast cells in the infiltrate are spindle-shaped or have atypical morphology or, of all mast cells in bone marrow aspirate smears, >25% are immature or atypical
(b)	Detection of an activating point mutation at codon 816 of *KIT* gene in bone marrow, blood, or other extracutaneous organ
c)	Mast cells in bone marrow, blood, or other extracutaneous organs with aberrant expression of CD2 and/or CD25 in addition to normal mast cell markers
(d)	Serum total tryptase persistently exceed 20 ng/mL (this parameter is invalid in the setting of an associated clonal myeloid disorder)

12. How is mastocytosis classified?

The classification of mastocytosis has undergone significant revision in recent years. Mastocytosis is a neoplasm of mast cells that involves one or multiple organs. Cutaneous mastocytosis, is limited to the skin, occurs predominantly in children, and has an excellent prognosis. It manifests predominantly as urticaria pigmentosa, and less commonly as telangiectasia macularis eruptiva perstans, diffuse cutaneous mastocytosis, or solitary masocytoma. In contrast, systemic mastocytosis (SM) typically occurs in adults, involves multiple organs, almost invariably including the bone marrow, with additional involvement of the spleen, liver, and/or GI tract. SM does not spontaneously resolve, and has a variable clinical course. In the WHO 2016 classification, SM is subdivided into categories of increasingly poor prognosis: indolent SM, smoldering SM, SM with associated hematologic neoplasm (SM-AHN), aggressive SM, and mast cell leukemia (Table 12.3).

Indolent SM is a limited clonal expansion of mast cells that may be symptomatic, with a low rate of pro-

Table 12.3 Classification of mast cell disorders

1. Cutaneous mastocytosis	
(a)	Urticaria pigmentosa
(b)	Diffuse cutaneous mastocytosis
(c)	Solitary mastocytoma of skin
2. Systemic mastocytosis	
(a)	ISM: systemic mastocytosis without C findings, no evidence of associated non-MC lineage disease
(b)	SSM: ISM with two or more B findings and no C findings
(c)	SM-AHN: meets criteria for both SM and another clonal hematologic neoplasm
(d)	ASM: SM with one or more C findings, no evidence of MCL
(f)	MCL
3. MC sarcoma: unifocal MC tumor with destructive growth and characteristic histology; no evidence of SM	
"B findings"	
1.	>30% BM infiltration by MCs in focal, dense aggregates and/or serum total tryptase >20 ng/mL
2.	Signs of myelodysplasia or meloproliferation in non-MC lineage(s), not meeting criteria for a hematopoietic neoplasm, with normal or slightly abnormal blood counts
3.	Hepatomegaly and/or splenomegaly without functional impairment, and/or lymphadenopathy
"C findings"	
1.	One or more cytopenia(s) without obvious non-MC malignancy
2.	Palpable hepatomegaly with impairment of liver function, ascites, and/or portal hypertension
3.	Osteolytic lesions and/or pathologic fractures
4.	Palpable splenomegaly with hypersplenism
5.	Malabsorption with weight loss due to GI MC infiltrates

ISM indolent systemic mastocytosis, *MC* mast cell, *SSM* smoldering systemic mastocytosis, *SM-AHN* systemic mastocytosis with an associated clonal hematologic neoplasm, *SM* systemic mastocytosis, *ASM* aggressive systemic mastocytosis, *MCL* mast cell leukemia, *GI* gastrointestinal

gression (<2% in 5 years) to more aggressive disease. Smoldering SM is a *KIT*-mutant neoplastic process involving mast cells and other myeloid lineages, with a high extramedullary burden of mast cells. There must be two or more B findings and no C findings (Table 12.3). SM-AHN is defined by the presence of a non-mast-cell hematopoietic neoplasm in addition to SM, the prognosis of which is often determined by the non-mast-cell neoplasm. Aggressive SM is defined by evidence of organ damage (at least one C finding). Lastly, the exceedingly rare mast cell sarcoma, which has been reported in a broad range of anatomic locations but not yet in the GI tract, may arise as a late transformation event from cutaneous mastocytosis. The morphology of these tumors bears little resemblance to mast cells and these neoplasms are frequently misdiagnosed.

The vast majority (90%) of adult-onset mastocytosis is associated with *KIT* D816V mutation, which grants mast cells independence from stem cell factor and resistance to imatinib. While this mutation is highly prevalent, other molecular alterations (*TET2, ASXL1, DNMT3A*, among others) may also play an important role and are likely responsible for the heterogeneous clinical course in these patients.

Some patients do not meet the formal criteria for SM (Table 12.2) but have symptoms of mast cell activation and a clonal population demonstrated by a *KIT* D816 mutation or an aberrant CD25 expression on mast cells. These patients are currently assigned a provisional diagnosis of "monoclonal mast cell activation syndrome" (MMAS), an entity which is discussed but not formally included in the revised WHO 2017 classification. Thus far, the predilection of these patients to develop into mastocytosis is unknown. Lastly, some patients have symptoms attributable to mast cell activation, often in the setting of a baseline serum tryptase between 11.4 ng/mL (upper limit of normal) and 20.0 ng/mL (minor criterion for SM), and no evidence of a clonal mast cell population. The disease of these patients is categorized in an evolving entity referred to as non-clonal idiopathic mast cell activation syndrome.

References: [81–87]

13. What endoscopic and histologic features suggest systemic mastocytosis in the luminal GI tract?

GI tract mucosal involvement by systemic mastocytosis in symptomatic patients has been described in detail. The most commonly involved sites of the GI tract are the colon and ileum, followed by stomach, and rarely, the esophagus. The endoscopic impression of involved areas may reveal mucosal nodularity, granularity or erythema, or, in nearly half of involved biopsies, an entirely normal appearance; likely reflecting the wide range of mucosal disease burden.

Biopsies from the upper GI tract tend to show aggregates of spindled to ovoid mast cells scattered throughout the lamina propria (Figs. 12.10a–c and 12.11a, b). In the colon, mast cell aggregates in the lamina propria often show a strikingly superficial subepithelial distribution (Fig. 12.12a). Importantly, the disease is patchy in distribution; one quarter of involved biopsies showed only focal involvement by a single discrete aggregate of mast cells in one tissue fragment. Given the above, multiple biopsies from various regions of the GI tract are necessary for sufficient sensitivity for diagnosis. As noted previously, a prominent secondary eosinophilic infiltrate can obfuscate the underlying mast cell infiltrate (Fig. 12.12b). Prominent eosinophilia along with the neoplastic mast cells is reported in 44% of lower GI tract biopsies, 16% of duodenal biopsies, but none of the gastric biopsies. In the GI tract, immunohistochemistry for Kit has much greater sensitivity than mast cell tryptase immunostaining, toluidine blue, or Giemsa (Figs. 12.10b, c, 12.11b and 12.12c). Aberrant coexpression of CD25 by immunohistochemistry confirms the neoplastic

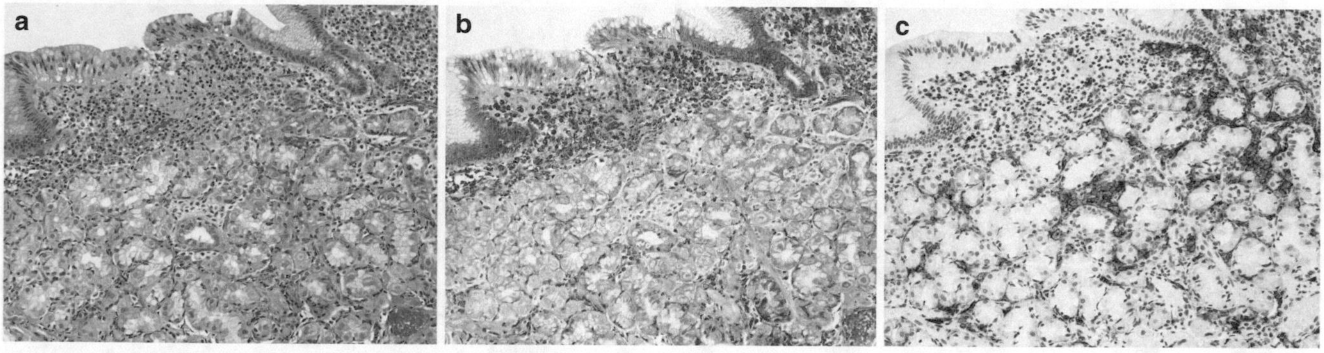

Fig. 12.10 Gastric involvement by systemic mastocytosis is difficult to detect on routine H&E stain (**a**). Characteristically, neoplastic mast cells are frequently negative or only weakly stained for the metachromatic cytoplasmic granules with Giemsa (**b**). Immunohistochemical stain for Kit reveals an abnormally clustered population of mast cells that inconspicuously infiltrate between the gastric glands (**c**)

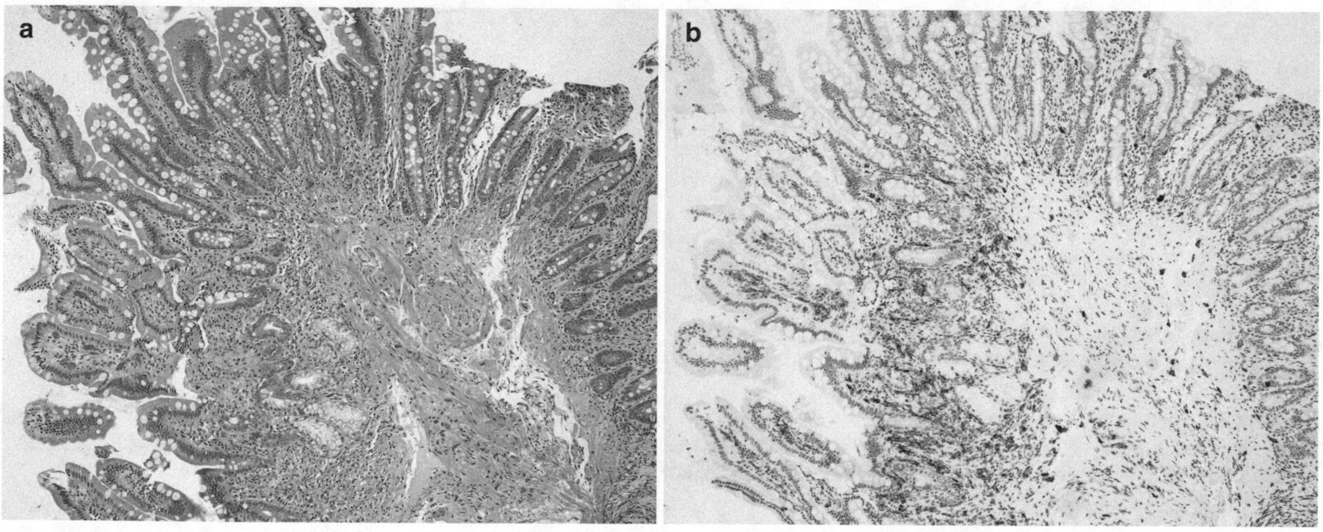

Fig. 12.11 Mastocytosis tends to have a subtle appearance in the duodenum on routine H&E stain (**a**), which can be highlighted by Kit immunohistochemistry (**b**)

nature of the mast cells (Fig. 12.12d). Importantly, mast cell number is not a clinically useful histologic feature to evaluate systemic mastocytosis or mast cell activation syndrome.

Reference: [59]

14. **What is the differential diagnosis for a histiocytic infiltrate in the luminal GI tract?**

Histiocytes are mononuclear myeloid cells of monocyte/macrophage lineage. Their microscopic appearance can be quite variable, which in turn affects the differential diagnosis. At rest, histiocytes have a round to oval nuclear contour, fine chromatin, and moderate to abundant pale or amphophilic cytoplasm. Upon activation, their nuclei can enlarge and acquire irregular nuclear contours and distinct nucleoli. When in clusters, their cytoplasmic borders are quite indistinct, giving them a syncytial appearance. Given their capacity for phagocytosis, the cytoplasmic characteristics vary depending on what the cell ingests: aggregates of glycolipids ("ceroid-laden" macrophages), abundant cell membrane constituents in a micellar distribution ("foamy" or "xanthomatous" macrophages), as well as pigments such as hemosiderin, bile, melanin, Hamazaki–Wesenberg bodies, and foreign materials such as tattoo pigment, contaminants from intravenous drug use, or metal particles from a dental amalgam or artificial bone. Thus, the histologic differential of histiocytic infiltrates can be far-ranging, and include disparate entities such as metastatic/locally invasive malignancies such as adenocarcinomas (lobular breast, signet-ring-cell, lung, renal, prostate) and melanoma. In most cases, these non-histiocytic mimics can be readily distinguished from true histiocytes by their growth pattern, relatively distinct cytoplasmic membranes, and/or nuclear atypia, in comparison to adjacent, nonneoplas-

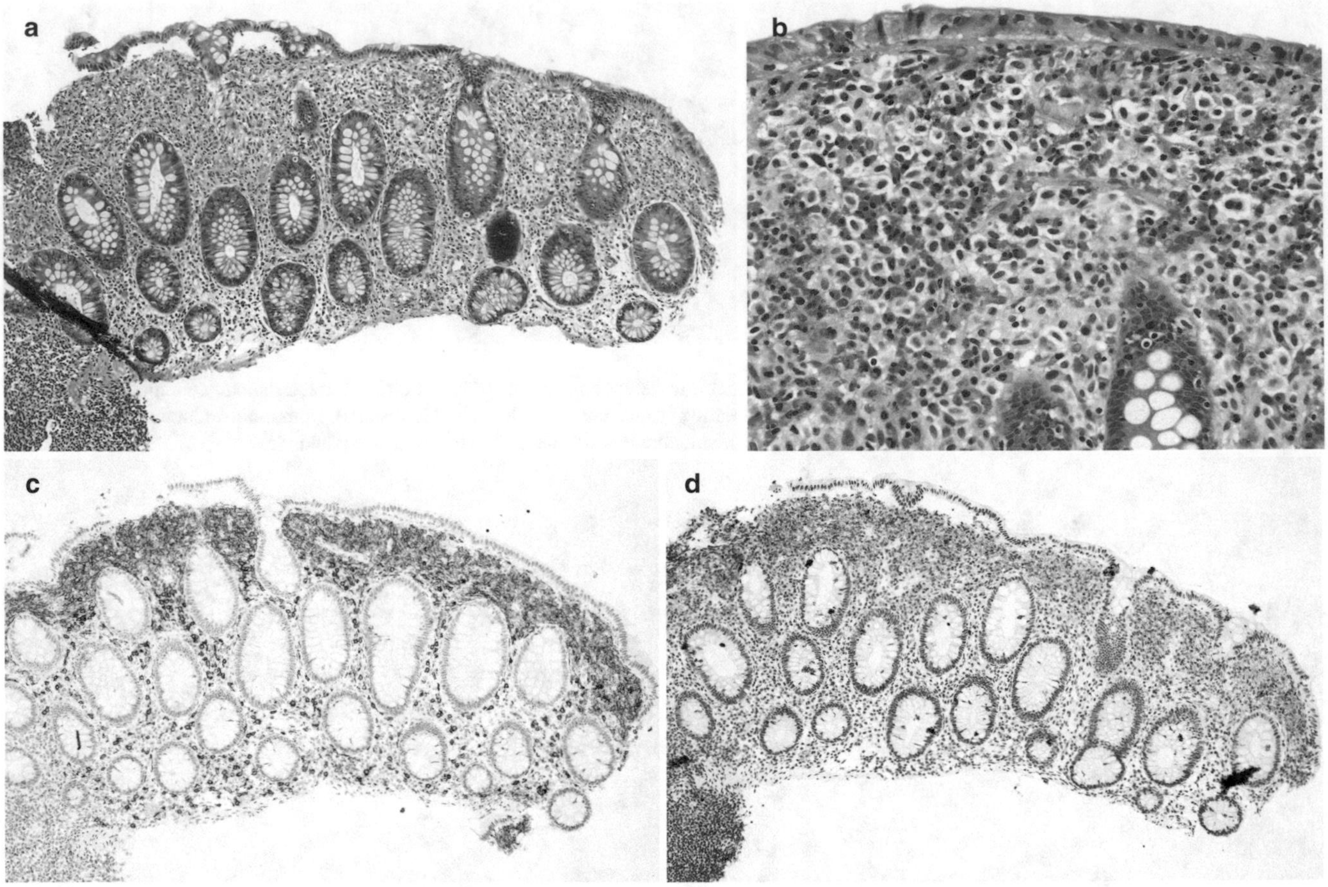

Fig. 12.12 Colonic involvement by systemic mastocytosis tends to be more densely superficial and subepithelial (**a**). Accompanying eosinophils can be so numerous as to obfuscate the presence of the neoplastic mast cells (**b**). Immunohistochemistry for Kit can be helpful to highlight the mast cell infiltrate (**c**). Aberrant coexpression of CD25 confirms their neoplastic nature (**d**)

tic histiocytes that are usually present. However, the distinction can become difficult in limited biopsies and in cases where true histiocytes are intimately admixed with the non-histiocytic lineage. In these settings, judicious use of immunohistochemical stains will usually resolve any diagnostic dilemma.

A true histiocytic infiltrate also has a broad range of potential clinical implications. Prominent histiocytic infiltrates can be seen in nonspecific inflammatory reactions such as lamina propria muciphages in response to ruptured crypts in the colorectum (Fig. 12.13a), melanosis coli associated with chronic laxative use (Fig. 12.13b), xanthoma (Fig. 12.13c), sometimes as distinct nodules or polyps in gastric or colonic malakoplakia (Fig. 12.14a–d), crystal-storing histiocytosis associated with B-cell lymphoproliferative disorders (Fig. 12.15a–c), and infections such as syphilis (Fig. 12.16a, b), Whipple disease, and atypical mycobacterial infection (see Chap. 10). Neoplastic histiocytic infiltration including histiocytic sarcoma and other primary histiocytic processes are discussed in more detail in the following.

15. What is the differential diagnosis for granulomas in the GI tract?

The differential diagnosis of epithelioid granulomas in the GI tract includes Crohn disease (Fig. 12.17a, b), drug reaction, sarcoidosis, chronic granulomatous disease, connective tissue disorders/vasculitides, bacterial (Yersinia, mycobacteria, etc.) or fungal (mucormycosis, histoplasmosis, blastomycosis, candidiasis, aspergillosis, etc.) infections, or as a reaction to helminth eggs (Fig. 12.18a–d). In Crohn disease, granulomas may occur at any anatomic location of the GI tract, and at any depth within the visceral wall. Crohn-related granulomas are more frequent in children than adults and like many of the features discussed in this chapter, the likelihood of detection increases with the extent of disease and the number of biopsies taken. These range in size from microgranulomas (5–18 cells) to large, sarcoid-like granulomas (25–90 cells). Occasionally, Schaumann bodies may be seen (Fig. 12.17b). Granulomas in Crohn disease are tightly formed, round, well-circumscribed without necrosis and usually without other admixed inflammatory cells. The latter feature is helpful in distin-

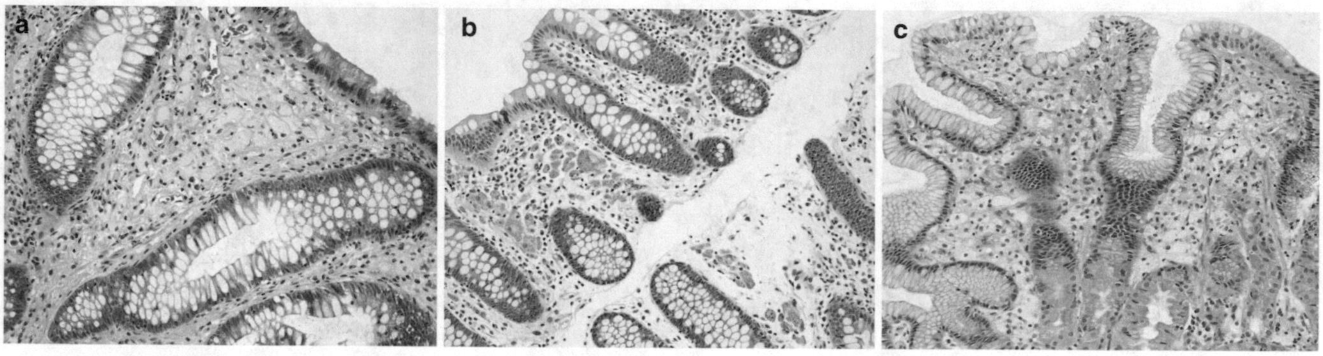

Fig. 12.13 (**a**) Muciphages are histiocytes that have accumulated mucin in their cytoplasm from damaged epithelium. Occasionally, their presence may raise the suspicion for mycobacterial or fungal infection, which may require special stains for the distinction. (**b**) Pigmented lamina propria histiocytes seen in melanosis coli, which should not be confused with metastatic melanoma. (**c**) A case of gastric xanthoma showing localized nondestructive infiltration of the lamina propria by epithelioid histiocytes with abundant foamy cytoplasm, reflecting lipid accumulation within intracytoplasmic vesicles, thought to be the result of prior injury

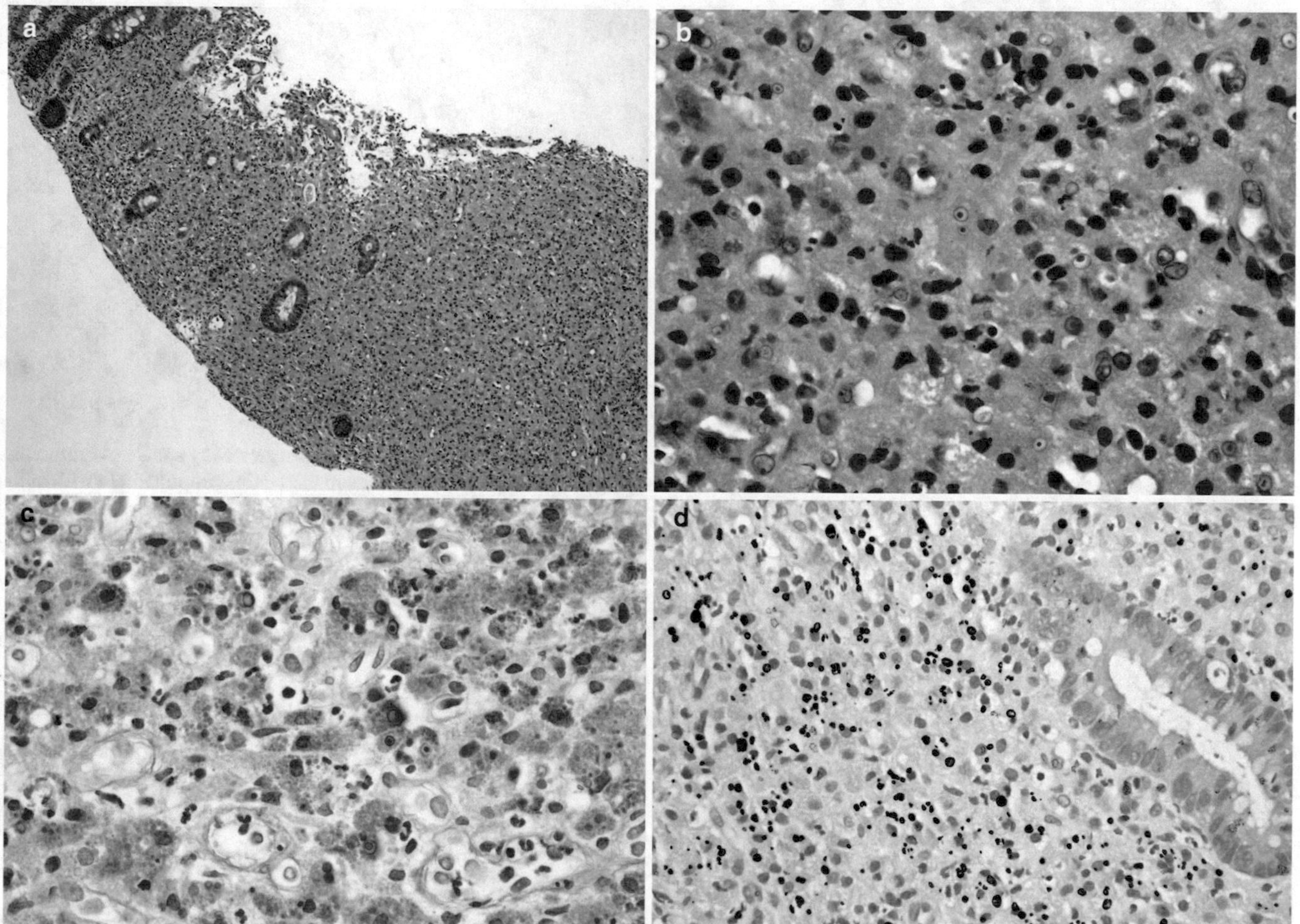

Fig. 12.14 A case of colonic malakoplakia showing sheets of epithelioid histiocytes with partial mucosal destruction (**a**). Frequent targetoid inclusions (Michaelis–Gutman bodies) are present (**b**), which are highlighted by PAS (**c**) and von Kossa (**d**) stains

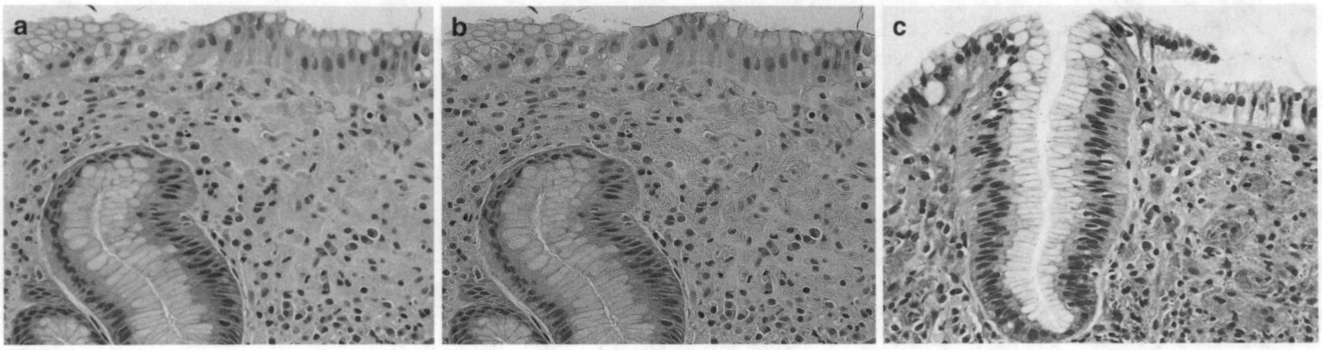

Fig. 12.15 Crystal-storing histiocytosis seen in a case of gastric MALT lymphoma in the background of Helicobacter gastritis (**a**). The histiocytes can be highlighted by removing the condenser (**b**) or on Giemsa stain (**c**). Note the presence of Helicobacter organisms on Giemsa stain

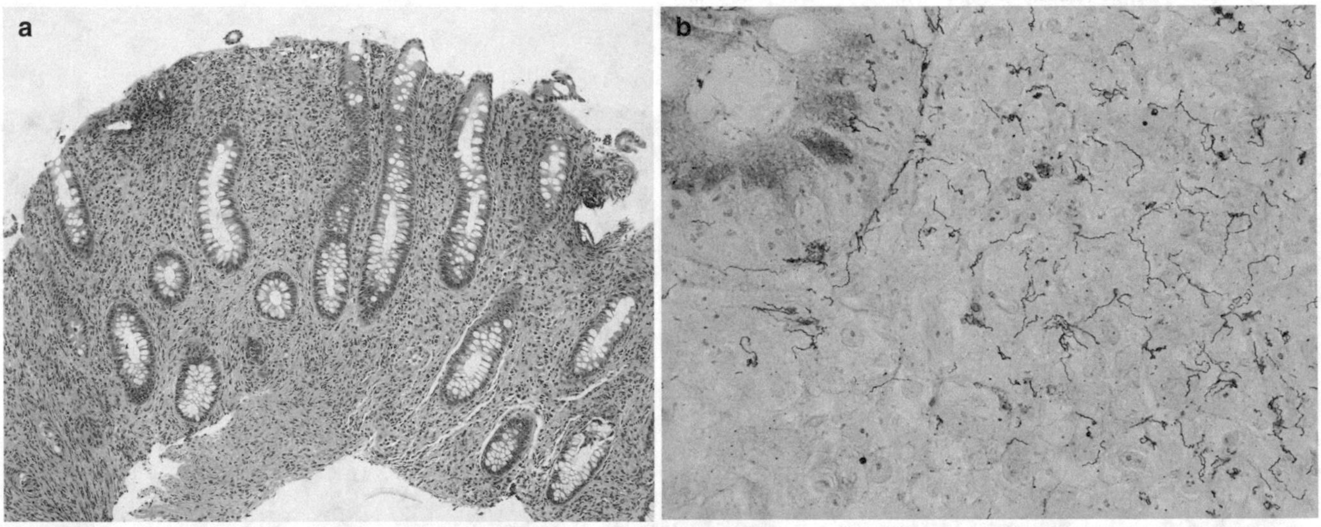

Fig. 12.16 A case of syphilitic proctitis showing diffuse lamina propria infiltrates with abundant histiocytes and relatively sparse plasma cells, often without the deep crypt branching as seen in IBD (**a**). Steiner stain highlights innumerable spirochetes in the lamina propria, often with infiltration of the epithelium and vascular spaces (**b**)

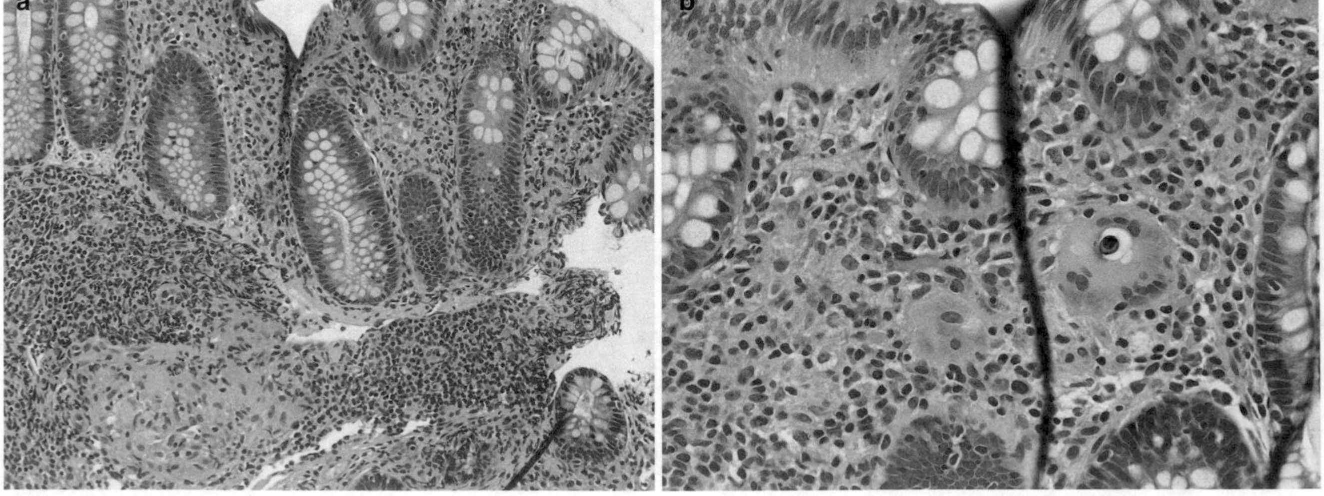

Fig. 12.17 Epithelioid granulomas may be seen in Crohn disease (**a**) and in this setting may occasionally include Schaumann bodies (**b**)

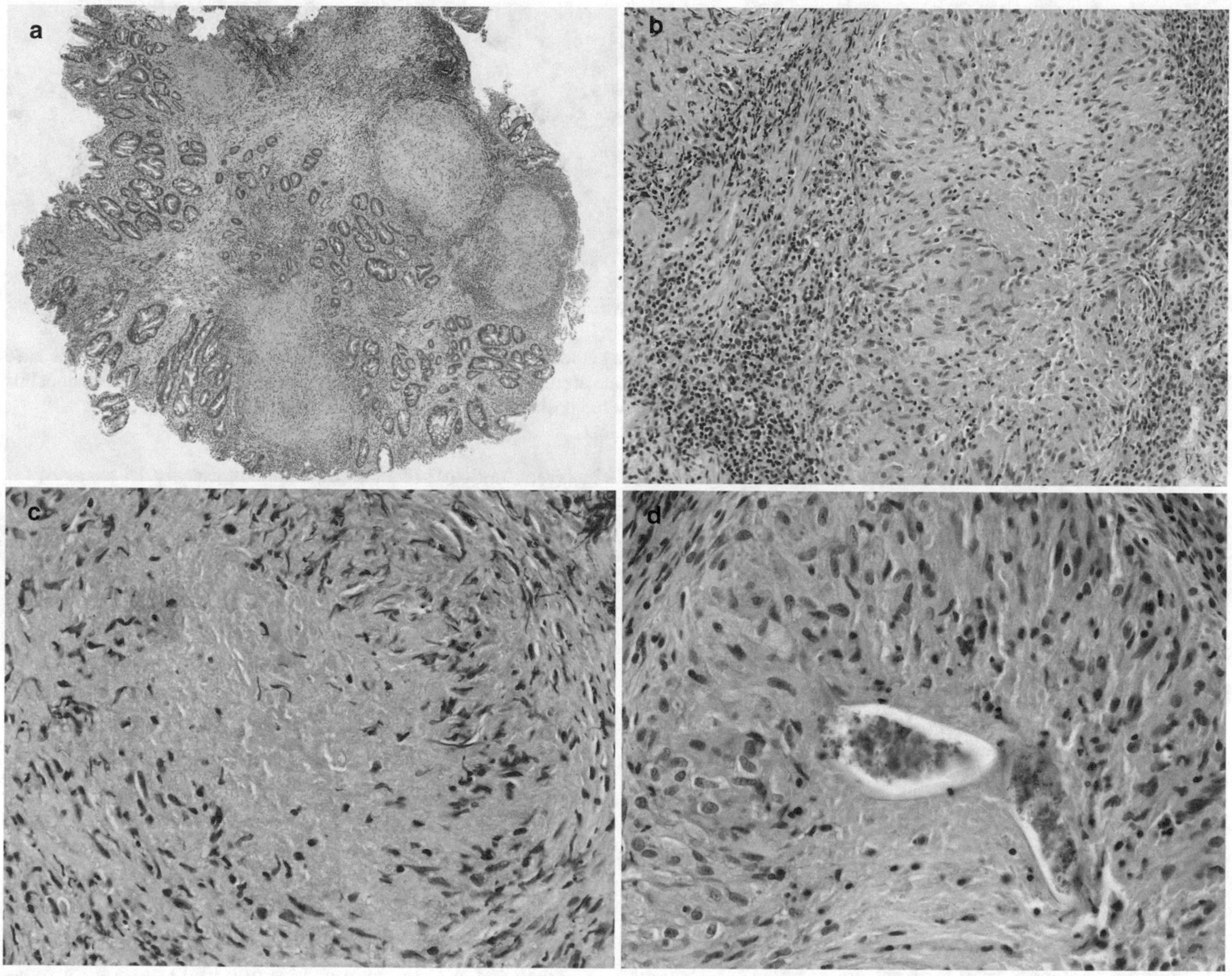

Fig. 12.18 When granulomas are large as seen in this rectal polyp (**a**), they should be scrutinized closely. Higher magnification examination reveals peripheral palisading of the histiocytes with central fibrinoid necrosis (**b**) and a single round refractile structure (**c**). Deeper levels confirmed the presence of degenerative Schistosomal eggs with lateral spine consistent with S. mansoni (**d**)

guishing Crohn-like granulomas from the loose histiocytic reaction around ruptured crypts in ulcerative colitis ("crypt granulomas").

References: [7, 8]

16. **What primary histiocytic disorders involve the GI tract?**

Langerhans cell histiocytosis (LCH) is a clonal proliferation of Langerhans cells defined by expression of CD1a, langerin, and S100, and the presence of Birbeck granules on ultrastructural studies. Approximately half of cases show *BRAF* V600E mutation. The majority of cases occur in children, most often seen in bone and soft tissue, less frequently the liver and spleen. Involvement of the GI tract is quite rare, with vastly different implications in children and adults.

In children, GI tract involvement by LCH is most commonly seen in male patients <2 years of age, presenting with intractable emesis, diarrhea, and failure to thrive. Endoscopy shows superficial erosions and hemorrhagic ulcers throughout the GI tract. Nearly all patients with GI involvement have multisystem disease, and majority of patients in this setting die within 18 months of diagnosis. In sharp contrast, when seen in adults, LCH is most commonly seen in asymptomatic females as a small isolated polyp, probably analogous to the newly described Langerhans cell histiocytoma of the skin. Regardless of clinical setting, the histology of LCH is identical at all sites, with a locally infiltrative lesion comprised of sheets of large cells with ovoid to reniform nuclear contours, nuclear grooves, fine chromatin with a single centrally located nucleolus, and a large amount of pale eosinophilic cytoplasm with a syncytial appearance. Since the infiltrate

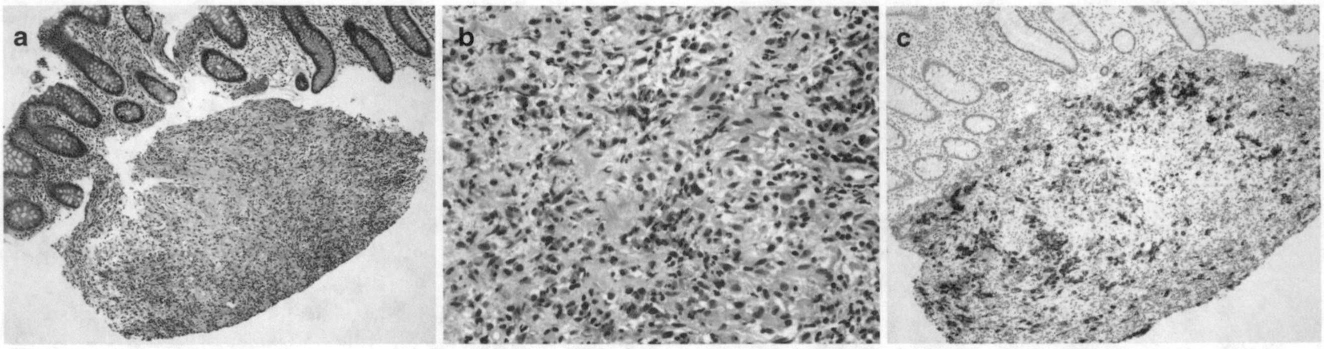

Fig. 12.19 Langerhans cell histiocytosis presented as a 5-mm ascending colon sessile polyp in a 54-year-old man (**a**). The lesional cells have ovoid or elongated nuclei, fine chromatin, inconspicuous nucleoli, and pale eosinophilic cytoplasm, and are admixed with numerous eosinophils and scattered lymphocytes (**b**). Immunohistochemically, the lesional cells are positive for CD1a (**c**), langerin and S100

may be prominent in the superficial lamina propria, the low-power histologic appearance can be similar to systemic mastocytosis in the colon. There is often an accompanying infiltrate of eosinophils, neutrophils, lymphocytes, and plasma cells. Despite this, the histology of LCH is unlikely to be a source of diagnostic confusion as the nuclear features are distinct, and immunostains for Kit, CD1a, and langerin are robust markers helpful for definitive diagnosis (Fig. 12.19a–c).

Malakoplakia ("soft plaque") is an inflammatory pseudotumorous process that is the result of ineffective macrophage microbicidal activity, typically in response to a Gram-negative bacterium. After the genitourinary tract, the GI tract is the second most commonly involved organ system, amongst which the colon is the most frequent site of involvement. Depending on the extent of disease, patients may present with fever, abdominal pain, and diarrhea, or malakoplakia may be diagnosed incidentally on screening colonoscopy. On endoscopic exam, malakoplakia typically appears as friable yellowish polyps to large masses. Histology is remarkable for an infiltrate of large, bland epithelioid histiocytes, with admixed lymphocytes, plasma cells, neutrophils, and eosinophils. The infiltrate can be destructive. Targetoid intracytoplasmic bodies (Michaelis–Gutman bodies) confirm the diagnosis, which can be highlighted by periodic acid–Schiff (PAS) stain and stains for iron and calcium (Fig. 12.14a–d). Michaelis–Gutman bodies are thought to represent calcified remnants of phagolysosomes that contained bacteria. In support of this, careful exam can sometimes identify coliform bacteria within phagolysosomes (von Hansemann bodies).

Rosai–Dorfman disease is a proliferation of histiocytes of uncertain neoplastic nature, typically involving lymph nodes of young, black males. Extranodal Rosai–Dorfman disease has a ubiquitous anatomic distribution; most common sites being skin, bone, upper respiratory tract, and soft tissue. Only approximately 15 cases of GI tract involvement have been reported in the literature. The histiocytes are large, epithelioid cells with round nuclei and abundant cytoplasm that demonstrate emperipolesis (presence of an intact lymphocyte within the cytoplasm). The cytoplasm of the lesional cells stains diffusely with S100.

Erdheim–Chester disease (ECD) is a neoplastic proliferation of histiocytes, commonly foamy histiocytes, with Touton giant cells and a fibrotic background. ECD is less common than LCH, and similarly, involvement of the GI tract is rare. ECD can present at any age, and involve any organ, with skeletal involvement in nearly all cases, and an overall poor prognosis. ECD frequently harbors activating mutations in MAPK genes (*BRAF* V600E >50%; *NRAS* ~ 4%) and also recurrent mutations in *PI3KCA* pathway genes. While ECD has a poor overall prognosis, vemurafenib has shown therapeutic promise in the *BRAF*-mutant cases.

Juvenile xanthogranuloma (JXG) of the GI tract is exceptionally rare and found in the setting of systemic disease. JXG histology is usually distinguished from LCH because the histiocytes are lipid-laden, similar to those seen in a xanthoma, but as a more nodular distribution and with the presence of admixed lymphocytes, eosinophils, and Touton giant cells. In cases where histology overlaps with LCH, immunohistochemical stains will demonstrate strong, diffuse positivity for factor XIIIa, with negative CD1a expression.

Histiocytic sarcoma is a rare neoplasm that may occur in the GI tract. While most occur in adults, patients span all ages of life. GI tract involvement frequently presents with obstruction, often accompanied by systemic "B symptoms" (fever, weight loss). The etiology is unknown, but histiocytic sarcomas show a curious association with B-cell lymphoproliferative disorders and mediastinal germ cell tumors. The tumor is com-

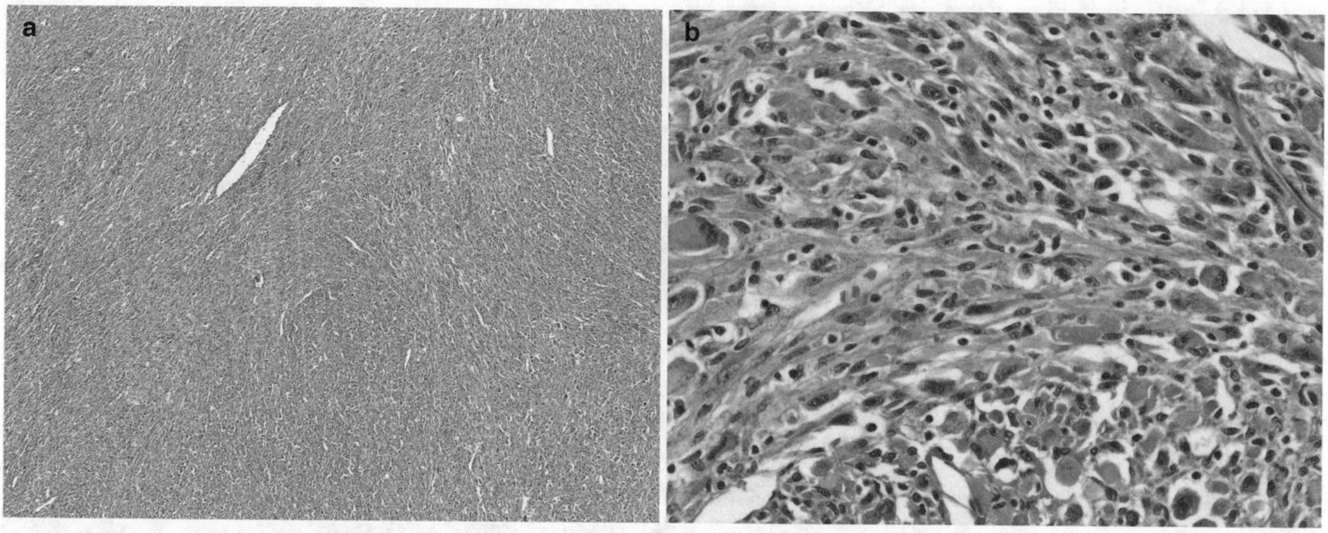

Fig. 12.20 Histiocytic sarcoma showing a sheet-like destructive growth pattern (**a**). The lesion consists of spindled to pleomorphic epithelioid histiocytic cells with significant nuclear atypia, prominent nucleoli, and abundant intratumoral lymphocytes (**b**)

prised of large discohesive cells with a mass-forming, tissue-destructive growth pattern. Tumor cells are frequently pleomorphic (but can be monomorphic), with round to oval irregularly folded nuclei, vesicular chromatin, and frequent multinucleated forms (Fig. 12.20a, b). A high proportion of these tumors have activating mutations in genes involved in the MAPK pathway, a feature that is shared with neoplasms of dendritic cells. References: [88–96]

Case Presentation

Case 1

Learning Objectives

1. To recognize common endoscopic and histologic features of the disease
2. To understand the common immunostaining pattern of the disease
3. To understand the most common molecular mutation profile of the disease

Case History

A 45-year-old male with a history of hypertension and a family history of colon cancer underwent screening colonoscopy. On colonoscopy, some unusual pale, yellowish thickened folds were noted throughout the right colon (Fig. 12.21a), which were biopsied.

Histologic Findings

Microscopic evaluation of the biopsies demonstrated clusters of spindled cells in the colon mucosa (Fig. 12.21b), which were more concentrated in the superficial lamina propria beneath the surface lining epithelium.

Differential Diagnosis

- Langerhans histiocytosis
- Systemic mastocytosis
- Spindle cell malignant neoplasm
- Malakoplakia

IHC and Other Ancillary Studies

Immunostains demonstrated the cells to be positive for Kit (Fig. 12.21c) and CD25 (Fig. 12.21d). Further molecular study showed positive result for *KIT* D816V mutation.

Final Diagnosis

Systemic mastocytosis.

Follow-Up

The patient had remained asymptomatic for 5 years without therapy. His serum tryptase levels had remained normal during follow-up.

Take-Home Messages

1. Systemic mastocytosis can be symptomatic and asymptomatic. The colon and ileum are the most commonly

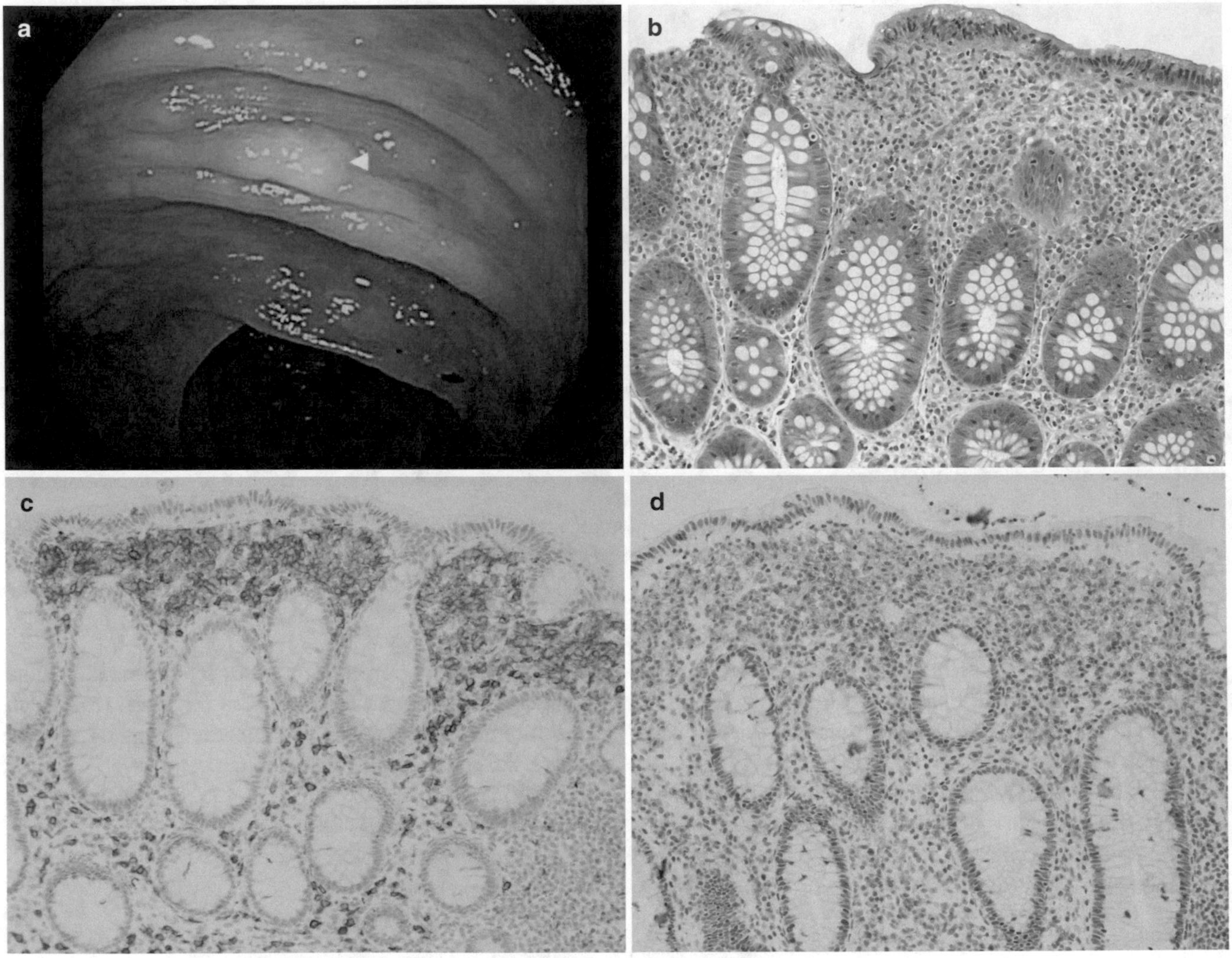

Fig. 12.21 (Case 1) (**a**) Colonoscopy showing pale yellowish thickening of the colonic folds, scattered throughout the right colon. (**b**) Biopsy showing a monotonous bland spindle cell population expanding the superficial lamina propria. Immunohistochemistry showing expression of Kit (**c**) with coexpression of CD25 (**d**)

involved sites of the GI tract, followed by stomach, and rarely, the esophagus.

2. The disease is patchy in distribution; one quarter of involved biopsies show only focal involvement by a single discrete aggregate of mast cells in one tissue fragment. Sometimes, a prominent secondary eosinophilic infiltrate can obfuscate the underlying mast cell infiltrate. This seems to occur more often in lower GI tract biopsies than upper ones.
3. Immunohistochemistry for Kit has much greater sensitivity than mast cell tryptase, and aberrant coexpression of CD25 by immunohistochemistry confirms the neoplastic nature of the mast cells.
4. The vast majority (90%) of adult onset mastocytosis is associated with *KIT* D816V mutation, which grants mast cells independence from stem cell factor and resistance to imatinib.
5. Incidental finding of mast cell aggregates in GI biopsies may not reflect a generalized disease.
   References: [59, 80, 84]

Case 2

Learning Objectives

1. To understand the differential diagnosis of histiocytic infiltration in GI tract
2. To understand the characteristic histologic findings of the disease
3. To be aware of some useful stains for confirming the diagnosis

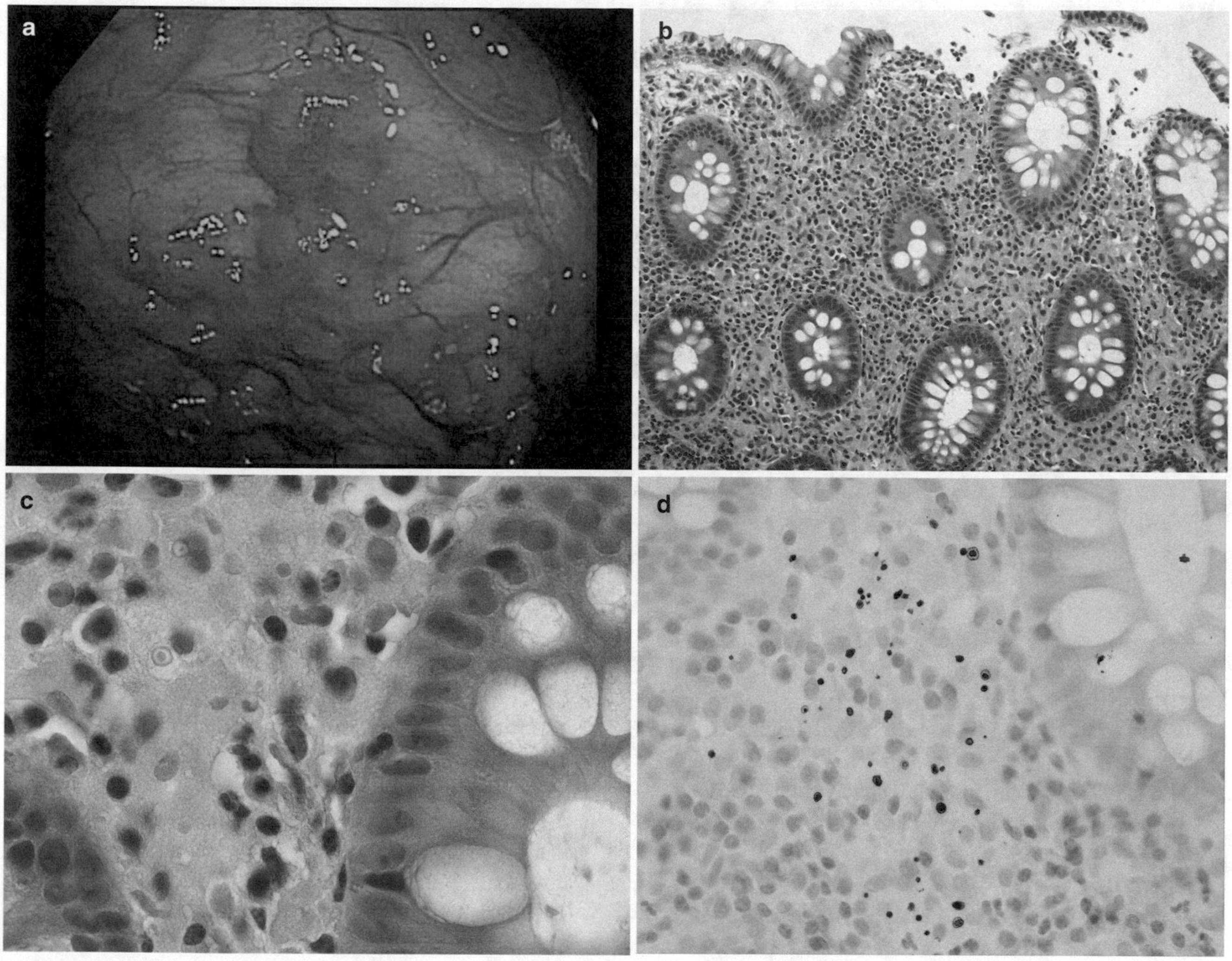

Fig. 12.22 (Case 2) (**a**) Colonoscopy showing soft, irregular mucosal irregularities throughout the colon. (**b**) Biopsy showing numerous epithelioid histiocytes in the lamina propria. (**c**) A subset of cells containing targetoid inclusions (Michaelis–Gutman bodies). (**d**) von Kossa stain for calcium highlighting the Michaelis–Gutman bodies

Case History

A 73-year-old female with a history of diverticulosis underwent screening colonoscopy. Numerous soft, irregular mucosal irregularities were seen (Fig. 12.22a). Biopsies were obtained.

Histologic Findings

Biopsies revealed a diffuse population of epithelioid histiocytes with targetoid Michaelis–Guttmann bodies (Fig. 12.22b, c) highlighted on von Kossa stain (Fig. 12.22d).

Differential Diagnosis

- Malakoplakia
- Langerhans cell histiocytosis
- Fungal infection
- Metastatic malignant epithelioid neoplasm

Final Diagnosis

Malakoplakia.

Take-Home Messages

1. Malakoplakia is an inflammatory pseudotumorous process that is the result of ineffective macrophage microbicidal activity, typically in response to a Gram-negative bacterium.
2. Histologically, it may be confused with malignancy including carcinoma and sarcoma.
3. The finding of targetoid intracytoplasmic bodies (Michaelis–Gutman bodies) confirms the diagnosis, which can be highlighted by PAS and stains for iron and calcium.

   Reference: [97]

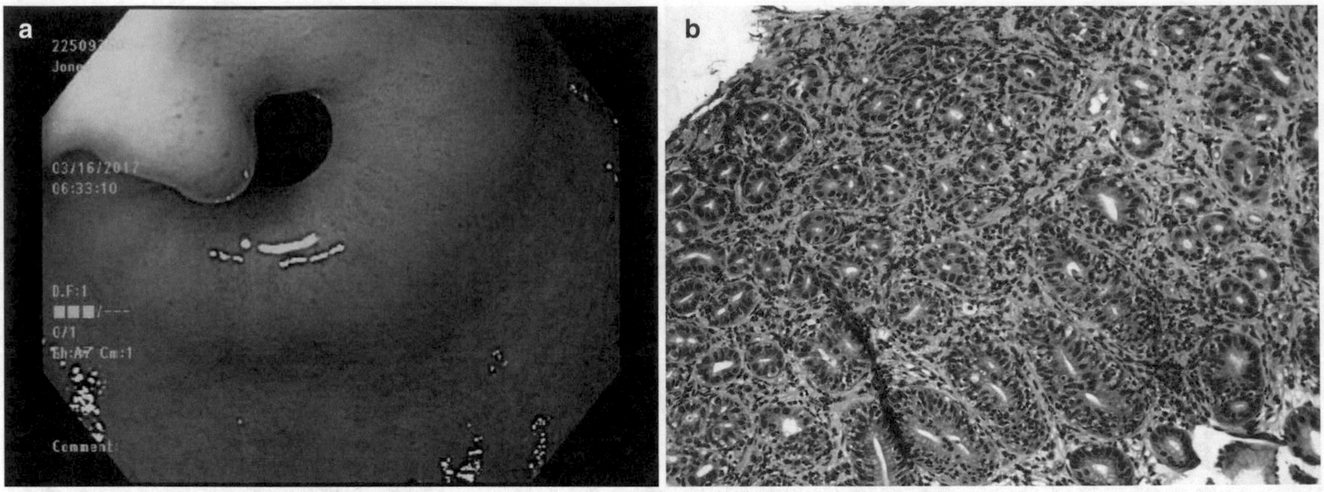

Fig. 12.23 (Case 3) (**a**) Endoscopy showing flattening of the gastric rugal folds and pinpoint petechiae. (**b**) Biopsy showing numerous eosinophils infiltrating the lamina propria and gastric glands

Case 3

Learning Objectives

1. To understand common clinical presentation of the disease
2. To understand the histologic features of the disease
3. To understand the differential diagnosis of the disease

Case History

A 64-year-old female with a history of rheumatoid arthritis was recently prescribed to use Remicade. She presented with nausea and early satiety. Endoscopy revealed flattening of the rugal folds and pinpoint petechiae (Fig. 12.23a).

Histologic Findings

Biopsy revealed diffuse expansion of the lamina propria by eosinophils, with scattered superficial erosions. Eosinophilic infiltration of gastric glands was evident (Fig. 12.23b). Immunostain for Helicobacter was negative.

Differential Diagnosis

- Langerhans cell histiocytosis
- Systemic mastocytosis
- Eosinophilic gastritis
- Anisakis infection

Final Diagnosis

Eosinophilic gastritis.

Follow-Up

At follow-up, the patient's gastritis resolved after a change in medication and cession of Remicade. She was thus diagnosed with Remicade hypersensitivity.

Take-Home Messages

1. Tissue eosinophilia in the GI tract is usually encountered in the setting of drug reaction, food allergy, infections, IBD, and rarely due to an idiopathic primary eosinophilic gastritis/gastroenteritis.
2. Primary idiopathic eosinophilic gastroenteritis may present with nonspecific upper GI symptoms such as vomiting and/or diarrhea, obstruction, or occasionally with ileus and pseudo-obstruction. Patients with serosal involvement may develop eosinophilic ascites.
3. The designation of "eosinophilic gastritis/enteritis" is best reserved for samples in which tissue eosinophilia is marked with significant clusters/aggregates and is associated with intraepithelial infiltration and epithelial injury, or the infiltration extends deep into the muscularis mucosae and/or submucosa.
4. Unlike eosinophilic esophagitis where a diagnostic cutoff of 15/HPF is used, the cutoff values of eosinophil count are not well established for eosinophilic gastritis, enteritis, and colitis. For the diagnosis of eosinophilic gastritis, the following criteria have been proposed by some authors: $\geq$30 eosinophils/HPF in at least five separate, most concentrated HPFs. It also requires to rule out other causes of eosinophilia including *H. pylori* infection. A threshold of 20 eosinophils/HPF has also been used by some authors for the diagnosis of eosinophilic colitis, but this number would have a significant overlap with the eosinophil density in the normal colon, particularly the proximal colon.

References: [7, 45–48, 98, 99]

References

1. Lwin T, Melton SD, Genta RM. Eosinophilic gastritis: histopathological characterization and quantification of the normal gastric eosinophil content. Mod Pathol. 2011;24:556–63.
2. DeBrosse CW, Case JW, Putnam PE, Collins MH, Rothenberg ME. Quantity and distribution of eosinophils in the gastrointestinal tract of children. Pediatr Dev Pathol. 2006;9:210–8.
3. Ronkainen J, Talley NJ, Aro P, Storskrubb T, Johansson SE, Lind T, Bolling-Sternevald E, Vieth M, Stolte M, Walker MM, Agréus L. Prevalence of oesophageal eosinophils and eosinophilic oesophagitis in adults: the population-based Kalixanda study. Gut. 2007;56:615–20.
4. Lowichik A, Weinberg AG. A quantitative evaluation of mucosal eosinophils in the pediatric gastrointestinal tract. Mod Pathol. 1996;9:110–4.
5. Polydorides AD, Banner BF, Hannaway PJ, Yantiss RK. Evaluation of site-specific and seasonal variation in colonic mucosal eosinophils. Hum Pathol. 2008;39:832–6.
6. Pascal RR, Gramlich TL, Parker KM, Gansler TS. Geographic variations in eosinophil concentration in normal colonic mucosa. Mod Pathol. 1997;10:363–5.
7. Yantiss RK. Eosinophils in the GI tract: how many is too many and what do they mean? Mod Pathol. 2015;28(Suppl 1):S7–21.
8. Conner JR, Kirsch R. The pathology and causes of tissue eosinophilia in the gastrointestinal tract. Histopathology. 2017;71:177–99.
9. Hirano I, Moy N, Heckman MG, Thomas CS, Gonsalves N, Achem SR. Endoscopic assessment of the oesophageal features of eosinophilic oesophagitis: validation of a novel classification and grading system. Gut. 2013;62:489–95.
10. Dellon ES, Gebhart JH, Higgins LL, Hathorn KE, Woosley JT, Shaheen NJ. The esophageal biopsy "pull" sign: a highly specific and treatment-responsive endoscopic finding in eosinophilic esophagitis (with video). Gastrointest Endosc. 2016;83:92–100.
11. Kim HP, Vance RB, Shaheen NJ, Dellon ES. The prevalence and diagnostic utility of endoscopic features of eosinophilic esophagitis: a meta-analysis. Clin Gastroenterol Hepatol. 2012;10:988–996.e5.
12. Gonsalves N, Policarpio-Nicolas M, Zhang Q, Rao MS, Hirano I. Histopathologic variability and endoscopic correlates in adults with eosinophilic esophagitis. Gastrointest Endosc. 2006;64:313–9.
13. Collins MH, Martin LJ, Alexander ES, Boyd JT, Sheridan R, He H, Pentiuk S, Putnam PE, Abonia JP, Mukkada VA, Franciosi JP, Rothenberg ME. Newly developed and validated eosinophilic esophagitis histology scoring system and evidence that it outperforms peak eosinophil count for disease diagnosis and monitoring. Dis Esophagus. 2017;30:1–8.
14. Liacouras CA, Furuta GT, Hirano I, Atkins D, Attwood SE, Bonis PA, Burks AW, Chehade M, Collins MH, Dellon ES, Dohil R, Falk GW, Gonsalves N, Gupta SK, Katzka DA, Lucendo AJ, Markowitz JE, Noel RJ, Odze RD, Putnam PE, Richter JE, Romero Y, Ruchelli E, Sampson HA, Schoepfer A, Shaheen NJ, Sicherer SH, Spechler S, Spergel JM, Straumann A, Wershil BK, Rothenberg ME, Aceves SS. Eosinophilic esophagitis: updated consensus recommendations for children and adults. J Allergy Clin Immunol. 2011;128:3–20.e6.
15. Wang J, Park JY, Huang R, Souza RF, Spechler SJ, Cheng E. Obtaining adequate lamina propria for subepithelial fibrosis evaluation in pediatric eosinophilic esophagitis. Gastrointest Endosc. 2018;87:1207–1214.e3.
16. Molina-Infante J, Bredenoord AJ, Cheng E, Dellon ES, Furuta GT, Gupta SK, Hirano I, Katzka DA, Moawad FJ, Rothenberg ME, Schoepfer A, Spechler SJ, Wen T, Straumann A, Lucendo AJ, PPI-REE Task Force of the European Society of Eosinophilic Oesophagitis (EUREOS). Proton pump inhibitor-responsive oesophageal eosinophilia: an entity challenging current diagnostic criteria for eosinophilic oesophagitis. Gut. 2016;65:524–31.
17. Molina-Infante J, Hirano I, Spechler SJ, PPI-REE Task Force of the European Society of Eosinophilic Oesophagitis (EUREOS). Clarifying misunderstandings and misinterpretations about proton pump inhibitor-responsive oesophageal eosinophilia. Gut. 2017;66:1173–4.
18. Cunnion KM, Willis LK, Minto HB, Burch TC, Werner AL, Shah TA, Krishna NK, Nyalwidhe JO, Maples KM. Eosinophil quantitated urine kinetic: a novel assay for assessment of eosinophilic esophagitis. Ann Allergy Asthma Immunol. 2016;116:435–9.
19. Safroneeva E, Straumann A, Coslovsky M, Zwahlen M, Kuehni CE, Panczak R, Haas NA, Alexander JA, Dellon ES, Gonsalves N, Hirano I, Leung J, Bussmann C, Collins MH, Newbury RO, De Petris G, Smyrk TC, Woosley JT, Yan P, Yang GY, Romero Y, Katzka DA, Furuta GT, Gupta SK, Aceves SS, Chehade M, Spergel JM, Schoepfer AM, International Eosinophilic Esophagitis Activity Index Study Group. Symptoms have modest accuracy in detecting endoscopic and histologic remission in adults with eosinophilic esophagitis. Gastroenterology. 2016;150:581–590.e4.
20. Mansoor E, Cooper GS. The 2010–2015 prevalence of eosinophilic esophagitis in the USA: a population-based study. Dig Dis Sci. 2016;61:2928–34.
21. Krupp NL, Sehra S, Slaven JE, Kaplan MH, Gupta S, Tepper RS. Increased prevalence of airway reactivity in children with eosinophilic esophagitis. Pediatr Pulmonol. 2016;51:478–83.
22. Blanchard C, Wang N, Stringer KF, Mishra A, Fulkerson PC, Abonia JP, Jameson SC, Kirby C, Konikoff MR, Collins MH, Cohen MB, Akers R, Hogan SP, Assa'ad AH, Putnam PE, Aronow BJ, Rothenberg ME. Eotaxin-3 and a uniquely conserved gene-expression profile in eosinophilic esophagitis. J Clin Invest. 2006;116:536–47.
23. Alexander ES, Martin LJ, Collins MH, Kottyan LC, Sucharew H, He H, Mukkada VA, Succop PA, Abonia JP, Foote H, Eby MD, Grotjan TM, Greenler AJ, Dellon ES, Demain JG, Furuta GT, Gurian LE, Harley JB, Hopp RJ, Kagalwalla A, Kaul A, Nadeau KC, Noel RJ, Putnam PE, von Tiehl KF, Rothenberg ME. Twin and family studies reveal strong environmental and weaker genetic cues explaining heritability of eosinophilic esophagitis. J Allergy Clin Immunol. 2014;134:1084–1092.e1.
24. Markowitz JE, Spergel JM, Ruchelli E, Liacouras CA. Elemental diet is an effective treatment for eosinophilic esophagitis in children and adolescents. Am J Gastroenterol. 2003;98:777–82.
25. Peterson KA, Byrne KR, Vinson LA, Ying J, Boynton KK, Fang JC, Gleich GJ, Adler DG, Clayton F. Elemental diet induces histologic response in adult eosinophilic esophagitis. Am J Gastroenterol. 2013;108:759–66.
26. Warners MJ, Vlieg-Boerstra BJ, Verheij J, van Rhijn BD, Van Ampting MT, Harthoorn LF, de Jonge WJ, Smout AJ, Bredenoord AJ. Elemental diet decreases inflammation and improves symptoms in adult eosinophilic oesophagitis patients. Aliment Pharmacol Ther. 2017;45:777–87.
27. Molina-Infante J, Arias A, Barrio J, Rodriguez-Sanchez J, Sanchez-Cazalilla M, Lucendo AJ. Four-food group elimination diet for adult eosinophilic esophagitis: a prospective multicenter study. J Allergy Clin Immunol. 2014;134:1093–1099.e1.
28. Rodriguez-Sanchez J, Gomez Torrijos E, Lopez Viedma B, de la Santa BE, Martin Davila F, Garcia Rodriguez C, Feo Brito F, Olmedo Camacho J, Reales Figueroa P, Molina-Infante J. Efficacy of IgE-targeted vs empiric six-food elimination diets for adult eosinophilic oesophagitis. Allergy. 2014;69:936–42.
29. Arias A, Gonzalez-Cervera J, Tenias JM, Lucendo AJ. Efficacy of dietary interventions for inducing histologic remission in patients with eosinophilic esophagitis: a systematic review and meta-analysis. Gastroenterology. 2014;146:1639–48.

30. Fogg MI, Ruchelli E, Spergel JM. Pollen and eosinophilic esophagitis. J Allergy Clin Immunol. 2003;112:796–7.
31. van Rhijn BD, Verheij J, van den Bergh Weerman MA, Verseijden C, van den Wijngaard RM, de Jonge WJ, Smout AJ, Bredenoord AJ. Histological response to fluticasone propionate in patients with eosinophilic esophagitis is associated with improved functional esophageal mucosal integrity. Am J Gastroenterol. 2015;110:1289–97.
32. Mangla S, Goldin AH, Singal G, Hornick JL, Hsu Blatman KS, Burakoff R, Chan WW. Endoscopic features and eosinophil density are associated with food impaction in adults with esophageal eosinophilia. Dig Dis Sci. 2016;61:2578–84.
33. Assa'ad AH, Gupta SK, Collins MH, Thomson M, Heath AT, Smith DA, Perschy TL, Jurgensen CH, Ortega HG, Aceves SS. An antibody against IL-5 reduces numbers of esophageal intraepithelial eosinophils in children with eosinophilic esophagitis. Gastroenterology. 2011;141:1593–604.
34. Straumann A, Blanchard C, Radonjic-Hoesli S, Bussmann C, Hruz P, Safroneeva E, Simon D, Schoepfer AM, Simon HU. A new eosinophilic esophagitis (EoE)-like disease without tissue eosinophilia found in EoE families. Allergy. 2016;71:889–900.
35. O'Shea KM, Aceves SS, Dellon ES, Gupta SK, Spergel JM, Furuta GT, Rothenberg ME. Pathophysiology of eosinophilic esophagitis. Gastroenterology. 2018;154:333–45.
36. Kitajima M, Lee HC, Nakayama T, Ziegler SF. TSLP enhances the function of helper type 2 cells. Eur J Immunol. 2011;41:1862–71.
37. Litosh VA, Rochman M, Rymer JK, Porollo A, Kottyan LC, Rothenberg ME. Calpain-14 and its association with eosinophilic esophagitis. J Allergy Clin Immunol. 2017;139:1762–1771.e7.
38. Rieder F, Nonevski I, Ma J, Ouyang Z, West G, Protheroe C, DePetris G, et al. T-helper 2 cytokines, transforming growth factor beta1, and eosinophil products induce fibrogenesis and alter muscle motility in patients with eosinophilic esophagitis. Gastroenterology. 2014;146:1266–1277.e1–9.
39. Eluri S, Runge TM, Cotton CC, Burk CM, Wolf WA, Woosley JT, Shaheen NJ, Dellon ES. The extremely narrow-caliber esophagus is a treatment-resistant subphenotype of eosinophilic esophagitis. Gastrointest Endosc. 2016;83:1142–8.
40. Aceves SS. Unmet therapeutic needs in eosinophilic esophagitis. Dig Dis. 2014;32:143–8.
41. Clayton F, Fang JC, Gleich GJ, Lucendo AJ, Olalla JM, Vinson LA, Lowichik A, Chen X, Emerson L, Cox K, O'Gorman MA, Peterson KA. Eosinophilic esophagitis in adults is associated with IgG4 and not mediated by IgE. Gastroenterology. 2014;147:602–9.
42. Shah SC, Tepler A, Peek RM Jr, Colombel JF, Hirano I, Narula N. Association between Helicobacter pylori exposure and decreased odds of eosinophilic esophagitis: a systematic review and meta-analysis. Clin Gastroenterol Hepatol. 2019;17:2185–2198.e3.
43. Rothenberg ME. Eosinophilic gastrointestinal disorders (EGID). J Allergy Clin Immunol. 2004;113:11–28; quiz 29.
44. Pusztaszeri MP, Genta RM, Cryer BL. Drug-induced injury in the gastrointestinal tract: clinical and pathologic considerations. Nat Clin Pract Gastroenterol Hepatol. 2007;4:442–53.
45. Muraoka A, Suehiro I, Fujii M, Nagata K, Kusunoki H, Kumon Y, Shirasaka D, Hosooka T, Murakami K. Acute gastric anisakiasis: 28 cases during the last 10 years. Dig Dis Sci. 1996;41:2362–5.
46. Rivasi F, Pampiglione S, Boldorini R, Cardinale L. Histopathology of gastric and duodenal Strongyloides stercoralis locations in fifteen immunocompromised subjects. Arch Pathol Lab Med. 2006;130:1792–8.
47. Genta RM, Lew GM, Graham DY. Changes in the gastric mucosa following eradication of Helicobacter pylori. Mod Pathol. 1993;6:281–9.
48. Nanagas VC, Kovalszki A. Gastrointestinal manifestations of hypereosinophilic syndromes and mast cell disorders: a comprehensive review. Clin Rev Allergy Immunol. 2019;57:194–212.
49. Barak N, Hart J, Sitrin MD. Enalapril-induced eosinophilic gastroenteritis. J Clin Gastroenterol. 2001;33:157–8.
50. Brown IS, Smith J, Rosty C. Gastrointestinal pathology in celiac disease: a case series of 150 consecutive newly diagnosed patients. Am J Clin Pathol. 2012;138:42–9.
51. Casella G, Villanacci V, Fisogni S, Cambareri AR, Di Bella C, Corazzi N, Gorla S, Baldini V, Bassotti G. Colonic left-side increase of eosinophils: a clue to drug-related colitis in adults. Aliment Pharmacol Ther. 2009;29:535–41.
52. Bridges AJ, Marshall JB, Diaz-Arias AA. Acute eosinophilic colitis and hypersensitivity reaction associated with naproxen therapy. Am J Med. 1990;89:526–7.
53. Jimenez-Saenz M, Gonzalez-Campora R, Linares-Santiago E, Herrerias-Gutierrez JM. Bleeding colonic ulcer and eosinophilic colitis: a rare complication of nonsteroidal anti-inflammatory drugs. J Clin Gastroenterol. 2006;40:84–5.
54. Anttila VJ, Valtonen M. Carbamazepine-induced eosinophilic colitis. Epilepsia. 1992;33:119–21.
55. Friedberg JW, Frankenburg FR, Burk J, Johnson W. Clozapine-caused eosinophilic colitis. Ann Clin Psychiatry. 1995;7:97–8.
56. Saeed SA, Integlia MJ, Pleskow RG, Calenda KA, Rohrer RJ, Dayal Y, Grand RJ. Tacrolimus-associated eosinophilic gastroenterocolitis in pediatric liver transplant recipients: role of potential food allergies in pathogenesis. Pediatr Transplant. 2006;10:730–5.
57. Star KV, Ho VT, Wang HH, Odze RD. Histologic features in colon biopsies can discriminate mycophenolate from GVHD-induced colitis. Am J Surg Pathol. 2013;37:1319–28.
58. Lange P, Oun H, Fuller S, Turney JH. Eosinophilic colitis due to rifampicin. Lancet. 1994;344:1296–7.
59. Doyle LA, Sepehr GJ, Hamilton MJ, Akin C, Castells MC, Hornick JL. A clinicopathologic study of 24 cases of systemic mastocytosis involving the gastrointestinal tract and assessment of mucosal mast cell density in irritable bowel syndrome and asymptomatic patients. Am J Surg Pathol. 2014;38:832–43.
60. Dvorak AM, Monahan RA, Osage JE, Dickersin GR. Crohn's disease: transmission electron microscopic studies. II. Immunologic inflammatory response: alterations of mast cells, basophils, eosinophils, and the microvasculature. Hum Pathol. 1980;11:606–19.
61. Dvorak AM. Ultrastructural evidence for release of major basic protein-containing crystalline cores of eosinophil granules in vivo: cytotoxic potential in Crohn's disease. J Immunol. 1980;125:460–2.
62. Saitoh O, Kojima K, Sugi K, Matsuse R, Uchida K, Tabata K, Nakagawa K, Kayazawa M, Hirata I, Katsu K. Fecal eosinophil granule-derived proteins reflect disease activity in inflammatory bowel disease. Am J Gastroenterol. 1999;94:3513–20.
63. Peterson CG, Sangfelt P, Wagner M, Hansson T, Lettesjo H, Carlson M. Fecal levels of leukocyte markers reflect disease activity in patients with ulcerative colitis. Scand J Clin Lab Invest. 2007;67:810–20.
64. Dubucquoi S, Janin A, Klein O, Desreumaux P, Quandalle P, Cortot A, Capron M, Colombel JF. Activated eosinophils and interleukin 5 expression in early recurrence of Crohn's disease. Gut. 1995;37:242–6.
65. Masterson JC, McNamee EN, Fillon SA, Hosford L, Harris R, Fernando SD, Jedlicka P, Iwamoto R, Jacobsen E, Protheroe C, Eltzschig HK, Colgan SP, Arita M, Lee JJ, Furuta GT. Eosinophil-mediated signalling attenuates inflammatory responses in experimental colitis. Gut. 2015;64:1236–47.
66. Ahrens R, Waddell A, Seidu L, Blanchard C, Carey R, Forbes E, Lampinen M, Wilson T, Cohen E, Stringer K, Ballard E, Munitz A, Xu H, Lee N, Lee JJ, Rothenberg ME, Denson L, Hogan SP. Intestinal macrophage/epithelial cell-derived CCL11/eotaxin-1 mediates eosinophil recruitment and function in pediatric ulcerative colitis. J Immunol. 2008;181:7390–9.
67. Maltby S, Wohlfarth C, Gold M, Zbytnuik L, Hughes MR, McNagny KM. CD34 is required for infiltration of eosinophils into

the colon and pathology associated with DSS-induced ulcerative colitis. Am J Pathol. 2010;177:1244–54.
68. Hahn HP, Hornick JL. Immunoreactivity for CD25 in gastrointestinal mucosal mast cells is specific for systemic mastocytosis. Am J Surg Pathol. 2007;31:1669–76.
69. Sokol H, Georgin-Lavialle S, Canioni D, Barete S, Damaj G, Soucie E, Bruneau J, Chandesris MO, Suarez F, Launay JM, Aouba A, Grandpeix-Guyodo C, Lanternier F, Grosbois B, de Gennes C, Cathébras P, Fain O, Hoyeau-Idrissi N, Dubreuil P, Lortholary O, Beaugerie L, Ranque B, Hermine O. Gastrointestinal manifestations in mastocytosis: a study of 83 patients. J Allergy Clin Immunol. 2013;132:866–873.e1–3.
70. Drossman DA, Dumitrascu DL. Rome III: new standard for functional gastrointestinal disorders. J Gastrointestin Liver Dis. 2006;15:237–41.
71. Manning AP, Thompson WG, Heaton KW, Morris AF. Towards positive diagnosis of the irritable bowel. Br Med J. 1978;2:653–4.
72. Barbara G, Stanghellini V, De Giorgio R, Cremon C, Cottrell GS, Santini D, Pasquinelli G, Morselli-Labate AM, Grady EF, Bunnett NW, Collins SM, Corinaldesi R. Activated mast cells in proximity to colonic nerves correlate with abdominal pain in irritable bowel syndrome. Gastroenterology. 2004;126:693–702.
73. Barbara G, Wang B, Stanghellini V, de Giorgio R, Cremon C, Di Nardo G, Trevisani M, Campi B, Geppetti P, Tonini M, Bunnett NW, Grundy D, Corinaldesi R. Mast cell-dependent excitation of visceral-nociceptive sensory neurons in irritable bowel syndrome. Gastroenterology. 2007;132:26–37.
74. Jakate S, Demeo M, John R, Tobin M, Keshavarzian A. Mastocytic enterocolitis: increased mucosal mast cells in chronic intractable diarrhea. Arch Pathol Lab Med. 2006;130:362–7.
75. Akhavein MA, Patel NR, Muniyappa PK, Glover SC. Allergic mastocytic gastroenteritis and colitis: an unexplained etiology in chronic abdominal pain and gastrointestinal dysmotility. Gastroenterol Res Pract. 2012;2012:950582.
76. Carter MC, Metcalfe DD, Komarow HD. Mastocytosis. Immunol Allergy Clin N Am. 2014;34:181–96.
77. Castells M, Austen KF. Mastocytosis: mediator-related signs and symptoms. Int Arch Allergy Immunol. 2002;127:147–52.
78. Cohen SS, Skovbo S, Vestergaard H, Kristensen T, Moller M, Bindslev-Jensen C, Fryzek JP, Broesby-Olsen S. Epidemiology of systemic mastocytosis in Denmark. Br J Haematol. 2014;166:521–8.
79. Jensen RT. Gastrointestinal abnormalities and involvement in systemic mastocytosis. Hematol Oncol Clin North Am. 2000;14:579–623.
80. Johncilla M, Jessurun J, Brown I, Hornick JL, Bellizzi AM, Shia J, Yantiss RK. Are enterocolic mucosal mast cell aggregates clinically relevant in patients without suspected or established systemic mastocytosis? Am J Surg Pathol. 2018;42:1390–5.
81. Caplan RM. The natural course of urticaria pigmentosa. Analysis and follow-up of 112 cases. Arch Dermatol. 1963;87:146–57.
82. Escribano L, Alvarez-Twose I, Sánchez-Muñoz L, Garcia-Montero A, Núñez R, Almeida J, Jara-Acevedo M, Teodósio C, García-Cosío M, Bellas C, Orfao A. Prognosis in adult indolent systemic mastocytosis: a long-term study of the Spanish Network on Mastocytosis in a series of 145 patients. J Allergy Clin Immunol. 2009;124:514–21.
83. Ryan RJ, Akin C, Castells M, Wills M, Selig MK, Nielsen GP, Ferry JA, Hornick JL. Mast cell sarcoma: a rare and potentially under-recognized diagnostic entity with specific therapeutic implications. Mod Pathol. 2013;26:533–43.
84. Piao X, Bernstein A. A point mutation in the catalytic domain of c-kit induces growth factor independence, tumorigenicity, and differentiation of mast cells. Blood. 1996;87(8):3117–23.
85. Jawhar M, Schwaab J, Naumann N, Horny HP, Sotlar K, Haferlach T, Metzgeroth G, Fabarius A, Valent P, Hofmann WK, Cross NCP, Meggendorfer M, Reiter A. Response and progression on midostaurin in advanced systemic mastocytosis: KIT D816V and other molecular markers. Blood. 2017;130:137–45.
86. Falchi L, Verstovsek S. Kit mutations: new insights and diagnostic value. Immunol Allergy Clin N Am. 2018;38:411–28.
87. Hamilton MJ. Nonclonal mast cell activation syndrome: a growing body of evidence. Immunol Allergy Clin N Am. 2018;38: 469–81.
88. Geissmann F, Thomas C, Emile JF, Micheau M, Canioni D, Cerf-Bensussan N, Lazarovits AI, Brousse N, The French Langerhans Cell Histiocytosis Study Group. Digestive tract involvement in Langerhans cell histiocytosis. J Pediatr. 1996;129:836–45.
89. Hait E, Liang M, Degar B, Glickman J, Fox VL. Gastrointestinal tract involvement in Langerhans cell histiocytosis: case report and literature review. Pediatrics. 2006;118:e1593–9.
90. Sharma S, Gupta M. A colonic polyp due to Langerhans cell histiocytosis: a lesion not to be confused with metastatic malignant melanoma. Histopathology. 2006;49:438–9.
91. Singhi AD, Montgomery EA. Gastrointestinal tract Langerhans cell histiocytosis: a clinicopathologic study of 12 patients. Am J Surg Pathol. 2011;35:305–10.
92. Dupeux M, Boccara O, Frassati-Biaggi A, Hélias-Rodzewicz Z, Leclerc-Mercier S, Bodemer C, Molina TJ, Emile JF, Fraitag S. Langerhans cell histiocytoma: a benign histiocytic neoplasm of diverse lines of terminal differentiation. Am J Dermatopathol. 2019;41:29–36.
93. Foucar E, Rosai J, Dorfman R. Sinus histiocytosis with massive lymphadenopathy (Rosai-Dorfman disease): review of the entity. Semin Diagn Pathol. 1990;7:19–73.
94. Rosai J, Dorfman RF. Sinus histiocytosis with massive lymphadenopathy: a pseudolymphomatous benign disorder: analysis of 34 cases. Cancer. 1972;30:1174–88.
95. Campochiaro C, Tomelleri A, Cavalli G, Berti A, Dagna L. Erdheim-Chester disease. Eur J Intern Med. 2015;26:223–9.
96. Dehner LP. Juvenile xanthogranulomas in the first two decades of life: a clinicopathologic study of 174 cases with cutaneous and extracutaneous manifestations. Am J Surg Pathol. 2003;27:579–93.
97. De Petris G, Leung ST. Pseudoneoplasms of the gastrointestinal tract. Arch Pathol Lab Med. 2010;134:378–92.
98. Turner KO, Sinkre RA, Neumann WL, Genta RM. Primary colonic eosinophilia and eosinophilic colitis in adults. Am J Surg Pathol. 2017;41:225–33.
99. Hurrell JM, Genta RM, Melton SD. Histopathologic diagnosis of eosinophilic conditions in the gastrointestinal tract. Adv Anat Pathol. 2011;18:335–48.

Motility Disorders of the Gastrointestinal Tract

13

Raffaella Morotti and Dhanpat Jain

List of Frequently Asked Questions

1. What kind of tissue specimens are ideal if you anticipate a motility disorder of the gastrointestinal tract?
2. How to triage tissues for special studies if a biopsy or resection specimen is sent to the pathology lab?
3. What special stains are useful for the work-up of mobility disorders?
4. What is the role of electron microscopy in evaluation of motility disorders?
5. What is the clinical information that pathologist should seek while working up cases of motility disorders?
6. How are gastrointestinal motility disorders classified and what are the distinctive pathologic features?
7. What are various systemic disorders that are associated with motility disorders?
8. What are the histopathologic features of scleroderma involvement of the bowel?
9. What are the common histopathologic findings in cases of achalasia cardia?
10. What is postinfectious intestinal pseudo-obstruction?
11. What are the infiltrative disorders that lead to intestinal pseudo-obstruction?
12. How do you evaluate resection specimens from patients with chronic idiopathic constipation and intestinal pseudo-obstruction?
13. What medications are known to be associated with motility disorders?
14. What is the most common presentation of Hirschsprung disease and what biopsy type is preferred and adequate for the diagnosis?
15. How do you triage biopsy tissues in a suspected case of Hirschsprung disease?
16. In a suspected case of Hirschsprung disease how do you evaluate the biopsies and what special stains are useful?
17. What is the role of intraoperative consultation during pull-through surgery for a Hirschsprung disease patient?
18. How do you evaluate the resections performed for a Hirschsprung disease?
19. Is persistence of symptoms frequent after surgical resection for Hirschsprung disease and what are the implications?
20. What is intestinal neuronal dysplasia?
21. What is hypoganglionosis and how do you evaluate the number of ganglia in the gastrointestinal tract and what does it mean?
22. Abnormalities of which components of neurohormonal apparatus of the gastrointestinal tract lead to bowel dysmotility?

Frequently Asked Questions

1. What kind of tissue specimens are ideal if you anticipate a motility disorder of the gastrointestinal tract?

A variety of specimens, as discussed below, are evaluated for motility disorders. Examination of full-thickness seromuscular biopsies or resection specimens are ideal, although this is not always feasible. In many disorders, the diagnosis is established based on clinical findings. Mucosal biopsies have a very limited role, barring few exceptions, and are seldom performed.

The role of different types of specimens in the evaluation of motility disorders of the gastrointestinal (GI) tract.

1. Suction mucosal biopsies. The mucosal biopsies are either normal or show only nonspecific findings, and thus, are of limited value in the workup of GI motility disorders except Hirschsprung disease. Their role is largely to exclude a primary mucosal pathology. In some disorders such as irritable bowel syndrome (IBS) a variety of mucosal changes have been described, but these lack diagnostic specificity and their evaluation is largely

R. Morotti (✉) · D. Jain
Yale University School of Medicine, New Haven, CT, USA
e-mail: raffaella.morotti@yale.edu

H. L. Wang, Z. E. Chen (eds.), *Practical Gastrointestinal Pathology*, Practical Anatomic Pathology,
https://doi.org/10.1007/978-3-030-51268-2_13

limited to research. On the other hand, suction mucosal biopsies of the rectum, which provide deeper tissue compared to conventional endoscopic biopsies, have become the standard method of practice in the diagnostic workup of Hirschsprung disease (see later).

2. Full thickness/seromuscular biopsy. An appropriate diagnostic workup of GI motility disorders often requires a full thickness biopsy. Full thickness biopsies with immunohistochemical (IHC) analysis and electron microscopy (EM) have shown to be useful in identifying myopathic or neuropathic changes. However, the appropriate site and number of biopsies needed to establish a diagnosis in this regard have not been established. Biopsies can be obtained laparoscopically or by open surgery. In general, for patients with localized disease, samples from the most affected/dilated segment of bowel along with uninvolved areas for comparison are considered most helpful. For generalized disease, biopsies from the first available loop of the jejunum, about 15 cm distal to the ligament of Trietz, has been suggested since this coincides with the location to measure small bowel motor activity by manometry. A sample size of 1–1.5 cm^2 is generally considered adequate. Some disorders tend to be patchy, so multiple samples are recommended, but hardly ever obtained in clinical practice. Thus, the specimen may confirm, but does not exclude the diagnosis of a neuromuscular disorder. The surgeons can help by selecting tissues from areas most likely to yield positive histology, namely, the dilated thin segments of bowel wall showing abnormal contractility. Some also like to take a control biopsy from the unaffected segment for comparison. Most of these biopsies tend to be taken longitudinally so that when it is embedded on edge only the circular muscle is seen in cross section. Ideally, if a square of muscularis propria is taken, it is worth taking a transverse section from both ends across the longitudinal muscle, and then cutting the rest longitudinally so that both muscle coats can be assessed with ease. Whenever feasible, some tissue should be frozen, and some immediately fixed in gluteraldehyde for EM. The biopsy should then be immediately fixed in neutral buffered formalin, pinned to a cork or sylgard board with the mucosal surface in contact with the board to allow good fixation of the muscle layers. Care should be taken not to stretch the biopsy. As mentioned above, ideally, both longitudinal and transverse sections should be obtained from the biopsy. Special stains can be decided after evaluation of initial hematoxylin and eosin (H&E) stains. For studying neural networks and interstitial cells of Cajal (ICC), whole mount or en face sections offer a distinct advantage. However, these studies require special expertise and are largely limited to research.

3. Resection specimens. Resections for GI motility disorders performed for treatment provide the best specimens for diagnostic workup. Small bowel and large bowel resections are handled similarly. The specimens should be fixed immediately after cleansing of the lumen and after taking frozen samples for histochemistry and tissues fixed in gluteraldehyde for potential EM. From the large bowel, samples should be obtained from the ascending colon, transverse colon, left/sigmoid colon, and rectum. Sections from the intestines should be obtained from the transverse and longitudinal axis; although, in general, transverse sections are more informative. Longitudinal sections can produce an erroneous impression of thinning or thickening of the longitudinal muscle layer, depending on whether tenia coli have been included in the sections or not. Resections for achalasia and gastroparesis should be handled similarly.

References: [1–4]

2. How to triage tissues for special studies if a biopsy or resection specimen is sent to the pathology lab?

The specimens should be fixed immediately. If there is enough tissue, frozen samples for histochemistry, and tissue fixed in glutaraldehyde for EM should be kept. However, for laboratories that do not have access to EM, this can be omitted as the role of EM has been declining over the years, while at the same time molecular diagnostics is becoming readily applicable in clinical practice.

3. What special stains are useful for the workup of motility disorders?

A variety of histochemical and IHC stains are helpful in the workup of motility disorders and need to be chosen after the intial evalutionof the H&E stain, clinical setting, and differential diagnosis.

Histochemical stains Connective tissue stains, such as trichrome or Verhoeff-van Gieson, are helpful in delineating the pattern of fibrosis. Periodic acid-Schiff (PAS) stain, with and without diastase, highlights polyglucosamine inclusion bodies, whereas Congo red is useful for identifying amyloid. In many cases, amyloid deposition is suspected on H&E stain, while in some it can be subtle. The role of acetylcholinesterase (AchE) stain in the workup of Hirschsprung disease is discussed in detail later in the chapter. Modified Gomori trichrome, cytochrome C and succinic dehydrogenase stains are useful to demonstrate mitochondrial abnormalities in patients with mitochondrial myopathies, and require frozen tissues. Silver staining techniques, for studying the neural networks, are now obsolete and have been replaced by IHC stains.

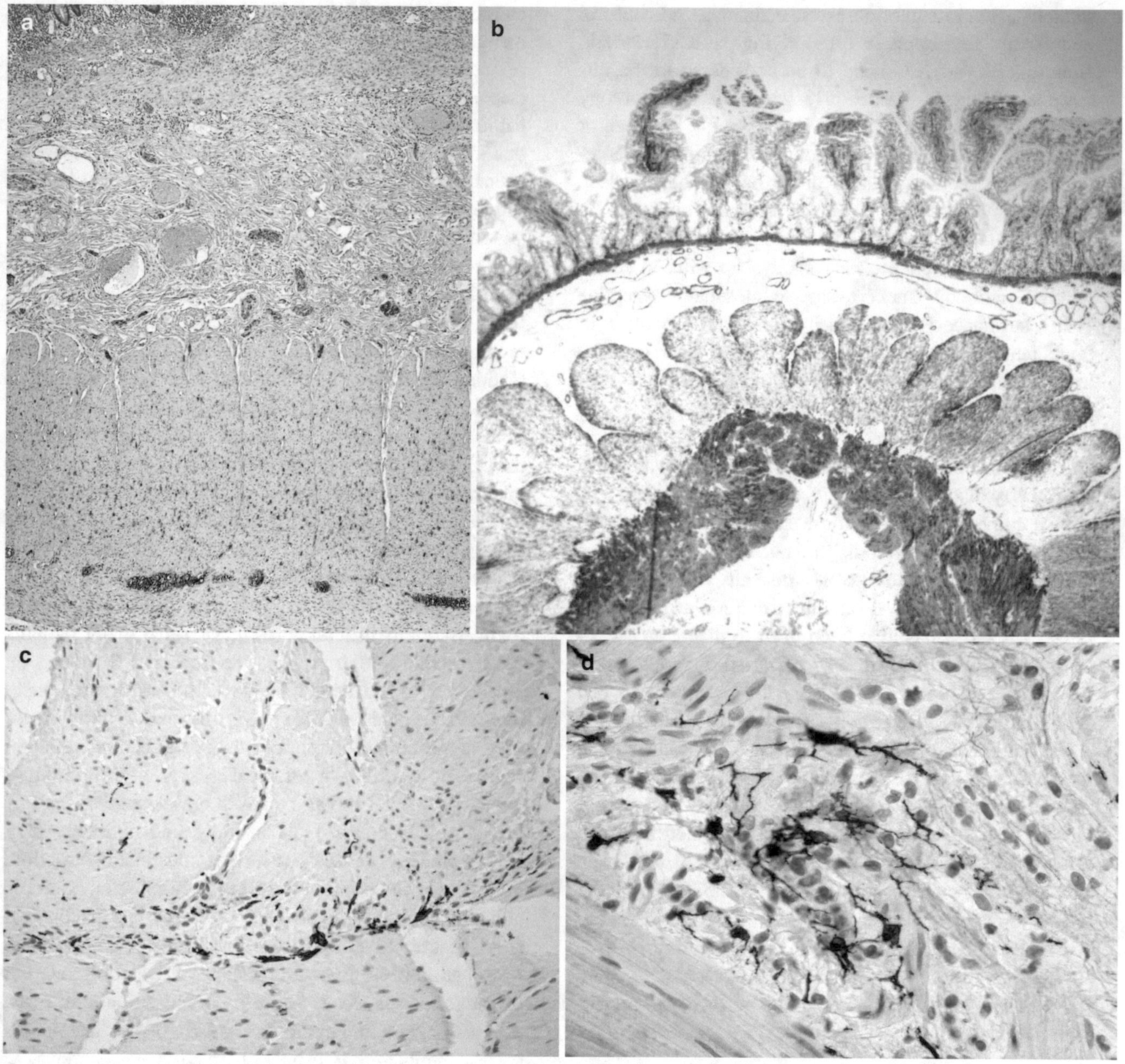

Fig. 13.1 (**a**) S-100 stain to show the myenteric and submucosal plexuses. (**b**) SMA immunostain to show loss of staining in the inner circular muscle layer of the muscularis propria of the small bowel. (**c**) DOG1 stain showing the distribution of ICCs around the myenteric plexuses. (**d**) High power showing dendritic morphology of the ICCs in a tangential section

IHC stains A variety of IHC stains are helpful in evaluating cases in which routine histological examination is either normal, nonspecific, or nondiagnostic. These include stains to highlight myofilaments, neural plexus, ganglion cells, ICCs, viral infections, and neurohormonal peptides. For highlighting the neural plexus, one can use S-100, PGP 9.5, or NSE (Fig 13.1a). Antibodies suggested to be useful for identification of myofilaments include alpha smooth muscle actin (αSMA), smoothelin, caldesmon, and desmin. Of these, αSMA staining is the most useful (Fig 13.1b), whereas others such as smooth muscle myosin heavy chain, smoothelin, and histone deacetylase 8 remain of unclear signfincance. These stains may show decreased expression in the muscle layers despite normal staining with αSMA. Desmin myopathy is often a systemic disease diagnosed with skeletal muscle biopsies. ICCs are difficult to appreciate on H&E stained tissue and require c-kit (CD117) or DOG1 (Ano1) stains. DOG1 is superior to c-kit since it does not stain mast cells (Fig 13.1c, d). However, most studies that evaluated ICCs (quantitative or qualitative) have been performed using the c-kit antibody. Quantitation of ICCs and evaluation of their network are difficult on routine tissue sections. It requires experience and appropriate controls. Whole mount and en face

sections using immunofluorescence staining and confocal microscopy are important for studying the ICC network. Abnormalities of ICC need to be considered in the differential diagnosis, particularly when routine histology is unremarkable (Fig 13.2a–f). Although the presence or absence of ICC is usually appreciated on routine formalin-fixed tissue sections, subtle abnormalities of the deep muscular/submucosal ICC plexus are better evaluated on frozen tissue, with immunofluorescence. A more detailed evaluation of the enteric nervous system with an elaborate IHC antibody panel (vasoactive intestinal polypeptide (VIP), substance P/related tachykinins, nitric oxide synthase, neuropeptide Y, calcitonin gene-related and peptide) has not been validated for routine clinical use.
References: [5–11]

4. **What is the role of electron microscopy in evaluation of motility disorders?**

EM can be valuable in some cases, particularly when light microscopy is nondiagnostic. Many degenerative changes in the muscle cells, neurons, or mitochondria are best identified on ultrastructural examination (Fig 13.2f). EM has also been used to diagnose a variety of lysosomal storage disorders and different tissue types have been used for diagnostic purposes. In one such study, foamy ganglion cells were identified in the Auerbach plexus on routine sections (Fig 13.3a, b) and then confirmed with ultrastructure to show zebra bodies. Rectal biopsies have been used in the past to diagnose storage disease, especially those involving neurons, as it allows easier access to these cells compared to a brain biopsy. Often other tissues like skin, conjuctiva, blood, or marrow are used where possible or applicable. More so, EM for clinical practice is now available in only limited institutions and increasingly molecular tests are used for making diagnosis of genetic disorders.
Reference: [12]

5. **What is the clinical information that pathologist should seek while working up cases of motility disorders?**

Diagnosis of motility disorders is challenging for both clinicians and pathologists. Thus, the diagnostic approach to patients with GI dysmotility requires careful evaluation of the patient's clinical presentation, family history, medication use, exposure to toxins, imaging and physical findings, and pathologic features. The age of onset of symptoms, family history, duration of symptoms, associated systemic disorders, other organ involvments, history of medication or use of recreational drugs, and results of functional bowel studies are all important information that the pathologist should seek when handling cases of motility disorders. Clinically, early onset of symptoms in childhood or in the neonatal period suggests a developmental or congenital etiology, whereas the vast majority of motility disorders diagnosed in adults are acquired (secondary). Many disorders, particularly chronic idiopathic intestinal pseudo-obstruction, have an insidious onset. Thus, the chronic nature of the disease may not be overtly obvious. A positive family history may help in suggesting an inherited disorder; however, it is often negative since the disease in the affected family members may be mild or subclinical, and they may not seek clinical attention. The presence of other associated abnormalities (e.g., external opthalmoplegia), dilatation of other segments of GI tract or other viscera (e.g., duodenum, gallbladder, or urinary bladder) also help point toward an inherited form of visceral myopathy. Careful evaluation of associated symptoms or signs can often help determine the primary cause of bowel dysmotility. Occasionally, the underlying systemic disorder may be diagnosed only after pathologic evaluation of the bowel specimen, as in some collagen-vascular disorders such as scleroderma, while diabetes and hypothyroidism are often diagnosed clinically. A positive history of medication use, or exposure to toxin, is often difficult to evaluate since many patients consume multiple drugs, and the impact of the drugs on bowel motility may not be well known, or previously reported. A positive history of a preceding viral illness may suggest a possible infectious/postinfectious cause of pseudo-obstruction. In some cases, serology for circulating anti-neuronal and anti-smooth muscle antibodies may be helpful. Endoscopy, laparotomy, and radiology may help exclude mechanical causes of intestinal obstruction. Functional evaluation of the GI motlity using manometry, although not essential, also helps differentiate mechanical from functional obstruction. It also helps differentiate neuropathic from myopathic causes of dysmotility. Other investigations, such as neurologic and autonomic tests, may also play a role in the diagnostic workup. The majority of patients with intestinal obstruction are secondary to mechanical causes (e.g., adhesions, extrinsic compression, or internal hernia). At present, molecular and genetic tests play a very limited role in the diagnostic workup of motility disorders; although, with increasing use of molecular diagnostics one can anticipate that these may play an important role in the diagnosis of inherited disorders, particularly unsuspected mitochondrial disorders. Serum lactate and thymidine phosphorylase activities, brain MRI, and muscle biopsies, are all essential in the diagnosis of mitochondrial disorders. Recently, alteration in *FLNA* and *ACTG2* genes have been linked to certain forms of intestinal psuedo-obstruction. It is anticipated that genetic tests are likely to be used more frequently in the future for the diagnosis of GI motility disorders.
References: [13–20]

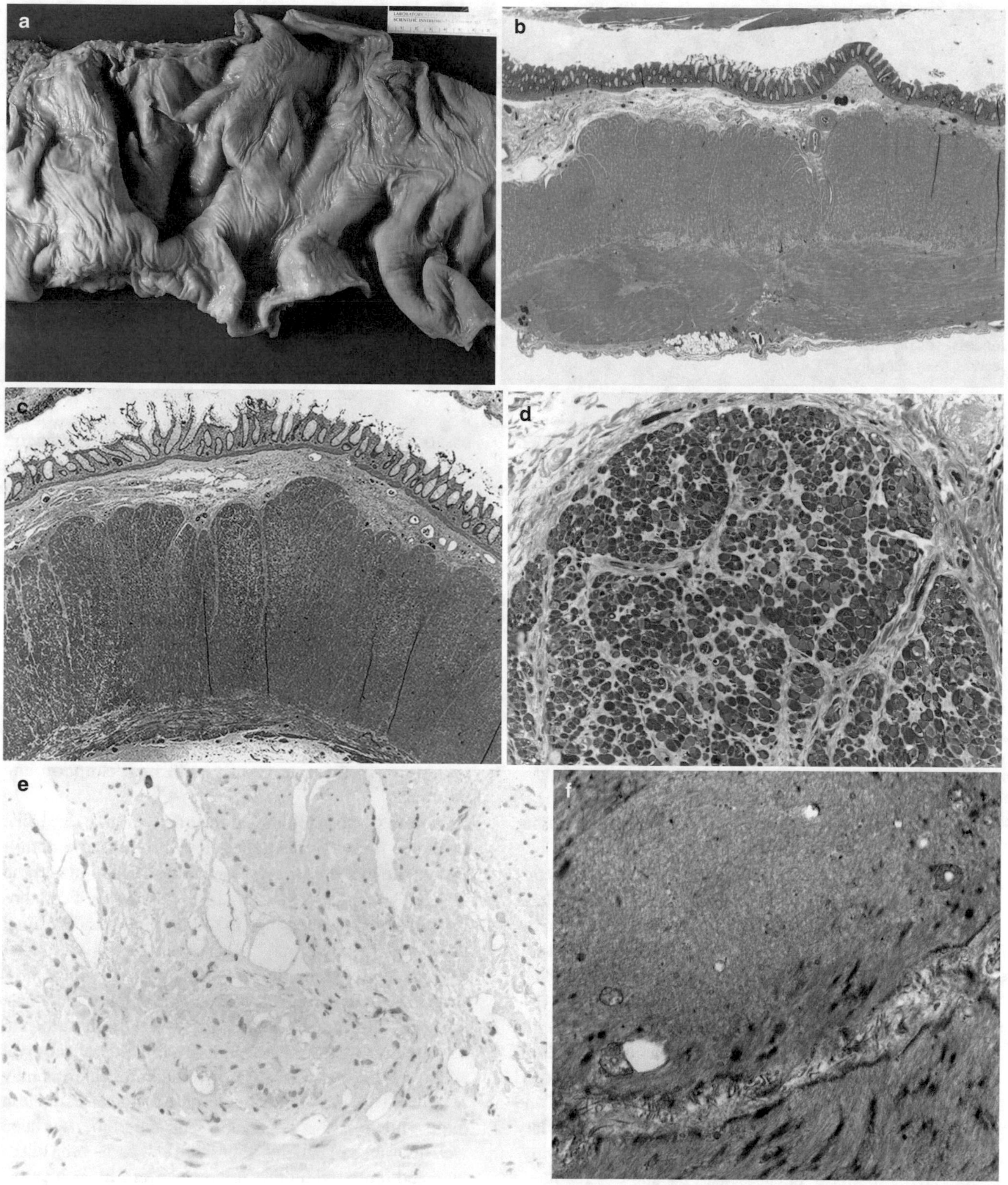

Fig. 13.2 A case of visceral myopathy with loss of ICC. (**a**) Gross photograph of the large bowel showing marked dilation. (**b**) Low magnification of the H&E stain showing marked thickening of both layers of the muscularis propria, normal mucosa, and normal appearing submucosal and myenteric plexuses. (**c**, **d**) Trichrome stain at low and higher magnifications showing interstitial fibrosis of the inner layer of muscularis propria with atrophy of the muscle fibers. (**e**) DOG1 stain showing complete loss of ICCs. (**f**) Electron micrograph of the muscle cells showing disorganized myofilaments

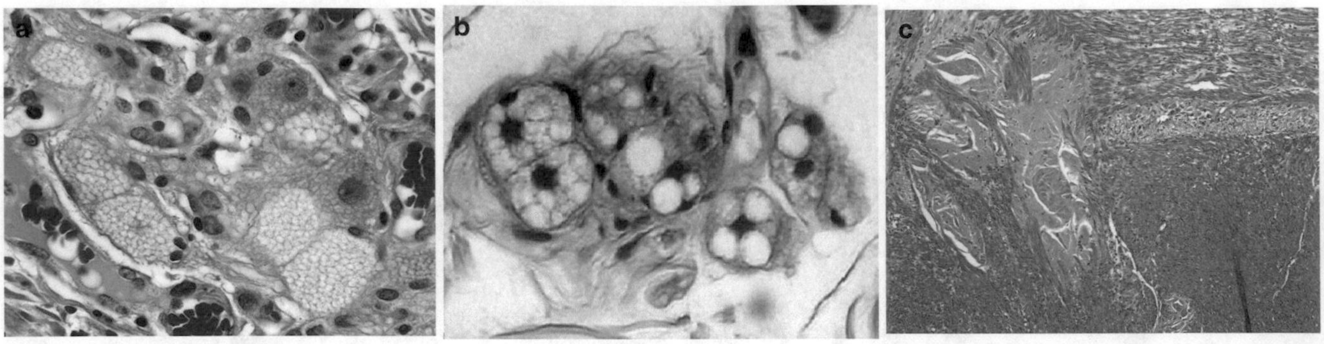

Fig. 13.3 (**a**) Ganglion cells of Auerbach plexus appear markedly foamy due to accumulation of globotriaosylceramide (GL3) in lysosomes secondary to deficiency in lysosomal α-galactosidase A (Fabry disease) (from Politei et al. [12], with permission). (**b**) Vacuolated cytoplasm of submucosal and myenteric plexus ganglion cells (From Politei et al. [12], with permission). (**c**) A case of amyloid deposition in the wall of the bowel leading to dysmotility

6. **How are gastrointestinal motility disorders classified and what are the distinctive pathologic features?**

   The most commonly used system for the classification of GI neuromuscular disorders based on pathology is the "London classification" and a modified version is shown in Table 13.1. GI motility disorders are classified under the broad categories of visceral neuropathy and visceral myopathies resulting from neural or muscular anomalies, respectively. Mixed neuromuscular forms exist. In all groups, sporadic and familial forms have been well characterized in addition to primary and secondary forms (Table 13.1). Familial visceral myopathies and neuropathies have been also classified on the basis of mode of transmission and clinical findings (Table 13.2).

7. **What are the various systemic disorders that are associated with motility disorders?**

   A variety of systemic disorders and medications/toxins have been associated with intestinal dysmotility. These may have a neuropathic or myopathic phenotype, or show mixed features, similar to idiopathic cases. The systemic disorders more frequently associated with dysmotility are listed in Table 13.3.

   Scleroderma, or a virtually identical disease but without the rest of the systemic manifestations of scleroderma, is likely the most common cause of intestinal pseudo-obstruction and discussed later. Amyloidosis and hypothyroidism are other rare causes of secondary pseudo-obstruction. It is usually not worth doing amyloid stains routinely in cases with pseudo-obstruction if there is no other indication of amyloid clinically or histologically in the mucosa, submucosa, or vessels, as it is invariably seen in advanced disease. However, it is necessary to ensure that none of these changes are present on the H&E stain and that the patient has nothing to suggest the disease clinically. Patients with amyloid deposition in the muscularis propria (myopathy) or myenteric plexus (neuropathy) may present with intestinal pseudo-obstruction. Primary amyloidosis with deposition of monoclonal immunoglobulin light chain (AL amyloidosis) is the most common type. AA-type amyloid with deposition of serum amyloid A protein is often deposited in the myenteric plexus, whereas AL-type amyloid is more often deposited in the muscularis mucosae, submucosa, and the muscularis propria (Fig 13.3c). Pseudo-obstruction is more frequently associated with AL amyloidosis while the AA form presents usually with malabsorption and diarrhea.

   A variety of neurological disorders (Table 13.3) like myotonic muscular dystrophy, Parkinson disease, familial autonomic dysfunction and Shy–Drager syndrome may be associated with dysmotility, but no specific pathologic changes are identified in these conditions. Intestinal pseudo-obstruction may also occur in patients with hypoparathyroidism, hypothyroidism, and pheochromocytoma. However, diabetes is by far the commonest endocrine disorder associated with bowel dysmotility and this may result from autonomic dysfunction, electrolyte abnormalities, and vasculopathy. Radiation enteritis may also result in intestinal pseudo-obstruction. Destruction of ganglion cells, as a paraneoplastic syndrome, has been well described in patients with small cell carcinoma of the lung and rarely with other tumors as well. In such cases, neuronal autoantibodies have been detected, and ganglionic destruction is likely to be immune-mediated.

   References: [21–26]

Table 13.1 Modified London classification of GI neuromuscular disorders

Primary neuropathy	Primary myopathy

Absent neurons
  Aganglionosis (Hirschsprung disease)
Decreased number of neurons
  Hypoganglionosis
Increased number of neurons
  Intestinal neuronal dysplasia-type B
  Ganglioneuromatosis
Degenerative neuropathies
Inflammatory neuropathies (not sure if accepted now – they are considered myopathies)
  Lymphocytic ganglionitis
  Eosinophilic ganglionitis
Abnormal content in neurons
  Intraneuronal inclusion disease
  Megamitochondria
Abnormal neuronal coding
Relative immaturity of neurons
Abnormal enteric glia
  Increased number of glia
  Decreased number of glia
	Muscularis propria malformations
	  Focal absence of enteric muscle coats
	  Segmental fusion of enteric muscle coats
	  Presence of additional muscle coats
	  Colonic desmosis (absent connective tissue scaffold)
	Muscle cell degeneration
	  Degenerative leiomyopathy
	    Sporadic
	    Familial
	  Inflammatory myopathies
	    Lymphocytic leiomyositis
	    Eosinophilic leiomyositis
	Muscle hyperplasia/hypertrophy
	  Muscularis mucosae hyperplasia
	Abnormal content in myocytes
	  Filament protein abnormalities
	    Alpha actin myopathy
	    Desmin myopathy
	  Inclusion bodies
	    Polyglucosan bodies
	    Amphophilic "M" bodies

Secondary neuropathy	**Secondary myopathy**

Systemic disorders
  Paraneoplastic inflammatory neuropathy
  Diabetic neuropathy
  Chagasic neuropathy
  Connective tissue disorder-associated neuropathy
  Storage disease
  Amyloidosis
Local disorders
  Crohn disease
	Systemic disorders
	  Desmin myopathy
	  Muscular dystrophies
	  Mitochondrial cytopathies
	  Metabolic storage disorders
	  Amyloidosis
	  Progressive systemic sclerosis
	  Other collagen vascular disorders
	  Cystic fibrosis
	Local disorders
	  Obstructive/post-irradiation muscle failure

8. **What are the histopathologic features of scleroderma involvement of the bowel?**

Patients with scleroderma or progressive systemic sclerosis may show significant involvement of the bowel, which may become severe enough to require surgical resection. Clinically, esophageal involvement usually predominates. The inner circular layer of the bowel wall is often preferentially involved, in contrast to primary visceral myopathy in which the outer longitudinal muscle layer is typically most involved, but this is not always true. In scleroderma, collagen replacement of the muscle layer tends to be nearly complete, unlike the delicate and incomplete type of interstitial fibrosis characteristic of primary visceral myopathy (Fig 13.4a, b). Fibrosis may cause muscle weakness resulting in diverticula and the formation of squared-mouth ostia. Mucosal changes are nonspecific. They are typically secondary to the underlying motility problem (e.g., reflux esophagitis and villous blunting due to bacterial overgrowth in the small bowel).
References: [27–29]

9. **What are the common histopathologic findings in cases of achalasia cardia?**

Achalasia is a motor disorder of the esophagus characterized by failure of the lower esophageal sphincter to relax in response to swallowing. The main histological abnormality in achalasia is related to the widespread, often total, loss of myenteric ganglion cells in the myenteric plexus, although numerous secondary changes are often present, presumably due to prolonged stasis and reflux. The diagnosis is established based on clinical basis and mucosal biopsies are only performed to evaluate secondary changes or evolving neoplasia. Pathologist sometimes get resection specimens of the esophagus when all other options have failed or complications including neoplasia have developed. Grossly, the esophagus is dilated and the extent of dilatation depends on the severity and duration of disease (Fig 13.5a). It often contains stagnant and foul-smelling partially digested food. The distal end is typically narrowed and stenotic.

While the distal esophagus shows complete loss of ganglion cells in the myenteric plexus (Fig 13.5b), some preservation of the ganglion cells may be present in the more proximal portions of the esophagus. Some degree of neural hyperplasia often accompanies the neuronal loss. A variable amount of chronic inflammation often admixed with eosinophils, and plasma cells can be seen, especially in the early sages of the disease. Mast cells may also be noted surrounding the myenteric plexus and residual ganglion cells. In end-stage disease, the degree of inflammation may become minimal or disappear completely. Occasionally, lymphocytes may infiltrate the cytoplasm of ganglion cells (ganglionitis). The majority of chronic inflammatory cells are CD8 positive T cells.

Other changes frequently present are related to distal esophageal obstruction, and include muscularis propria hypertrophy, muscularis propria eosinophilia, and dystrophic calcification. Hypertrophied muscle may also show degenerative changes, including cytoplasmic vacuolation

Table 13.2 Classification of familial visceral myopathy and neuropathy

Type	Mode of transmission	Age of onset	Symptoms	GI lesions	Main findings	Extraintestinal involvement
Visceral myopathy						
I	AD	After 1st decade of life	Varied; dysphagia, constipation, and/or CIIP	Dilatation of esophagus, duodenum, colon	Involvement of both layers of muscularis propria	Dilation of bladder, uterine inertia, mydriasis
II	AR	Teenagers	Severe abdominal pain, CIIP	Dilation of stomach, mild dilatation of small intestine, small bowel diverticulosis	Involvement of both layers of muscularis propria	Ptosis and external opthalmoplegia, mild degeneration of striated muscle
III	AR	Middle age	CIIP	Mild dilation of entire GI tract	Involvement of both layers of muscularis propria	None
IV	?AR	Childhood	CIIP	Gastroparesis, narrowed small bowel, normal esophagus and colon	More severe involvement of outer layers of muscularis propria	None
Visceral neuropathy						
I	AD	Any age	Abdominal pain diarrhea, abdominal distension, gastroparesis, CIIP	Segmental dilation of jejunum and ileum, proximal small intestine is always involved	Reduction and degeneration of myenteric plexus, loss and degenerative changes in neurons	None
II	AR	Infancy	Hypertrophic pyloric stenosis, short dilated small intestine, intestinal malrotation		Decreased neurons	CNS malformation with heterotopia and absence of operculum, patent ductus arteriosus

AD autosomal dominant, *AR* autosomal recessive, *CIIP* chronic idiopathic intestinal pseudo-obstruction, *CNS* central nervous system, *GI* gastrointestinal

Table 13.3 Secondary chronic intestinal pseudo-obstruction

A. Associated with systemic disorders
1. Progressive systemic sclerosis/polymyositis
2. Systemic lupus erythematosus
3. Progressive muscular dystrophy
4. Myotonic dystrophy
5. Fabry disease
6. Parkinson disease
7. Multiple sclerosis
B. Endocrine and metabolic disorders
1. Diabetes mellitus
2. Hypothyroidism
3. Hypoparathyroidism
4. Pheochromocytoma
5. Acute intermittent porphyria
C. Infiltrative disorders
1. Amyloidosis
2. Diffuse lymphoid infiltration
3. Eosinophilic gastroenteritis
D. Paraneoplastic
1. Small cell carcinoma
2. Others
F. Infections
1. Trypanosoma Cruizi (Chagas disease)
2. Herpes virus
3. Cytomegalovirus
4. Epstein–Barr virus
5. Lyme disease

and liquefactive necrosis. The branches of the vagus nerve within the adventitia are unremarkable in most cases, although degenerative changes in the vagus nerve and in dorsal motor nuclei have been described as well. The squamous mucosa also shows secondary changes, including diffuse hyperplasia, increased intraepithelial lymphocytes ("lymphocytic esophagitis"), papillomatosis, basal cell hyperplasia, and an increase in nonspecific lamina propria inflammation (Fig 13.5c). Some of these changes mimic reflux esophagitis, although sustained lower esophageal pressure does not allow regurgitation of gastric contents in untreated cases. Following esophagomyotomy, gastroesophageal reflux develops in up to 50% of patients, and can lead to the development of Barrett esophagus in some cases.
References: [30–39]

10. What is postinfectious intestinal pseudo-obstruction?

About 3.7–36% of patients following resolution of an acute infection develop some chronic GI symptoms, including bowel dysmotility. The common bacterial infections leading to postinfection dysmotility include Salmonella, Shigella, and Campylobacter. While this may occur secondary to some of the neurotropic viruses that can infect the intestinal ganglia, this may also occur after resolution of the infection as well. Most of these

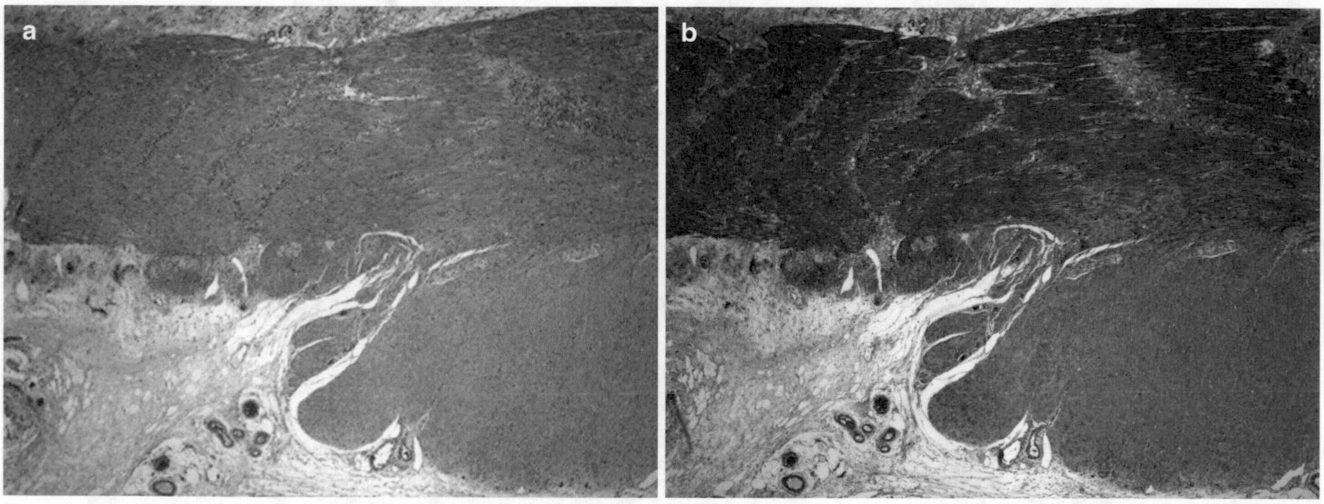

Fig. 13.4 Atrophy of outer muscle layer with complete disappearance in a case of scleroderma. (**a**) H&E stain. (**b**) Trichrome stain

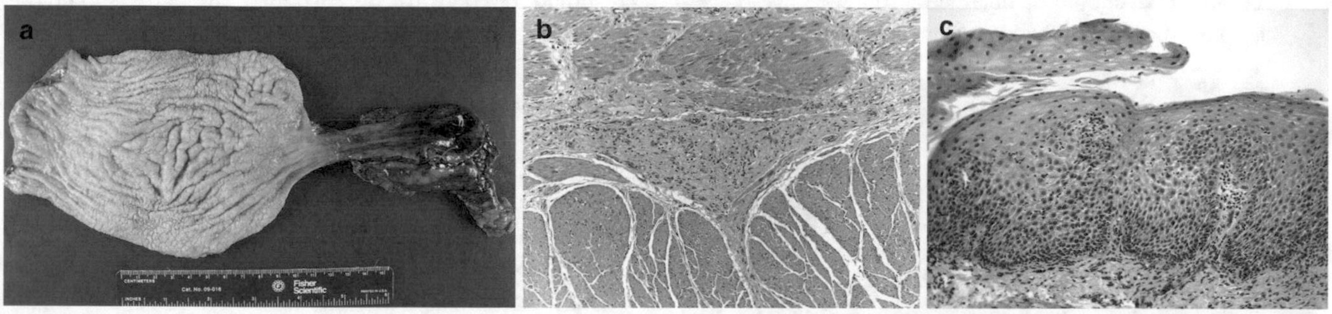

Fig. 13.5 (**a**) Gross photograph showing marked proximal dilatation with severe narrowing of the distal esophagus typical of achalasia cardia. (**b**) Histology of the same case showing complete absence of ganglion cells near the gastroesophageal junction. (**c**) The squamous mucosa in the same case showing increased intraepithelial lymphocytes (lymphocytic esophagitis), which has been associated with motility disorders of the esophagus

conditions are self-limited, although the symptoms may last for many months. The infectious organisms have usually disappeared by this time and pathologically the changes are fairly nonspecific. Besides mild peri-ganglionic lymphocytic infiltrate one may not see much on histology (Fig. 13.6).

Reference: [40]

11. **What are the infiltrative disorders that lead to intestinal pseudo-obstruction?**

A variety of neoplastic and non-neoplastic disorders may lead to motility disorder. Infiltration of the bowel wall with cellular elements or noncellular elements can interfere with the neuromuscular functions of bowel. Of these, in practice amyloidosis remains one of the most common diseases that may not be clinically evident and may require a tissue diagnosis (see Question 7).

Amongst cellular infiltates, bowel dysmotilty has been associated with infiltration due to lymphocytes, eosinophils, and mast cells. Rare cases of chronic instestinal pseudo-obstruction, predominantly found in children, are due to an idiopathic form of lymphocytic leiomyositis. Patients may present with episodes of bowel obstruction with radiographic evidence of bowel obstruction without occlusive lesions. Histologically, they are characterized by infiltration of polyclonal lymphocytes in the muscularis propria without any significant abnormalities in the mucosa or submucosa (Fig 13.7a). However, the muscle fibers appear to be morphologically intact. The myenteric plexus shows no abnormality of neurons or axons. The diagnosis is therefore made on a full-thickness biopsy. The lymphocytic infiltrate is composed of CD3, CD4, CD8 T lymphocytes. Macrophages may be present, but B lymphocytes are absent. Whether this represents yet undefined smooth muscle disorder, or is autoimmune in nature, remains to be determined.

Eosinophilic gastroenteritis (deep muscular form) and eosinophilic myenteric ganglionitis have been associated with bowel dysmotility (Fig 13.7c). Eosinophilic myenteric ganglionitis has been mainly described in children, with only rare reports in adults (Fig 13.7b). Increased mast cells have also been reported in bowel dysmotility, and are believed to interact with the neural apparatus causing dysmotility.

References: [2, 41–44]

12. **How do you evaluate resection specimens from patients with chronic idiopathic constipation and intestinal pseudo-obstruction?**

Small bowel and large bowel resections are handled similarly (see Question 1). The specimens should be fixed immediately after cleansing of the lumen. Frozen samples for histochemistry, and tissues fixed in gluteraldehyde for potential EM, should be obtained. From the large bowel, samples should be obtained from the ascending colon, transverse colon, left/sigmoid colon, and rectum. Sections from the intestines should be obtained from the transverse and longitudinal axis, although in general, transverse sections are more informative. Longitudinal sections can produce an erroneous impression of thinning or thickening of the longitudinal muscle layer, depending on whether tenia coli have been included in the section or not. Resections for achalasia and gastroparesis should be handled similarly. A good gross examination of the resected specimen should be performed, and one should look for any gross abnormalties in the luminal diameter (narrowing or dilatation), thickness of muscular wall, presence of diverticula or adhesions. In some cases an abnormal layering of muscle, which can be identified both grossly and microscopically, especially an extra outer layer in the muscularis propria, has been reported associated with intestinal dysmotility.

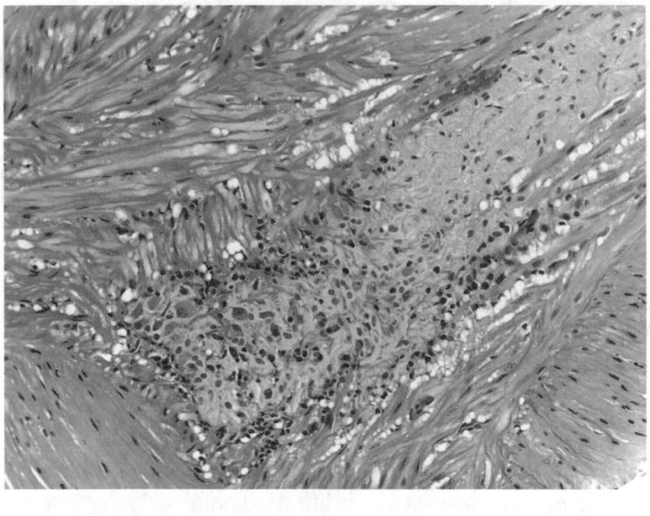

Fig. 13.6 Lymphocytic inflammation in and around myenteric ganglia in a case of post-Varicella intestinal pseudo-obstruction

On routine histology, careful examination of the mucosal changes and the neuromuscular apparatus should be performed. Particular attention should be given to the thickness of the muscle layers, myocyte morphology, pattern of fibrosis, number and morphology of ganglion cells, number and distribution of ICCs, presence or absence of neural plexus hypertrophy or atrophy, and the presence or absence of inflammation involving the neuromuscular apparatus. Inflammation surrounding the neural plexus, and ganglionitis, may point toward an infectious or para-neoplastic/autoimmune neuropathy, whereas dense lymphocytic inflammation limited to the muscular layers may suggest autoimmune leiomyositis. However, one should be cautious when evaluating inflammation within the neuromuscular apparatus, since secondary involvement (e.g., inflammatory bowel disease) is more common than primary involvement. Intranuclear inclusions in ganglion cells, and cytoplasmic inclusions in smooth muscle fibers, are associated with certain motility disorders. Neural hypertrophy and atrophy, although nonspecific, may indicate involvement of the neuromuscular appara-

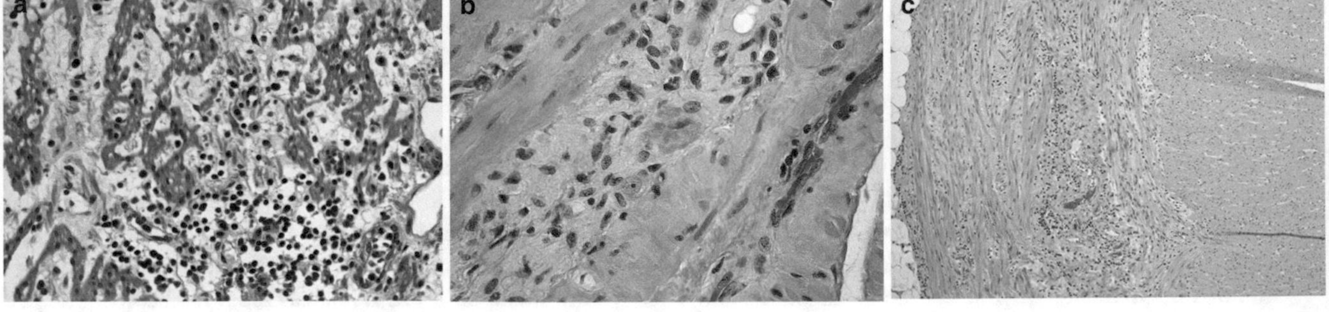

Fig. 13.7 (**a**) Dense lymphocytic inflammation in a case of lymphocytic leiomyositis. (**b**) Infiltration of eosinophils in the myenteric ganglia in a case of eosinophilic myenteric ganglionitis. (**c**) A case showing an eosinophilic infiltrate in the muscularis propria without involvement of the mucosa

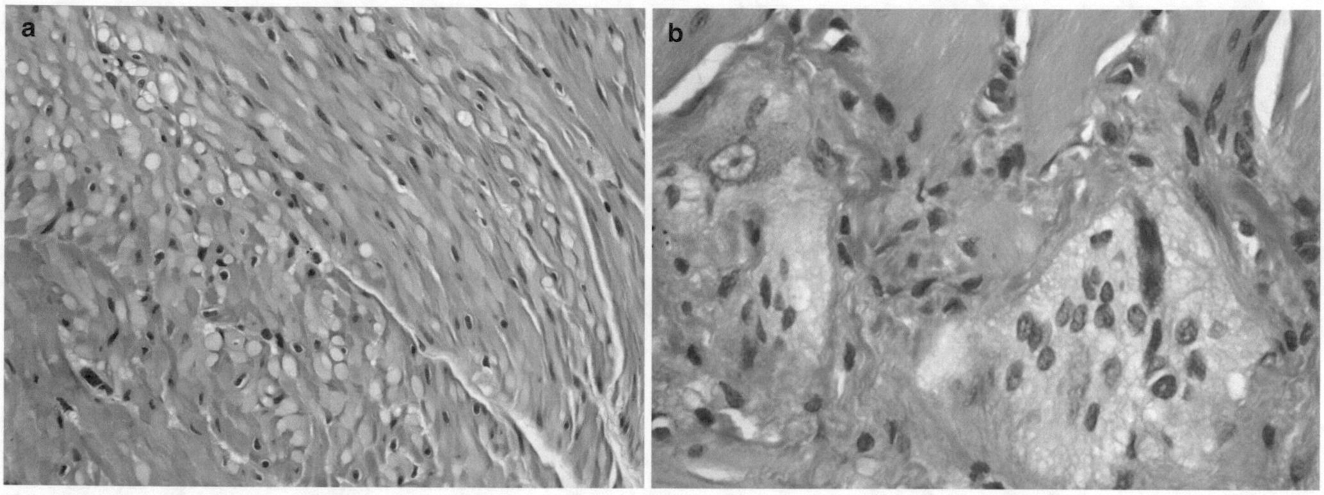

Fig. 13.8 (**a**) Cytoplasmic clearing in the myocytes, which is patchy and represents artifact. (**b**) Cytoplasmic eosinophilia and smudgy nucleus in a ganglion cell mimicking degenerative changes

tus and an underlying motility disorder. Artifactual cytoplasmic vacuolation and nuclear pyknosis in muscle and ganglion cells, which are not uncommon in resection specimens performed for a variety of conditions, should be differentiated from true pathology (Fig 13.8a, b). True degenerative changes in the muscle are often diffuse/extensive, accompanied by thinning or hypertrophy of the muscle and interstitial fibrosis, whereas the artifacts tends to be focal/patchy.

Accurate diagnosis of GI motility disorders requires correlation of various clinical and laboratory data in order to establish diagnosis. For example, one study that looked at 21 cases of intestinal pseudo-obstruction showed myopathic changes in 9 (43%), neuropathic changes in 2 (9.5%), and mixed changes in 2 (9.5%) cases. Abnormalities of ICC were found in 10 (48%) cases. In eight cases, routine histology failed to show any changes but abnormal numbers of ICCs and ganglion cells were found on IHC analysis in two and four cases, respectively. Neuropathic forms are more common in some studies; however, validity of many diagnoses based on quantitative changes in ganglia can be questioned. Recent recommendations and guidelines suggested by the international working group is likely to circumvent some of these issues. However, this group of disorders still remains frustrating despite extensive and sometime expensive workup in many cases. While a number of changes are sometimes identified, their significance in the pathophysiology and nature (primary vs. secondary) remain unclear. The underlying molecular mechanisms and etiopathogenesis of many disorders remain poorly understood. Thus, it is not surprising that the therapeutic options are also limited and very little progress has been made so far. It is antcipated that with standardizaion of the methodology, diagnostic criteria, and application of evolving technologies in the field of proteomics and genomics, our understanding of these disorders may advance significantly leading to better diagnosis and treatment.

References: [4, 17, 20, 45–47]

Table 13.4 Pharmacologic agents and toxins associated with intestinal dysmotility

1. Tricyclic antidepressants
2. Phenothiazines
3. Ganglionic blockers
4. Clonidine
5. Anti-Parkinsonism medication
6. Opiates (narcotic bowel syndrome)
7. Amanita phalloides toxin

13. What medications are known to be associated with motility disorders?

Certain drugs, particularly the antineoplastic drugs such as the vinca alkaloids, as well as others, such as the phenothiazines, tricyclic antidepressants, and anticholinergics, may produce severe intestinal motor dysfunction in addition to stercoral ulceration (Table 13.4). It is postulated that these drugs act as neurotoxins, damaging the myenteric plexus. Use or ingestion of some of the naturally occurring toxins such as Amanita phalloides may also result in intestinal pseudo-obstruction. Recently, immune check-point inhibitor Nivolumab has been reported to be associated with intestinal pseudo-obstruction.

Chronic ingestion of certain laxatives, such as the anthraquinones, has been found to be associated with loss of argyrophilic neurons, marked axonal fragmentation, and glial cell proliferation in some patients with severe constipation. Although these changes have been ascribed to the laxatives, it is possible that they represent a primary disorder of the enteric plexus, which was responsible for the ingestion of the laxatives in the first place. Additional features seen more commonly in these patients are melanosis coli and rectal ulceration (cathartic ulcers).

References: [48–53]

14. What is the most common presentation of Hirschsprung disease and what biopsy type is preferred and adequate for the diagnosis?

Hirschsprung disease (HSCR) is characterized by the congenital absence of ganglion cells in the myenteric and submucosal plexuses of the terminal rectum (classic disease). The aganglionosis may extend to involve variable length of contiguous rectosigmoid and proximal colon, and rarely the entire large bowel (total aganglionosis). The majority (90%) of cases present in the neonatal period with failure to pass meconium in the first 24 h of life. Less common presentation include sign of intestinal obstruction, vomiting, abdominal distention relieved by enemas or rectal stimulation, or severe constipation. Diarrhea, explosive stool, and abdominal distension may result from HSCR-associated enterocolitis, which remains the most common cause of mortality.

Diagnosis of HSCR requires documentation of absence of ganglion cells in the myenteric ganglia, which is feasible only with the full-thickness seromuscular biopsies or resection specimens. However, absence of ganglion cells in the submucosal plexus correlates with absence of ganglion cells in the myenteric ganglia and can be evaluated with rectal suction biopsies that can be obtained at bedside without general anesthesia. The diagnostic accuracy of rectal suction biospy is fairly high with a sensitivity of 96% and a specificity of 99% in some studies. Nowadays suction biopsies have become the diagnostic procedure of choice in the workup of patients suspected with HSCR. Seromuscular biopsies, instead, are limited to only rare and challenging cases, where some form of dysmotility disorder is suspected and the rectal suction biopsies remain nondiagnostic. In older children with severe constipation, full-thickness biopsy is preferred over suction biopsies in most institutions.

Criteria for adequacy of suction biopsy include: site of biopsy set at 2–3 cm above the dentate line and presence of adequate amount of submucosa. As a general guide, the thickness of submucosa should be approximately equal to the thickness of the mucosa. Several studies have demonstrated that enteric ganglia in the distal 1–2 cm of rectum are physiologically sparse, therefore the standard of practice is to provide biopsy samples above that zone. Number of biopsies varies amongst institutions and some groups favor taking biopsies routinely from multiple levels in the rectum.

References: [3, 54, 55]

15. How do you triage biopsy tissues in a suspected case of Hirschsprung disease?

The choice of biopsy triage depends on how many biopsy fragments are available. Priority should be given to routine H&E stained sections, but if multiple fragments are provided one should be kept frozen for AchE staining (see below). EM has no role in the workup of suspected HSCR cases.

16. In a suspected case of Hirschsprung disease how do you evaluate the biopsies and what special stains are useful?

H&E remains the most valuable stain in the workup of biopsies for suspected HSCR. Presence of ganglion cells in the submucosal ganglia virtually excludes the diagnosis of HSCR, which can be easily recognized in most cases. Since ganglion cells can be sparse in submucosa, multiple levels must be examined in biopsies before deeming it devoid of ganglion cells. The practice varies amongst institutions. Some would recommend cutting multiple serial sections upfront (Fig 13.9a, b), with staining of alternate sections with H&E sections and preserving the unstained sections for possible immunostains. Some institutions recommend exhausting the entire biopsy tissue, while most would consider 75–100 H&E stained levels as adequate. Some institutions initially stain only a few sections and proceed with multiple serial sections only if they fail to show ganglion cells or directly proceed to IHC for calretinin.

The challenges are when the histologic appearance of ganglion cells is not typical (immature ganglion cells) or other cells are present that can mimic ganglion cells (e.g., plasma cells, histiocytes, or endothelial cells). Traditionally, the most relied upon ancillary technique for diagnosing HSCR is AchE histochemical stain performed on fresh frozen tissue. Biopsies of patients with HSCR show increased density and thickness of AchE positive nerves in muscularis mucosa plus/minus lamina propria, while normally the staining in nerve fibers is limited in the submucosa and muscularis mucosae (Fig 13.9c). AchE stain, however, may add complexity to the diagnostic workup, not only because it requires frozen sections, but it is also a technically challenging stain to perform. Satisfactory results are obtained in histology laboratories that perform sufficient number of stains with adequate controls.

In recent years, calretinin immunostain has been shown to be equally reliable, if not superior to AchE stain and has the advantage that it can be performed on

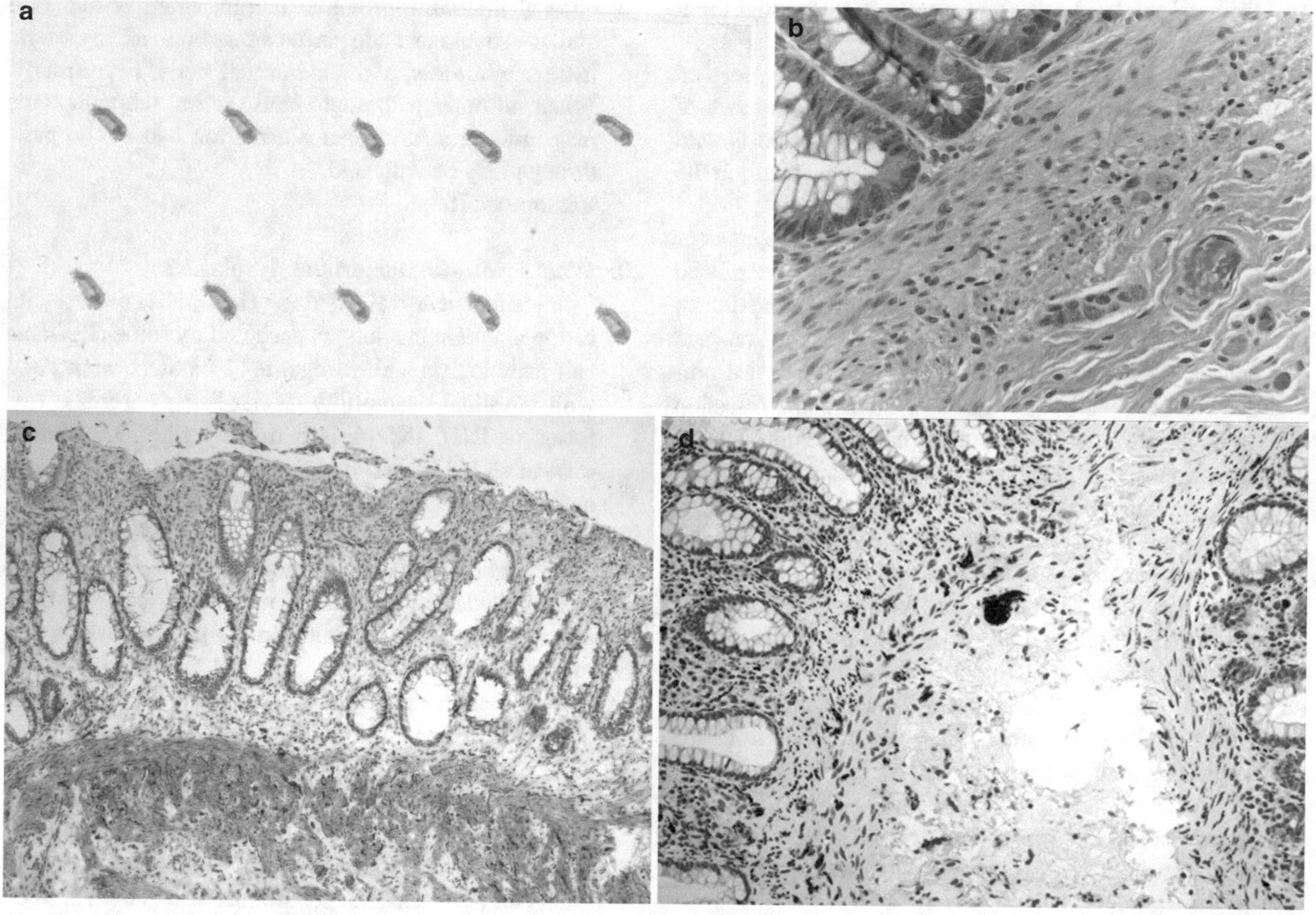

Fig. 13.9 (**a**) Low magnification showing multiple serial sections in a case of Hirschsprung disease put on the same slide. (**b**) Higher magnification of the submucosal plexus showing presence of a few ganglion cells ruling out Hirschsprung disease. (**c**) AchE stain showing a normal staining pattern of the submucosal nerves, but none in the lamina propria. (**d**) Calretinin stain showing a normal staining pattern in the nerves and ganglion cells

formalin-fixed paraffin-embedded sections. Calretinin immunostain normally shows dense, granular staining in nerves of the muscularis mucosae, superficial submucosa, and focally in lamina propria. Ganglion cells also show strong immunolabeling (Fig 13.9d). Biopsies from HSCR patients show complete absence of ganglion cells in addition to lack of staining in the nerves. Mast cells, which are also positive for calretinin, often serve as internal control. The only issue with calretinin stain is that it is a negative stain that is diagnostic of HSCR, and hence many institutions still prefer to do both AchE and calretinin stains to confirm HSCR, when possible. This topic is discussed in detail in Chap. 1.

An ancillary criterion supportive of the diagnosis of HSCR is the presence of hypertrophic nerves. In HSCR both density and caliber (>40 micron) of submucosal nerves are increased. Hypertrophic nerves can be seen in association with ganglion cells and this finding is considered indicative of transition zone. Identification of hypertrophic nerves therefore can be asked during a pull-through surgery (see below), during intraoperative consultation.

References: [56–59]

17. **What is the role of intraoperative consultation during pull-through surgery for a Hirschsprung disease patient?**

The surgical approach to HSCR disease has evolved from three- and two-stage procedures to a single-stage procedure, of which the transanal (Swenson and Soave) approach is the most frequently used. At the time of surgery, seromuscular biopsies are usually obtained as intraoperative frozen sections to assure that a properly ganglionated segment is reached before either an anastomosis is performed for a one-stage procedure or an ostomy is performed for subsequent hookup.

18. How do you evaluate the resections performed for a Hirschsprung disease?

The goals of examination of the resections performed in a patient with HSCR are to confirm the presence of aganglionosis, define the extent of aganglionosis, and the presence of adequate number of ganglion cells at the proximal anastomosic site.

The resected HSCR specimen consists of a segment of dilated colon of variable length tapering to a narrowed rectal segment. The tapering portion between the dilated and narrowed segments represents the transition zone and the narrowed segment represents the aganglionated portion (Fig 13.10a, b). The goals of examining a resection specimen are largely to document and define the extent of aganglionosis, and the presence of an adequate number of ganglia at the proximal resection margin. One easy way to achieve this is to obtain transverse (en face) sections from the proximal and distal margins, and then take a longitudinal strip along the entire length of the specimen. This may be submitted as multiple sequential sections, or as a "swiss roll," in a single block keeping the orientation of the proximal and distal segments. Alternatively, one may submit multiple sequential transvese sections from the entire specimhn, at 1 cm intervals.

19. Is persistence of symptoms frequent after surgical resection for Hirschsprung disease and what are the implications?

Despite corrective surgery, obstructive symptoms may persist in 10–15% of patients. Failure to resect the transition zone, which has less than adequate number of ganglion cells (so-called transition zone pull-through) is one of the reported etiologies. Intraoperative frozen section evaluation of the proximal resection margin is recommended to reduce the likelihood of transition zone pull-through. One should ensure that adequate number of ganglion cells are present throughout the circumference of the entire proximal margin submitted en face and one should exclude partial aganglionosis, myenteric hypoganglionosis, and submucosal nerve hypertrophy. When no other pathologic cause exists the symptoms may indicate a functional obstruction and a redo pull-through may be indicated.
References: [60, 61]

20. What is intestinal neuronal dysplasia?

Intestinal neuronal dysplasia (IND) is a controversial histopathologic phenotype, accepted by some clinicians and pathologists and disregarded by others, associated with intestinal dysmotility. Meier-Ruge described two forms of IND. IND-A is extremely rare, constituting <5% of all IND cases. It is characterized by sympathetic aplasia, myenteric hyperplasia, and colonic inflammation. Mucosal biopsy generally shows ulceration and inflammation similar to ulcerative colitis. Typical features include hyperplasia of myenteric ganglion cells and increased AchE staining in the lamina propria and muscularis mucosae.

IND-B is characterized by marked neural hypertrophy and an increased number of large ganglion cells in the submucosal neural plexuses. It constitutes about 95% of all IND cases. The diagnostic criteria for IND-B have changed over time. Currently, it requires the presence of giant submucosal ganglia, which is defined as >8 ganglion cell cross sections per submucosal ganglion. Such "giant" ganglia should constitute >20% of all ganglia and at least 25 submucosal ganglia should be evaluated. Ancillary criteria include increase in AchE positive fibers in the muscularis mucosae and/or lamina propria and ectopic ganglion cells located in the lamina propria or muscularis mucosae. Calretinin stain is positive in neurons and nerve trunk, which differentiates this from HSCR, but apparently is less sensitive than H&E stained sections. The validity of the diagnostic criteria for IND

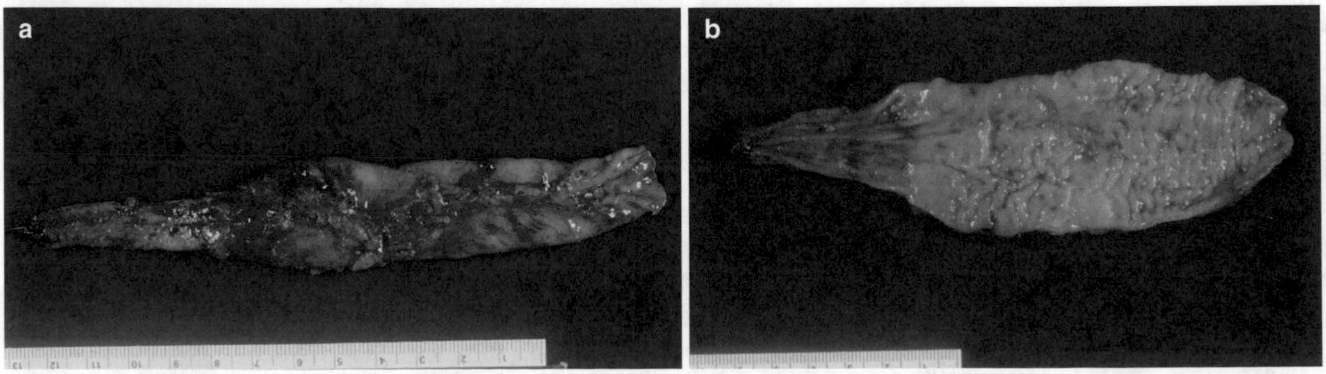

Fig. 13.10 (**a**) Gross specimen of Hirschsprung disease showing narrowed distal end and dilated proximal segment. (**b**) Opened up specimen showing the same with no specific mucosal abnormalities on gross examination

has been frequently challenged, and it is suggested that IND may merely represent a secondary phenomenon and not a primary disorder. It is also recommended that a diagnosis of IND-B should be made only in children older than 1, and less than 4 years of age after exclusion of other causes of dysmotility. There is no consensus on the treatment of patients with IND-B, which varies from a conservative medical treatment to anal sphincter myomectomy to more aggressive surgical resection.
References: [55, 62–67]

21. **What is hypoganglionosis and how do you evaluate the number of ganglia in the gastrointestinal tract and what does it mean?**

Hypoganglionosis is a rare disorder and constitutes about 3–5% of all pediatric motility disorders. Most cases present in children, although rare cases in adults are also reported. Hypoganglionosis can be diffuse, localized, or segmental. Isolated hypoganglionosis of the colon is even rarer. Clinical features mimic HSCR, chronic constipation or intestinal pseudo-obstruction. Histologically, it is characterized by decreased number of myenteric ganglia accompanied by decreased AchE staining in the lamina propria nerves and hypertrophy of the muscularis mucosae. Evaluating the increase or decrease in the number of ganglion cells in the intestinal neuronal plexus remains far more challenging and controversial compared to mere evaluation of their presence or absence. The challenges and controversies associated with the diagnosis of IND characterized by increased number of ganglion cells have already been discussed above. The evaluation of decreased number of ganglion cells for the diagnosis of hypoganglionosis remains equally challenging and controversial. A variety of criteria have been used in the literature, including (1) ≥10 fold reduction in the number of ganglion cells compared with age-matched controls, (2) <10 ganglion cells/mm and/or <2 ganglia/mm length of bowel, or (3) ≤20 Hu C/D positive ganglion cells/cm of bowel. It goes without saying that the thickness of the sections, segment of bowel analyzed, stains used, experience of the pathologist, and sampling variability contribute to varying results and the associated controversies.
References: [68–76]

22. **Abnormalities of which components of neurohormonal apparatus of the gastrointestinal tract lead to bowel dysmotility?**

GI motility disorders are classified under the broad categories of visceral neuropathies and myopathies resulting from neural or muscular anomalies. Mixed neuromuscular forms exist far more commonly than we recognize. In all groups sporadic and familial forms have been described, in addition to primary and secondary forms. An attempt to an all-inclusive classification is shown in Table 13.1.

The proposed classification of the inherited visceral myopathies used in the past included four types based on the inheritance pattern and clinical features. Type I with autosomal dominant transmission has megaduodenum, megacolon, and megacystis. Type II, autosomal recessive, has ptosis and ophtalmoplegia with diverticula of stomach and small bowel. Type III, also autosomal recessive, has dilatation of the entire GI tract from esophagus to rectum. Type IV is extremely rare and poorly characterized. It involves the stomach and small bowel, but spares the esophagus and colon. However, newer primary inherited forms of visceral myopathies have been described since this classification, which likely needs to be further expanded.

Primary visceral neuropathies (excluding HSCR and IND described above) that may have specific histopathologic findings include neuronal inclusion disorders and neuromyopathies associated with mitochondrial disorders.

Case Presentation

Case 1

Learning Objectives

1. Type of biopsies for the diagnosis of HSCR in older children
2. Pathology workup and adequacy for number of sections
3. Immunostains to assist in the diagnosis

Case History

A 2-year-old boy presented with severe constipation. A barium enema showed diffuse dilatation of the rectum, but normal rectosigmoid ratio. While the findings were not completely supportive for the diagnosis of HSCR, given the severity of the symptoms a suction rectal biopsy was carried on to rule it out. Two biopsy fragments were obtained and were put in formalin to be sent to the pathology lab.

Pathology

Both rectal suction biopsy fragments were processed for H&E stains. Unfortunately, no tissue could be kept frozen. While the biopsies were considered adequate for assessment, initial sections did not show any convincing ganglion cells, but neural hypertrophy was absent. As a next step multiple serial sections (10 slides with 100 sections were obtained) (Fig 13.9a). A calretinin immunostain was performed, although no AchE stain could be performed due to lack of frozen tissue. Careful examination of the serial sections showed few ganglion cells on only three levels of the H&E stained section (Fig 13.11a). The calretinin stain showed granular staining in the nerve fibers in the submucosa and muscularis mucosae, and also highlighted a few ganglion cells (Fig 13.11b). Bcl2 and ALK1 stains were performed that also highlighted a few ganglion cells (Fig 13.11c, d).

Differential Diagnosis and Discussion

While rectal suction biopsies are considered standard of care for the diagnosis of HSCR in the neonate, there is debate if the amount of tissue obtained is sufficient for the diagnosis in infants and older children. This case is an example of a suction biopsy obtained at bedside in an older child. It includes an amount of submucosa equal to the amount of mucosa and appears adequate. However, the majority of pediatric surgeons still favor a full-thickness or seromuscular biopsy in older children. The initial section failed to show any convincing ganglion cells; however, these were identified on subsequent levels. As discussed earlier, the number of serial levels obtained to rule out HSCR varies from institution to institution. A seminal paper compared the practice of different Children Hospitals in the handling of rectal biopsy to rule out HSCR. At present, there is no uniformity in the number of levels deemed to be sufficient for a diagnosis of HSCR with some institutions still favoring complete exhaustion of the block before rendering a diagnosis of HSCR. The presence of a single ganglion cell will rule out HSCR, as seen in this case.

A number of immunostains can be used to confirm the presence of ganglion cells, particularly when the morphology of the ganglion cells is not the most characteristic. The immunostain most widely accepted is calretinin, and in most institutions it has replaced the use of AchE histochemical stain. Calretinin not only highlights the ganglion cells, but also shows a delicate pattern of nerve fibers present in muscularis mucosae that extend into the lamina propria (neuritic pattern), which is absent in HSCR. Mast cells also stain with calretinin and can be used as an internal control. Mast cells are smaller in size, usually single, dispersed in both lamina propria and submucosa, and can be easily differentiated from

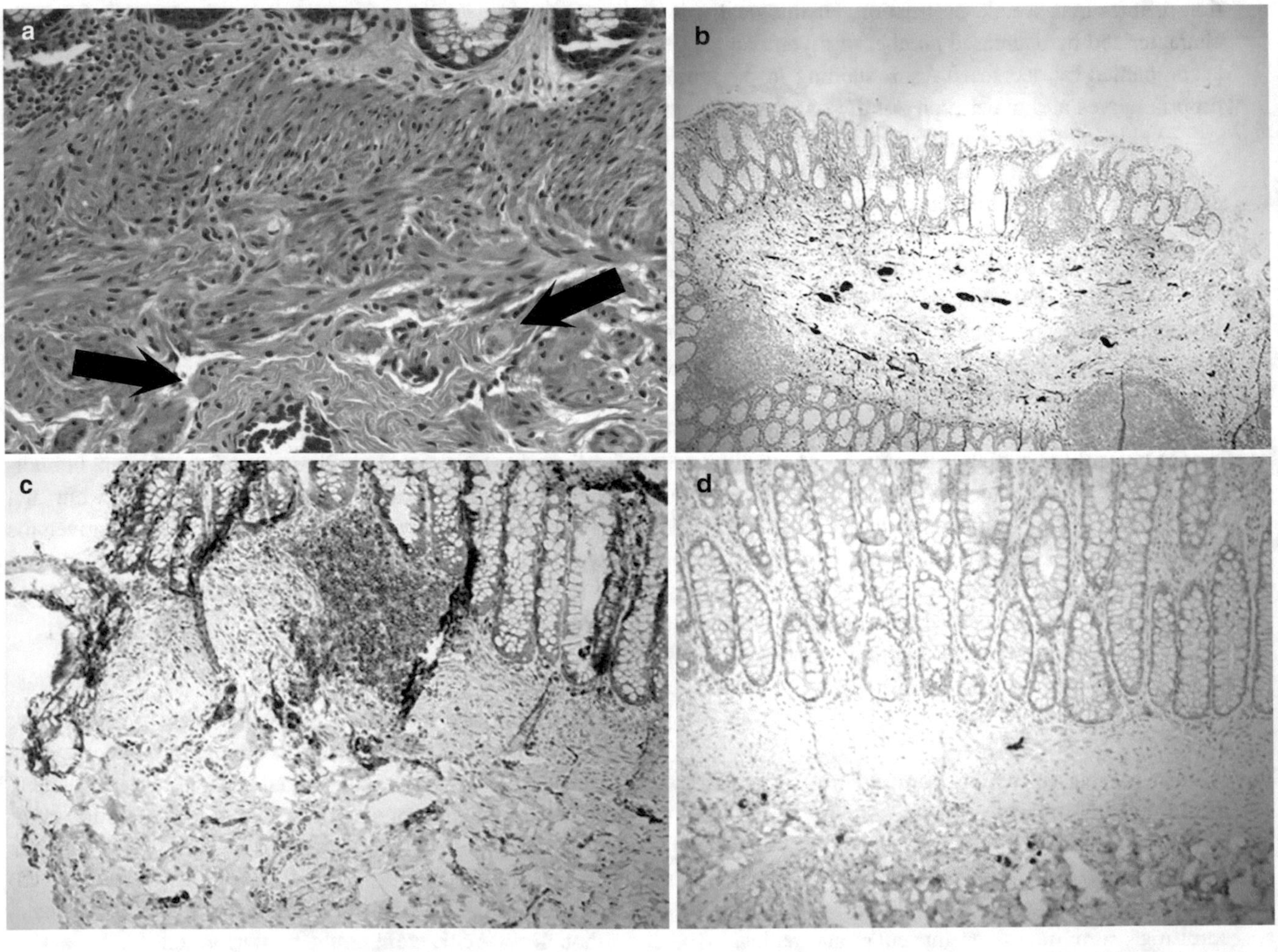

Fig. 13.11 (Case 1) (**a**) Biopsy showing a few cells suggestive of ganglion cells that were present only on few sections (arrows). (**b**) Calretinin immunostain in the rectal biopsy showing granular staining in the submucosal and lamina propria nerves and highlighting a few submucosal ganglion cells. (**c**) Bcl2 immunostain showing the presence of ganglion cells in the submucosa, which are present underneath a lymphoid aggregate in this biopsy. (**d**) ALK1 immunostain showing the presence of ganglion cells in the submucosa. These findings rule out the possibility of HSCR

ganglion cells. Besides calretinin many other immunostains (Bcl2, ALK1, neu1, etc.) have been reported in the literature that stain ganglion cells and the use depends on availability of the antibody and personal choice.

In this case, while the diagnosis of HSCR was excluded, a possiblity of "allied disorders of HSCR" remains in the differential diagnosis. Various conditions considered under the umbrella of "allied disorders of HSCR" include conditions that clinically present very similar to HSCR, but histologically show the presence of ganglion cells (Table 13.5). Many of these entities remain poorly characterized with poorly defined and controversial criteria (see Questions 20 and 21). In this case, the possibilities of hypoganglionosis and internal sphincter achalasia (also called ultra-short segment of Hirschsprung disease) need to be considered as possible diagnoses. These diagnoses can be established only with a combination of clinical features, evaluation of full-thickness biopsies/resection specimen, anorectal manometry, and follow-up.

Final Diagnosis

Findings not supportive of Hirschsprung disease, but the possibilities of hypoganglionosis and internal sphincter achalasia need to be considered.

References: [56, 77, 78]

Case 2

Learning Objectives

1. To become familiar with clinical presentation and workup of patients suspected to have HSCR
2. To become familiar with the handling and histologic findings of suction rectal biopsies
3. To become familiar with surgical procedures and pathology handling of resection specimens for HSCR

Case History

A 9-day-old male, born at term, did not pass meconium for the first 48 h of life and presented with distended abdomen. The initial hypaque enema was consistent with meconium plug and turned out to be therapeutic. The infant did not tolerate oral intake and became distended again. Repeat hypaque enema showed distended colon suspicious for HSCR (Fig. 13.12).

Table 13.5 Allied disorders of Hirschsprung disease

Diseases with intestinal ganglion cell abnormality	
	Immature ganglion cells
	Isolated hypoganglionosis
	Intestinal neuronal dysplasia
Diseases without intestinal ganglion cell abnormalities	
	Megacystis microcolon intestinal hypoperistalsis syndrome
	Segmental dilatation of intestine
	Internal anal sphincter achalasia
	Chronic idiopathic intestinal pseudo-obstruction

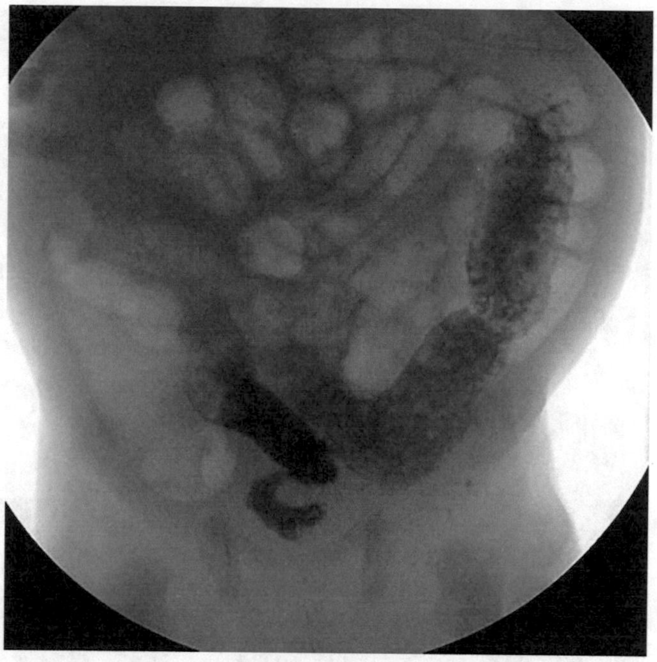

Fig. 13.12 (Case 2) Fluoroscopic appearance of rectum instilled with water-soluble contrast showing dilatation of the rectosigmoid and descending colon with filling defect due to accumulation of feces

Pathology

The infant underwent rectal suction biopsy that provided three biopsy fragments obtained 2 cm above the pectinate line. Two of the biopsy fragments were fixed in formalin and serial H&E sections were obtained, in addition to alternate unstained sections for calretinin immunostain. The third fragment was frozen and subsequently processed for AchE stain. The initial master slide and subsequent H&E serial sections failed to reveal any ganglion cells and the biopsy was considered to be adequate (Fig 13.13a). Immunostain for calretinin failed to show any staining in the nerves or highlight any ganglion cells (Fig 13.13b). The AchE stain showed delicate fibers in the lamina propria, muscularis mucosae, and superficial submucosa (Fig 13.13c). All the findings led to a diagnosis of HSCR.

The infant underwent a pull-through with request of intraoperative evaluation of ganglion cell at proximal anastomotic margin. The resected specimen had a suture at the distal margin, which was just slightly narrower compared to the proximal end (Fig 13.13d). The narrowed segment corresponded to the aganglionotic segment and the dilated segment showed progressively more ganglion cells in both Meissner and Auerbach plexuses confirming good number of ganglion cells at the proximal margin.

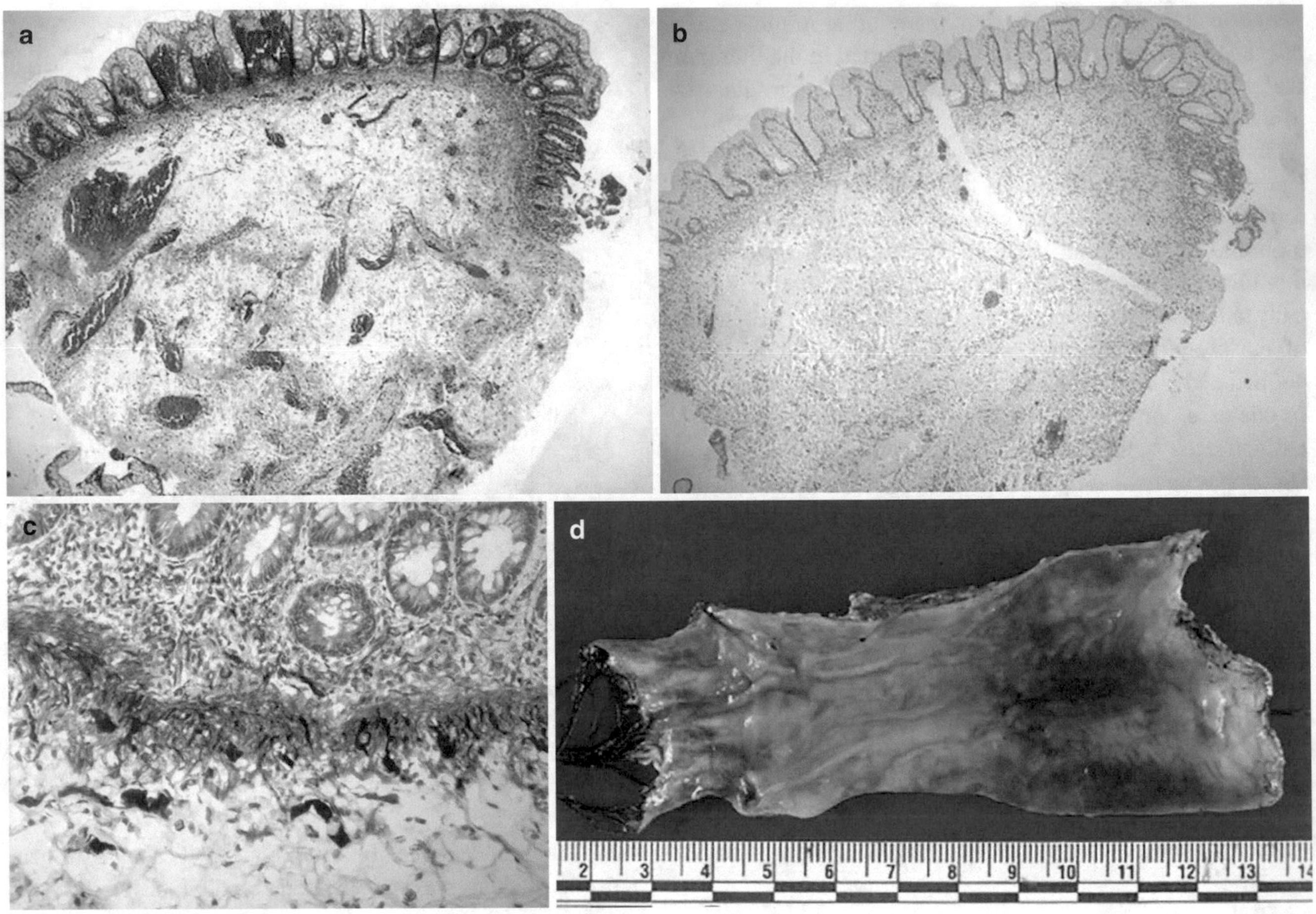

Fig. 13.13 (Case 2) (**a**) An adequate suction rectal biopsy showing a good amount of submucosa for evaluation of Meissner plexus ganglion cells, which were not identified in multiple (approximately 100) serial levels. In addition, neural hypertrophy is present. (**b**) Immunostain for calretinin showed no staining in neuritis and failed to highlight any ganglion cells. (**c**) AchE stain showed ropy brown staining in neuritis in the submucosa, muscularis mucosae and lamina propria, supporting a diagnosis of HSCR. (**d**) The gross specimen of the rectum after the resection and pull-through procedure showing the distal narrowing in aganglionic segment, a transitional zone and proximal dilated segment

Differential Diagnosis and Discussion

The diagnosis in this case is very clear and consistent with HSCR. The handling of the biopsies was ideal in this case with tissues kept frozen for AchE stain. The intraoperative frozen section of full-thickness biopsies and the resection specimen confirmed the diagnosis. Proper handling of the resection specimen is also shown in this case.

Final Diagnosis

Hirschsprung disease (short segment).

Case 3

Learning Objectives

1. To become familiar with clinical presentation and workup of patients suspected to have intestinal pseudo-obstruction
2. To become familiar with the handling and histologic findings in bowel resection of intestine for motility disorder
3. To integrate clinical and pathologic findings for diagnosis and differential diagnosis

Case History

The patient was a 60-year-old female with long-standing history of chronic constipation and bouts of abdominal distension suggestive of intestinal pseudo-obstruction. Clinical workup ruled out any mechanical causes of obstruction. The symptoms had become persistent and all prokinetic medical therapies had failed. Patient had a hysterectomy at age 35 for excessive uterine bleeding that revealed multiple uterine fibroids. She denied use of any recreational drugs. There was a family history of colon cancer in father at the age of 80 years and endometrial carcinoma in older sister of the patient. She had diabetes mellitus type-II and hypertension, for which she was getting treated. The patient finally underwent a near total colectomy with a diagnosis of intestinal pseudo-obstruction and to rule out visceral myopathy or neuropathy.

Pathology

The colon was markedly dilated and the muscular propria appeared thick, especially near the sigmoid colon. The sigmoid colon showed a few diverticula (Fig 13.14a). The mucosal folds throughout the colon and the small bowel grossly appeared normal. Multiple transverse and few longitudinal sections were obtained from the ascending, transverse, descending, and the sigmoid colon. The sections revealed slight fullness of lamina propria with lymphoplasmacytic cells and rare branched crypts (Fig 13.14b). There was fairly extensive melanosis coli (Fig 13.14c). The muscularis propria appeared thickened microscopically as well; however, the morphology of the smooth muscle cells was normal (Fig 13.14d). The submucosal and myenteric plexuses appeared within normal limits with ganglion cells readily identified. The ganglion cells and nerve bundles were highlighted with Bcl2, S-100, and calretinin stains, and appeared normal in morphology. DOG1 immunostain revealed normal population of ICCs (Fig 13.14e). There was no evidence of interstitial fibrosis as highlighted with trichrome stain. Immunostain for SMA showed normal staining in the smooth muscle layers of the large bowel, but showed decreased staining in the inner circular layer of the terminal ileum (Fig 13.14f). Microscopy from the sigmoid colon confirmed few uncomplicated diverticula.

Differential Diagnosis and Discussion

The mucosal changes are nonspecific and likely the result of long-standing bacterial stasis and the melanosis coli is likely related to chronic laxative use. The neuromuscular apparatus appears within normal limits on histology. Calretinin, Bcl2, and S-100 stains show normal staining patterns. The findings fail to show any specific myopathic or neuropathic changes. There were multiple adhesions around the sigmoid colon that could have contributed to mechanical obstruction following prior abdominal surgery. This case highlights several features commonly encountered in cases of motility disorders. Melanosis coli is a common finding as many of these patients have a long-standing history of laxatives use. This should be differentiated from brown-bowel syndrome, which is associated with intestinal dysmotility and is characterized by extensive deposition of dark brown lipofuscin pigment in the smooth muscle cells (Fig. 13.15). Brown-bowel syndrome has been associated with malnutrition and vitamin E deficiency. Decreased staining for SMA in the inner layer of small bowel muscularis propria has been reported to be associated with visceral myopathies. However, subsequent studies and our own experience suggest that this is not an uncommon nonspecific finding in the sections taken from the terminal ileum. Presence of peritoneal adhesions, often resulting from prior abdominal procedures/surgeries or intestinal perforation is often overlooked at pathologic examination. These can lead to mechanical obstruction. However, this patient's symptoms seem to have preceded her abdominal surgery, and the adhesions are unlikely to be the primary cause for the obstructive symptoms, although they could have contributed to worsening of the symptoms. While presence of multiple squared-mouth diverticula throughout the intestines is often associated with primary motility disorders of the bowel, presence of acquired-type diverticula in the sigmoid colon is unusual for visceral myopathy or neuropathy, especially the inherited types. Presence of acquired diverticula in the sigmoid also implies increased intraluminal pressure, which makes the possibility of a primary myopathy or neuropathy very unlikely. Lack of any family history or involvement of any other hollow viscera also makes the possibility of congenital or inherited forms of visceral myopathy or neuropathy very unlikely.

Final Diagosis

Final diagnosis in this case was colonic diverticulosis with no evidence of any primary visceral myopathy or neuropathy. A comment was also made about melanosis coli and extensive adhesions.

References: [79–82]

Case 4

Learning Objectives

1. To become familiar with clinical presentation and pathologic findings in patients suspected to have gastroparesis
2. To become familiar with the handling and pathologic findings in patients suspected to have gastroparesis
3. To integrate clinical and pathologic findings for diagnosis and differential diagnosis of neuromuscular disorders involving stomach

Clinical History

The patient was a 60-year-old male with a long-standing history of diabetes type II, for which he has been on oral antihyperglycemics. Over the years, he developed upper GI symptoms that included early satiety, nausea, abdominal distension, and bloating, which have become progressively worse. He had bouts of vomiting every month along with abdominal pain. He underwent upper GI endoscopy with gastric biopsies, which were unrevealing. Gastric emptying studies showed delayed gastric emptying. He had been on a variety of medications for his diabetes, hypertension, abdominal pain, and nausea. His symptoms progressed and repeat endoscopy and subsequently imaging studies showed a 3-cm submucosal lesion suggestive of a gastrointestinal stromal tumor (GIST) in the antrum. The patient eventually underwent a subtotal gastrectomy with Rou-en-Y anastomosis.

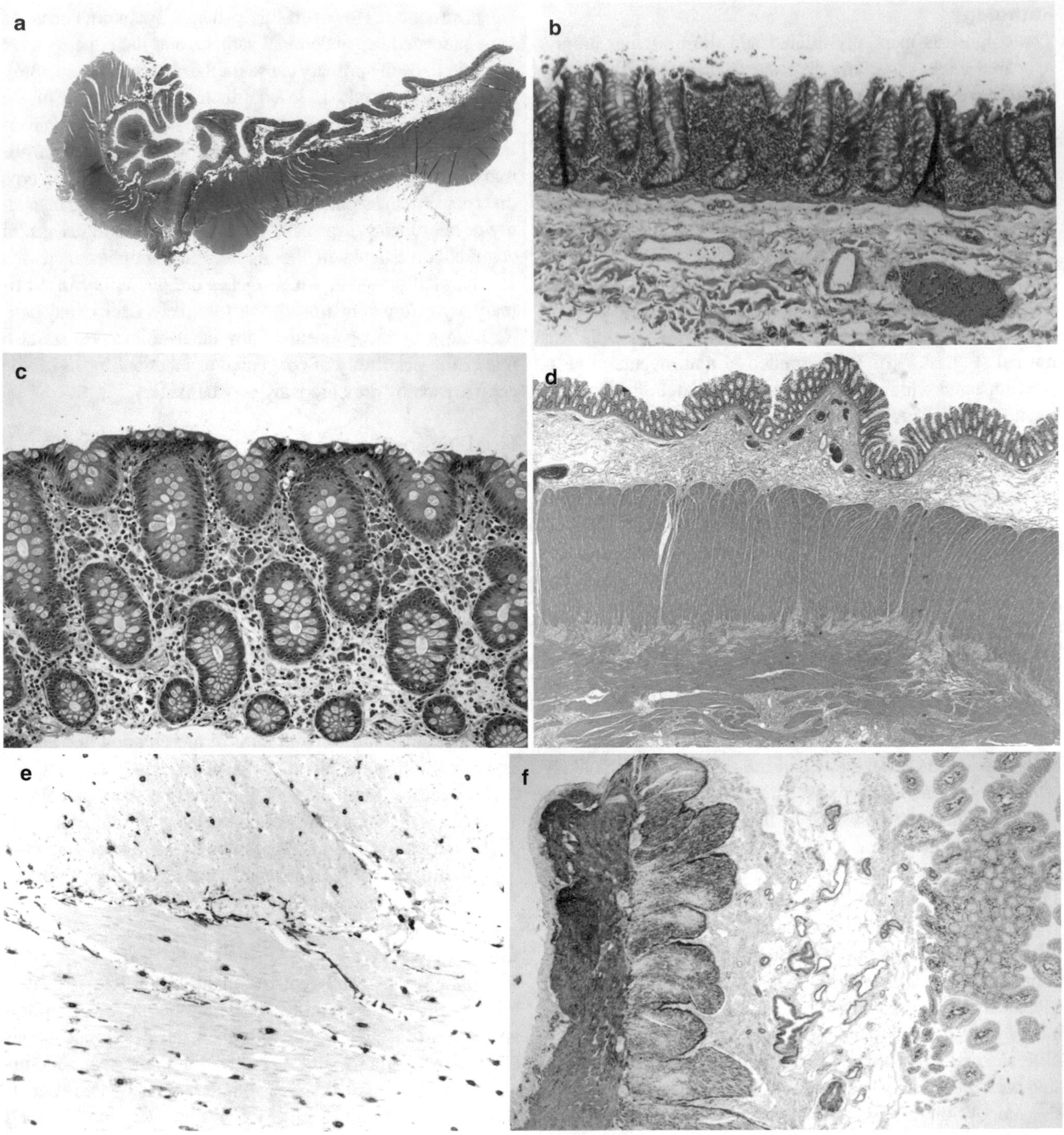

Fig. 13.14 (Case 3) (**a**) Low-power view of the section showing thickened muscularis propria, involving both layers of the muscularis propria. A diverticulum is evident at this magnification. (**b**) The higher power of the mucosa showing lamina propria fullness due to lymphoplasmacytic cells. Occasional branching crypts were seen, but basal lymphoplasmacytosis or Paneth cell metaplasia were not seen. (**c**) Higher magnification of the mucosa showing melanosis coli. (**d**) Low magnification showing hypertrophy of the muscularis propria. (**e**) C-kit immunostain showing the presence of ICCs. Numerous mast cells were also seen, which served as an internal control. (**f**) SMA immunostain showing loss of staining in the inner circular muscle layer of the muscularis propria of the small bowel

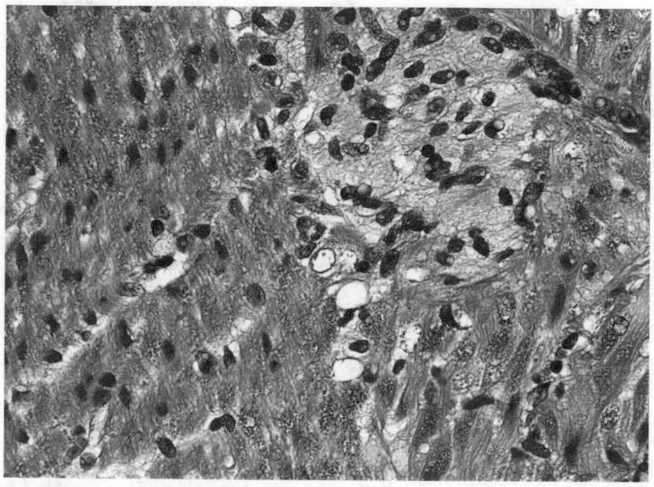

Fig. 13.15 Smooth muscle cells of the muscularis propria showing accumulation of dark brown lipofuscin pigment in a case of brown-bowel syndrome

Pathology

The stomach was dilated and showed foul-smelling contents (Fig 13.16a). After washing of the luminal contents and fixation, gross examination revealed an unremarkable mucosal pattern (Fig 13.16b). The submucosal lesion was identified, submitted entirely, and confirmed to be a c-kit positive GIST with very low malignant risk. In addition, multiple longitudinal and transverse sections along the length of the stomach were randomly taken from various sites including the antrum, body, fundus, and cardia. There was no mucosal pathology identified. Special attention was paid to the neuromuscular apparatus of the stomach in view of the clinical history. The muscle fibers appeared normal on low magnification. However, on closer examination scattered eosinophilic hyaline inclusions were identified scattered in the muscularis propria in the smooth muscle cells (Fig 13.16c). Ganglion cells were present throughout the submucosal and myenteric plexuses, and appeared normal, although focal inflammation was seen around the nerves and ganglia (Fig 13.16d). The neural plexus appeared normal. Immunostains for S-100 and calretinin to highlight nerves and ganglion cells appeared normal. DOG1 stain highlighted ICCs that were present and appeared normal in distribution (Fig 13.16e). Trichrome stain failed to show any fibrosis in the muscle layers. No evidence of amyloid deposition or cellular infiltrate (eosinophils or lymphocytes) was seen. Overall, the findings were considered nonspecific and consistent with changes described with gastroparesis. Changes of primary visceral myopathy or neuropathy were not seen.

Differential Diagnosis and Discussion

Surgical resection is not a standard approach for the management of patients with gastroparesis. However, occasionally one encounters resections for gastroparesis either associated with other disease requiring resection or gastroparesis resistant to other therapies. Gastroparesis can be idiopathic or associated with systemic disorders or medications (Table 13.6). In this case, diabetes is a very likely cause for the gastroparesis. The main issue during pathologic evaluation of such specimens is largely to exclude other causes of dysmotility, especially visceral myopathy or neuropathy and treatable infiltrative disorders like amyloidosis or eosinophilic gastritis. Very few studies have described pathologic changes in gastroparesis, which remain very nonspecific. The changes include a decrease in nerve fibers, reduced number of ganglion cells, mild inflammatory changes in the nerve plexuses and ganglia, reduced number of ICC, fibrosis in muscular layers, and degenerative changes in the muscle including the presence of cytoplasmic hyaline inclusions (M-bodies). However, the finding of M-bodies is nonspecific and has been reported in a wide range of GI motility disorders. The quantitative changes in neural apparatus are often subtle, require time-consuming morphometric analysis, and are largely reserved for research. It is also unclear if these changes are secondary or primary. When ganglion cells and nerve fibers are normal, they are easily identified on H&E stains. In clinical practice besides commenting on obvious findings, there is very little one can do in such cases. However, the histology is important in excluding most of the conditions in the differential diagnosis, which can be largely excluded on H&E stain alone. Immunostains like DOG1 and/or c-kit are useful to exclude abnormalities of ICC, which cannot be evaluated on H&E stains.

Final Diagnosis

The final diagnosis in this case included GIST with low malignant risk and comment about eosinophilic inclusions in the muscularis propria that are nonspecific, but consistent with gastroparesis.

References: [83–87]

Case 5

Learning Objectives

1. To become familiar with indications for esophageal biopsies in patients with achalasia
2. To become familiar with the histologic findings in the squamous mucosa in patients with achalasia
3. To integrate clinical and pathologic findings for diagnosis and differential diagnosis

Case History

A 45-year-old man with a long-standing history of achalasia underwent upper endoscopy for the long-standing symptoms of heartburn and chest pain, which revealed a tongue of salmon-colored mucosa in the distal esophagus and some

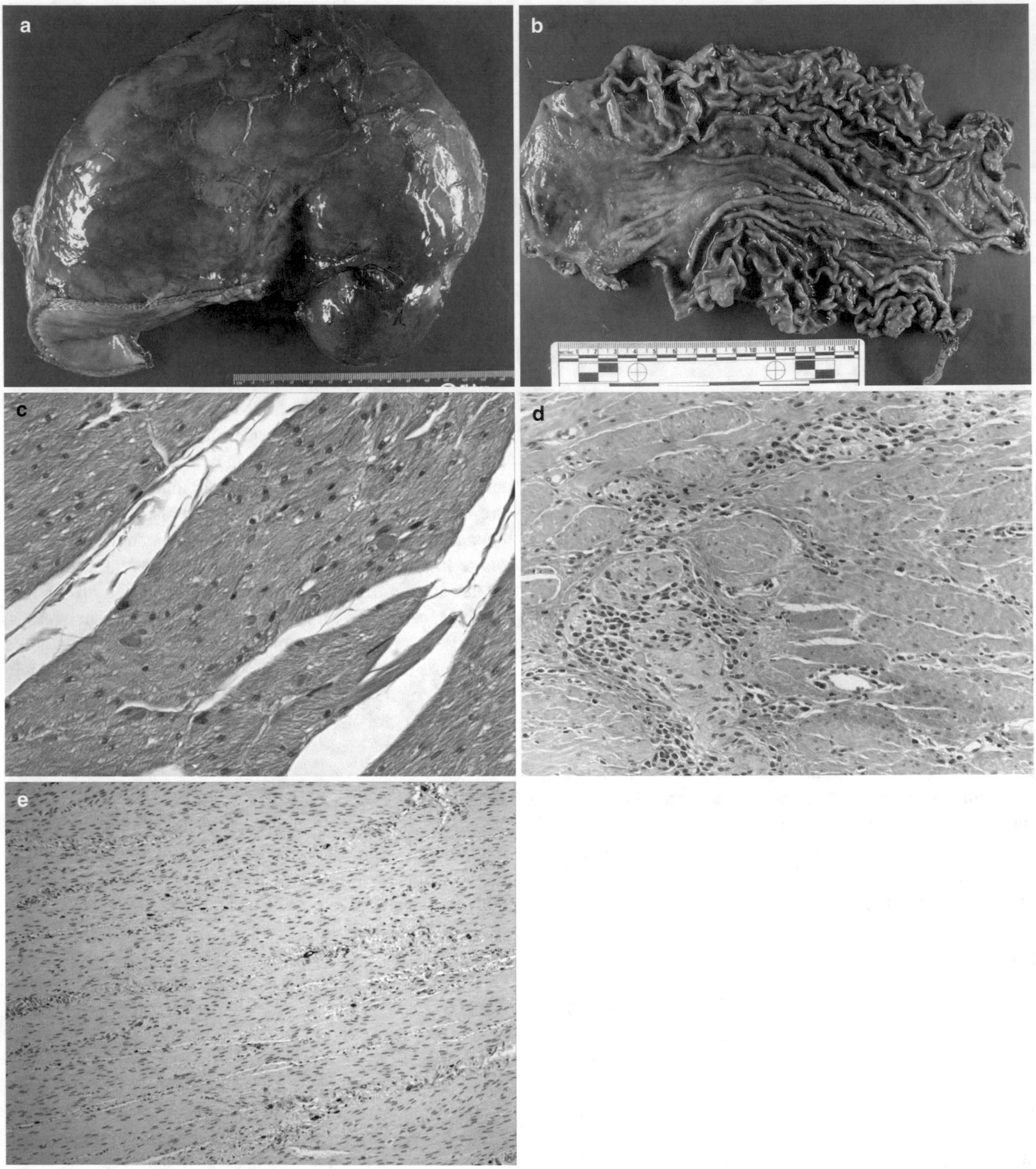

Fig. 13.16 (Case 4) (**a**) The resected specimen shows slightly dilated stomach. (**b**) Opened up specimen of subtotal gastrectomy showing no specific mucosal abnormality. (**c**) High power of the muscularis propria showing cytoplasmic hyaline inclusions (M-bodies), frequently seen in gastroparesis, but are nonspecific. (**d**) Inflammation around the neural plexus and ganglion cells. (**e**) DOG1 immunostain showing the presence of ICCs without obvious abnormalities

Table 13.6 Various causes of gastroparesis

Type	Causes
Idiopathic	Unknown etiology
Associated with other disorders	Diabetes mellitus type 1 and type 2
	Amyloidosis
	Connective tissue disorders (e.g., scleroderma and systemic lupus erythematosus)
	Neurologic disorders (e.g., Parkinson disease, and dysautonomia)
	Renal insufficiency
	Cirrhosis
Postviral infection	Norovirus, Epstein–Barr virus, cytomegalovirus and herpesvirus
Postsurgical	Fundoplication and vagotomy
Paraneoplastic	Small cell carcinoma
Medications	Opioids, antibiotics, antiarrhythmics, and anticonvulsants

irregularity of the squamous mucosa. Patient has been diagnosed with achalasia with the help of manometry and imaging studies 10 years ago. He underwent Heller myotomy to relieve the obstructive symptoms, which seemed to have worked so far. Multiple biopsies were taken from the gastroesophageal junction and abnormal-looking areas in the distal esophagus.

Pathology

The biopsies revealed squamous mucosa with reactive hyperplasia and mild lamina propria inflammation. Many intraepithelial lymphocytes were seen along with intercellular edema evidenced by dilated intercellular spaces. Junctional columnar mucosa showed focal intestinal metaplasia. No dysplasia or carcinoma was seen.

Differential Diagnosis and Discussion

Achalasia cardia is characterized by absence or marked reduction of ganglion cells in the myenteric plexus of the esophagus, especially in distal esophagus and gastroesophageal junction. The diagnosis is made reliably on clinical grounds, with history, endoscopy, manometry, and imaging. Biopsies are not required for establishing the diagnosis. However, patients with achalasia are at risk for developing squamous cell carcinoma as well as adenocarcinoma. Barrett esophagus also remains a concern after myotomy. Endoscopic surveillance and biopsies in patients with achalasia are performed to exclude evolving neoplasia. The histologic changes in such cases are often nonspecific as seen here, and the key is to evaluate the possibility of Barrett esophagus and associated complication, and squamous dysplasia/neoplasia. The squamous mucosa tends to show squamous hyperplasia, pseudo-epitheliomatous hyperplasia, intercellular edema, and/or lymphocytic esophagitis.

Final Diagnosis

Squamous mucosa with mild nonspecific inflammatory and reactive changes. Presence of intestinal metaplasia was consistent with the endoscopic findings of Barrett esophagus. The patient was scheduled for follow-up in 1 year, largely due to his symptoms.
Reference: [34]

References

1. Knowles CH, De Giorgio R, Kapur RP, Bruder E, Farrugia G, Geboes K, et al. The London Classification of gastrointestinal neuromuscular pathology: report on behalf of the Gastro 2009 International Working Group. Gut. 2010;59(7):882–7.
2. Kirsch R, Riddell RH. Histopathological alterations in irritable bowel syndrome. Mod Pathol. 2006;19(12):1638–45.
3. Lindberg G, Tornblom H, Iwarzon M, Nyberg B, Martin JE, Veress B. Full-thickness biopsy findings in chronic intestinal pseudo-obstruction and enteric dysmotility. Gut. 2009;58(8):1084–90.
4. Keller J, Bassotti G, Clarke J, Dinning P, Fox M, Grover M, et al. Expert consensus document: advances in the diagnosis and classification of gastric and intestinal motility disorders. Nat Rev Gastroenterol Hepatol. 2018;15(5):291–308.
5. Sipponen T, Karikoski R, Nuutinen H, Markkola A, Kaitila I. Three-generation familial visceral myopathy with alpha-actin-positive inclusion bodies in intestinal smooth muscle. J Clin Gastroenterol. 2009;43(5):437–43.
6. Magi GE, Mariotti F, Berardi S, Piccinini A, Vullo C, Palumbo Piccionello A, et al. Loss of alpha-smooth muscle actin expression associated with chronic intestinal pseudo-obstruction in a young Miniature Bull Terrier. Acta Vet Scand. 2018;60(1):25.
7. Wedel T, Spiegler J, Soellner S, Roblick UJ, Schiedeck TH, Bruch HP, et al. Enteric nerves and interstitial cells of Cajal are altered in patients with slow-transit constipation and megacolon. Gastroenterology. 2002;123(5):1459–67.
8. Ariza A, Coll J, Fernandez-Figueras MT, Lopez MD, Mate JL, Garcia O, et al. Desmin myopathy: a multisystem disorder involving skeletal, cardiac, and smooth muscle. Hum Pathol. 1995;26(9):1032–7.
9. Nemeth L, Yoneda A, Kader M, Devaney D, Puri P. Three-dimensional morphology of gut innervation in total intestinal aganglionosis using whole-mount preparation. J Pediatr Surg. 2001;36(2):291–5.
10. He CL, Burgart L, Wang L, Pemberton J, Young-Fadok T, Szurszewski J, et al. Decreased interstitial cell of cajal volume in patients with slow-transit constipation. Gastroenterology. 2000;118(1):14–21.
11. Feldstein AE, Miller SM, El-Youssef M, Rodeberg D, Lindor NM, Burgart LJ, et al. Chronic intestinal pseudoobstruction associated with altered interstitial cells of cajal networks. J Pediatr Gastroenterol Nutr. 2003;36(4):492–7.
12. Politei J, Durand C, Schenone AB, Torres A, Mukdsi J, Thurberg BL. Chronic intestinal pseudo-obstruction. Did you search for lysosomal storage diseases? Mol Genet Metab Rep. 2017; 11:8–11.
13. Cogliandro RF, De Giorgio R, Barbara G, Cogliandro L, Concordia A, Corinaldesi R, et al. Chronic intestinal pseudo-obstruction. Best Pract Res Clin Gastroenterol. 2007;21(4):657–69.
14. Kebede D, Barthel JS, Singh A. Transient gastroparesis associated with cutaneous herpes zoster. Dig Dis Sci. 1987;32(3):318–22.
15. Pai NB, Murthy RS, Kumar HT, Gerst PH. Association of acute colonic pseudo-obstruction (Ogilvie's syndrome) with herpes zoster. Am Surg. 1990;56(11):691–4.

16. De Giorgio R, Sarnelli G, Corinaldesi R, Stanghellini V. Advances in our understanding of the pathology of chronic intestinal pseudo-obstruction. Gut. 2004;53(11):1549–52.
17. Ruuska TH, Karikoski R, Smith VV, Milla PJ. Acquired myopathic intestinal pseudo-obstruction may be due to autoimmune enteric leiomyositis. Gastroenterology. 2002;122(4):1133–9.
18. Amiot A, Tchikviladze M, Joly F, Slama A, Hatem DC, Jardel C, et al. Frequency of mitochondrial defects in patients with chronic intestinal pseudo-obstruction. Gastroenterology. 2009;137(1):101–9.
19. Milunsky A, Baldwin C, Zhang X, Primack D, Curnow A, Milunsky J. Diagnosis of chronic intestinal pseudo-obstruction and megacystis by sequencing the ACTG2 gene. J Pediatr Gastroenterol Nutr. 2017;65(4):384–7.
20. Kapur RP, Robertson SP, Hannibal MC, Finn LS, Morgan T, van Kogelenberg M, et al. Diffuse abnormal layering of small intestinal smooth muscle is present in patients with FLNA mutations and x-linked intestinal pseudo-obstruction. Am J Surg Pathol. 2010;34(10):1528–43.
21. Iida T, Hirayama D, Sudo G, Mitsuhashi K, Igarashi H, Yamashita K, et al. Chronic intestinal pseudo-obstruction due to al amyloidosis: a case report and literature review. Clin J Gastroenterol. 2019;12(2):176–81.
22. Tada S, Iida M, Yao T, Kitamoto T, Fujishima M. Intestinal pseudo-obstruction in patients with amyloidosis: clinicopathologic differences between chemical types of amyloid protein. Gut. 1993;34(10):1412–7.
23. Liapis K, Michelis FV, Delimpasi S, Karmiris T. Intestinal pseudo-obstruction associated with amyloidosis. Amyloid. 2011;18(2):76–8.
24. Lennon VA, Sas DF, Busk MF, Scheithauer B, Malagelada JR, Camilleri M, et al. Enteric neuronal autoantibodies in pseudoobstruction with small-cell lung carcinoma. Gastroenterology. 1991;100(1):137–42.
25. Kulling D, Reed CE, Verne GN, Cotton PB, Tarnasky PR. Intestinal pseudo-obstruction as a paraneoplastic manifestation of malignant thymoma. Am J Gastroenterol. 1997;92(9):1564–6.
26. Lee HR, Lennon VA, Camilleri M, Prather CM. Paraneoplastic gastrointestinal motor dysfunction: clinical and laboratory characteristics. Am J Gastroenterol. 2001;96(2):373–9.
27. Rohrmann CA Jr, Ricci MT, Krishnamurthy S, Schuffler MD. Radiologic and histologic differentiation of neuromuscular disorders of the gastrointestinal tract: visceral myopathies, visceral neuropathies, and progressive systemic sclerosis. AJR Am J Roentgenol. 1984;143(5):933–41.
28. Krishnamurthy S, Schuffler MD. Pathology of neuromuscular disorders of the small intestine and colon. Gastroenterology. 1987;93(3):610–39.
29. Venizelos ID, Shousha S, Bull TB, Parkins RA. Chronic intestinal pseudo-obstruction in two patients. Overlap of features of systemic sclerosis and visceral myopathy. Histopathology. 1988;12(5):533–40.
30. Goldblum JR, Whyte RI, Orringer MB, Appelman HD. Achalasia. A morphologic study of 42 resected specimens. Am J Surg Pathol. 1994;18(4):327–37.
31. Cassella RR, Brown AL Jr, Sayre GP, Ellis FH Jr. Achalasia of the esophagus: pathologic and etiologic considerations. Ann Surg. 1964;160:474–87.
32. Goldblum JR, Rice TW, Richter JE. Histopathologic features in esophagomyotomy specimens from patients with achalasia. Gastroenterology. 1996;111(3):648–54.
33. Clark SB, Rice TW, Tubbs RR, Richter JE, Goldblum JR. The nature of the myenteric infiltrate in achalasia: an immunohistochemical analysis. Am J Surg Pathol. 2000;24(8):1153–8.
34. Gockel I, Bohl JR, Doostkam S, Eckardt VF, Junginger T. Spectrum of histopathologic findings in patients with achalasia reflects different etiologies. J Gastroenterol Hepatol. 2006;21(4):727–33.
35. Villanacci V, Annese V, Cuttitta A, Fisogni S, Scaramuzzi G, De Santo E, et al. An immunohistochemical study of the myenteric plexus in idiopathic achalasia. J Clin Gastroenterol. 2010;44(6):407–10.
36. Lehman MB, Clark SB, Ormsby AH, Rice TW, Richter JE, Goldblum JR. Squamous mucosal alterations in esophagectomy specimens from patients with end-stage achalasia. Am J Surg Pathol. 2001;25(11):1413–8.
37. Csendes A. Results of surgical treatment of achalasia of the esophagus. Hepatogastroenterology. 1991;38(6):474–80.
38. Peracchia A, Segalin A, Bardini R, Ruol A, Bonavina L, Baessato M. Esophageal carcinoma and achalasia: prevalence, incidence and results of treatment. Hepatogastroenterology. 1991;38(6):514–6.
39. Jamieson GG. Gastro-esophageal reflux following myotomy for achalasia. Hepatogastroenterology. 1991;38(6):506–9.
40. De Giorgio R, Ricciardiello L, Naponelli V, Selgrad M, Piazzi G, Felicani C, et al. Chronic intestinal pseudo-obstruction related to viral infections. Transplant Proc. 2010;42(1):9–14.
41. McDonald GB, Schuffler MD, Kadin ME, Tytgat GN. Intestinal pseudoobstruction caused by diffuse lymphoid infiltration of the small intestine. Gastroenterology. 1985;89(4):882–9.
42. Chander B, Fiedler P, Jain D. Eosinophilic myenteric ganglionitis: a case of intestinal pseudo-obstruction in a 93-year-old female. J Clin Gastroenterol. 2011;45(4):314–6.
43. Schappi MG, Smith VV, Milla PJ, Lindley KJ. Eosinophilic myenteric ganglionitis is associated with functional intestinal obstruction. Gut. 2003;52(5):752–5.
44. De Giorgio R, Barbara G, Stanghellini V, De Ponti F, Salvioli B, Tonini M, et al. Clinical and morphofunctional features of idiopathic myenteric ganglionitis underlying severe intestinal motor dysfunction: a study of three cases. Am J Gastroenterol. 2002;97(9):2454–9.
45. Angkathunyakul N, Treepongkaruna S, Molagool S, Ruangwattanapaisarn N. Abnormal layering of muscularis propria as a cause of chronic intestinal pseudo-obstruction: a case report and literature review. World J Gastroenterol. 2015;21(22):7059–64.
46. Schobinger-Clement S, Gerber HA, Stallmach T. Autoaggressive inflammation of the myenteric plexus resulting in intestinal pseudoobstruction. Am J Surg Pathol. 1999;23(5):602–6.
47. Amiot A, Cazals-Hatem D, Joly F, Lavergne-Slove A, Peuchmaur M, Bouhnik Y, et al. The role of immunohistochemistry in idiopathic chronic intestinal pseudoobstruction (CIPO): a case-control study. Am J Surg Pathol. 2009;33(5):749–58.
48. Howard LM, Markus H. Pseudo-obstruction secondary to anticholinergic drugs in Parkinson's disease. Postgrad Med J. 1992;68(795):70–1.
49. George CF. Drugs causing intestinal obstruction: a review. J R Soc Med. 1980;73(3):200–4.
50. Diezi M, Nydegger A, Di Paolo ER, Kuchler H, Beck-Popovic M. Vincristine and intestinal pseudo-obstruction in children: report of 5 cases, literature review, and suggested management. J Pediatr Hematol Oncol. 2010;32(4):e126–30.
51. Fragulidis G, Pantiora E, Michalaki V, Kontis E, Primetis E, Vezakis A, et al. Immune-related intestinal pseudo-obstruction associated with nivolumab treatment in a lung cancer patient. J Oncol Pharm Pract. 2019;25(2):487–91.
52. De Ponti F, De Giorgio R. The cathartic colon? Aliment Pharmacol Ther. 2002;16(3):643–4.
53. Joo JS, Ehrenpreis ED, Gonzalez L, Kaye M, Breno S, Wexner SD, et al. Alterations in colonic anatomy induced by chronic stimu-

lant laxatives: the cathartic colon revisited. J Clin Gastroenterol. 1998;26(4):283–6.
54. Reyes-Mugica M. Hirschpung disease. Path Case Rev. 2000;5:51–9.
55. Puri P. Intestinal neuronal dysplasia. Semin Pediatr Surg. 2003;12(4):259–64.
56. Qualman SJ, Jaffe R, Bove KE, Monforte-Munoz H. Diagnosis of hirschsprung disease using the rectal biopsy: multi-institutional survey. Pediatr Dev Pathol. 1999;2(6):588–96.
57. Montedonico S, Caceres P, Munoz N, Yanez H, Ramirez R, Fadda B. Histochemical staining for intestinal dysganglionosis: over 30 years experience with more than 1,500 biopsies. Pediatr Surg Int. 2011;27(5):479–86.
58. Vanderwinden JM, Rumessen JJ, Liu H, Descamps D, De Laet MH, Vanderhaeghen JJ. Interstitial cells of Cajal in human colon and in Hirschsprung's disease. Gastroenterology. 1996;111(4):901–10.
59. Horisawa M, Watanabe Y, Torihashi S. Distribution of c-Kit immunopositive cells in normal human colon and in Hirschsprung's disease. J Pediatr Surg. 1998;33(8):1209–14.
60. Kapur RP. Histology of the transition zone in hirschsprung disease. Am J Surg Pathol. 2016;40(12):1637–46.
61. Dickie BH, Webb KM, Eradi B, Levitt MA. The problematic Soave cuff in Hirschsprung disease: manifestations and treatment. J Pediatr Surg. 2014;49(1):77–80; discussion -1.
62. Fadda B, Maier WA, Meier-Ruge W, Scharli A, Daum R. Neuronal intestinal dysplasia. Critical 10-years' analysis of clinical and biopsy diagnosis. Z Kinderchir. 1983;38(5):305–11.
63. Rajalakshmi T, Makhija P, Babu MK, Kini U. Intestinal neuronal dysplasia type A. Indian J Pediatr. 2003;70(10):839–41.
64. Lake B. Intestinal neuronal dysplasia: a little local difficulity? Pediatr Pathol Lab Med. 1997;17:687.
65. Meier-Ruge WA, Longo-Bauer CH. Morphometric determination of the methodological criteria for the diagnosis of intestinal neuronal dysplasia (IND B). Pathol Res Pract. 1997;193(7): 465–9.
66. Meier-Ruge WA, Bruder E, Kapur RP. Intestinal neuronal dysplasia type B: one giant ganglion is not good enough. Pediatr Dev Pathol. 2006;9(6):444–52.
67. Terra SA, de Arruda Lourencao PL, Silva MG, Miot HA, Rodrigues MAM. A critical appraisal of the morphological criteria for diagnosing intestinal neuronal dysplasia type B. Mod Pathol. 2017;30(7):978–85.
68. Dingemann J, Puri P. Isolated hypoganglionosis: systematic review of a rare intestinal innervation defect. Pediatr Surg Int. 2010;26(11):1111–5.
69. Qadir I, Salick MM, Barakzai A, Zafar H. Isolated adult hypoganglionosis presenting as sigmoid volvulus: a case report. J Med Case Reports. 2011;5:445.
70. Aldossary MY, Privitera A, Elzamzami O, Alturki N, Sabr K. A rare case of adult-onset rectosigmoid hypoganglionosis. Am J Case Rep. 2018;19:557–61.
71. Kwok AM, Still AB, Hart K. Acquired segmental colonic hypoganglionosis in an adult Caucasian male: a case report. World J Gastrointest Surg. 2019;11(2):101–11.
72. Meier-Ruge WA, Brunner LA. Morphometric assessment of Hirschsprung's disease: associated hypoganglionosis of the colonic myenteric plexus. Pediatr Dev Pathol. 2001;4(1):53–61.
73. Swaminathan M, Kapur RP. Counting myenteric ganglion cells in histologic sections: an empirical approach. Hum Pathol. 2010;41(8):1097–108.
74. Muto M, Matsufuji H, Taguchi T, Tomomasa T, Nio M, Tamai H, et al. Japanese clinical practice guidelines for allied disorders of Hirschsprung's disease, 2017. Pediatr Int. 2018;60(5):400–10.
75. Meier-Ruge WA, Brunner LA, Engert J, Heminghaus M, Holschneider AM, Jordan P, et al. A correlative morphometric and clinical investigation of hypoganglionosis of the colon in children. Eur J Pediatr Surg. 1999;9(2):67–74.
76. Martucciello G, Pini Prato A, Puri P, Holschneider AM, Meier-Ruge W, Jasonni V, et al. Controversies concerning diagnostic guidelines for anomalies of the enteric nervous system: a report from the fourth International Symposium on Hirschsprung's disease and related neurocristopathies. J Pediatr Surg. 2005;40(10):1527–31.
77. Qiu J, Yang G, Lin A. Allied disorders of Hirschsprung's disease. Tech Coloproctol. 2019;23:509–11.
78. Murakami J. Clinical practice guidelines for allied disorders of Hirschsprung's disease. Pediatr Int. 2018;60(5):399.
79. Hitzman JL, Weiland LH, Oftedahl GL, Lie JT. Ceroidosis in the "Brown bowel syndrome". Mayo Clin Proc. 1979;54(4):251–7.
80. Asher C, Mavinamane S. Brown bowel syndrome. Br J Hosp Med (Lond). 2013;74(2):111.
81. Gamba E, Carr NJ, Bateman AC. Deficient alpha smooth muscle actin expression as a cause of intestinal pseudo-obstruction: fact or fiction? J Clin Pathol. 2004;57(11):1168–71.
82. Smith VV, Lake BD, Kamm MA, Nicholls RJ. Intestinal pseudo-obstruction with deficient smooth muscle alpha-actin. Histopathology. 1992;21(6):535–42.
83. Onyimba FU, Clarke JO. Helping patients with gastroparesis. Med Clin North Am. 2019;103(1):71–87.
84. Harberson J, Thomas RM, Harbison SP, Parkman HP. Gastric neuromuscular pathology in gastroparesis: analysis of full-thickness antral biopsies. Dig Dis Sci. 2010;55(2):359–70.
85. Omer E, Kedar A, Nagarajarao HS, Nikitina Y, Vedanarayanan V, Subramony C, et al. Cajal cell counts are important predictors of outcomes in drug rcfractory gastroparesis patients with neurostimulation. J Clin Gastroenterol. 2019;53(5):366–72.
86. Heckert J, Thomas RM, Parkman HP. Gastric neuromuscular histology in patients with refractory gastroparesis: relationships to etiology, gastric emptying, and response to gastric electric stimulation. Neurogastroenterol Motil. 2017;29:e13068.
87. Bashashati M, Moraveji S, Torabi A, Sarosiek I, Davis BR, Diaz J, et al. Pathological findings of the antral and pyloric smooth muscle in patients with gastroparesis-like syndrome compared to gastroparesis: similarities and differences. Dig Dis Sci. 2017;62(10):2828–33.

Non-syndromic Epithelial Polyps of the Gastrointestinal Tract

14

Dorina Gui, Hanlin L. Wang, and Kristin A. Olson

List of Frequently Asked Questions

1. What are the diagnostic features of squamous papilloma of the esophagus?
2. Is squamous papilloma of the esophagus associated with human papillomavirus and does it carry any malignant risk?
3. What are the diagnostic features and clinical significance of glycogenic acanthosis of the esophagus?
4. How is hyperplastic polyp of the stomach distinguished from fundic gland polyp?
5. Do hyperplastic polyp and fundic gland polyp of the stomach have malignant risk?
6. How are the subtypes of gastric adenoma differentiated from one another and their potential clinical significance?
7. How is hyperplastic polyp of the stomach distinguished from pyloric gland adenoma?
8. What are the diagnostic features of gastritis/colitis cystica profunda/polyposa?
9. How is Brunner gland hyperplasia distinguished from normal Brunner glands?
10. How is Brunner gland hyperplasia distinguished from pyloric gland adenoma of the duodenum?
11. What are the characteristic features of heterotopic gastric mucosa and heterotopic pancreatic tissue?
12. What is the clinical significance of an adenomatous polyp at the ampulla as compared to elsewhere in the small bowel?
13. What are the diagnostic features of an inflammatory polyp?
14. What should one do if an inflammatory polyp shows atypical stromal cells?
15. What is inflammatory cap polyp/polyposis?
16. What is filiform polyposis?
17. What are the diagnostic features of mucosal prolapse?
18. What are the diagnostic features of inflammatory cloacogenic polyp?
19. What are the diagnostic features of inflammatory myoglandular polyp?
20. Is there any clinical significance to the hyperplastic polyp subtypes of the large intestine?
21. How is sessile serrated lesion distinguished from hyperplastic polyp?
22. How is traditional serrated adenoma distinguished from sessile serrated lesion and tubulovillous adenoma?
23. Does sessile serrated lesion have any malignant potential, and what is the clinical significance of cytologic dysplasia in these polyps?
24. Is there any clinical significance to subclassify an adenomatous polyp as tubular, villous, or tubulovillous?
25. Is there any clinical significance of a squamous morule or minute clusters of neuroendocrine cell proliferation found in a colonic adenoma?
26. What are the morphological features to determine high-grade dysplasia in an adenomatous polyp?
27. What are the morphological features that help distinguish "pseudoinvasion" from true invasion?
28. What should one do if an adenomatous component is found extending into submucosal lymphoid follicles?
29. How can colonic polyps be stratified in terms of risk of progression to adenocarcinoma, and how should the patients be surveilled?
30. What histologic characteristics must be included in the pathology report for an adenomatous polyp with invasive adenocarcinoma?
31. What are the diagnostic features of different appendiceal polyps?

D. Gui (✉) · K. A. Olson
University of California at Davis School of Medicine, Sacramento, CA, USA
e-mail: dgui@ucdavis.edu

H. L. Wang
University of California at Los Angeles David Geffen School of Medicine, Los Angeles, CA, USA

H. L. Wang, Z. E. Chen (eds.), *Practical Gastrointestinal Pathology*, Practical Anatomic Pathology,
https://doi.org/10.1007/978-3-030-51268-2_14

32. What is the clinical significance of different appendiceal polyps?
33. Can juvenile polyp and Peutz-Jeghers polyp be non-syndromic?

Frequently Asked Questions

1. **What are the diagnostic features of squamous papilloma of the esophagus?**

   Endoscopically, the typical appearance is that of a whitish nodule/polyp (usually <0.5 cm) occurring in the middle to lower third of the esophagus. Most of the squamous papillomas of the esophagus (SPE) are solitary and the reported prevalence ranges between 0.07% and 0.45%. Histologically, it consists of finger-like fronds of acanthotic stratified squamous papillae covering delicate fibrovascular cores (Fig. 14.1). The squamous cells typically lack cytologic atypia or features of koilocytosis. Based on the predominant shape of the squamous papillae, SPEs can be classified into three types: exophytic (50%), endophytic (37%), and spiked (13%).
   References: [1, 2]

2. **Is squamous papilloma of the esophagus associated with human papillomavirus and does it carry any malignant risk?**

   Proposed etiologic factors for SPE include gastroesophageal reflux disease (GERD), mucosal trauma, and HPV. A study by Takeshita et al. in 2006 showed 10.5% of SPEs to be positive for HPV by PCR, which were located in the middle third of the esophagus of female patients only. The study group consisted of 35 Japanese patients including 21 females and 14 males. In contrast, studies from Europe, Canada, and United States report a male predominance and a high prevalence in the lower third esophagus. A meta-analysis performed by K. Syrjanen and S. Syrjanen in 2012 showed that 30.9% of reported SPE cases tested HPV-positive (genotypes detected: 6/11, 16/18, 31, 33, 35). The data for this analysis were derived from 39 studies covering 427 SPEs from different geographic regions.

   While the malignant potential of the SPEs is still unclear, the chronic infection with HPV can induce progression to dysplasia and carcinoma, especially for high-risk genotypes such as 16, 18, 31, and 81. A study by Pantham et al. indicated that the incidence of SPE had increased fourfold over the past 14 years and approximately half of the tested patients were positive for high-risk HPV, which may suggest a potential risk for esophageal squamous cell cancer.

   However, our anecdotal experience suggests that SPE is not a high risk lesion and we have never seen a case with malignant transformation in our practice. In fact, our recent study of 78 SPE cases using the highly sensitive and specific RNA in situ hybridization technology failed to demonstrate the presence of HPV RNA in these lesions (unpublished data).
   References: [2–6]

3. **What are the diagnostic features and clinical significance of glycogenic acanthosis of the esophagus?**

   Glycogenic acanthosis presents endoscopically as white plaques (up to 1 cm in size), mostly in the distal third of the esophagus. Rarely these plaques coalesce into larger ones that can be mistaken as Candida plaques or leukoplakia. Histologically, the lesion is comprised of hyperplastic squamous epithelium with enlarged, vacuolated, and glycogen-filled cells (Fig. 14.2), which are PAS-positive and PAS with diastase-negative. Although

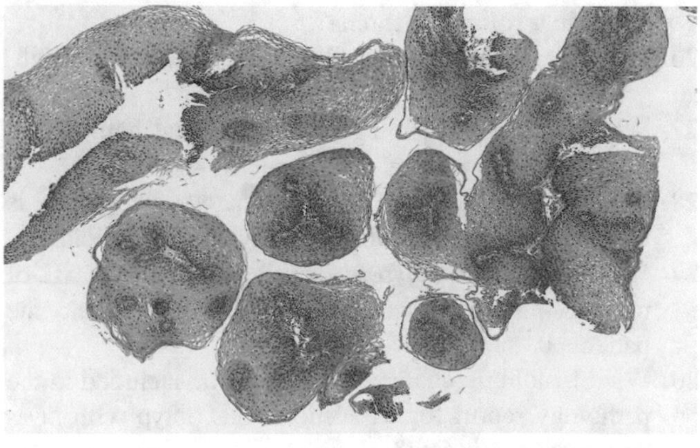

Fig. 14.1 Esophageal squamous papilloma showing papillary proliferation of acanthotic squamous epithelium covering delicate fibrovascular cores. There is no significant cytologic atypia. No koilocytosis is seen

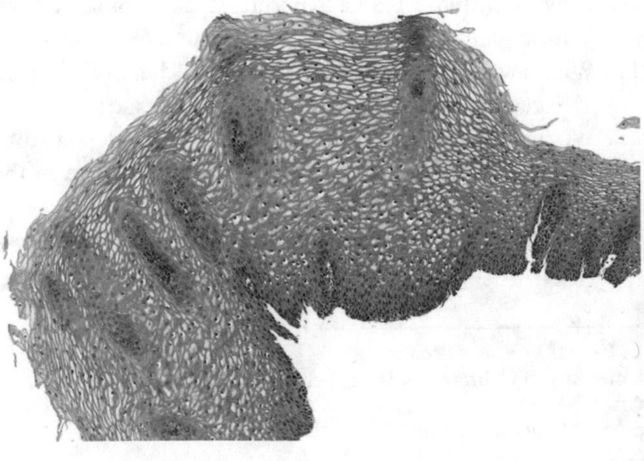

Fig. 14.2 Glycogenic acanthosis showing hyperplastic squamous epithelium with abundant vacuolated (glycogen-filled) cytoplasm

the etiology and pathogenesis are unknown, there are few studies suggesting that glycogenic acanthosis may be related to GERD while others bring up the point that the antireflux therapy improved GERD symptoms but failed to eradicate glycogenic acanthosis. Glycogenic acanthosis in its diffuse form is emphasized in the literature as a feature of Cowden syndrome, which can be seen in up to 80% of patients with Cowden syndrome associated with *PTEN* mutation.

References: [7–12]

4. How is hyperplastic polyp of the stomach distinguished from fundic gland polyp?

Hyperplastic polyps are the most common gastric polyps, representing up to 71% of all gastric polyps as per a 5-year review by Morais et al. They are usually small, flat, or sessile, ranging from less than 0.5 to 3 cm, with rare cases measuring more than 10 cm. Hyperplastic polyps can occur anywhere in the stomach, with a slight preference for the antral region. Most cases are solitary but they can be multiple. It is believed that the polyps generally arise in response to chronic inflammation, and there is a strong association with various types of gastritis such as *Helicobacter pylori* gastritis and autoimmune gastritis, and gastroenteric anastomoses such as Billroth II gastrojejunostomy.

The histologic appearance is characterized by elongated, distorted, and cystically dilated foveolae lined by hyperplastic mucin-containing epithelium set in an inflamed stroma (Fig. 14.3a). The lamina propria of hyperplastic polyps is typically edematous and infiltrated by variable numbers of inflammatory cells (Fig. 14.3b). Proliferation of smooth muscle bundles in the lower portion may be seen in larger polyps, consistent with prolapse-related change. Surface erosion or ulceration with granulation tissue may occur (Fig. 14.3c), causing occult

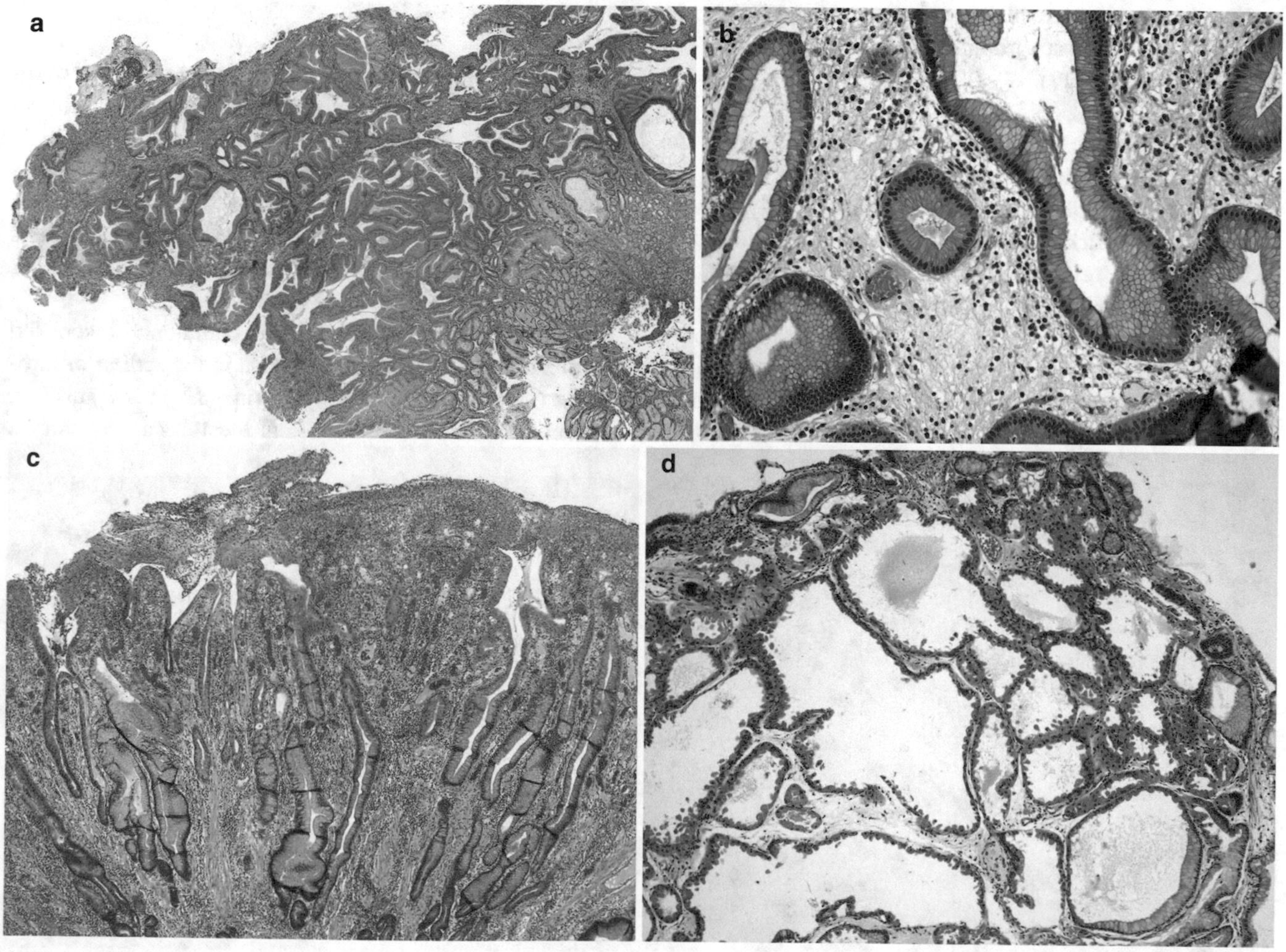

Fig. 14.3 Gastric hyperplastic polyp showing proliferation of distorted and cystically dilated foveolae (**a**), with edematous and inflamed lamina propria (**b**), and surface erosions (**c**). Fundic gland polyp showing cystically dilated oxyntic glands lined by hypertrophic parietal cells with cytoplasmic protrusions (**d**)

bleeding and anemia especially if they are large in size. Reactive fibroblasts and endothelial cells with prominent nuclear atypia (pseudosarcomatous change) may be seen in the areas with granulation tissue.

A rare variant is the inverted hyperplastic polyp, characterized by submucosal downward growth of the hyperplastic foveolar glands, with only a few cases reported in the literature. The histologic features suggest that these reported inverted hyperplastic polyps likely represent gastritis cystica profunda/polyposa associated with hyperplastic and metaplastic changes.

Fundic gland polyps occur in the gastric fundus and body and are usually multiple, representing 16–51% of all gastric epithelial polyps and having an increasing occurrence due to proton pump inhibitor (PPI) therapy. They are rarely larger than 1 cm. The characteristic histologic appearance is of cystically dilated oxyntic glands lined by hypertrophic or flattened parietal, chief, and mucous cells (Fig. 14.3d). They lack the hyperplastic foveolar epithelium as seen in hyperplastic polyps, and have little to no association with background mucosal disease.
References: [13–17]

5. **Do hyperplastic polyp and fundic gland polyp of the stomach have malignant risk?**

It was not long ago that hyperplastic polyps were viewed as markers of an abnormal gastric mucosa background rather than an isolated preneoplastic lesion. More recent studies show that unremoved gastric hyperplastic polyps can enlarge and undergo neoplastic transformation via hyperplasia-metaplasia-dysplasia-carcinoma sequence (Fig. 14.4a, b). Focal intestinal metaplasia is not an uncommon finding in hyperplastic polyps. The reported rates of dysplasia and carcinoma range from 1.5% to 10%, usually seen in polyps that are larger than 1 cm. *TP53* and *PIK3CA* mutations have been identified in dysplastic gastric hyperplastic polyps.

Sporadic fundic gland polyps frequently harbor mutations of the beta-catenin gene (*CTNNB1*) and are much less likely to have mutations of the adenomatous polyposis coli (*APC*) gene. Only rare sporadic cases show low-grade dysplasia, however. In contrast, familial fundic gland polyps seen in the setting of familial adenomatous polyposis (FAP) frequently harbor *APC* mutations. Low-grade dysplasia is more common in familial cases (see Fig. 14.1d in Chap. 15). However, progression to high-grade dysplasia or gastric adenocarcinoma is exceedingly rare in FAP patients. Fundic gland polyps are also common lesions in patients with gastric adenocarcinoma and proximal polyposis of the stomach (GAPPS), which also involves the *APC* gene (see Chap. 15, Question 19).
References: [18–22]

6. **How are the subtypes of gastric adenoma differentiated from one another and their potential clinical significance?**

Gastric adenomas can derive from deep gastric mucous glands (pyloric gland adenoma), from the surface foveolar epithelium (foveolar adenoma), from chief cells (oxyntic gland adenoma), or can contain goblet cells or Paneth cells (intestinal-type adenoma).

Pyloric gland adenomas are commonly associated with chronically damaged mucosa in the setting of atrophic (mostly autoimmune) gastritis, *H. pylori* gastritis, chemical gastritis, and intestinal metaplasia, and carry a

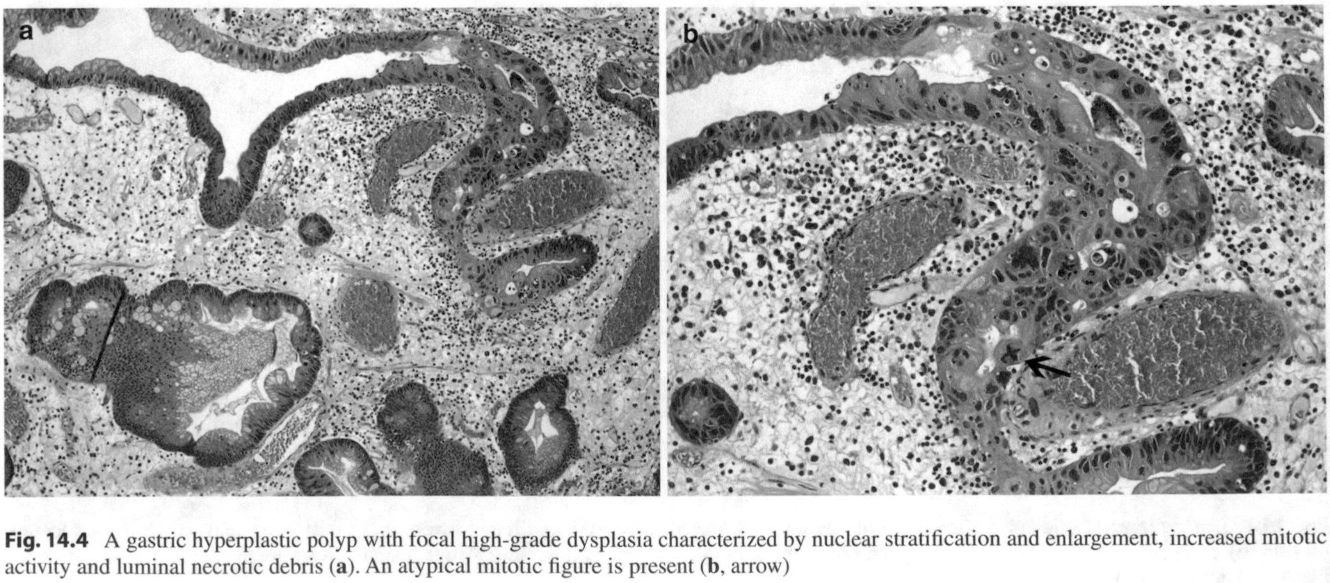

Fig. 14.4 A gastric hyperplastic polyp with focal high-grade dysplasia characterized by nuclear stratification and enlargement, increased mitotic activity and luminal necrotic debris (**a**). An atypical mitotic figure is present (**b**, arrow)

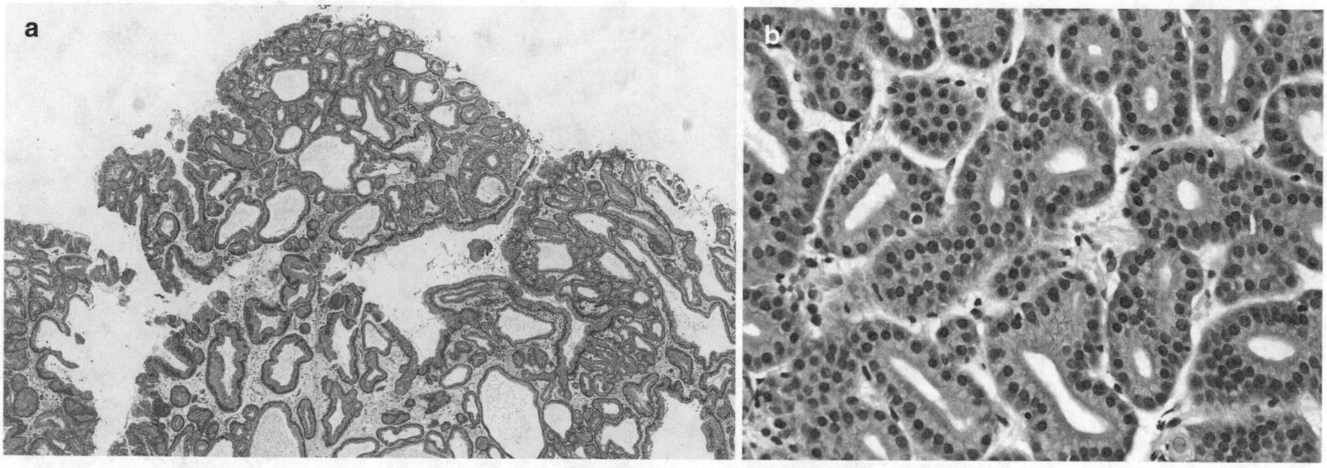

Fig. 14.5 Pyloric gland adenoma showing closely packed pyloric-type tubular glands (**a**). A few mildly dilated glands are also present. The lining epithelial cells are relatively uniform and lack well-defined apical mucin caps (**b**)

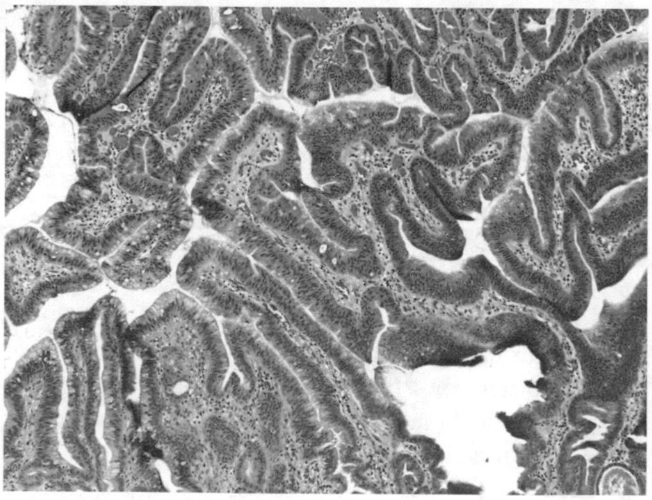

Fig. 14.6 Foveolar-type gastric adenoma characterized by low-grade dysplasia and apical mucin caps. No intestinal metaplasia is seen

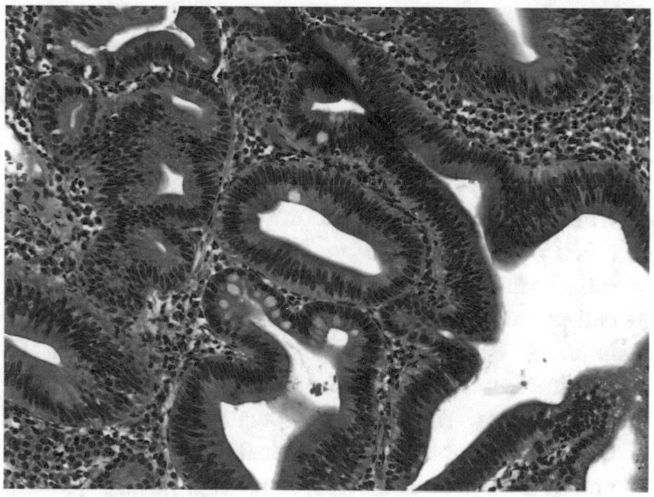

Fig. 14.7 Intestinal-type gastric adenoma resembling a tubular adenoma of the colorectum. Scattered goblet cells are present

high risk for progression to high-grade dysplasia and invasive adenocarcinoma. They are formed by closely packed pyloric-type tubular glands (Fig. 14.5a), but dilated glands may also be seen in larger polyps. The neoplastic cells are cuboidal to low columnar and lack well-defined apical mucin cap. They have relatively uniform round to oval nuclei, inconspicuous or occasional prominent nucleoli, and pale to eosinophilic, ground-glass-appearing cytoplasm (Fig. 14.5b). High-grade dysplasia is characterized by complex glands, crowded and enlarged nuclei, and loss of nuclear polarity. In addition to the stomach, pyloric gland adenomas also occur in the esophagus, gastroesophageal junction, duodenum, gallbladder and bile duct.

The foveolar-type gastric adenomas are rare, mostly occurring in the gastric body and fundus. They are formed by dysplastic foveolar cells with a distinctive apical mucin cap (PAS positive), have no association with chronic gastritis or intestinal metaplasia, and only rarely to almost never progress to high-grade dysplasia or adenocarcinoma. The lesions typically show low-grade nuclear atypia with stratified and elongated nuclei (Fig. 14.6).

Intestinal-type gastric adenomas are similar to those seen in the colorectum and small intestine. They form tubules lined by dysplastic intestinalized cells with elongated hyperchromatic nuclei (Fig. 14.7). Occasional goblet cells and/or Paneth cells may be present. The neoplastic

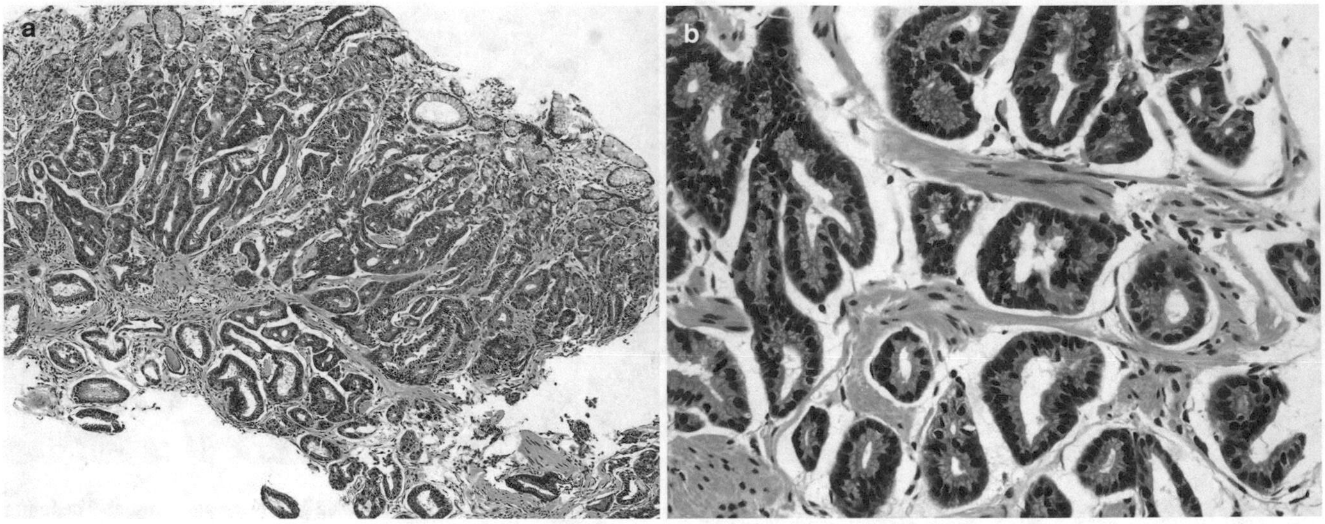

Fig. 14.8 Oxyntic gland adenoma of the stomach showing irregular, branching, and focally anastomosing glands separated by wisps of smooth muscle (**a**). The glands are lined by a mixture of chief (predominant), parietal and mucous neck cells with minimal (if any) nuclear atypia (**b**)

cells are usually columnar with no apical mucin cap. This type of adenoma typically arises in the background of intestinal metaplasia and has a high incidence of progression to high-grade dysplasia and invasive adenocarcinoma.

Previously classified as "gastric adenocarcinoma with chief cell differentiation" or "gastric adenocarcinoma of fundic gland type," oxyntic gland adenomas (also termed "oxyntic gland polyps/adenomas" or "chief cell-predominant gastric polyps" in the literature) occur in areas with oxyntic mucosa, predominantly in the proximal stomach. They are small, solitary polyps, typically <1 cm. There is no association with gastritis or intestinal metaplasia. Histologically, most oxyntic adenomas arise within the deeper zone of gastric mucosa. They are composed of irregular, dilated, branching, or anastomosing glands lined by a mixture of chief (predominant), parietal, and mucous neck cells. Mild nuclear atypia may be present, but there is no mitosis. The neoplastic glands are usually separated by radiating wisps of smooth muscle (Fig. 14.8a, b), but there is no desmoplasia. Some cases show submucosal extension, which remains debatable whether it presents true submucosal invasion (progression to adenocarcinoma of fundic gland type) or prolapse-type noninvasive change. The studies by Singhi et al. and Chan et al. showed that neither the patients included in their study groups nor the cases reported previously had recurrence or disease progression following endoscopic excision, supporting the benign nature of these lesions.

Table 14.1 MUC2, MUC5AC, and MUC6 expression by immunohistochemistry in gastric adenomas

	MUC2	MUC5AC	MUC6
Pyloric gland adenoma	Negative	*Positive*	*Positive*
Intestinal-type gastric adenoma	*Positive*	Negative	Negative
Foveolar-type gastric adenoma	Negative	*Positive*	Negative
Oxyntic gland adenoma	Negative	Negative	*Positive*

The distinction among different types of adenoma of the stomach relies on histology. Immunohistochemical stains for mucin markers (Table 14.1) can be useful but are rarely used in practice.
References: [23–26]

7. **How is hyperplastic polyp of the stomach distinguished from pyloric gland adenoma?**

These two types of polyp are different by morphology. Hyperplastic polyp is essentially a form of localized foveolar hyperplasia, characterized by a corkscrew appearance given by tortuous elongated pits lined by foveolar cells that extend deep down in the lamina propria. It has an inflamed and edematous stroma, with or without surface erosions/ulcerations. Pyloric gland adenoma is characterized by a closely packed collection of small pyloric gland-type tubules, lined by cuboidal to columnar cells with ground-glass-appearing cytoplasm. Cystically dilated glands are less common than in hyperplastic polyp.

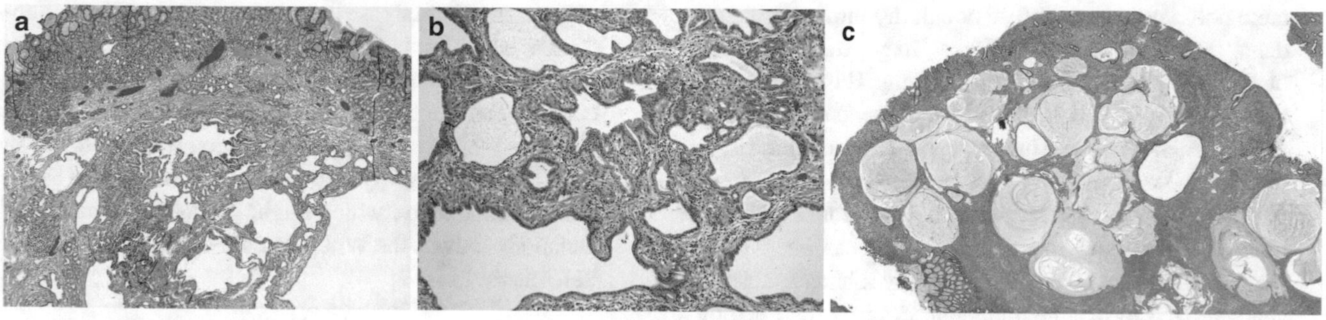

Fig. 14.9 Gastritis cystica profunda showing entrapped gastric glands in the submucosa (**a**), some of which are cystically dilated (**b**). A case of colitis cystica profunda showing cystically dilated colonic crypts in the submucosa with mucin accumulation and extravasation (**c**). The lining epithelial cells are atrophic-appearing

8. What are the diagnostic features of gastritis/colitis cystica profunda/polyposa?

Gastritis cystica profunda/polyposa may present as a polyp, a submucosal tumor, or giant gastric folds. It is referred to as "polyposa" when there is an identifiable lesion (localized) or "profunda" when there is lack of a discrete lesion (diffuse). Histologically, it represents ectopic entrapment of gastric glands in the deep portions of the gastric wall including the submucosa, muscularis propria, and even the subserosa (Fig. 14.9a, b). The entrapped glands are often dilated and may show hyperplastic, reactive, or atrophic changes. They are usually surrounded by a rim of lamina propria or disorganized smooth muscle bundles. While majority of these cases are associated with prior gastroenterostomy (with or without gastric resection), it has also been described in patients with no gastric surgical history.

When similar lesions occur in the colorectum, they are termed colitis cystica profunda/polyposa. Patients may have a history of mucosal injury such as that caused by inflammatory bowel disease (IBD), radiation, diverticulitis, prolapse, etc. The localized form can occur anywhere in the colon, but is more commonly seen in the rectum. Mucin extravasation, fibrosis, and dystrophic calcification/ossification may be seen in older lesions (Fig. 14.9c).

A major differential diagnosis for gastritis/colitis cystica profunda/polyposa is invasive well-differentiated or mucinous adenocarcinoma, particularly in the presence of extravasated mucin. Lack of infiltrative growth pattern, angulated or anastomosing glands, significant cytologic atypia, free-floating epithelial cells in mucin pools and desmoplasia, as well as the presence of lamina propria component and/or smooth muscle bundles are not features of invasive carcinoma.

References: [27–29]

9. How is Brunner gland hyperplasia distinguished from normal Brunner glands?

The Brunner glands are mucin-secreting glands mostly located in the duodenal submucosa. About one-third also normally occur in the lamina propria, with focal extension through the muscularis mucosae. They are more concentrated in the gastroduodenal junction area and diminish quantitatively toward distal duodenum. They are tubuloalveolar glands lined by cuboidal to columnar cells with basally situated nuclei, arranged in a lobular architecture containing fibrous septa.

Brunner gland hyperplasia is characterized by lobules of non-dysplastic, closely packed Brunner glands and ducts that are divided by strands of fibrous tissue and smooth muscle, with variable adipose tissue or lymphoid aggregates in the stroma (Fig. 14.10). The individual glands are morphologically indistinguishable from normal Brunner glands. It is usually an incidental finding endoscopically as a dis-

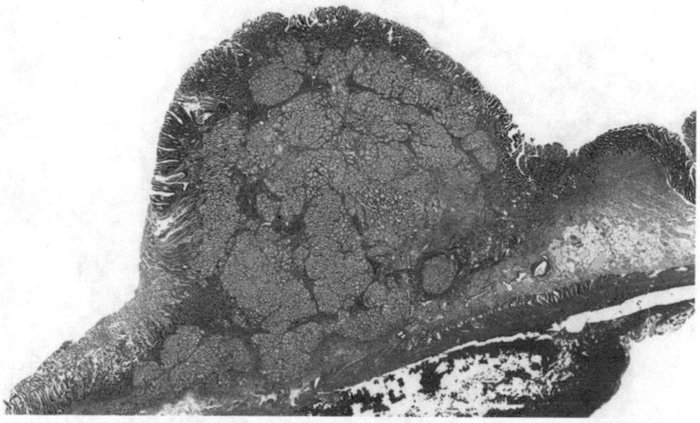

Fig. 14.10 Brunner gland hyperplasia showing closely packed Brunner glands mainly in the submucosa, giving rise to a polypoid appearance

crete polyp/nodule or diffuse nodularity involving the duodenal mucosa. Larger polyps may cause duodenal obstruction or gastrointestinal bleeding. This condition has been variably called Brunner gland adenoma or Brunner gland hamartoma in the literature, but Brunner gland hyperplasia is the currently preferred terminology.

Occasionally, cystic dilatation of Brunner glands or main draining duct may occur, which has been termed Brunner gland cyst. These are typically submucosal lesions characterized by a large unilocular cystic space lined by a single layer of bland epithelial cells morphologically identical to those lining the Brunner glands. Rarely, dysplasia is seen in Brunner gland cyst (Fig. 14.11a, b).
References: [30–33]

10. How is Brunner gland hyperplasia distinguished from pyloric gland adenoma of the duodenum?

In the absence of overt cytologic dysplasia, pyloric gland adenoma can be difficult to distinguish from Brunner gland hyperplasia. However, pyloric gland adenoma does not exhibit a lobular architecture and usually does not have intestinal mucosa on the surface. It is believed that duodenal pyloric gland adenoma likely occurs in heterotopic gastric mucosa.

A recent study by Hida et al. has demonstrated that the duodenal pyloric gland adenoma has an immunophenotype similar to that of Brunner gland hyperplasia: HGM (human gastric mucin) negative/MUC5AC negative/MUC6 positive/Pepsinogen-I negative). However, *GNAS* gene mutations have been identified in gastric and duodenal pyloric gland adenomas, but not in Brunner gland hyperplasia. Interestingly, the identical *GNAS* mutations have been identified in 28% cases of heterotopic gastric mucosa and 41% of gastric foveolar metaplasia in the duodenum, which further supports the hypothesis that duodenal pyloric gland adenomas may originate from *GNAS*-mutant cells in heterotopic gastric mucosa. Studies have also shown nuclear expression of β-catenin in 50–80% of cases of pyloric gland adenomas of the stomach and duodenum, which might suggest that the *GNAS* mutations activate the Wnt/β-catenin pathway.
References: [34–39]

11. What are the characteristic features of heterotopic gastric mucosa and heterotopic pancreatic tissue?

Heterotopic gastric mucosa can be seen throughout the gastrointestinal tract with a higher frequency in the esophagus (3.6–10%) and duodenum (0.5–11%), with a male predilection. It is also a common finding in the Meckel diverticulum. There are two histologic types of heterotopic gastric mucosa: one comprises oxyntic glands (Fig. 14.12a) with parietal cells and chief cells in addition to foveolar epithelium (thought to be congenital); and the other is composed only of foveolar epithelium without oxyntic glands (identical to gastric foveolar metaplasia). A few studies have shown that the presence of heterotopic or metaplasia gastric mucosa in the duodenum has no association with *H. pylori* infection. In the proximal esophagus, heterotopic gastric mucosa is commonly termed "inlet patch", while in the anorectal region the term "outlet patch" has been used.

Although gastric foveolar metaplasia (Fig. 14.12b) was initially thought to be a histologic marker of peptic duodenitis, it can virtually be seen in any condition that causes mucosal injury such as celiac disease or drug effect. In fact, it is a frequent nonspecific finding in duo-

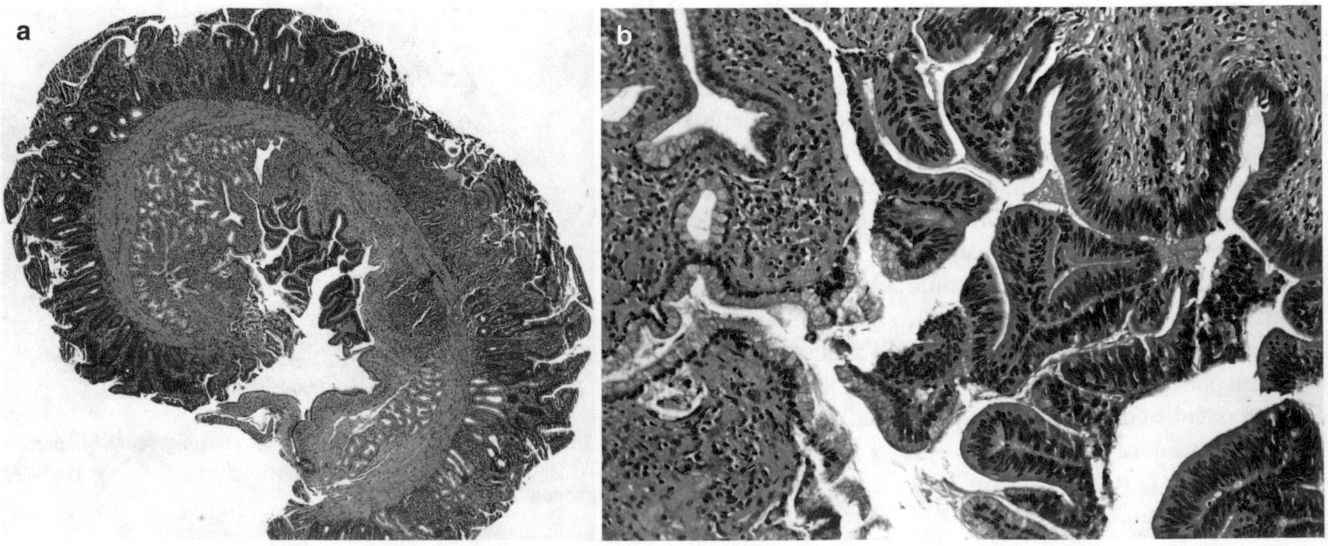

Fig. 14.11 Brunner gland cyst showing a cystic space associated with Brunner glands in the submucosa (**a**). Focal low-grade dysplasia is noted in this case (**b**)

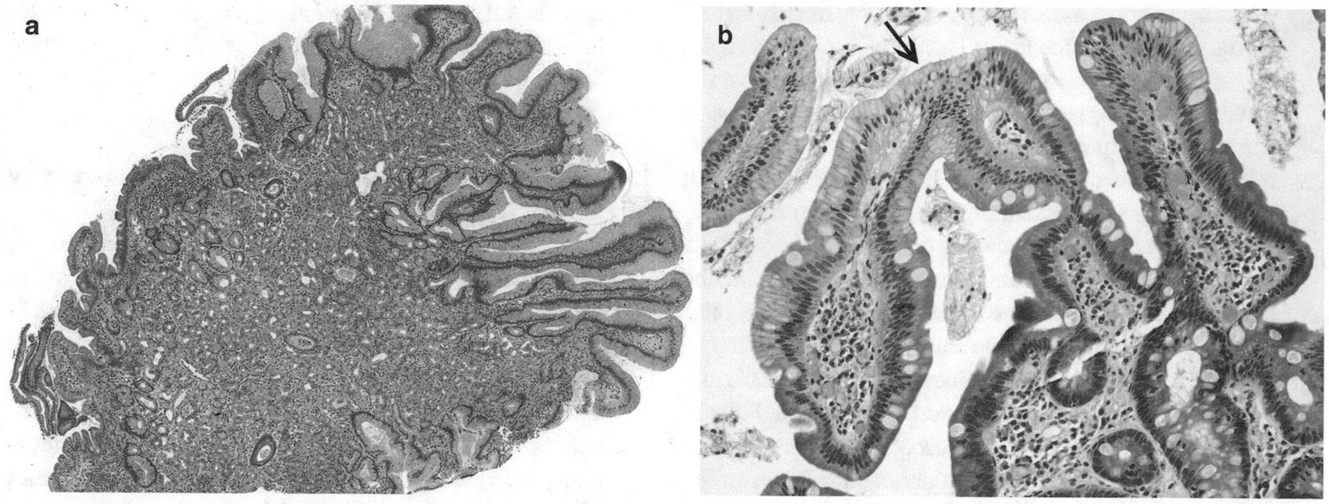

Fig. 14.12 Heterotopic gastric mucosa in the duodenum showing the presence of oxyntic glands and gastric foveolae (**a**). Residual duodenal mucosa is seen at the left lower corner. Gastric foveolar metaplasia is frequently seen in duodenal biopsies (**b**), which can be focal, patchy, or extensive (arrow). Oxyntic glands are absent

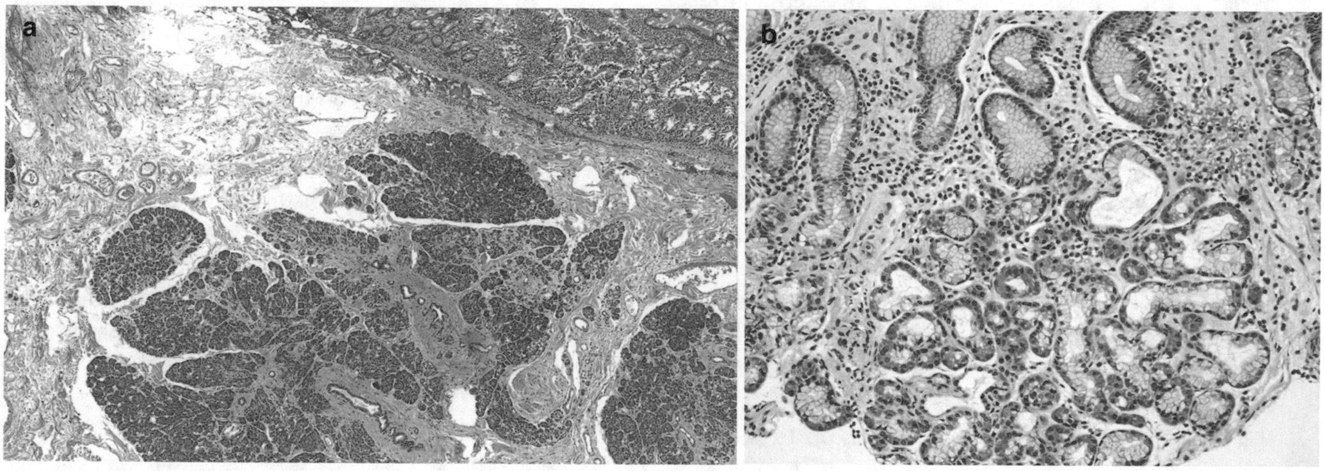

Fig. 14.13 Heterotopic pancreatic tissue found in the duodenal wall, consisting of normal-appearing pancreatic acini and ducts (**a**). Pancreatic acinar metaplasia seen in a biopsy from the gastric antrum showing an island of mucous glands with cells containing cytoplasmic eosinophilic granules, resembling pancreatic acini (**b**)

denal biopsies in the absence of *H. pylori* gastritis, indicating a history of prior mucosal injury.

Heterotopic pancreatic tissue (Fig. 14.13a) can occur anywhere in the gastrointestinal tract, most commonly in the duodenum, proximal jejunum and stomach. It may also be seen in the Meckel diverticulum. It can be classified into four types (Table 14.2). In the duodenum and para-ampullary region, heterotopic pancreatic tissue may present as a mural mass lesion mimicking a malignancy, and may cause stricture, obstruction, and intussusception.

A closely related lesion, adenomyoma of the ampulla of Vater, is believed to be a form of pancreatic heterotopia

Table 14.2 Classification of pancreatic heterotopia

Type	Original Heinrich classification (1909)	Modified Gasper-Fuentes classification (1973)
Type I (similar to the normal pancreas)	Acini, ducts, and islet cells	Acini, ducts, and islet cells
Type II	Acini and ducts (only exocrine components, no islets)	Ducts only (canalicular variety)
Type III	Ducts only	Acini only (exocrine pancreas)
Type IV	–	Islet cells only (endocrine pancreas)

with ducts only in association with smooth muscle hyperplasia. Another related lesion, pancreatic acinar metaplasia, is a common incidental finding in biopsies from the distal esophagus, gastroesophageal junction, and gastric antrum. It may also be seen in the setting of atrophic gastritis. It consists of a small cluster of mucous glands with interspersed cells containing cytoplasmic eosinophilic granules, resembling pancreatic acini (Fig. 14.13b). The lesion can be solitary or multiple, is usually located in the lower portion of the mucosa, and usually does not exhibit an endoscopically detectable abnormality. The finding of pancreatic acinar metaplasia does not appear to have any clinical significance. A recent study demonstrated that in the distal esophagus and gastroesophageal junction there is a significant association with chronic carditis, chronic proton pump inhibitor use, and chronic use of nonsteroidal anti-inflammatory drugs.

References: [19, 40–49]

12. **What is the clinical significance of an adenomatous polyp at the ampulla as compared to elsewhere in the small bowel?**

Ampullary adenomas have a higher rate of progression to carcinoma compared to adenomas arising in non-ampullary small bowel. Duodenal adenomas are easily detected via endoscopy while adenomas in the distal small bowel are only seldom detected before progressing to invasive carcinoma. They have a similar morphology to the adenomas arising in the colorectum and are also classified as: tubular, tubulovillous, and villous (Fig. 14.14a, b). The last two (tubulovillous and villous) are more common in the small bowel. As they grow larger, up to 60% of ampullary adenomas will harbor foci of high-grade dysplasia or invasive carcinoma. Adsay et al. classified primary ampullary carcinomas based on their locations as intra-ampullary (best prognosis), ampullary-ductal (worst prognosis), peri-ampullary-duodenal (intermediate prognosis), and not otherwise specified (papilla of Vater).

References: [50–54]

13. **What are the diagnostic features of an inflammatory polyp?**

Inflammatory polyps are usually seen in the large and small intestines, mostly found in patients with IBD (more common in ulcerative colitis compared to Crohn disease). They also occur in association with other inflammatory conditions, such as ischemic, infectious, and diverticular disease-associated enterocolitis. Also known as pseudopolyps, they are thought to originate from excessive reparatory changes of the mucosa following multiple episodes of inflammatory damage. Inflammatory polyps can be single or multiple, sessile or pedunculated, and variable in size (usually up to 1.5 cm). First described in 1968 by Hinrichs and Goldman, "giant" inflammatory polyps can reach 10 cm in length and can cause bleeding, abdominal pain via obstruction, and intussusception.

Histologically, inflammatory polyps may consist entirely or partially of granulation tissue with mixed inflammatory infiltrates in the lamina propria (Fig. 14.15a). When crypts are present, they can be relatively normal-appearing, distorted, dilated, and hyperplastic (Fig. 14.15b), and can be confused with juvenile polyps. Crypt abscesses, surface erosion or ulceration, and lymphoid aggregates can be seen. These lesions are not considered to be preneoplastic, but dysplasia may develop in IBD-related inflammatory polyps.

References: [55–57]

14. **What should one do if an inflammatory polyp shows atypical stromal cells?**

Inflammatory polyps may show spindled or epithelioid, giant or multinucleated stromal cells in inflamed

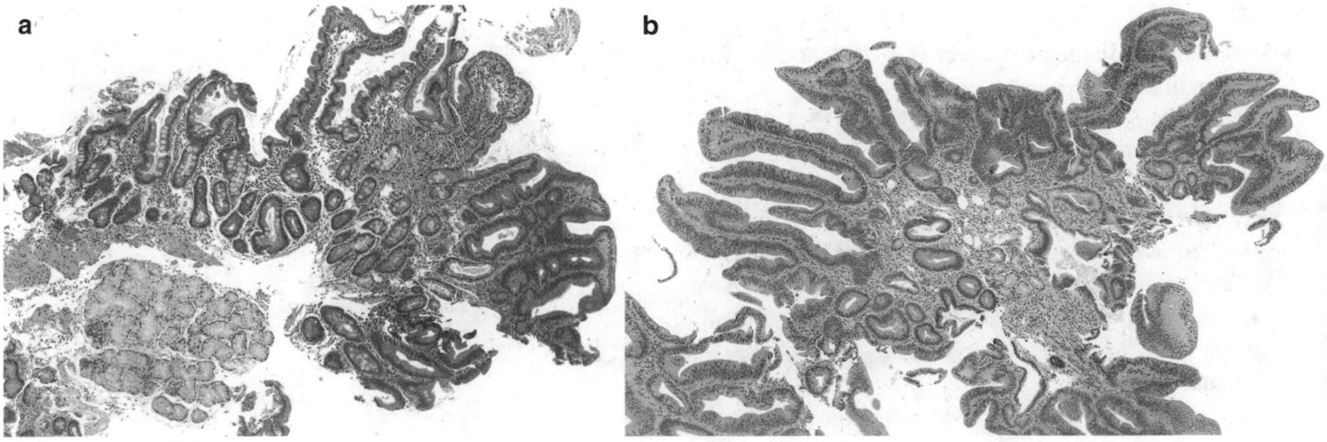

Fig. 14.14 Tubular (**a**) and villous (**b**) adenomas of the duodenum, histologically similar to those seen in the colorectum

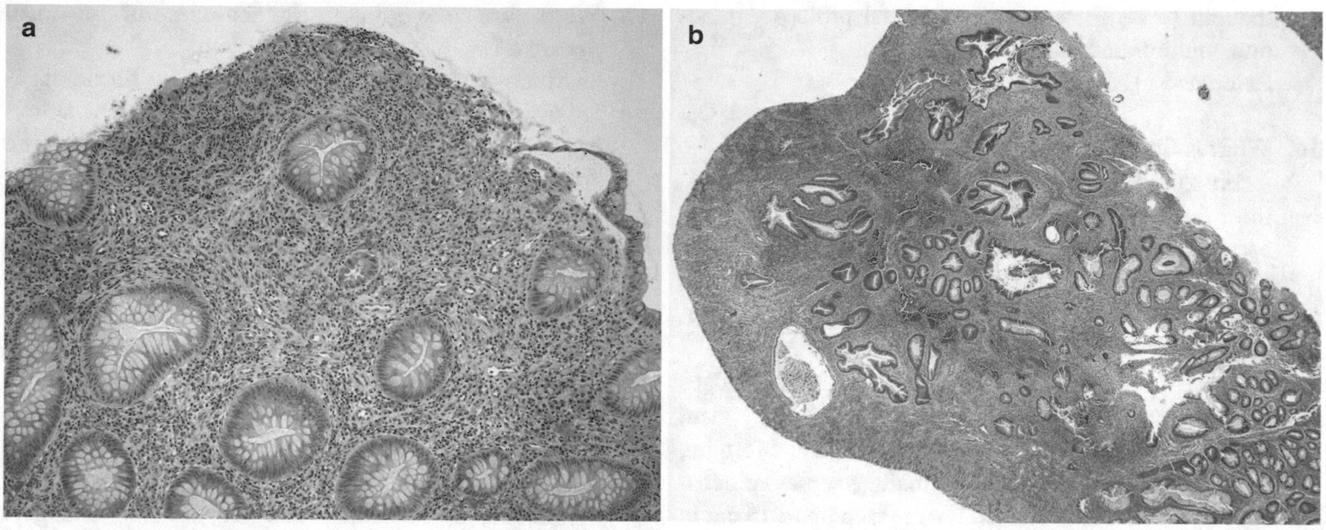

Fig. 14.15 Inflammatory polyp of the colon showing surface erosion with granulation tissue and inflammatory cell infiltrates in the lamina propria (**a**). The preserved crypts are only slightly distorted in this case. Distorted, dilated, and hyperplastic crypts can be prominent in inflammatory polyp (**b**), resembling juvenile polyp

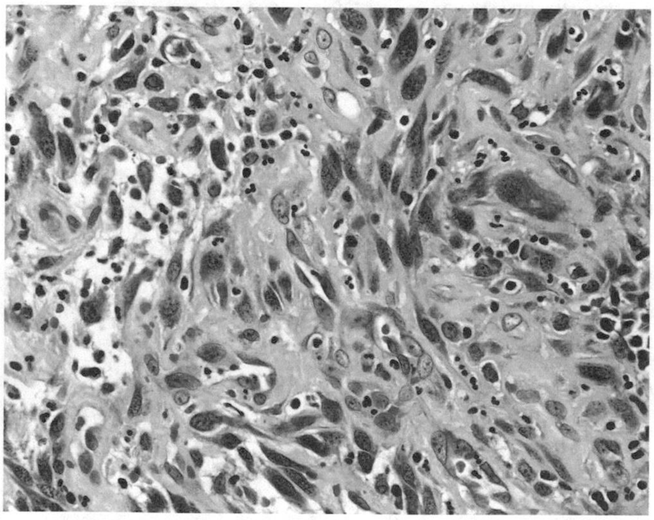

Fig. 14.16 A colonic inflammatory polyp showing pseudosarcomatous stromal cells

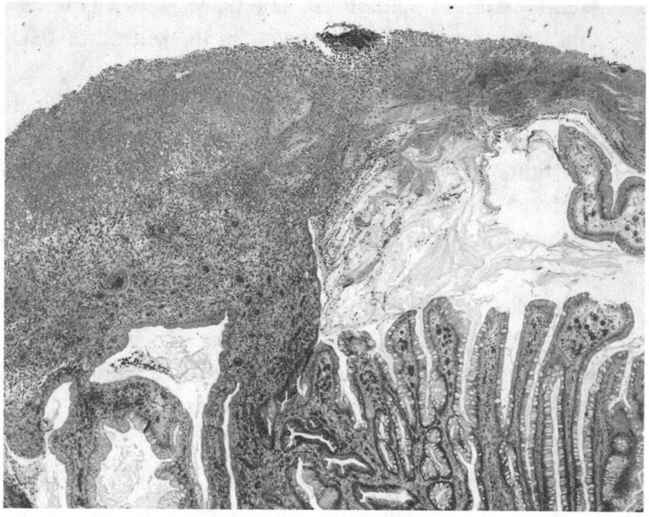

Fig. 14.17 An inflammatory cap polyp showing elongated colonic crypts with eroded surface and fibrinopurulent exudate

granulation tissue, which may mimic sarcomatous change or viral infection (Fig. 14.16). However, these pseudosarcomatous stromal cells lack atypical mitoses. Expression of myofibroblastic or endothelial immunomarkers can help distinguish them from true malignant cells in difficult cases.

15. **What is inflammatory cap polyp/polyposis?**

Inflammatory cap polyps most commonly occur in the rectum and sigmoid colon but have been reported to involve the entire colon and even the stomach. Patients may present with mucous diarrhea, severe constipation, and rectal bleeding. Endoscopically, these polyps range from few millimeters up to 2 cm, are sessile, semi-pedunculated or plaque-like, and are covered by adherent white fibrin caps.

Histologic examination shows elongated, dilated colonic crypts with abundant inflammatory cells in the lamina propria. The surface is ulcerated with granulation tissue covered by fibrinopurulent exudate that forms the characteristic overlying "cap" (Fig. 14.17). Smooth muscle bundles oriented perpendicularly to the muscularis mucosae can be seen in larger polyps (reminiscent of mucosal prolapse). In comparison to the normal colonic mucosa, the mucus cells in inflammatory cap polyps produce nonsulfated mucins.

Hypoproteinemia can be seen in patients with extensive cap polyposis due to impairment of epithelial barriers at the tip of the polyps caused by the downregulation of pore-sealing Claudin-7. The pathogenesis of cap polyposis has yet to be determined. It is

thought to be secondary to mucosal prolapse, infection, and inflammation.
References: [58–60]

16. **What is filiform polyposis?**

First used by Appelman et al. in 1974, the term filiform polyposis was used to describe the radiographic appearance of numerous, long, filamentous filling defects in an otherwise normal colon. It is a rare variant of inflammatory polyposis, composed of multiple, conglomerated slender worm- or finger-like projections that can be interconnected, forming mucosal bridges (Fig. 14.18a, b). It has been reported as a solitary giant polyp as well, diffusely involving the colon and forming a fungating mass mimicking a malignancy at colonoscopy or on imaging studies. It can reach up to 15 cm in length, with the most commonly affected sites being sigmoid colon and rectum.

Histologically, filiform polyps have a fibrovascular core and normal-appearing lamina propria, and are covered by normal epithelium. The pathogenesis is uncertain but majority of cases occur in the setting of IBD, particularly ulcerative colitis. However, there are rare reports of cases encountered in non-IBD patients, which may suggest that these polyps might not be related to a post-inflammatory reparative process. Some of these solitary non-IBD-related polyps have been called "colonic mucosubmucosal elongated polyp", which ususlly have thick-walled and congested blood vessels in the submucosa mimicking arteriovenous malformation. It has been hypothesized that filiform polyposis may represent a hamartomatous process in the colon similar to the neuromuscular and vascular hamartoma of the small bowel described by Fernando and McGovern.
References: [61–63]

17. **What are the diagnostic features of mucosal prolapse?**

Mucosal prolapse is characterized by fibromuscular hyperplasia within the lamina propria and splaying of the muscularis mucosae. Frequently, the splayed smooth muscle fibers encircle the elongated, dilated, or distorted crypts, which can assume a diamond-shaped appearance. Ectatic capillaries may be present. The mucosal surface may become architecturally villiform, or traumatized with erosion/ulceration (Fig. 14.19a, b). Endoscopically, a polypoid lesion, mucosal hyperemia, ulceration, or nodularity is often observed.

Peristalsis-associated traction and torsion of the mucosa drives the pathogenesis of mucosal prolapse, resulting in ischemia and reparative changes. Although mucosal prolapse can occur throughout the colon, it is particularly common as a component of solitary rectal ulcer syndrome – a loosely named condition that may not be solitary, rectal, or associated with an ulcer. In addition, some authors have proposed that mucosal prolapse is the unifying etiology for a few differently named polyps (such as inflammatory myoglandular polyp, inflammatory cloacogenic polyp, inflammatory cap polyp, diverticular disease-associated polyp), and that these entities simply represent a spectrum of mucosal prolapse-induced change. Others contend that the distinction between these entities should be preserved. Differential diagnosis of mucosal prolapse may include inflammatory polyp, ischemic colitis, adenoma, hyperplastic polyp, sessile serrated lesion, Peutz–Jeghers polyp, and IBD, depending on the most prominent features in a particular case.
References: [15, 64–67]

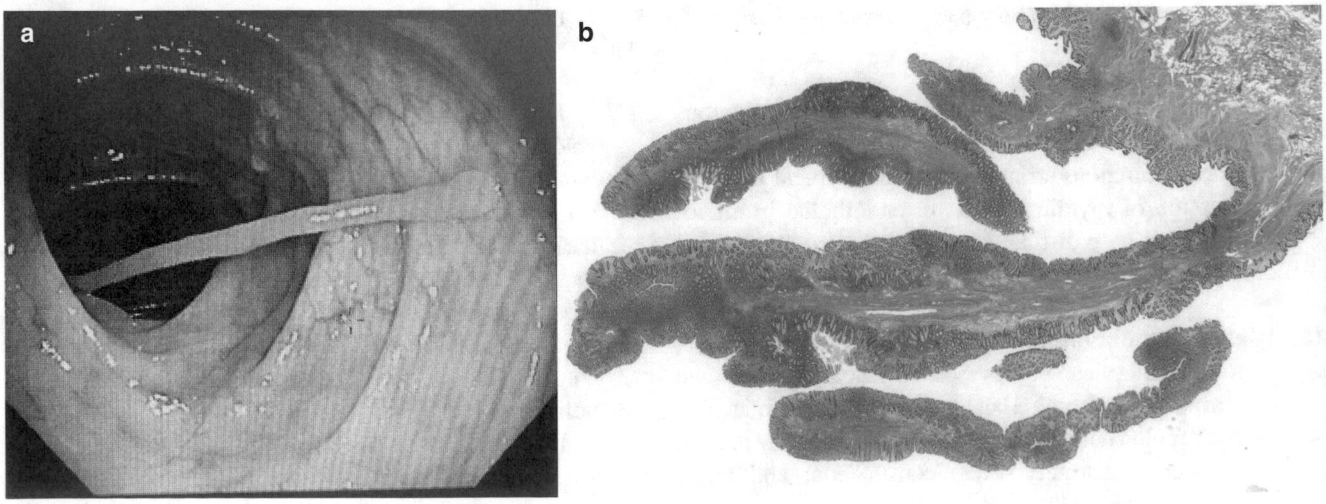

Fig. 14.18 Filiform polyps showing long, worm- or finger-like projections on colonoscopy (**a**) and histologic examination (**b**)

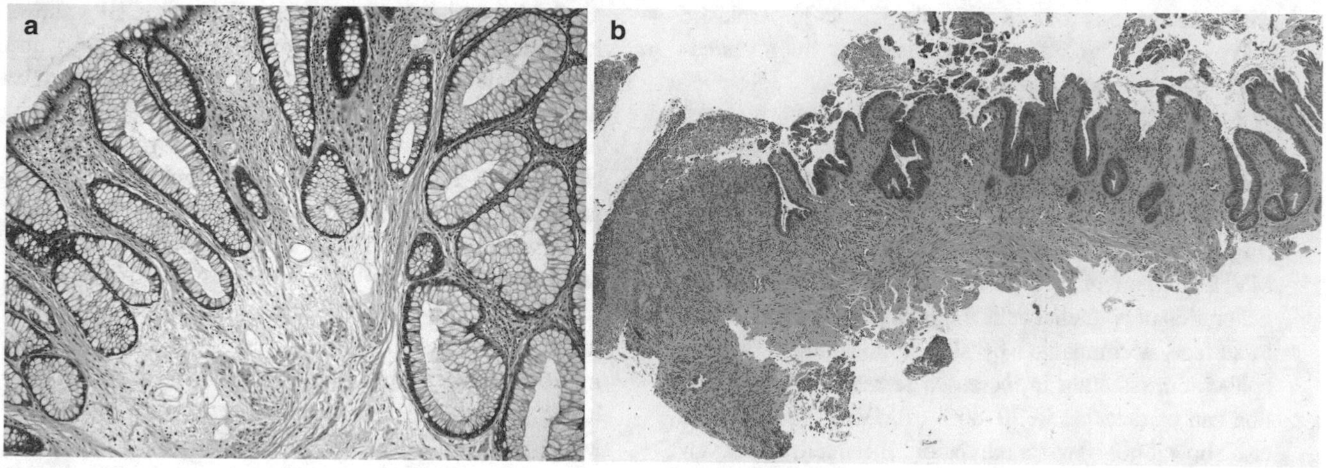

Fig. 14.19 Mucosal prolapse showing elongated and distorted colonic crypts with lamina propria extension of smooth muscle fibers from the muscularis mucosae (**a**). Ulceration, erosion, and lamina propria fibromuscular hyperplasia can be prominent (**b**)

18. What are the diagnostic features of inflammatory cloacogenic polyp?

The inflammatory cloacogenic polyp is variably surfaced by squamocolumnar transitional epithelium characteristic of its location at anorectal transitional zone. Classically, this polyp demonstrates a complex tubulovillous architecture, which can be confused with a tubulovillous adenoma (Fig. 14.20). However, no dysplastic cytologic features are present in this polyp. There are irregularly sized and spaced crypts, some with cystic dilation, surrounded by fibromuscular stroma, similar to that seen for mucosal prolapse. Superficial erosions/ulcers with fibrinopurulent exudate may be evident, accompanied by mixed inflammatory cells in the lamina propria. The classic endoscopic appearance is that of a solitary, pedunculated polyp in an individual with mucosal prolapse/solitary rectal ulcer syndrome, though associations with Crohn disease and coexistent adjacent adenocarcinoma have also been reported. This polyp has also been reported in children.

References: [65, 68, 69]

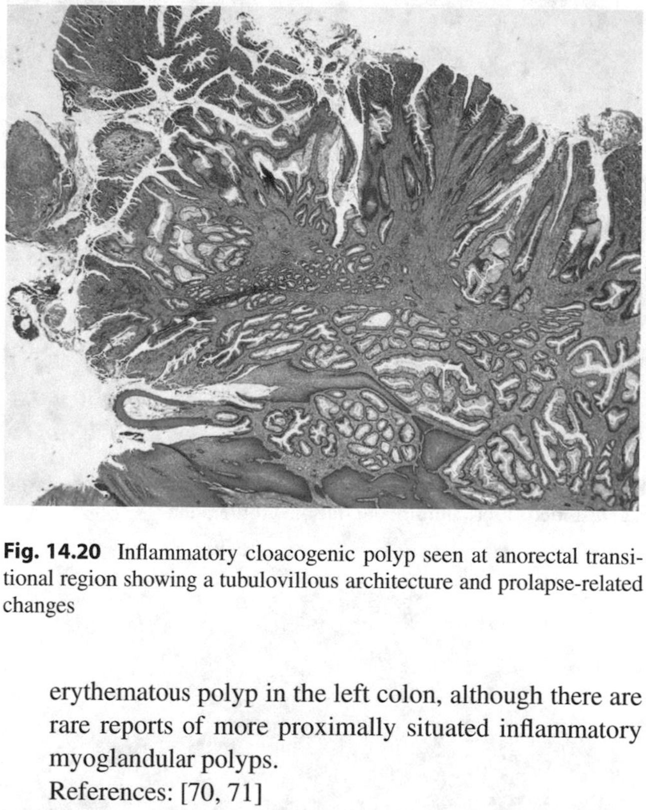

Fig. 14.20 Inflammatory cloacogenic polyp seen at anorectal transitional region showing a tubulovillous architecture and prolapse-related changes

19. What are the diagnostic features of inflammatory myoglandular polyp?

Inflammatory myoglandular polyp features hyperplastic, mucin-filled crypts with cystic dilation, inflamed granulation tissue, hemosiderin deposition and hemorrhage, and smooth muscle proliferation in the lamina propria. The smooth muscle may be arranged in a tree-like pattern similar to that seen in Peutz–Jeghers polyp (Fig. 14.21), and for that reason, some consider this entity hamartomatous rather than prolapse-induced. Overlying mucosal erosion is common in inflammatory myoglandular polyp, but is uncommon in Peutz–Jeghers polyp. The classic endoscopic appearance of inflammatory myoglandular polyp is of a pedunculated, smooth, erythematous polyp in the left colon, although there are rare reports of more proximally situated inflammatory myoglandular polyps.

References: [70, 71]

20. Is there any clinical significance to the hyperplastic polyp subtypes of the large intestine?

Hyperplastic polyps are predominantly found in the left colon and rectum. They are typically small (<0.5 cm) and asymptomatic. A classic hyperplastic polyp shows evenly spaced crypts with superficial serration ("saw-toothed" lumens) and pointed base (Fig. 14.22a). There should be no basal dilation but crypt branching may be present. The proliferation zone is limited to the base portion of the crypts. The basement membrane can be prominently thickened, which should not be confused with collagenous colitis. Histologically, hyperplastic polyps can be divided into three subtypes: microvesicular, goblet cell-rich, and mucin-poor.

Microvesicular hyperplastic polyp (MVHP) is the most common subtype. It has a distinct "sawtoothed" appearance in the upper two-thirds of the crypts, lined by microvesicular epithelial cells with fine apical vacuoles (Fig. 14.22b). The number of goblet cells is variable. MVHP is thought to arise as a consequence of delayed maturation of epithelial cells migrating from the crypt base to surface, accompanied by slower sloughing of surface epithelium, resulting in increased serration. *BRAF* mutation can be detected in 70–80% of MVHPs. Some cases also show CpG-island methylation. It remains controversial if MVHP is a precursor for sessile serrated lesion.

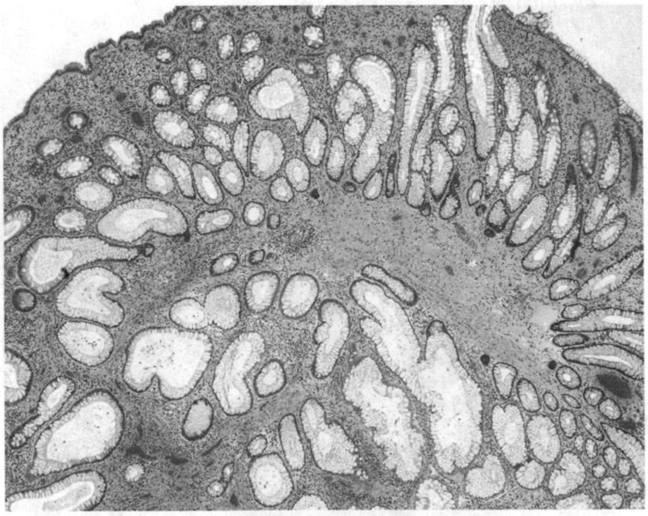

Fig. 14.21 Inflammatory myoglandular polyp showing hyperplastic and distorted crypts and smooth muscle proliferation

Goblet cell-rich hyperplastic polyp (GCHP) shows less prominent serration, more elongated crypts, and more numerous goblet cells. *KRAS* mutation can be detected in ~50% of GCHPs. Mucin-poor hyperplastic polyp (MCHP) is the least common subtype. The main characteristics are little to no mucin and mild reactive atypia with hyperchromatic nuclei, thought to be secondary to injury and regeneration. The molecular alterations are less clear in this subtype.

Because hyperplastic polyps can demonstrate a multitude of genetic and cell cycle regulatory abnormalities, some authors have suggested that they may harbor malignant potential. However, the United States Multi-Society Task Force on Colorectal Cancer has defined hyperplastic polyp of <1.0 cm to be innocuous; individuals with ≤20 hyperplastic polyps (all <1.0 cm) are considered to have normal colonoscopy. Only those with a hyperplastic polyp of ≥1.0 cm need closer surveillance colonoscopy (Table 14.3). Currently, there is no clinical significance to subtype hyperplastic polyps because their management is similarly conservative, with complete resection of all small rectosigmoid hyperplastic polyps deemed unnecessary by one expert panel. The most important facet of serrated polyp management is distinguishing hyperplastic polyp from sessile serrated lesion.

Hyperplastic polyp rarely occurs in the duodenum. Histologically, it resembles its colorectal counterpart, particularly MVHP. It is not associated with serrated polyposis. *BRAF* and *KRAS* mutations have been described in a subset of reported cases.

References: [72–78]

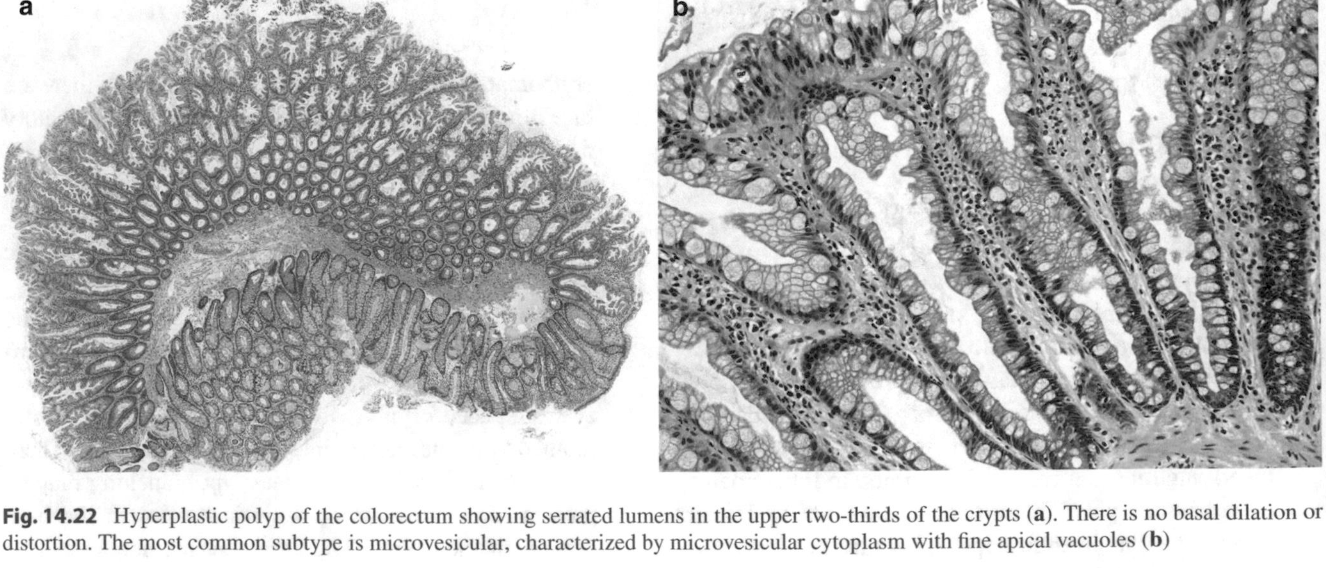

Fig. 14.22 Hyperplastic polyp of the colorectum showing serrated lumens in the upper two-thirds of the crypts (**a**). There is no basal dilation or distortion. The most common subtype is microvesicular, characterized by microvesicular cytoplasm with fine apical vacuoles (**b**)

Table 14.3 Recommended surveillance interval per most advanced finding at baseline colonoscopy by the United States Multi-Society Task Force on Colorectal Cancer [75][a]

Most advanced finding at baseline colonoscopy	Recommended surveillance interval (years)
Normal colonoscopy ≤20 hyperplastic polyps, <1.0 cm	10
1–2 adenomas, <1.0 cm	7–10
1–2 sessile serrated adenomas/polyps, <1.0 cm	5–10
3–4 adenomas, <1.0 cm 3–4 sessile serrated adenomas/polyps, <1.0 cm Hyperplastic polyp, ≥1.0 cm	3–5
5–10 adenomas, <1.0 cm Adenoma, ≥1.0 cm Adenoma with villous or tubulovillous histology Adenoma with high-grade dysplasia 5–10 sessile serrated adenomas/polyps, <1.0 cm Sessile serrated adenoma/polyp, ≥1.0 cm Sessile serrated adenoma/polyp with cytologic dysplasia Traditional serrated adenoma	3
>10 adenomas on single examination[b]	1
Piecemeal resection of adenoma, ≥2.0 cm	0.5 (6 months)
Serrated polyposis syndrome[c]	Specialized management

[a]All recommendations assume a complete examination to the cecum with bowel preparation adequate to detect lesions >0.5 cm in size, and assume a high confidence of complete resection
[b]Patients with >10 adenomas or lifetime >10 cumulative adenomas may need to be considered for genetic testing based on absolute/cumulative adenoma number, patient age, and other factors such as family history of colorectal cancer
[c]See Chap. 15, Question 18, for definition of serrated polyposis syndrome

21. How is sessile serrated lesion distinguished from hyperplastic polyp?

Sessile serrated lesion (SSL) was previously termed sessile serrated adenoma (SSA), sessile serrated polyp (SSP) or sessile serrated adenoma/polyp (SSA/P), and now is the recommended term by *WHO Classification of Tumours of the Digestive System* 5th edition (2019). However, the rationale for the name change by WHO is not overtly clear. Many pathologists in the United States may choose not to adopt the change and to continue the use of SSA/P in their practice to avoid confusion to clinicians.

SSLs or SSA/Ps are usually larger (>0.5 cm) than hyperplastic polyps, and more commonly seen in the right colon. The most important distinguishing feature is distorted architecture at the base of crypts characterized by horizontal widening ("lateralization") along the muscularis mucosae, contributing to the formation of a "boot" (L-shaped) or "anchor" (inverted T) appearance, or dilation of the base (Fig. 14.23a–c). Crypt herniation through the muscularis mucosae may occur. Increased serration and maturation is often seen at the crypt base, with Ki67-labeled proliferation occurring throughout the crypt. Crypt branching is not a specific feature of SSL, which can also be seen in hyperplastic polyp.

Despite these well-defined diagnostic criteria, there can be challenges in distinguishing between the SSL and the MVHP, as evidenced by the low-to-moderate interobserver agreement among gastrointestinal pathologists. This is in part because SSL and MVHP bracket two ends of a diagnostic spectrum, with ambiguity in the middle. The 5th edition of *WHO Classification of Tumours of the Digestive System* has adopted the recommendation by an expert panel, which requires only one unequivocal architecturally distorted serrated crypt (as described above) for the diagnosis of SSL. It is thus important to have well-oriented tissue sections so that all the crypt bases in a serrated polyp can be examined. When the specimen is tangentially sectioned and the muscularis mucosae is not well represented, deeper sections should be performed, which can be very helpful. There are a few immunomarkers (such as annexin A10 and Hes1) that may be potentially useful, but histologic evaluation is the current practice to separate SSLs from hyperplastic polyps. It should be emphasized that the diagnosis of SSL should not be biased by location and size. SSL can be small and can be found in the left colon and even the rectum, but care should be taken not to overdiagnose SSL in the setting of mucosal prolapse, particularly in the rectum.

Both SSL and hyperplastic polyp can show perineuriomatous stromal cell proliferation (mucosal perineurioma) in the lamina propria or lipomatous change in the submucosa. These additional findings have no clinical significance. The perineuriomatous stromal cell proliferation (Fig. 14.23d) is believed to be reactive rather than neoplastic.

References: [76, 79–82]

22. How is traditional serrated adenoma distinguished from sessile serrated lesion and tubulovillous adenoma?

Predominantly found in the left colon and rectum, traditional serrated adenoma (TSA) is usually an exophytic polyp characterized by villiform architecture, slit-like serration, and tall columnar cells with abundant intensely eosinophilic cytoplasm and stratified pencillate nuclei (Fig. 14.24a, b). Scattered goblet cells may be seen. TSA is less commonly seen in the proximal colon where it is usually a flat lesion. Another feature that can be seen in TSA is ectopic crypts, which are small crypts that bud into the lamina propria (Fig. 14.24c), perpendicular to the long axis of villi and without anchoring to the muscularis mucosae. TSA can show serrated dysplasia or conventional adenomatous dysplasia, has a relatively high frequency of *KRAS* and *BRAF* mutations as well as a low level of CpG-island methylation, and is considered to have malignant potential.

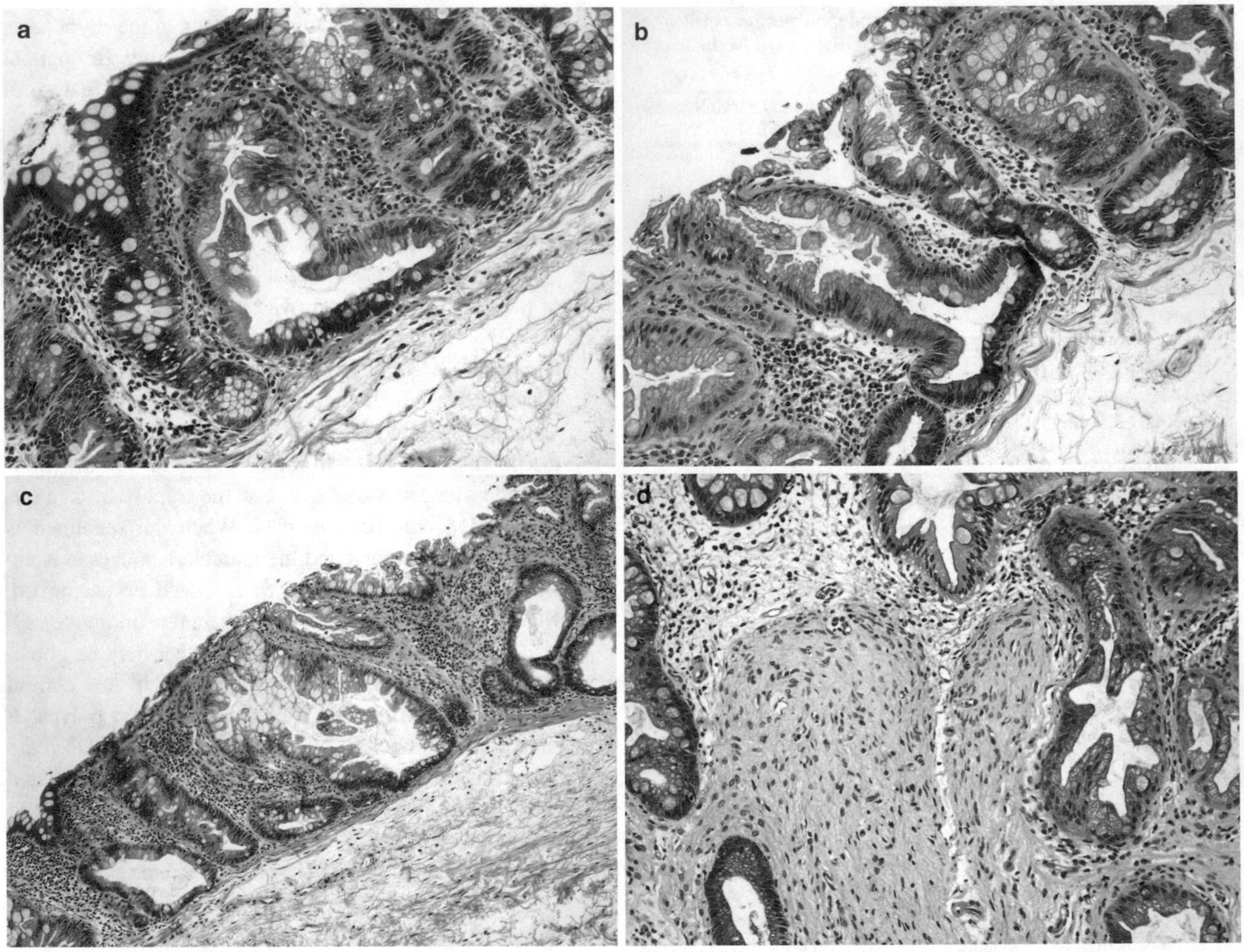

Fig. 14.23 Sessile serrated lesion (or sessile serrated adenoma/polyp) showing distorted crypt base, which may assume a "L" (**a**), inverted "T" (**b**), or dilated (**c**) architecture. Perineuriomatous stromal cell proliferation may be seen in the lamina propria (**d**)

Ectopic crypts, slit-like serration, cytoplasmic eosinophilia, and nuclear stratification are not characteristically seen in SSL. Of note, some studies have shown that TSAs can arise adjacent to hyperplastic polyps or SSLs, but it remains unclear as to whether TSA can truly arise from an SSL. TSA typically shows a villiform architecture and sometimes demonstrates conventional adenomatous cytologic dysplasia, similar to that seen in a tubulovillous adenoma (TVA). However, slit-like serration, cytoplasmic eosinophilia, and ectopic crypts are not typically seen in TVA. Moreover, the cytologic features of dysplasia seen in TVA are more prominent than those seen in TSA.

Serrated adenomas morphologically resembling TSA of the colorectum have also been reported in the stomach, the small intestine (mainly the duodenum), and even the esophagus. Serrated adenomas of the upper gastrointestinal tract are thought to be aggressive lesions, with >50% of reported cases having simultaneous invasive adenocarcinoma.

References: [79, 83–86]

23. Does sessile serrated lesion have any malignant potential, and what is the clinical significance of cytologic dysplasia in these polyps?

Despite the lack of morphologic dysplasia and the lack of direct evidence to show morphologic progression from SSL to adenocarcinoma, SSL is currently considered to be a type of "adenoma" in keeping with its molecularly premalignant nature. In contrast to the conventional adenoma-carcinoma pathway characterized by chromosomal instability, SSL is believed to participate in the "serrated neoplasia" pathway of colorectal cancer featuring methylation, *BRAF* mutation, and high microsatellite instability. It is speculated that SSL arises without cytologic dysplasia, later transforming (after what may be a long latent period) into an SSL with cytologic dysplasia, and then into an invasive adenocarcinoma. This transformation process appears to involve MLH-1 methylation, *RNF43* mutation, and *BRAF* mutation (see Chap. 15, Fig. 15.5d, e). Once cytologic dysplasia has developed, the SSL is considered an advanced lesion requiring complete endoscopic resection. The rate at which adenocarcinoma develops from an SSL

with cytologic dysplasia appears to be faster than that from a conventional adenoma. This rapid rate of cancer development may explain some of the "interval cancers" that arise during the interval between colonoscopies with current surveillance recommendations.
Reference: [87]

24. Is there any clinical significance to subclassify an adenomatous polyp as tubular, villous, or tubulovillous?

The current guidelines by the United States Multi-Society Task Force on Colorectal Cancer consider adenoma villosity in determining appropriate colon cancer surveillance intervals for affected patients. Specifically, an individual with one or more adenomas with villous features has a recommended surveillance interval of 3 years. Although the Task Force does not recommend quantifying the proportion of villous component, adenomatous polyps are traditionally classified into three subtypes: a small villous component (<25%) is allowable for a tubular adenoma; a >25% villous component is required for the diagnosis of tubulovillous adenoma; and >75% is required for villous adenoma. Villous architecture is defined as leaf- or finger-like projections of adenomatous epithelium overlying a small amount of lamina propria (Fig. 14.25a). Despite the concern for interobserver variability, tubulovillous or villous architecture has been considered as one of features of advanced adenoma that is associated with an increased risk of synchronous or metachronous adenomas and subsequent progression to adenocarcinoma, which thus requires complete removal and closer colonoscopic surveillance. The other features of advanced adenoma include a size ≥1.0 cm and the presence of high-grade dysplasia.

Conventional adenomas are most commonly seen in the colorectum, and less frequent in the small intestine and stomach. Non-syndromic adenomas are usually detected in individuals >50 years, but can also be seen in younger patients. Histologically, tubular adenoma shows enlarged, crowded, straight, or distorted but noncomplex crypts lined by dysplastic epithelial cells with hyperchromatic, stratified, and elongated (pencillate) nuclei. Increased apoptotic activity can be prominent (Fig. 14.25b, c). Loss of nuclear polarity may be seen. Paneth cells may be present, but goblet cells are usually reduced in number comparing to adjacent non-adenomatous colonic crypts.
References: [75, 88]

25. Is there any clinical significance of a squamous morule or minute clusters of neuroendocrine cell proliferation found in a colonic adenoma?

No, although care must be taken by the pathologist to not misinterpret this finding. Observed in both colonic adenomas and adenocarcinomas, the squamous morule

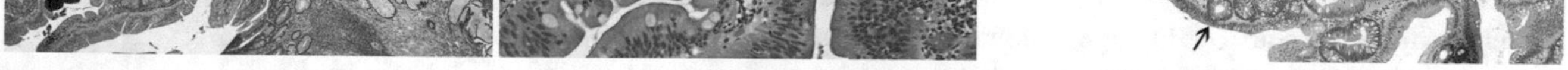

Fig. 14.24 Traditional serrated adenoma showing villiform architecture and slit-like serration (**a**), lined by tall columnar cells with abundant intensely eosinophilic cytoplasm and stratified pencillate nuclei (**b**). Ectopic crypts (arrows) can be frequent (**c**)

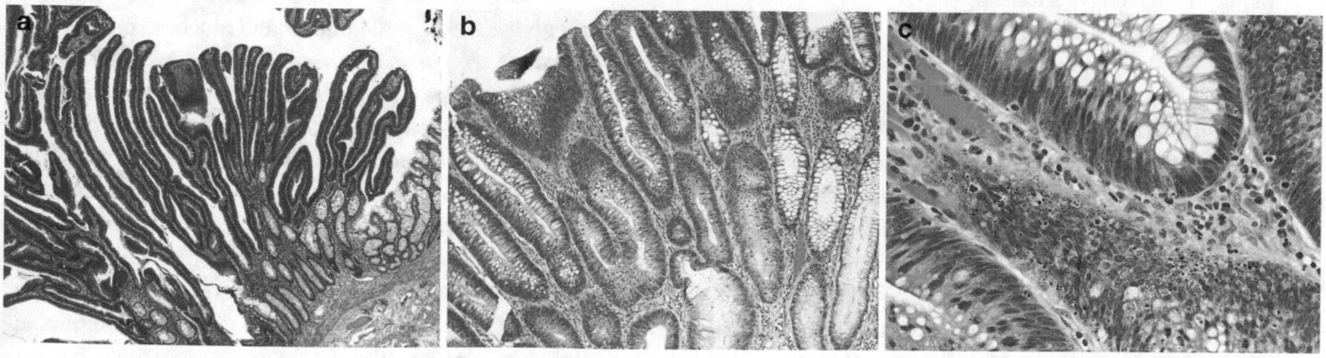

Fig. 14.25 Conventional adenomas with villous (**a**) and tubular (**b**) architecture. Apoptotic activity can be brisk in adenomatous epithelium (**c**)

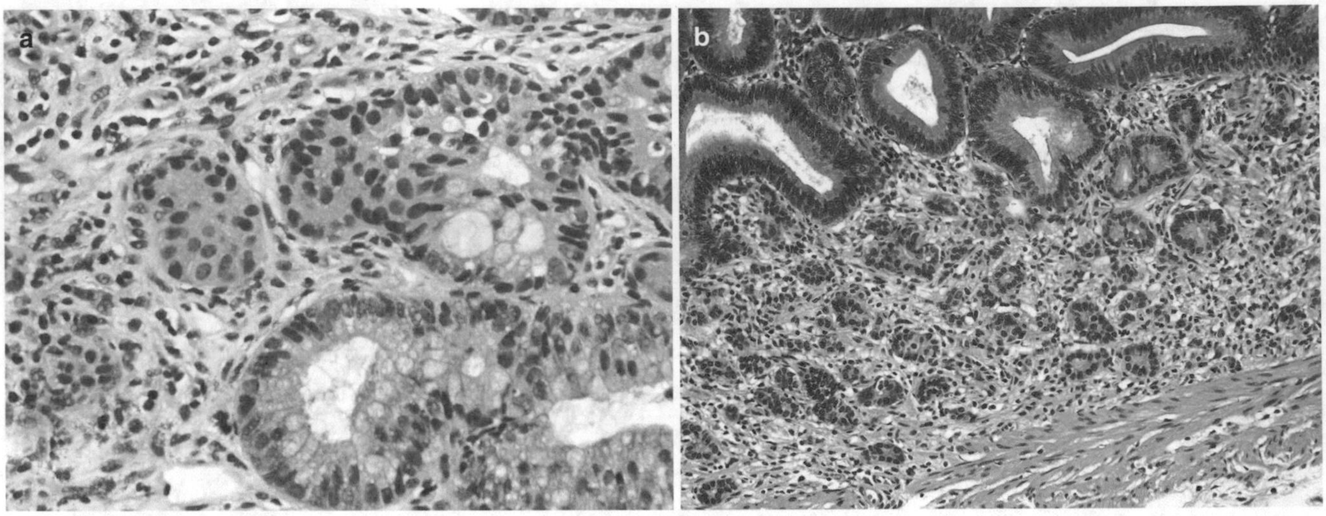

Fig. 14.26 Squamous morules (**a**) and minute clusters of neuroendocrine cells (**b**) seen in adenomas. The latter has been termed "composite intestinal adenoma-microcarcinoid"

is a small pseudo-cribriform or elongated or round solid nest of undifferentiated cells lacking keratinization and intercellular bridges (Fig. 14.26a). The cells have round to ovoid, often optically clear, nuclei and plentiful, lightly eosinophilic cytoplasm. Squamous morules tend to involve adenomatous glands, often resulting in partial replacement of the epithelium. The morules may protrude into the gland lumina or surrounding stroma, with the potential to mimic tumor budding, high-grade dysplasia, or invasive carcinoma. One study suggested the squamous morule immunophenotype included nuclear overexpression of cyclin D1 and beta-catenin (nuclear staining), as well as expression of 34βE12 and p63. The latter expression may be indicative of a basal/stem cell phenotype for these cells.

Rarely, minute clusters of neuroendocrine cells are present in the lower portion of the lamina propria underneath the adenomatous crypts (Fig. 14.26b). These lesions have been termed "composite intestinal adenoma-microcarcinoid". Although infiltration of the muscularis mucosae and submucosa by neuroendocrine cells may occur, these lesions are clinically indolent and do not require additional excision if the polyp is completely removed by endoscopy.

References: [89–95]

26. What are the morphological features to determine high-grade dysplasia in an adenomatous polyp?

By definition, all conventional adenomas should at least show low-grade dysplasia. As mentioned above, high-grade dysplasia is a feature of advanced adenoma, which is defined by architectural complexity and/or high-grade cytology. Architectural complexity may include cribriforming architecture, marked irregularity and back-to-back glands with effacement of the intervening lamina propria, which can be easily recognized at low-power view (Fig. 14.27a). Intraluminal necrosis may be seen. Cytologically, high-grade dysplasia features marked nuclear stratification with loss of nuclear polarity, marked nuclear enlargement and pleomorphism, round nuclear contour, vesicular chromatin, prominent nucleoli, and atypical mitotic figures (Fig. 14.27b). Appelman has described his criteria for high-grade dysplasia as "epithelium that is identical to what is found in a typical invasive carcinoma," while noting that "others might find that requirement too restrictive".

It should be emphasized that the high-grade category for colorectal adenomas includes not only adenocarcinoma in situ, but also intramucosal adenocarcinoma that shows histologic evidence of lamina propria invasion (Fig. 14.27c, d). In the colorectum, intramucosal carcinoma is staged as Tis and thought to have no metastatic potential, whereas in the esophagus, stomach, and small intestine, it is staged as T1a.

Reference: [96]

27. What are the morphological features that help distinguish "pseudoinvasion" from true invasion?

Pseudoinvasion, defined as the herniation of adenomatous glands through the muscularis mucosae into the submucosa, is the *sine qua non* of epithelial misplacement in polyps due to prolapse or peristalsis-related traumatization. Architecturally, misplaced glands typically show a distinct lobular arrangement (Fig. 14.28a), but haphazard single glands without a lobular pattern may also be seen. Deeper sections, if performed, may eventually reveal continuity of misplaced glands with the overlying mucosa. The herniated glands may become distended or mucin-filled, and may rupture leading to the formation of acellular mucin pools. The lining epithelium may become

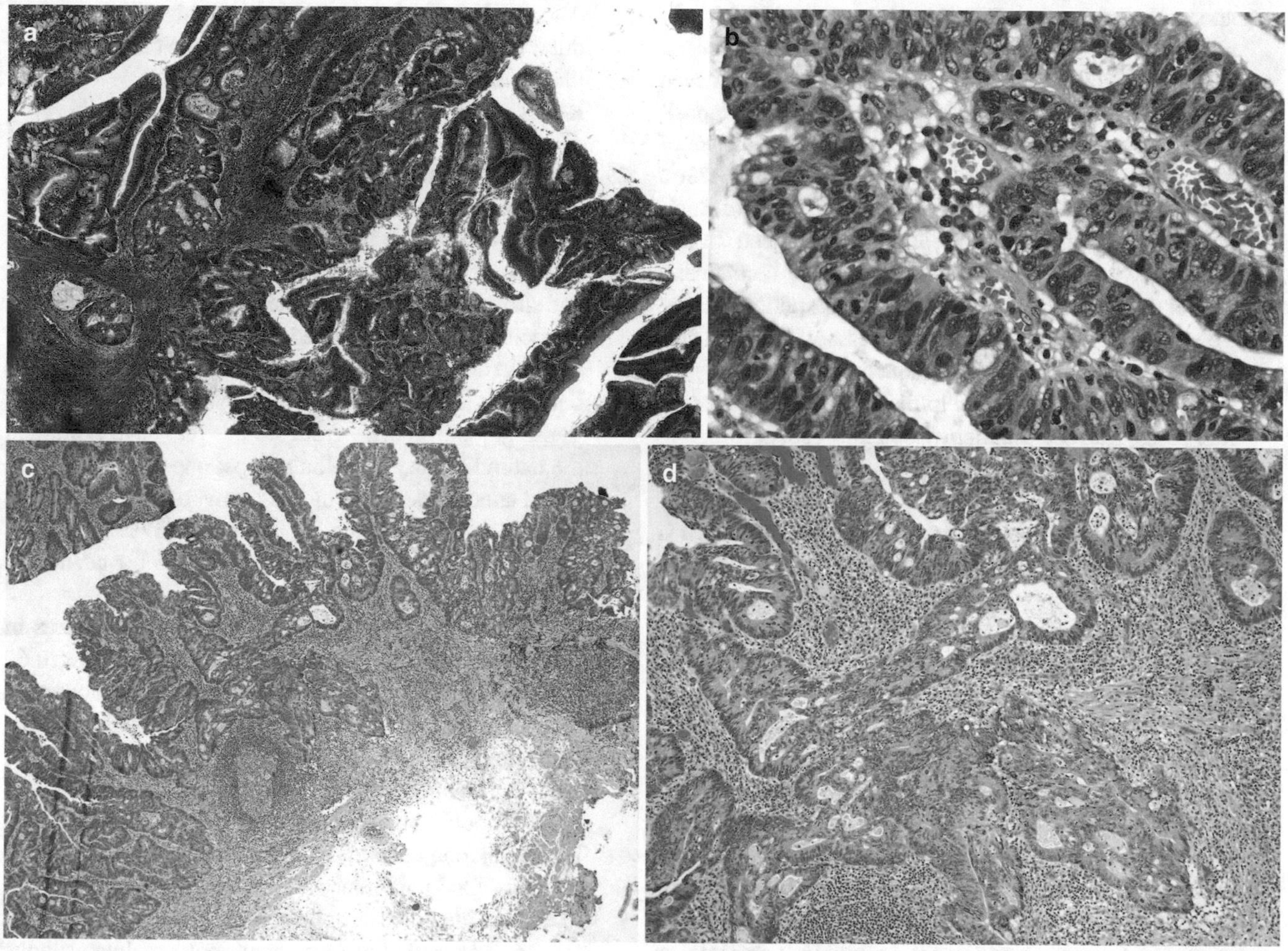

Fig. 14.27 High-grade dysplasia arising in an adenomatous polyp showing architectural complexity with a cribriform or back-to-back appearance (**a**). Marked cytologic atypia, such as nuclear enlargement, stratification and loss of polarity, is prominent (**b**). Intramucosal adenocarcinoma (**c**, **d**) is also in the category of high-grade dysplasia in the colorectum

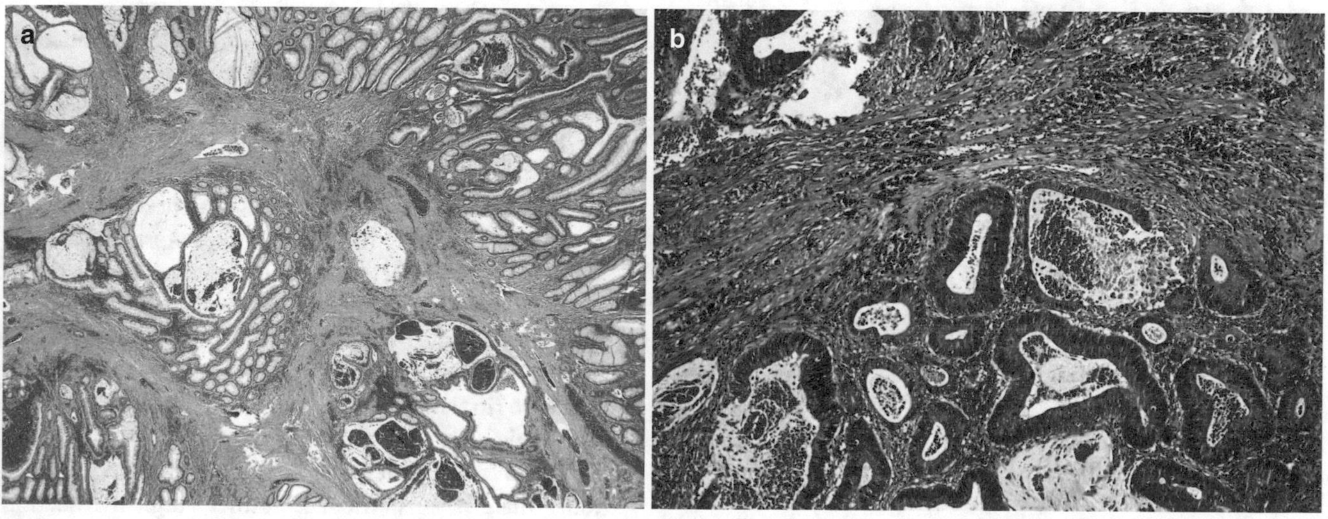

Fig. 14.28 Pseudoinvasion in an adenomatous polyp showing a lobular arrangement of misplaced crypts (**a**). It is associated with lamina propria components, hemorrhage, and hemosiderins (**b**). Ruptured crypts may be seen

attenuated or reactive. Consistently surrounding the misplaced glands is a rim of lamina propria component. Splayed smooth muscle fibers may be present, and even prominent. Fresh hemorrhage and hemosiderin deposition are common, and are considered direct evidence of recent trauma or torsion to the site (Fig. 14.28b). Histologic features characteristic of a true invasive carcinoma, such as stromal desmoplasia, are not seen. In difficult cases, such as misplaced high-grade component, deeper sections and consultation with an experienced gastrointestinal pathologist may be necessary. Evaluation of the distance of herniated component from the polypectomy margin may also be helpful in challenging cases. In rare cases, true and pseudoinvasion may coexist.

References: [97, 98]

28. What should one do if an adenomatous component is found extending into submucosal lymphoid follicles?

The lymphoglandular complex is found in the normal colon (Fig. 14.29), where a dense, spherical lymphoid aggregate is immediately subjacent to a discontinuity in the muscularis mucosae. Because of the anatomic discontinuity, herniation of colonic crypts into the lymphoid aggregate can readily occur, particularly in the setting of increased pressure or local trauma. In the left colon, for example, the increasingly solid stool in the fecal stream can cause colonic crypts to extrude through weakened areas in the muscularis mucosae to enter a subjacent lymphoid aggregate to form a lymphglandular complex. Dysplastic or neoplastic crypts within a lymphoglandular complex should be assessed with a skeptical eye, with particular thought given to the possibility of "pseudoinvasion." As described above, true invasion involving a lymphoglandular complex should also have classic diagnostic features such as stromal desmoplasia.

Reference: [99]

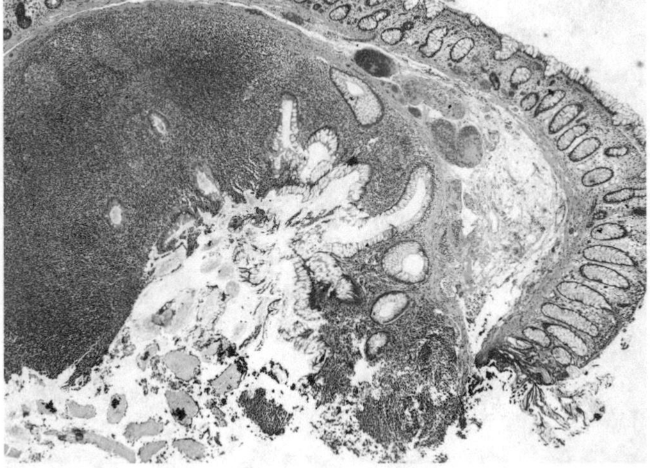

Fig. 14.29 Lymphoglandular complex showing a prominent benign lymphoid aggregate beneath the muscularis mucosae. Herniated colonic crypts are present within the aggregate. Herniated glands can be adenomatous when associated with an adenomatous polyp, which should not be confused with submucosal invasion

29. How can colonic polyps be stratified in terms of risk of progression to adenocarcinoma, and how should the patients be surveilled?

Current guidelines for colorectal cancer screening and surveillance from the American Gastroenterological Association and the United States Multi-Society Task Force on Colorectal Cancer incorporate polyp type, number, size, villosity, and degree of dysplasia (Table 14.3). These guidelines draw from studies that have examined the natural history of colon polyps; one such study proposed annual adenocarcinoma "conversion rates" of 3% for adenomas exceeding 1.0 cm in size, 17% for adenomas with a villous component, and 37% for adenomas with high-grade dysplasia.

Given the reduced incidence of advanced features in "diminutive" polyps (≤0.5 cm) and "small" polyps (0.6–0.9 cm), there has been growing interest in adopting a "predict, resect, and discard" approach during colonoscopy, in which select polyps are not submitted for histopathologic examination. Some studies have suggested this practice could be safely adopted with little risk to patients, ideally in conjunction with *in vivo* optical diagnostic methods. One particular study found that advanced features were identified in only 0.5% of diminutive adenomatous polyps and 1.5% of small polyps. Interestingly, however, sessile serrated lesions with cytologic dysplasia or adenocarcinoma have been shown in one study to be diminutive or small 54% of the time, and the advanced component typically flat rather than exophytic.

References: [75, 86, 100, 101]

30. What histologic characteristics must be included in the pathology report for an adenomatous polyp with invasive adenocarcinoma?

The College of American Pathologists (CAP) has established evidence-based guidelines on the reporting of invasive adenocarcinoma in an adenomatous polyp ("malignant polyp") following polypectomy. By definition, malignant polyps contain adenocarcinoma that invades into the submucosa or beyond, with an associated biological risk of metastasis. Pathology reports should include all elements that influence risk of adverse outcome (in the form of metastasis or local recurrence): histologic grade of carcinoma, lymphovascular invasion, and distance of invasive carcinoma from polypectomy margin. In particular, further surgical resection needs to be considered for high-grade (poorly differentiated) carcinoma, carcinoma present at or <0.1 cm from resection margin, and the presence of lymphovascular

invasion. Other important features to address in the pathology report include tumor budding and the depth of submucosa invasion. Studies have shown that high tumor budding, defined as ≥10 buds in 0.785 mm^2 area (equivalent to a 20× field for most microscopes), is a significant predictor for nodal metastasis. Submucosal invasion >0.1 cm in depth is also considered an adverse prognostic factor. The greatest dimension of the invasive component and the histologic type of carcinoma are also frequently requested by the clinical team, but their prognostic significance is currently not emphasized.
References: [102–104]

31. What are the diagnostic features of different appendiceal polyps?

Appendiceal polyps are morphologically similar to their colorectal counterparts, which have historically invited use of similar diagnostic terminologies such as hyperplastic polyp, sessile serrated lesion, sessile serrated lesion with dysplasia, and adenoma (tubular, tubulovillous, or villous). Dysplasia seen in serrated polyps can take the form of conventional adenoma or traditional serrated adenoma. The old term "cystadenoma" is no longer recommended for appendiceal lesions by the Peritoneal Surface Oncology Group International (PSOGI).

By definition, appendiceal polyps should remain confined to the mucosa with preservation of the muscularis mucosae, although there is a tendency for the lamina propria to shrink and the lymphoid follicles to atrophy. The lumen is often circumferentially involved by the polyp. Most conventional adenomatous appendiceal polyps are villous in nature and contain villi of varying heights, though their architecture can also be flat or undulating (Fig. 14.30). Should the muscularis mucosae be effaced, or the appendiceal wall be dissected by mucin, a diagnosis of low-grade appendiceal mucinous neoplasm (LAMN) or appendiceal adenocarcinoma must be considered.
Reference: [105]

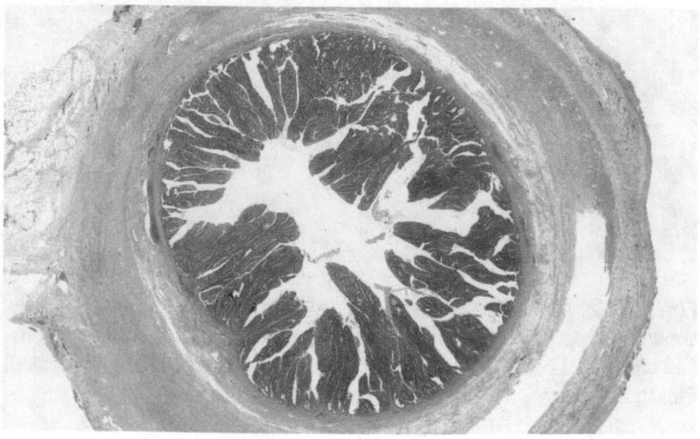

Fig. 14.30 A villous adenoma of the appendix that circumferentially involves the appendiceal lumen

32. What is the clinical significance of different appendiceal polyps?

Polyps at or adjacent to the appendiceal orifice are readily identified on colonoscopy, and can be removed during the procedure. Those polyps deeper within the appendiceal lumen will go endoscopically undetected in the asymptomatic patient given their cloistered location. Occasionally, appendiceal polyps may be incidentally identified with radiographic imaging, or may cause acute appendicitis that prompts appendectomy followed by histopathologic assessment and diagnosis. The gastroenterologist will then modify the colorectal cancer surveillance interval accordingly, with the appendiceal polyp presumptively treated as if it bestows a similar risk as its colorectal counterpart.

Interestingly, although our current approach to diagnostic classification of appendiceal polyps is similar to that used in the colorectum, there is some evidence of variability in the appendiceal polyp to carcinoma pathway. For example, one study shows that serrated appendiceal polyps demonstrate more *KRAS* mutations than *BRAF* mutations, which is contrary to the typical mutation profile seen in serrated colorectal polyps. Further clarification of these genetic differences and any associated clinical consequences would be of benefit before implementing changes to surveillance protocols.
Reference: [106]

33. Can juvenile polyp and Peutz–Jeghers polyp be non-syndromic?

Both juvenile polyp and Peutz–Jeghers polyp are hamartomatous and can be syndromic or sporadic. The definitions and histologic features of syndromic juvenile polyposis and Peutz–Jeghers polyposis are discussed in Chap. 15 (Questions 10, 11, 12, 13 and 14). Briefly, patients with <3 juvenile polyps and a negative family history are considered sporadic. It is the most common type of colon polyp in pediatric population but is not uncommon in adult patients. Sporadic juvenile polyps do not harbor the same genetic abnormalities as their syndromic counterparts. Patients with sporadic juvenile polyps do not have an increased risk for malignancy and thus do not require a specific follow-up. Sporadic Peutz–Jeghers polyp is considered extremely rare. Whether patients should undergo high-risk screening as for those with Peutz–Jeghers polyposis syndrome is currently unclear. Studies on a small number of patients showed that sporadic Peutz–Jeghers polyps might not carry the same risk of gastrointestinal neoplasia as Peutz–Jeghers polyposis. However, one study demonstrated that individuals with even one Peutz–Jeghers polyp may have a cumulative lifetime risk of cancer similar to those with syndromic polyps. Therefore, patients with sporadic polyps should also receive high-risk screening and close follow-up.
References: [107–109]

Case Presentation

Case 1

Learning Objectives
1. To learn the histologic features of the lesion
2. To generate the differential diagnosis

Case History
A 38-year-old male with a history of anal fissure treated with Botox injection in the past was admitted for hemoglobin of 7.9 g/dL. The patient reported minimal amounts of fresh red blood from the rectum.

Colonoscopy
A large (at least 3 cm) circumferential ulcer was found in the rectum. Biopsies were taken from the ulcer edge.

Histologic Findings
- Crypt architectural distortion.
- Diffuse fibrosis of the lamina propria, with strands of smooth muscle extending from thickened muscularis mucosae (Fig. 14.31).
- Areas of ulceration or erosion.

Differential Diagnosis
- Inflammatory bowel disease
- Ischemic colitis
- Inflammatory myoglandular polyp
- Mucosal prolapse (solitary rectal ulcer)

Final Diagnosis
Solitary rectal ulcer.

Take-Home Messages
1. Solitary rectal ulcer can be easily mistaken for inflammatory bowel disease or ischemic colitis.
2. Main histologic findings are those of mucosal prolapse.
3. The name is a misnomer: it can be multiple, can be seen outside the rectum, and may not be ulcerated.
   References: [71, 110–113]

Case 2

Learning Objectives
1. To learn the histologic features of the lesion
2. To generate the differential diagnosis

Case History
A 60-year-old male with a history of iron deficiency anemia, on oral iron (ferrous sulfate) supplement therapy.

Endoscopy
Erythematous, polypoid lesions in the gastric antrum with overlying exudate. Polypectomy was performed.

Histologic Findings
- Hyperplastic, tortuous, dilated gastric foveolae, with surface erosions and inflamed stroma (Fig. 14.3a).
- Clusters of black-brown crystalline material noted on mucosal surface (Fig. 14.32).

Differential Diagnosis
- Inflammatory polyp
- Menetrier disease
- Hyperplastic polyp

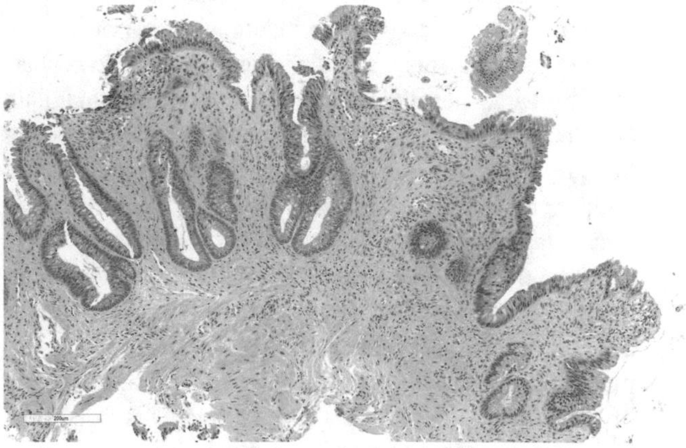

Fig. 14.31 (Case 1) A biopsy of the rectal ulcer edge showing crypt architectural distortion, lamina propria fibromuscular proliferation, and focal erosions

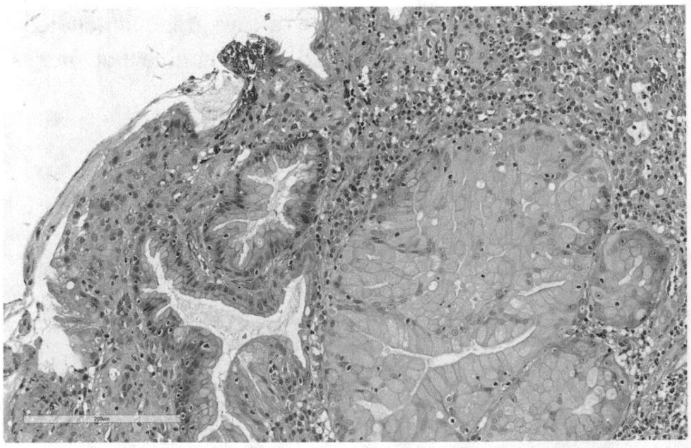

Fig. 14.32 (Case 2) Polypectomy of the gastric polypoid lesions showing hyperplastic foveolae with inflamed stroma, surface erosions, and clusters of black-brown crystalline material on the mucosal surface. Please also see Fig. 14.3a for low power view

- Pyloric gland adenoma
- Reactive gastropathy

Final Diagnosis

Hyperplastic polyp with iron deposition.

Take-Home Messages

1. Hyperplastic polyp can occur in association with various forms of chronic gastritis.
2. A small percentage (2–3%) of hyperplastic polyps of the stomach can show dysplasia (especially the larger ones).
3. Polypectomy is recommended for all gastric hyperplastic polyps greater than 0.5–1 cm.
   References: [15, 18, 21, 114, 115]

Case 3

Learning Objectives

1. To become familiar with the histologic features of the lesion
2. To generate the differential diagnosis

Case History

A 73-year-old male with a history of colon polyps.

Endoscopy

One sessile irregular distal cecal polyp (about 1.0 cm) removed with snare and cautery.

Histologic Findings

- Distorted crypts with dilated bases and horizontal widening.
- Elongated cells with pencillate, hyperchromatic, and pseudostratified nuclei (Fig. 14.33).

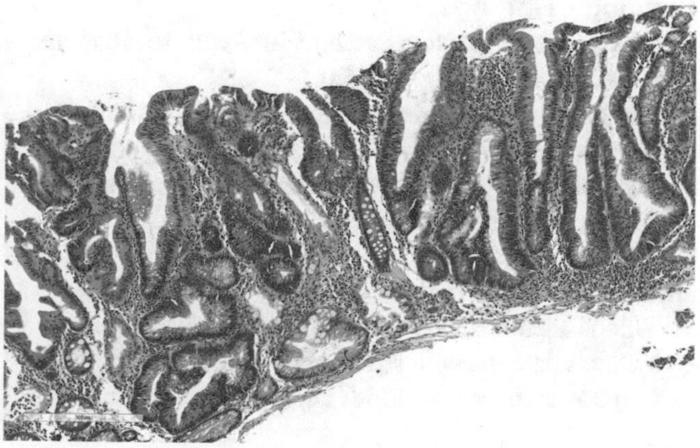

Fig. 14.33 (Case 3) Polypectomy of cecal polyp showing a few basally serrated/dilated crypts. Many crypts show elongated, hyperchromatic and pseudostratified nuclei, as well as goblet cell depletion

Differential Diagnosis

- Hyperplastic polyp
- Sessile serrated lesion with cytologic dysplasia
- Traditional serrated adenoma
- Tubular adenoma

Final Diagnosis

Sessile serrated lesion (or sessile serrated adenoma/polyp) with cytologic dysplasia.

Take-Home Messages

1. One distorted crypt base is sufficient to render the diagnosis of sessile serrated lesion (or sessile serrated adenoma/polyp).
2. It is important to recognize cytologic dysplasia in a serrated lesion because it is believed to carry a much higher risk for cancer development.
3. It is unnecessary to distinguish between low-grade and high-grade dysplasia in a serrated lesion.
   References: [76, 116, 117]

Case 4

Learning Objectives

1. To become familiar with the histologic features of lesion
2. To generate the differential diagnosis

Case History

A 59-year-old male presenting for colon cancer screening and for family history of colon cancer.

Endoscopy

One 3.0 cm, pedunculated polyp found at 20 cm from the anal verge, removed in two pieces with submucosal tattoo injection.

Histologic Findings

- Most of the polyp showed a tubulovillous architecture with features of low-grade dysplasia (Fig. 14.34a).
- Focal areas showed a cribriform architecture with luminal necrosis.
- The component with a cribriform architecture extended into the superficial submucosa, where large submucosal blood vessels were present (Fig. 14.34b).
- The distance of the component with a cribriform architecture to cauterized submucosal margin was 0.1 cm.
- No lymphovascular invasion identified.
- No significant tumor budding.

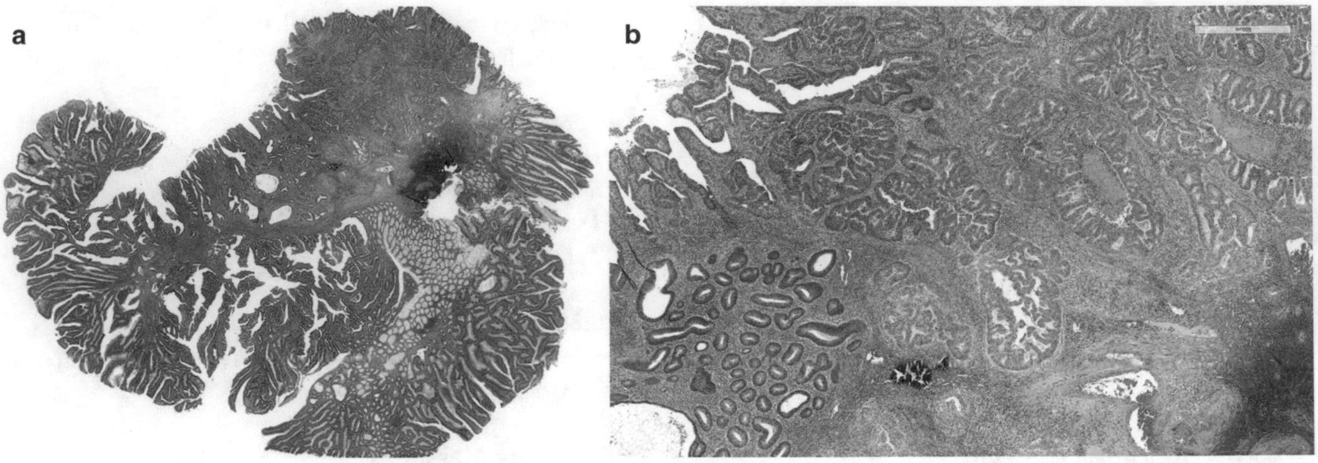

Fig. 14.34 (Case 4) Polypectomy from 20 cm of the colon showing a predominantly tubulovillous architecture (**a**). One area shows a cribriform architecture with luminal necrosis, with close contact with large submucosal blood vessels (**b**)

Differential Diagnosis

- Invasive moderately differentiated adenocarcinoma arising in a tubulovillous adenoma
- Tubulovillous adenoma with high-grade dysplasia
- Tubulovillous adenoma with pseudoinvasion

Final Diagnosis

Invasive moderately differentiated adenocarcinoma arising in a tubulovillous adenoma.

Follow-Up

An endoscopic ultrasound (EUS) performed at 3 months following polypectomy showed no lesions. Biopsy of prior polypectomy site was negative for residual adenoma or carcinoma.

Take-Home Messages

1. It can be difficult to differentiate between pseudoinvasion and invasive carcinoma, particularly when misplaced glands exhibit features of high-grade dysplasia. Features favoring true invasion may include stromal dysplasia, close proximity of neoplastic glands to submucosal large vessels, lack of surrounding lamina propria, lack of a lobular arrangement, and lack of evidence of traumatization such as hemorrhage and hemosiderin deposition.
2. It is important to assess high-risk histologic features in a malignant polyp, which mainly include differentiation, lymphovascular invasion, distance to polypectomy margin, and tumor budding.
3. Endoscopic resection with a negative margin (>0.1 cm) is an effective and safe intervention for malignant polyps, sparing surgery in >90% of the cases.

   References: [75, 87, 118, 119]

Case 5

Learning Objectives

1. To become familiar with this rare colorectal lesion
2. To generate the differential diagnosis

Case History

61-year-old male with a large polyp in the rectum referred for lower EUS for evaluation for cancer.

Endoscopy and EUS

The polyp was carpet-like with a large central protrusion and measured 6 × 5 × 4 cm. There was no grossly evident ulceration. EUS showed the lesion to be confined to the mucosa. Based on these findings, saline was injected around the bed of the polyp with lifting noted and the polyp was removed via piecemeal technique.

Histologic Findings

- Predominantly a villous architecture with focal architectural complexity (Fig. 14.35a).
- Minute clusters of bland and uniform cells coming off the base of neoplastic glands (Fig. 14.35b), which stained positive for synaptophysin (Fig. 14.35c). These cells occupied a distance of 0.3 cm.

Differential Diagnosis

- Villous adenoma with focal high-grade dysplasia
- Villous adenoma with squamous morules
- Composite intestinal villous adenoma-microcarcinoid

Final Diagnosis

Composite intestinal villous adenoma-microcarcinoid.

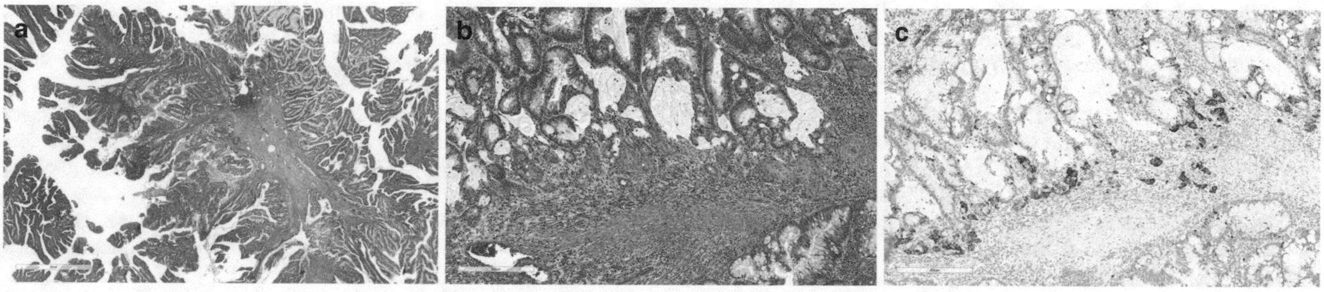

Fig. 14.35 (Case 5) Sections of the large rectal polyp showing predominantly a villous architecture (**a**). Architectural complexity is noted in a focal area, where minute clusters of bland and uniform cells are also seen at the base of neoplastic glands (**b**), which stain positive for synaptophysin (**c**)

Take-Home Messages

1. Microcarcinoid is a rare incidental finding in colorectal adenomas, which usually does not require additional treatment.
2. Given its location, microcarcinoid can be confused with high-grade dysplasia (intramucosal carcinoma) or even invasive carcinoma.
3. There are reported cases showing low-grade neuroendocrine tumors arising in intestinal adenomas, however.

References: [92–95, 120]

References

1. Wong MW, Bair MJ, Shih SC, Chu CH, Wang HY, Wang TE, et al. Using typical endoscopic features to diagnose esophageal squamous papilloma. World J Gastroenterol. 2016;22(7):2349–56.
2. Takeshita K, Murata S, Mitsufuji S, Wakabayashi N, Kataoka K, Tsuchihashi Y, et al. Clinicopathological characteristics of esophageal squamous papillomas in Japanese patients--with comparison of findings from Western countries. Acta Histochem Cytochem. 2006;39(1):23–30.
3. Carr NJ, Bratthauer GL, Lichy JH, Taubenberger JK, Monihan JM, Sobin LH. Squamous cell papillomas of the esophagus: a study of 23 lesions for human papillomavirus by in situ hybridization and the polymerase chain reaction. Hum Pathol. 1994;25(5):536–40.
4. Syrjanen K, Syrjanen S. Detection of human papillomavirus in sinonasal carcinoma: systematic review and meta-analysis. Hum Pathol. 2013;44(6):983–91.
5. Tiftikci A, Kutsal E, Altiok E, Ince U, Cicek B, Saruc M, et al. Analyzing esophageal squamous cell papillomas for the presence of human papilloma virus. Turk J Gastroenterol. 2017;28(3):176–8.
6. Pantham G, Ganesan S, Einstadter D, Jin G, Weinberg A, Fass R. Assessment of the incidence of squamous cell papilloma of the esophagus and the presence of high-risk human papilloma virus. Dis Esophagus. 2017;30(1):1–5.
7. Vadva MD, Triadafilopoulos G. Glycogenic acanthosis of the esophagus and gastroesophageal reflux. J Clin Gastroenterol. 1993;17(1):79–83.
8. Tsai SJ, Lin CC, Chang CW, Hung CY, Shieh TY, Wang HY, et al. Benign esophageal lesions: endoscopic and pathologic features. World J Gastroenterol. 2015;21(4):1091–8.
9. Kay PS, Soetikno RM, Mindelzun R, Young HS. Diffuse esophageal glycogenic acanthosis: an endoscopic marker of Cowden's disease. Am J Gastroenterol. 1997;92(6):1038–40.
10. Levi Z, Baris HN, Kedar I, Niv Y, Geller A, Gal E, et al. Upper and lower gastrointestinal findings in PTEN mutation-positive Cowden syndrome patients participating in an active surveillance program. Clin Transl Gastroenterol. 2011;2:e5.
11. McGarrity TJ, Wagner Baker MJ, Ruggiero FM, Thiboutot DM, Hampel H, Zhou XP, et al. GI polyposis and glycogenic acanthosis of the esophagus associated with PTEN mutation positive Cowden syndrome in the absence of cutaneous manifestations. Am J Gastroenterol. 2003;98(6):1429–34.
12. Modi RM, Arnold CA, Stanich PP. Diffuse esophageal glycogenic acanthosis and colon polyposis in a patient with Cowden syndrome. Clin Gastroenterol Hepatol. 2017;15(8):e131–e2.
13. Morais DJ, Yamanaka A, Zeitune JM, Andreollo NA. Gastric polyps: a retrospective analysis of 26,000 digestive endoscopies. Arq Gastroenterol. 2007;44(1):14–7.
14. Markowski AR, Markowska A, Guzinska-Ustymowicz K. Pathophysiological and clinical aspects of gastric hyperplastic polyps. World J Gastroenterol. 2016;22(40):8883–91.
15. Jain R, Chetty R. Gastric hyperplastic polyps: a review. Dig Dis Sci. 2009;54(9):1839–46.
16. Yamashita M, Hirokawa M, Nakasono M, Kiyoku H, Sano N, Fujii M, et al. Gastric inverted hyperplastic polyp: report of four cases and relation to gastritis cystica profunda. APMIS. 2002;110(10):717–23.
17. Castro R, Pimentel-Nunes P, Dinis-Ribeiro M. Evaluation and management of gastric epithelial polyps. Best Pract Res Clin Gastroenterol. 2017;31(4):381–7.
18. Abraham SC, Singh VK, Yardley JH, Wu TT. Hyperplastic polyps of the stomach: associations with histologic patterns of gastritis and gastric atrophy. Am J Surg Pathol. 2001;25(4):500–7.
19. Terada T. Heterotopic gastric mucosa of the gastrointestinal tract: a histopathologic study of 158 cases. Pathol Res Pract. 2011;207(3):148–50.
20. Salomao M, Luna AM, Sepulveda JL, Sepulveda AR. Mutational analysis by next generation sequencing of gastric type dysplasia occurring in hyperplastic polyps of the stomach: mutations in gastric hyperplastic polyps. Exp Mol Pathol. 2015;99(3):468–73.
21. Markowski AR, Guzinska-Ustymowicz K. Gastric hyperplastic polyp with focal cancer. Gastroenterol Rep. 2016;4(2):158–61.
22. Abraham SC, Park SJ, Mugartegui L, Hamilton SR, Wu TT. Sporadic fundic gland polyps with epithelial dysplasia: evidence for preferential targeting for mutations in the adenomatous polyposis coli gene. Am J Pathol. 2002;161(5):1735–42.
23. Chen ZM, Scudiere JR, Abraham SC, Montgomery E. Pyloric gland adenoma: an entity distinct from gastric foveolar type adenoma. Am J Surg Pathol. 2009;33:186–93.
24. Pezhouh MK, Park JY. Gastric pyloric gland adenoma. Arch Pathol Lab Med. 2015;139(6):823–6.

25. Singhi AD, Lazenby AJ, Montgomery EA. Gastric adenocarcinoma with chief cell differentiation: a proposal for reclassification as oxyntic gland polyp/adenoma. Am J Surg Pathol. 2012;36(7):1030–5.
26. Chan K, Brown IS, Kyle T, Lauwers GY, Kumarasinghe MP. Chief cell-predominant gastric polyps: a series of 12 cases with literature review. Histopathology. 2016;68(6):825–33.
27. Effenberger M, Steinle H, Offner FA, Vogel W, Millonig G. Holes in gastric mucosa in upper gastrointestinal endoscopy. Eur J Gastroenterol Hepatol. 2014;26(6):676–8.
28. Park JS, Myung SJ, Jung HY, Yang SK, Hong WS, Kim JH, et al. Endoscopic treatment of gastritis cystica polyposa found in an unoperated stomach. Gastrointest Endosc. 2001;54(1):101–3.
29. Yu XF, Guo LW, Chen ST, Teng LS. Gastritis cystica profunda in a previously unoperated stomach: a case report. World J Gastroenterol. 2015;21(12):3759–62.
30. Levine JA, Burgart LJ, Batts KP, Wang KK. Brunner's gland hamartomas: clinical presentation and pathological features of 27 cases. Am J Gastroenterol. 1995;90(2):290–4.
31. Gao YP, Zhu JS, Zheng WJ. Brunner's gland adenoma of duodenum: a case report and literature review. World J Gastroenterol. 2004;10(17):2616–7.
32. Rocco A, Borriello P, Compare D, De Colibus P, Pica L, Iacono A, et al. Large Brunner's gland adenoma: case report and literature review. World J Gastroenterol. 2006;12(12):1966–8.
33. Powers M, Sayuk GS, Wang HL. Brunner gland cyst: report of three cases. Int J Clin Exp Pathol. 2008;1(6):536–8.
34. Poeschl EM, Siebert F, Vieth M, Langner C. Pyloric gland adenoma arising in gastric heterotopia within the duodenal bulb. Endoscopy. 2011;43 Suppl 2 UCTN:E336–7.
35. Manabat M, Jackson M, Ngo K, Stawick L. Duodenal pyloric gland adenoma in a 59-year-old Asian male. Case Rep Gastrointest Med. 2018;2018:9287843.
36. Hida R, Yamamoto H, Hirahashi M, Kumagai R, Nishiyama K, Gi T, et al. Duodenal neoplasms of gastric phenotype: an immunohistochemical and genetic study with a practical approach to the classification. Am J Surg Pathol. 2017;41(3):343–53.
37. Hashimoto T, Ogawa R, Matsubara A, Taniguchi H, Sugano K, Ushiama M, et al. Familial adenomatous polyposis-associated and sporadic pyloric gland adenomas of the upper gastrointestinal tract share common genetic features. Histopathology. 2015;67(5):689–98.
38. Matsubara A, Ogawa R, Suzuki H, Oda I, Taniguchi H, Kanai Y, et al. Activating GNAS and KRAS mutations in gastric foveolar metaplasia, gastric heterotopia, and adenocarcinoma of the duodenum. Br J Cancer. 2015;112(8):1398–404.
39. Hidaka Y, Mitomi H, Saito T, Takahashi M, Lee SY, Matsumoto K, et al. Alteration in the Wnt/beta-catenin signaling pathway in gastric neoplasias of fundic gland (chief cell predominant) type. Hum Pathol. 2013;44(11):2438–48.
40. Borhan-Manesh F, Farnum JB. Incidence of heterotopic gastric mucosa in the upper oesophagus. Gut. 1991;32(9):968–72.
41. Mann NS, Mann SK, Rachut E. Heterotopic gastric tissue in the duodenal bulb. J Clin Gastroenterol. 2000;30(3):303–6.
42. Yu L, Yang Y, Cui L, Peng L, Sun G. Heterotopic gastric mucosa of the gastrointestinal tract: prevalence, histological features, and clinical characteristics. Scand J Gastroenterol. 2014;49(2):138–44.
43. Genta RM, Kinsey RS, Singhal A, Suterwala S. Gastric foveolar metaplasia and gastric heterotopia in the duodenum: no evidence of an etiologic role for Helicobacter pylori. Hum Pathol. 2010;41(11):1593–600.
44. Conlon N, Logan E, Veerappan S, McKiernan S, O'Briain S. Duodenal gastric heterotopia: further evidence of an association with fundic gland polyps. Hum Pathol. 2013;44(4):636–42.
45. Wlaz J, Madro A, Kazmierak W, Celinski K, Slomka M. Pancreatic and gastric heterotopy in the gastrointestinal tract. Postepy Hig Med Dosw (Online). 2014;68:1069–75.
46. Betzler A, Mees ST, Pump J, Scholch S, Zimmermann C, Aust DE, et al. Clinical impact of duodenal pancreatic heterotopia: is there a need for surgical treatment? BMC Surg. 2017;17(1):53.
47. Rezvani M, Menias C, Sandrasegaran K, Olpin JD, Elsayes KM, Shaaban AM. Heterotopic pancreas: histopathologic features, imaging findings, and complications. Radiographics. 2017;37(2):484–99.
48. Sathyanarayana SA, Deutsch GB, Bajaj J, Friedman B, Bansal R, Molmenti E, et al. Ectopic pancreas: a diagnostic dilemma. Int J Angiol. 2012;21(3):177–80.
49. Al Salihi S, Jaitly V, Saulino DM, DuPont AW, Ertan A, Everett JM, Younes M. Pancreatic acinar metaplasia in distal esophageal biopsies is associated with chronic nonsteroidal anti-inflammatory drug use. Arch Pathol Lab Med. 2019;143(4):510–2.
50. Genta RM, Feagins LA. Advanced precancerous lesions in the small bowel mucosa. Best Pract Res Clin Gastroenterol. 2013;27(2):225–33.
51. Perzin KH, Bridge MF. Adenomas of the small intestine: a clinicopathologic review of 51 cases and a study of their relationship to carcinoma. Cancer. 1981;48(3):799–819.
52. Maguire A, Sheahan K. Primary small bowel adenomas and adenocarcinomas: recent advances. Virchows Arch. 2018;473(3):265–73.
53. Raman SP, Fishman EK. Abnormalities of the distal common bile duct and ampulla: diagnostic approach and differential diagnosis using multiplanar reformations and 3D imaging. AJR Am J Roentgenol. 2014;203(1):17–28.
54. Adsay V, Ohike N, Tajiri T, Kim GE, Krasinskas A, Balci S, et al. Ampullary region carcinomas: definition and site specific classification with delineation of four clinicopathologically and prognostically distinct subsets in an analysis of 249 cases. Am J Surg Pathol. 2012;36(11):1592–608.
55. Hinrichs HR, Goldman H. Localized giant pseudopolyps of the colon. JAMA. 1968;205(4):248–9.
56. Wolf EM, Strasser C, Geboes K, Spuller E, Vieth M, Langner C. Localized giant inflammatory polyp of the colon in a patient without inflammatory bowel disease. Virchows Arch. 2011;459(2):245–6.
57. Politis DS, Katsanos KH, Tsianos EV, Christodoulou DK. Pseudopolyps in inflammatory bowel diseases: have we learned enough? World J Gastroenterol. 2017;23(9):1541–51.
58. De Petris G, Dhungel BM, Chen L, Pasha SF. Inflammatory "cap" polyposis: a case report of a rare nonneoplastic colonic polyposis. Int J Surg Pathol. 2014;22(4):378–82.
59. Arimura Y, Isshiki H, Hirayama D, Onodera K, Murakami K, Yamashita K, et al. Polypectomy to eradicate cap polyposis with protein-losing enteropathy. Am J Gastroenterol. 2014;109(10):1689–91.
60. Konishi T, Watanabe T, Takei Y, Kojima T, Nagawa H. Cap polyposis: an inflammatory disorder or a spectrum of mucosal prolapse syndrome? Gut. 2005;54(9):1342–3.
61. Lim YJ, Choi JH, Yang CH. What is the clinical relevance of filiform polyposis? Gut Liver. 2012;6(4):524–6.
62. Oakley GJ 3rd, Schraut WH, Peel R, Krasinskas A. Diffuse filiform polyposis with unique histology mimicking familial adenomatous polyposis in a patient without inflammatory bowel disease. Arch Pathol Lab Med. 2007;131(12):1821–4.
63. Shiomi T, Kameyama K, Kawano Y, Shimizu Y, Takabayashi T, Okada Y. Neuromuscular and vascular hamartoma of the cecum. Virchows Arch. 2002;440(3):338–40.
64. Madigan MR, Morson BC. Solitary ulcer of the rectum. Gut. 1969;10(11):871–81.
65. Lobert PF, Appelman HD. Inflammatory cloacogenic polyp: a unique inflammatory lesion of the anal transitional zone. Am J Surg Pathol. 1981;5(8):761–6.

66. du Boulay CE, Fairbrother J, Isaacson PG. Mucosal prolapse syndrome: a unifying concept for solitary ulcer syndrome and related disorders. J Clin Pathol. 1983;36(11):1264–8.
67. Tjandra JJ, Fazio VW, Petras RE, Lavery IC, Oakley JR, Milsom JW, et al. Clinical and pathologic factors associated with delayed diagnosis in solitary rectal ulcer syndrome. Dis Colon Rectum. 1993;36(2):146–53.
68. Saul SH. Inflammatory cloacogenic polyp: relationship to solitary rectal ulcer syndrome/mucosal prolapse and other bowel disorders. Hum Pathol. 1987;18(11):1120–5.
69. Poon KK, Mills S, Booth IW, Murphy MS. Inflammatory cloacogenic polyp: an unrecognized cause of hematochezia and tenesmus in childhood. J Pediatr. 1997;130(2):327–9.
70. Nakamura S, Kino I, Akagi T. Inflammatory myoglandular polyps of the colon and rectum: a clinicopathological study of 32 pedunculated polyps, distinct from other types of polyps. Am J Surg Pathol. 1992;16(8):772–9.
71. Meniconi RL, Caronna R, Benedetti M, Fanello G, Ciardi A, Schiratti M, et al. Inflammatory myoglandular polyp of the cecum: case report and review of literature. BMC Gastroenterol. 2010;10:10.
72. Torlakovic E, Skovlund E, Snover DC, Torlakovic G, Nesland JM. Morphologic reappraisal of serrated colorectal polyps. Am J Surg Pathol. 2003;27(1):65–81.
73. Jass JR. Classification of colorectal cancer based on correlation of clinical, morphological and molecular features. Histopathology. 2007;50(1):113–30.
74. Yang S, Farraye FA, Mack C, Posnik O, O'Brien MJ. BRAF and KRAS mutations in hyperplastic polyps and serrated adenomas of the colorectum: relationship to histology and CpG island methylation status. Am J Surg Pathol. 2004;28(11):1452–9.
75. Gupta S, Lieberman D, Anderson JC, Burke CA, Dominitz JA, Kaltenbach T, Robertson DJ, Shaukat A, Syngal S, Rex DK. Recommendations for follow-up after colonoscopy and polypectomy: a consensus update by the US Multi-Society Task Force on colorectal cancer. Gastroenterology. 2020;115(3):415–34.
76. Rex DK, Ahnen DJ, Baron JA, Batts KP, Burke CA, Burt RW, et al. Serrated lesions of the colorectum: review and recommendations from an expert panel. Am J Gastroenterol. 2012;107(9):1315–29; quiz 4, 30.
77. Ponugoti P, Lin J, Odze R, Snover D, Kahi C, Rex DK. Prevalence of sessile serrated adenoma/polyp in hyperplastic-appearing diminutive rectosigmoid polyps. Gastrointest Endosc. 2017;85(3):622–7.
78. Rosty C, Buchanan DD, Walters RJ, Carr NJ, Bothman JW, Young JP, Brown IS. Hyperplastic polyp of the duodenum: a report of 9 cases with immunohistochemical and molecular findings. Hum Pathol. 2011;42(12):1953–9.
79. Torlakovic EE, Gomez JD, Driman DK, Parfitt JR, Wang C, Benerjee T, et al. Sessile serrated adenoma (SSA) vs. traditional serrated adenoma (TSA). Am J Surg Pathol. 2008;32(1):21–9.
80. Khalid O, Radaideh S, Cummings OW, O'Brien MJ, Goldblum JR, Rex DK. Reinterpretation of histology of proximal colon polyps called hyperplastic in 2001. World J Gastroenterol. 2009;15(30):3767–70.
81. Farris AB, Misdraji J, Srivastava A, Muzikansky A, Deshpande V, Lauwers GY, et al. Sessile serrated adenoma: challenging discrimination from other serrated colonic polyps. Am J Surg Pathol. 2008;32(1):30–5.
82. Huang CC, Frankel WL, Doukides T, Zhou XP, Zhao W, Yearsley MM. Prolapse-related changes are a confounding factor in misdiagnosis of sessile serrated adenomas in the rectum. Hum Pathol. 2013;44(4):480–6.
83. Haramis AP, Begthel H, van den Born M, van Es J, Jonkheer S, Offerhaus GJ, et al. De novo crypt formation and juvenile polyposis on BMP inhibition in mouse intestine. Science. 2004;303(5664):1684–6.
84. Wiland HO, Shadrach B, Allende D, Carver P, Goldblum JR, Liu X, et al. Morphologic and molecular characterization of traditional serrated adenomas of the distal colon and rectum. Am J Surg Pathol. 2014;38(9):1290–7.
85. Rubio CA. Traditional serrated adenomas of the upper digestive tract. J Clin Pathol. 2016;69(1):1–5.
86. Rosty C, Campbell C, Clendenning M, Bettington M, Buchanan DD, Brown IS. Do serrated neoplasms of the small intestine represent a distinct entity? Pathological findings and molecular alterations in a series of 13 cases. Histopathology. 2015;66(3):333–42.
87. Bettington M, Walker N, Rosty C, Brown I, Clouston A, McKeone D, et al. Clinicopathological and molecular features of sessile serrated adenomas with dysplasia or carcinoma. Gut. 2017;66(1):97–106.
88. Hamilton SR, Bosman FT, Boffetta P, Ilyas M, Morreau H. Carcinoma of the colon and rectum. In: Bosnan FT, Carneiro F, Hruban RH, Theise ND, editors. WHo classification of tumours of the digestive system. Lyon: IARC Press; 2010. p. 134–46.
89. Lee HE, Chandan VS, Lee CT, Wu TT. Squamoid morules in the pseudoinvasive foci of colonic polyp morphologically mimic invasive carcinoma. Hum Pathol. 2017;68:54–60.
90. Ueo T, Kashima K, Daa T, Kondo Y, Sasaki A, Yokoyama S. Immunohistochemical analysis of morules in colonic neoplasms: morules are morphologically and qualitatively different from squamous metaplasia. Pathobiology. 2005;72(5):269–78.
91. Reis-Filho JS, Preto A, Soares P, Ricardo S, Cameselle-Teijeiro J, Sobrinho-Simoes M. p63 expression in solid cell nests of the thyroid: further evidence for a stem cell origin. Mod Pathol. 2003;16(1):43–8.
92. Fu Z, Saade R, Koo BH, Jennings TA, Lee H. Incidence of composite intestinal adenoma-microcarcinoid in 158 surgically resected polyps and its association with squamous morule. Ann Diagn Pathol. 2019;42:69–74.
93. Kim MJ, Lee EJ, Kim DS, Lee DH, Youk EG, Kim HJ. Composite intestinal adenoma-microcarcinoid in the colon and rectum: a case series and historical review. Diagn Pathol. 2017;12(1):78.
94. Lin J, Goldblum JR, Bennett AE, Bronner MP, Liu X. Composite intestinal adenoma-microcarcinoid. Am J Surg Pathol. 2012;36(2):292–5.
95. Salaria SN, Abu Alfa AK, Alsaigh NY, Montgomery E, Arnold CA. Composite intestinal adenoma-microcarcinoid clues to diagnosing an under-recognised mimic of invasive adenocarcinoma. J Clin Pathol. 2013;66(4):302–6.
96. Rex DK, Goldblum JR. Pro: villous elements and high-grade dysplasia help guide post-polypectomy colonoscopic surveillance. Am J Gastroenterol. 2008;103(6):1327–9.
97. Yantiss RK, Goldman H, Odze RD. Hyperplastic polyp with epithelial misplacement (inverted hyperplastic polyp): a clinicopathologic and immunohistochemical study of 19 cases. Mod Pathol. 2001;14(9):869–75.
98. Panarelli NC, Somarathna T, Samowitz WS, Kornacki S, Sanders SA, Novelli MR, et al. Diagnostic challenges caused by endoscopic biopsy of colonic polyps: a systematic evaluation of epithelial misplacement with review of problematic polyps from the Bowel Cancer Screening Program, United Kingdom. Am J Surg Pathol. 2016;40(8):1075–83.
99. O'Leary AD, Sweeney EC. Lymphoglandular complexes of the colon: structure and distribution. Histopathology. 1986;10(3):267–83.
100. Eide TJ. Risk of colorectal cancer in adenoma-bearing individuals within a defined population. Int J Cancer. 1986;38(2):173–6.
101. Gupta N, Bansal A, Rao D, Early DS, Jonnalagadda S, Wani SB, et al. Prevalence of advanced histological features in diminutive and small colon polyps. Gastrointest Endosc. 2012;75(5):1022–30.

102. Cooper HS. Pathologic issues in the treatment of endoscopically removed malignant colorectal polyps. J Natl Compr Canc Netw. 2007;5(9):991–6.
103. Ueno H, Mochizuki H, Hashiguchi Y, Shimazaki H, Aida S, Hase K, et al. Risk factors for an adverse outcome in early invasive colorectal carcinoma. Gastroenterology. 2004;127(2):385–94.
104. Bosch SL, Teerenstra S, de Wilt JH, Cunningham C, Nagtegaal ID. Predicting lymph node metastasis in pT1 colorectal cancer: a systematic review of risk factors providing rationale for therapy decisions. Endoscopy. 2013;45(10):827–34.
105. Carr NJ, Cecil TD, Mohamed F, Sobin LH, Sugarbaker PH, Gonzalez-Moreno S, et al. A consensus for classification and pathologic reporting of pseudomyxoma peritonei and associated appendiceal neoplasia: the results of the Peritoneal Surface Oncology Group International (PSOGI) Modified Delphi Process. Am J Surg Pathol. 2016;40(1):14–26.
106. Pai RK, Hartman DJ, Gonzalo DH, Lai KK, Downs-Kelly E, Goldblum JR, et al. Serrated lesions of the appendix frequently harbor KRAS mutations and not BRAF mutations indicating a distinctly different serrated neoplastic pathway in the appendix. Hum Pathol. 2014;45(2):227–35.
107. Patel R, Hyer W. Practical management of polyposis syndromes. Frontline Gastroenterol. 2019;10(4):379–87.
108. Culver EL, McIntyre AS. Sporadic duodenal polyps: classification, investigation, and management. Endoscopy. 2011;43(2):144–55.
109. Burkart AL, Sheridan T, Lewin M, Fenton H, Ali NJ, Montgomery E. Do sporadic Peutz-Jeghers polyps exist? Experience of a large teaching hospital. Am J Surg Pathol. 2007;31(8):1209–14.
110. Abid S, Khawaja A, Bhimani SA, Ahmad Z, Hamid S, Jafri W. The clinical, endoscopic and histological spectrum of the solitary rectal ulcer syndrome: a single-center experience of 116 cases. BMC Gastroenterol. 2012;12:72.
111. Brosens LA, Montgomery EA, Bhagavan BS, Offerhaus GJ, Giardiello FM. Mucosal prolapse syndrome presenting as rectal polyposis. J Clin Pathol. 2009;62(11):1034–6.
112. Libanio D, Meireles C, Afonso LP, Henrique R, Pimentel-Nunes P, Dinis-Ribeiro M. Mucosal prolapse polyp mimicking rectal malignancy: a case report. GE Port J Gastroenterol. 2016;23(4):214–7.
113. Zhu QC, Shen RR, Qin HL, Wang Y. Solitary rectal ulcer syndrome: clinical features, pathophysiology, diagnosis and treatment strategies. World J Gastroenterol. 2014;20(3):738–44.
114. Abraham SC, Yardley JH, Wu TT. Erosive injury to the upper gastrointestinal tract in patients receiving iron medication: an underrecognized entity. Am J Surg Pathol. 1999;23(10):1241–7.
115. ASGE Standards of Practice Committee, Evans JA, Chandrasekhara V, Chathadi KV, Decker GA, Early DS, et al. The role of endoscopy in the management of premalignant and malignant conditions of the stomach. Gastrointest Endosc. 2015;82(1):1–8.
116. Niv Y. Changing pathological diagnosis from hyperplastic polyp to sessile serrated adenoma: systematic review and meta-analysis. Eur J Gastroenterol Hepatol. 2017;29(12):1327–31.
117. Sandmeier D, Seelentag W, Bouzourene H. Serrated polyps of the colorectum: is sessile serrated adenoma distinguishable from hyperplastic polyp in a daily practice? Virchows Arch. 2007;450(6):613–8.
118. Raju GS, Lum PJ, Ross WA, Thirumurthi S, Miller E, Lynch PM, et al. Outcome of EMR as an alternative to surgery in patients with complex colon polyps. Gastrointest Endosc. 2016;84(2):315–25.
119. Yantiss RK, Bosenberg MW, Antonioli DA, Odze RD. Utility of MMP-1, p53, E-cadherin, and collagen IV immunohistochemical stains in the differential diagnosis of adenomas with misplaced epithelium versus adenomas with invasive adenocarcinoma. Am J Surg Pathol. 2002;26(2):206–15.
120. Estrella JS, Taggart MW, Rashid A, Abraham SC. Low-grade neuroendocrine tumors arising in intestinal adenomas: evidence for alterations in the adenomatous polyposis coli/beta-catenin pathway. Hum Pathol. 2014;45(10):2051–8.

Syndromic Epithelial Polyps of the Gastrointestinal Tract

15

Michael Lee, Zongming Eric Chen, and Hanlin L. Wang

List of Frequently Asked Questions

1. What are the genetic and clinical features of familial adenomatous polyposis (FAP)?
2. What are the common gross and histologic features of FAP?
3. If a patient has numerous adenomatous polyps in the colon and a gastrointestinal syndrome is suspected, what is the clinical testing algorithm?
4. How do you distinguish each FAP variant (Turcot syndrome, Gardner syndrome, attenuated FAP)?
5. What are the prognostic and treatment implications in patients with FAP syndrome?
6. What is the molecular etiology behind Lynch syndrome?
7. What are the clinical and histologic features of Lynch syndrome-associated polyps?
8. How do you differentiate colorectal cancers of sporadic mismatch repair deficiency from hereditary Lynch syndrome based on immunohistochemical and molecular studies?
9. What are the prognostic and treatment implications of Lynch syndrome?
10. When should you raise a suspicion for Peutz–Jeghers syndrome?
11. Which histologic features distinguish a Peutz-Jeghers polyp from a juvenile polyp?
12. Which clinical features distinguish Peutz–Jeghers polyps from juvenile polyps?
13. What are the prognostic implications in Peutz–Jeghers syndrome patients?
14. When do you need to raise a suspicion for juvenile polyposis?
15. How do you differentiate Cowden/PTEN hamartoma syndrome from Cronkhite–Canada syndrome?
16. What are the major and minor diagnostic criteria for Cowden/PTEN hamartoma syndrome?
17. What is MUTYH-associated polyposis and how do you differentiate it from FAP?
18. What is serrated polyposis syndrome?
19. What is gastric adenocarcinoma and proximal polyposis of the stomach (GAPPS)?

M. Lee (✉)
Columbia University Vagelos College of Physicians and Surgeons, New York, NY, USA
e-mail: mjl2197@cumc.columbia.edu

Z. E. Chen
Mayo Clinic, Rochester, MN, USA

H. L. Wang
University of California at Los Angeles David Geffen School of Medicine, Los Angeles, CA, USA

Frequently Asked Questions

1. What are the genetic and clinical features of familial adenomatous polyposis (FAP)?

Familial adenomatous polyposis (FAP) is an autosomal dominant disorder caused by a germline mutation in the adenomatous polyposis coli (*APC*) gene, located on chromosome 5q21.

- APC is a tumor suppressor that manages the cell cycle by shutting off transcription in the Wnt signaling pathway by regulating β-catenin.
- Since FAP patients have inherited a germline mutation in *APC*, a somatic mutation or loss of heterozygosity in the remaining allele leads to the clinical manifestations of FAP. This is the two-hit hypothesis.
- Mutations occur at different sites along the *APC* gene, therefore phenotypic variations are possible.

FAP is the most common syndromic gastrointestinal epithelial polyposis syndrome. The frequency ranges from 1 in 5000 to 30,000 people.

- Approximately 10–30% of patients develop FAP without a family history because of a spontaneous *APC* mutation or mosaicism.

H. L. Wang, Z. E. Chen (eds.), *Practical Gastrointestinal Pathology*, Practical Anatomic Pathology,
https://doi.org/10.1007/978-3-030-51268-2_15

- Patients present with gastrointestinal bleeding and abdominal pain, and colonoscopy demonstrates hundreds of polyps diffusely covering the length of the colon. Some patients have thousands of polyps. These adenomas harbor a 100% risk of transformation into adenocarcinoma by the age of 60 and cases have been diagnosed in patients as young as 17 years old. Most patients develop colorectal carcinoma (CRC) by the third decade of life.
- FAP-related and sporadic adenomas have a similar distribution, predominantly on the left side with a predilection for the sigmoid colon and rectum. Extra-colonic polyps include duodenal adenomas at or near the ampulla, jejunal/ileal adenomas, gastric fundic gland polyps with or without dysplasia, and gastric adenomas. They can lead to small intestinal and gastric adenocarcinomas. Duodenal cancer is one of the leading causes of death in FAP patients.
- The *MUTYH* gene transcribes a DNA repair enzyme, MYH glycosylase, which fixes mismatched base pairs by excision. Mutations in the *MUTYH* gene lead to clinical features resembling FAP. Approximately 10–20% of patients with the clinical impression of FAP but lacking a germline *APC* mutation, harbor a *MUTYH* mutation (see Question 17).

References: [1–9]

2. **What are the common gross and histologic features of FAP?**

FAP patients have hundreds or thousands of polyps throughout the length of their colon (Fig. 15.1a, b).

- Tubular adenomas are pedunculated or sessile and resemble their sporadic counterparts with pencillate, elongated, and hyperchromatic nuclei along the epithelial surface and crypts (Fig. 15.1c).
- Most adenomas are tubular; however, varying degrees of villous architecture can be seen. Adenomas are also seen in the duodenum at or near the ampulla of Vater, and in the stomach, jejunum, and ileum.
- FAP patients are more likely to have gastric fundic gland polyps (FGP). Higher rates of dysplasia are seen in FGPs within the context of FAP (Fig. 15.1d) than a

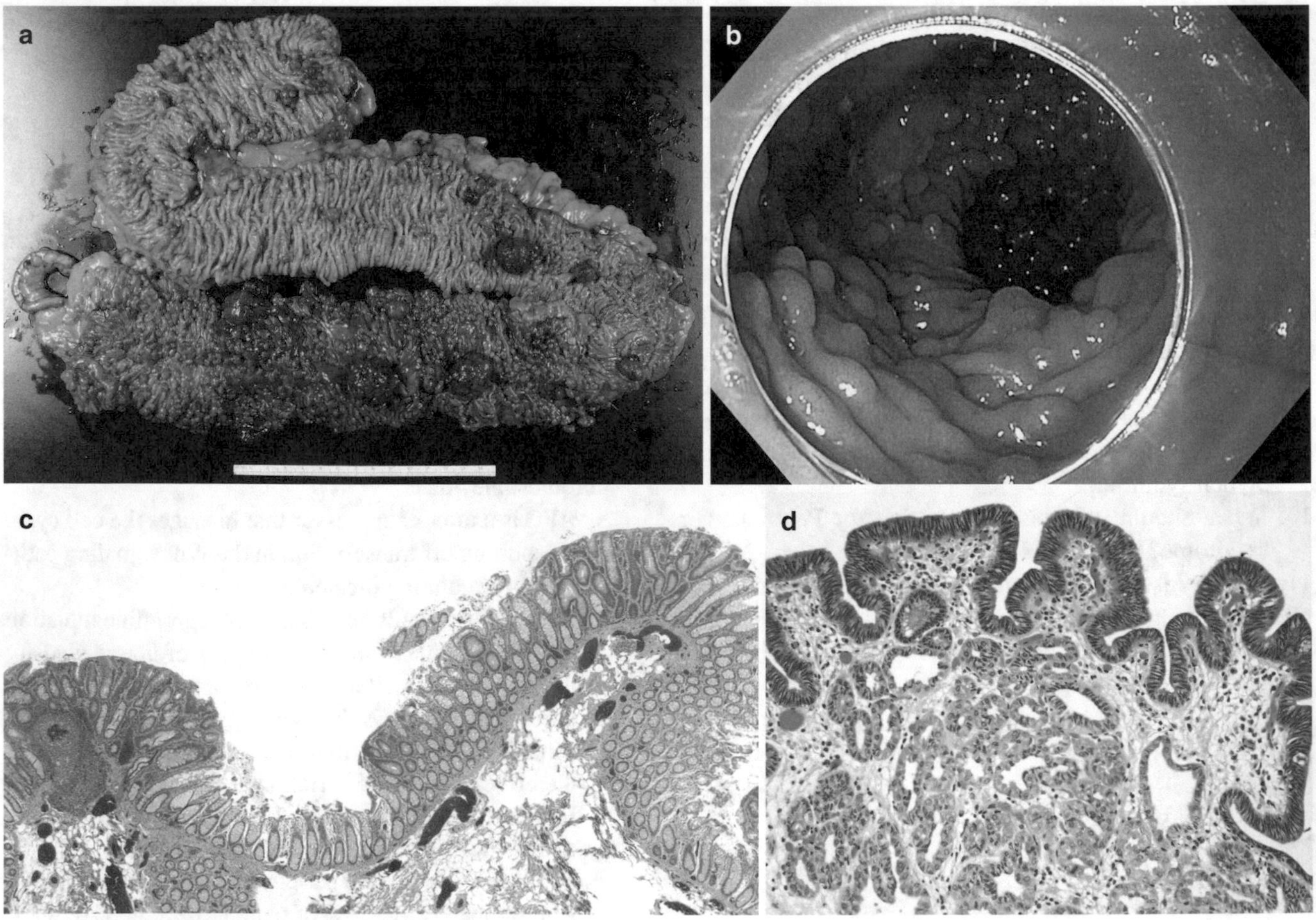

Fig. 15.1 Gross (**a**) and endoscopic (**b**) photos of an FAP case showing numerous polyps in the colon. Histologic examination of colonic polyps (**c**) shows multiple tubular adenomas. Histologic examination of a gastric polyp (**d**) shows a fundic gland polyp with low-grade dysplasia involving the surface foveolar epithelium

sporadic FGP, which are seen in patients who use proton pump inhibitors. Dysplasia seen in FGP is typically low grade or indefinite at most. Progression to high-grade dysplasia or invasive adenocarcinoma is exceedingly rare.

Since all FAP patients develop CRC by the sixth decade of life, treatment is aimed at prevention.

- Patients begin annual screening sigmoidoscopies and colonoscopies at age 10 with upper gastrointestinal endoscopies at age 20.
- By the second decade, a total colectomy with an ileorectal anastomosis may be performed as a prophylactic measure.
- FAP patients are also at risk for other tumors, which include desmoid tumor (fibromatosis), hepatoblastoma, and brain cancer (see Question 4). Therefore, a total colectomy is not always a guarantee in reducing a patient's mortality risk.

References: [4, 7, 10–13]

3. If a patient has numerous adenomatous polyps in the colon and a gastrointestinal syndrome is suspected, what is the clinical testing algorithm?

See Fig. 15.2 for diagnostic algorithm for syndromic epithelial adenomatous polyposis.

References: [9, 14–20]

4. How do you distinguish each FAP variant (Turcot syndrome, Gardner syndrome, attenuated FAP)?

Turcot syndrome is a gastrointestinal polyposis syndrome with an increased risk for colorectal and brain cancer.

- Turcot syndrome patients have FAP symptoms and malignant central nervous system (CNS) tumors, medulloblastoma being the most common.
- FAP-associated medulloblastomas are usually seen in patients younger than 20 years of age, caused by an *APC* mutation between codons 697 and 1224.
- Patients with Lynch syndrome (formerly termed "hereditary nonpolyposis colorectal cancer syndrome") can also have CNS tumors, more commonly glioblastoma multiforme due to mutation in one of the DNA mismatch repair (MMR) genes (see below).

Gardner syndrome patients have FAP findings and lesions outside of the gastrointestinal tract including:

- Desmoid tumor, biliary dysplasia/adenocarcinoma, hepatoblastoma, osteoma of the long bones, skull and mandible, impacted or supernumerary teeth, congenital hypertrophy of retinal pigment epithelium (CHRPE), epidermoid cyst, papillary thyroid carcinoma, nasopharyngeal angiofibroma, and endocrine neoplasia (i.e., pancreas, adrenal, and pituitary glands).

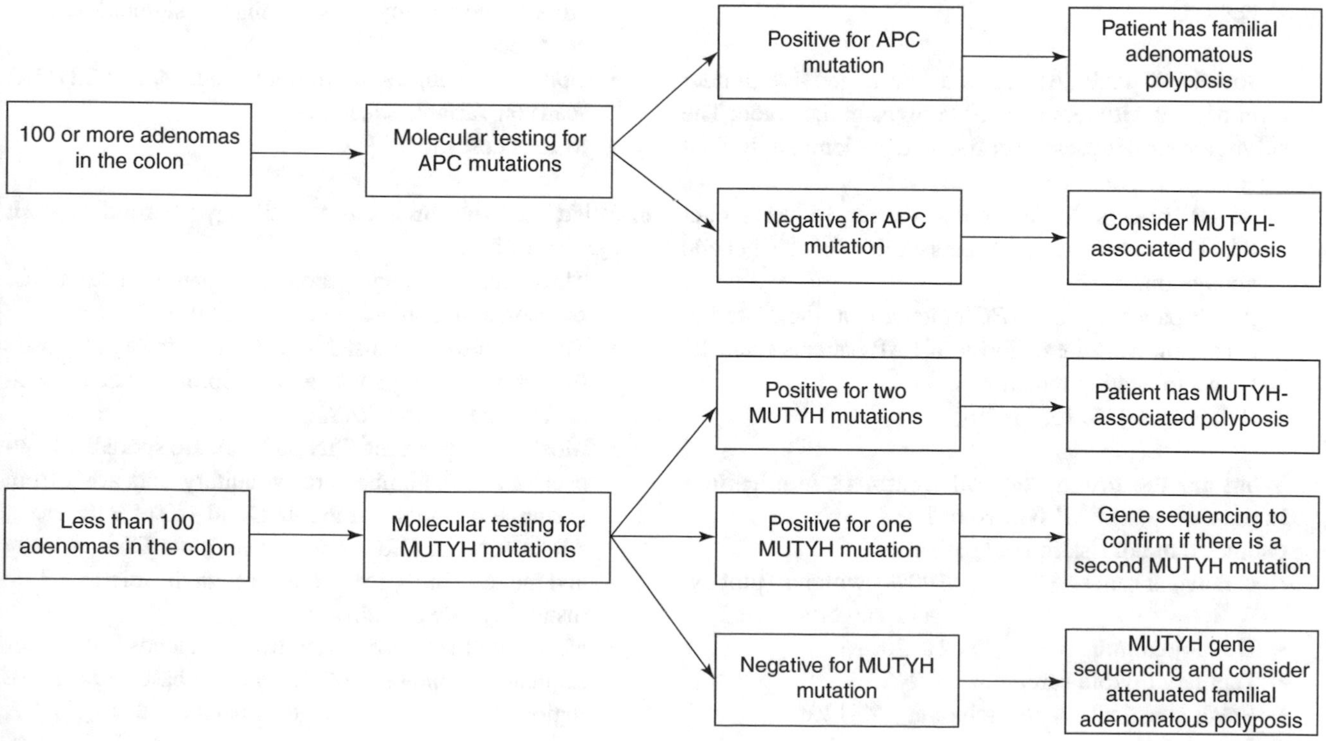

Fig. 15.2 Diagnostic algorithm for syndromic epithelial adenomatous polyposis

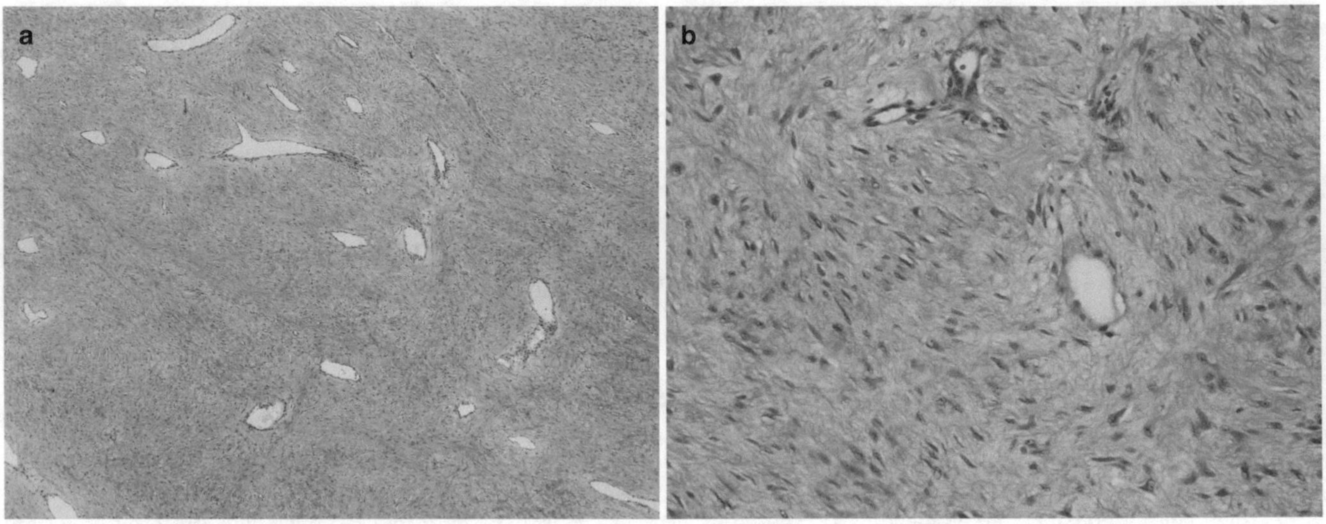

Fig. 15.3 Histology of fibromatosis (desmoid tumor) in an FAP patient showing spindle cell proliferation with prominent vasculature at low-power view (**a**). A higher-power view (**b**) shows no significant nuclear atypia. No mitotic figures are seen in this field

- Desmoid tumors are fibroblastic/myofibroblastic tumors in the abdomen or limbs, composed of spindled cells of uniform morphology arranged in long fascicles and a variable collagenous background with scattered blood vessels (Fig. 15.3a, b). There is usually minimal, if any, nuclear atypia, and mitotic figures are rare. These tumors typically show an infiltrative growth pattern with poorly defined borders.

Attenuated FAP (AFAP) is a less aggressive, milder form of FAP with less than 100 polyps in the colon. The polyps are smaller, sessile or flat, and predominantly right sided.

- AFAP patients develop colon cancer 15 years later than FAP patients and 10 years earlier than the general population.
- AFAP patients show *APC* mutations at the 5′ and 3′ ends; however, the majority of FAP patients typically have a truncating mutation in 5q.

References: [15, 16, 21–29]

5. What are the prognostic and treatment implications in patients with FAP syndrome?

Estimated tumor risk in FAP patients:

- Colorectal cancer 100% without prophylactic surgery
- Desmoid tumor 10–20%
- Papillary thyroid carcinoma 2–25%
- Small intestinal adenocarcinoma 4–12%
- Pancreatic adenocarcinoma 2%
- Hepatoblastoma 1.5%
- Brain tumors <1%
- Gastric adenocarcinoma 0.5%

Screening and treatment options:

- FAP – sigmoidoscopy or colonoscopy every 1–2 years, starting at age 10–11.
- AFAP – sigmoidoscopy or colonoscopy every 1–2 years, beginning at age 18–20.
- Once polyps are discovered, annual colonoscopies until prophylactic colectomy.
- After colectomy, screening sigmoidoscopies commence.
- Upper endoscopies, thyroid ultrasounds, and CT/MRI scans on variable schedules.

References: [30–32]

6. What is the molecular etiology behind Lynch syndrome?

There are two major molecular pathways to CRC: chromosomal and microsatellite instability.

- The chromosomal instability (CIN) pathway is caused by loss of heterozygosity and aneuploidy in genes such as *APC*, *p53*, and *KRAS*.
- Most CRCs from the CIN pathway are sporadic; however, a small number are hereditary and arise from germline mutations of the *APC* and *MUTYH* genes.
- About 85% of CRCs arise through the CIN pathway and the remaining 15% arise through the microsatellite instability (MSI) pathway.
- Microsatellites are repetitive stretches of DNA sequences, composed of one or more base pairs. These regions are susceptible to mistakes during DNA replication.
- The protein products of MMR genes fix mistakes in the microsatellites; otherwise, the length of the micro-

satellite sequence is changed by an insertion or deletion causing MSI and frameshift mutations.
- MSI in genes responsible for cell growth causes neoplasia.
- The MMR genes and their protein products include MLH1, PMS2, MSH2, MSH6, and MSH3. For single base pair errors, MSH2 binds to the mismatched DNA sequence as a heterodimer with MSH6. For longer base pair errors of 2–8 nucleotides, MSH2 binds with MSH3. Then, the MLH1 and PMS2 heterodimer binds and completes the excision of mismatched base pairs.

MMR gene mutations and subsequent MSI can be germline or sporadic.
- Lynch syndrome is an autosomal dominant disorder characterized by a germline mutation in one of the MMR genes.
- About 90% of germline mutations affect *MLH1* or *MSH2*. Since there is another functioning allele, mismatch repair function is retained until a somatic mutation hits the second allele.
- Mutations of adjacent genes that affect or extend into an MMR gene can also lead to Lynch syndrome. One of the examples is an *EPCAM* mutation affecting *MSH2*.
- Lynch syndrome patients are younger (approximately 45 years of age) than the general population when diagnosed with CRC and roughly 80% will develop CRC in their lifetimes.
- MSI also places Lynch syndrome patients at risk for cancers of the endometrium, pancreas, biliary tract, stomach, small intestine, ovaries, renal pelvis, and brain.

Sporadic MMR deficiency leading to MSI occurs through hypermethylation of cytosine-guanosine dinucleotides, also called CpG islands.
- Hypermethylation of CpG islands silences promoter regions causing downregulation of genes, this leads to biallelic transcriptional silencing of the *MLH1* gene.
- About half of sporadic MSI CRCs also have a *BRAF* mutation. Their histologic precursor is the sessile serrated adenoma/polyp (now the preferred term by *WHO Classification of Digestive System Tumours*, 5th edition, is "sessile serrated lesion" – see Chap. 14, Questions 21, 22 and 23).

References: [33–44]

7. What are the clinical and histologic features of Lynch syndrome-associated polyps?

Lynch syndrome patients show similar rates of colonic adenomas as the general population and they are histologically indistinguishable from their sporadic, conventional counterparts.
- Grossly, they are more likely to be flat or sessile lesions.
- Adenomas occur in younger patients and transform to adenocarcinoma at a faster rate.
- One study showed that 88% of adenomas in Lynch syndrome show loss of nuclear expression in one of the MMR proteins (Fig. 15.4a, b). However, using MMR immunohistochemistry as a screening method

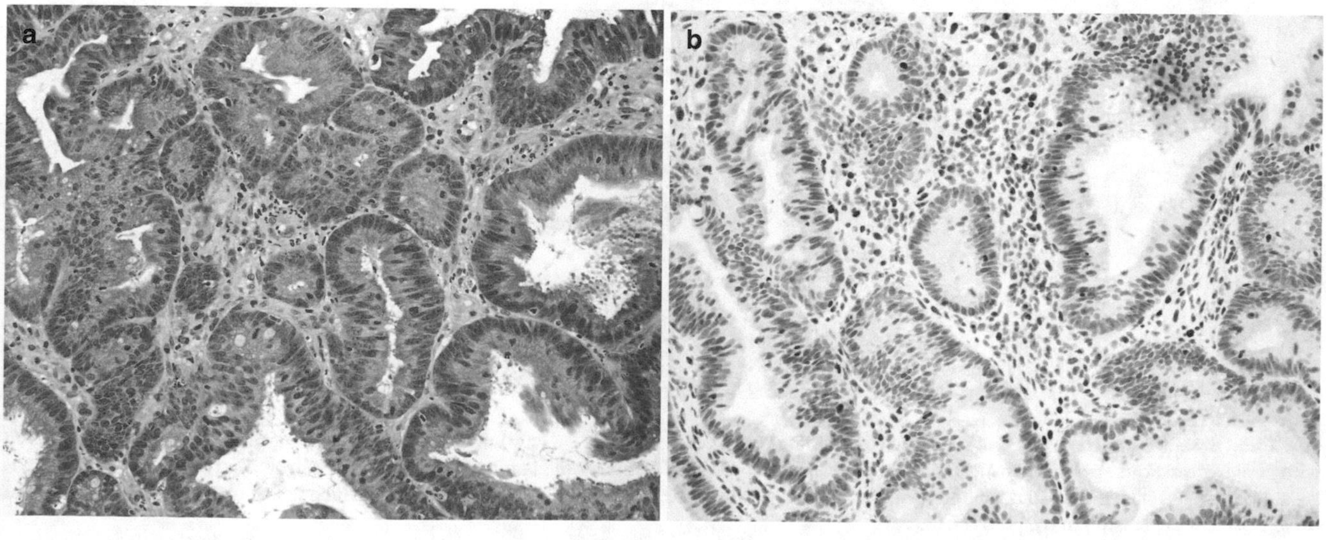

Fig. 15.4 An ordinary tubular adenoma of the colon (**a**) endoscopically removed from a patient with Lynch syndrome shows loss of nuclear expression of MSH6 protein by immunohistochemistry (**b**). The lamina propria stromal and inflammatory cells demonstrate positive staining, which serve as internal controls. The other three MMR proteins (MLH1, MSH2, and PMS2) show intact nuclear expression in adenomatous cells

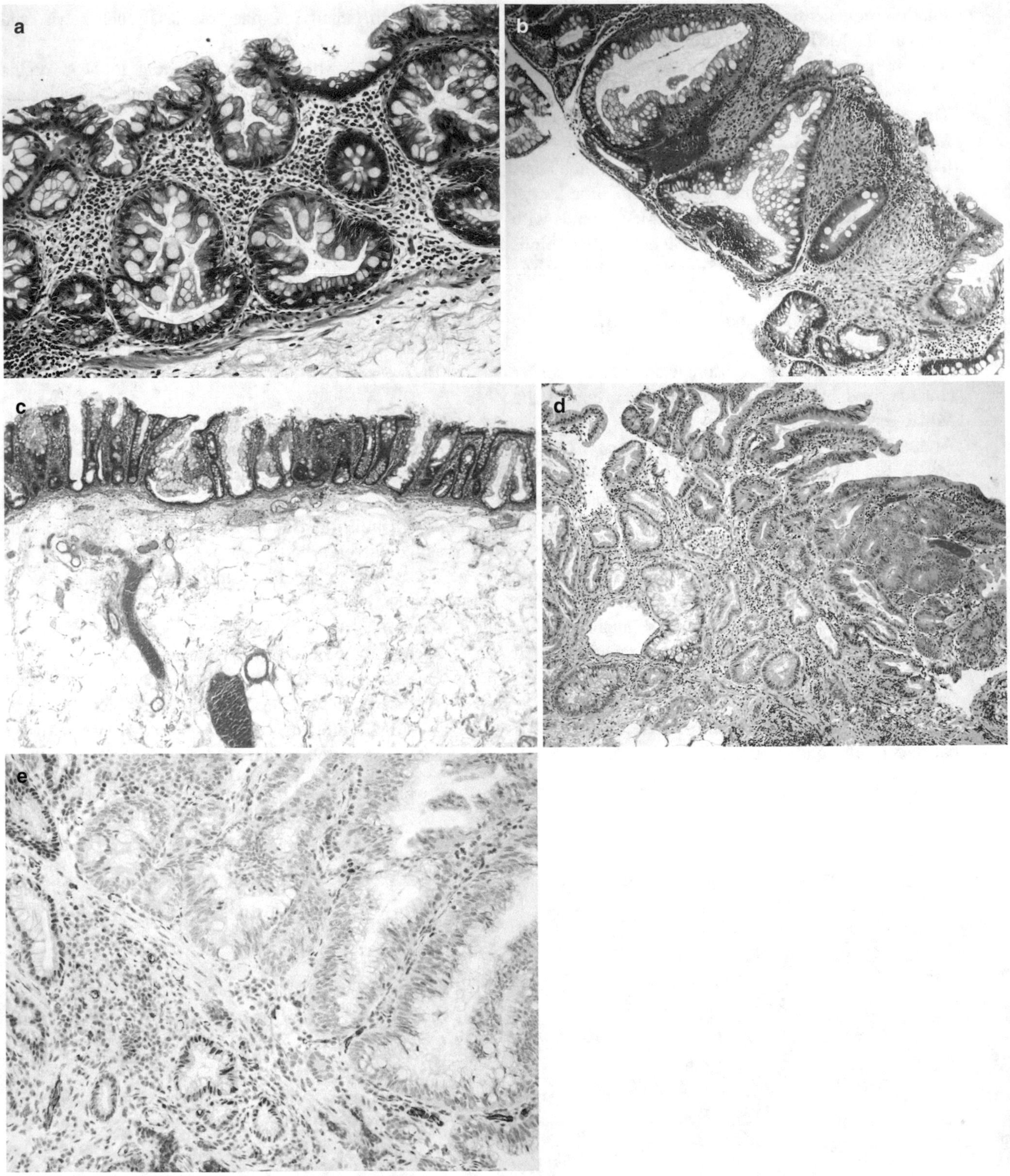

Fig. 15.5 Sessile serrated lesion (sessile serrated adenoma/polyp) characterized by basal dilatation of serrated crypts (**a**). It may be associated with perineuriomatous stroma characterized by a bland spindle cell proliferation in the lamina propria between serrated crypts (**b**), or with submucosal lipomatous change (**c**). Conventional cytologic dysplasia can be seen in sessile serrated lesions (**d**), which is usually associated with loss of MLH1 nuclear expression in dysplastic cells (**e**)

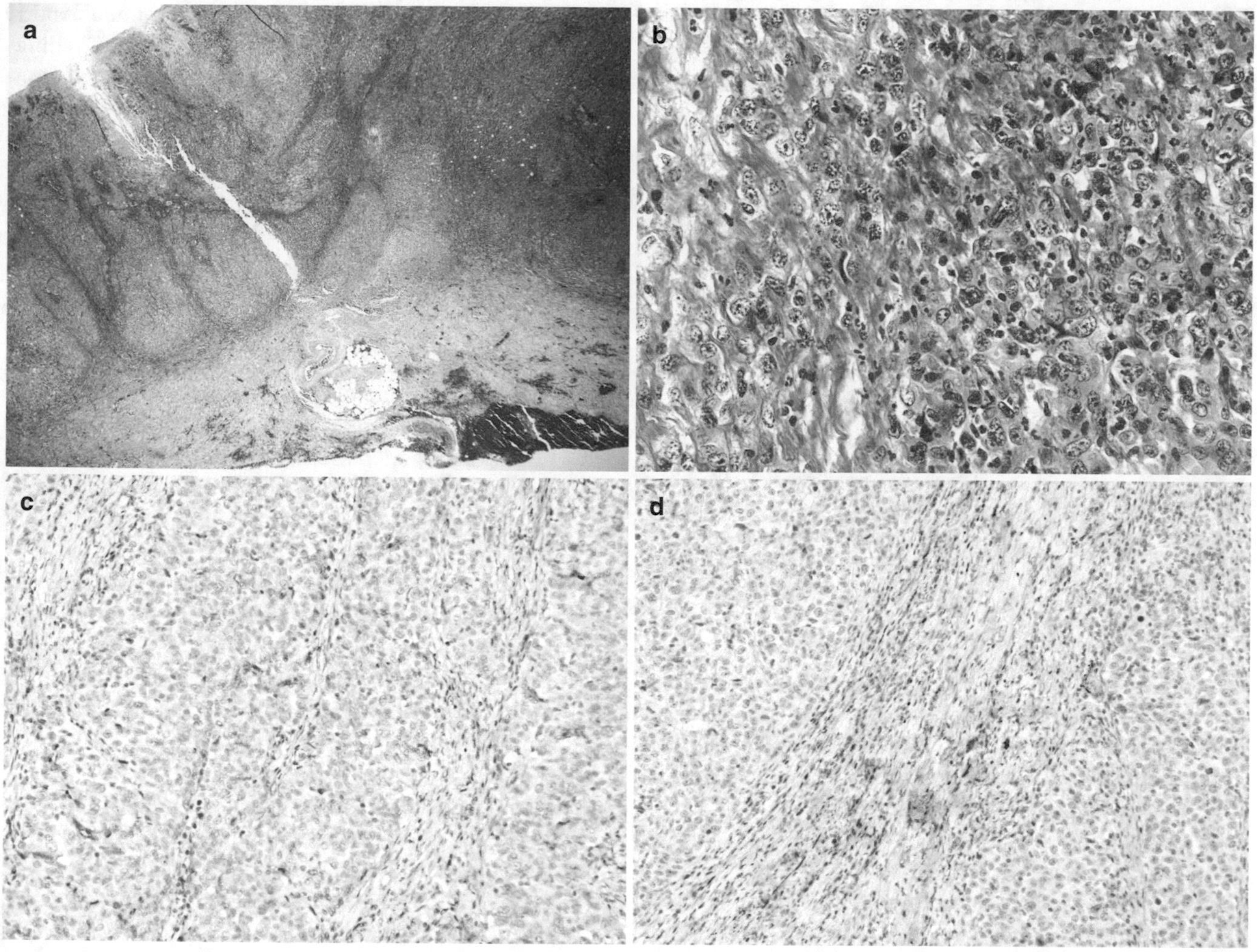

Fig. 15.6 A medullary carcinoma of the colon showing sheets of tumor cells with a pushing border (**a**), no glandular formation, and numerous intratumoral lymphocytes (**b**). Tumor cells show loss of nuclear expression of MLH1 (**c**) and PMS2 (**d**) proteins by immunohistochemistry

for Lynch syndrome in young patients (<40 years old) with adenomas is not recommended.

Patients along the sporadic MSI pathway have sessile serrated adenomas/polyps (or sessile serrated lesions), mostly in the right colon.

- Microscopically, there are serrations throughout the length of the crypt with dilation at the base or with lateral extension along the muscularis mucosae (resembling an L-shaped boot or an inverted T) (Fig. 15.5a). There may be associated perineuriomatous stromal cell proliferation (mucosal perineurioma; Fig. 15.5b) or submucosal lipomatous change (submucosal lipoma; Fig. 15.5c).
- The architectural abnormality of sessile serrated lesions can be accompanied by traditional features of cytologic dysplasia (i.e., hyperchromatic, elongated, pencillate, and stratified nuclei) (Fig. 15.5d), which is usually associated with loss of MLH1 nuclear expression (Fig. 15.5e). This is considered to be a critical step toward CRC development. Histologically, cytologic dysplasia can be low grade or high grade, but this stratification is not critical and appears unnecessary.
- MSI CRCs demonstrate unique histologic features regardless of whether it is sporadic or syndromic, which include right colon predilection, Crohn-like peritumoral lymphoid response, tumor-infiltrating lymphocytes, mucinous, signet ring cell, poorly differentiated or medullary morphologies (Fig. 15.6a–d).

References: [42, 45–49]

8. **How do you differentiate colorectal cancers of sporadic mismatch repair deficiency from hereditary Lynch syndrome based on immunohistochemical and molecular studies?**

Immunohistochemistry for the MMR proteins (MLH1, PMS2, MSH2, and MSH6) show distinct patterns for sporadic and germline MSI CRCs (Table 15.1).

Table 15.1 Common MMR immunohistochemical patterns and their interpretation

MLH1	PMS2	MSH2	MSH6	Interpretation
+	+	+	+	Sporadic CRC
–	–	+	+	Sporadic (*MLH1* promoter hypermethylation) or Lynch syndrome (germline *MLH1* mutation)
+	–	+	+	Lynch syndrome (germline *PMS2* mutation)
+	+	–	–	Lynch syndrome (germline *MSH2* mutation)
+	+	+	–	Lynch syndrome (germline *MSH6* mutation or sporadic CRC with treatment effect)
–	+	+	+	Lynch syndrome (germline *MLH1* mutation)
+	+	–	+	Lynch syndrome (germline *MSH2* mutation)
–	–	–	–	Null pattern (usually germline *MSH2* mutation with concurrent *MLH1* promoter hypermethylation)

CRC colorectal carcinoma

- Both germline mutation of the *MLH1* gene and hypermethylation silencing of the *MLH1* promoter lead to loss of expression of MLH1 protein in tumor cell nuclei. Since MLH1 pairs with PMS2 as a heterodimer, nuclear immunoreactivity for PMS2 is also lost.
- A germline mutation in *MSH2* will show loss of nuclear staining for both MSH2 and MSH6.
- However, germline mutations of either *PMS2* or *MSH6* will only show loss of nuclear staining in that mutated protein without affecting the expression of its heterodimer partner.
- Lymphocytes and normal crypt epithelial nuclei serve as an internal positive control for each MMR immunomarker.

Therefore, loss of nuclear expression of MSH6 alone, PMS2 alone, or MSH2 paired with MSH6 indicates Lynch syndrome. However, paired negative MLH1 and PMS2 immunostains do not determine whether the patient has sporadic or hereditary MSI-CRC. In that case, additional testing will be necessary.

- Positive *BRAF* mutation and/or MLH1 promoter hypermethylation indicate that the CRC is sporadic. On the other hand, lack of *BRAF* mutation and/or MLH1 promoter hypermethylation indicate Lynch syndrome.
- There are varying screening algorithms and final confirmation may also require direct sequencing of the MMR genes for germline mutations.

Alternatively, MSI can be tested by polymerase chain reaction (PCR). There are multiple microsatellite regions in the genome.

- BAT25 and BAT26 are areas with mononucleotide repeats; D5S346, D17S250, and S2S123 have dinucleotide repeats. These five loci are tested and comprise a reference standard called the Bethesda panel. There are additional, less common loci that can also be examined.
- The test requires DNA extraction from both normal and neoplastic tissues. Either fresh or formalin-fixed paraffin-embedded tissue can be used. PCR amplifies and compares the length of the microsatellite regions in both normal and neoplastic tissues.
- Any change in microsatellite length (shorter or longer) means that the tumor is microsatellite-unstable. The results are reported as MSI-high if two or more of the five loci are found to be unstable, MSI-low if only one locus is unstable, and microsatellite stable (MSS) if zero loci are unstable.
- Molecular testing with an MSI-high result does not distinguish whether an MSI-CRC is sporadic or Lynch syndrome.
- In practice, MMR immunohistochemistry is preferred over MSI PCR, which also has the advantage to evaluate which specific gene is mutated.

Most Lynch syndrome patients have a germline mutation in *MLH1* or *MSH2*. There are rare cases where MMR immunohistochemistry shows a loss of expression and MSI PCR demonstrates MSI-high, but DNA sequencing cannot identify a germline mutation. This Lynch-like syndrome appears to be caused by biallelic somatic inactivation in one of the MMR genes. Somatic genetic testing may be considered for those cases.
References: [33, 40, 42, 50–59]

9. **What are the prognostic and treatment implications of Lynch syndrome?**
   - Lynch syndrome tumors progress through the adenoma-carcinoma sequence at a faster rate (within 2–3 years instead of >10 years in the general population) and should have screening colonoscopies on a more frequent basis.
   - These CRCs are predominantly right sided, affecting younger patients with an increased risk of synchronous and metachronous malignancies.
   - They are at a higher risk for a second CRC and extracolonic malignancies as described above. The risk for endometrial carcinoma is 50–60%.
   - Some studies show better CRC survival rates in Lynch syndrome compared to sporadic CIN-related CRC in the general population. However, this may be due to earlier detection and treatment.

- Since Lynch syndrome patients have a genetic predisposition for CRC with an autosomal dominant pattern of inheritance, genetic counseling for family members is necessary.
  References: [60–65]

10. When should you raise a suspicion for Peutz–Jeghers syndrome?

Peutz–Jeghers polyps (PJP) can be sporadic or part of Peutz–Jeghers syndrome (PJS).

- PJS should be suspected in the following scenarios:
  - At least three PJPs confirmed by histology.
  - At least one PJP and characteristic mucocutaneous pigmented lesions (brown or dark-blue macules of the lips, buccal mucosa, hands, feet, nose, etc.).
  - There is a PJP or pigmented mucocutaneous lesions in a patient with a family history of PJS.
- Patients present in the first three decades of life with pigmented mucocutaneous lesions, PJPs of the stomach, small intestine, and colon. Approximately, 95% of PJS patients have polyps in the small intestine, and about 25% have polyps in the colon and stomach.
- PJS patients are susceptible to intestinal intussusception, polyp prolapse, bleeding, and an increased risk of gastrointestinal and extra-gastrointestinal tumors (see Question 13).
- PJS is caused by mutations in the serine threonine kinase (*STK11*) gene, a tumor suppressor that regulates cellular proliferation, polarization, and apoptosis.
  - PJS is diagnosed by PCR and sequencing of the *STK11* coding regions or probe amplification to detect *STK11* deletions or duplications.
  References: [66–73]

11. Which histologic features distinguish a Peutz-Jeghers polyp from a juvenile polyp?

PJPs have a lobulated and villous architecture with an arborizing pattern of smooth muscle, and cystically dilated or hyperplastic crypts/pits (Fig. 15.7a–c).

- The smooth muscle bundles that traverse between the crypts/pits separate them into discrete lobules.
- Dysplasia and carcinoma can be seen in the context of PJS but it is not common.
- Rectal prolapse also demonstrates smooth muscle strands within the lamina propria, which may be mistaken for a PJP. In rectal prolapse, the smooth muscle strands are seen diffusely throughout the lamina propria and surround most of the crypts instead of the distinct arborizing bundles of smooth muscle imparting the lobulated appearance of PJP.
- The lobulated architecture may not be evident in gastric PJPs, which may resemble conventional gastric hyperplastic polyps. In the absence of intestinal PJPs and the appropriate clinical context, one should be cautious to suggest a diagnosis of PJS based on gastric polyps alone.
- Epithelial misplacement (pseudoinvasion) is relatively common in PJPs, which should not be confused with invasive carcinoma.

- Juvenile polyps have cystically dilated, irregular, branching, and tortuous crypts filled with mucin or neutrophil clusters (Fig. 15.8a).

- The lamina propria is edematous with a mixture of lymphocytes, eosinophils, and neutrophils.
- The surface of the polyp is often eroded with granulation tissue and reactive changes.
- Larger polyps can twist or outgrow their blood supply leading to vascular congestion, dilated blood vessels, and hemosiderin laden macrophages in the lamina propria.
  References: [66–68, 70, 73–78]

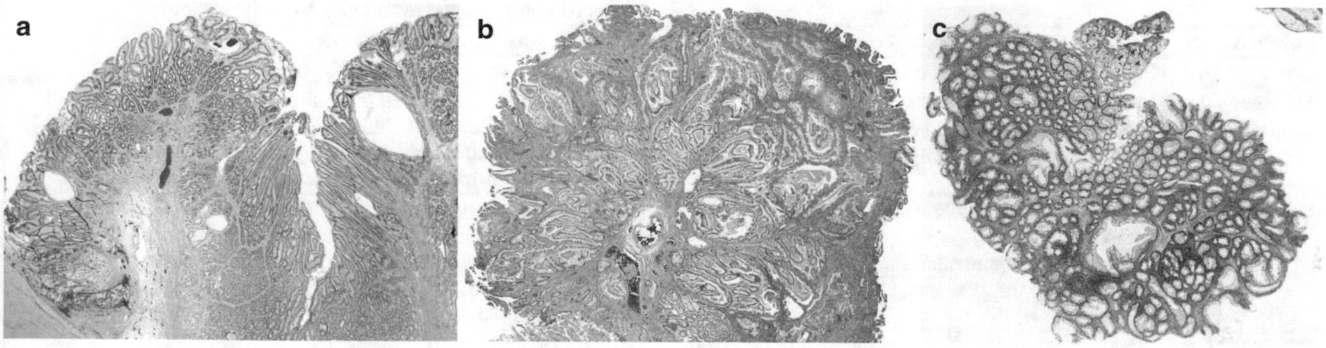

Fig. 15.7 Peutz–Jeghers polyps seen in the stomach (**a**), jejunum (**b**), and colon (**c**)

12. Which clinical features distinguish Peutz–Jeghers polyps from juvenile polyps?

See Table 15.2 for a comparison between PJP and juvenile polyp.

References: [66–70, 73–80]

13. What are the prognostic implications in Peutz–Jeghers syndrome patients?

PJS patients are at increased risk for gastrointestinal and non-gastrointestinal malignancies.

- Increased risk of colorectal, small intestinal, gastric, pancreatic, breast, esophageal, lung, uterine, and ovarian cancers.
- At risk for large cell calcifying Sertoli tumor of the testis, sex cord tumor with annular tubules of the ovary, and cervical adenoma malignum.
- Cumulative risk of each carcinoma varies by organ system.
- Endoscopy and colonoscopy every 2–3 years starting at age 18.
- Mammography every year starting at age 18.
- Pancreatic ultrasound every other year is debatable.

References: [68, 71–73, 81–83]

14. When do you need to raise a suspicion for juvenile polyposis?

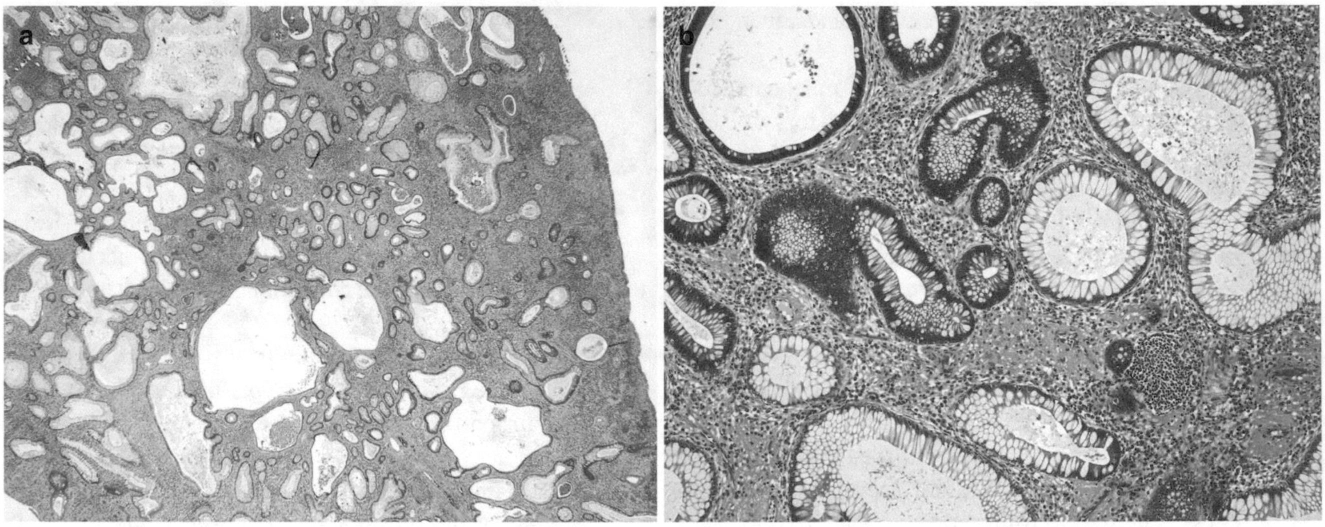

Fig. 15.8 Juvenile polyp of the colon showing cystically dilated crypts and an eroded surface (**a**). Low-grade dysplasia is seen in this juvenile polyp (**b**)

Table 15.2 Peutz–Jeghers polyp versus Juvenile polyp

	Peutz–Jeghers polyp	Juvenile polyp
Genetics	Mutations in *STK11* gene in >90% of patients Autosomal dominant	JPC: *BMPR1A*, *SMAD4*, and *ENG* gene mutations GJP: *SMAD4* and *BMPR1A* mutations JPI: Germline deletion of 10q23 involving *BMPR1A* and *PTEN* Autosomal dominant
Incidence	Variable, ranging from 1 in 25,000 to 200,000 births, usually presenting in the second or third decade of life	Variable, sporadic juvenile polyps seen in 2% of children and are common in the first decade of life but can also be seen in adults Juvenile polyposis is rare and variable in incidence
Location	Stomach, small intestine, and colon	Stomach, small intestine, and colon
Gross	Pedunculated or sessile polyp	Round with a smooth, erythematous, eroded cap on the surface
Microscopic features	Lobulated architecture, arborizing pattern of smooth muscle, cystically dilated or hyperplastic crypts/pits with increased lamina propria inflammatory cells	Cystically dilated, irregular, branching, and tortuous crypts filled with mucin or neutrophil clusters Edematous and inflamed lamina propria with a mixture of lymphocytes, eosinophils, and neutrophils
Behavior	Dysplasia can occur in PJPs but is extremely uncommon Some polyps acquire additional mutations in β-catenin and TP53 and progress along the adenoma-carcinoma sequence	Some may show atypical features: villiform, multilobulated, complex branching architecture, epithelial component greater than stroma, and mild cytologic atypia Dysplasia (Fig. 15.8b) is more commonly seen than that in PJPs, particularly in those with atypical features as described above
Complications	Intussusception, bleeding, and increased risk for GI and extra-GI tumors, mucocutaneous pigmented lesions	Rectal bleeding, polyp prolapse, increased risk for GI malignancies, particularly CRC

JPC juvenile polyposis coli, *GJP* generalized juvenile polyposis, *JPI* juvenile polyposis of infancy, *GI* gastrointestinal

Juvenile polyps can be sporadic or part of a syndromic inherited polyposis: juvenile polyposis coli (JPC), generalized juvenile polyposis (GJP), and juvenile polyposis of infancy (JPI).

- JPC patients have three or more juvenile polyps without a family history or any number of juvenile polyps with a family history. They have an increased risk of CRC.
- GJP patients have numerous juvenile polyps (ranging from 50 to 200) throughout the length of the stomach, small intestine, colon, and rectum. They have an increased of risk of upper and lower gastrointestinal tract cancers.
- JPI occurs in the pediatric population within the first 2 years of age with juvenile polyps throughout the length of the stomach, small intestine, colon, and rectum.
  - Protein-losing enteropathy, diarrhea, and rectal prolapse often lead to death before the age of 2.
- Suspicion for juvenile polyposis should be raised in patients who meet the criteria for these categories.
- Patients with less than three juvenile polyps and a negative family history are considered to be sporadic with no concern of malignancy.

References: [78, 84–88]

15. How do you differentiate Cowden/PTEN hamartoma syndrome from Cronkhite–Canada syndrome?

See Table 15.3 for a comparison of Cowden versus Cronkhite–Canada syndromes.

References: [73, 89–98]

16. What are the major and minor diagnostic criteria for Cowden/PTEN hamartoma syndrome?

Diagnosis requires either two major criteria, one major and two minor criteria, three minor criteria or a germline PTEN mutation (Figs. 15.9 and 15.10).

Major diagnostic criteria for PTEN hamartoma syndrome:

- Breast cancer, non-medullary thyroid cancer, endometrial cancer, macrocephaly, three or more gastrointestinal hamartomas, mucocutaneous lesions (acral keratosis, oral papillomas, trichilemmomas, papillomas, pigmented freckles on the glans penis).

Minor diagnostic criteria for PTEN hamartoma syndrome:

- Colon cancer, renal cancer, glycogenic acanthosis of the esophagus, three or more lipomas, autism, intellectual disability, testicular lipomatosis, vascular anomalies (arteriovenous malformations or hemangiomas).

References: [99–101]

17. What is MUTYH-associated polyposis and how do you differentiate it from FAP?

- The *MUTYH* gene transcribes a DNA repair enzyme, MYH glycosylase, which fixes mismatched base pairs by excision. Mutations in the *MUTYH* gene lead to clinical features resembling FAP. MUTYH-associated polyposis (MAP) has an autosomal recessive pattern of inheritance.

Table 15.3 Cowden syndrome versus Cronkhite–Canada syndrome

	Cowden syndrome	Cronkhite–Canada syndrome
Genetics	Autosomal dominant, germline mutation of the *PTEN* gene (chromosome 10q23) (Fig. 15.9a)	Unknown, not hereditary
Incidence	Estimated 1 in 200,000–250,000 populations Most patients show symptoms before the second decade	Very rare, approximately 500 cases to date Usually seen in the fifth decade of life
Location/ Features	Stomach, small intestine and colon – hamartomatous polyps Esophagus – diffuse glycogenic acanthosis (Fig. 15.9b) Breast – fibroadenoma, carcinoma, fibrocystic change Thyroid – goiter, follicular adenoma, carcinoma Mucocutaneous lesions – facial trichilemmomas, oral papilloma, acral keratosis Others – macrocephaly, gangliocytoma of the cerebellum, genitourinary defects, renal cell carcinoma, endometrial carcinoma	Ectodermal disorders – alopecia, hyperpigmented macules on the torso, face, palms and soles, cataracts, nail dystrophy Stomach, small intestine and colon – hamartomatous polyps (Fig. 15.10a, b)
Microscopic features	Variable in the gastrointestinal tract – hamartomatous or juvenile polyps, adenomas, ganglioneuromas (Fig. 15.9c), colonic intramucosal lipomas, diffuse esophageal glycogenic acanthosis, fibromas	Colonic polyps resemble juvenile polyps with cystically dilated crypts, inflamed and edematous lamina propria, with or without dysplasia Non-polypoid, intervening mucosa also shows cystic dilatation of the crypts with lamina propria inflammation and edema
Behavior	Colorectal adenocarcinoma seen in approximately 9% of Cowden syndrome patients with *PTEN* mutations	Cases of dysplasia and carcinoma are reported but unclear if sporadic or syndromic High mortality rate (50–60%) due to diarrhea, malnutrition, gastrointestinal bleeding, and infection

- There usually are between 15 and 100 adenomas in the colon and rectum, serrated polyps may also be seen (Fig. 15.11a, b).
- Patients are at increased risk for CRC.
- Approximately 10–20% of patients with the clinical impression of FAP, and lacking a germline *APC* mutation, harbor a *MUTYH* mutation.
- Diagnosed by genetic testing and/or sequencing for the most common mutations in the *MUTYH* gene.

References: [9, 18, 24, 102]

18. What is serrated polyposis syndrome?

Serrated polyposis syndrom (SPS) is a relatively new, poorly characterized disease entity with ongoing research.

Diagnostic criteria for SPS:

- Five or more serrated polyps/lesions proximal to the rectum, all being ≥0.5 cm in size, with two or more being ≥1.0 cm.
- More than 20 serrated polyps/lesions of any size throughout the large intestine, with five or more being proximal to the rectum.
- Serrated polyps/lesions can be either sessile serrated lesions (sessile serrated adenomas/polyps) with or without cytologic dysplasia, hyperplastic polyps, or traditional serrated adenomas.
- The polyp count is cumulative over multiple colonoscopies.

The molecular profile of SPS is unclear and may be variable. Different pathways have been hypothesized:

- *BRAF* or *KRAS* mutations.
- *APC* mutations and chromosomal instability.
- Microsatellite instability (MSI-H) and loss of function in mismatch repair proteins.
- Inactivation of MGMT causing MSI-L and loss of heterozygosity in tumor suppressor genes.
- Germline mutation of *RNF43*, a Wnt pathway inhibitor, was proposed as a rare cause.

The frequency and incidence are unclear because of evolving and changing diagnostic criteria.

- It may represent multiple disorders on a clinical spectrum with overlapping characteristics.

SPS is believed to be associated with an increased risk for CRC. However, the phenotypic expression of SPS may vary:

- Goblet cell-rich or microvesicular hyperplastic polyps have a minimal risk for progression to CRC.

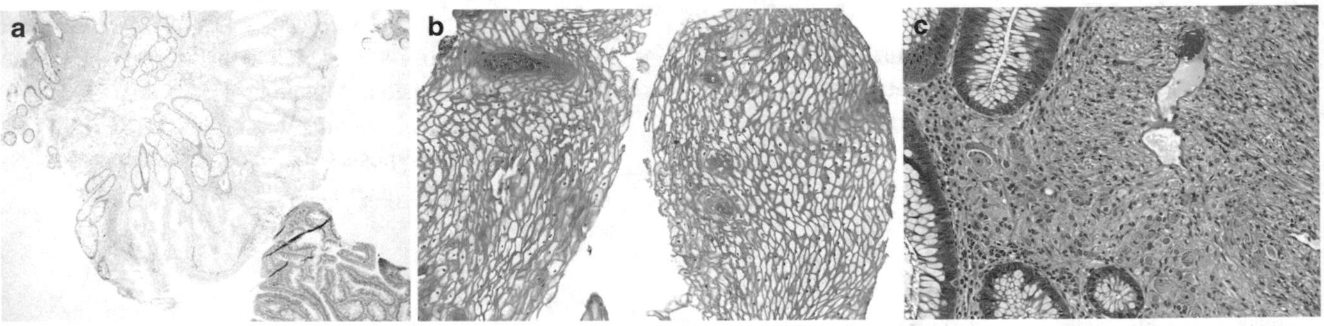

Fig. 15.9 Immunohistochemistry showing loss of PTEN protein expression in a hamartomatous polyp of the colon (**a**). The immunoreactivity is retained in the adjacent normal colonic mucosa. Glycogenic acanthosis of the esophagus featuring cytoplasmic clearing in squamous epithelium (**b**). A ganglioneuroma of the colon showing spindle cell proliferation with a variable number of ganglion cells in the mucosa (**c**)

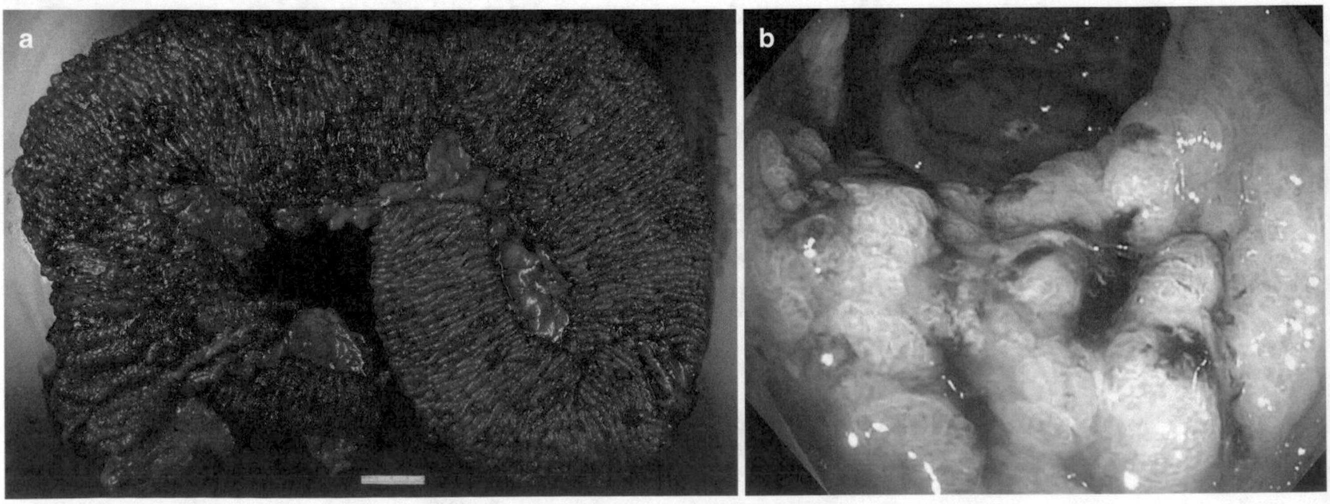

Fig. 15.10 Gross (**a**) and endoscopic (**b**) photos for a case of Cronkhite–Canada syndrome

- Multiple sessile serrated adenomas/polyps with or without cytologic dysplasia or traditional serrated adenomas have a higher risk for CRC.
  References: [103–109]

19. What is gastric adenocarcinoma and proximal polyposis of the stomach (GAPPS)?

GAPPS is characterized by >100 gastric polyps carpeting the mucosal surface of the stomach (Fig. 15.12a).

- Most polyps are small, usually <1.0 cm.
- It spares the antrum and relatively spares the lesser curvature, but diffusely involves the body and fundus.
- Small intestine and colon are uninvolved.
- Microscopically, it shows various types of lesions including fundic gland polyps (Fig. 15.12b), hyperplastic polyps, adenomas (Fig. 15.12c) and adenocarcinomas. Focal dysplasia may be seen in fundic gland polyps.
- Some of the polypoid lesions in GAPPS may not be typical histologically. These have been described as "fundic gland-like polyps" and "hyperproliferative aberrant pits." The former resembles a fundic gland polyp but lacks the typical cystically dilated glands. The latter shows disorganized proliferation of oxyntic glands in the superficial portion of the mucosa around the gastric pits and shows an increased proliferation index on Ki67 immunostaining.
- It is a rare disease with a wide age range from 10 to 75 years. The youngest patient with gastric adenocarcinoma was 33 years old.
  Autosomal dominant pattern of inheritance.
- GAPPS patients harbor a point mutation in the Ying Yang 1 binding motif of the promoter 1B region in the *APC* gene.
- Even though the *APC* gene is involved, there is no association with other epithelial polyposis syndromes of the gastrointestinal tract.

Treatment plans for patients include surveillance endoscopies and prophylactic or therapeutic gastrectomies.

References: [110–114]

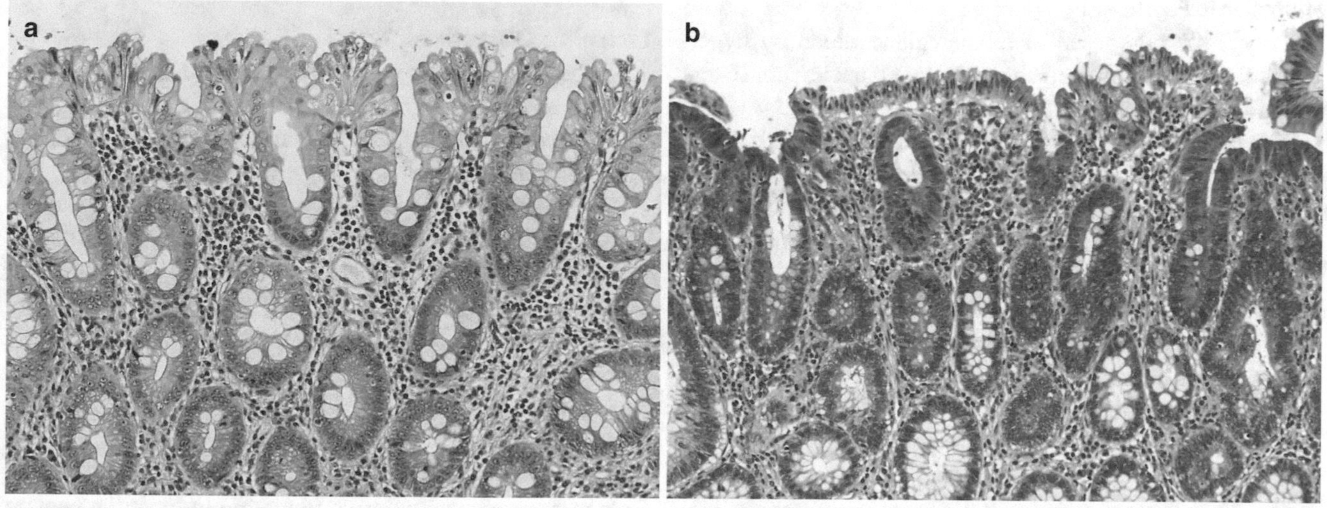

Fig. 15.11 A serrated polyp seen in a patient with MUTYH-associated polyposis (**a**). Note the unique pattern of nuclei in the superficial epithelium. Tubular adenomas are also seen in the same patient (**b**)

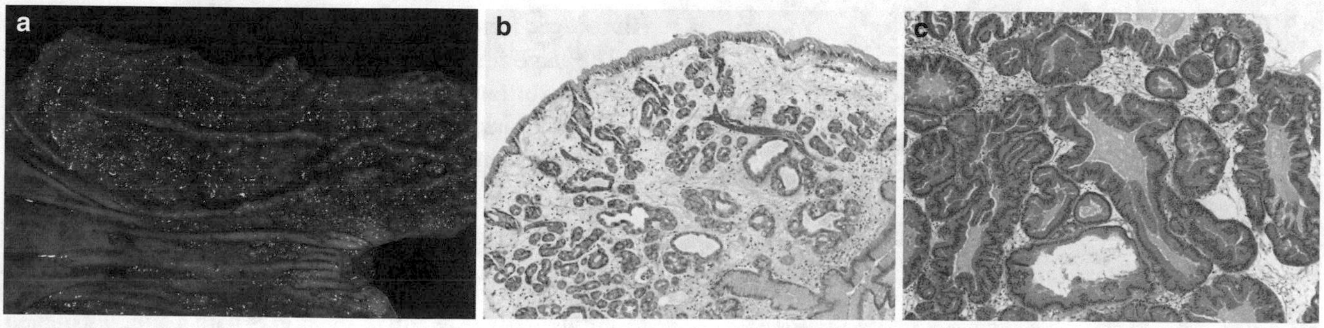

Fig. 15.12 Gross photo of the stomach from a patient with GAPPS showing numerous polyps involving the proximal portion of the stomach (**a**). Various types of polyps including fundic gland polyps (**b**) and pyloric gland adenomas (**c**) are seen in this patient

Case Presentation

Case 1

Learning Objectives

1. To become familiar with the clinical and endoscopic features of the syndrome
2. To become familiar with the microscopic features of the syndrome
3. To generate a differential diagnosis and understand the diagnostic algorithm for syndromic epithelial polyposis

Case History

A 20-year-old male presented with abdominal pain and gastrointestinal bleeding.

Gross

Colonoscopy showed numerous polyps (>100) throughout the length of the colon, but more concentrated distally. The polyps ranged in size from 2 mm to 3 cm. A few polyps (including the 3 cm polyp) were biopsied. Following endoscopic biopsies, the patient underwent total colectomy (Fig. 15.13).

Histologic Findings

- Polyps are composed of tubular glands lined by hyperchromatic, pencillate, and elongated nuclei consistent with tubular adenomas.
- The large polyp shows a complex architecture with cribriforming glands, comedonecrosis, glands and single cells invading beyond the muscularis mucosae into the submucosa representing a pT1 invasive adenocarcinoma.

Differential Diagnosis

- Familial adenomatous polyposis (FAP)
- Attenuated familial adenomatous polyposis (AFAP)
- Lynch syndrome

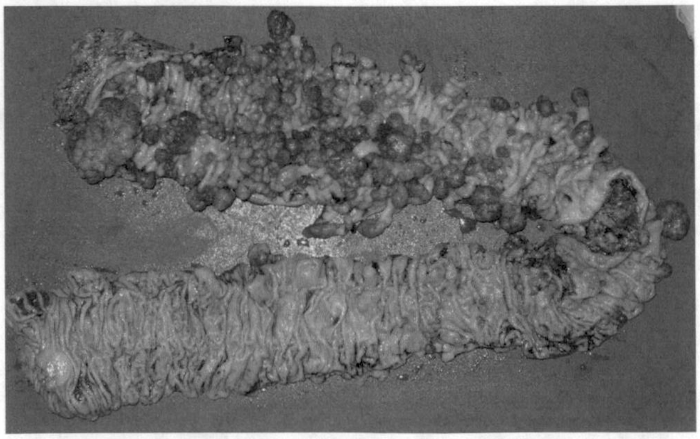

Fig. 15.13 (Case 1) Gross photo of the total colectomy specimen showing numerous polyps

IHC and Other Ancillary Studies

Molecular testing was positive for an *APC* mutation.

Final Diagnosis

Familial adenomatous polyposis (FAP).

Take Home Messages

1. FAP demonstrates more than 100 polyps composed of tubular adenomas throughout the length of the colon and rectum.
2. Within this clinical context, if molecular testing reveals an *APC* mutation, it is diagnostic of FAP.
3. If the *APC* mutation test is negative, follow the diagnostic algorithm shown in Fig. 15.2 to rule out AFAP and MUTYH-associated polyposis.
4. FAP patients with extra-intestinal manifestations such as brain tumors, desmoid tumors, etc. raise the possibility of Turcot and Gardner syndrome.

References: [1–13]

Case 2

Learning Objectives

1. To become familiar with the clinical and endoscopic features of the syndrome
2. To become familiar with the microscopic features of the syndrome
3. To generate a differential diagnosis and understand the diagnostic algorithm for syndromic epithelial polyposis

Case History

A 55-year-old female presented with abdominal pain, weight loss, and gastrointestinal bleeding.

Gross

Colonoscopy showed a large, fungating mass at the hepatic flexure. There were also two small polyps in the ascending colon.

Histologic Findings

- The large fungating mass shows a complex architecture with cribriforming glands, comedonecrosis, with neoplastic glands invading into the submucosa consistent with an invasive adenocarcinoma.
- There is a band of lymphocytic infiltrates surrounding the periphery of the tumor with a broad, advancing tumor edge.
- The small ascending colon polyps show serrations throughout the length of the crypts with a laterally dilated base. Conventional cytologic features of a tubular ade-

noma are absent. These features are consistent with sessile serrated lesions.

Differential Diagnosis

- Sporadic CRC, chromosomal instability pathway (CIN)
- Sporadic CRC, microsatellite instability pathway (MSI)
- Lynch syndrome

IHC and Other Ancillary Studies

- Immunohistochemical stains for MMR proteins demonstrated positive, retained nuclear expression of MSH2 and MSH6. There was loss of nuclear expression in MLH1 and PMS2.
- Molecular studies were positive for *BRAF* mutation.

Final Diagnosis

Sporadic colorectal cancer, microsatellite instability pathway (MSI).

Take Home Messages

1. Immunohistochemistry for MMR proteins or PCR for MSI should be performed on all newly diagnosed CRCs to rule out microsatellite unstable cancers.
2. Loss of nuclear expression for MLH1 and PMS2 by MMR IHC raises the possibility of sporadic or hereditary MSI CRC.
3. A positive *BRAF* mutation or MLH1 promoter hypermethylation confirms that the MSI CRC is sporadic.

References: [33–50]

Case 3

Learning Objectives

1. To become familiar with the clinical and endoscopic features of the syndrome
2. To become familiar with the microscopic features of the syndrome
3. To generate a differential diagnosis and understand the diagnostic algorithm for syndromic epithelial polyposis

Case History

A 19-year-old male presented with abdominal pain and gastrointestinal bleeding. Physical examination showed brown spots and patches on the skin of the hands and feet. There were also hyperpigmented lesions on the gums and buccal mucosa.

Gross

Colonoscopy showed scattered pendunculated and sessile polyps throughout the stomach, small intestine, and colon. There were 15 polyps in total and all were <2.0 cm in greatest dimension.

Histologic Findings

- The polyps showed a lobulated architecture with an arborizing pattern of smooth muscle, cystically dilated or hyperplastic crypts/pits with increased lamina propria inflammatory cells.
- Cytologic and architectural features of dysplasia are absent.

Differential Diagnosis

- Juvenile polyposis
- Peutz–Jeghers syndrome
- Cronkhite–Canada syndrome

IHC and Other Ancillary Studies

- Molecular testing revealed a mutation in the *STK11* gene.

Final Diagnosis

Peutz–Jeghers syndrome.

Take Home Messages

1. PJS patients may initially present with bowel obstruction due to intussusception.
2. PJS is characterized by pigmented mucocutaneous lesions and Peutz–Jeghers polyps in the stomach, small intestine, and/or colon.
3. Typical polyps show an arborizing pattern of smooth muscle giving the polyp a lobulated appearance. Crypts and pits are cystically dilated with an inflamed lamina propria.
4. Patients are at a high risk for gastrointestinal and extra-intestinal malignancies.

References: [66–72]

Case 4

Learning Objectives

1. To become familiar with the clinical and endoscopic features of the syndrome
2. To become familiar with the microscopic features of the syndrome
3. To generate a differential diagnosis and understand the diagnostic algorithm for syndromic epithelial polyposis

Case History

A 47-year-old female presented with abdominal pain.

Gross

Endoscopy and gastrectomy showed numerous polyps (>100) throughout the proximal stomach. The antrum was spared and appeared uninvolved. Colonoscopy was unremarkable.

Histologic Findings

- Some of the gastric polyps had dilated oxyntic glands consistent with fundic gland polyps, while others showed polypoid oxyntic mucosa with no apparently dilated glands consistent with fundic gland-like polyps (Fig. 15.14). Polypoid foveolar hyperplasia was also seen, consistent with hyperplastic polyp.
- A few larger fundic glands polyps showed hyperchromatic and elongated nuclei with an increased nuclear-to-cytoplasmic ratio, consistent with low-grade dysplasia.

Differential Diagnosis

- Gastric adenocarcinoma and proximal polyposis of the stomach (GAPPS)
- Familial adenomatous polyposis (FAP)
- Juvenile polyposis

IHC and Other Ancillary Studies

Not performed.

Final Diagnosis

Gastric adenocarcinoma and proximal polyposis of the stomach (GAPPS).

Take Home Messages

1. The proximal stomach is carpeted by fundic gland and hyperplastic polyps with or without dysplasia.
2. The gastric antrum, small bowel, and colon are spared.
3. GAPPS patients have a point mutation in the Ying Yang 1 binding motif of the promoter 1B region in the *APC* gene. This test is not routinely available currently, however.

References: [110–114]

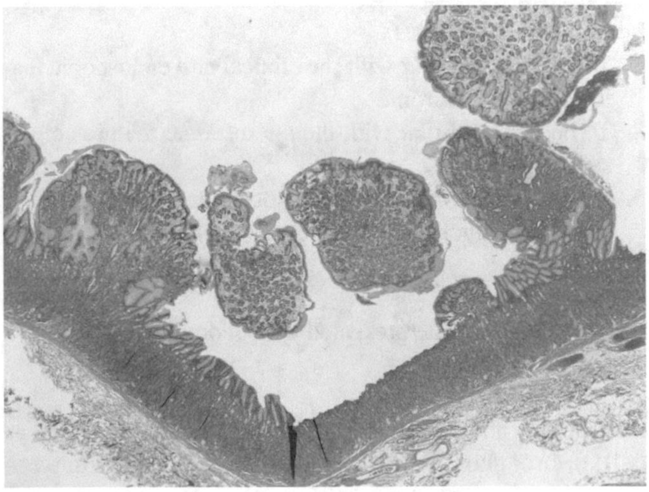

Fig. 15.14 (Case 4) Numerous fundic gland polyps and fundic gland-like polyps are seen in gastrectomy specimen

Case 5

Learning Objectives

1. To become familiar with the clinical and endoscopic features of the syndrome
2. To become familiar with the microscopic features of the syndrome
3. To generate a differential diagnosis and understand the diagnostic algorithm for syndromic epithelial polyposis

Case History

A 28-year-old male presented with abdominal pain. His past medical history was significant for multiple facial trichilemmomas. On physical examination, his head appeared large (macrocephaly).

Gross

Upper endoscopy showed multiple small, pale nodules in the esophagus. There were scattered polyps in the stomach and small intestine. Colonoscopy showed scattered polyps throughout the colon.

Histologic Findings

- The esophagus biopsy showed squamous epithelium with increased cytoplasmic vacuolization in the superficial layers, consistent with glycogenic acanthosis.
- The stomach, small bowel and colonic polyps were variable in appearance. Some had cystically dilated glands with an inflamed lamina propria resembling juvenile polyps, while others showed bland spindle cell proliferation in the lamina propria with scattered ganglion cells consistent with ganglioneuromas.
- A few tubular adenomas and an intramucosal lipoma were also seen in the colon.

Differential Diagnosis

- Peutz–Jeghers syndrome
- Cronkhite–Canada syndrome
- Cowden/PTEN hamartoma syndrome

IHC and Other Ancillary Studies

Molecular testing confirmed a germline mutation in the *PTEN* gene.

Final Diagnosis

Cowden/PTEN hamartoma syndrome.

Take Home Messages

1. Cowden syndrome is a disorder characterized by hamartomas in all three germ cell layers.
2. The findings of gastrointestinal hamartomatous polyps and extra-gastrointestinal lesions should raise the possibility of Cowden syndrome.

3. Patients should be screened for gastrointestinal and extra-gastrointestinal malignancies.

References: [73, 74, 89–92]

References

1. Ellis CN. Colonic adenomatous polyposis syndromes: clinical management. Clin Colon Rectal Surg. 2008;21(4):256–62. https://doi.org/10.1055/s-0028-1089940.
2. Lal G, Gallinger S. Familial adenomatous polyposis. Semin Surg Oncol. 18(4):314–23. https://doi.org/10.1002/(SICI)1098-2388(200006)18:4<314::AID-SSU6>3.0.CO;2-9.
3. Plawski A, Banasiewicz T, Borun P, et al. Familial adenomatous polyposis of the colon. Hered Cancer Clin Pract. 2013;11(1):15. https://doi.org/10.1186/1897-4287-11-15.
4. Bussey HJR. Familial polyposis coli: family studies, histopathology, differential diagnosis, and results of treatment. Baltimore, London: Johns Hopkins University Press; 1975.
5. Groden J, Thliveris A, Samowitz W, et al. Identification and characterization of the familial adenomatous polyposis coli gene. Cell. 1991;66(3):589–600.
6. Kinzler KW, Nilbert MC, Su LK, et al. Identification of FAP locus genes from chromosome 5q21. Science. 1991;253(5020):661–5.
7. Arvanitis ML, Jagelman DG, Fazio VW, Lavery IC, McGannon E. Mortality in patients with familial adenomatous polyposis. Dis Colon Rectum. 1990;33(8):639–42.
8. Petersen GM, Slack J, Nakamura Y. Screening guidelines and premorbid diagnosis of familial adenomatous polyposis using linkage. Gastroenterology. 1991;100(6):1658–64.
9. Yamaguchi S, Ogata H, Katsumata D, et al. MUTYH-associated colorectal cancer and adenomatous polyposis. Surg Today. 2014;44(4):593–600. https://doi.org/10.1007/s00595-013-0592-7.
10. Iwama T, Mishima Y, Okamoto N, Inoue J. Association of congenital hypertrophy of the retinal pigment epithelium with familial adenomatous polyposis. Br J Surg. 1990;77(3):273–6.
11. Matsumoto T, Iida M, Tada S, Mibu R, Yao T, Fujishima M. Early detection of nonpolypoid cancers in the rectal remnant in patients with familial adenomatous polyposis/Gardner's syndrome. Cancer. 1994;74(1):12–5.
12. Bertoni G, Sassatelli R, Nigrisoli E, et al. High prevalence of adenomas and microadenomas of the duodenal papilla and periampullary region in patients with familial adenomatous polyposis. Eur J Gastroenterol Hepatol. 1996;8(12):1201–6.
13. Iwama T, Mishima Y. Mortality in young first-degree relatives of patients with familial adenomatous polyposis. Cancer. 1994;73(8):2065–8.
14. Syngal S, Brand RE, Church JM, et al. ACG clinical guideline: genetic testing and management of hereditary gastrointestinal cancer syndromes. Am J Gastroenterol. 2015;110(2):223–62; quiz 263. https://doi.org/10.1038/ajg.2014.435.
15. Knudsen AL, Bisgaard ML, Bülow S. Attenuated familial adenomatous polyposis (AFAP): a review of the literature. Fam Cancer. 2003;2(1):43–55.
16. Hernegger GS, Moore HG, Guillem JG. Attenuated familial adenomatous polyposis: an evolving and poorly understood entity. Dis Colon Rectum. 2002;45(1):127–134–136.
17. Spier I, Aretz S. Gastrointestinal polyposis syndromes. Internist. 2012;53(4):371–2, 374–376, 378–380 passim. https://doi.org/10.1007/s00108-011-2984-3.
18. Sereno M, Merino M, López-Gómez M, et al. MYH polyposis syndrome: clinical findings, genetics issues and management. Clin Transl Oncol Off Publ Fed Span Oncol Soc Natl Cancer Inst Mex. 2014;16(8):675–9. https://doi.org/10.1007/s12094-014-1171-0.
19. Burt RW. Screening and survival in familial adenomatous polyposis. J Clin Gastroenterol. 2016;50(1):3–4. https://doi.org/10.1097/MCG.0000000000000438.
20. Hegde M, Ferber M, Mao R, Samowitz W, Ganguly A, Committee a WG of the AC of MG and G (ACMG) LQA. ACMG technical standards and guidelines for genetic testing for inherited colorectal cancer (Lynch syndrome, familial adenomatous polyposis, and MYH-associated polyposis). Genet Med. 2014;16(1):101–16. https://doi.org/10.1038/gim.2013.166.
21. Bilkay U, Erdem O, Ozek C, et al. Benign osteoma with Gardner syndrome: review of the literature and report of a case. J Craniofac Surg. 2004;15(3):506–9.
22. Attard TM, Giglio P, Koppula S, Snyder C, Lynch HT. Brain tumors in individuals with familial adenomatous polyposis: a cancer registry experience and pooled case report analysis. Cancer. 2007;109(4):761–6. https://doi.org/10.1002/cncr.22475.
23. Wimmer K, Kratz CP. Constitutional mismatch repair-deficiency syndrome. Haematologica. 2010;95(5):699–701. https://doi.org/10.3324/haematol.2009.021626.
24. Galiatsatos P, Foulkes WD. Familial adenomatous polyposis. Am J Gastroenterol. 2006;101(2):385–98. https://doi.org/10.1111/j.1572-0241.2006.00375.x.
25. Gardner EJ. Follow-up study of a family group exhibiting dominant inheritance for a syndrome including intestinal polyps, osteomas, fibromas and epidermal cysts. Am J Hum Genet. 1962;14:376–90.
26. Burt R, Neklason DW. Genetic testing for inherited colon cancer. Gastroenterology. 2005;128(6):1696–716.
27. Turcot J, Despres JP, St Pierre F. Malignant tumors of the central nervous system associated with familial polyposis of the colon: report of two cases. Dis Colon Rectum. 1959;2:465–8.
28. Gardner EJ, Richards RC. Multiple cutaneous and subcutaneous lesions occurring simultaneously with hereditary polyposis and osteomatosis. Am J Hum Genet. 1953;5(2):139–47.
29. Dipro S, Al-Otaibi F, Alzahrani A, Ulhaq A, Al Shail E. Turcot syndrome: a synchronous clinical presentation of glioblastoma multiforme and adenocarcinoma of the colon. Case Rep Oncol Med. 2012;2012 https://doi.org/10.1155/2012/720273.
30. American Society of Clinical Oncology. Familial adenomatous polyposis. https://www.cancer.net/cancer-types/familial-adenomatous-polyposis. Accessed 12 May 2018.
31. Parc Y, Piquard A, Dozois RR, Parc R, Tiret E. Long-term outcome of familial adenomatous polyposis patients after restorative coloproctectomy. Ann Surg. 2004;239(3):378–82. https://doi.org/10.1097/01.sla.0000114216.90947.f6.
32. Campos FG. Surgical treatment of familial adenomatous polyposis: dilemmas and current recommendations. World J Gastroenterol. 2014;20(44):16620–9. https://doi.org/10.3748/wjg.v20.i44.16620.
33. Domingo E, Laiho P, Ollikainen M, et al. BRAF screening as a low-cost effective strategy for simplifying HNPCC genetic testing. J Med Genet. 2004;41(9):664–8. https://doi.org/10.1136/jmg.2004.020651.
34. Malkhosyan S, Rampino N, Yamamoto H, Perucho M. Frameshift mutator mutations. Nature. 1996;382(6591):499–500. https://doi.org/10.1038/382499a0.
35. Lynch HT, de la Chapelle A. Genetic susceptibility to non-polyposis colorectal cancer. J Med Genet. 1999;36(11):801–18.
36. Jang E, Chung DC. Hereditary colon cancer: lynch syndrome. Gut Liver. 2010;4(2):151–60. https://doi.org/10.5009/gnl.2010.4.2.151.
37. Moreira L, Balaguer F, Lindor N, et al. Identification of Lynch syndrome among patients with colorectal cancer. JAMA. 2012;308(15):1555–65. https://doi.org/10.1001/jama.2012.13088.

38. Markowitz S, Wang J, Myeroff L, et al. Inactivation of the type II TGF-beta receptor in colon cancer cells with microsatellite instability. Science. 1995;268(5215):1336–8.
39. Herman JG, Umar A, Polyak K, et al. Incidence and functional consequences of hMLH1 promoter hypermethylation in colorectal carcinoma. Proc Natl Acad Sci U S A. 1998;95(12):6870–5.
40. Loughrey MB, Waring PM, Tan A, et al. Incorporation of somatic BRAF mutation testing into an algorithm for the investigation of hereditary non-polyposis colorectal cancer. Fam Cancer. 2007;6(3):301–10. https://doi.org/10.1007/s10689-007-9124-1.
41. Kane MF, Loda M, Gaida GM, et al. Methylation of the hMLH1 promoter correlates with lack of expression of hMLH1 in sporadic colon tumors and mismatch repair-defective human tumor cell lines. Cancer Res. 1997;57(5):808–11.
42. Bedeir A, Krasinskas AM. Molecular diagnostics of colorectal cancer. Arch Pathol Lab Med. 2011;135(5):578–87. https://doi.org/10.1043/2010-0613-RAIR.1.
43. Marra G, Schär P. Recognition of DNA alterations by the mismatch repair system. Biochem J. 1999;338(Pt 1):1–13.
44. Chung DC, Rustgi AK. The hereditary nonpolyposis colorectal cancer syndrome: genetics and clinical implications. Ann Intern Med. 2003;138(7):560–70.
45. Yearsley M, Hampel H, Lehman A, Nakagawa H, de la Chapelle A, Frankel WL. Histologic features distinguish microsatellite-high from microsatellite-low and microsatellite-stable colorectal carcinomas, but do not differentiate germline mutations from methylation of the MLH1 promoter. Hum Pathol. 2006;37(7):831–8. https://doi.org/10.1016/j.humpath.2006.02.009.
46. Mecklin JP, Sipponen P, Järvinen HJ. Histopathology of colorectal carcinomas and adenomas in cancer family syndrome. Dis Colon Rectum. 1986;29(12):849–53.
47. Hemminger JA, Pearlman R, Haraldsdottir S, et al. Histology of colorectal adenocarcinoma with double somatic mismatch repair mutations is indistinguishable from those caused by Lynch syndrome. Hum Pathol. 2018;78(8):125–30. https://doi.org/10.1016/j.humpath.2018.04.017.
48. Halvarsson B, Lindblom A, Johansson L, Lagerstedt K, Nilbert M. Loss of mismatch repair protein immunostaining in colorectal adenomas from patients with hereditary nonpolyposis colorectal cancer. Mod Pathol. 2005;18(8):1095–101. https://doi.org/10.1038/modpathol.3800392.
49. Jass JR, Smyrk TC, Stewart SM, Lane MR, Lanspa SJ, Lynch HT. Pathology of hereditary non-polyposis colorectal cancer. Anticancer Res. 1994;14(4B):1631–4.
50. Wei C, Chen J, Pande M, Lynch PM, Frazier ML. A pilot study comparing protein expression in different segments of the normal colon and rectum and in normal colon versus adenoma in patients with Lynch syndrome. J Cancer Res Clin Oncol. 2013;139(7):1241–50. https://doi.org/10.1007/s00432-013-1437-x.
51. Shia J, Holck S, Depetris G, Greenson JK, Klimstra DS. Lynch syndrome-associated neoplasms: a discussion on histopathology and immunohistochemistry. Fam Cancer. 2013;12(2):241–60. https://doi.org/10.1007/s10689-013-9612-4.
52. Walsh MD, Buchanan DD, Pearson S-A, et al. Immunohistochemical testing of conventional adenomas for loss of expression of mismatch repair proteins in Lynch syndrome mutation carriers: a case series from the Australasian site of the colon cancer family registry. Mod Pathol. 2012;25(5):722–30. https://doi.org/10.1038/modpathol.2011.209.
53. Warrier SK, Trainer AH, Lynch AC, et al. Preoperative diagnosis of Lynch syndrome with DNA mismatch repair immunohistochemistry on a diagnostic biopsy. Dis Colon Rectum. 2011;54(12):1480–7. https://doi.org/10.1097/DCR.0b013e318231db1f.
54. Umar A, Boland CR, Terdiman JP, et al. Revised Bethesda guidelines for hereditary nonpolyposis colorectal cancer (Lynch syndrome) and microsatellite instability. J Natl Cancer Inst. 2004;96(4):261–8.
55. Boland CR, Thibodeau SN, Hamilton SR, et al. A National Cancer Institute Workshop on Microsatellite Instability for cancer detection and familial predisposition: development of international criteria for the determination of microsatellite instability in colorectal cancer. Cancer Res. 1998;58(22):5248–57.
56. Wang HL, Kim CJ, Koo J, et al. Practical immunohistochemistry in neoplastic pathology of the gastrointestinal tract, liver, biliary tract, and pancreas. Arch Pathol Lab Med. 2017;141(9):1155–80. https://doi.org/10.5858/arpa.2016-0489-RA.
57. Radu OM, Nikiforova MN, Farkas LM, Krasinskas AM. Challenging cases encountered in colorectal cancer screening for Lynch syndrome reveal novel findings: nucleolar MSH6 staining and impact of prior chemoradiation therapy. Hum Pathol. 2011;42(9):1247–58. https://doi.org/10.1016/j.humpath.2010.11.016.
58. Bao F, Panarelli NC, Rennert H, Sherr DL, Yantiss RK. Neoadjuvant therapy induces loss of MSH6 expression in colorectal carcinoma. Am J Surg Pathol. 2010;34(12):1798–804. https://doi.org/10.1097/PAS.0b013e3181f906cc.
59. Hagen CE, Lefferts J, Hornick JL, Srivastava A. "Null pattern" of immunoreactivity in a Lynch syndrome-associated colon cancer due to germline MSH2 mutation and somatic MLH1 hypermethylation. Am J Surg Pathol. 2011;35(12):1902–5. https://doi.org/10.1097/PAS.0b013e318237c6ab.
60. Møller P, Seppälä T, Bernstein I, et al. Cancer incidence and survival in Lynch syndrome patients receiving colonoscopic and gynaecological surveillance: first report from the prospective Lynch syndrome database. Gut. 2017;66(3):464–72. gutjnl-2015-309675. https://doi.org/10.1136/gutjnl-2015-309675.
61. Cohen SA, Leininger A. The genetic basis of Lynch syndrome and its implications for clinical practice and risk management. Appl Clin Genet. 2014;7:147–58. https://doi.org/10.2147/TACG.S51483.
62. Pylvänäinen K, Lehtinen T, Kellokumpu I, Järvinen H, Mecklin J-P. Causes of death of mutation carriers in Finnish Lynch syndrome families. Fam Cancer. 2012;11(3):467–71. https://doi.org/10.1007/s10689-012-9537-3.
63. Lynch HT, Lynch PM. Colorectal cancer: update on the clinical management of Lynch syndrome. Nat Rev Gastroenterol Hepatol. 2013;10(6):323–4. https://doi.org/10.1038/nrgastro.2013.70.
64. Vasen HFA, Blanco I, Aktan-Collan K, et al. Revised guidelines for the clinical management of Lynch syndrome (HNPCC): recommendations by a group of European experts. Gut. 2013;62(6):812–23. https://doi.org/10.1136/gutjnl-2012-304356.
65. de Vos tot Nederveen Cappel WH, Järvinen HJ, Lynch PM, Engel C, Mecklin J-P, Vasen HFA. Colorectal surveillance in Lynch syndrome families. Fam Cancer. 2013;12(2):261–5. https://doi.org/10.1007/s10689-013-9631-1.
66. Tse JY, Wu S, Shinagare SA, et al. Peutz-Jeghers syndrome: a critical look at colonic Peutz-Jeghers polyps. Mod Pathol. 2013;26(9):1235–40. https://doi.org/10.1038/modpathol.2013.44.
67. Latchford AR, Phillips RKS. Gastrointestinal polyps and cancer in Peutz-Jeghers syndrome: clinical aspects. Fam Cancer. 2011;10(3):455–61. https://doi.org/10.1007/s10689-011-9442-1.
68. Giardiello FM, Trimbath JD. Peutz-Jeghers syndrome and management recommendations. Clin Gastroenterol Hepatol. 2006;4(4):408–15. https://doi.org/10.1016/j.cgh.2005.11.005.
69. McGarrity TJ, Kulin HE, Zaino RJ. Peutz-Jeghers syndrome. Am J Gastroenterol. 2000;95(3):596–604. https://doi.org/10.1111/j.1572-0241.2000.01831.x.
70. Miyaki M, Iijima T, Hosono K, et al. Somatic mutations of LKB1 and beta-catenin genes in gastrointestinal polyps from patients with Peutz-Jeghers syndrome. Cancer Res. 2000;60(22):6311–3.

71. Lim W, Olschwang S, Keller JJ, et al. Relative frequency and morphology of cancers in STK11 mutation carriers. Gastroenterology. 2004;126(7):1788–94.
72. Giardiello FM, Brensinger JD, Tersmette AC, et al. Very high risk of cancer in familial Peutz-Jeghers syndrome. Gastroenterology. 2000;119(6):1447–53.
73. Wirtzfeld DA, Petrelli NJ, Rodriguez-Bigas MA. Hamartomatous polyposis syndromes: molecular genetics, neoplastic risk, and surveillance recommendations. Ann Surg Oncol. 2001;8(4):319–27.
74. Ngeow J, Heald B, Rybicki LA, et al. Prevalence of germline PTEN, BMPR1A, SMAD4, STK11, and ENG mutations in patients with moderate-load colorectal polyps. Gastroenterology. 2013;144(7):1402–9, 1409–5. https://doi.org/10.1053/j.gastro.2013.02.001.
75. Calva-Cerqueira D, Chinnathambi S, Pechman B, Bair J, Larsen-Haidle J, Howe JR. The rate of germline mutations and large deletions of SMAD4 and BMPR1A in juvenile polyposis. Clin Genet. 2009;75(1):79–85. https://doi.org/10.1111/j.1399-0004.2008.01091.x.
76. Schreibman IR, Baker M, Amos C, McGarrity TJ. The hamartomatous polyposis syndromes: a clinical and molecular review. Am J Gastroenterol. 2005;100(2):476–90. https://doi.org/10.1111/j.1572-0241.2005.40237.x.
77. Goodman ZD, Yardley JH, Milligan FD. Pathogenesis of colonic polyps in multiple juvenile polyposis: report of a case associated with gastric polyps and carcinoma of the rectum. Cancer. 1979;43(5):1906–13.
78. Grosfeld JL, West KW. Generalized juvenile polyposis coli: clinical management based on long-term observations. Arch Surg Chic Ill 1960. 1986;121(5):530–4.
79. Howe JR, Haidle JL, Lal G, et al. ENG mutations in MADH4/BMPR1A mutation negative patients with juvenile polyposis. Clin Genet. 2007;71(1):91–2. https://doi.org/10.1111/j.1399-0004.2007.00734.x.
80. Delnatte C, Sanlaville D, Mougenot J-F, et al. Contiguous gene deletion within chromosome arm 10q is associated with juvenile polyposis of infancy, reflecting cooperation between the BMPR1A and PTEN tumor-suppressor genes. Am J Hum Genet. 2006;78(6):1066–74. https://doi.org/10.1086/504301.
81. Mangili G, Taccagni G, Garavaglia E, Carnelli M, Montoli S. An unusual admixture of neoplastic and metaplastic lesions of the female genital tract in the Peutz-Jeghers syndrome. Gynecol Oncol. 2004;92(1):337–42.
82. van Lier MGF, Wagner A, Mathus-Vliegen EMH, Kuipers EJ, Steyerberg EW, van Leerdam ME. High cancer risk in Peutz–Jeghers syndrome: a systematic review and surveillance recommendations. Am J Gastroenterol. 2010;105(6):1258–64. https://doi.org/10.1038/ajg.2009.725.
83. Scully RE. Sex cord tumor with annular tubules a distinctive ovarian tumor of the Peutz-Jeghers syndrome. Cancer. 25(5):1107–21. https://doi.org/10.1002/1097-0142(197005)25:5<1107::AID-CNCR2820250516>3.0.CO;2-7.
84. Oliveira PH, Cunha C, Almeida S, et al. Juvenile polyposis of infancy in a child with deletion of BMPR1A and PTEN genes: surgical approach. J Pediatr Surg. 2013;48(1):e33–7. https://doi.org/10.1016/j.jpedsurg.2012.09.067.
85. Giardiello FM, Hamilton SR, Kern SE, et al. Colorectal neoplasia in juvenile polyposis or juvenile polyps. Arch Dis Child. 1991;66(8):971–5.
86. Friedl W, Uhlhaas S, Schulmann K, et al. Juvenile polyposis: massive gastric polyposis is more common in MADH4 mutation carriers than in BMPR1A mutation carriers. Hum Genet. 2002;111(1):108–11. https://doi.org/10.1007/s00439-002-0748-9.
87. Chow E, Macrae F. A review of juvenile polyposis syndrome. J Gastroenterol Hepatol. 2005;20(11):1634–40. https://doi.org/10.1111/j.1440-1746.2005.03865.x.
88. Latchford AR, Neale K, Phillips RKS, Clark SK. Juvenile polyposis syndrome: a study of genotype, phenotype, and long-term outcome. Dis Colon Rectum. 2012;55(10):1038–43. https://doi.org/10.1097/DCR.0b013e31826278b3.
89. Stanich PP, Pilarski R, Rock J, Frankel WL, El-Dika S, Meyer MM. Colonic manifestations of PTEN hamartoma tumor syndrome: case series and systematic review. World J Gastroenterol. 2014;20(7):1833–8. https://doi.org/10.3748/wjg.v20.i7.1833.
90. Stanich PP, Owens VL, Sweetser S, et al. Colonic polyposis and neoplasia in Cowden syndrome. Mayo Clin Proc. 2011;86(6):489–92. https://doi.org/10.4065/mcp.2010.0816.
91. Shaco-Levy R, Jasperson KW, Martin K, et al. Morphologic characterization of hamartomatous gastrointestinal polyps in Cowden syndrome, Peutz-Jeghers syndrome, and juvenile polyposis syndrome. Hum Pathol. 2016;49(3):39–48. https://doi.org/10.1016/j.humpath.2015.10.002.
92. Chi SG, Kim HJ, Park BJ, et al. Mutational abrogation of the PTEN/MMAC1 gene in gastrointestinal polyps in patients with Cowden disease. Gastroenterology. 1998;115(5):1084–9.
93. Heald B, Mester J, Rybicki L, Orloff MS, Burke CA, Eng C. Frequent gastrointestinal polyps and colorectal adenocarcinomas in a prospective series of PTEN mutation carriers. Gastroenterology. 2010;139(6):1927–33. https://doi.org/10.1053/j.gastro.2010.06.061.
94. Tan M-H, Mester JL, Ngeow J, Rybicki LA, Orloff MS, Eng C. Lifetime cancer risks in individuals with germline PTEN mutations. Clin Cancer Res. 2012;18(2):400–7. https://doi.org/10.1158/1078-0432.CCR-11-2283.
95. Ward EM, Wolfsen HC. The non-inherited gastrointestinal polyposis syndromes. Aliment Pharmacol Ther. 2002;16(3):333–42.
96. Burke AP, Sobin LH. The pathology of Cronkhite-Canada polyps: a comparison to juvenile polyposis. Am J Surg Pathol. 1989;13(11):940–6.
97. Slavik T, Montgomery EA. Cronkhite–Canada syndrome six decades on: the many faces of an enigmatic disease. J Clin Pathol. 2014;67(10):891–7. https://doi.org/10.1136/jclinpath-2014-202488.
98. Sweetser S, Ahlquist DA, Osborn NK, et al. Clinicopathologic features and treatment outcomes in Cronkhite-Canada syndrome: support for autoimmunity. Dig Dis Sci. 2012;57(2):496–502. https://doi.org/10.1007/s10620-011-1874-9.
99. Pilarski R, Burt R, Kohlman W, Pho L, Shannon KM, Swisher E. Cowden syndrome and the PTEN hamartoma tumor syndrome: systematic review and revised diagnostic criteria. J Natl Cancer Inst. 2013;105(21):1607–16. https://doi.org/10.1093/jnci/djt277.
100. Eng C. PTEN Hamartoma tumor syndrome. In: Adam MP, Ardinger HH, Pagon RA, et al., editors. GeneReviews®. Seattle, WA: University of Washington; 1993. http://www.ncbi.nlm.nih.gov/books/NBK1488/.
101. Salem OS, Steck WD. Cowden's disease (multiple hamartoma and neoplasia syndrome): a case report and review of the English literature. J Am Acad Dermatol. 1983;8(5):686–96.
102. Sieber OM, Lipton L, Crabtree M, et al. Multiple colorectal adenomas, classic adenomatous polyposis, and germ-line mutations in MYH. N Engl J Med. 2003;348(9):791–9. https://doi.org/10.1056/NEJMoa025283.
103. Rosty C, Buchanan DD, Walsh MD, et al. Phenotype and polyp landscape in serrated polyposis syndrome: a series of 100 patients from genetics clinics. Am J Surg Pathol. 2012;36(6):876–82. https://doi.org/10.1097/PAS.0b013e31824e133f.

104. Rashid A, Houlihan PS, Booker S, Petersen GM, Giardiello FM, Hamilton SR. Phenotypic and molecular characteristics of hyperplastic polyposis. Gastroenterology. 2000;119(2):323–32.
105. Torlakovic E, Snover DC. Serrated adenomatous polyposis in humans. Gastroenterology. 1996;110(3):748–55.
106. Huang CS, O'brien MJ, Yang S, Farraye FA. Hyperplastic polyps, serrated adenomas, and the serrated polyp neoplasia pathway. Am J Gastroenterol. 2004;99(11):2242–55. https://doi.org/10.1111/j.1572-0241.2004.40131.x.
107. Jass JR, Iino H, Ruszkiewicz A, et al. Neoplastic progression occurs through mutator pathways in hyperplastic polyposis of the colorectum. Gut. 2000;47(1):43–9.
108. Rashid A, Issa JPJ. CpG island methylation in gastroenterologic neoplasia: a maturing field. Gastroenterology. 2004;127(5):1578–88.
109. Quintana I, Mejias-Luque R, Terradas M, et al. Evidence suggests that gemline RNF43 mutations are a rare cause of serrated polyposis. Gut. 2018;67(12):2230–2. https://doi.org/10.1136/gutjnl-2017-315733.
110. de Boer WB, Ee H, Kumarasinghe MP. Neoplastic lesions of gastric adenocarcinoma and proximal polyposis syndrome (GAPPS) are gastric phenotype. Am J Surg Pathol. 2018;42(1):1–8. https://doi.org/10.1097/PAS.0000000000000924.
111. Li J, Woods SL, Healey S, et al. Point mutations in exon 1B of APC reveal gastric adenocarcinoma and proximal polyposis of the stomach as a familial adenomatous polyposis variant. Am J Hum Genet. 2016;98(5):830–42. https://doi.org/10.1016/j.ajhg.2016.03.001.
112. Beer A, Streubel B, Asari R, Dejaco C, Oberhuber G. Gastric adenocarcinoma and proximal polyposis of the stomach (GAPPS): a rare recently described gastric polyposis syndrome – report of a case. Z Gastroenterol. 2017;55(11):1131–4. https://doi.org/10.1055/s-0043-117182.
113. Worthley DL, Phillips KD, Wayte N, et al. Gastric adenocarcinoma and proximal polyposis of the stomach (GAPPS): a new autosomal dominant syndrome. Gut. 2012;61(5):774–9. https://doi.org/10.1136/gutjnl-2011-300348.
114. Repak R, Kohoutova D, Podhola M, et al. The first European family with gastric adenocarcinoma and proximal polyposis of the stomach: case report and review of the literature. Gastrointest Endosc. 2016;84(4):718–25. https://doi.org/10.1016/j.gie.2016.06.023.

Mesenchymal Lesions Often Presenting as Polyps of the Gastrointestinal Tract

16

Ari Kassardjian, David Borzik, Aaron W. James, and Sarah M. Dry

List of Frequently Asked Questions

1. What is the endoscopic differential for an esophageal fibrovascular polyp?
2. What other entities should be considered before diagnosing a fibrovascular polyp of the esophagus?
3. What is the endoscopic appearance of a xanthoma?
4. Are any special stains required to make the diagnosis of xanthoma?
5. What is the differential diagnosis for a xanthoma?
6. How does a Schwann cell hamartoma differ from a schwannoma or neurofibroma?
7. Where does Schwann cell hamartoma usually arise?
8. What are the histologic and clinical features of a granular cell tumor?
9. Are granular cell tumors always benign?
10. What are the histologic and clinical features of calcifying fibrous pseudotumor/reactive nodular fibrous pseudotumor (CFPT/RNFP)?
11. Are there any clinically aggressive lesions that can mimic CFPT/RNFP?
12. Do ganglioneuromas arise as solitary or multiple lesions??
13. What other lesions are in the differential diagnosis for ganglioneuroma?
14. What tumors are in the differential diagnosis of mucosal perineurioma and how can one distinguish these histologically?
15. Where does mucosal perineurioma typically arise?
16. What mutations are often seen in inflammatory fibroid polyp and why is this interesting?
17. Where does inflammatory fibroid polyp usually occur?
18. How can inflammatory fibroid polyp be distinguished from other entities in the differential diagnosis?
19. What immunostains may be useful in the diagnosis of glomus tumor?
20. What is the differential diagnosis for glomus tumor?
21. What entities are in the differential diagnosis for leiomyoma?
22. What histologic features indicate leiomyosarcoma rather than leiomyoma?
23. Where does lipoma commonly arise?
24. How can one distinguish a lipoma from a well-differentiated liposarcoma?
25. What are the characteristic presentation and histologic findings of lymphangioma?

A. Kassardjian · S. M. Dry (✉)
University of California at Los Angeles David Geffen School of Medicine, Los Angeles, CA, USA
e-mail: SDry@mednet.ucla.edu

D. Borzik · A. W. James
Johns Hopkins University School of Medicine, Baltimore, MD, USA

Frequently Asked Questions

1. What is the endoscopic differential for an esophageal fibrovascular polyp?

On endoscopic exam, fibrovascular polyps (FVPs) are smooth, pedunculated, and "sausage-shaped" masses that are often found in the cervical esophagus, in the cricopharyngeal region. Given this location, prolapse of a soft fleshy mass into the oral cavity is a characteristic finding. The gross/endoscopic differential consists of other intraluminal polypoid lesions that may be found in the esophagus, which includes a wide range of benign and malignant lesions. Our list is not exhaustive but represents more common lesions the pathologist is likely to encounter:

- Leiomyoma
- Squamous papilloma
- Hemangioma
- Granular cell tumor
- Carcinoid tumor

H. L. Wang, Z. E. Chen (eds.), *Practical Gastrointestinal Pathology*, Practical Anatomic Pathology,
https://doi.org/10.1007/978-3-030-51268-2_16

2. **What other entities should be considered before diagnosing a fibrovascular polyp of the esophagus?**
   - FVPs are composed of adipose and fibrovascular tissue in varying proportions, with a mucosal lining of squamous epithelium. Myxoid change may be seen. Mucosal ulceration is a common finding. Depending on the histologic appearance, the differential diagnosis may include an inflammatory fibroid polyp (IFP), hemangioma, or adipose tumors such as lipoma or well-differentiated liposarcoma.
   - IFP is a rare entity which most commonly occurs in the gastric antrum rather than the esophagus. IFP has a histologic appearance of bland spindle cells with abundant inflammatory cells including numerous eosinophils (see below).
   - Adipose tumors may be considered if fat tissue predominates, including lipoma or well-differentiated liposarcoma.
   - Lipomas do not contain a core of mature fibromyxoid tissue as seen in FVPs.
   - Like well-differentiated liposarcoma (WDLPS), FVPs may be large (usually 2–4 cm in diameter but can extend to 25 cm). FVPs do not include the atypical, enlarged, and hyperchromatic stromal cells present in WDLPS and do not show MDM2 amplification. WDLPS is rare in this location (see below and Chap. 20 for further discussion).

   References: [1–4]

3. **What is the endoscopic appearance of a xanthoma?**
   - Xanthomas are multiple or solitary, well-demarcated, pale yellow plaques.
   - Virtually all are <1.0 cm in diameter, with most lesions being <0.5 cm.
   - In the GI tract, the most common location is the gastric antral mucosa and submucosa.
   - These are most often an incidental finding during endoscopy.

4. **Are any special stains required to make the diagnosis of xanthoma?**
   - Xanthomas are morphologically distinct entities and so rarely require special stains or immunohistochemical stains.
   - The histology consists of foamy, lipid-rich histiocytes (Fig. 16.1).
   - Histiocytes demonstrate distinct cell membranes; abundant eosinophilic to clear, granular, or vacuolated cytoplasm; and medium-sized centrally placed nuclei.
     - No nuclear atypia is present.
     - As expected based on their histiocytic identity, lesional cells stain positively for CD68, CD163, and PU.1 and are negative for cytokeratins.

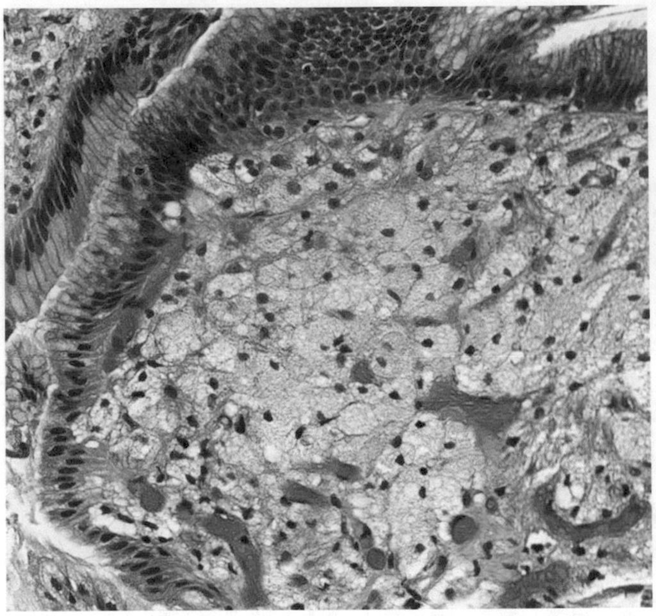

Fig. 16.1 Gastric xanthoma demonstrating accumulation of foamy, lipid-rich histiocytes within the lamina propria

   - While xanthomas do not typically present a diagnostic challenge, the vacuolated cytoplasm may sometimes mimic malignant cells seen in clear cell carcinoid tumors or signet ring carcinomas. Distinguishing immunohistochemical and histochemical features are described below:
     - Carcinoid: Positive for chromogranin and synaptophysin; negative for mucicarmine, CK7, CK20, and CD68
     - Signet ring adenocarcinoma: Positive for cytokeratin, EMA, CEA, and mucicarmine; negative for CD68
   - Xanthomas contain neutral fat and will thus be negative for PAS. In contrast, a PAS stain will be positive in signet ring adenocarcinoma.

5. **What is the differential diagnosis for a xanthoma?**
   - Submucosal lipoma: Mature adipose tissue rather than histiocytes.
   - Russell body gastritis: Lamina propria is expanded by plasma cells with cytoplasmic Russell bodies rather than histiocytes.
   - Signet ring cell gastric adenocarcinoma: Mucicarmine- and keratin-positive infiltrative cells. Nuclei are larger and more hyperchromatic than histiocytes and typically show some pleomorphism. Usually there are at least some cells with an eccentrically placed nucleus creating the so-called "signet ring" appearance.
   - Clear cell carcinoid: Cells are arranged in nests with abundant vascular stroma and stain positively for neuroendocrine markers (i.e., synaptophysin, chromogranin).

- Metastatic clear cell renal cell carcinoma: Enlarged epithelial cells with clear to eosinophilic cytoplasm, nuclear atypia, a background of hemorrhage, and prominent delicate vasculature.
- Certain infectious states, such as Whipple disease, mycobacterium avium-intracellulare infection, and histoplasmosis, will expand the lamina propria with abundant histiocytes and may impart a clear to foamy appearance. Special stains, such as PAS, AFB, and GMS, will be helpful.

References: [5–13]

6. How does a Schwann cell hamartoma differ from a schwannoma or neurofibroma (Table 16.1)?

- Distinguishing schwannomas from Schwann cell hamartomas is often challenging. Both lesions show bland spindle cells composed exclusively of Schwann cells arranged in vague fascicles which are diffusely and strongly positive for S100.

Table 16.1 Unique features of GI schwannoma and neurofibroma to distinguish from Schwann cell hamartoma

Tumor	Features to distinguish from Schwann cell hamartoma
Schwannoma	Peripheral cuff-like lymphoid aggregates with germinal centers Centered in the muscularis propria Commonly arise in the stomach
Neurofibroma	Composed of Schwann cells, fibroblasts, and perineurial-like cells Positive for S100 and CD34 and with NFP-positive axons Commonly arise in stomach and jejunum High association with NF1

  - Schwann cell hamartomas involve the lamina propria and surround the colonic crypts (Fig. 16.2a, b).
  - Schwannomas are centered in the muscularis propria, typically arising in the stomach.
  - GI schwannomas are rarely found in the colon, which is where virtually all Schwann cell hamartomas are encountered.
  - Unlike schwannomas from the central nervous system and peripheral soft tissue, Verocay bodies, vascular hyalinization, and foamy histiocytes are absent in both GI schwannomas and Schwann cell hamartomas. Nuclear palisading is rarely encountered.
  - GI schwannomas are notable for the presence of peripheral cuff-like lymphoid aggregates with germinal centers, a feature not seen in Schwann cell hamartomas (see Chap. 20).
- Colorectal neurofibroma is another important differential diagnosis of Schwann cell hamartomas. Although histologically they may look very similar, Schwann cell hamartomas are composed of a pure Schwann cell population. In contrast, neurofibromas are composed of Schwann cells, fibroblasts, and perineurial-like cells and thus show more cellular heterogeneity and nuclear variability.
  - Schwann cell hamartomas show strong diffuse staining for S100 in almost all cells, a paucity of positive axons by neurofilament protein (NFP) staining, and are negative for CD34. In contrast, and in keeping with the fact that they are composed of numerous cell types from the peripheral nerve and nerve sheath, neurofibromas show a mixture of S100- and CD34-positive cells and a higher concentration of NFP-positive axons (see Chap. 20).

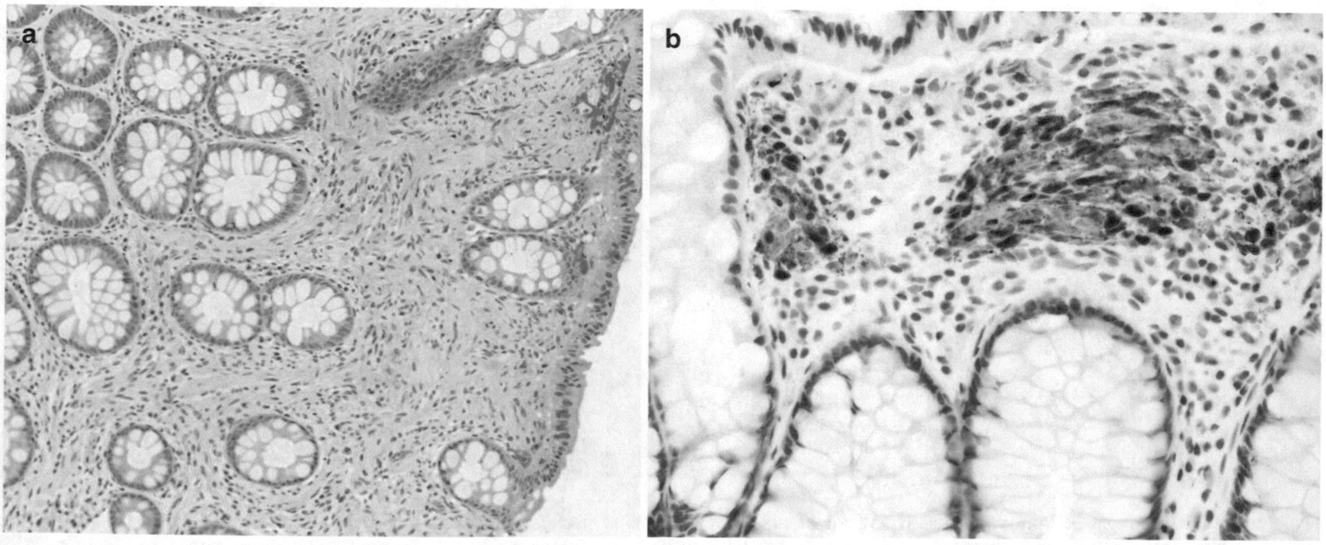

Fig. 16.2 (**a**) Schwann cell hamartoma composed of bland spindle cells involving the lamina propria and surrounding the colonic crypts. (**b**) Spindle cells stain positive for S100 by immunohistochemistry

- GI neurofibroma has a high association with neurofibromatosis type 1 (NF1). There are diverse clinical manifestations of NF1, including multiple cutaneous neurofibromas. A GI neurofibroma as the primary clinical presentation of NF1 without skin manifestations is exceedingly rare; however, the clinical features of NF1 may be subtle. NF1 clinically may be overlooked by inexperienced clinicians or until the patient is diagnosed with a tumor, such as a plexiform neurofibroma, which is highly associated with NF1.
- When making a diagnosis of a GI neurofibroma in a patient without a history of NF1, the pathology report should indicate that NF1 should be excluded clinically.
- Schwann cell hamartomas are not associated with syndromic states. Clinical or endoscopic follow-up is not necessary after diagnosis.
- Neurofibromas are typically found in the stomach and jejunum and are rarely colonic where Schwann cell hamartomas are commonly encountered.

7. **Where does Schwann cell hamartoma usually arise?**
   - Schwann cell hamartomas are characterized by a diffuse, ill-defined proliferation of spindle cells within the lamina propria surrounding the colonic crypts.
   - They are most commonly encountered in the left colon with greatest concentration in the rectosigmoid; however, these polyps may arise anywhere in the colon.
   - They are usually small (1–6 mm) and are typically an incidental finding at colonoscopy (Table 16.1).

   References: [14–17]

8. **What are the histologic and clinical features of a granular cell tumor?**
   - Granular cell tumor cells are arranged in ribbons or nests and may be divided by fibrous septa or arranged in large sheets (Fig. 16.3a). Tumor cells are round to polygonal with plump eosinophilic, fine to coarsely granular cytoplasm (Fig. 16.3b). Nuclei may range from small and dark to large and vesicular. Mild to moderate nuclear atypia may be present and by itself does not indicate malignancy.
   - Older lesions may show desmoplasia, producing scattered nests of tumor cells dispersed in a background of dense collagen (Fig. 16.3c).
   - Granular cell tumors are often associated with pseudoepitheliomatous hyperplasia (Fig. 16.3a).
     - Pseudoepitheliomatous hyperplasia of the overlying epithelium is characterized by a pseudo-invasive growth pattern consisting of strands of epithelium extending to the underlying connective tissue. This may be confused with a well-differentiated squamous cell carcinoma.

9. **Are granular cell tumors always benign?**
   - The vast majority of granular cell tumors are benign; however, a small subset (1–2%) show clinical features of malignancy such as local recurrence and distant metastasis. Even a histologically bland granular cell tumor may behave aggressively.
   - Histologic criteria are not entirely predictive of clinical behavior. Efforts to identify specific histologic criteria have been complicated by the relative rarity of granular cell tumors with atypical histologic features or aggressive clinical behavior. As a result, there are

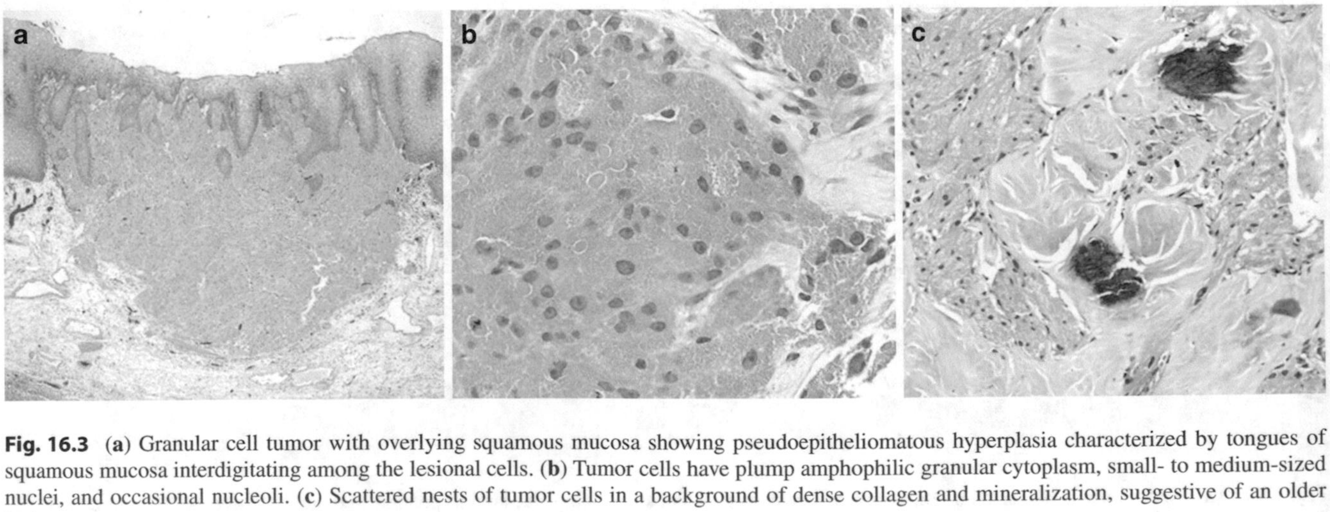

Fig. 16.3 (**a**) Granular cell tumor with overlying squamous mucosa showing pseudoepitheliomatous hyperplasia characterized by tongues of squamous mucosa interdigitating among the lesional cells. (**b**) Tumor cells have plump amphophilic granular cytoplasm, small- to medium-sized nuclei, and occasional nucleoli. (**c**) Scattered nests of tumor cells in a background of dense collagen and mineralization, suggestive of an older lesion

few large clinical series with adequate clinical follow-up.
- Fanburg-Smith and colleagues studied a series of 73 tumors, 55% of which had clinical follow-up for 1–17 years. Using six histologic criteria, they characterized tumors with one to two of these features as "atypical" and three and more histologic features as "malignant." All the "atypical" tumors followed a benign clinical course. Of those patients with malignant granular cell tumors with clinical follow-up, 40% died of disease and 30% were alive with disease (local recurrence or distant metastases) at last follow-up. Overall, approximately one-third developed local recurrences and half developed distant metastases. The histologic features are:
  - Necrosis
  - Spindling
  - Vesicular nuclei with large nucleoli
  - Increased mitotic activity (>2/10 HPF)
  - High N:C ratio
  - Marked nuclear pleomorphism
- In addition to histologic criteria, an elevated Ki67 proliferation index and aberrant p53 staining may be useful; however, normal staining does not preclude malignancy.

  References: [18–20]

10. What are the histologic and clinical features of calcifying fibrous pseudotumor/reactive nodular fibrous pseudotumor (CFPT/RNFP)?

- Architecturally, these lesions are well circumscribed, nonencapsulated, and hypocellular, composed of bland spindled cells in dense, birefringent, collagenous stroma (Fig. 16.4a–c).
- No necrosis, atypia, or mitotic activity should be present.
- There is often an accompanying lymphoplasmacytic infiltrate with or without germinal centers.
- The immunohistochemical staining pattern of CFPT/RNFP is relatively nonspecific:
  - Positive staining is seen for factor XIIIa.
  - Variable CD34 expression is seen.
  - No staining is present for ALK (or ALK1), SMA, MSA, desmin, or S100.
- Characteristic feature: Dystrophic or psammomatous calcifications.
- These lesions can occur in any parts of the GI tract, including the mesentery, but stomach and small bowel are the most common sites. They can range from a few millimeters to several centimeters in size.

11. Are there any clinically aggressive lesions that can mimic CFPT/RNFP?

- A number of spindle cell tumors with a collagenous stroma have some degree of histologic overlap with CFPT/RNFP but should be distinguished on morphologic grounds. Immunohistochemical stains may be helpful in some cases.
  - Intra-abdominal (desmoid) fibromatosis (see Chap. 20). Distinguishing features of fibromatosis include bland spindle cells with scant cytoplasm arranged in broad fascicles in a background of collagenous stroma. An infiltrative border is virtually always present. Medium-sized gaping vessels, some with muscular walls, are present. CD34 immunostaining is negative. Diffuse nuclear beta-catenin immunostaining, when present, is consistent with desmoid fibromatosis.
  - Inflammatory myofibroblastic tumor (IMT) (see Chap. 20). As the name suggests, the lesion is comprised of fibroblasts, myofibroblasts, and inflammatory cells. The myofibroblastic component consists of spindled to stellate cells arranged in a storiform or fascicular pattern, commonly showing

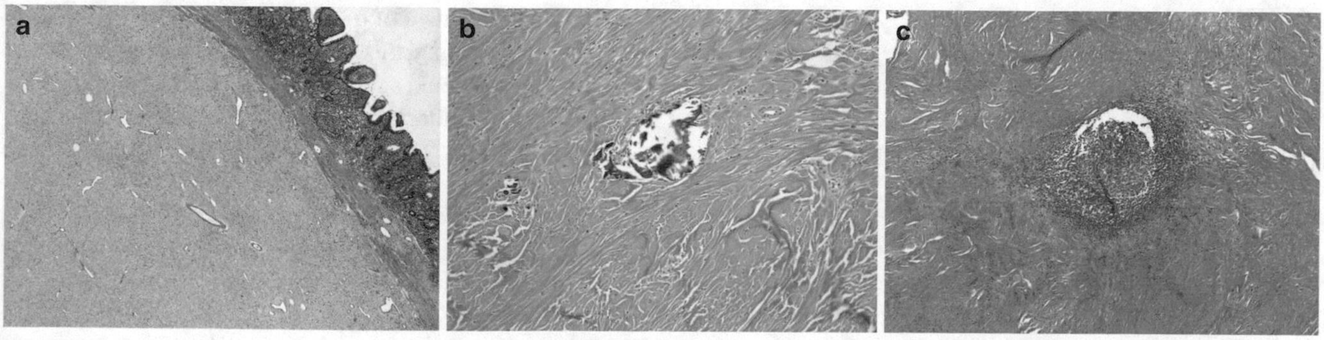

Fig. 16.4 Calcifying fibrous pseudotumor/reactive nodular fibrous pseudotumor. (**a**) Low power view showing a well-circumscribed, hypocellular, and collagenous lesion. The overlying mucosa is spared. (**b**) Higher power view showing collagenous stroma and focal calcifications. (**c**) Scattered lymphoid follicles are present. Though described under different names in the literature, these two lesions likely represent a same or similar clinicopathologic entity

prominent nucleoli, scattered mitosis, and varying degrees of atypia. The inflammatory component consists of lymphocytes, plasma cells, histiocytes, and eosinophils. Keloid-type collagen may be present. IMT is frequently positive for ALK (57%) and desmin (79%) and negative for CD34.

- Gastrointestinal stromal tumor (GIST) (see Chap. 19). A spindle cell GIST with bland cytomorphology may have a sclerotic stroma with dystrophic calcification and thus some histologic overlap with CFPT/RNFP. Distinguishing features of GIST include c-kit (CD117) and DOG1 immunoreactivity, as well as *KIT* or *PDGFRA* mutations. Features more consistent with CFPT/RFNP include multinodular growth, psammomatous calcification, patchy chronic inflammation, and prominent hyalinized stroma.
- Solitary fibrous tumor (SFT). SFT may be hyalinized but should have increased cellularity in comparison to CFPT/RNFP. Other distinguishing features of SFT include characteristic ropy collagen, hemangiopericytomatous (staghorn-type) blood vessels, and diffuse nuclear STAT6 immunoreactivity. Both SFT and CFPT/RNFP are CD34 positive.

References: [21–35]

12. Do ganglioneuromas arise as solitary or multiple lesions?

- In the GI tract, there are three different clinical presentations:
  - Solitary polypoid ganglioneuroma (most common)
    Single polyp
    Sporadic, not associated with any syndromes
    Middle to older adults
    Colon by far the most common site
  - Ganglioneuromatous polyposis
    Multiple polyps.
    Ganglioneuromatous polyps may be focal or diffuse.
    Upper and lower GI tract affected.
    Associated with Cowden syndrome (PTEN hamartoma tumor syndrome, germline mutations in the *PTEN* gene): a mixed polyposis syndrome. The patients may have:
    - Adenomas
    - Hyperplastic polyps
    - Inflammatory polyps
    - Hamartomatous polyps
    - Ganglioneuromatous polyps

    If one identifies multiple ganglioneuromatous polyps, or mixture of ganglioneuromas with other types of polyps, the pathology report should suggest the possibility that the patient has Cowden syndrome, as these patients are at a much higher risk for colorectal, breast, and thyroid cancers.
  - Ganglioneuromatosis (diffuse, not polypoid, involvement)
    Associated with both multiple endocrine neoplasia type 2 (MEN2) and neurofibromatosis type 1 (NF1).
    MEN2 usually involves the intestines or esophagus and may present in childhood or adulthood. Abdominal pain, constipation, and diarrhea are common symptoms. Megacolon may occur. Recommendation within the pathology report to exclude MEN2 is important to ensure screening for medullary thyroid carcinoma.
    NF1 may also show additional diverse GI tumors, including somatostatinoma, multiple GISTs (usually of small bowel), gangliocytic paraganglioma of the duodenum, and visceral neurofibroma. Patients typically show other clinical diagnostic features of NF1, such as multiple neurofibromas, plexiform neurofibromas, Lisch nodules, etc.
- Histology shows an admixture of Schwann cells and ganglion cells set in a collagenous stroma; the ganglion cells may be numerous or focal. Immunohistochemistry is not usually needed, as the combination of Schwann cells and ganglion cells is specific. If immunostains are used, the Schwann cells will be diffusely and strongly positive for S100, while the ganglion cells will be positive for S100, NSE, and synaptophysin.
- Solitary polypoid gangliomas and ganglioneuromatous polyposis of the GI tract both arise in the mucosa with usually limited extension into submucosa. Colonic crypts are surrounded by lesional tissue and not destroyed (Fig. 16.5a, b).
- GI tract ganglioneuromatosis shows more infiltration and less polypoid growth.
  - In MEN2B, the neoplasm involves both the myenteric and submucosal plexi, with infiltration through the muscularis propria and minimal involvement of the mucosa.
  - In NF1 patients, the neoplasm is centered in the mucosa and submucosa (Fig. 16.6a, b).
- GI tract solitary polypoid ganglioneuromas and GI ganglioneuromatous polyposis are benign. These tumors do not metastasize.
- Patients with GI tract ganglioneuromatosis may experience intestinal obstruction or chronic constipation which may require excision.

13. What other lesions are in the differential diagnosis for ganglioneuroma?

- If ganglion cells are present, essentially none.
- In a small biopsy without ganglion cells, differentials may include:

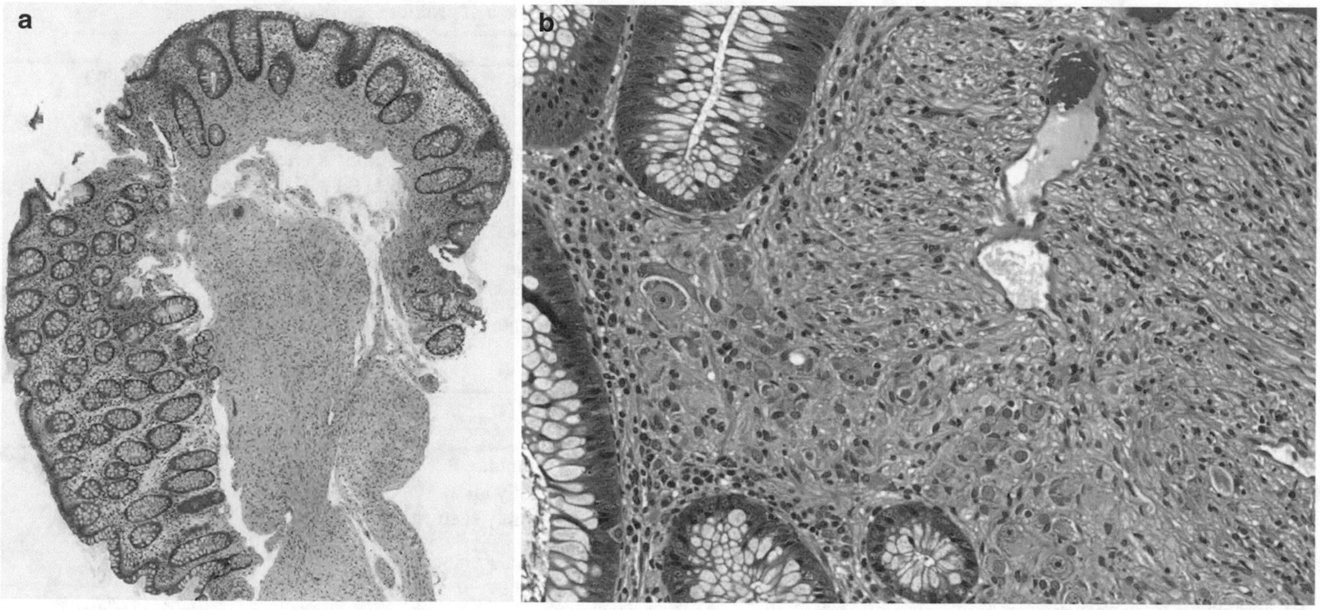

Fig. 16.5 (**a**) Solitary polypoid ganglioneuroma of the colon involving the mucosa and possibly the superficial submucosa. (**b**) Higher power view showing an admixture of Schwann cells and ganglion cells

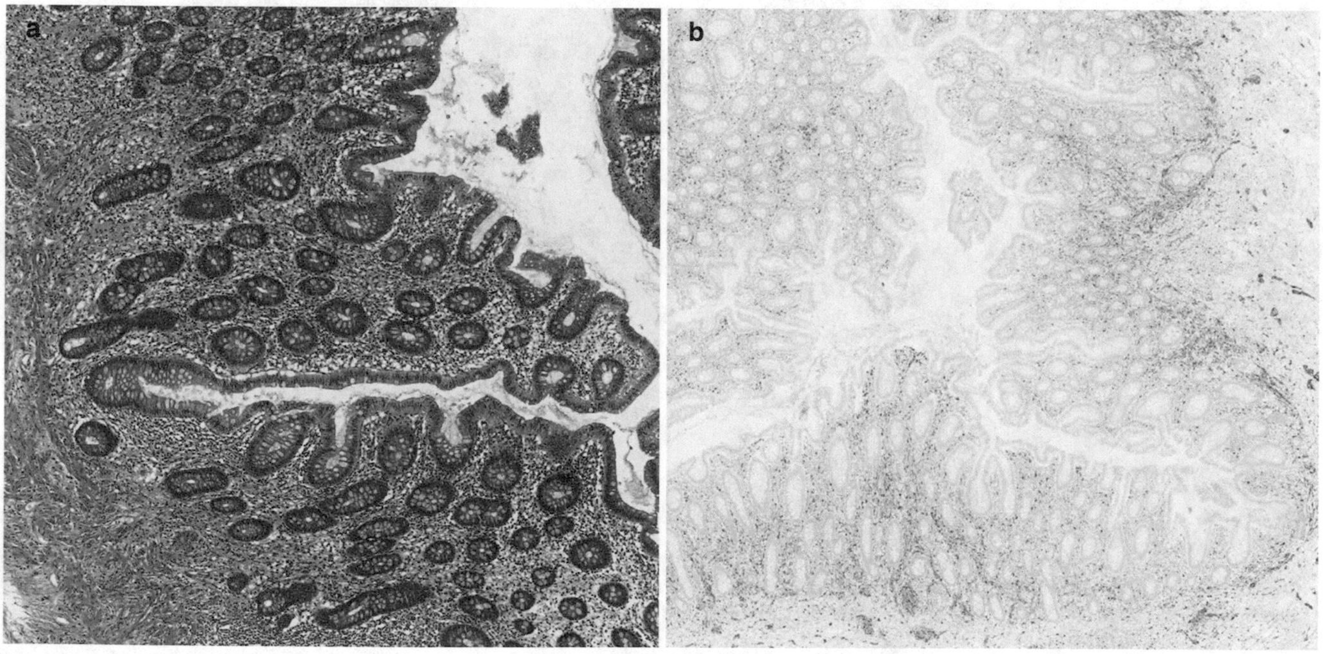

Fig. 16.6 (**a**) Diffuse ganglioneuromatosis is centered in the mucosa and submucosa in a NF1 patient, highlighted by S100 immunohistochemical stain (**b**)

- Schwann cell hamartoma (usually located in colon)
- Perineurioma (negative for S100, positive for EMA/claudin-1/GLUT-1)
- Schwannoma (usually arising from muscularis propria and most common in the stomach)
- Neurofibroma (positive for both S100 and CD34)

References: [36–38]

14. What tumors are in the differential diagnosis of mucosal perineurioma and how can one distinguish these histologically?

- Mucosal perineurioma can be distinguished from other benign spindle cell proliferations on the basis of histology, location, and immunohistochemical staining (Table 16.2; Fig. 16.7a, b).

Table 16.2 Distinction between mucosal perineurioma and other types of benign spindle cell proliferation in the GI tract

Lesion	Histology	Location	IHC
Mucosal perineurioma	Circumscribed expansion of the lamina propria by uniform, bland spindled cells with oval to elongated nuclei, indistinct cytoplasm. Distortion, entrapment, or hyperplasia of adjacent crypts with an intact mucosal surface. Crypts may resemble a hyperplastic polyp or a sessile serrated adenoma/polyp (Fig. 16.7a, b). An inflammatory component is absent. No nuclear pleomorphism, atypia, or mitotic figures	Lamina propria. Virtually all in colorectum	Perineurial markers (EMA, GLUT-1, claudin-1, and collagen type IV) are positive, and S100 is negative. EMA staining is often patchy and weak, while GLUT-1 and claudin-1 typically show diffuse strong staining
Schwannoma	Usually uniformly cellular, Verocay bodies rarely seen, peripheral lymphoid cuff characteristic, degenerative-type atypia may be seen	Intramural. Majority in the stomach	S100 positive, perineurial markers negative
Ganglioneuroma	Ganglion cells and spindled cells	Virtually all in colorectum	S100 positive, perineurial markers negative
Schwann cell hamartoma	Not associated with hyperplastic/serrated crypts	Confined to lamina propria. Virtually all in colorectum; rarely seen at gastroesophageal junction	S100 positive, perineurial markers negative

IHC immunohistochemistry

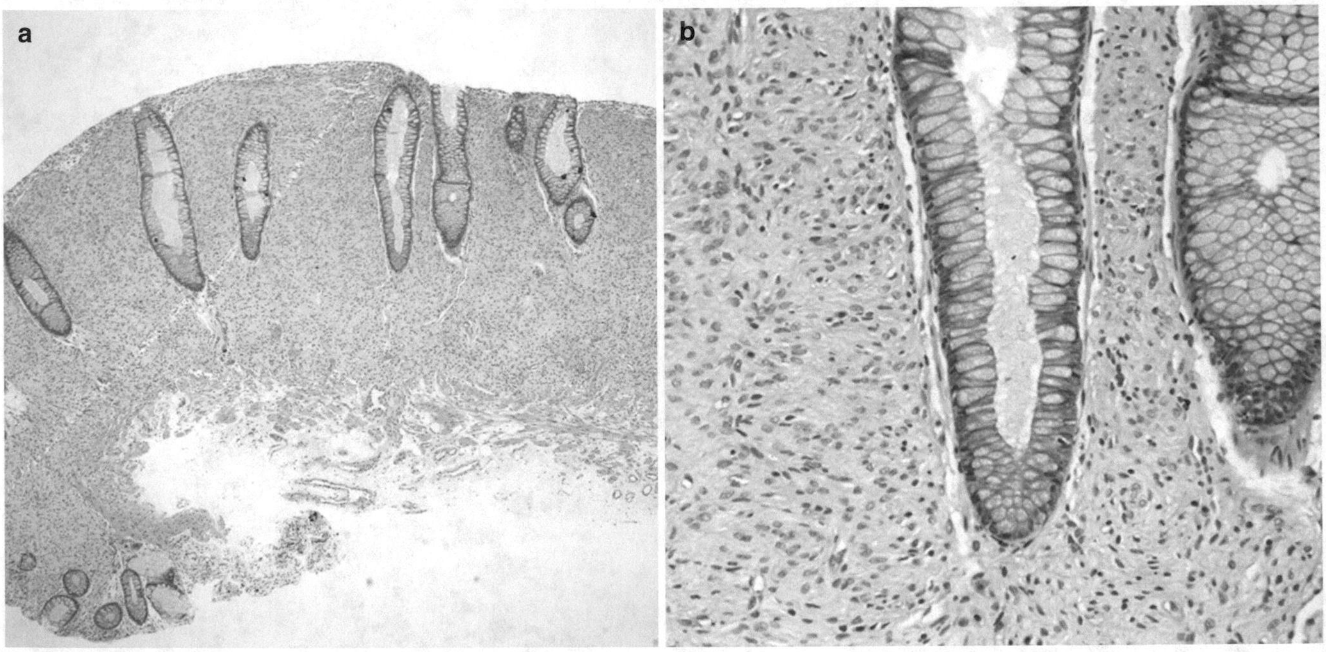

Fig. 16.7 (**a**) Mucosal perineurioma expanding the lamina propria with uniform sheets of spindled cells. Note the associated serrated epithelium, which is frequently seen. (**b**) Higher power view showing bland spindled cells with oval nuclei

15. **Where does mucosal perineurioma typically arise?**
    - Virtually all occur in the colon or rectum of adults (average age 60), equally in males and females.
    - Prior name for these was "benign fibroblastic polyp."
    - Depending on how cases are selected, molecular studies of the epithelial component, but not the spindled component, show the same *BRAF* V600E mutation seen in sessile serrated adenoma/polyps or hyperplastic polyps in 50–100% of lesions with epithelial serrations. While this relationship currently is uncertain, some authors believe the perineuriomatous stroma could represent a reactive response to the underlying hyperplastic polyp or sessile serrated adenoma/polyp. If true, this would affect the patient's risk for subsequent colon cancer development and thus would affect current screening recommendations. Further research is required to clarify this.

    References: [39–45]

16. **What mutations are often seen in inflammatory fibroid polyp and why is this interesting?**
   - The etiology of IFP has been long debated. Originally, it was hypothesized to be a reactive/granulomatous lesion. Recent systematic and molecular studies have postulated that IFPs are within the spectrum of mesenchymal tumors similar to a subset of GIST because of their shared immunoreactivity for CD34 as well as similar gain of function *PDGFRA* mutations.
     - The *PDGFRA* mutation is a key element in the pathogenesis of IFPs. Recognition of the *PDGFRA* mutation has changed the perception regarding these polyps, which are now considered to represent true neoplasms rather than reactive lesions.
     - The *PDGFRA* gene maps to chromosome 4q12 and encodes a transmembrane glycoprotein of type III receptor tyrosine kinase. This protein is highly homologous to KIT. Normally, PDGFRA kinase is activated by its ligands, platelet-derived growth factors, but mutations can lead to ligand-independent kinase activation.
     - It has been reported that 70% of IFPs contain mutations in exons 12 and 18 of the *PDGFRA* gene.
     - Interestingly, the specific exon involved in the *PDGFRA* activating mutations is associated with the IFP anatomic location; exon 12 mutations are more often associated with small intestinal lesions, whereas exon 18 mutations are associated with gastric IFPs.

17. **Where does inflammatory fibroid polyp usually occur?**
   - IFP is a rare benign lesion of the GI tract. It is a solitary, nonencapsulated, polypoid lesion. Although they arise in the submucosa, most examples extend into the overlying mucosa (Fig. 16.8a).
     - At least 1000 IFPs have been described thus far in the literature, of which 70% have been gastric in origin (0.1% of all gastric polyps), arising mainly from the antrum, followed by the ileum (23%).
     - Outside of the stomach and ileum, the incidence of GI tract IFPs is low, but cases have been reported throughout the GI tract.
     - Clinical presentation depends on the site of involvement. Gastric and colonic IFPs are typically identified incidentally at endoscopy, whereas small intestinal lesions are often encountered in the setting of intussusception.

18. **How can inflammatory fibroid polyp be distinguished from other entities in the differential diagnosis?**
   - GI tract tumors characterized by spindle and stellate cells set in a background of an inflammatory and myxoid stroma can be diagnostically challenging. The differential diagnosis for IFPs may include GIST, IMT, and mucosal perineurioma (Table 16.3).
   - IFPs are composed of uniform spindled cells and mixed inflammatory cells with increased eosinophils. The spindle cells have amphophilic cytoplasm and pale nuclei, ranging from ovoid to spindle shape, that display variable collagen deposition within a loose collagenous to myxoid stroma (Fig. 16.8b).
     - A characteristic finding and often a clue to the diagnosis is the presence of concentric cuffing of vessels by the spindle cells, referred to as an "onion skinning" appearance.
     - The proliferating stromal cells in IFPs are diffusely positive for CD34 (Fig. 16.8c), fascin, and cyclin D1 and are frequently immunoreactive for calponin, SMA, and CD35. These findings suggest

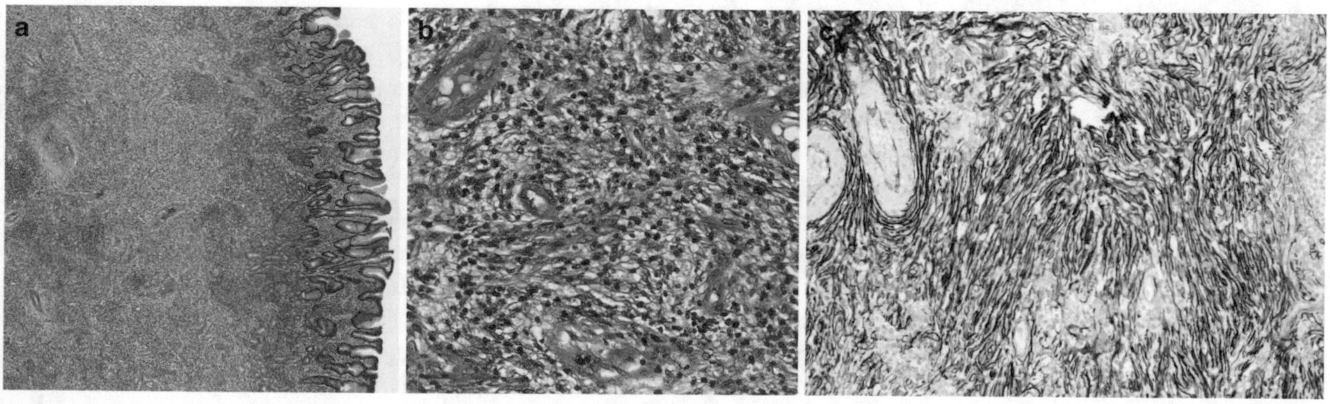

Fig. 16.8 (**a**) Inflammatory fibroid polyp centered in the submucosa with extension into the overlying mucosa. (**b**) Higher power view showing uniform spindled cells and mixed inflammatory cells including prominent eosinophils. (**c**) Spindled cells are immunohistochemically positive for CD34

Table 16.3 Unique features of GIST, IMT, and mucosal perineurioma to distinguish from IFP

Tumor	Features to distinguish from IFP
GIST	Arise from the interstitial cells of Cajal within the muscularis propria Minimal background inflammatory cells with very few eosinophils c-Kit and DOG1 positive Gain-of-function mutations in the *KIT* gene
IMT	Inflammatory infiltrate predominantly lymphoplasmacytic with very few eosinophils CD34 negative and ALK positive
Mucosal perineurioma	Almost always in the rectosigmoid colon Minimal to no background inflammatory cells Often associated with sessile serrated adenoma/polyp or hyperplastic polyp EMA and GLUT-1 positive, CD34 negative

GIST gastrointestinal stromal tumor, *IMT* inflammatory myofibroblastic tumor, *IFP* inflammatory fibroid polyp

that the proliferating stromal cells are of dendritic cell origin with myofibroblastic differentiation. IFPs are negative for HMB-45, desmin, h-caldesmon, S100, EMA, ALK, DOG1, and c-kit.
  - IFPs are benign lesion with no risk of malignant transformation and an excellent prognosis even in cases that extend beyond the muscularis propria.
- GISTs are the most common mesenchymal tumors of the GI tract and are commonly found in the stomach and small intestine. In contrast to IFPs which arise in the submucosa, GISTs arise from the interstitial cells of Cajal within the muscularis propria layer of the GI tract (see Chap. 19).
  - Morphologically, GISTs are cellular tumors composed of spindle or epithelioid cells and can show a wide variety of histologic features with minimal background inflammatory cells.
  - Immunohistochemically, GISTs are c-kit, DOG1, and CD34 positive with some cases staining for SMA, desmin, and S100.
  - Gain-of-function mutations have been found in the *KIT* gene (80–85% of cases) and in the *PDGFRA* gene (5%). Similar to IFPs, *PDGFRA* mutations are found mostly in exon 12 and exon 18.
  - The most reliable prognostic factors for GIST are size of the primary tumor and the mitotic index. Additionally, recurrence and survival rates can be affected by the location of the primary GIST lesion (e.g., small bowel and colorectal primary GIST have worse prognosis than gastric GISTs).
  - *PDGFRA* mutations (almost always in gastric primaries) appear to be a favorable prognostic factor for low risk of recurrence.
- IMT is another key differential of IFPs. They can arise anywhere in the wall of GI tract. The stomach and small intestine are the most common locations. Similar to IFPs, IMTs feature prominent inflammatory infiltrates admixed with spindle-shaped fibroblasts/myofibroblasts set in a collagenous, fibrovascular, or myxoid stroma. The inflammatory infiltrate, however, is predominantly lymphoplasmacytic with very few eosinophils (see Chap. 20).
  - IMTs have been reported in a variety of organs, including lung, lymph nodes, spleen, liver, urinary bladder, and mesentery. Unlike IMTs, IFPs are restricted to the gastrointestinal tract.
  - Immunohistochemically, IMTs are negative for CD34, c-kit, and S100 and positive for SMA and cytokeratins which may be helpful in distinguishing IMTs from other soft tissue neoplasms.
  - 50–60% of IMTs carry translocations involving the *ALK* gene on chromosome 2p23 resulting in constitutive activation of the ALK tyrosine kinase. By immunohistochemistry, ALK has been detected in about 60–70% of cases, a finding that is helpful in both the diagnosis and prognosis.
  - In general, IMTs follow a benign course with a favorable outcome after they are surgically removed. In some cases, they can be invasive, recur locally, or metastasize (<5%).
  - Epithelioid variant of IMT is almost exclusively seen in the omentum or mesentery, with marked male predominance. It is characterized by vesicular nuclear and prominent large nucleoli in loose sheets set in a myxoid stroma. Mitoses may be readily seen. Abundant mixed inflammatory cells and a prominent neutrophilic infiltrate may be present. ALK-RANBP2 fusion is seen in epithelioid variant and thought to result in the characteristic ALK membrane staining.
- Mucosal perineurioma, also known as benign fibroblastic polyp, is another differential of IFPs (see above). These are incidental lesions detected in adult patients undergoing screening colonoscopy. They present as small, solitary, asymptomatic polyps almost always encountered in the rectosigmoid colon.
  - Mucosal perineuriomas lack the prominent inflammation, concentric perivascular, and periglandular arrangement of the spindle cells and the edematous or myxoid change commonly seen in IFPs. Although a vague, concentric, periglandular, and perivascular arrangement of the spindle cells has been noted in perineuriomas, this is typically not the predominant pattern and is considered a nonspecific histologic finding.

- Mucosal perineuriomas are often associated with sessile serrated adenoma/polyp or hyperplastic polyp.
- Immunohistochemically, mucosal perineuriomas are strongly and diffusely positive for GLUT-1 and weakly, patchy positive for EMA. They are negative for CD34, c-kit, S100, desmin, SMA, keratins, and cyclin D1.
- Similar to IFPs, mucosal perineuriomas are benign lesions and have an excellent prognosis after complete excision.

References: [27, 29, 45–52]

19. What immunostains may be useful in the diagnosis of glomus tumor?

- Glomus tumors stain for SMA, calponin, MSA, and type IV collagen (Table 16.4).

20. What is the differential diagnosis for glomus tumor?

- Glomus tumors are composed of epithelioid cells with small round nuclei and distinct cell borders, growing in nests and trabeculae surrounded by a thin vascular network (Fig. 16.9a, b).
- Epithelioid GIST (see Chap. 19).
  - GISTs with epithelioid cytomorphology may arise in a similar location as glomus tumors of the GI tract, usually the stomach, and both tumors can have clear cytoplasm. Glomus tumors demonstrate characteristic cytomorphology showing round lesional cells with distinct cell borders and uniform nuclei. Epithelioid GISTs have indistinct cell borders and often have more oval or spindled cells.
  - The immunohistochemical profile of GIST includes positive staining for c-kit (95%) and DOG1 (95%), while SMA is frequently negative (13–47% depending on location). Glomus tumors are negative for c-kit and DOG1 and are positive for SMA (99%), type IV collagen (94–100%), and CD34 (18–32%).
  - Most GISTs are characterized by activating mutation in *KIT* (80–85%) or *PDGFRA* (5–7%), while mutations in these genes are absent in glomus tumors.

    MIR143-NOTCH fusion has been shown to drive tumorigenesis of >50% of glomus tumors, regardless of location or degree of malignancy.
- Vascular tumors.
  - Glomus tumors are highly vascular and occasionally are misidentified as either an epithelioid hemangioma or, rarely, epithelioid angiosarcoma.
  - Glomus tumor cells are negative for endothelial markers (CD31, ERG), while CD34 is often patchy positive.
- Well-differentiated neuroendocrine tumor (NET).
  - These lesions are the closest morphological mimicker of glomus tumor, being composed of epithelioid cells with round nuclei and inconspicuous nucleoli, growing in nests and trabeculae surrounded by a thin vascular network.
  - Immunohistochemistry is most helpful, with NET virtually all positive for synaptophysin and chromogranin and negative for SMA. Weak synaptophysin immunoreactivity can be seen in glomus tumors, however (Fig. 16.9c).

References: [53–62]

Table 16.4 Useful immunostains for the diagnosis of granular cell tumor

SMA	99%
MSA	95%
Calponin	100%
CD34	18–32%
S100	2%
Collagen type IV	94–100%
Keratins, desmin, CD31	Negative

SMA smooth muscle actin, *MSA* muscle-specific actin

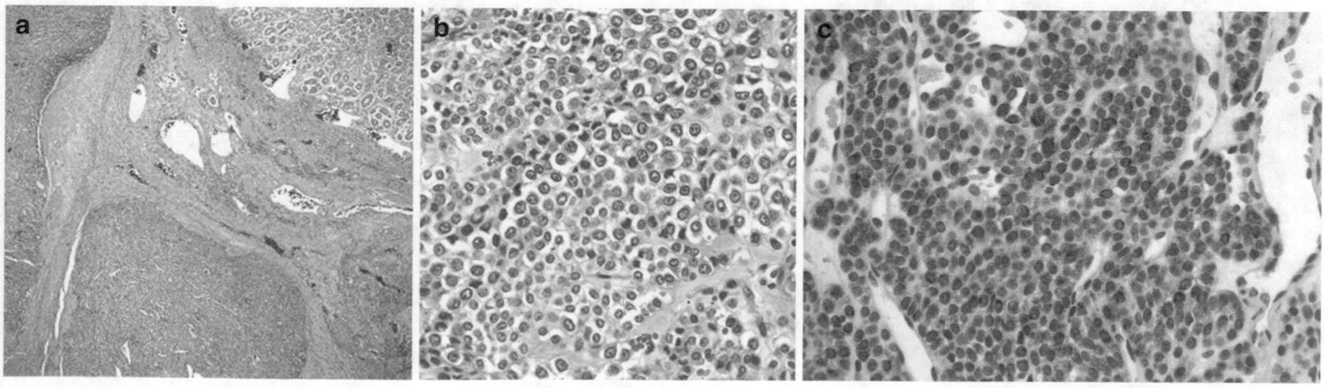

Fig. 16.9 Glomus tumor of the stomach. (**a**) Low power showing nodular growth pattern and relation to mucosa. (**b**) Higher power view showing epithelioid cells with round nuclei and distinct cell borders. (**c**) Weak synaptophysin immunoreactivity can be detected in glomus tumor cells

21. What entities are in the differential diagnosis for leiomyoma?

- Leiomyoma is the second most common mesenchymal neoplasm of the GI tract, after GIST (Table 16.5).

Table 16.5 Unique features of GIST, GI schwannoma, and IFP- and EBV-associated smooth muscle neoplasm to distinguish from leiomyoma

Tumor	Features that distinguish from leiomyoma
GIST	Arise from the interstitial cells of Cajal within the muscularis propria Much more common in stomach and small intestine c-Kit and DOG1 positive Mutations in the *KIT* or *PDGFRA* genes
GI schwannoma	Peripheral cuff-like lymphoid aggregates with germinal centers Centered in the muscularis propria Commonly arise in the stomach S100 and GFAP positive
IFP	Submucosa/mucosa of stomach and small bowel Marked inflammatory infiltrate, many eosinophils CD34, SMA positive; desmin negative
EBV-associated smooth muscle neoplasm	Arises in immunosuppressed patients Multifocal lesion Presence of variable numbers of intratumoral lymphocytes Primitive small ovoid blue cell areas or more mature-appearing smooth muscle cells may be seen EBV EBER is strongly and diffusely positive

GIST gastrointestinal stromal tumor, *IFP* inflammatory fibroid polyp

The two main differential diagnoses include GIST and schwannoma. A much rarer entity that can highly mimic leiomyoma is an EBV-associated smooth muscle tumor.

- Leiomyomas are most commonly seen in the esophagus and colorectum. It is the most common mesenchymal neoplasm in the esophagus. In the esophagus, the mid-esophagus and the gastroesophageal (GE) junction are the most common sites.
- In the esophagus, leiomyomas arise from the muscularis propria, may result in a single or multiple luminal polypoid projections, and may grow to large size (>10 cm) with resultant mediastinal compression.
- Leiomyomas of the colorectum arise from the muscularis mucosae and usually present incidentally as polyps on colonoscopy (Fig. 16.10a).
- GISTs usually occur in an inverse anatomic location compared to leiomyomas.
  - GISTs are much more common in the stomach and small intestine and more commonly arise from the muscularis propria.
  - Histologically, leiomyomas are less cellular and have abundant eosinophilic cytoplasm compared to GISTs.
  - Immunohistochemically, leiomyomas are negative for CD34, c-kit, and DOG1 and positive for SMA, caldesmon, and desmin.
  - One diagnostic pitfall to be aware of is that numerous c-kit-positive mast cells are often present within leiomyomas. Furthermore,

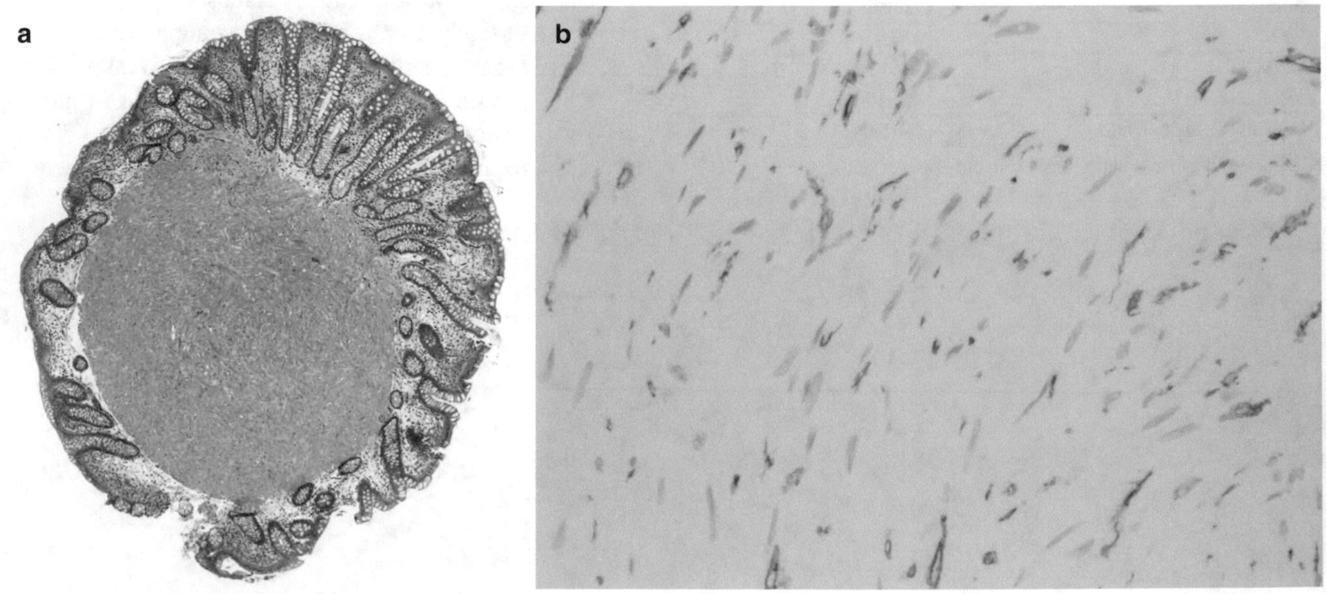

Fig. 16.10 Leiomyoma of the colorectum incidentally detected as a small polyp on colonoscopy. (**a**) The tumor arises from the muscularis mucosae and grows into the submucosa. (**b**) Numerous colonized interstitial cells of Cajal can be detected by c-kit or DOG1 immunohistochemistry

numerous c-kit- and DOG1-positive spindle cell (dendritic-like) elements are often present between smooth muscle cells, believed to represent colonization by Cajal cells (Fig. 16.10b). This should not be confused with GISTs because the tumor cells proper (the smooth muscle cells) are negative for these GIST markers.
  - Leiomyomas are wild type for *KIT* and *PDGFRA* mutations.
- GI tract schwannomas are composed of fascicles of bland spindle cells with plump nuclei and fibrillary eosinophilic cytoplasm.
  - GI schwannomas are notable for the presence of peripheral cuff-like lymphoid aggregates with germinal centers, a feature not seen in leiomyomas.
  - They are typically found in the stomach, although the colon and rectum is the second most common site. Leiomyomas are most common in the esophagus and colorectum.
  - These tumors are often incidentally discovered during routine colonoscopy. However, if large enough, they can cause GI bleeding, abdominal pain/discomfort, and obstructive symptoms.
  - Immunohistochemical staining is very helpful. Schwannomas are strongly positive for S100 and GFAP and negative for SMA, desmin, c-kit, and DOG1.
- IFPs usually arise in the submucosa of the stomach and small bowel, which are unusual sites for leiomyoma.
  - Lesional cells are ovoid, spindled, or epithelioid cells with scant cytoplasm set in a myxoid to edematous stroma.
  - Unlike leiomyoma, IFPs show a marked intratumoral inflammatory infiltrate consisting predominantly of eosinophils as well as lymphocytes and histiocytes.
  - IFPs are positive for CD34. A minority of cases are positive for SMA, but they are negative for desmin, c-kit, DOG1, and S100.
- EBV-associated smooth muscle neoplasm is an uncommon neoplasm affecting both adult and pediatric populations. It has been reported to occur at numerous visceral sites and soft tissue and often presents as multifocal lesions (see Chap. 20).
  - It arises in immunosuppressed patients.
  - The clinical findings are related to the site of tumor manifestation. The main presentation in these patients is pain and organ dysfunction.
  - Histology can be quite variable within the same tumor and between tumors within the same patient.
  - Unique histologic features include the presence of variable numbers of intratumoral lymphocytes. The lymphocytic infiltrate is composed primarily of T-cells. Distinct histologic features within or between tumors may be seen, with some areas showing primitive small ovoid blue cells, while other areas have the appearance of well-differentiated/mature smooth muscle cells.
  - Immunohistochemical staining is positive for SMA in all histologic types. Desmin is often positive in the more mature-appearing areas and overall more variable in expression.
  - EBV EBER is strongly and diffusely positive and is diagnostic.

22. **What histologic features indicate leiomyosarcoma rather than leiomyoma?**
- Histologic features indicate leiomyosarcoma including infiltrative growth, marked nuclear atypia, pleomorphism, and brisk mitotic activity (>10/10 HPFs) (Fig. 16.11a).
- Coagulative tumor necrosis can often be seen in leiomyosarcomas.
- Grossly, leiomyosarcomas often present as large transmural masses with grossly obvious necrosis.
  - It is difficult to estimate the prevalence of true leiomyosarcomas of the GI tract in the post-GIST era because the older literature predates analyses of c-kit expression and *KIT* mutations to allow their accurate separation from GISTs. Large case series since 2000 have reported fewer than 100 GI tract leiomyosarcomas.
- Leiomyomas are composed of fascicles of uniform, spindled, well-differentiated smooth muscle cells with abundant eosinophilic cytoplasm, minimal to no nuclear atypia, and infrequent mitotic activity (Fig. 16.11b). Coagulative necrosis should not be seen in leiomyomas. Occasionally, degenerative atypia can be seen similar to the changes seen in leiomyoma with bizarre nuclei (previously known as atypical leiomyoma/symplastic leiomyoma) of the uterus.
  - Leiomyomas are common smooth muscle tumors mainly found in the esophagus, GE junction, and colon, typically arising in association with the muscularis mucosae (colon) or muscularis propria (esophagus/GE junction).
  - Colonic leiomyomas are typically small, usually an incidental finding in patients undergoing screening colonoscopy.
  - Grossly, leiomyomas are firm, well-circumscribed, tan-white masses with a whorled cut surface similar to leiomyomas in other sites.

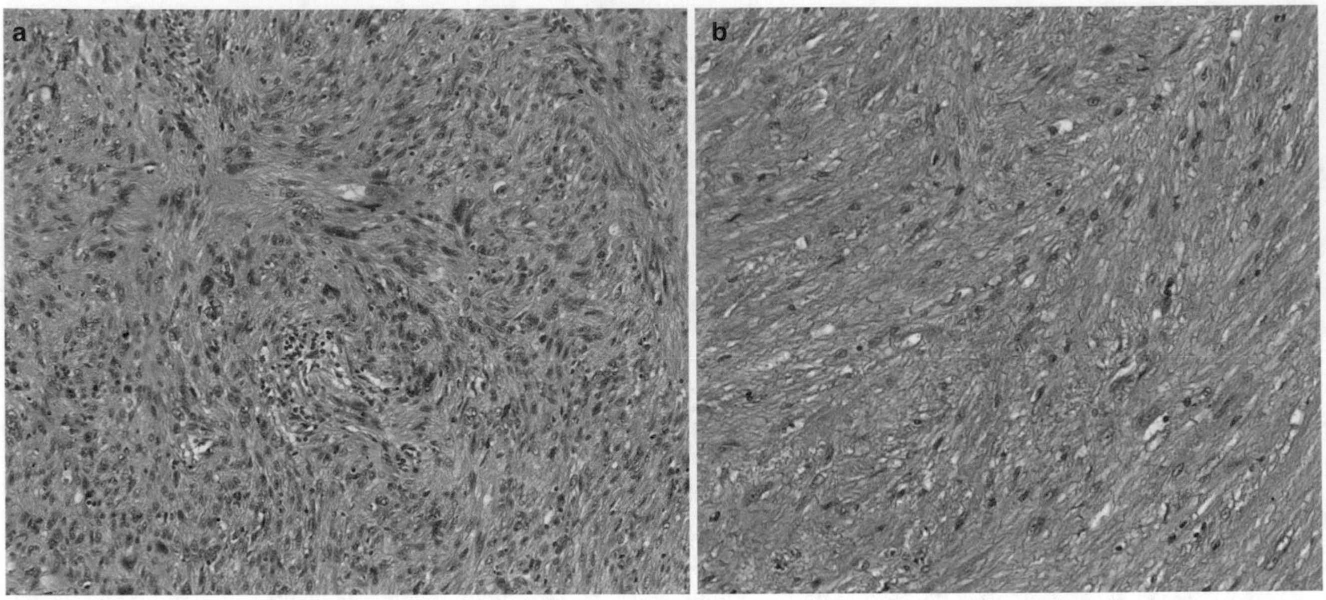

Fig. 16.11 (a) Leiomyosarcoma showing marked nuclear atypia, nuclear pleomorphism, and brisk mitotic activity. (b) In contrast, leiomyoma is composed of fascicles of uniform, spindled, well-differentiated smooth muscle cells

- Leiomyomas are benign lesions with no risk of malignant transformation and have an excellent prognosis after complete excision. Rare recurrence can occur, however.

  References: [63–72]

23. Where does lipoma commonly arise?

- Lipomas are common benign neoplasms of mature adipocytes that can be found throughout the GI tract.
  - Approximately 70% of GI tract lipomas are located in the colon, the most common site being the cecum and ascending colon, followed by the small intestine (20–25%) and stomach (5%).
  - The vast majority of colonic lipomas are located in the submucosa; the remainder of these tumors are subserosal or intramucosal in origin.

24. How can one distinguish a lipoma from a well-differentiated liposarcoma?

- Liposarcomas are one of the most common soft tissue sarcomas of adults. They commonly occur in deep soft tissues of the extremities and retroperitoneum.
- Unlike lipomas, the GI tract does not represent a typical location for primary liposarcomas.
- Rare cases of primary liposarcoma have been reported in different parts of the GI tract, such as esophagus, stomach, and small intestine. Primary liposarcomas of the colon are extremely rare.
- The GI tract can be secondarily involved as a site for metastases from liposarcomas located in the retroperitoneum and extremities.
- Histologic features typically allow distinction between lipoma and liposarcoma.
  - Well-differentiated liposarcomas (WDLS) are often larger and more deeply seated than lipomas and contain variably thickened fibrous septa containing atypical and hyperchromatic stromal spindle cells.
  - Lipoblasts may or may not be present and are not required for the diagnosis of WDLS.
  - Lipomas can get large and extrude into the intestinal lumen, leading to traumatic and inflammatory changes, resulting in necrosis, ulceration, and hemorrhage. Secondary changes including nuclear enlargement, hyperchromasia, fat necrosis, lipoblasts, and foamy macrophages may be observed, mimicking a WDLS.
- Cytogenetics and molecular testing offer new powerful tools for differentiating benign and malignant lipomatous tumors.
  - WDLS is characterized by ring and giant marker chromosomes, sometimes as a sole finding or occasionally in association with other numerical or structural chromosomal changes.
  - The giant marker and ring chromosomes contain amplified sequences of 12q13–15. This structural abnormality results in the consistent amplification of *MDM2* and the frequent amplification of adjacent genes, like *CDK4*.
  - The high specificity and sensitivity of detection of *MDM2* and *CDK4* amplification in WDLS and dedifferentiated liposarcoma have been demon-

strated, which help identify and separate WDLS from various benign lipomatous lesions.

- MDM2 FISH has a higher sensitivity (100%) and specificity (100%) compared with MDM2 immunohistochemistry (65% sensitivity and 89% specificity) in needle core biopsies. FISH is the gold standard in the diagnosis of WDLS.
- Immunostaining of MDM2 and CDK4 proteins in lipomatous tumors can be used as a screening tool due to its lower cost and rapid turnaround time, with reflex testing by FISH if immunostaining is negative. However, FISH should be the first-line test in all cases in which WDLS is a plausible diagnosis.

References: [73, 74]

25. What are the characteristic presentation and histologic findings of lymphangioma?

- Lymphangiomas are benign hamartomatous masses consisting of dilated endothelial-lined spaces with a connective tissue scaffold interspersed with lymphocytes.
- Usually submucosal in location, these lesions can arise anywhere in the body except the central nervous system.
- Considered a disease of childhood, 90% of lymphangiomas occur in children under 2 years of age.
- In the GI tract, pediatric lymphangiomas typically arise in the mesentery and present with obstruction, while adult lymphangiomas form masses intraluminally.

26. How does one distinguish a lymphangioma from lymphangiomatosis?

- These entities have differing etiologies. Lymphangioma is thought to be a benign congenital malformation of lymphatic vasculature that forms a mass lesion. Thus, it often occurs in childhood but can remain undetected until adulthood.
- Intestinal lymphangiectasia is a dilation of existing lymphatics, which does not form a mass lesion. It can be seen in association with a variety of conditions such as sarcoidosis, Waldenstrom macroglobulinemia, neoplasms, or inflammatory conditions. Most cases are asymptomatic and represent incidental endoscopic findings. However, protein-losing enteropathy or occult GI bleeding may occur in some patients.
- Histologically, lymphangioma and lymphangiectasia of the small intestine are difficult to separate. Involvement of the mucosa and submucosa are seen in both conditions. However, lymphangiomas appear to have a distinct circumferential lining of endothelial cells invested in smooth muscle fibers and may have dense lymphoid aggregates. In contrast, lymphangiectasia appears to lack a complete, distinct endothelial lining or smooth muscle component (Fig. 16.12a, b).
- Lymphangiomas can present diffusely, involving either a single organ or multiple organ systems. This more generalized process is termed lymphangiomatosis, which is also thought to be a congenital condition that leads to abnormal development of the lymphatic system.

References: [75–78]

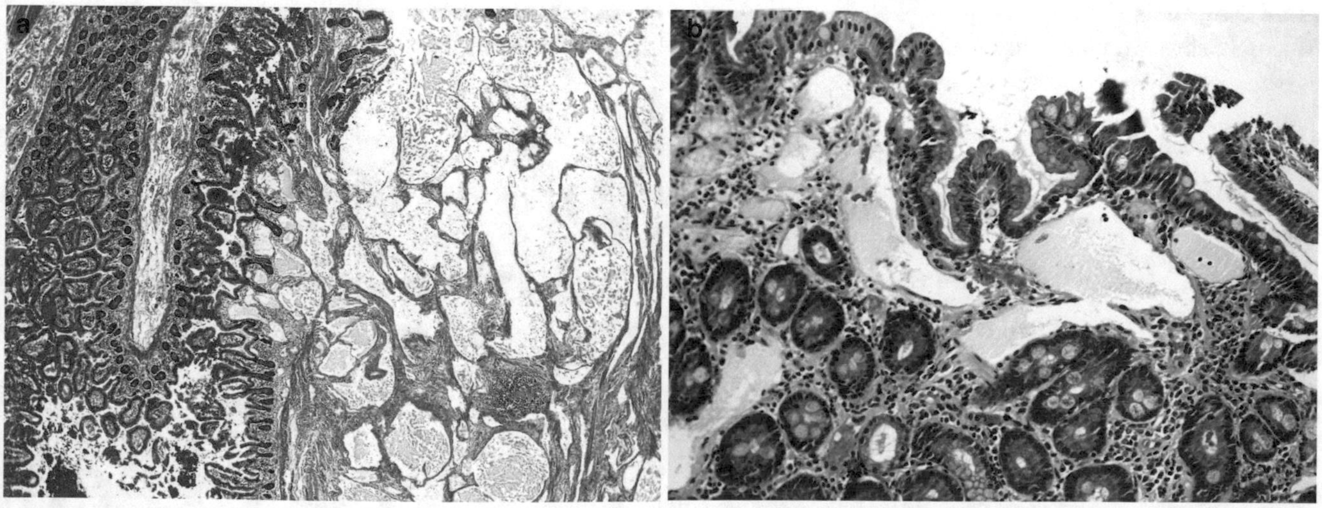

Fig. 16.12 (**a**) Lymphangioma of the small intestine showing collections of dilated lymphatics mainly seen in the submucosa. Involvement of the mucosa is also noted. Invested smooth muscle fibers and a lymphoid aggregate are appreciated at this power. (**b**) Intestinal lymphangiectasia showing dilated lymphatics with proteinaceous fluid involving the mucosa. Focal gastric foveolar metaplasia is noted in this case. It should be mentioned that rare dilated lacteals within the tips of villi are not an uncommon incidental finding in duodenal biopsies, which may not have clinical significance in many cases

Case Presentation

Case 1

Learning Objectives

1. To become familiar with histologic features of the tumor
2. To become familiar with the immunohistochemical features of the tumor
3. To generate the differential diagnosis

Case History

A 60-year-old female undergoing screening colonoscopy has a 0.5 cm sigmoid polyp.

Histologic Findings

- Diffuse, ill-defined proliferation of spindle cells within the lamina propria, surrounding the colonic crypts (Fig. 16.13a).
- Lesional cells are uniform, bland, spindled to wavy with eosinophilic cytoplasm (Fig. 16.13b).
- Mitoses are absent.

Differential Diagnosis

- Schwannoma
- Schwann cell hamartoma
- Mucosal perineurioma

Immunohistochemistry and Other Ancillary Studies

- Tumor cells show diffuse, strong S100 positivity (Fig. 16.13c).

Final Diagnosis

Mucosal Schwann cell hamartoma.

Take-Home Messages

- Schwann cell hamartoma is not associated with hyperplastic or serrated changes in the colonic crypts, unlike mucosal perineurioma.
- Schwannoma of the GI tract arises most commonly in the stomach from the muscularis propria, unlike mucosal Schwann cell hamartoma which is most common in the colorectum and arises in the mucosa.
- S100 is strongly and diffusely positive and can be helpful in confirming the diagnosis.

References: [16, 79]

Case 2

Learning Objectives

1. To become familiar with the histologic features of the tumor
2. To become familiar with the immunohistochemical features of the tumor
3. To understand the different clinical presentations of the tumor

Case History

A 35-year-old female with NF1 and a history of fecal occult blood undergoes colonoscopy with findings of multiple prominent folds throughout the colon, which are biopsied.

Histologic Findings

- Admixture of spindled cells with rare ganglion cells seen diffusely involving the lamina propria (Fig. 16.14a, b).
- Collagenous stroma.
- Mitoses are absent.

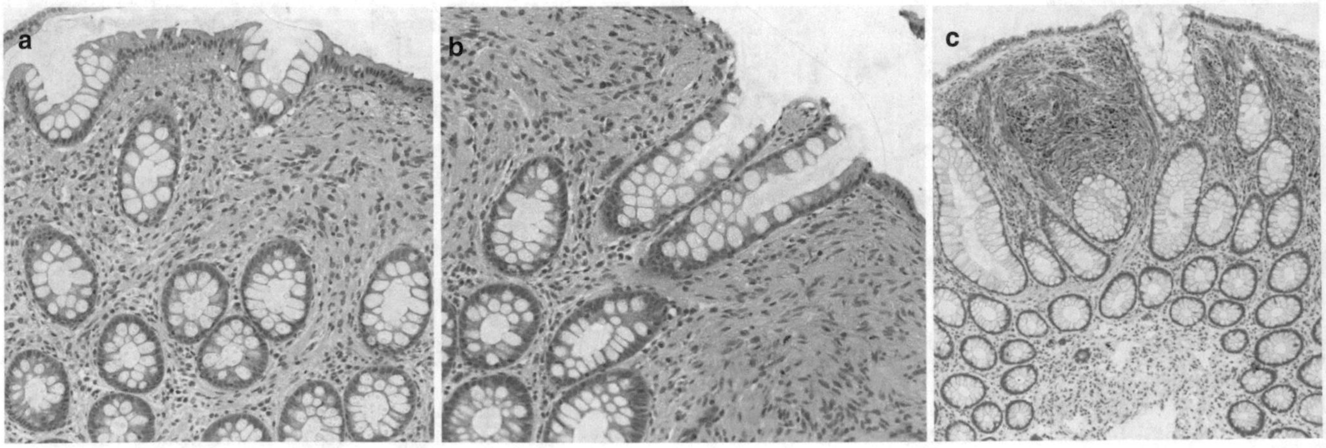

Fig. 16.13 (**a**) Schwann cell hamartoma with diffuse, ill-defined proliferation of spindle cells within the lamina propria, surrounding the colonic crypts. (**b**) Lesional cells are uniform, bland, spindled, to wavy with eosinophilic cytoplasm. (**c**) Lesional cells showing diffuse and strong S100 positivity

Differential Diagnosis

- Ganglioneuroma
- Ganglioneuromatous polyposis
- Ganglioneuromatosis

Immunohistochemistry and Other Ancillary Studies

Spindle cells show diffuse and strong S100 positivity (Fig. 16.14c).

Final Diagnosis

Diffuse ganglioneuromatosis.

Take-Home Messages

- Ganglioneuromatous lesions in the GI tract include solitary polypoid ganglioneuroma, ganglioneuromatous polyposis, and ganglioneuromatosis.
- Ganglioneuromatous polyposis is associated with Cowden syndrome (PTEN hamartoma tumor syndrome), and patients often show a mixture of polyp types including adenomas, hyperplastic polyps, inflammatory polyps, hamartomatous polyps, and ganglioneuromatous polyps.
- Ganglioneuromatosis is characterized by diffuse involvement of the GI tract and is associated with MEN2 (usually involving the submucosa and muscularis propria with minimal involvement of the mucosa) and NF1 (usually centered in the mucosa and submucosa).
- Immunohistochemistry is not usually required as the histologic combination of spindled cells and ganglion cells is characteristic.

References: [36, 37, 80]

Case 3

Learning Objectives

1. To become familiar with the histologic and immunohistochemical features of the tumor
2. To generate the differential diagnosis
3. To understand the different clinical presentations of the tumor

Case History

A 55-year-old male undergoing screening colonoscopy has a 0.5 cm rectal polyp.

Histologic Findings

- Spindled cells with ample eosinophilic cytoplasm present in fascicles beneath the colonic crypts. They appear to arise from the muscularis mucosae and extend up in between the colonic crypts (Fig. 16.15a).
- Nuclei are plump with blunt ends and show minimal pleomorphism (Fig. 16.15b).
- Mitoses are not appreciated.

Differential Diagnosis

- GIST
- Mucosal Schwann cell hamartoma
- Leiomyoma

Immunohistochemistry and Other Ancillary Studies

- Spindle cells show diffuse and strong SMA and desmin positivity (Fig. 16.15c).
- Spindle cells are negative for c-kit, DOG1, and S100.

Final Diagnosis

Leiomyoma.

Take-Home Messages

- Leiomyomas of the GI tract show the inverse anatomic presentation as GIST, being most common in the colorectum, mid-esophagus, and GE junction and rarely in the stomach and small bowel.
- In the colorectum, leiomyomas mainly arise from the muscularis mucosae, with some being described attached to the serosa, while esophageal and GE junction leiomyomas are intramural and appear to arise from the muscularis propria.

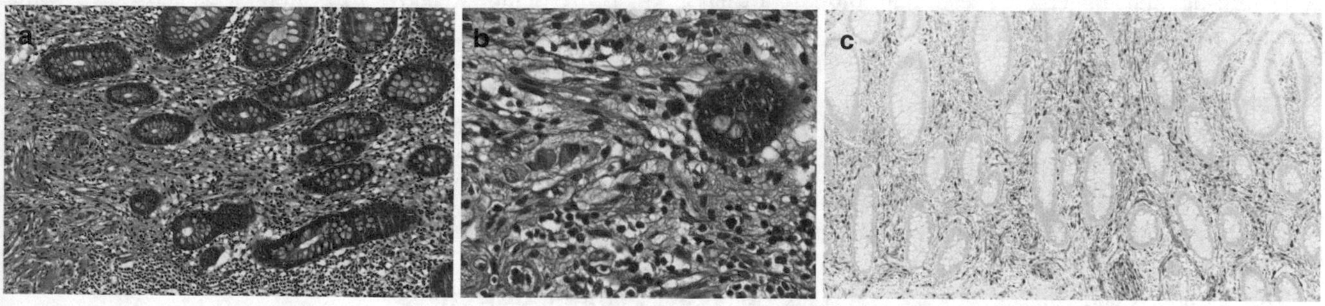

Fig. 16.14 (**a, b**) Diffuse ganglioneuromatosis showing an admixture of spindled cells with rare ganglion cells diffusely involving the lamina propria. (**c**) Lesional cells demonstrating diffuse and strong S100 positivity

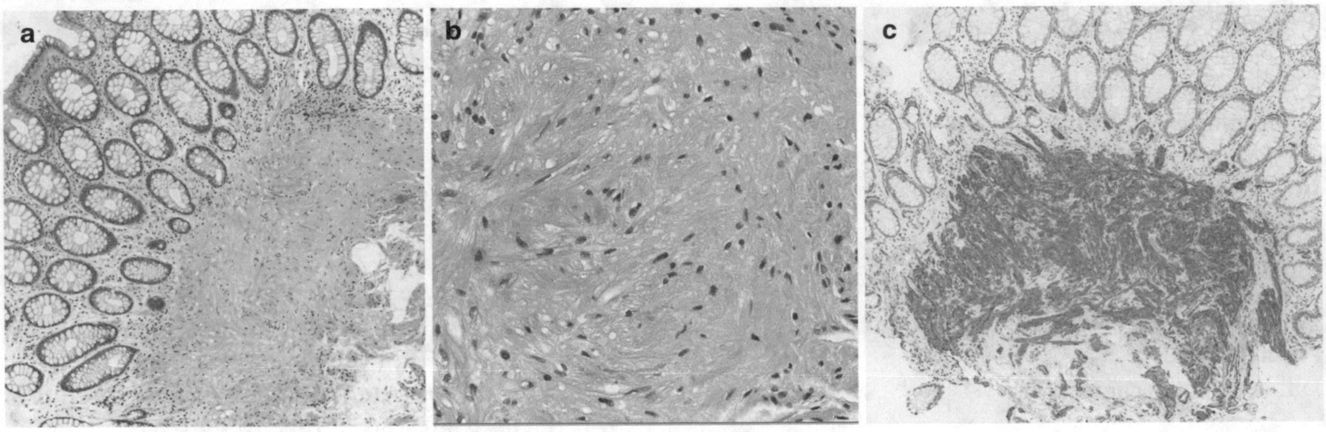

Fig. 16.15 (**a**) Leiomyoma showing spindled cells with ample eosinophilic cytoplasm present in fascicles, which appear to originate from the muscularis mucosae with extension into the deeper lamina propria and submucosa. (**b**) Lesional cells exhibiting plump nuclei with blunt ends and minimal pleomorphism. (**c**) Lesional cells demonstrating diffuse and strong SMA positivity

- Immunohistochemistry may be helpful in distinguishing leiomyoma from tumors in the differential diagnosis such as GIST (positive for c-kit and DOG1, which are negative in leiomyoma), mucosal Schwann cell hamartoma (positive for S100, which is negative in leiomyoma), and rare tumors such as EBV-associated smooth muscle tumors (usually positive for SMA and may be positive for desmin, similar to leiomyoma, but also positive for EBV-EBER, which is negative in leiomyoma).

References: [63–66]

Case 4

Learning Objectives

1. To become familiar with the histologic and immunohistochemical features of the tumor
2. To generate the differential diagnosis
3. To understand the different clinical presentations of the tumor

Case History

A 62-year-old male undergoing screening colonoscopy has a 0.3 cm transverse colon polyp.

Histologic Findings

- Circumscribed expansion of lamina propria by uniform, bland spindle cells with eosinophilic cytoplasm that are arranged haphazardly and whorl around crypts (Fig. 16.16a).
- Nuclei are oval to elongated, with fine chromatin, no nucleoli, and no pleomorphism (Fig. 16.16b).
- The entrapped and adjacent colonic crypts are distorted and hyperplastic/serrated-appearing, similar to those seen in sessile serrated adenoma/polyp (Fig. 16.16c).

Differential Diagnosis

- Mucosal perineurioma
- Mucosal Schwann cell hamartoma
- Leiomyoma

Immunohistochemistry and Other Ancillary Studies

- Spindle cells show diffuse and strong staining for GLUT-1 and weak patchy staining for EMA (Fig. 16.16d).
- Spindle cells are negative for S100, c-kit, and DOG1.

Final Diagnosis

Mucosal perineurioma.

Take-Home Messages

- Mucosal perineuriomas are benign polyps that in older literature were called benign fibroblastic polyps.
- *BRAF* mutations, identical to those seen in sessile serrated adenomas/polyps and hyperplastic polyps, are seen in the epithelial component but not in the spindle cell component, leading some authors to hypothesize that the perineuriomatous component is a reactive response to the epithelial serrated lesion.
- EMA immunoreactivity is often weak and focal, while other perineural markers such as GLUT-1 and claudin-1 are usually strong and diffuse.

References: [39–45]

Case 5

Learning Objectives

1. To become familiar with the histologic and immunohistochemical features of the tumor

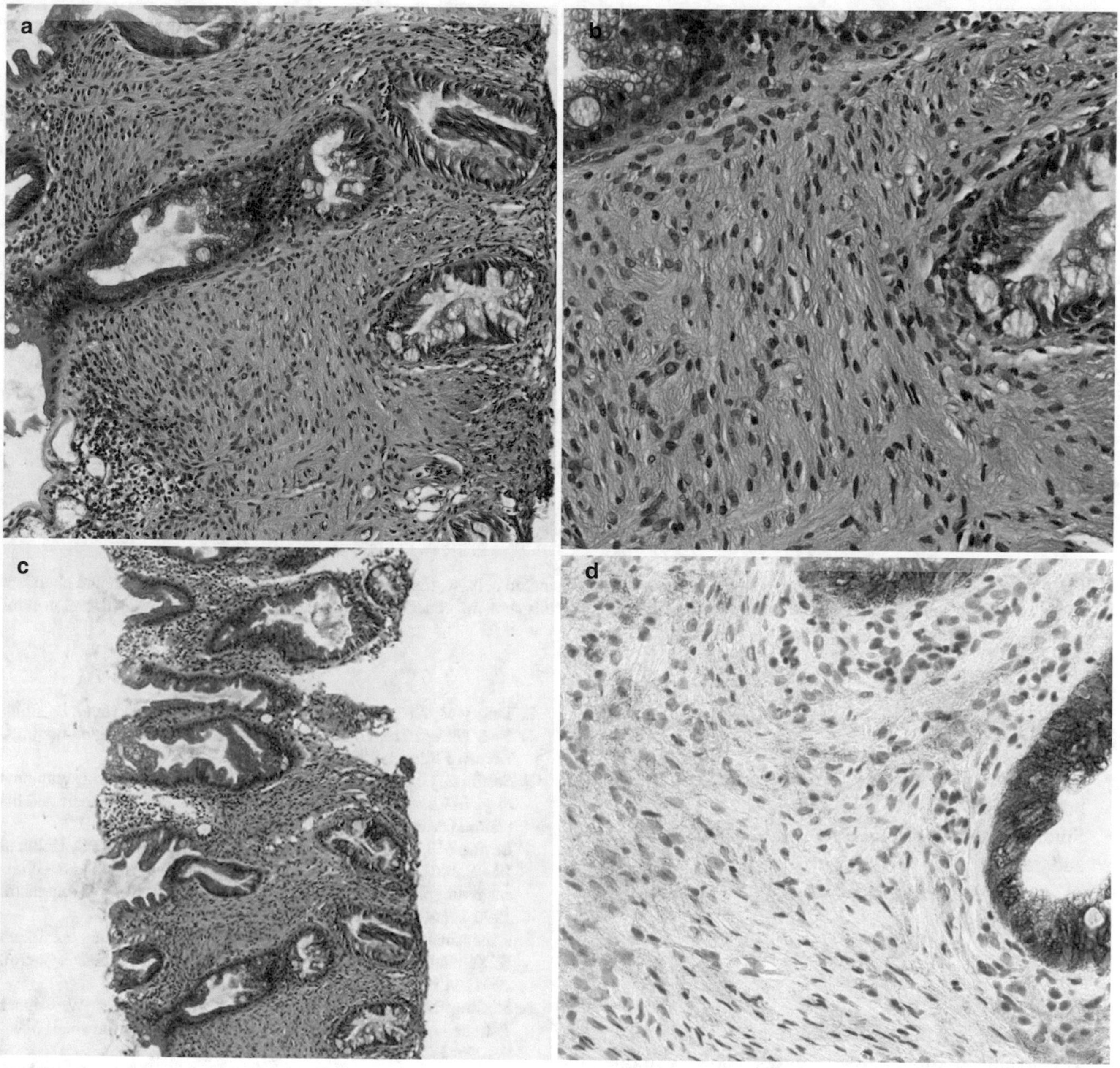

Fig. 16.16 (**a**) Mucosal perineurioma showing a circumscribed expansion of the lamina propria by haphazardly arranged uniform, bland spindle cells with eosinophilic cytoplasm. (**b**) Lesional cells have oval to elongated nuclei with fine chromatin, no nucleoli, and no pleomorphism. (**c**) The lesion distorts or entraps adjacent crypts, which often show serrated change. (**d**) Lesional cells show weak patchy staining for EMA

2. To generate the differential diagnosis
3. To understand the different clinical presentations of the tumor

Case History

A 55-year-old male with GERD undergoes upper endoscopy and is found to have a 1.0 cm polyp in the gastric antrum.

Histologic Findings

- Uniform delicate spindled cells within a loose collagenous to myxoid stroma and abundant mixed inflammatory cells including numerous eosinophils (Fig. 16.17a).
- Focally, the spindle cells show concentric cuffing of blood vessels (so-called "onion skinning" appearance) (Fig. 16.17b).

Differential Diagnosis

- GIST
- Inflammatory myofibroblastic tumor
- Mucosal perineurioma
- Inflammatory fibroid polyp

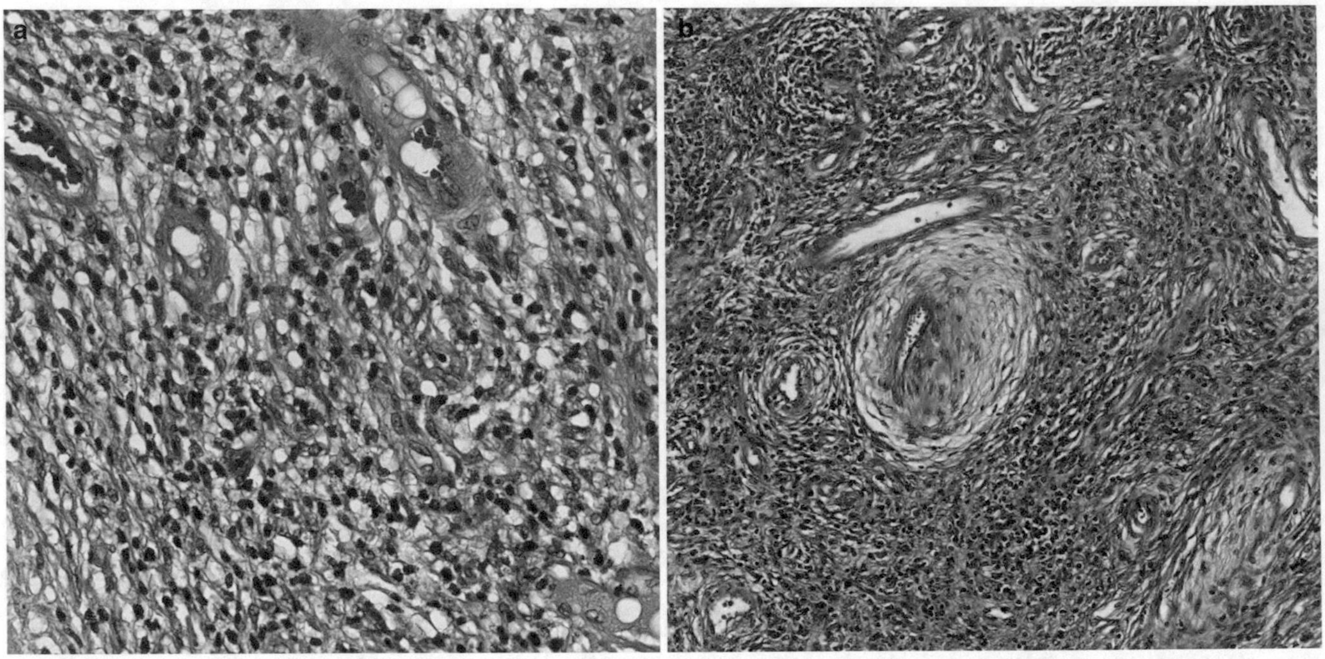

Fig. 16.17 (**a**) Inflammatory fibroid polyp contains uniform delicate spindled cells within a loose collagenous to myxoid stroma and abundant mixed inflammatory cells including numerous eosinophils. (**b**) Spindle cells showing concentric cuffing of blood vessels (so-called "onion skinning" appearance)

Immunohistochemistry and Other Ancillary Studies

- Spindle cells are diffusely positive for CD34 and patchy positive for SMA.
- Spindle cells are negative for c-kit, DOG1, S100, ALK, and desmin.

Final Diagnosis

Inflammatory fibroid polyp.

Take-Home Messages

- IFPs are benign polyps that most commonly arise in the gastric antrum (about 70% of cases) and less frequently in the small bowel and are centered in the submucosa.
- IFPs show similar gain-of-function mutations in the *PDGFRA* gene as GISTs.
- IFPs arise in the submucosa and typically show abundant eosinophils, whereas IMTs tend to occur within the abdomen/pelvis (external to the GI tract) and typically show abundant lymphocytes and plasma cells.

References: [46–50]

References

1. Levine MS, Buck JL, Pantongrag-Brown L, Buetow PC, Hallman JR, Sobin LH. Leiomyosarcoma of the esophagus: radiographic findings in 10 patients. AJR Am J Roentgenol. 1996;167(1):27–32.
2. Jang KM, Lee KS, Lee SJ, Kim EA, Kim TS, Hand D, Shim YM. The spectrum of benign esophageal lesions: imaging findings. Korean J Radiol. 2002;3(3):199–210.
3. Sestini S, Gisabella M, Pastorino U, Bille A. Presenting symptoms of giant fibrovascular polyp of the oesophagus: case report and literature review. Ann R Coll Surg Engl. 2016;98(5):e71–3.
4. Levine MS, Buck JL, Pantongrag-Brown L, Buetow PC, Hallman JR, Sobin LH. Fibrovascular polyps of the esophagus: clinical radiographic findings in 16 patients. AJR Am J Roentgenol. 1996;166(4):781–7.
5. Gencosmanoglu R, Sen-Oran E, Kurtkaya-Yapicier O, Tozun N. Xanthelasmas of the upper gastrointestinal tract. J Gastroenterol. 2004;39(3):215–9.
6. Melling N, Bruder E, Dimmler A, Hohenberger W, Aigner T. Localised massive tumourous xanthomatosis of the small intestine. Int J Colorectal Dis. 2007;22(11):1401–4.
7. Neto FA, Ferreira MC, Bertoncello LC, Neto AA, de Aveiro WC, Bento CA, Cecchino GN, Rocha MA. Gastric lipoma presenting as a giant bulging mass in an oligosymptomatic patient: a case report. J Med Case Reports. 2012;6:317.
8. Zhang H, Jin Z, Cui R. Russell body gastritis/duodenitis: a case series and description of immunoglobulin light chain restriction. Clin Res Hepatol Gastroenterol. 2014;38(5):e89–97.
9. Karabagli P, Gokturk HS. Russell body gastritis: case report and review of the literature. J Gastrointestin Liver Dis. 2012;21(1):97–100.
10. Hu B, El Hajj N, Sittler S, Lammert N, Barnes R, Meloni-Ehrig A. Gastric cancer: classification, histology and application of molecular pathology. J Gastrointest Oncol. 2012;3(3): 251–61.
11. Chetty R, Serra S. Lipid-rich and clear cell neuroendocrine tumors ("carcinoids") of the appendix: potential confusion with goblet cell carcinoid. Am J Surg Pathol. 2010;34(3):401–4.
12. Truong LD, Shen SS. Immunohistochemical diagnosis of renal neoplasms. Arch Pathol Lab Med. 2011;135(1):92–109.
13. Dutly F, Altwegg M. Whipple's disease and "Tropheryma whippelii". Clin Microbiol Rev. 2001;14(3):561–83.

14. Hou YY, Tan YS, Xu JF, Wang XN, Lu SH, Ji Y, et al. Schwannoma of the gastrointestinal tract: a clinicopathological, immunohistochemical and ultrastructural study of 33 cases. Histopathology. 2006;48:536–45.
15. Miettinen M, Shekitka KM, Sobin LH. Schwannomas in the colon and rectum: a clinicopathologic and immunohistochemical study of 20 cases. Am J Surg Pathol. 2001;25:846–55.
16. Gibson JA, Hornick JL. Mucosal Schwann cell "hamartoma": clinicopathologic study of 26 neural colorectal polyps distinct from neurofibromas and mucosal neuromas. Am J Surg Pathol. 2009;33:781–7.
17. Fuller CE, Williams GT. Gastrointestinal manifestations of type 1 neurofibromatosis (von Recklinghausen's disease). Histopathology. 1991;19:1–11.
18. Fanburg-Smith JC, Meis-Kindblom JM, Fante R, Kindblom LG. Malignant granular cell tumor of soft tissue: diagnostic criteria and clinicopathologic correlation. Am J Surg Pathol. 1998;22(7):779–94.
19. Ordonez NG, Mackay B. Granular cell tumor: a review of the pathology and histogenesis. Ultrastruct Pathol. 1999;23(4):207–22.
20. Ordonez NG. Granular cell tumor: a review and update. Adv Anat Pathol. 1999;6(4):186–203.
21. Fetsch JF, Montgomery EA, Meis JM. Calcifying fibrous pseudotumor. Am J Surg Pathol. 1993;17(5):502–8.
22. Nascimento AF, Ruiz R, Hornick JL, Fletcher CD. Calcifying fibrous 'pseudotumor': clinicopathologic study of 15 cases and analysis of its relationship to inflammatory myofibroblastic tumor. Int J Surg Pathol. 2002;10(3):189–96.
23. Hill KA, Gonzalez-crussi F, Chou PM. Calcifying fibrous pseudotumor versus inflammatory myofibroblastic tumor: a histological and immunohistochemical comparison. Mod Pathol. 2001;14(8):784–90.
24. Chorti A, Papavramidis TS, Michalopoulos A. Calcifying fibrous tumor: review of 157 patients reported in international literature. Medicine (Baltimore). 2016;95(20):e3690.
25. Bhattacharya B, Dilworth HP, Iacobuzio-Donahue C, Ricci F, Weber K, Furlong MA, Fisher C, Montgomery E. Nuclear beta-catenin expression distinguishes deep fibromatosis from other benign and malignant fibroblastic and myofibroblastic lesions. Am J Surg Pathol. 2005;29(5):653–9.
26. Montgomery E, Torbenson MS, Kaushal M, Fisher C, Abraham SC. Beta-catenin immunohistochemistry separates mesenteric fibromatosis from gastrointestinal stromal tumor and sclerosing mesenteritis. Am J Surg Pathol. 2002;26(10):1296–301.
27. Coffin CM, Hornick JL, Fletcher CD. Inflammatory myofibroblastic tumor: comparison of clinicopathologic, histologic, and immunohistochemical features including ALK expression in atypical and aggressive cases. Am J Surg Pathol. 2007;31:509–20.
28. Coffin CM, Watterson J, Priest JR, Dehner LP. Extrapulmonary inflammatory myofibroblastic tumor (inflammatory pseudotumor). A clinicopathologic and immunohistochemical study of 84 cases. Am J Surg Pathol. 1995;19:859–72.
29. Marino-Enriquez A, Wang WL, Roy A, Lopez-Terrada D, Lazar AJ, Fletcher CD, Coffin CM, Hornick JL. Epithelioid inflammatory myofibroblastic sarcoma: an aggressive intra-abdominal variant of inflammatory myofibroblastic tumor with nuclear membrane or perinuclear ALK. Am J Surg Pathol. 2011;35:135–44.
30. Jung SH, Suh KS, Kang DY, Kang DW, Kim YB, Kim ES. Expression of DOG1, PDGFRA, and p16 in gastrointestinal stromal tumors. Gut Liver. 2011;5(2):171–80.
31. Kang GH, Srivastava A, Kim YE, Park HJ, Park CK, Sohn TS, Kim S, Kang DY, Kim KM. DOG1 and PKC-θ are useful in the diagnosis of KIT-negative gastrointestinal stromal tumors. Mod Pathol. 2011;24(6):866–75.
32. Riddle ND, Gonzalez RJ, Bridge JA, Antonia S, Bui MM. A CD117 and CD34 immunoreactive sarcoma masquerading as a gastrointestinal stromal tumor: diagnostic pitfalls of ancillary studies in sarcoma. Cancer Control. 2011;18(3):152–9.
33. Doyle LA, Vivero M, Fletcher CD, Mertens F, Hornick JL. Nuclear expression of STAT6 distinguishes solitary fibrous tumor from histologic mimics. Mod Pathol. 2014;27(3):390–5.
34. Emanuel P, Qin L, Harpaz N. Calcifying fibrous tumor of small intestine. Ann Diagn Pathol. 2008;12(2):138–41.
35. Yantiss RK, Nielsen GP, Lauwers GY, Rosenberg AE. Reactive nodular fibrous pseudotumor of the gastrointestinal tract and mesentery: a clinicopathologic study of five cases. Am J Surg Pathol. 2003;27(4):532–40.
36. Antonescu, Christine R, Scheithauer, Bernd W, Woodruff, James M. Tumors of the peripheral nervous system. 2013. Silver Spring, Maryland, 20910. American Registry Pathology. Fourth Series.
37. Iwamuro M, Omote R, Tanaka T, Sunada N, Nada T, Kondo Y, Nose S, Kawaguchi M, Otsuka F, Okada H. Diffuse intestinal ganglioneuromatosis showing multiple large bowel ulcers in a patient with neurofibromatosis. Intern Med. 2017;56(24):3287–91.
38. Shetika KM, Sobin LH. Ganglioneuromas of the gastrointestinal tract. Relation to von Recklinghausen disease and other multiple tumor syndromes. Am J Surg Pathol. 1994;18(3):250–7.
39. Agaimy A, Stoehr R, Vieth M, Hartmann A. Benign serrated colorectal fibroblastic polyps/intramucosal perineuriomas are true mixed epithelial-stromal polyps (hybrid hyperplastic polyp/mucosal perineurioma) with frequent BRAF mutations. Am J Surg Pathol. 2010;34(11):1663–71.
40. Erlenbach-Wunsch K, Bihl M, Hatymann A, Groisman GM, Vieth M, Agaimy A. Serrated epithelial colorectal polyps (hyperplastic polyps, sessile serrated adenomas) with perineurial stroma: clinicopathological and molecular analysis of a new series. Ann Diagn Pathol. 2018;35:48–52.
41. Groisman GM, Polack-Charcon S, Appelman HD. Fibroblastic polyp of the colon: clinicopathological analysis of 10 cases with emphasis on its common association with serrated crypts. Histopathology. 2006;48(4):431–7.
42. Groisman GM, Polak-Charcon S. Fibroblastic polyp of the colon and colonic perineurioma: 2 names for a single entity? Am J Surg Pathol. 2008;32(7):1088–94.
43. Groisman GM, Hershkovitz D, Vieth M, Sabo E. Colonic perineuriomas with and without crypt serration: a comparative study. Am J Surg Pathol. 2013;37(5):745–51.
44. Hornick JL, Fletcher CD. Intestinal perineuriomas: clinicopathologic definition of a new anatomic subset in a series of 10 cases. Am J Surg Pathol. 2005;29(7):859–65.
45. Pai RK, Mojtahed A, Rouse RV, Soetikno RM, Kaltenbach T, Ma L, Arber DA, Plesec TP, Goldblum JR. Histologic and molecular analyses of colonic perineurial-like proliferations in serrated polyps: perineurial-like stromal proliferations are seen is sessile adenomas. Am J Surg Pathol. 2011;35(9):1373–80.
46. Schildhaus HU, Caviar T, Binot E, Büttner R, Wardelmann E, Merkelbach-Bruse S. Inflammatory fibroid polyps harbour mutations in the platelet-derived growth factor receptor alpha (PDGFRA) gene. J Pathol. 2008;216:176–82.
47. Lasota J, Wang ZF, Sobin LH, Miettinen M. Gain-of-function PDGFRA mutations, earlier reported in gastrointestinal stromal tumors, are common in small intestinal inflammatory fibroid polyps. A study of 60 cases. Mod Pathol. 2009;22:1049–56.
48. Huss S, Wardelmann E, Goltz D, Binot E, Hartmann W, Merkelbach-Bruse S, et al. Activating PDGFRA mutations in inflammatory fibroid polyps occur in exons 12, 14 and 18 and are associated with tumour localization. Histopathology. 2012;61:59–68.
49. Wysocki AP, Taylor G, Windsor JA. Inflammatory fibroid polyps of the duodenum: a review of the literature. Dig Surg. 2007;24(3):162–8.
50. Pantanowitz L, Antonioli DA, Pinkus GS, Shahsafaei A, Odze RD. Inflammatory fibroid polyps of the gastrointestinal tract: evidence for a dendritic cell origin. Am J Surg Pathol. 2004;28(1):107–14.

51. Subramanian S, West RB, Corless CL, Ou W, Rubin BP, Chu KM, et al. Gastrointestinal stromal tumors (GISTs) with KIT and PDGFRA mutations have distinct gene expression profiles. Oncogene. 2004;23:7780–90.
52. Huber AR, Shikle JF. Benign fibroblastic polyps of the colon. Arch Pathol Lab Med. 2009;133(11):1872–6.
53. Mravic M, LaChaud G, Nguyen A, Scott MA, Dry SM, James AW. Clinical and histopathological diagnosis of glomus tumor: an institutional experience of 138 cases. Int J Surg Pathol. 2015;23(3):181–8.
54. Folpe AL, Fanburg-Smith JC, Miettinen M, Weiss SW. Atypical and malignant glomus tumors: analysis of 52 cases, with a proposal for the reclassification of glomus tumors. Am J Surg Pathol. 2001;25(1):1–12.
55. Wang ZB, Yuan J, Shi HY. Features of gastric glomus tumor: a clinicopathologic, immunohistochemical and molecular retrospective study. Int J Clin Exp Pathol. 2014;7(4):1438–48.
56. Shen J, Shrestha S, Yen YH, Asatrian G, Mravic M, Soo C, Ting K, Dry SM, Peault B, James AW. Pericyte antigens in perivascular soft tissue tumors. Int J Surg Pathol. 2015;23(8):638–48.
57. Miettinen M, Sobin LH, Sarlomo-Rikala M. Immunohistochemical spectrum of GISTs at different sites and their differential diagnosis with a reference to CD117 (KIT). Mod Pathol. 2000;13(10): 1134–42.
58. Kindblom LG, Remotti HE, Aldenborg F, Meis-Kindblom JM. Gastrointestinal pacemaker cell tumor (GIPACT): gastrointestinal stromal tumors show phenotypic characteristics of the interstitial cells of Cajal. Am J Pathol. 1998;152(5):1259–69.
59. Corless CL, Fletcher JA, Heinrich MC. Biology of gastrointestinal stromal tumors. J Clin Oncol. 2004;22(18):3813–25.
60. Mosquera JM, Sboner A, Zhang L, Chen CL, Sung YS, Chen HW, Agaram NP, Briskin D, Basha BM, Singer S, Rubin MA, Tuschi T, Antonescu CR. Novel MIR 143-NOTCH fusions in benign and malignant tumors. Genes Chromosomes Cancer. 2013;52(11):1075–87.
61. Wilson BS, Lloyd RV. Detection of chromogranin in neuroendocrine cells with a monoclonal antibody. Am J Pathol. 1984;115(3):458–68.
62. Wiedenmann B, Franke WW, Kuhn C, Moll R, Gould VE. Synaptophysin: a marker protein for neuroendocrine cells and neoplasms. Proc Natl Acad Sci U S A. 1986;83(10):3500–4.
63. Abraham SC, Krasinskas AM, Hofstetter WL, Swisher SG, Wu TT. “Seedling” mesenchymal tumors (gastrointestinal stromal tumors and leiomyomas) are common incidental tumors of the esophagogastric junction. Am J Surg Pathol. 2007;31(11):1629–35.
64. Miettinen M, Furlong M, Sarlomo-rikala M, Burke A, Sobin LH, Lasota J. Gastrointestinal stromal tumors, intramural leiomyomas, and leiomyosarcomas in the rectum and anus: a clinicopathologic, immunohistochemical and molecular genetic study of 14 cases. Am J Surg Pathol. 2001;25(9):1121–33.
65. Nozu K, Minamikawa S, Yamada S, Oka M, Yanagita M, Morisada N, Fujinaga S, Nagano C, Gotoh Y, Takahashi E, Morishita T, Yamamura T, Ninchoji T, Kaito H, Morioka I, Nakanishi K, Vorechovsky I, Iijima K. Characterization of continuous gene deletions in COL4A6 and COL4A5 in Alport syndrome-diffuse leiomyomatosis. J Hum Genet. 2017;62(7):733–5.
66. Deyrup AT, Lee VK, Hill CE, Cheuk W, Toh HC, Kesavan S, Chan EW, Weiss SW. Epstein-Barr virus-associated smooth muscle tumors are distinctive mesenchymal tumors reflecting multiple infection events: a clinicopathologic and molecular analysis of 29 tumors from 19 patients. Am J Surg Pathol. 2006;30(1): 75–82.
67. Deyrup AT. Epstein-Barr virus associated epithelial and mesenchymal neoplasms. Hum Pathol. 2008;39(4):473–83.
68. Miettinen M, Sarlome-Rikala M, Sobin LH, Lasota J. Esophageal stromal tumors: a clinicopathologic, immunohistochemical, and molecular genetic study of 17 cases and comparison with esophageal leiomyomas and leiomyosarcomas. Am J Surg Pathol. 2000;24(2):211–22.
69. Miettinen M, Sarlomo-Rikala M, Sobin LH, Lasota J. Gastrointestinal stromal tumors and leiomyosarcomas in the colon: a clinicopathologic immunohistochemical, and molecular genetic study of 44 cases. Am J Surg Pathol. 2000;24(10):1339–52.
70. Miettinen M, Sobin LH, Lasota J. True smooth muscle tumors of the small intestine: a clinicopathologic, immunohistochemical, and molecular genetic study of 25 cases. Am J Surg Pathol. 2009;33(3):430–6.
71. Deshpande A, Nelson D, Corless CL, Deshpande V, O'Brien MJ. Leiomyoma of the gastrointestinal tract with interstitial cells of Cajal: a mimic of gastrointestinal stromal tumor. Am J Surg Pathol. 2014;38(1):72–7.
72. Miettinen M, Wang ZF, Lasota J. DOG1 antibody in the differential diagnosis of gastrointestinal stromal tumors: a study of 1840 cases. Am J Surg Pathol. 2009;33(9):1401–8.
73. D'Annibale M, Cosimelli M, Covello R, Stasi E. Liposarcoma of the colon presenting as an endoluminal mass. World J Surg Oncol. 2009;7 https://doi.org/10.1186/1477-7819-7-78.
74. Goldblum JR, Weiss SW, Folpe AL. Enzinger and Weiss's soft tissue tumors. 6th ed. 2013. p. 784–854. doi:978-0323088343.
75. Levey DS, MacCormack LM, Sartoris DJ, Haghighi P, Resnick D, Thorne R. Cystic angiomatosis: case report and review of the literature. Skeletal Radiol. 1996;25(3):287–93.
76. Em M, Moran CA, Munden RF. Generalized lymphangiomatosis. AJR Am J Roentgenol. 2004;182(4):1068.
77. Fang YF, Qiu LF, Du Y, Jiang ZN, Gao M. Small intestinal hemolymphangioma with bleeding: a case report. World J Gastroenterol. 2012;18(17):2145–6.
78. Lawless ME, Lloyd KA, Swanson PE, Upton MP, Yeh MM. Lymphangiomatous lesions of the gastrointestinal tract: a clinicopathologic study and comparison between adults and children. Am J Clin Pathol. 2015;144(4):563–9.
79. Pasquini P, Baiocchini A, Falasca L, Anniball D, Gimbo G, Pace F, Del Nonno F. Mucosal Schwann cell “Hamartoma”: a new entity? World J Gastroenterol. 2009;15(18):2287–9.
80. Shekitka KM, Sobin LH. Ganglioneuromas of the gastrointestinal tract. Relation to Von Recklinghausen disease and other multiple tumor syndromes. Am J Surg Pathol. 1994;18(3):2350–7.

Neuroendocrine Neoplasms of the Gastrointestinal Tract

17

Brent K. Larson and Deepti Dhall

List of Frequently Asked Questions

1. What are neuroendocrine neoplasms?
2. How are neuroendocrine tumors (NETs) defined, and how are they diagnosed?
3. How are neuroendocrine carcinomas (NECs) defined, and how are they diagnosed?
4. How can NETs be differentiated from NECs?
5. How are NETs graded?
6. How are neuroendocrine neoplasms staged?
7. What are differential diagnostic considerations for neuroendocrine neoplasms?
8. Are there any site-specific markers for gastrointestinal NETs that can be used to identify the site of origin of neuroendocrine neoplasms of unknown primary?
9. What is the utility of immunohistochemistry for hormone products in diagnosing NETs?
10. What are mixed adenoneuroendocrine carcinomas?
11. What is gastric neuroendocrine cell hyperplasia, and how is it differentiated from gastric NET?
12. How are gastric NETs classified?
13. What types of NETs occur in the duodenum?
14. What are the characteristics of ileal NETs?
15. What are the characteristics of appendiceal NETs?
16. What are the characteristics of rectal NETs?
17. Are there any characteristic molecular features of NETs?

B. K. Larson
Cedars-Sinai Medical Center, Los Angeles, CA, USA
e-mail: brent.larson@cshs.org

D. Dhall (✉)
The University of Alabama at Birmingham School of Medicine, Birmingham, AL, USA

Frequently Asked Questions

1. What are neuroendocrine neoplasms?

With the exception of paragangliomas, neuroendocrine neoplasms are generally epithelial tumors with neuroendocrine differentiation. This category encompasses two discrete neoplasms: well-differentiated neuroendocrine tumors (NETs) and poorly differentiated neuroendocrine carcinomas (NECs). They can arise from numerous sites in the body, including the respiratory system, the pancreas, and the luminal gastrointestinal tract.

2. How are neuroendocrine tumors (NETs) defined, and how are they diagnosed?

NETs are well-differentiated neuroendocrine neoplasms, composed of cells with features similar to those of normal neuroendocrine cells. They are uncommon tumors, accounting for less than 1% of gastrointestinal malignancies, though they are increasing in incidence and prevalence. They are typically arranged in nests or trabecula, with rarer architectural patterns including broad sheets or pseudoglandular structures. The tumor cells have uniform cytological features, with moderate eosinophilic granular cytoplasm and round-to-ovoid nuclei with smooth nuclear membranes, finely granular (so-called salt-and-pepper) chromatin, and indistinct nucleoli.

Chromogranin A and synaptophysin are immunohistochemical markers of neuroendocrine differentiation that can be used to confirm a diagnosis of NET, though if the morphological features are classical, they are not needed. Chromogranin A is the most specific marker for neuroendocrine differentiation but is not very sensitive. Rates of positivity vary based on anatomical location, with the highest expression at over 80% in NETs of the tubular gastrointestinal tract proximal to the colon, and somewhat lower sensitivities in the colon and rectum, in the range of 40–60%. Synaptophysin is less specific for NETs, as its expression can be seen in other tumors, such as glomus tumors.

H. L. Wang, Z. E. Chen (eds.), *Practical Gastrointestinal Pathology*, Practical Anatomic Pathology,
https://doi.org/10.1007/978-3-030-51268-2_17

Although the histological features of NETs are similar at all sites throughout the body, the clinical features, tumor biology, and prognosis of NETs are site-specific. Depending on their cell of origin, NETs may secrete bioactive amine or peptide hormones that can cause clinical symptoms and syndromes. Although typically indolent compared to carcinomas, they frequently present at an advanced stage of disease. NETs have historically been referred to as "carcinoid tumors," though this term is technically only applicable to a subset of NETs and may lead to confusion and so is now discouraged. They have also historically been divided embryologically into foregut (gastric, pulmonary, duodenal, and pancreatic) tumors, midgut (jejunal, ileal, appendiceal, and cecal) tumors, and hindgut (colonic and rectal) tumors, as proposed by Williams and Sandler in 1963. Tumors grouped by this classification share some clinical and histological features. Midgut NETs have a propensity for nested architecture and brightly eosinophilic cytoplasmic granules and are frequently associated with the carcinoid syndrome. On the other hand, foregut and hindgut NETs commonly show trabecular architecture. This classification also correlates well with differential expression of transcription factors, which can be used to determine the site of origin of metastatic NETs of unknown primary.
References: [1–4]

3. **How are neuroendocrine carcinomas (NECs) defined, and how are they diagnosed?**

NECs are poorly differentiated, high-grade malignant neoplasms. They are classically divided into two types, small cell carcinoma (SCC) and large cell neuroendocrine carcinoma (LCNEC), based on their morphological features, though they frequently show mixed features. In SCC, cells are arranged in a diffuse, sheet-like pattern, though organoid or rosette-like arrangements may focally be present. The cells are small to intermediate sized with scant cytoplasm, though a minority of cells is allowed to have more moderate cytoplasm. They have a high nucleus-to-cytoplasm ratio with round to fusiform nuclei. Confluent necrosis, numerous apoptotic cells, and abundant mitotic figures are present (Fig. 17.1). If the morphological pattern is classical and easily discernible, confirmatory immunohistochemical staining may not be necessary.

LCNECs have variable growth patterns, including diffuse, nested, or trabecular patterns. They are composed of large polygonal tumor cells with abundant eosinophilic cytoplasm, coarse or vesicular chromatin, and prominent nucleoli. Given their similar cytomorphological appearance to other carcinomas, evidence of glandular or squamous differentiation must be excluded, and immunohistochemical confirmation with two markers of neuroendocrine differentiation (synaptophysin and chromogranin A) is recommended.

In one study, gastrointestinal NECs arising from squamous mucosa (esophagus and anus) were more frequently SCC, while those arising from glandular mucosa were more likely to be LCNEC or showed mixed morphological features.
Reference: [5]

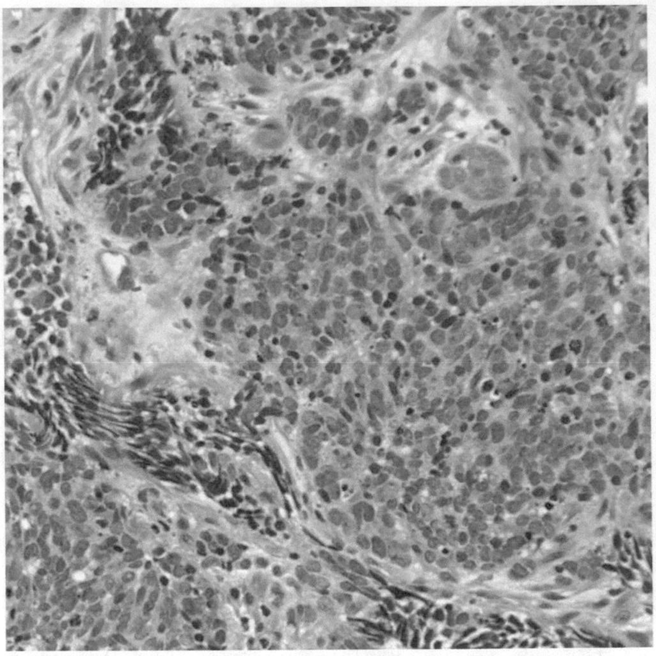

Fig. 17.1 Small cell carcinoma of the rectum. Tumor cells show fine nuclear chromatin, inconspicuous nucleoli, nuclear molding, readily identifiable mitotic figures, and abundant apoptotic cells

4. **How can NETs be differentiated from NECs?**

Distinguishing high grade (G3) NETs from NECs is primarily accomplished by recognizing the classical morphological patterns, as described in the preceding sections. However, in certain situations, this differentiation may be difficult, such as when an NET demonstrates a more prominent infiltrative or sheet-like growth pattern than usual or contains foci of necrosis, leading to the tumor potentially being mistaken for a NEC.

Small biopsies or biopsies with extensive crush artifact can also be problematic. Though difficult to interpret, Ki-67 immunohistochemistry can be useful for making the distinction in these circumstances, as NECs typically show a Ki-67 proliferative index of >50% whereas G3 NETs are less likely. However, borderline cases do exist because NECs may occasionally show a Ki-67 index of 20–50%. Thus, Ki-67 cannot be reliably used to distinguish a NEC from a G3 NET. Immunohistochemical staining for somatostatin receptor may also be helpful, as NETs typically express somatostatin receptor, while NECs show lower expression or lack it entirely. In addition, NECs may show loss of RB expression or aberrant p53 expression (either overexpression or complete absence) due to mutations of these genes, which may aid in the differential diagnosis. In some instances, definite determination between NET and NEC may be impossible, especially on core biopsy: the

clinical course ultimately determines the nature of a neuroendocrine neoplasm.
References: [6, 7]

5. How are NETs graded?

Until recently, grading schemes, including the World Health Organization (WHO) 2010 classification, divided neuroendocrine neoplasms into three grades (G1, G2, and G3) based on the mitotic count and Ki-67 index, in which NECs composed the G3 category. In 2017, after multiple published studies demonstrated different behaviors of pancreatic neuroendocrine neoplasms with high proliferative activity in combination with the degree of differentiation, a new scheme was adopted that uniformly applied to all gastrointestinal neuroendocrine neoplasms (Table 17.1). In this system, NETs are graded as G1, G2, and G3, whereas NEC are considered high grade, by definition.

Table 17.1 Summary of grading of neuroendocrine tumors at all sites of the gastrointestinal tract

Grade	Mitotic count (per 2 mm^2)[a]	Ki-67 proliferative index (%)[b]
Grade 1 (low grade)	<2	<3
Grade 2 (intermediate grade)	2–20	3–20
Grade 3 (high grade)	>20	>20%

[a]At least 10 mm^2 should be counted in most mitotically active areas. Only clearly identifiable mitotic figures should be counted. The number of high-power fields (40×) needed for 10 mm^2 depends on microscopes used. For example, 42 high-power fields need to be counted for a microscope with a field diameter of 0.55 mm at 40×
[b]A minimum of 500 tumor cells needs to be counted

Once the diagnosis of NET is established based on the morphological features previously outlined, grade is assigned based on the mitotic activity and Ki-67 proliferative index (Fig. 17.2), which is considered the most reliable predictor of prognosis. The mitotic count is assessed over 10 mm^2 of contiguous high-power fields and averaged to express the number of mitoses per 2 mm^2. The Ki-67 proliferative index is calculated by counting 500–2000 cells with all stained nuclei of any intensity and any pattern counted as positive. Both the mitotic count and Ki-67 proliferative index should be evaluated in "hot spot" regions with the highest proliferative activity. In the event that the mitotic rate and Ki-67 pro-

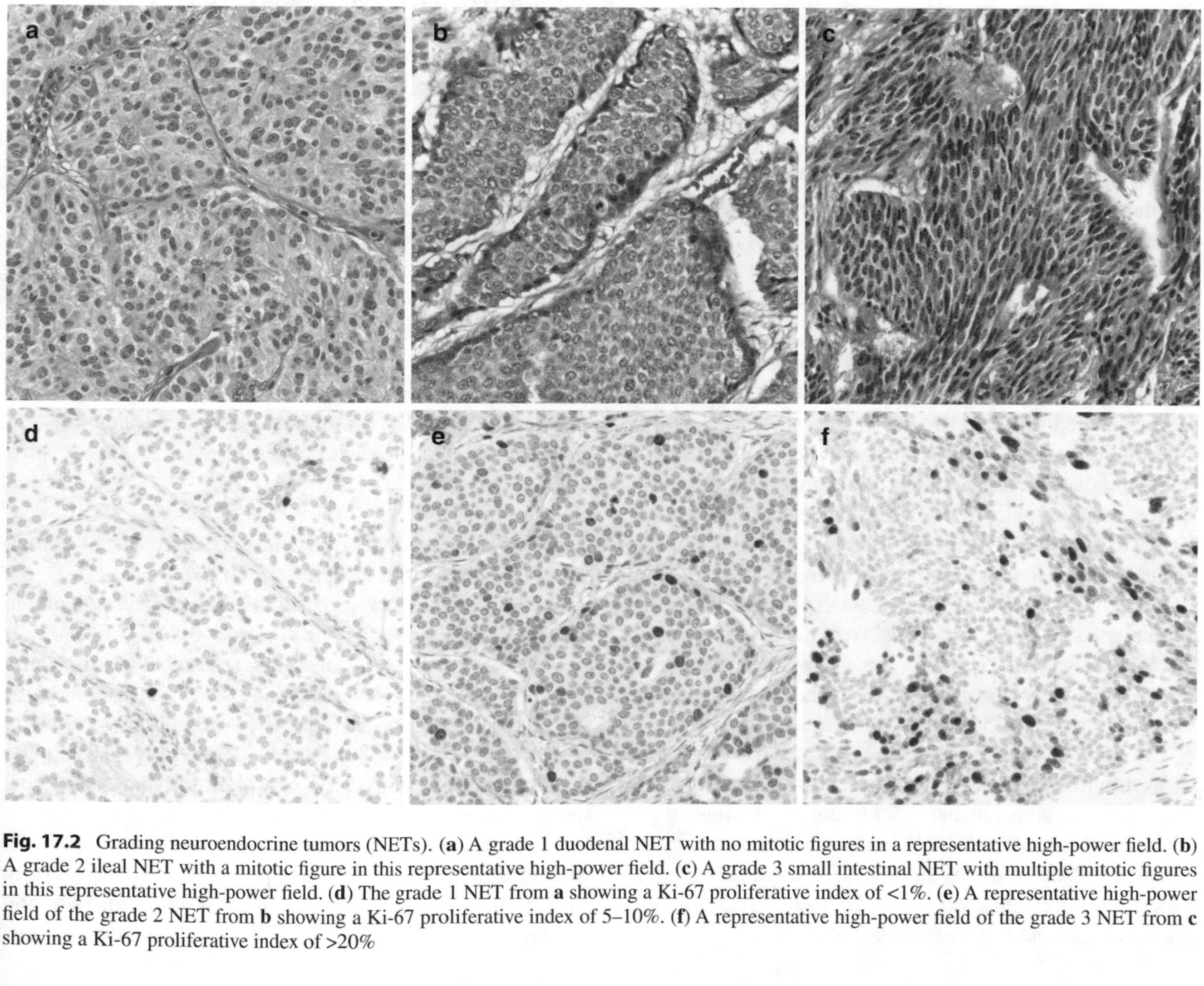

Fig. 17.2 Grading neuroendocrine tumors (NETs). (**a**) A grade 1 duodenal NET with no mitotic figures in a representative high-power field. (**b**) A grade 2 ileal NET with a mitotic figure in this representative high-power field. (**c**) A grade 3 small intestinal NET with multiple mitotic figures in this representative high-power field. (**d**) The grade 1 NET from **a** showing a Ki-67 proliferative index of <1%. (**e**) A representative high-power field of the grade 2 NET from **b** showing a Ki-67 proliferative index of 5–10%. (**f**) A representative high-power field of the grade 3 NET from **c** showing a Ki-67 proliferative index of >20%

liferative index lead to different grade assignments, the higher of the two is considered the final grade.

For assessment of the Ki-67 proliferative index, it was thought until recently that an overall "eyeball" assessment was acceptable. However, this gestalt visual inspection method has been shown to have very low accuracy, especially when considering borderline cases. In a recent comparison of four different counting methods including eyeballing, a visual cell count through a microscope, a manual count of a camera-captured printed image, and an automated cell count via a digital image analysis system, the manual cell count on a printed image was found to have the highest accuracy and lowest interobserver variability, making it now the preferred method for evaluating the Ki-67 proliferative rate. Ki-67 immunostaining also highlights inter- and intratumoral heterogeneity in primary and metastatic tumors and throughout the course of disease. Therefore, it is recommended to perform Ki-67 immunostaining not only on primary NETs but also on metastases. It has also been shown that Ki-67 staining on NET core biopsies provides a reliable proliferative index for prognostication of NET metastasis to the liver.

References: [8–11]

6. **How are neuroendocrine neoplasms staged?**

Staging of NETs varies by site throughout the gastrointestinal tract. In general, both size and depth of invasion play a part in the primary tumor stage. See Table 17.2 for a detailed explanation of staging for primary NETs at each primary site in the gastrointestinal tract. NECs are staged using the staging systems for other primary carcinomas at each primary site of the gastrointestinal tract and do not use the staging systems for NETs.

7. **What are differential diagnostic considerations for neuroendocrine neoplasms?**

NETs have a fairly characteristic appearance. Other tumors with trabecular or organoid arrangement and bland nuclei may be encountered in the gastrointestinal tract, though they are exceedingly rare. Metastatic polygonal cell tumors, such as hepatocellular carcinoma, adrenocortical carcinoma, or renal cell carcinoma, typically have greater nuclear irregularities, though a history of these neoplasms and immunohistochemistry are helpful. Glomus tumors very rarely involve the gastrointestinal tract (mostly in the stomach) and have similar trabecular architecture, though not typically the same densely collagenized stroma. If an NET has a prominent pseudoglandular pattern, it may be mistaken for adenocarcinoma, though adenocarcinoma usually has greater nuclear atypia.

The differential for NECs is broad. Sarcomas of the tubular gastrointestinal tract should be considered, particularly including gastrointestinal stromal tumor and malignant gastrointestinal neuroectodermal tumors in this location. Poorly cohesive LCNEC may be mistaken for large cell lymphomas. Broad-spectrum keratins may be useful to exclude these diagnoses, particularly on small biopsies.

Before diagnosing NEC, other poorly differentiated carcinomas, such as poorly differentiated squamous cell carcinoma or poorly differentiated adenocarcinoma, must be excluded. The presence of more than occasional intracytoplasmic mucin and significant nuclear pleomorphism/atypia favors the diagnosis of adenocarcinoma or mixed adenoneuroendocrine carcinoma (see below).

8. **Are there any site-specific markers for gastrointestinal NETs that can be used to identify the site of origin of neuroendocrine neoplasms of unknown primary?**

Some immunohistochemical markers may aid in the identification of the primary site of metastatic NETs of unknown origin. Most of these antibodies are directed against transcription factors and are most helpful for identifying the broad embryological categories of primary tumors as outlined by Williams and Sandler.

Midgut NETs (those of the jejunum, ileum, cecum, and appendix) are typically strongly positive for homeobox protein CDX2. They are usually negative for transcription termination factor 1 (TTF1), insulin gene enhancer protein islet-1 (ISL1), and paired box proteins 6 and 8 (PAX6 and PAX8).

Hindgut NETs (mainly composed of rectal NETs, though the rare colonic NETs are included) are typically strongly and diffusely positive for special AT-rich sequence-binding protein 2 (SATB2). However, the majority of appendiceal NETs show similarly strong and diffuse SATB2 positivity. Jejunal and ileal NETs may show SATB2 positivity, though staining is typically weak and patchy. Rectal NETs may also show strong positivity for CDX2, like midgut NETs.

Duodenal and rectal NETs have a unique profile among gastrointestinal NETs that is similar to pancreatic NETs. PAX6, PAX8 (polyclonal), and ISL1 are typically positive in duodenal and rectal NETs.

Immunohistochemical stains are not useful for determining the site of origin of NECs. Gastrointestinal tract primary NECs may show TTF1 positivity, and CDX2 may be positive, regardless of the site of origin.

References: [4, 12–15]

9. **What is the utility of immunohistochemistry for hormone products in diagnosing NETs?**

While the secretory products of normal neuroendocrine cells distributed throughout the gastrointestinal tract are well known, correlation of immunohistochemical staining and serum measurements is less precise. Many NETs show ectopic hormone secretion and may show immunohistochemical positivity for multiple hormones, though only one may be detected in serum, or the NET may be entirely nonfunctional. Immunohistochemical staining may also rarely be negative for products that have been measured to be elevated in serum, which may be due to abnormal proteins not recognized by the antibodies. Immunohistochemical staining for hormone products may be useful in select circumstances, such as con-

Table 17.2 Summary of staging of neuroendocrine tumors at different sites of the gastrointestinal tract

Stage	Stomach	Duodenum	Ampulla	Jejunum and ileum	Appendix	Colon and rectum
pT1	Invades the lamina propria or submucosa and ≤1 cm in size	Invades the lamina propria or submucosa and ≤1 cm in size	Confined to sphincter of Oddi and ≤1 cm in size	Invades the lamina propria or submucosa and ≤1 cm in size	≤2 cm in size	Invades lamina propria or submucosa and pT1a: <1 cm in size pT1b: 1–2 cm in size
pT2	Invades muscularis propria or >1 cm in size	Invades muscularis propria or >1 cm in size	Invades duodenal submucosa or muscularis propria or >1 cm in size	Invades muscularis propria or >1 cm in size	>2 cm and ≤4 cm in size	Invades muscularis propria or >2 cm
pT3	Invades subserosal tissue	Invades pancreas or peripancreatic tissue	Invades pancreas or peripancreatic tissue	Invades subserosal tissue	>4 cm or Invades subserosal tissue or Invades mesoappendix	Invades subserosal tissue
pT4	Invades serosa/visceral peritoneum or Invades adjacent organs or structures	Invades serosa/visceral peritoneum or Invades adjacent organs or structures	Invades serosa/visceral peritoneum or Invades adjacent organs or structures	Invades serosa/visceral peritoneum or Invades adjacent organs or structures	Invades serosa/visceral peritoneum or Invades adjacent organs or structures	Invades serosa/visceral peritoneum or Invades adjacent organs or structures
pN1	Regional lymph node metastases	Regional lymph node metastases	Regional lymph node metastases	Regional lymph node metastases in <12 lymph nodes	Regional lymph node metastases	Regional lymph node metastases
pN2	Not applicable	Not applicable	Not applicable	Regional lymph node metastases in ≥12 lymph or Mesenteric masses (>2 cm in size)	Not applicable	Not applicable
pM1a	Metastasis confined to liver	Metastasis confined to liver	Metastasis confined to liver	Metastasis confined to liver	Metastasis confined to liver	Metastasis confined to liver
pM1b	Metastasis to ≥1 extra-hepatic site	Metastasis to ≥1 extra-hepatic site	Metastasis to ≥1 extra-hepatic site	Metastasis to ≥1 extra-hepatic site	Metastasis to ≥1 extra-hepatic site	Metastasis to ≥1 extra-hepatic site
pM1c	Metastasis to liver and Metastasis to ≥1 extra-hepatic site	Metastasis to liver and Metastasis to ≥1 extra-hepatic site	Metastasis to liver and Metastasis to ≥1 extra-hepatic site	Metastasis to liver and Metastasis to ≥1 extra-hepatic site	Metastasis to liver and Metastasis to ≥1 extra-hepatic site	Metastasis to liver and Metastasis to ≥1 extra-hepatic site

Adapted from Amin et al.

firming that an NET is the source of hormone elevations or as an aid for diagnosis of uncommon NET variants (e.g., using somatostatin immunostaining to confirm the diagnosis of a duodenal somatostatinoma).
Reference: [16]

10. What are mixed adenoneuroendocrine carcinomas?

Mixed adenoneuroendocrine carcinomas (MANECs) are tumors composed of both morphologically recognizable adenocarcinoma and NEC components. Each component must account for at least 30% of the neoplasm as a whole, as defined by the WHO in 2010. La Rosa and coauthors have recently proposed changing this terminology to "mixed neuroendocrine-nonneuroendocrine neoplasms" (MiNENs) to more completely encompass this heterogeneous group. The MiNEN category incorporates all grades of neuroendocrine neoplasms (both NET and NEC) combined with different subtypes of carcinoma, including adenocarcinoma-NEC, squamous cell carcinoma-NEC, and adenocarcinoma-NET. MiNEN is the currently recommended terminology by WHO. Again, to qualify the diagnosis, both neuroendocrine and nonneuroendocrine components should be morphologically and immunohistochemically recognizable and each constitutes ≥30% of the neoplasm. Preinvasive precursor lesions, such as adenoma, should not be considered part of MiNEN.

While MANECs are rare as a whole, at least one-third of NECs will show some component of adenocarcinoma after thorough sampling. The NEC component of mixed tumors is

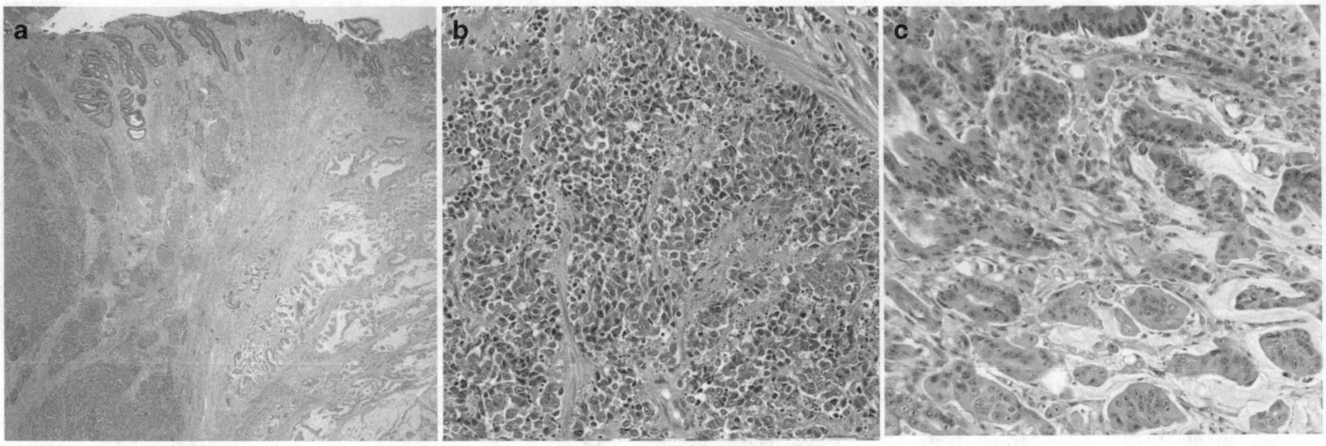

Fig. 17.3 Mixed adenoneuroendocrine carcinoma (MANEC). (**a**) A tumor in the right colon composed of a high-grade neuroendocrine carcinoma (NEC) component (left) and conventional and mucinous adenocarcinoma component (right) admixed and in close proximity, diagnostic of MANEC. (**b**) The NEC component shows high nucleus-to-cytoplasm ratios, markedly irregular nuclear contours, variably prominent nucleoli, numerous mitotic figures, and patchy necrosis. (**c**) The adenocarcinoma component shows infiltrative glands and cell clusters floating in mucin pools

often present in the deeper portions of the tumor, and sampling bias is frequent in biopsy samples. The NEC component of MANEC is more frequently of LCNEC or mixed morphology than SCC alone (Fig. 17.3). While the NEC component is most likely to metastasize to lymph nodes and the liver, both components may be present, with adenocarcinoma alone being the metastatic component in a very small subset of cases.

Although, by definition, at least 30% of both components are required to be labeled as a MANEC, smaller components of NEC may drive the prognosis. In such cases, it is advisable to diagnose adenocarcinoma with a focal NEC component and state the percentage of the NEC component. In adenocarcinoma or other types of carcinoma without morphological features of neuroendocrine differentiation, patchy expression of neuroendocrine markers may be seen that is of unclear prognostic significance. These lesions should not be diagnosed as MANEC. References: [5, 17–20]

11. What is gastric neuroendocrine cell hyperplasia, and how is it differentiated from gastric NET?

Neuroendocrine cell hyperplasia refers to enterochromaffin-like (ECL) cell proliferation in the stomach, especially occurring in a background of autoimmune (atrophic) gastritis. ECL cells are predominantly present in the gastric body and fundus. They are seen at the bases of the gastric pits, though scattered cells can be present in the neck region. Under normal physiological conditions, gastrin secreted by antral G cells stimulates the ECL cells to release histamine, which in turn stimulates parietal cells to secrete hydrochloric acid. In autoimmune gastritis, anti-parietal cell or anti-intrinsic factor antibodies lead to widespread destruction of parietal cells and subsequently decreased hydrochloric acid production (hypochlorhydria or achlorhydria). This loss of hydrochloric acid removes critical negative feedback on antral G cells, leading to hypergastrinemia, which in turn leads to ECL cell proliferation.

The spectrum of ECL proliferation ranges from simple hyperplasia to gastric NETs, as described by a landmark publication from Solcia and coauthors in 1988. Linear ECL cell hyperplasia is defined as at least two groups of five or more adjacent neuroendocrine cells lining a gastric pit per millimeter. This finding is not easily appreciated on routine hematoxylin and eosin staining and is best visualized with immunohistochemical (chromogranin) staining. Micronodular ECL cell hyperplasia consists of clusters of five or more neuroendocrine cells, bounded by a basement membrane, measuring <150 μm (or less than the diameter of a gastric pit). These clusters may be grouped or scattered throughout the mucosa. When five or more of these clusters aggregate, it is termed adenomatoid hyperplasia. Dysplasia occurs when these micronodules fuse with concomitant loss of basement membrane or an individual micronodule becomes >150 μm. An intramucosal aggregation of ≥500 μm or new stroma formation signifies microinvasion, and these lesions are designated as micro-NETs. These lesions are frequently undetected at endoscopy. Larger lesions (≥5 mm) or lesions of any size that invade the muscularis mucosae or submucosa are invasive NETs.
Reference: [21]

12. How are gastric NETs classified?

Gastric NETs are subclassified into four subtypes. Each type has a different mechanism of tumorigenesis, different clinical behavior, and different management implications (see Table 17.3 for a summary).

The majority (70–80%) of gastric NETs are type 1 NETs. These are derived from the ECL cells of the gastric body and are associated with autoimmune gastritis, in which ECL cell hyperplasia leads to dysplasia and to NET development (Fig. 17.4). The diagnosis of type 1 NETs is made by identifying the histological features of NET in background of atro-

Table 17.3 Gastric neuroendocrine tumor types

	Type 1	Type 2	Type 3	Type 4
Associated disorder	Autoimmune (atrophic) gastritis	Zollinger-Ellison syndrome, MEN1	None	Dysfunctional parietal cells
Background mucosa	ECL cell hyperplasia, parietal cell atrophy	ECL cell hyperplasia, parietal cell hyperplasia	Normal	ECL cell hyperplasia, parietal cell hyperplasia
Site	Body, fundus	Body, fundus	Throughout the stomach	Body, fundus
Serum gastrin	Elevated	Elevated	Normal	Elevated
Hydrochloric acid secretion	Achlorhydria	Hyperchlorhydria	Normal	Achlorhydria

MEN1 multiple endocrine neoplasia type 1, *ECL* enterochromaffin-like

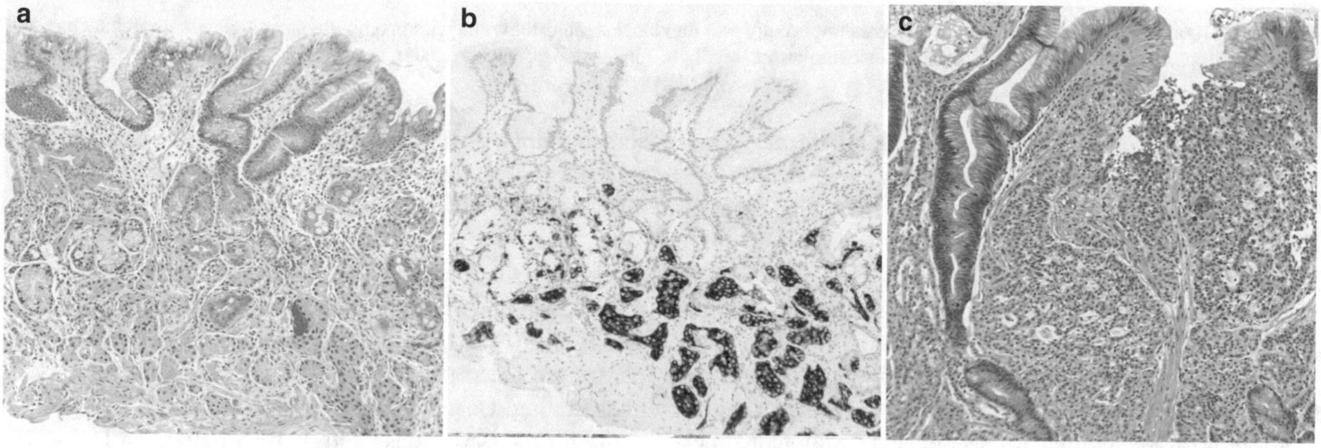

Fig. 17.4 Type 1 gastric neuroendocrine tumor arising in a background of autoimmune (atrophic) gastritis. (**a**) Gastric body mucosa showing a lymphoplasmacytic infiltrate, parietal cell atrophy, pyloric metaplasia, and intestinal metaplasia, all typical features of autoimmune (atrophic) gastritis. (**b**) Chromogranin A immunostain highlights neuroendocrine cell dysplasia consisting of confluent and irregularly shaped neuroendocrine cell nests. (**c**) A large, well-circumscribed neuroendocrine cell aggregate arising in a background of autoimmune (atrophic) gastritis, the size and confluent growth pattern of which qualify it as a type 1 gastric NET

phic metaplastic gastritis and ECL cell hyperplasia. These type 1 NETs have an indolent clinical course, with only rare reports of regional lymph node or distal metastases. Endoscopic surveillance with endoscopic resection is the typical management for these tumors, though definitive resection is suggested for the rare cases that are >2 cm in size, show lymphovascular invasion, invade the muscularis propria, or have a Ki-67 proliferative index indicating intermediate grade (G2).

Type 2 gastric NETs are caused by gastrinomas seen with Zollinger-Ellison syndrome. Zollinger-Ellison syndrome-associated gastrinomas are classically found in the "gastrinoma triangle," the anatomical triangle formed by the junction of the cystic duct with the common hepatic duct, the transition from the second to the third portion of the duodenum, and the head of the pancreas. However, contemporary studies reveal that type 2 gastric NETs account for only a minority of Zollinger-Ellison syndrome diagnoses (see the section on duodenal NETs below). Most patients with type 2 gastric NETs have multiple endocrine neoplasia (MEN) syndrome, type I (MEN1). Whether sporadic or syndromic, these gastrinomas cause gastrin hypersecretion with resultant proliferation of body and fundus ECL cells. The metastatic potential of type 2 gastric NETs is low, though marginally higher than type 1 gastric NETs. The diagnosis is based on identification of the morphological features of an NET (frequently multiple) in a background of normal mucosa or mucosa with parietal cell hyperplasia. Serum measurements reveal hypergastrinemia and hyperchlorhydria (pH <2).

Type 3 gastric NETs arise sporadically. They have morphology typical of NETs and arise in a background of normal mucosa and normal serum gastrin levels. They are commonly larger than 1 cm at the time of diagnosis, with consequently higher rates of metastasis and worse overall survival (75–80% at 5 years, compared to 90–95% for type 1 gastric NETs).

There are rare reports to suggest a type 4 gastric NET that consists of multiple small lesions arising in a background of parietal cell hyperplasia and hypertrophy. The parietal cells display vacuolated cytoplasm and harbor structural abnormalities that prevent the hydrochloric acid from being secreted. Consequently, achlorhydria, hypergastrinemia, and ECL cell hyperplasia ensue, leading to the development of these NETs. References: [22–31]

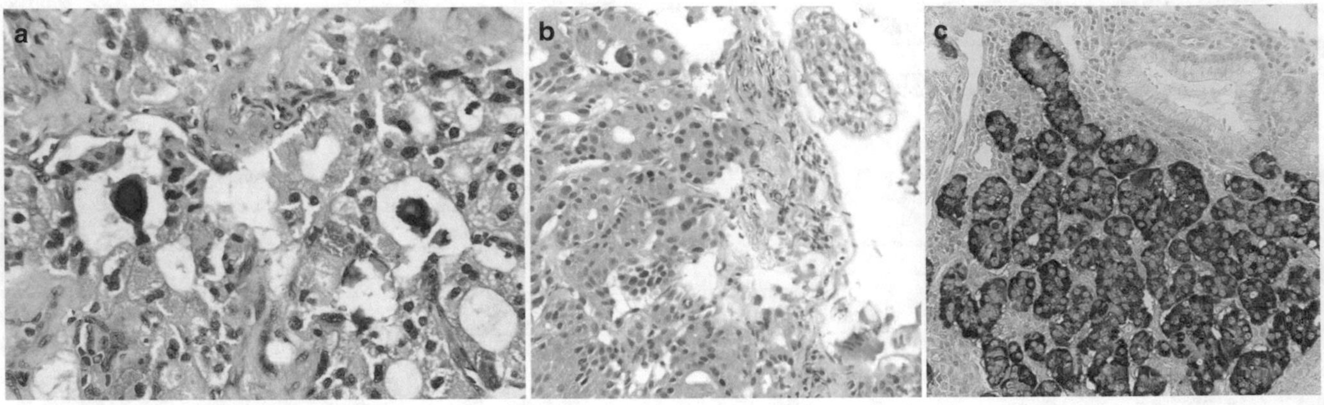

Fig. 17.5 Duodenal somatostatinoma. (**a**) Typical morphology of a duodenal somatostatinoma with prominent pseudoglandular architecture and psammomatous calcification. (**b**) Strong and diffuse immunoreactivity to somatostatin demonstrated in tumor cells

13. What types of NETs occur in the duodenum?

In addition to conventional NETs, the duodenum and periampullary area give rise to several particular types of NET, including some that are virtually exclusive to these locations.

Somatostatinomas are primarily located at the ampulla and in the duodenum (26% of duodenal NETs) with a lesser proportion of biologically distinct tumors in the pancreas. They arise from the somatostatin-producing D cells. They are characterized by prominent pseudoglandular/tubular architecture. The lumens of these structures may contain densely eosinophilic proteinaceous secretions. Psammomatous calcifications can be numerous throughout the tumor and are found in up to 68% of duodenal somatostatinomas. PAS with diastase predigestion highlights the secretions as brightly fuchsinophilic and also highlights a microvillous brush border on the pseudoglandular structures. Because of these peculiar morphological features, somatostatinomas may be mistaken for adenocarcinomas. The lack of significant cytological atypia and the presence of psammomatous calcifications should be an indication of the correct diagnosis, which can be confirmed by immunohistochemistry. Synaptophysin and chromogranin A immunostains are usually positive, and somatostatin immunostaining is diffusely positive (Fig. 17.5). Unlike pancreatic somatostatinomas that frequently present with somatostatin syndrome (the symptom constellation including cholelithiasis, diabetes mellitus, weight loss, and diarrhea), duodenal somatostatinomas are almost always asymptomatic upon discovery or only present due to biliary obstruction at the ampulla. The majority of duodenal somatostatinomas are sporadic, but a large subset (up to 43%) are associated with neurofibromatosis type 1 (NF1). These NF1-associated somatostatinomas have a particular predilection for the ampulla. Rare cases are also associated with MEN type 1, in which cases the somatostatinomas are often small, incidentally discovered upon resection for treatment of Zollinger-Ellison syndrome, and may be associated with somatostatin cell hyperplasia. Duodenal/ampullary somatostatinomas average 1.8 cm and may have lymph node metastases, though liver metastases or death from disease are rare.

Gastrin cell neoplasms predominantly arise in the proximal duodenum, with far fewer, biologically distinct tumors arising in the pancreas. Sporadic duodenal gastrin cell neoplasms are predominantly unifocal and may be secretory or nonsecreting. Gastrin cell neoplasms with secretory activity are termed "gastrinomas" and, with sufficient gastrin secretion, are responsible for Zollinger-Ellison syndrome, in which excessive gastrin secretion leads to gastric parietal cell and ECL cell hyperplasia with subsequent gastric and duodenal ulcers. Gastrinomas can be very small, with 74% of duodenal gastrinomas being smaller than 1 cm. And despite their small size, 60–80% of gastrin cell neoplasms have lymph node metastases at presentation. Between 25% and 33% of gastrinomas arise in the setting of MEN1. These are almost always secretory, located in the duodenum rather than the pancreas, and unlike sporadic gastrinomas are most commonly multifocal and arise in a background of duodenal gastrin cell hyperplasia. Morphologically, both sporadic and syndromic gastrin cell neoplasms show morphological features typical of gastrointestinal NETs, with predominantly trabecular architecture and fibrotic stroma. Patchy pseudoglandular formation may be seen, though this is not typically a prominent feature as in somatostatinomas, and a small subset of syndromic gastrinomas may have associated psammomatous calcifications. MEN1-associated gastrinomas have a much higher rate of lymph node and liver metastases than sporadic tumors (75% versus 6% and 20% versus 0, respectively, in one large series). Some authors propose that 28% of gastrinomas may be lymph nodal primary tumors based on an inability to localize a primary tumor and superior prognosis after resection compared to cases with known duodenal or pancreatic primaries. However, extensive tissue examination with correlative hormone immunohistochemistry has shown that duodenal gastri-

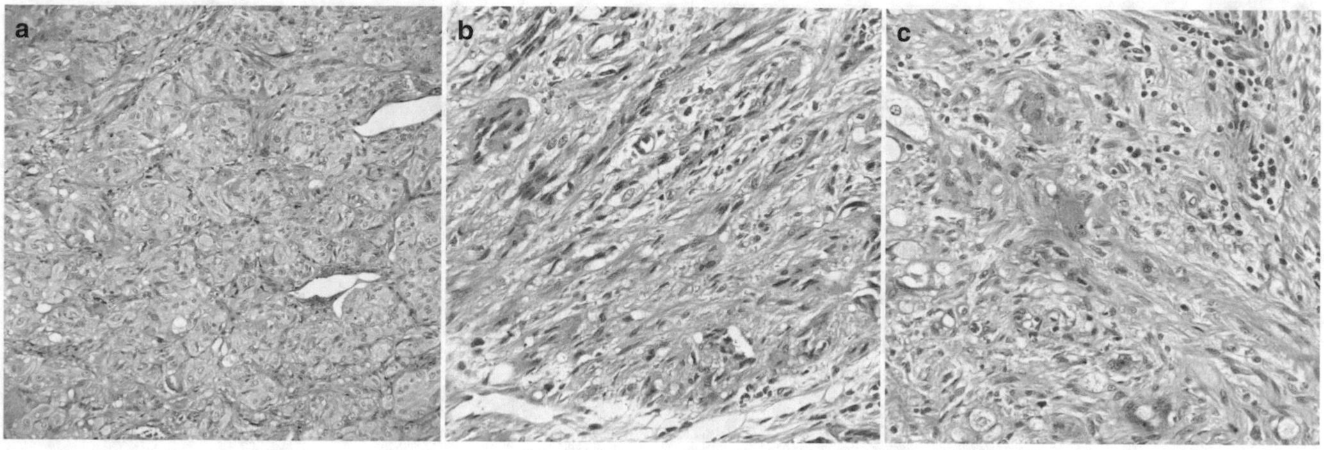

Fig. 17.6 Gangliocytic paraganglioma. (**a**) An area of prominent epithelioid component, arranged in trabecula. (**b**) Another area of the same mass predominantly showing a spindle cell component. (**c**) Scattered ganglion cells interspersed in the spindle cell area

nomas even <1 mm in size are capable of producing much larger lymph node metastases. This would explain why surgery removing bulky peripancreatic and/or periduodenal lymph nodal disease without an identifiable primary improves prognosis and suggests that many (if not all) of these instances are due to microscopic, unidentifiable gastrointestinal primary tumors.

Gangliocytic paraganglioma is a rare, unique tumor nearly exclusive to the second part of the duodenum and ampulla. It is composed of an admixture of three cell types (Fig. 17.6). Epithelioid cells are arranged in nests, trabecula, or pseudoglands, with palely eosinophilic cytoplasm and ovoid nuclei with fine chromatin and inconspicuous nucleoli. Ganglion cells may be clustered or scattered and are characterized by abundant eosinophilic cytoplasm with Nissl bodies and round nuclei with prominent nucleoli. Bland spindle cells are the third cell type and may be arranged haphazardly or in fascicles. The three components may be present in variable amounts and may not all be evident on small biopsies. Neuroendocrine markers, such as synaptophysin and chromogranin A, or pancytokeratin can highlight the epithelioid cells, which are also frequently positive for pancreatic polypeptide and somatostatin. Ganglion cells are highlighted by synaptophysin and neurofilament. Spindle cells are positive for S100 protein and neurofilament. Depending on which component is most prevalent in the sampled tissue, differential diagnostic considerations include NET, ganglioneuroma, paraganglioma, schwannoma, leiomyoma, and gastrointestinal stromal tumor. Before diagnosing any of these in the duodenum/ampulla, one should make a careful examination for the three components of gangliocytic paraganglioma, with immunohistochemistry applied as necessary to highlight the components. Up to 11% of gangliocytic paragangliomas may have metastases to regional lymph nodes, though only up to 1% may have liver metastases, and there is only a single reported case of death from disease. Extension into the submucosa or sphincter of Oddi and size >3.1 cm are associated with a significantly increased risk of lymph node metastases. No histological features have been shown to predict metastasis or aggressive behavior, and no necrosis or significant cytological atypia is typically seen, even in cases with metastases.

References: [32–42]

14. What are the characteristics of ileal NETs?

While the ileum is a common site for NETs, this category also includes biologically similar tumors that occur in the jejunum and cecum (the "midgut carcinoids" as originally proposed by Williams and Sandler). They are predominantly derived from ECL cells and are characterized morphologically by solid nests of cells with brightly eosinophilic cytoplasmic granules (Fig. 17.7). They are typically strongly and diffusely positive for CDX2.

Ileal NETs are graded similarly to other gastrointestinal NETs (see Question 5). However, detailed multivariate analysis has suggested that a Ki-67 proliferative rate cutoff of 5%, rather than 3%, may better predict aggressive tumor behavior. Recent studies using modern imaging and endoscopic techniques indicate up to 54% of small intestinal NETs are multifocal at presentation, though this feature does not seem to have an impact on survival or recurrence.

Although typically small, with an average size of 1.8 cm, ileal NETs are frequently metastatic at the time of diagnosis. Tumors <2 cm can produce significant mesenteric tumor deposits, including some many times larger than the primary tumor. Recent studies indicate that these tumor deposits are more prognostically significant even than lymph node metastases. This led to the addition of an N2 stage in the eighth edition of the *AJCC Cancer Staging Manual* for jejunal and ileal NETs, which includes tumors with ≥12 positive lymph nodes or mesenteric masses measuring >2 cm (Table 17.2). However, more recent investigation indicates that the num-

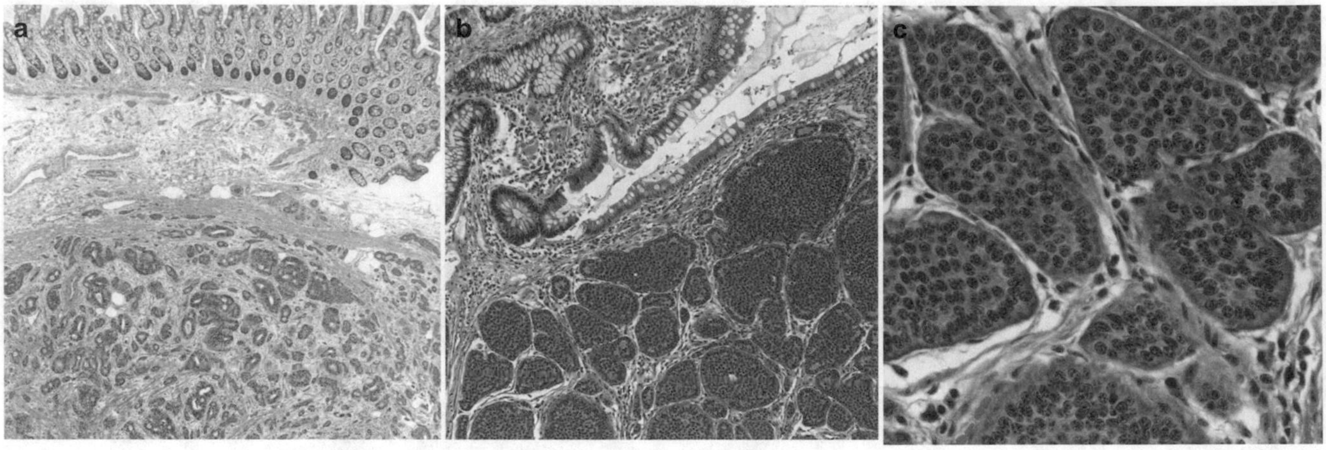

Fig. 17.7 Typical morphological features of midgut neuroendocrine tumor. (**a**) An ileal NET presenting as a submucosal proliferation with nests, trabecula, cords, and pseudoglandular architecture set in fibrotic stroma. (**b**) Predominantly nested architecture. (**c**) High magnification showing a moderate amount of eosinophilic granular cytoplasm, round nuclei, stippled chromatin, and inconspicuous nucleoli

ber, rather than size, of mesenteric deposits has a greater impact on prognosis.

Serotonin secretion is typically subclinical until a large metastatic tumor burden, particularly in the liver, leads to the carcinoid syndrome. Carcinoid syndrome appears in 20–30% of patients with metastases and is composed of diarrhea, flushing, and bronchoconstriction. Of patients with carcinoid syndrome, 25–50% develop carcinoid heart disease, in which effects of elevated serum serotonin lead to right heart endocardial fibrosis, subsequent tricuspid and pulmonic valve dysfunction, and right heart failure. Significant mesenteric and retroperitoneal fibrosis is also associated with advanced disease and significant serum serotonin elevation in rare cases, which can lead to adhesions, obstruction, and ischemia.
References: [4, 12, 43–52]

15. What are the characteristics of appendiceal NETs?

Prognostication is particularly important in appendiceal NETs, as they are frequently identified incidentally at the time of laparoscopic appendectomy, prompting the question of whether additional intervention is necessary. In addition to histological grading and staging, which are broadly important in all gastrointestinal NETs, tumor size, location, depth of invasion, and histology play key roles in management decisions.

Size is a particularly clear indicator of whether a right hemicolectomy with appropriate lymphadenectomy is warranted or not. For NETs <1 cm, appendectomy with clear margins is curative. NETs >2 cm have a risk of lymph node metastases ranging from 25% to 40%, and right hemicolectomy is recommended. For NETs measuring between 1 and 2 cm with a reported lymph node positivity rate of up to 10%, the necessity of a right hemicolectomy is less clear.

In these intermediate-sized NETs, the location of the tumor can provide additional guidance. Tumors limited to the appendiceal tip or otherwise clearly completely resected may be cured with appendectomy alone. >3 mm infiltration of tumor into the mesoappendix has also been suggested to reflect more aggressive biology and a higher probability of lymph-vascular invasion, suggesting consideration for right hemicolectomy. While less well documented, intermediate histological grade (G2) and the presence of lymphovascular invasion have also been suggested to confer a worse prognosis and warrant consideration of right hemicolectomy.

While the majority of appendiceal NETs derive from enterochromaffin (EC) cells, a subset is derived from the glucagon-like peptide-, pancreatic polypeptide-, and peptide YY-secreting L cells that are quantitatively less abundant in the appendix than in more distal parts of the gastrointestinal tract. L cell NETs are typically incidental findings at appendectomy. If detected grossly, they may appear as <1 cm nodules near the distal tip of the appendix. Histologically, they are composed of cords, thin trabecula, or tubular structures. They have no or minimal mitotic activity. While synaptophysin is positive by immunohistochemistry, most widely available chromogranin immunohistochemical stains (which stain for chromogranin A) are negative. Positivity for glucagon is a helpful adjunct to confirm the diagnosis. Due to their small size and minimal invasion at the time of diagnosis, L cell NETs have an indolent prognosis, when compared to EC NETs of similar size.

L cell NETs composed exclusively or predominantly of a tubular pattern have historically been described as "tubular carcinoids" (Fig. 17.8). The currently recommended terminology by WHO is "tubular NET" for this lesion. The tubular structures may show inspissated mucin, which is a diagnostic pitfall that may lead these to be mistaken for adenocarcinoma or goblet cell adenocarcinoma, though no intracellular mucin is present. They have a similar immunohistochemical profile to other L cell NETs. Tubular carcinoids described in the literature are uniformly benign. Please see Chap. 8, Question 9, for more discussion on this topic.
References: [51, 53–55]

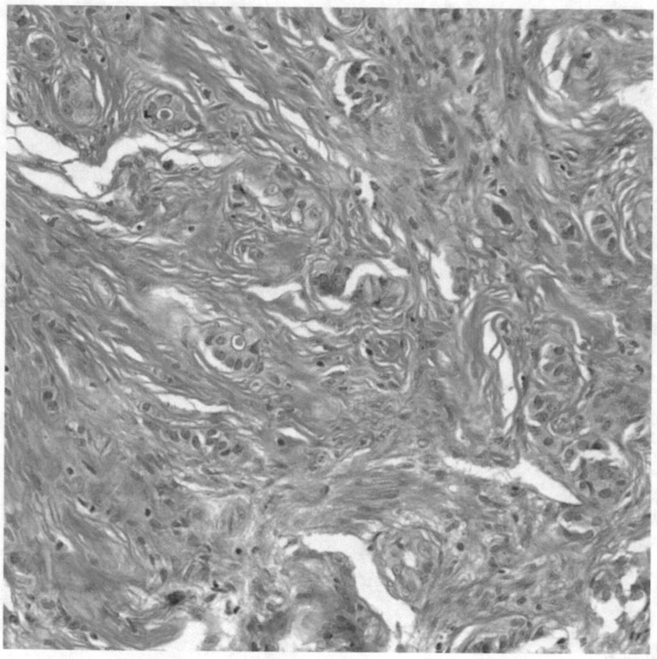

Fig. 17.8 An L cell neuroendocrine tumor of the appendix with predominantly tubular architecture (so-called "tubular carcinoid" or "tubular NET")

16. What are the characteristics of rectal NETs?

Rectal NETs can be subdivided into two types based on histological pattern and secretory products: serotonin-producing EC cell NETs and glucagon-like peptide-, pancreatic polypeptide-, and peptide YY-producing L cell NETs.

L cell NETs are characterized by predominantly trabecular or ribbon-like architecture and are the type most commonly found in the rectum (Fig. 17.9). In contrast, EC cell NETs predominantly show solid nests. However, staining for pancreatic polypeptide and serotonin does not correlate well with the morphological pattern, and immunohistochemical staining is not mutually exclusive between these two NET types. L cell rectal NETs are regarded as of uncertain malignant potential, in comparison to other gastrointestinal NETs, which are generally considered malignant. In one recent study, non-L cell immunophenotype and large tumor size (>1 cm) were associated with tumor grade and stage, both of which were independently poor prognostic indicators, although small L cell NETs may have lymph node metastases.

Only 30% of rectal NETs are positive for chromogranin A. Large majorities show diffuse, moderate to strong staining for ISL1 (89%) and polyclonal PAX8 (79%), similar to pancreatic NETs. CDX2 positivity is reported in only approximately 30% of rectal NETs, with CDX2-positive cases often showing patchy and weak staining. In contrast, rectal NETs often show strong and diffuse positivity for SATB2. Rectal NETs also display high levels (97%) of positivity for prostatic acid phosphatase.

References: [12, 15, 56, 57]

17. Are there any characteristic molecular features of NETs?

NETs have only a small number of recurrent molecular alterations, with the most common mutation being in *CDKN1B* in approximately 10% of small intestinal NETs. This mutation most frequently coexists with chromosome 18 loss of heterozygosity, the single most common genomic alteration in small intestinal NETs at 55%. Amplifications on chromosomes 4, 5, and 20 are also well described. New evidence suggests that methylation may play a key role in driving NET biology, as tumors with high methylation have a worse prognosis than tumors with chromosome 18 losses and low methylation rates.

In NETs, greater understanding of molecular mechanisms has led to recent treatment innovations. NETs have long been noted to have a rich capillary network, and targeting the vascular endothelial growth factor pathway has been shown to extend progression-free survival in a clinical trial. Inhibition of the mammalian target of rapamycin (mTOR) pathway, affecting both proliferation and angiogenesis, has also shown promise against gastrointestinal NETs in a late phase clinical trial. Recent studies have shown that grade 3 NETs and NECs have a high expression of programmed death-ligand 1 (PD-L1) on tumor cells and tumor-infiltrating lymphocytes, suggesting that these tumors could be promising targets for immunotherapeutic agents involved in PD-L1 blockade.

Microsatellite instability has been detected in 12–15% of NECs and MANECs, highly correlated with extensive gene methylation (CpG island methylator phenotype), a rate similar to that in adenocarcinomas of the gastrointestinal tract. *BRAF* V600E mutations are frequent in these microsatellite-unstable NECs and MANECs. The microsatellite-unstable subset of NECs and MANECs is also associated with a significantly better prognosis, with a median survival of 60 months in microsatellite-unstable carcinomas compared to 5.5 months in microsatellite-stable carcinomas.

A greater understanding of the genomic landscape of NECs and MANECs has led to strong evidence that the neuroendocrine component of these carcinomas is derived from glandular adenomas or adenocarcinomas, rather than from NETs. Loss of heterozygosity at the same loci for *APC* and *TP53* genes has been demonstrated in the adenocarcinoma and NEC components of MANECs. In sequencing studies, identical *BRAF*, *KRAS*, and *TP53* mutations are frequently seen in the adenocarcinoma and NEC components of colorectal MANECs. Gastric MANECs have shown similar alterations. Alterations in these genes are common in typical colorectal adenocarcinomas and suggest derivation from glandular dysplasia/neoplasia. The NEC components of gastrointestinal MANECs then typically show additional mutations, most commonly of the retinoblastoma (*RB*) gene or related genes.

References: [58–68]

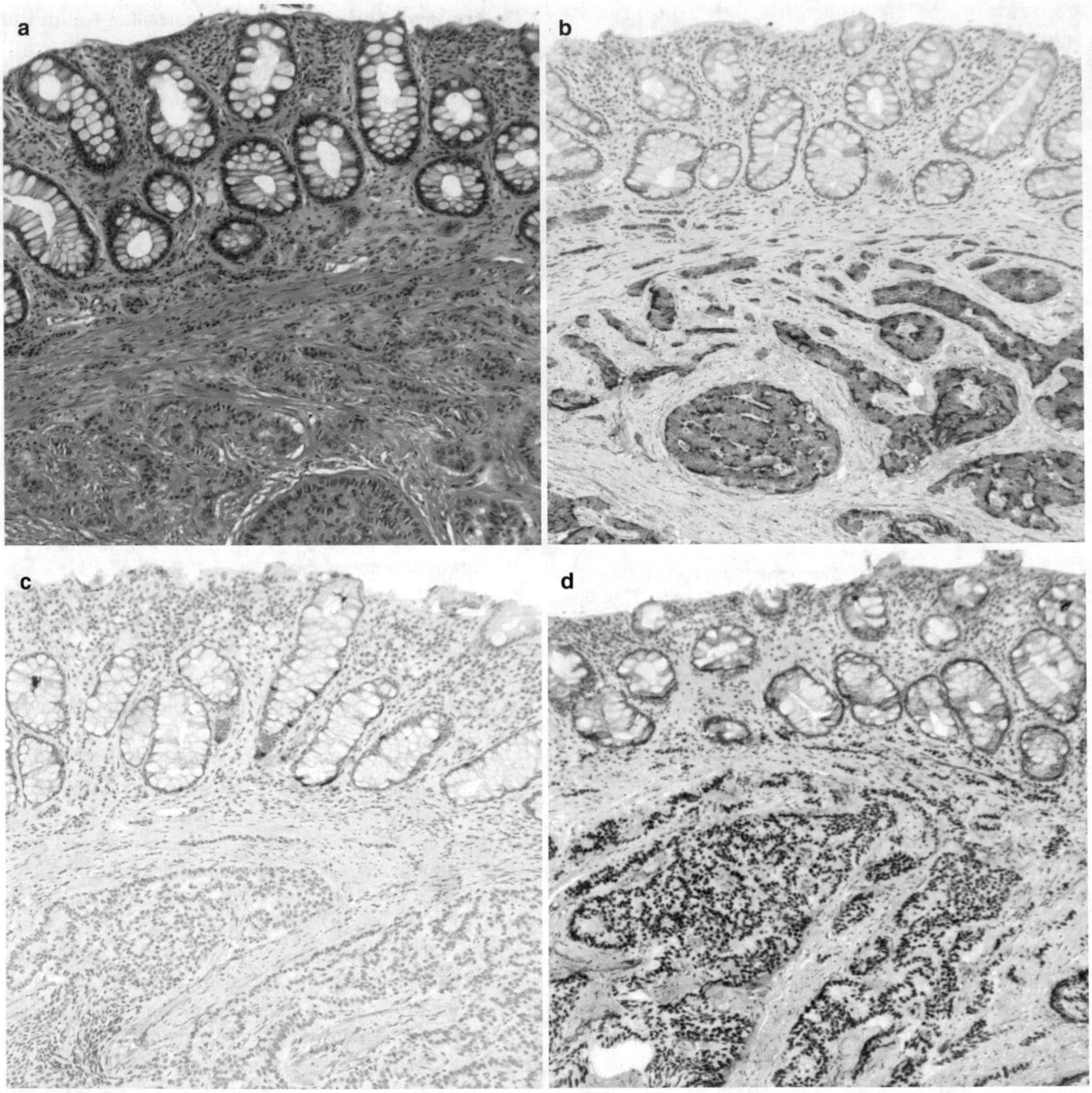

Fig. 17.9 Typical features of rectal neuroendocrine tumor. (**a**) A rectal NET presenting as a predominantly submucosal proliferation of neuroendocrine cells arranged in cords, trabecula, and nests. (**b**) Strong and diffuse synaptophysin positivity seen in tumor cells. (**c**) Negativity for chromogranin A. (**d**) Strong and diffuse nuclear ISL1 positivity

Case Presentation

Case 1

A gastric biopsy shows a monotonous, nested epithelioid cellular proliferation in the deep lamina propria. The cells have a nested architecture, moderate amount of cytoplasm, round nuclei with inconspicuous nucleoli, and stippled chromatin, typical of an NET (Fig. 17.10). Synaptophysin and chromogranin A are positive, confirming neuroendocrine differentiation.

But is this proliferation an NET, neuroendocrine cell hyperplasia, or dysplasia? Neuroendocrine cell hyperplasia is characterized by linear arrangements of neuroendocrine cells present within gastric pits but increased in number. Nodular neuroendocrine cell hyperplasia consists of small

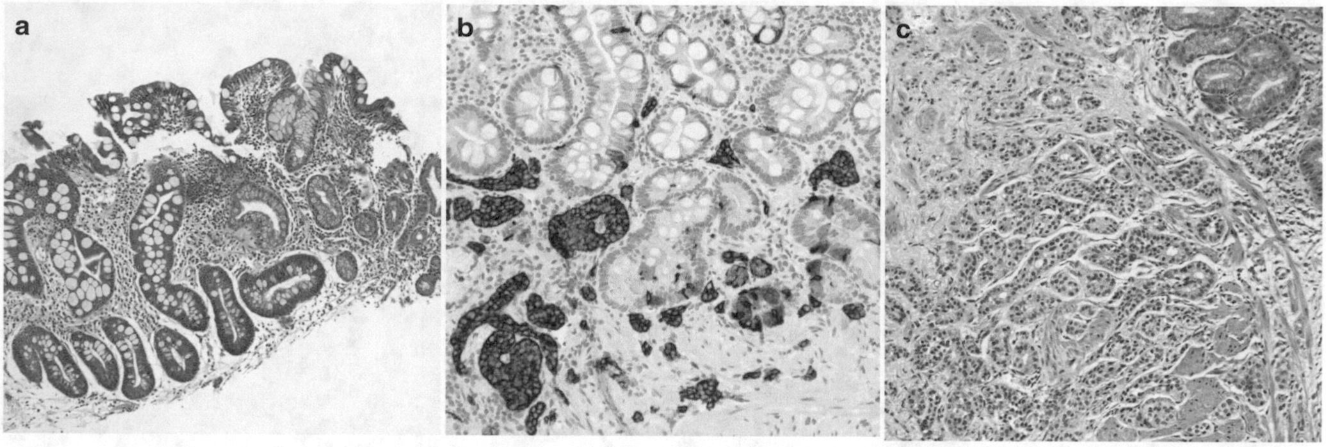

Fig. 17.10 (Case 1) (**a**) Atrophic gastric corpus mucosa with extensive intestinal metaplasia, pyloric metaplasia, lamina propria lymphoplasmacytic infiltrate, and parietal cell atrophy. (**b**) Nodular neuroendocrine cell hyperplasia and dysplasia consistent with autoimmune (atrophic) gastritis. (**c**) NET with confluent growth and infiltration into the submucosa

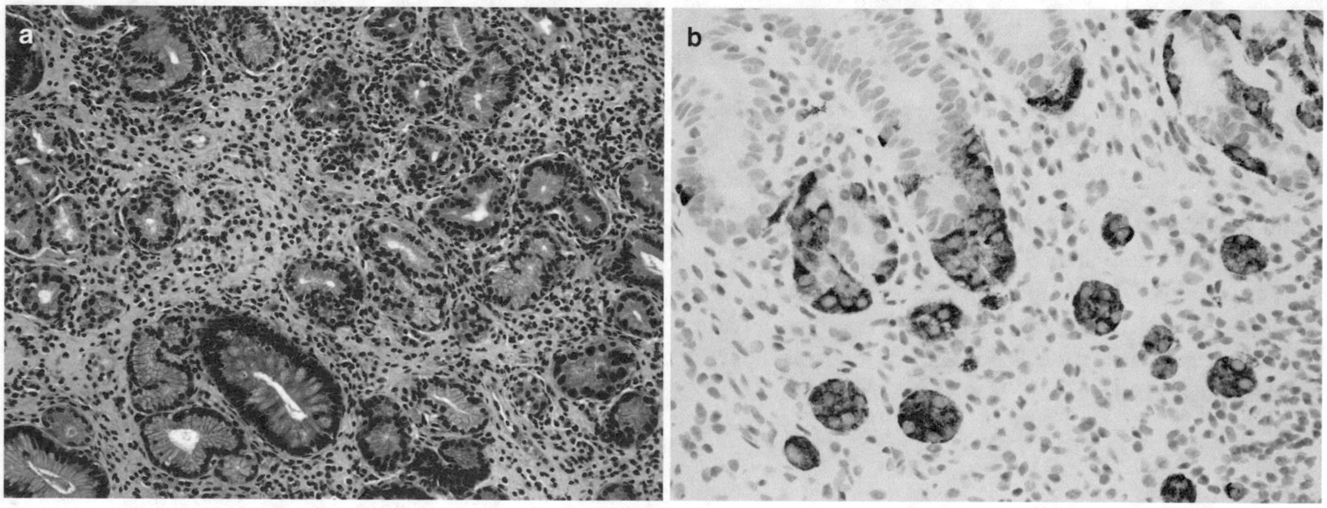

Fig. 17.11 (Case 1) Additional biopsies of the gastric body further showing features of atrophic gastritis (**a**) and linear and nodular neuroendocrine cell hyperplasia as highlighted by chromogranin immunostain (**b**). The findings support the diagnosis of low-grade gastric NET, type 1

aggregates of five or more neuroendocrine cells. Adenomatoid hyperplasia is characterized by five or more of these nodules aggregated near each other. Finally, dysplasia occurs when these neuroendocrine nests become confluent and/or enlarged to ≥150 μm. The proliferation in this case is a discrete mass with new stroma formation and measures >500 μm, all features of NET.

Biopsies of the background mucosa of the gastric antrum show mild chronic inactive gastritis. The background corpus mucosa shows moderate chronic gastritis, patchy intestinal and pyloric metaplasia, and marked parietal cell atrophy. The findings of corpus-predominant inflammation, metaplasia, and parietal cell atrophy in the background mucosa raise the possibility of autoimmune (atrophic) gastritis. Careful microscopic examination reveals no *Helicobacter* organisms (confirmed by immunohistochemistry) and a gastrin immunostain on the sections labeled as coming from the gastric corpus confirm a lack of G cells, thereby confirming that the biopsies are from atrophic body mucosa and not antral mucosa. A chromogranin A immunostain highlights linear and nodular neuroendocrine cell hyperplasia, further suggesting the possibility of autoimmune (atrophic) gastritis (Fig. 17.11).

The lack of identified *Helicobacter* organisms and the pattern of corpus-predominant chronic inactive gastritis rather than antral-predominant chronic active gastritis exclude *Helicobacter*-associated gastritis. The presence of parietal cell atrophy rather than parietal cell hyperplasia excludes Zollinger-Ellison syndrome (and type 2 gastric NET). Altogether, the background features are strongly suggestive of a type 1 gastric NET: an NET arising in the background of autoimmune atrophic gastritis. This case is reported with a note to correlate with serological testing for anti-parietal cell and anti-intrinsic factor antibodies to confirm the diagnosis of autoimmune gastritis and

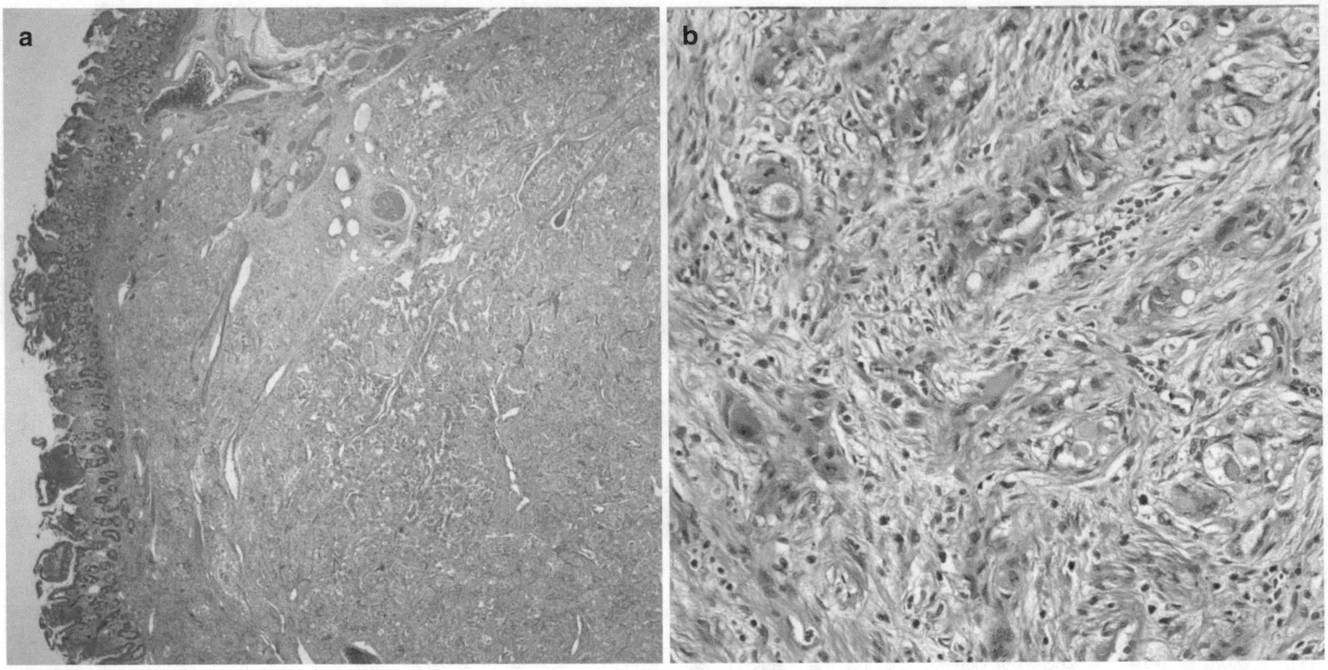

Fig. 17.12 (Case 2) (**a**) Low-power examination showing a nested proliferation in the submucosa. (**b**) High-power examination revealing an admixture of nests of epithelioid cells, scattered ganglion cells, and intervening spindle cells, diagnostic of gangliocytic paraganglioma

report the high likelihood that this NET represents a type 1 gastric NET. This information is important to convey to the clinician, as type 1 NETs have indolent biology with lower risks of nodal and distant metastases than type 2 and type 3 gastric NETs, and endoscopic surveillance with mucosal resection may be an adequate treatment.

Case 2

A mucosal biopsy from the ampulla of Vater shows an epithelioid cellular proliferation in the lamina propria. Careful inspection shows rare ganglion cells intimately admixed and scattered with spindle cell areas (Fig. 17.12). This characteristic triphasic morphology is diagnostic of gangliocytic paraganglioma.

The second part of the duodenum and the ampulla of Vater are the classical location for gangliocytic paraganglioma, and, though very rare, this diagnosis should always be kept in mind from biopsies of nodules, polyps, or masses in this area. In the current case, careful examination of the hematoxylin- and eosin-stained sections readily reveals all three of the characteristic cells. However, in small biopsies, one or more of the cell types may be sparse or entirely absent (unsampled). Thus, a high index of suspicion at this site is necessary. Immunohistochemistry may be used to highlight rare cells: a practical panel may include pancytokeratin to highlight the epithelioid cells, synaptophysin to highlight the ganglion cells, and S100 protein to highlight the spindle cells.

If the characteristic morphology is not recognized, these tumors can easily be misdiagnosed as ganglioneuromas (if an epithelioid component is not identified), paragangliomas (if the ganglion cell component is not identified), or spindle cell neoplasms (schwannomas, smooth muscle tumors, or even gastrointestinal stromal tumors, if epithelioid and ganglion cell components are not identified). If the epithelioid cell component is prominent, the fact that these frequently stain positively for synaptophysin and chromogranin A makes NET a frequent misdiagnosis. Furthermore, the same location is notable for several unique NETs, such as somatostatinoma and gastrinoma.

While gangliocytic paragangliomas typically behave in an indolent fashion, even with lymph node metastases, it is important to exclude some of the above entities with decidedly more aggressive prognoses. NETs at this location may also suggest wider syndromes, such as the association of somatostatinomas with NF1 and of gastrinomas with MEN1.

Case 3

A small intestinal resection is performed for a submucosal/intramural tumor. The tumor is composed primarily of trabecula and nests of epithelioid cells with a moderate amount of cytoplasm, finely granular chromatin, and inconspicuous nucleoli (Fig. 17.13). Synaptophysin and chromogranin A immunostains are diffusely positive, confirming neuroendocrine differentiation. Mitotic figures are readily

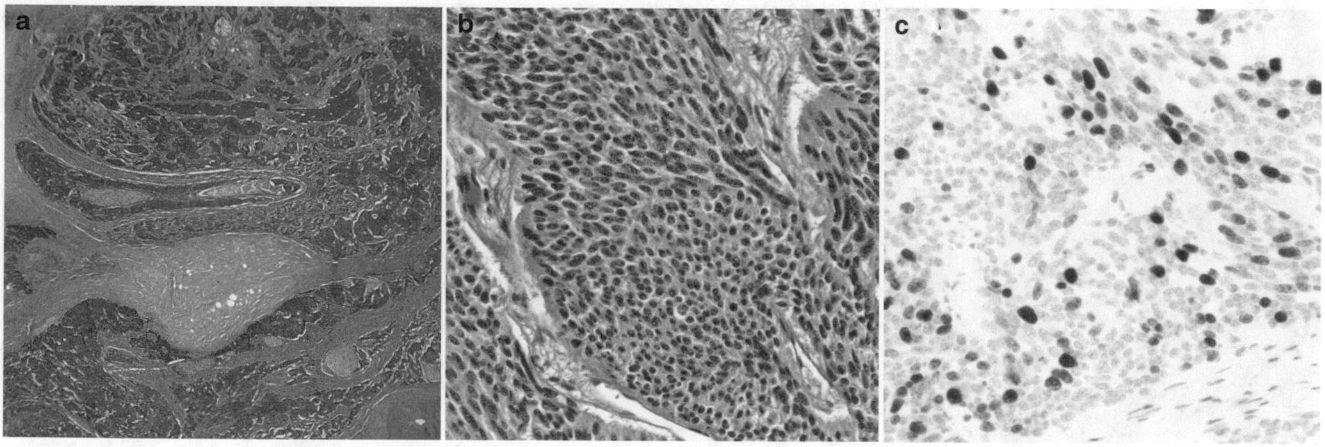

Fig. 17.13 (Case 3) (**a**) Low-power view showing nested and trabecular architecture with significant stromal fibrosis and perineural invasion. (**b**) Although the tumor cells are somewhat spindled in this case, they have moderate cytoplasm, inconspicuous nucleoli, and finely granular chromatin, all features of an NET. (**c**) Although well-differentiated morphologically, the tumor shows a Ki-67 proliferative rate in excess of 20%

identified, and a count of 10 mm^2 reveals 22 mitotic figures per 2 mm^2. Ki-67 immunostain shows 30% of 1300 tumor cells counted staining positively in the area of highest positivity.

Now that the diagnosis of a neuroendocrine neoplasm is established, the primary question becomes: Is this a high-grade (G3) NET or a NEC? Both NETs and NECs may have mitotic rates >20 per 2 mm^2, and both may have Ki-67 proliferative indexes of >20%. Differentiating the two resides in the morphological appearance. The tumor described above shows classical features of an NET. NECs are, by definition, poorly differentiated showing morphological features not seen in the current case. SCCs show a high nucleus-to-cytoplasm ratio, nuclear molding, smooth chromatin, necrosis, and abundant apoptosis. LCNECs show vesicular or coarse chromatin, prominent nucleoli, abundant cytoplasm, and necrosis. Immunohistochemistry may be helpful as supportive evidence. NECs are more likely to show aberrant staining for p53, loss of RB protein, and negative staining for somatostatin receptor 2.

Although high-grade NETs appear to be rare in the gastrointestinal tract, reports from other organs indicate a prognosis intermediate between G2 NETs and NECs. More investigation is necessary as to the implications of this diagnosis in the tubular gastrointestinal tract, but accurate diagnosis is the first step toward determining prognostic differences and differences in therapeutic efficacy.
Reference: [6]

Case 4

A portion of terminal ileum is resected for a large mesenteric mass and lymphadenopathy. Gross examination reveals an 11.5 cm well-circumscribed mass near the root of the mesentery, multiple enlarged lymph nodes, and a 1.5 cm submucosal mass with focal overlying mucosal ulceration. Microscopic examination of the submucosal mass shows features typical of an NET, including trabecular architecture, moderate cytoplasm, eosinophilic cytoplasmic granules, finely granular chromatin, and inconspicuous nucleoli predominantly involving the submucosa with extension through the muscularis propria and to the serosal surface. Identical features are seen in abundant representative sections of the mesenteric mass (Fig. 17.14). Five lymph nodes are positive, though the large mesenteric mass shows no obvious residual lymphoid tissue after extensive sampling. Chromogranin A and synaptophysin immunostains confirm the diagnosis of NET. Mitotic rate and Ki-67 proliferative index are both low, indicating low grade (G1).

Can such a small ileal tumor produce such a large mesenteric mass? Should the possibility of an occult, unsampled primary be considered? Small intestinal primary NETs even <2 cm may produce significant lymphadenopathy and mesenteric masses. In a case like this, there is no reason to doubt that the sampled submucosal mass represents the primary. Should there be any doubt, positive CDX2 immunostaining in the mesenteric mass, combined with negative TTF1, PAX6, PAX8, ISL1, and/or SATB2, would be consistent with an ileal primary.

But what is the nature of this large mesenteric mass? Is it a large nodal metastasis, lymphovascular invasion, or perineural invasion? No surrounding residual lymph nodal tissue or vascular smooth muscle is identified, excluding classification as a lymph node metastasis or lymphovascular invasion. While small entrapped vessels and nerves may be seen, the size and gross configuration (well circumscribed) of this lesion best qualifies it as a mesenteric mass rather than perineural invasion or lymphovascular invasion. In the current version of the AJCC staging manual, mesenteric masses >2 cm in size qualify as N2 disease. The finding of the large mesenteric mass in this case upstages the tumor to pT4N2.
Reference: [49]

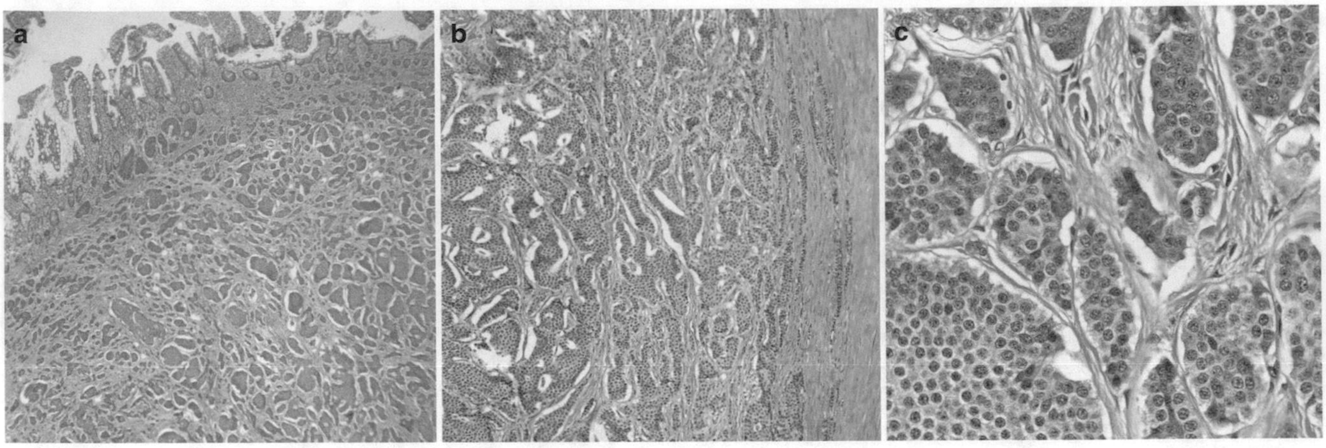

Fig. 17.14 (Case 4) (**a**) A small intestinal tumor composed of nests, cords, and trabecula of tumor cells set in fibrotic stroma filling the submucosa. (**b**) A discrete mesenteric mass with a thick fibrotic capsule present, which is separate from the mural tumor in part A. There is no discernible lymphoid tissue or surrounding vascular smooth muscle to indicate a lymph node metastasis or vascular invasion. (**c**) High-power examination showing the classical features of an NET, including moderate cytoplasm and round nuclei with fine granular cytoplasm and inconspicuous nucleoli

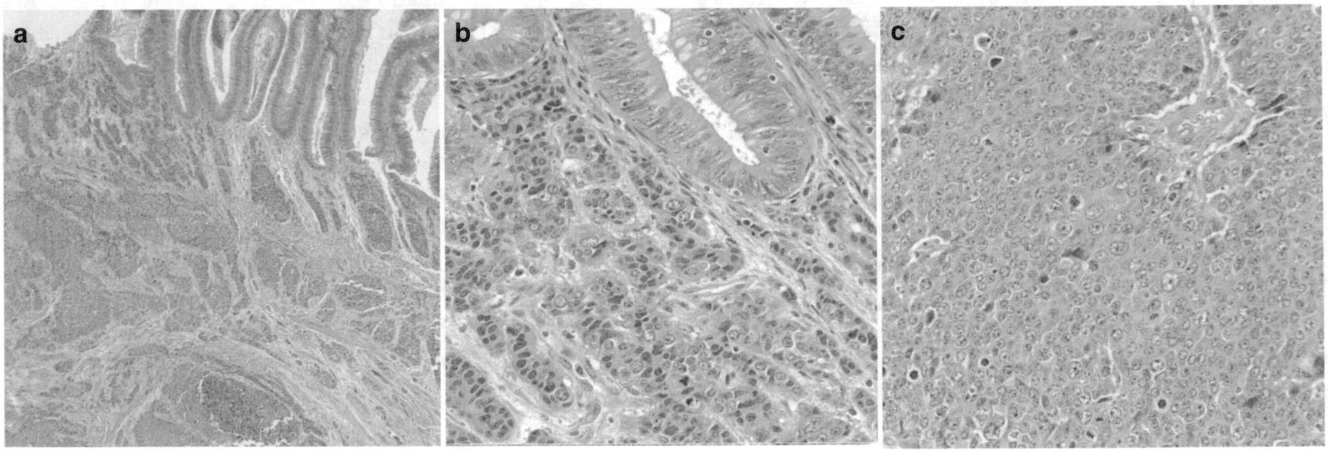

Fig. 17.15 (Case 5) (**a**) The top portion of the photomicrograph shows villiform surface projections lined by low-grade neoplastic epithelium overlying solid nests and trabecula of more poorly differentiated cells. (**b**) High-power examination showing glandular epithelium with scattered apical mucin-containing cells and elongated, hyperchromatic, and pseudostratified nuclei. The glandular component is directly adjacent to invasive carcinoma arranged in trabecula and cords, typical morphology for neuroendocrine neoplasms. (**c**) High-power examination of the invasive component showing neoplastic cells with a high nucleus-to-cytoplasm ratio, irregular nuclear contours, vesicular chromatin, variably prominent nucleoli, and brisk mitotic activity. With confirmation of neuroendocrine differentiation by immunohistochemistry, this component is labeled as NEC. The entire tumor can thus be labeled as a mixed neuroendocrine-nonneuroendocrine neoplasm (MiNEN)

Case 5

An abdominoperineal resection is performed for a low rectal mass. Histological examination shows that the superficial half of the mass is composed of villous adenoma with pseudostratified columnar cells having apical intracellular mucin and elongated, hyperchromatic nuclei. Immediately deep to the villous adenoma are nests and trabecula of cells with high nucleus-to-cytoplasm ratios, vesicular chromatin, and variably prominent nucleoli (Fig. 17.15). Mitotic figures are abundant. Due to the nested and trabecular architecture, immunostains for synaptophysin and chromogranin A are performed, which are diffusely positive in the portion of the tumor with this architecture. The villous component is negative for both immunostains. Ki-67 proliferative index in the neuroendocrine component is 80%.

What is the explanation for half of the tumor showing positivity for neuroendocrine markers? Is this NET or NEC? Although the nested and trabecular architecture of the tumor may raise the possibility of NET, high-power examination reveals nuclear atypia, a high nucleus-to-cytoplasm ratio, and chromatin patterns suggestive of LCNEC. This tumor would be best classified as NEC arising in a villous adenoma.

The recent proposal by La Rosa and colleagues creates the expansive category of mixed neuroendocrine-nonneuroendocrine neoplasms (MiNEN), which captures all tumors composed of ≥30% each of neuroendocrine and nonneuroendocrine elements. This classification includes neuroendocrine neoplasms of all types (NET, LCNEC, and SCC) and all grades and includes any glandular component, whether invasive or adenomatous. While broad, this proposal best reflects the heterogeneity of these mixed neoplasms and has been adopted by the current WHO tumor classification. In the current case, the designation of MiNEN best fits the histological findings and appropriately flags the potentially aggressive nature of the lesion.
Reference: [18]

References

1. Dasari A, Shen C, Halperin D, et al. Trends in the incidence, prevalence, and survival outcomes in patients with neuroendocrine tumors in the United States. JAMA Oncol. 2017;3(10):1335–42.
2. Kimura N, Pilichowska M, Okamoto H, Kimura I, Aunis D. Immunohistochemical expression of chromogranins A and B, prohormone convertases 2 and 3, and amidating enzyme in carcinoid tumors and pancreatic endocrine tumors. Mod Pathol. 2000;13(2):140–6.
3. Chejfec G, Falkmer S, Grimelius L, et al. Synaptophysin. A new marker for pancreatic neuroendocrine tumors. Am J Surg Pathol. 1987;11(4):241–7.
4. Williams ED, Sandler M. The classification of carcinoid tumours. Lancet. 1963;1(7275):238–9.
5. Shia J, Tang LH, Weiser MR, et al. Is nonsmall cell type high-grade neuroendocrine carcinoma of the tubular gastrointestinal tract a distinct disease entity? Am J Surg Pathol. 2008;32(5):719–31.
6. Tang LH, Basturk O, Sue JJ, Klimstra DS. A practical approach to the classification of WHO grade 3 (G3) well-differentiated neuroendocrine tumor (WD-NET) and poorly differentiated neuroendocrine carcinoma (PD-NEC) of the pancreas. Am J Surg Pathol. 2016;40(9):1192–202.
7. Wang Y, Wang W, Jin K, et al. Somatostatin receptor expression indicates improved prognosis in gastroenteropancreatic neuroendocrine neoplasm, and octreotide long-acting release is effective and safe in Chinese patients with advanced gastroenteropancreatic neuroendocrine tumors. Oncol Lett. 2017;13(3):1165–74.
8. Amin MB, Edge SB, Greene FL, et al., editors. AJCC Cancer staging manual. 8th ed. Chicago, IL: American College of Surgeons; 2017. p. 351–406.
9. Reid MD, Bagci P, Ohike N, et al. Calculation of the Ki67 index in pancreatic neuroendocrine tumors: a comparative analysis of four counting methodologies. Mod Pathol. 2015;28(5):686–94.
10. Klöppel G, La Rosa S. Ki67 labeling index: assessment and prognostic role in gastroenteropancreatic neuroendocrine neoplasms. Virchows Arch. 2018;472:341–9.
11. Yang Z, Tang LH, Klimstra DS. Effect of tumor heterogeneity on the assessment of Ki67 labeling index in well-differentiated neuroendocrine tumors metastatic to the liver: implications for prognostic stratification. Am J Surg Pathol. 2011;35(6):853–60.
12. Bellizzi AM. Assigning site of origin in metastatic neuroendocrine neoplasms: a clinically significant application of diagnostic immunohistochemistry. Adv Anat Pathol. 2013;20(5):285–314.
13. Li Z, Yuan J, Wei L, et al. SATB2 is a sensitive marker for lower gastrointestinal well-differentiated neuroendocrine tumors. Int J Clin Exp Pathol. 2015;8(6):7072–82.
14. Mohanty S, Bhardwaj N, Lugo H, et al. Diagnostic utility of SATB2 in determining the site of origin of well-differentiated neuroendocrine tumors. Pancreas. 2018;47(3):348.
15. Koo J, Zhou X, Moschiano E, De Peralta-Venturina M, Mertens RB, Dhall D. The immunohistochemical expression of islet 1 and PAX8 by rectal neuroendocrine tumors should be taken into account in the differential diagnosis of metastatic neuroendocrine tumors of unknown primary origin. Endocr Pathol. 2013;24(4):184–90.
16. Uccella S, La Rosa S, Volante M, Papotti M. Immunohistochemical biomarkers of gastrointestinal, pancreatic, pulmonary, and thymic neuroendocrine neoplasms. Endocr Pathol. 2018;29(2):150–68.
17. Klimstra DS, Capella C, Arnold R, et al. Neuroendocrine neoplasms of the colon and rectum. In: Bosman FT, Carneiro F, Hruban RH, Theise N, editors. WHO classification of tumours of the digestive tract. 4th ed. Lyon, France: IARC Press; 2010. p. 714–177.
18. La Rosa S, Sessa F, Uccella S. Mixed neuroendocrine-nonneuroendocrine neoplasms (MiNENs): unifying the concept of a heterogeneous group of neoplasms. Endocr Pathol. 2016;27(4):284–311.
19. De Mestier L, Cros J, Neuzillet C, et al. Digestive system mixed neuroendocrine-nonneuroendocrine neoplasms. Neuroendocrinology. 2017;105(4):412–25.
20. Li Y, Yau A, Schaeffer D, et al. Colorectal glandular-neuroendocrine mixed tumor: pathologic spectrum and clinical implications. Am J Surg Pathol. 2011;35(3):413–25.
21. Solcia E, Bordi C, Creutzfeldt W, et al. Histopathological classification of nonantral gastric endocrine growths in man. Digestion. 1988;41(4):185–200.
22. Scherübel H, Cadiot G, Jensen RT, Rösch T, Stölzel U, Klöppel G. Neuroendocrine tumors of the stomach (gastric carcinoids) are on the rise: small tumors, small problems? Endoscopy. 2010;42(8):664–71.
23. Gladdy RA, Strong VE, Coit D, et al. Defining surgical indications for type I gastric carcinoid tumor. Ann Surg Oncol. 2009;16(11):3154–60.
24. Lupinacci RM, Dias AR, Mello ES, Kondo A. Minute type I gastric carcinoid with regional lymph node metastasis. Int J Surg Pathol. 2013;21(2):169–72.
25. Grozinsky-Glasberg S, Thomas D, Strosberg JR, et al. Metastatic type 1 gastric carcinoid: a real threat or just a myth? World J Gastroenterol. 2013;19(46):8687–95.
26. Modlin IM, Kidd M, Latich I, Zikusoka MN, Shapiro MD. Current status of gastrointestinal carcinoids. Gastroenterology. 2005;128(6):1717–51.
27. Hung OY, Maithel SK, Willingham FF, Farris AB 3rd, Kauh JS. Hypergastrinemia, type 1 gastric carcinoid tumors: diagnosis and management. J Clin Oncol. 2011;29(25):e713–5.
28. Borch K, Ahrén B, Ahlman H, Falkmer S, Granérus G, Grimelius L. Gastric carcinoids: biologic behavior and prognosis after differential treatments in relation to type. Ann Surg. 2005;242(1):64–73.
29. Ooi A, Ota M, Katsuda S, Nakanishi I, Sugawara H, Takahashi I. An unusual case of multiple gastric carcinoids associated with diffuse endocrine cell hyperplasia and parietal cell hypertrophy. Endocr Pathol. 1995;6(3):229–37.
30. Abraham SC, Carney JA, Ooi A, Choti MA, Argani P. Achlorhydria, parietal cell hyperplasia, and multiple gastric carcinoids: a new disorder. Am J Surg Pathol. 2005;29(7):969–75.
31. Nakata K, Aishima S, Ichimiya H, et al. Unusual multiple gastric carcinoids with hypergastrinemia: report of a case. Surg Today. 2010;40(3):267–71.
32. Garbrecht N, Anlauf M, Schmitt A, et al. Somatostatin-producing neuroendocrine tumors of the duodenum and pancreas: incidence,

types, biological behavior, association with inherited syndromes, and functional activity. Endocr Relat Cancer. 2008;15(1):229–41.
33. Tanaka S, Yamasaki S, Matsushita H, et al. Duodenal somatostatinoma: a case report and review of 31 cases with special reference to the relationship between tumor size and metastasis. Pathol Int. 2000;50(2):146–52.
34. Anlauf M, Perren A, Meyer CL, et al. Precursor lesions in patients with multiple endocrine neoplasia type 1-associated duodenal gastrinomas. Gastroenterology. 2005;128(5):1187–98.
35. Williams GT. Endocrine tumours of the gastrointestinal tract-selected topics. Histopathology. 2007;50(1):30–41.
36. Donow C, Pipeleers-Marichal M, Schröder S, Stamm B, Heitz PU, Klöppel G. Surgical pathology of gastrinoma. Site, size, multicentricity, association of multiple endocrine neoplasia type 1, and malignancy. Cancer. 1991;68(6):1329–34.
37. Anlauf M, Garbrecht N, Henopp T, et al. Sporadic versus hereditary gastrinomas of the duodenum and pancreas: distinct clinico-pathological and epidemiological features. World J Gastroenterol. 2006;12(34):5440–6.
38. Rosentraeger MJ, Garbrecht N, Anlauf M, et al. Syndromic versus non-syndromic sporadic gastrin-producing neuroendocrine tumors of the duodenum: comparison of pathological features and biological behavior. Virchows Arch. 2016;468(3):277–87.
39. Chen Y, Deshpande V, Ferrone C, et al. Primary lymph node gastrinoma: a single institution experience. Surgery. 2017;162(5):1088–94.
40. Anlauf M, Enosawa T, Henopp T, et al. Primary lymph node gastrinoma or occult duodenal microgastrinoma with lymph node metastasis in an MEN1 patient: the need for a systematic search for the primary tumor. Am J Surg Pathol. 2008;32(7):1101–5.
41. Okubo Y, Yoshioka E, Suzuki M, et al. Diagnosis, pathological findings, and clinical management of gangliocytic paraganglioma: a systematic review. Front Oncol. 2018;8:291.
42. Li B, Li Y, Tian XY, Luo BN, Li Z. Malignant gangliocytic paraganglioma of the duodenum with distant metastases and a lethal course. World J Gastroenterol. 2014;20(41):15454–61.
43. Burke AP, Thomas RM, Elsayed AM, Sobin LH. Carcinoids of the jejunum and ileum: an immunohistochemical and clinicopathologic study of 167 cases. Cancer. 1997;79(6):1086–93.
44. Panzuto F, Campana D, Fazio N, et al. Risk factors for disease progression in advanced jejunoileal neuroendocrine tumors. Neuroendocrinology. 2012;96(1):32–40.
45. Choi AB, Maxwell JE, Keck KJ, et al. Is multifocality an indicator of aggressive behavior in small bowel neuroendocrine tumors? Pancreas. 2017;46(9):1115–20.
46. Gangi A, Siegel E, Barmparas G, et al. Multifocality in small bowel neuroendocrine tumors. J Gastrointest Surg. 2018;22(2):303–9.
47. Gonzalez RS, Liu EH, Alvarez JR, Ayers GD, Washington MK, Shi C. Should mesenteric tumor deposits be included in staging of well-differentiated small intestine neuroendocrine tumors? Mod Pathol. 2014;27(9):1288–95.
48. Fata CR, Gonzalez RS, Liu E, Cates JM, Shi C. Mesenteric tumor deposits in midgut small intestinal neuroendocrine tumors are a stronger indication than lymph node metastasis for liver metastasis and poor prognosis. Am J Surg Pathol. 2017;41(1):128–33.
49. Woltering EA, Bergsland EK, Beyer DT, et al. Neuroendocrine tumors of the jejunum and ileum. In: Amin MB, Edge SB, Greene FL, et al., editors. AJCC Cancer staging manual. 8th ed. Chicago, IL: American College of Surgeons; 2017. p. 375–87.
50. Gonzalez RS, Cates JMM, Shi C. Number, not size, of mesenteric tumor deposits affects prognosis of small intestinal well-differentiated neuroendocrine tumors. Mod Pathol. 2018;31(10):1560–6.
51. Pape UF, Perren A, Niederle B, et al. ENETS Consensus Guidelines for the management of patients with neuroendocrine neoplasms from the jejuno-ileum and the appendix including goblet cell carcinomas. Neuroendocrinology. 2012;95(2):135–56.
52. Daskalakis K, Karakatsanis A, Stålberg P, Norlén O, Hellman P. Clinical signs of fibrosis in small intestinal neuroendocrine tumours. Br J Surg. 2017;104(1):69–75.
53. Iwafuchi M, Watanabe H, Ajoka Y, Shimoda T, Iwashita A, Ito S. Immunohistochemical and ultrastructural studies of twelve argentaffin and six argyrophil carcinoids of the appendix vermiformis. Hum Pathol. 1990;21(7):773–80.
54. Burke AP, Sobin LH, Federspiel BH, Shekitka KM, Helwig EB. Goblet cell carcinoids and related tumors of the vermiform appendix. Am J Clin Pathol. 1990;94(1):27–35.
55. Warkel RL, Cooper PH, Helwig EB. Adenocarcinoid, a mucin-producing carcinoid tumor of the appendix: a study of 39 cases. Cancer. 1978;42(6):2781–93.
56. Koo J, Mertens RB, Mirocha JM, Wang HL, Dhall D. Value of islet 1 and PAX8 in identifying metastatic neuroendocrine tumors of pancreatic origin. Mod Pathol. 2012;25(6):893–901.
57. Kim JY, Kim KS, Kim KJ, et al. Non-L-cell immunophenotype and large tumor size in rectal neuroendocrine tumors are associated with aggressive clinical behavior and worse prognosis. Am J Surg Pathol. 2015;39(5):632–43.
58. Karpathakis A, Dibra H, Pipinikas C, et al. Prognostic impact of novel molecular subtypes of small intestinal neuroendocrine tumor. Clin Cancer Res. 2016;22(1):250–8.
59. Yao JC, Phan A, Hoff PM, et al. Targeting vascular endothelial growth factor in advanced carcinoid tumor: a random assignment phase II study of depot octreotide with bevacizumab and pegylated interferon alpha-2b. J Clin Oncol. 2008;26(8):1316–23.
60. Pavel ME, Hainsworth JD, Baudin E, et al. Everolimus plus octreotide long-acting repeatable for the treatment of advanced neuroendocrine tumours associated with carcinoid syndrome (RADIANT-2): a randomised, placebo-controlled, phase 3 study. Lancet. 2011;378(9808):2005–12.
61. Cavalcanti E, Armentano R, Valentini AM, Chieppa M, Caruso ML. Role of PD-L1 expression as a biomarker for GEP neuroendocrine neoplasm grading. Cell Death Dis. 2017;8(8):e3004.
62. Sahnane N, Furlan D, Monti M, et al. Microsatellite unstable gastrointestinal neuroendocrine carcinomas: a new clinicopathologic entity. Endocr Relat Cancer. 2015;22(1):35–45.
63. La Rosa S, Marando A, Furlan D, Sahnane N, Capella C. Colorectal poorly differentiated neuroendocrine carcinomas and mixed adenoneuroendocrine carcinomas: insights into the diagnostic immunophenotype, assessment of methylation profile, and search for prognostic markers. Am J Surg Pathol. 2012;36(4):601–11.
64. Vortmeyer AO, Lubensky IA, Merino MHJ, et al. Concordance of genetic alterations in poorly differentiated colorectal neuroendocrine carcinomas and associated adenocarcinomas. J Natl Cancer Inst. 1997;89(19):1448–53.
65. Karkouche R, Bachet JB, Sandrini J, et al. Colorectal neuroendocrine carcinomas and adenocarcinomas share oncogenic pathways. A clinico-pathologic study of 12 cases. Eur J Gastroenterol Hepatol. 2012;24(12):1430–7.
66. Scardoni M, Vittoria E, Volante M, et al. Mixed adenoneuroendocrine carcinomas of the gastrointestinal tract: targeted next-generation sequencing suggests a monoclonal origin of the two components. Neuroendocrinology. 2014;100(4):310–6.
67. Woischke C, Schaaf CW, Yang HM, et al. In-depth mutational analyses of colorectal neuroendocrine carcinomas with adenoma or adenocarcinoma components. Mod Pathol. 2017;30(1):95–103.
68. Takizawa N, Ohishi Y, Hirahashi M, et al. Molecular characteristics of colorectal neuroendocrine carcinoma; similarities with adenocarcinoma rather than neuroendocrine tumor. Hum Pathol. 2015;46(12):1890–900.

Carcinomas of the Gastrointestinal Tract

18

Eric Swanson, Jolanta Jedrzkiewicz, Hanlin L. Wang, and Wade Samowitz

List of Frequently Asked Questions

1. How are carcinomas of the gastrointestinal (GI) tract classified?
2. What are the general gross and histologic features of adenocarcinomas of the GI tract? How are they graded histologically?
3. What are the general gross and histologic features of squamous cell carcinomas of the GI tract? How are they graded histologically?
4. How to determine if a tumor is a primary of the distal esophagus, gastroesophageal junction, or proximal stomach?
5. Can histologic grading of the tumors on biopsies influence management?
6. What are the common predisposing conditions for adenocarcinomas of the GI tract?
7. What is the definition of high-grade dysplasia in the GI tract?
8. How is invasive adenocarcinoma diagnosed in the colorectum?
9. How do you differentiate true submucosal invasion from submucosal misplacement (pseudoinvasion)?
10. What to report when diagnosing a malignant colorectal polyp?
11. What are the common subtypes of adenocarcinomas in the GI tract?
12. What are the uncommon subtypes of adenocarcinomas in the GI tract?
13. Do salivary gland tumors occur in the GI tract?
14. What should be considered when diagnosing diffuse-type adenocarcinoma of the stomach?
15. Does the staging system for carcinomas differ depending on the gastrointestinal site?
16. How is tumor involvement of the serosal surface (pT4a) evaluated?
17. What should be considered as a radial margin at different sites of the GI tract for resection specimens?
18. What is the significance of mesorectal envelop evaluation and how is it evaluated?
19. What distance from margin to tumor is adequate to achieve a negative margin?
20. What are the minimal numbers of regional lymph nodes at different sites of the GI tract required for adequate pN staging?
21. How to diagnose tumor deposits?
22. What is the significance of isolated tumor cells in a lymph node?
23. What is the significance of acellular mucin in pTNM staging or present at surgical margin?
24. What is tumor budding and its significance?
25. What is the significance of large venous invasion versus small lymphovascular invasion?
26. What is the significance of perineural invasion?
27. How is tumor regression in response to neoadjuvant therapies assessed in a resection specimen?
28. What is lymphoglandular complex and how to distinguish it from invasive adenocarcinoma?
29. What is a colorectal-type adenocarcinoma of the appendix?
30. What is the definition of adenocarcinoma of the ampulla of Vater?
31. What are the histologic features of conventional squamous cell carcinoma versus verrucous carcinoma of the anus?
32. How to distinguish in situ from invasive squamous cell carcinoma?

E. Swanson (✉)
Scripps Health, La Jolla, CA, USA
e-mail: Swanson.Eric@scrippshealth.org

J. Jedrzkiewicz · W. Samowitz
University of Utah, Salt Lake City, UT, USA

H. L. Wang
University of California at Los Angeles, Los Angeles, CA, USA

H. L. Wang, Z. E. Chen (eds.), *Practical Gastrointestinal Pathology*, Practical Anatomic Pathology,
https://doi.org/10.1007/978-3-030-51268-2_18

33. What is the significance of p16 positivity in squamous lesions of the anus?
34. How is anorectal squamous cell carcinoma treated compared with adenocarcinoma?
35. What is anal canal adenocarcinoma?
36. What are useful immunohistochemical markers for GI carcinomas?
37. What are the common metastatic lesions encountered in the GI tract, and how do you diagnose them?
38. When to perform and how to report Her2 testing on gastric and GEJ adenocarcinomas?
39. What is the current recommendation for MMR deficiency testing and what is the significance of MMR deficiency?
40. What are the common tests used to evaluate for MMR deficiency?
41. How are MMR immunostains interpreted?
42. What are some pitfalls in the interpretation of MMR protein immunohistochemical testing?
43. When an abnormal MMR protein test result is seen, what are the next steps taken to determine the significance of the findings?
44. What colorectal tumor morphologic subtypes are likely to be associated with MMR deficiency?
45. What molecular tests may be performed on metastatic (stage IV) colorectal adenocarcinoma?
46. What is the role of Her2 testing in colorectal adenocarcinoma?
47. What is the significance of PIK3CA mutations in colorectal adenocarcinoma?
48. What is the significance of PTEN expression in colorectal adenocarcinoma?
49. How to report programmed death-ligand 1 (PD-L1) immunostaining results?

Frequently Asked Questions

1. **How are carcinomas of the gastrointestinal (GI) tract classified?**
   - Carcinomas of the GI tract are classified based on location, histomorphology, immunophenotype, and molecular phenotype according to the WHO tumor classification, but histomorphology remains the gold standard.
   - The most common types of carcinoma in the GI tract are adenocarcinoma and squamous cell carcinoma. Variants of these two broad categories, as well as other rare types of carcinoma, are listed in Table 18.1.
   - Neuroendocrine carcinomas are included in Table 18.1 but discussed in Chap. 17.
   - Carcinomas unique to the appendix and anus are also included in Table 18.1 but discussed in Chaps. 8 and 9, respectively.

   Reference: [1]

2. **What are the general gross and histologic features of adenocarcinomas of the GI tract? How are they graded histologically?**
   - Grossly, adenocarcinomas may present as exophytic, polypoid, or fungating mass lesions; cratered ulceration often with heaped-up edges; or diffuse infiltration of the visceral wall with wall thickening, loss of distensibility, and/or stricturing (Fig. 18.1a–c).
   - The term "linitis plastica" has been used to describe diffuse-type adenocarcinoma of the stomach that infiltrates the entirety or majority of the stomach, which results in diffuse thickening and stiffness of the gastric wall (leather bottle stomach). The rugal folds may become prominent or flattened (Fig. 18.1d).
   - Early-stage carcinomas may present as small nodules, polyps, irregular plaques, or superficial erosions.
   - Histologically, adenocarcinomas are primarily characterized by neoplastic gland formation. Intracytoplasmic mucin, luminal mucin, and extracellular mucin pools may be seen. Cytologic atypia is typically present with enlarged, crowded nuclei, nuclear pleomorphism, and brisk mitotic activity.
   - Nonmucinous adenocarcinoma is graded based on the degree of gland formation (Fig. 18.2a–c).
     - Well-differentiated adenocarcinoma
       Carcinoma with >95% glandular morphology
     - Moderately differentiated adenocarcinoma
       Carcinoma with 50–95% glandular morphology
     - Poorly differentiated adenocarcinoma
       Carcinoma with <50% glandular morphology
   - Very well-differentiated adenocarcinomas of the stomach and bowel are tumors that show minimal or low-grade cytologic features of malignancy and may lack desmoplastic reaction. The diagnosis is based on deeply invasive growth and/or abnormal architectural features such as anastomosing, spiky, distended, and abortive glands. Examples include low-grade tubuloglandular adenocarcinoma of the colorectum (rarely seen in the terminal ileum) in the setting of inflammatory bowel disease (Fig. 18.3a, b) and very well-differentiated gastric carcinoma of the intestinal type (Fig. 18.4a, b).
     - In biopsy specimens, low-grade tubuloglandular adenocarcinoma of the colorectum may only show features of low-grade dysplasia or indefinite for dysplasia (see Chap. 6, Case 5).
     - In biopsy specimens, very well-differentiated gastric carcinoma of the intestinal type may show intestinal metaplasia in the upper portion of the mucosa and abnormally shaped glands in the lower portion. A "crawling" pattern of lateral spread is characteristic.
   - Very well-differentiated adenocarcinoma must be differentiated from benign deeply misplaced glands of

Table 18.1 WHO classification of carcinomas of the GI tract

Esophagus	Stomach	Small intestine	Ampulla	Appendix	Colon and rectum	Anal canal
Adenocarcinoma[a]	Adenocarcinoma[b]	Adenocarcinoma	Adenocarcinoma	Adenocarcinoma	Adenocarcinoma	Adenocarcinoma
	Tubular adenocarcinoma		Intestinal-type adenocarcinoma	LAMN		Mucosal-type adenocarcinoma
	Papillary adenocarcinoma		Pancreatobiliary-type adenocarcinoma	HAMN		Anal gland adenocarcinoma
	Micropapillary adenocarcinoma		Adenocarcinoma with mixed types	Goblet cell adenocarcinoma	Micropapillary adenocarcinoma	Fistula-associated adenocarcinoma
	Poorly cohesive carcinoma[c]	Poorly cohesive carcinoma[c]	Poorly cohesive carcinoma[c]	Signet-ring cell carcinoma	Poorly cohesive carcinoma[c]	Extramucosal-type adenocarcinoma, non-anal gland type and non-fistula-associated
	Mucinous adenocarcinoma	Mucinous adenocarcinoma	Mucinous adenocarcinoma	Mucinous adenocarcinoma	Mucinous adenocarcinoma	Mucinous adenocarcinoma
	Adenocarcinoma with lymphoid stroma[d]	Medullary carcinoma	Medullary carcinoma	Medullary carcinoma	Medullary carcinoma	
	Hepatoid adenocarcinoma				Serrated adenocarcinoma	
	Adenocarcinoma of fundic gland type				Adenoma-like adenocarcinoma	
	Mixed adenocarcinoma[e]				Carcinoma with sarcomatoid components	
Squamous cell carcinoma	Squamous cell carcinoma	Squamous cell carcinoma	Squamous cell carcinoma		Squamous cell carcinoma	Squamous cell carcinoma
Verrucous squamous cell carcinoma						Verrucous squamous cell carcinoma
Basaloid squamous cell carcinoma						Basaloid squamous cell carcinoma
Spindle cell squamous cell carcinoma						
Adenosquamous carcinoma	Adenosquamous carcinoma	Adenosquamous carcinoma	Adenosquamous carcinoma	Adenosquamous carcinoma	Adenosquamous carcinoma	
Mucoepidermoid carcinoma						Basal cell carcinoma
Adenoid cystic carcinoma						Paget disease
Undifferentiated carcinoma	Undifferentiated carcinoma	Undifferentiated carcinoma	Undifferentiated carcinoma	Undifferentiated carcinoma	Undifferentiated carcinoma	Undifferentiated carcinoma
Lymphoepithelioma-like carcinoma						
Small cell neuroendocrine carcinoma	Small cell neuroendocrine carcinoma	Small cell neuroendocrine carcinoma	Small cell neuroendocrine carcinoma	Small cell neuroendocrine carcinoma	Small cell neuroendocrine carcinoma	Small cell neuroendocrine carcinoma
Large cell neuroendocrine carcinoma	Large cell neuroendocrine carcinoma	Large cell neuroendocrine carcinoma	Large cell neuroendocrine carcinoma	Large cell neuroendocrine carcinoma	Large cell neuroendocrine carcinoma	Large cell neuroendocrine carcinoma

(continued)

Table 18.1 (continued)

Esophagus	Stomach	Small intestine	Ampulla	Appendix	Colon and rectum	Anal canal
MiNEN	MiNEN	MiNEN	MiNEN	MiNEN	MiNEN	MiNEN
	Gastroblastoma					

MiNEN mixed neuroendocrine-non-neuroendocrine neoplasm, *LAMN* low-grade appendiceal mucinous neoplasm, *HAMN* high-grade appendiceal mucinous neoplasm

[a]Also including adenocarcinoma of the gastroesophageal junction (GEJ). Like adenocarcinomas in other locations, adenocarcinomas of the esophagus and GEJ may also show tubular, papillary, mucinous, and signet-ring cell patterns, but these patterns are not described as subtypes in the WHO tumor classification

[b]Adenocarcinomas of the stomach may also be classified as intestinal, diffuse, and mixed types (Lauren classification). The diffuse type is equivalent to poorly cohesive carcinoma, which also includes signet-ring cell carcinoma if >50% of tumor cells are signet-ring cells. The mixed type consists of approximately equal amounts of intestinal and diffuse components

[c]Poorly cohesive carcinoma or poorly cohesive cell carcinoma can be of either signet-ring cell type (signet-ring cell carcinoma) or non-signet-ring cell type

[d]Synonymous to medullary carcinoma

[e]Mixed adenocarcinoma of the stomach is defined by having two or more distinct histologic components, such as glandular (tubular or papillary) and poorly cohesive components. It is believed to be clonal with diverse morphologic phenotypes, and is thought to have a worse prognosis than carcinomas that have only one component

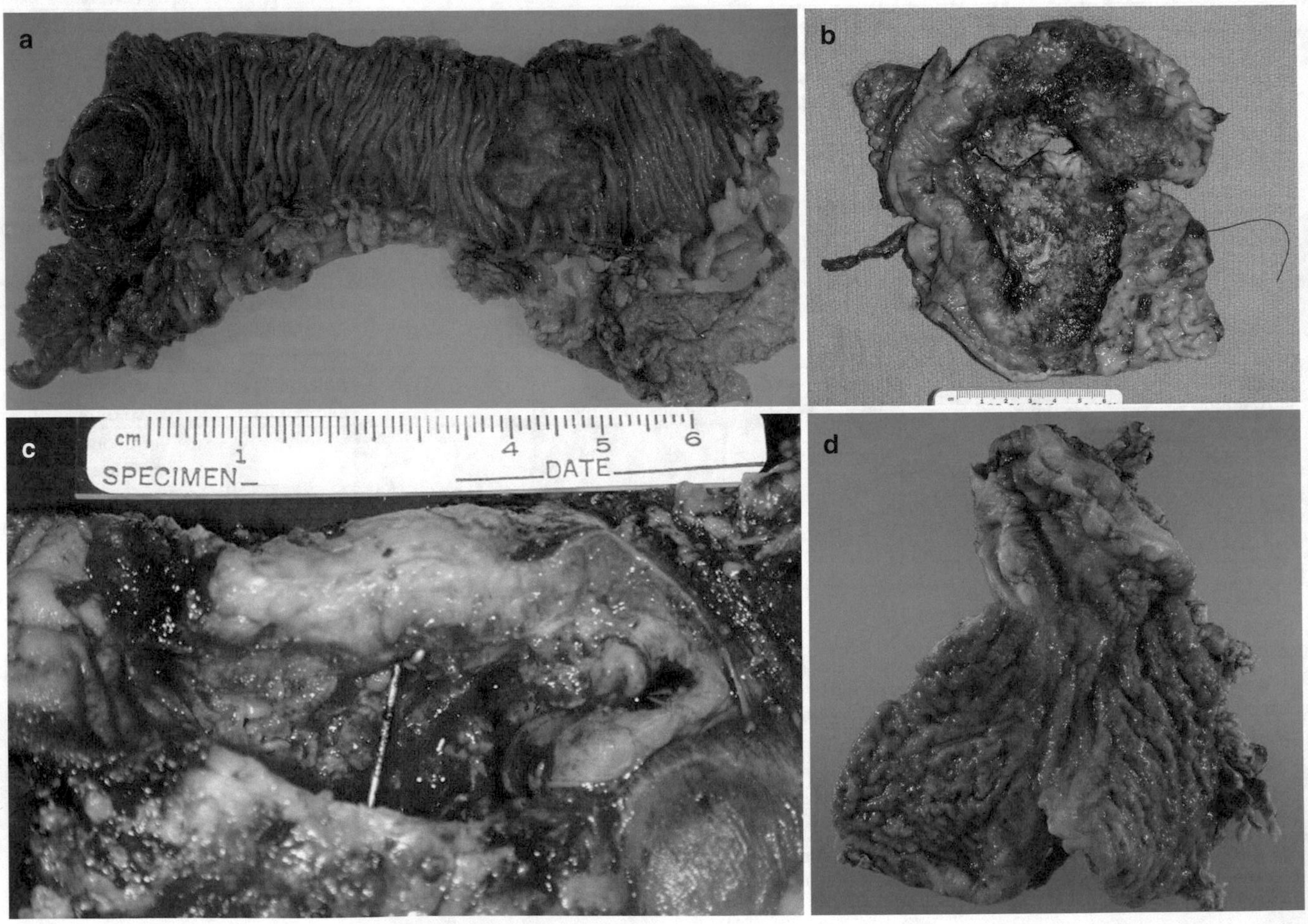

Fig. 18.1 (**a**) Right hemicolectomy showing an exophytic adenocarcinoma in the ascending colon. (**b**) Partial gastrectomy showing an ulcerated adenocarcinoma with heaped-up edges. (**c**) Segmental colectomy showing an adenocarcinoma diffusely infiltrating the colon wall causing wall thickening and stricturing. (**d**) Total gastrectomy showing features of linitis plastica with diffuse wall thickening and prominent rugal folds

gastritis or colitis cystica profunda based on growth patterns, glandular architecture, and cytology.

- The criteria for grading mucinous adenocarcinoma are less well standardized. The grading system for nonmucinous adenocarcinoma based on glandular formation as described above is not generally applicable to histologic variants including mucinous adenocarcinoma. Some studies have advocated that the histology be correlated with the microsatellite status to determine tumor grade. If a mucinous carcinoma is microsatellite unstable, it would be considered low grade. Conversely, if the tumor is microsatellite stable, it would be high

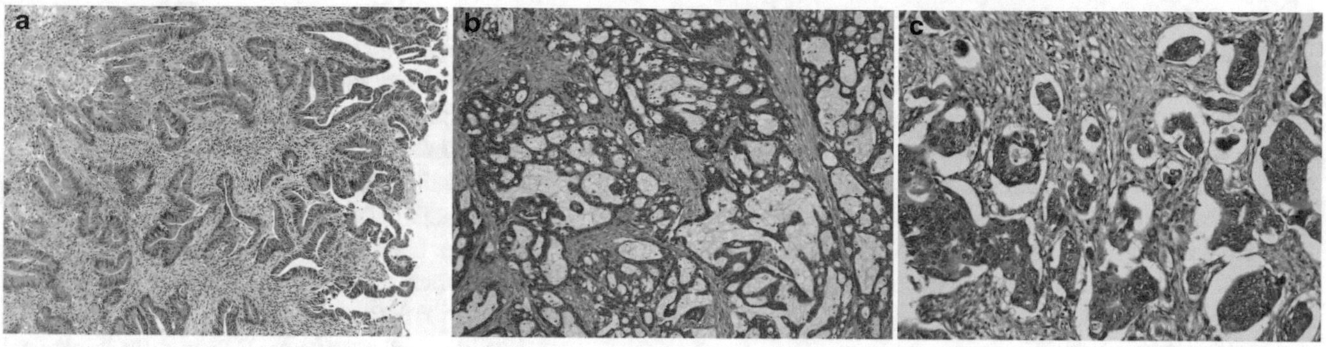

Fig. 18.2 (**a**) Well-differentiated adenocarcinoma showing a simple glandular architecture. (**b**) Moderately differentiated adenocarcinoma showing a complex glandular architecture. Note the presence of luminal mucin. (**c**) Poorly differentiated adenocarcinoma showing no overt glandular formation

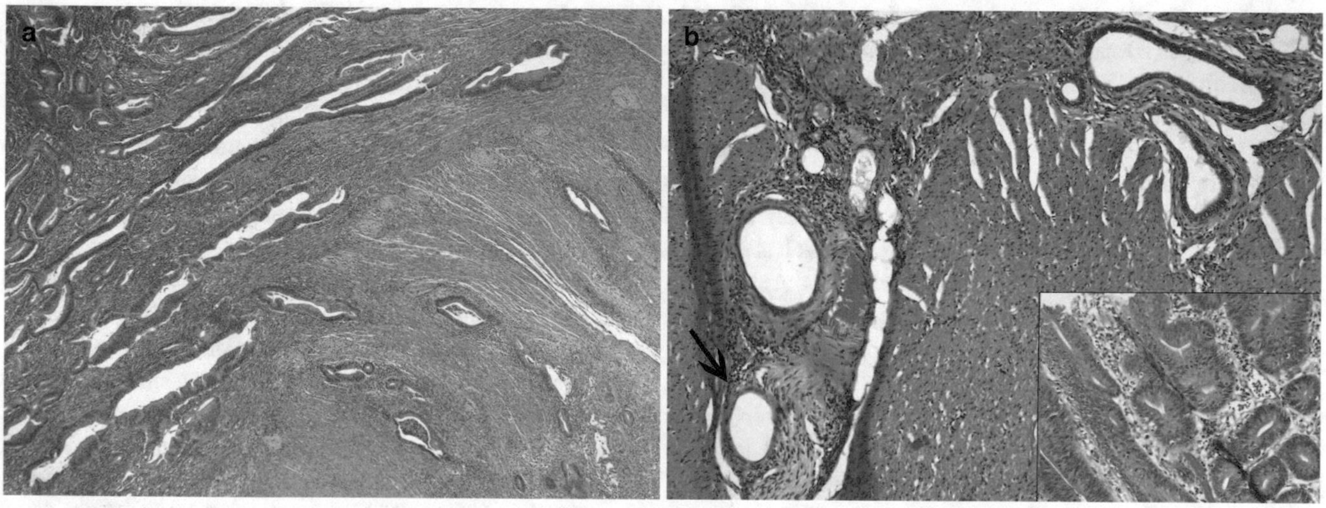

Fig. 18.3 (**a**, **b**) Examples of very well-differentiated colonic adenocarcinoma arising in the setting of inflammatory bowel disease. Neoplastic glands show simple tubular structures and low-grade cytology infiltrating the bowel wall but without significant desmoplasia. Focal perineural invasion is noted in example **b** (arrow). The overlying mucosa shows features of low-grade dysplasia (inset of example **b**)

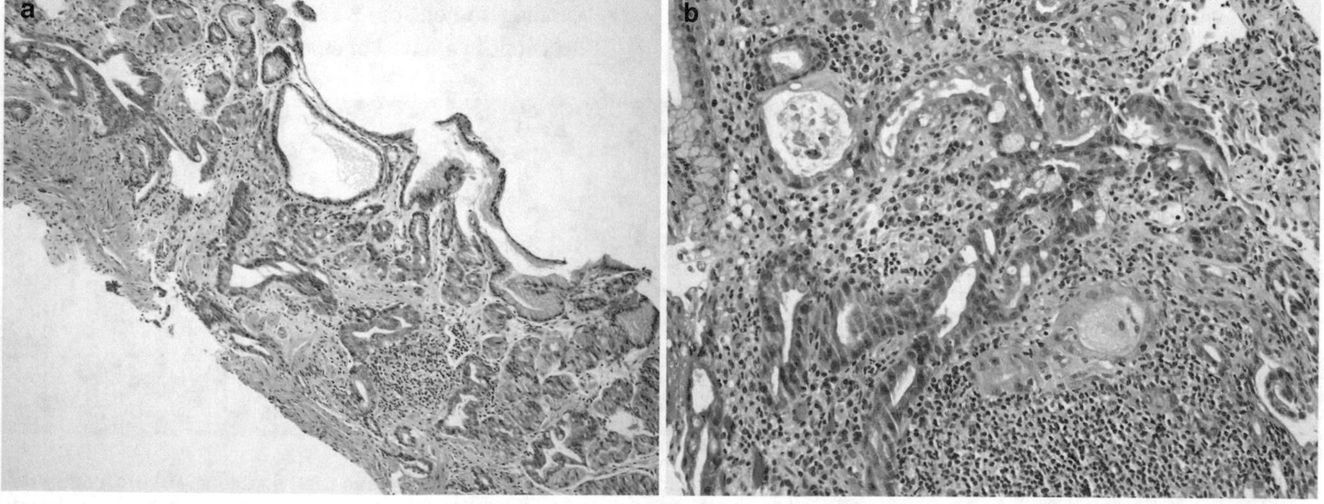

Fig. 18.4 (**a**, **b**) An example of very well-differentiated gastric adenocarcinoma. Neoplastic glands are seen in the lower portion of the gastric mucosa with a lateral "crawling" or anastomosing pattern

grade. Recent literature, however, suggests that grading based on microsatellite status may not be sufficient. More recently, a new grading system has been proposed for mucinous adenocarcinoma of the appendix. This system also grades mucinous adenocarcinoma as well, moderately, and poorly differentiated based on cytologic features, tumor cellularity, invasion, and signet-ring cells, which appears to correlate well with patients' outcomes (see Chap. 8, Question 22 and Table 18.8).
References: [2–6]

3. **What are the general gross and histologic features of squamous cell carcinomas of the GI tract? How are they graded histologically?**
   - In the GI tract, squamous cell carcinoma is most commonly found in the esophagus and anus. It is included in the WHO carcinoma classifications of the stomach, small bowel, appendix, and colorectum, but it is exceedingly rare in these locations.
   - Grossly, squamous cell carcinomas may present as exophytic mass lesions that are protruding, ulcerative, and/or infiltrative. They may also show a diffusely infiltrative pattern without forming a discrete mass lesion.
   - Histologically, squamous cell carcinomas are graded based on the degree of cytologic atypia, mitotic activity, and keratinization (Fig. 18.5a–c).
     – Grade 1 (well-differentiated) squamous cell carcinoma shows sheets of enlarged tumor cells with prominent cytoplasmic keratinization and keratin pearl formation. There is no or only a minor component of non-keratinizing basal-type cells. Cytologic atypia is minimal and mitotic activity is low. The invasive margin is pushing.
     – Grade 2 (moderately differentiated) squamous cell carcinoma shows a mixture of non-keratinizing basal-type tumor cells and keratinizing tumor cells with less ordered arrangement. Surface parakeratosis may be present, but keratin pearls are typically absent or infrequent. Mitotic figures are easily identifiable.
     – Grade 3 (poorly differentiated) squamous cell carcinoma shows large or small nests of predominantly non-keratinizing basal-type tumor cells with a pavement-like arrangement. Central necrosis may be present. Punctuating keratinizing or parakeratotic tumor cells are occasionally seen.
   - Currently, human papillomavirus (HPV) is considered to be an unlikely risk factor for the development of esophageal squamous cell carcinoma. However, the etiological relationship between HPV (mainly HPV16) and anal squamous cell carcinoma has been well established.
   References: [1, 7]

4. **How to determine if a tumor is a primary of the distal esophagus, gastroesophageal junction, or proximal stomach?**
   - Adenocarcinomas that lie entirely above the GEJ are considered esophageal carcinomas.
   - Squamous cell carcinomas that are seen at the GEJ are also considered to be esophageal carcinomas.
   - Adenocarcinomas that lie entirely below the GEJ are considered gastric carcinomas.
   - Adenocarcinomas that cross the GEJ are considered GEJ carcinomas, without consideration of where the bulk of the tumor is located. For staging purposes, however, the AJCC eighth edition classifies adenocarcinomas that involve the GEJ with epicenter within the proximal 2 cm of the proximal stomach (cardia) to be staged as adenocarcinoma of the esophagus. Tumors that involve the GEJ with epicenter >2 cm distal from the GEJ are staged as gastric adenocarcinomas.
   References: [1, 7]

5. **Can histologic grading of the tumors on biopsies influence management?**
   - Grading tumors on a biopsy can influence treatment decisions in a subset of cases. Endoscopic local resection

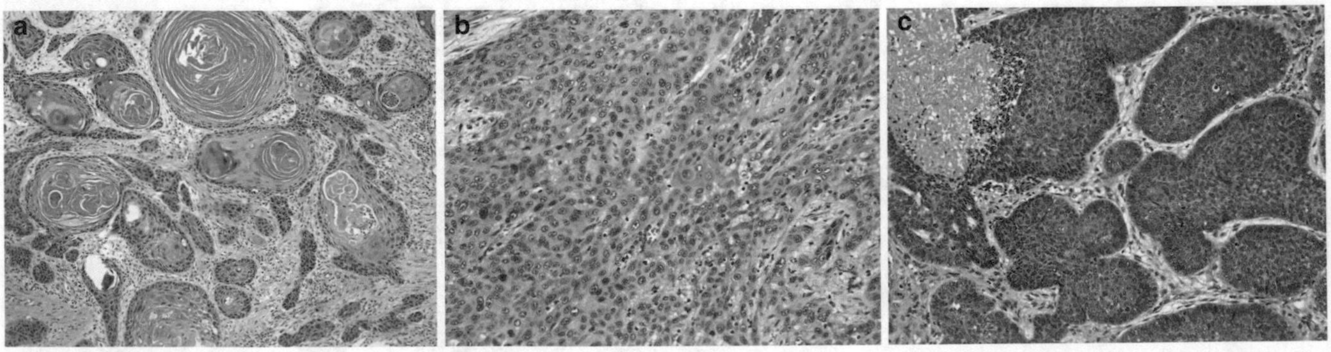

Fig. 18.5 (**a**) Well-differentiated squamous cell carcinoma showing prominent keratinization with keratin pearl formation. (**b**) Moderately differentiated squamous cell carcinoma showing more prominent cytologic atypia and less prominent keratinization. (**c**) Poorly differentiated squamous cell carcinoma showing basaloid features and necrosis

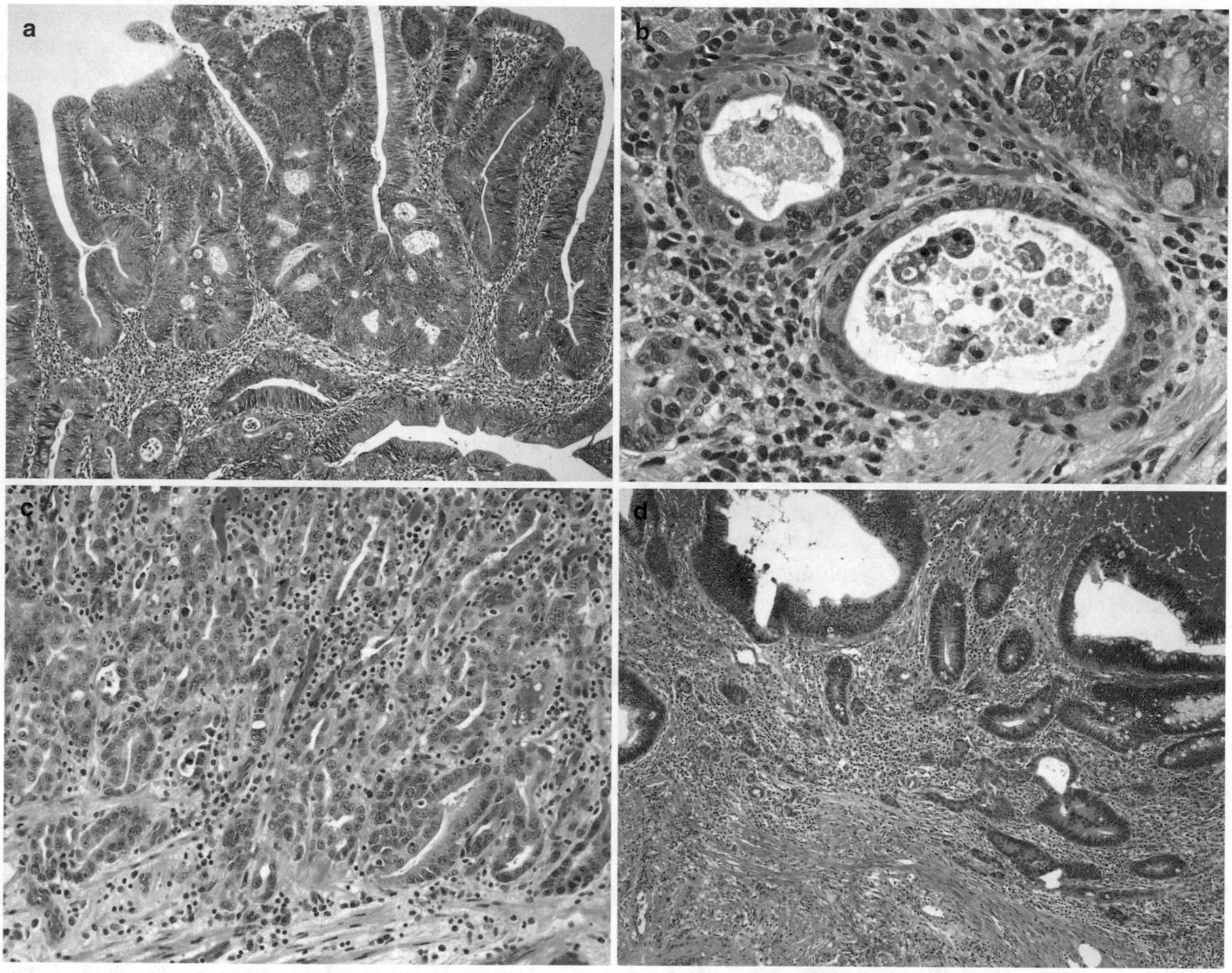

Fig. 18.6 (**a**) High-grade dysplasia arising in a tubular adenoma of the colon, characterized by a cribriform architecture. (**b**) High-grade dysplasia arising in Barrett mucosa, characterized by round nuclei and intraluminal necrotic debris. (**c**) Intramucosal adenocarcinoma arising in Barrett mucosa. (**d**) Intramucosal adenocarcinoma arising in a colonic adenoma

(endoscopic mucosal resection, endoscopic submucosal dissection, endoscopic polypectomy) may be sufficient treatment for early-stage well- or moderately differentiated adenocarcinomas. However, poorly differentiated carcinomas may require more extensive surgery.

- Tumor grade on a biopsy from a mass lesion may not represent the overall tumor grade because of sampling variability and tumor heterogeneity, which are known pitfalls.

  References: [8–10]

6. **What are the common predisposing conditions for adenocarcinomas of the GI tract?**
   - Genetic syndromes such as familial adenomatous polyposis, Lynch syndrome, Peutz-Jeghers syndrome, serrated polyposis, and gastric adenocarcinoma and proximal polyposis of the stomach (see Chap. 15)
   - Germline mutations of the *CDH1* gene for hereditary diffuse gastric cancer
   - Inflammatory bowel disease for intestinal adenocarcinoma
   - Barrett esophagus for esophageal adenocarcinoma
   - Sporadic gastric and intestinal adenomas, including sessile serrated adenoma/polyp of the colorectum, for gastric and intestinal adenocarcinomas
   - *H. pylori* gastritis and atrophic gastritis with intestinal metaplasia for gastric adenocarcinoma
   - Hyperplastic polyp of the stomach for gastric adenocarcinoma
   - Celiac disease for small intestinal adenocarcinoma

7. **What is the definition of high-grade dysplasia in the GI tract?**
   - High-grade dysplasia can be seen in Barrett esophagus, inflammatory bowel disease, and various adeno-

matous polyps in the GI tract. It usually arises from low-grade dysplasia or adenomatous epithelium such as an adenomatous polyp and may be focal, multifocal, or extensive. The dysplastic cells are confined to the epithelial cell layer without invasion through the basement membrane. It is synonymous with intraepithelial carcinoma or adenocarcinoma in situ (staged as pTis) and regarded as the immediate precursor to invasive adenocarcinoma.

- High-grade dysplasia is characterized by architectural complexity and/or cytologic atypia. Architecturally, high-grade areas typically show increased glandular density with crowded glands that have a cribriform or back-to-back pattern (Fig. 18.6a). Cytologically, cells with high-grade dysplasia exhibit rounded nuclei, coarse chromatin, prominent nucleoli, and loss of nuclear polarity with nuclei no longer being oriented perpendicular to the basement membrane. Necrotic debris within the lumina of dysplastic glands may be seen (Fig. 18.6b).
- Invasion through the basement membrane into the lamina propria or muscularis mucosae is considered intramucosal adenocarcinoma, which is generally considered single cell infiltration into the lamina propria, small clusters of cells budding out of the dysplastic glands, or a complex anastomosing glandular pattern with lateral crawling. This is staged as pT1a in the esophagus, stomach, and small bowel (Fig. 18.6c).
- In the colorectum and appendix, intramucosal adenocarcinoma (including invasion into the muscularis mucosae) is still considered carcinoma in situ and staged as pTis (Fig. 18.6d). The rationale is that the intramucosal adenocarcinoma of the colorectum and appendix has a negligible potential of metastasis. If a polypoid lesion in these locations is completely excised, intramucosal carcinoma carries virtually no risk of progression. Therefore, only submucosal invasion is considered invasive carcinoma in the colorectal and appendiceal regions (see Question 8).
  - Special considerations are given to colorectal intramucosal poorly differentiated carcinomas. The outcome data for these cases are extremely limited but suggest conservative management.

  References: [7, 11–13]

8. **How is invasive adenocarcinoma diagnosed in the colorectum?**
   - As discussed above, tumor invasion limited to the mucosa of the colorectum is staged as carcinoma in situ. The term invasive adenocarcinoma is reserved to tumors showing histologic evidence of at least submucosal invasion.
   - Invasive tumor may be comprised of infiltrative neoplastic glands or single tumor cells.
   - Desmoplastic stroma is a hallmark of submucosal invasion in an endoscopic biopsy or polypectomy specimen. It is proteoglycan-rich with loose spindled myofibroblasts/fibroblasts and an amphophilic hue (Fig. 18.7). Close approximation of neoplastic cells to medium-sized vessels, which normally should not be seen in the mucosa, may be observed. A pitfall is lamina propria fibrosis, which may be seen in a larger, usually villous or tubulovillous adenoma, due to mechanical injury. This is typically seen in the superficial portion of the polyp, which may contain dilated vessels.
   - Invasion through the muscularis mucosae into the submucosa can also be assessed in well-oriented specimens, which may show abrupt destruction of the muscularis mucosae by tumor cells. Immunostaining for smooth muscle actin (SMA) or desmin to highlight the muscularis mucosae may help in difficult cases. However, assessment of invasion through the muscularis mucosae may be unreliable due to poor orientation of the specimen. Multiple deeper sections may help in those cases.
     - Duplication of the muscularis mucosae may also occur, which may interfere with the assessment of submucosal invasion. This is more commonly seen in the setting of Barrett esophagus. A comparison of the depth/location of a neoplastic gland(s) with that of a nonneoplastic gland can be helpful.

9. **How do you differentiate true submucosal invasion from submucosal misplacement (pseudoinvasion)?**
   - Epithelial misplacement or herniation into the submucosa (so-called pseudoinvasion) can be seen in larger adenomatous polyps due to mechanical traumatization such as torsion, prolapse, prior biopsy, or other types of injury.

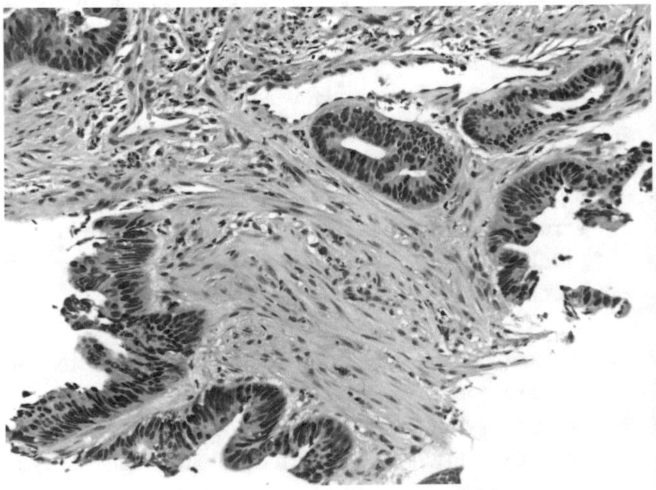

Fig. 18.7 Neoplastic glands in desmoplastic stroma are a diagnostic feature of invasive adenocarcinoma on biopsy specimens

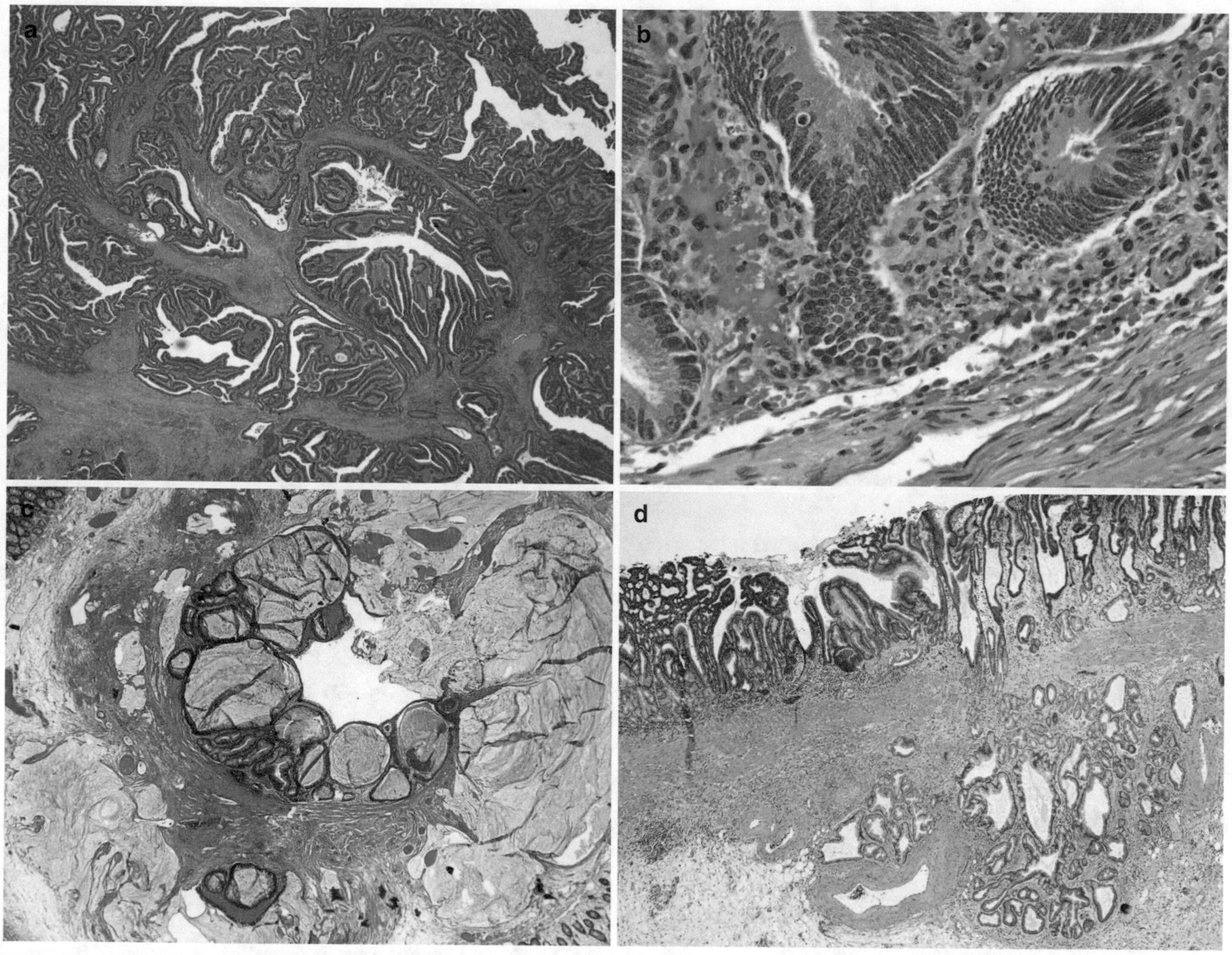

Fig. 18.8 Misplaced adenomatous glands in the submucosa showing a lobular configuration (**a**), typically surrounded by a rim of lamina propria components with hemorrhage and hemosiderin (**b**). (**c**) Misplaced adenomatous glands are associated with mucin pools with no floating neoplastic cells. (**d**) Benign misplaced gastric glands seen in a case of gastritis cystica profunda

- Features associated with pseudoinvasion include a lobular pattern at low power view, the presence of lamina propria components around neoplastic glands, the presence of hemorrhage and hemosiderin, and the lack of desmoplasia (Fig. 18.8a, b). Extravasated mucin may be present, which usually forms acellular mucin pools but can be lined by misplaced epithelial cells at the periphery (Fig. 18.8c). Pseudoinvasion is also favored if the cytoarchitectural features of herniated glands are similar to those of the overlying adenoma, as invasive carcinoma typically takes on a higher-grade appearance. It should be mentioned, however, that the herniated components can show high-grade features, which may pose a diagnostic challenge. Pseudoinvasion and bona fide invasive adenocarcinoma may also coexist within the same polyp. The main distinctive histologic features between pseudo- and true invasion are summarized in Table 18.2.

Table 18.2 Distinction between pseudoinvasion and true submucosal invasion

Pseudoinvasion	True invasion
Lobular pattern or well-circumscribed aggregates of glands	Irregular glands, small clusters, or single cells
Rim of lamina propria components around neoplastic glands	Desmoplasia
Presence of hemorrhage and/or hemosiderin	Higher-grade cytoarchitectural features comparing to surface adenoma
Similar cytoarchitectural features of herniated glands to surface adenoma	Cytologically malignant cells floating in mucin pools

- Misplacement of nonneoplastic epithelium into the deeper layers of the GI tract can also occur as a consequence of increased intraluminal pressure. Examples include gastritis or colitis cystica profunda (Fig. 18.8d).
- This topic is also discussed in Chap. 14, Question 27. References: [14, 15]

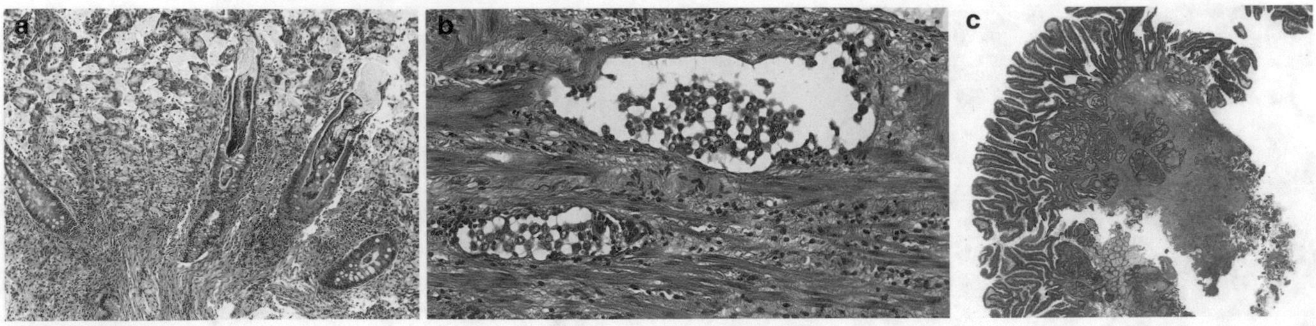

Fig. 18.9 (**a**) Malignant polyp with a poorly differentiated histology. (**b**) Malignant polyp with lymphovascular invasion. (**c**) Malignant polyp with positive polypectomy margin

10. What to report when diagnosing a malignant colorectal polyp?

- Malignant polyps are polyps harboring adenocarcinoma with submucosal invasion.
- Malignant polyps removed by endoscopic polypectomy require evaluation for the presence of histologic features that would increase the risk of nodal metastasis or local recurrence, determining the need for further surgical treatment.
- It is important to assess tumor grade, lymphovascular invasion, and margin status. Poorly differentiated histology, the presence of lymphovascular invasion, and positive polypectomy margin (defined as ≤1 mm from deep cauterized margin) are considered high-risk features and indications for consideration of further surgical resection (Fig. 18.9a–c).
- Other proposed high-risk features that may convey an adverse outcome include high tumor budding (see Question 24) and depth of submucosal invasion (>1 mm).
- It is therefore important that polypectomy specimens be received in one intact piece. It should be inked at the cauterized base, although the stalk may retract and thus be difficult to identify. The specimen is either bisected or serially sectioned depending on its size and entirely submitted. Sectioning should follow the vertical plane of the stalk to maximize the histologic evaluation of polypectomy margin and submucosal involvement. If the specimen is received in multiple pieces, however, margin evaluation may become impossible. Inability to assess margin status due to piecemeal resection may also be considered as a risk factor.
- Currently, a formal staging protocol for reporting malignant polyps is recommended but not required by the College of American Pathologists (CAP) for accreditation purpose.

  References: [13, 16, 17]

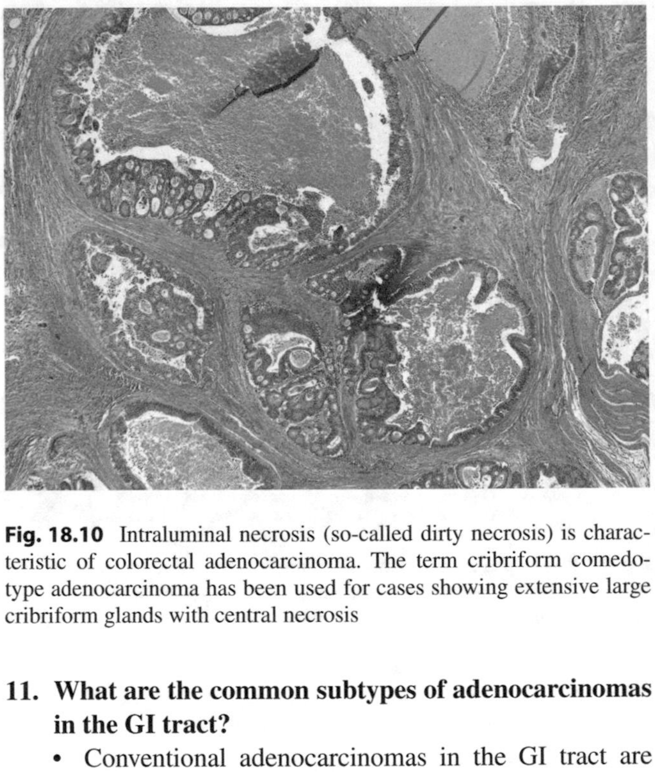

Fig. 18.10 Intraluminal necrosis (so-called dirty necrosis) is characteristic of colorectal adenocarcinoma. The term cribriform comedo-type adenocarcinoma has been used for cases showing extensive large cribriform glands with central necrosis

11. What are the common subtypes of adenocarcinomas in the GI tract?

- Conventional adenocarcinomas in the GI tract are typically gland-forming tumors with desmoplasia. A cribriform architecture and intraluminal necrosis ("dirty necrosis") are commonly seen in colorectal adenocarcinomas, which is a relatively unique feature to this location. Rarely, a colorectal adenocarcinoma may show extensive large cribriform glands with central necrosis, recapitulating cribriform carcinoma of the mammary and salivary glands. This has been termed "cribriform comedo-type adenocarcinoma" in the literature (Fig. 18.10).
- Common subtypes of adenocarcinoma of the GI tract include:
  - *Signet-ring cell carcinoma* is composed of cells showing prominent intracytoplasmic mucin, which displaces the nucleus toward the periphery of the

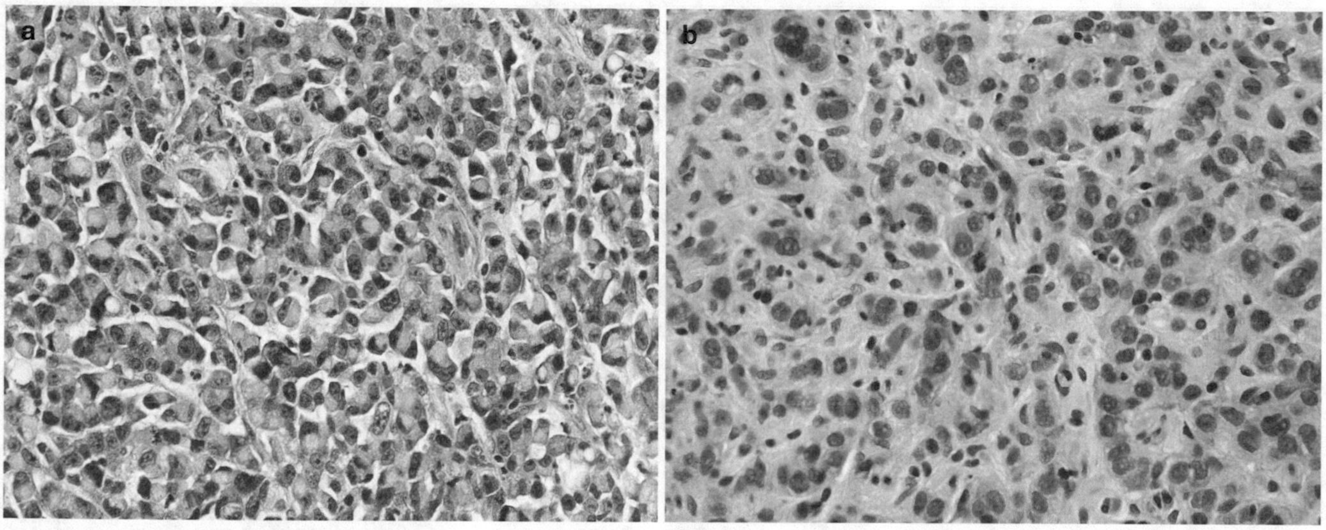

Fig. 18.11 (**a**) Gastric poorly cohesive carcinoma, signet-ring cell type. (**b**) Gastric poorly cohesive carcinoma, non-signet-ring cell type

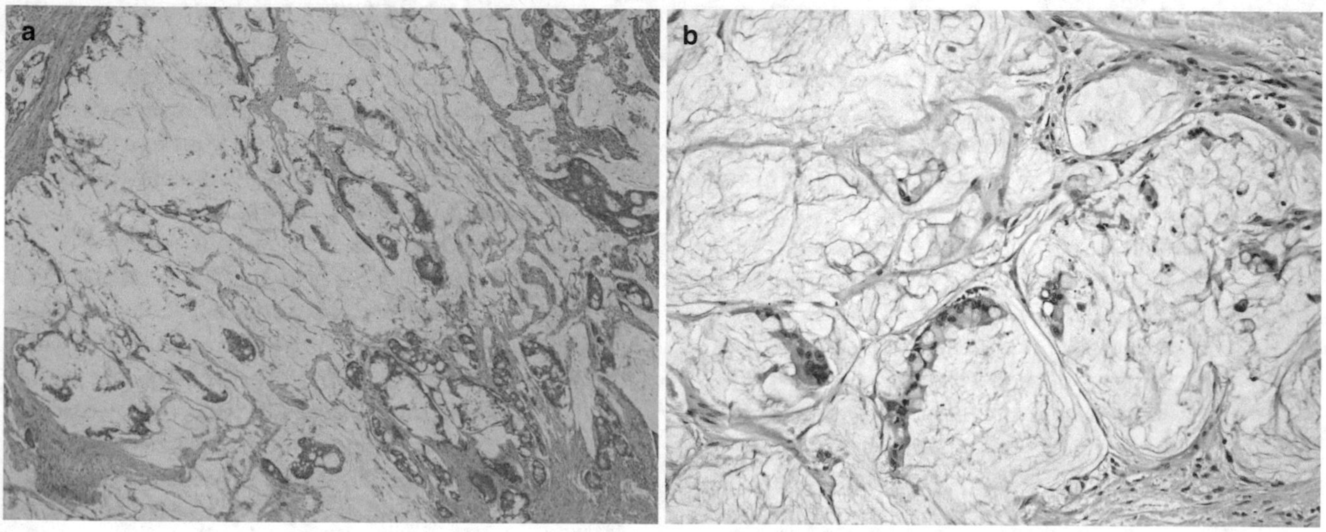

Fig. 18.12 (**a**) Mucinous adenocarcinoma of the colon showing abundant extracellular mucin dissecting the bowel wall. (**b**) Higher power view showing strips and clusters of neoplastic epithelial cells in mucin pools

cytoplasm. By definition, signet-ring cells constitute >50% of the overall tumor volume. Signet-ring cells may float within mucin pools or infiltrate tissue, as either single individual cells or small aggregates (Fig. 18.11a). A subset of these tumors show a high level of microsatellite instability (MSI-high) that results from DNA mismatch repair (MMR) protein deficiency. This subtype is included in the WHO carcinoma classification under the category of poorly cohesive carcinoma, which also includes non-signet-ring cell type (Fig. 18.11b).

– *Mucinous carcinoma* shows abundant extracellular mucin production with a mucinous component constituting >50% of the overall tumor volume. The mucin pools contain malignant epithelial cells typically arranged in glandular structures, strips of tumor cells, individual tumor cells, or scattered signet-ring cells depending on the level of tumor differentiation (Fig. 18.12a, b). A subset of mucinous carcinomas are MSI-high.

– *Medullary carcinoma* is also known as adenocarcinoma with lymphoid stroma or lymphoepithelioma-like carcinoma. It is characterized by large malignant cells with abundant cytoplasm, vesicular nuclei, and prominent nucleoli growing in solid, syncytial sheets with a pushing border. Nested or trabecular patterns may also be seen. Glandular structures are usually absent or poorly developed if present. These tumors characteristically have numerous tumor-infiltrating and background lymphocytes. The vast majority of these tumors are MSI-high. This

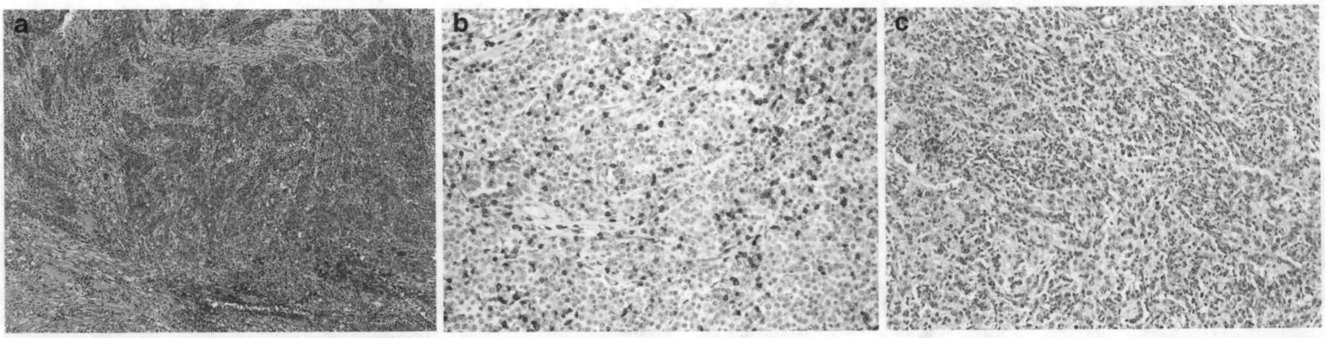

Fig. 18.13 (**a**) Medullary carcinoma (adenocarcinoma with lymphoid stroma) arising in the stomach showing poorly differentiated tumor growing in nests with abundant lymphocytes in the background. (**b**) A case of medullary carcinoma of the colon showing sheets of poorly differentiated tumor cells with abundant intratumoral T-lymphocytes as demonstrated by immunostaining for CD3. (**c**) A case of gastric medullary carcinoma with frequent tumor cells positive for EBV as demonstrated by in situ hybridization. (Courtesy of Dr. Lihong Chen of Fujian Medical University, China)

tumor is associated with EBV in many cases (Fig. 18.13a–c). The prognosis is reported to be more favorable compared to other types of carcinomas.

EBV-associated gastric carcinoma accounts for nearly 10% of gastric carcinomas worldwide. It tends to occur in the remnant stomach. In addition to lymphoepithelioma-like histology, it can also be moderately differentiated with varying degrees of lymphocytic infiltration. It carries a relatively favorable prognosis compared to other types of gastric carcinoma, with lower frequencies of lymphovascular invasion and nodal metastasis.

– *Adenosquamous carcinoma* has a conventional adenocarcinoma component along with a squamous carcinoma component consisting of more than occasional small foci of squamous differentiation. These tumors may either be mixed haphazardly with dual differentiation of malignant cells or collision-type tumors with two distinct components adjoining each other. By definition, the diagnosis requires at least 25% of squamous component in the tumor, but any amount of glandular differentiation would suffice. Therefore, the diagnosis should be made on a resection specimen although a biopsy may suggest the possibility. Although this type of carcinoma is not listed in the carcinoma classification of the anus, the epithelium near the dentate line of the anus is theoretically capable of undergoing both glandular and squamous differentiation (Fig. 18.14).

References: [18–25]

12. **What are the uncommon subtypes of adenocarcinomas in the GI tract?**

- *Serrated adenocarcinoma* is only included in the WHO carcinoma classification of the colon and rectum. It is defined as tubular adenocarcinoma with luminal serrations. It most commonly occurs in the right colon, reportedly arising from a sessile serrated lesion. The malignant cells typically have vesicular nuclei, abundant eosinophilic cytoplasm, tufting, and tumor cell clusters or chains floating in a mucinous background without much necrosis (Fig. 18.15a). These tumors can have *BRAF* mutations and CpG island hypermethylation and can be MSI-high or MSI-low.
- *Micropapillary adenocarcinoma* is included in the WHO carcinoma classification of the stomach and colorectum. It is characterized by small clusters of malignant cells without fibrovascular cores, embedded within lacunar-like clear spaces separated by thin fibrous septa. These small clusters of tumor cells display an inside out appearance (reverse polarity) on EMA immunostain. Associated leukocytes can be prominent. The diagnosis of this subtype requires at least 5% of the tumor showing a micropapillary histology. These tumors tend to show an unfavorable prognosis with frequent lymphovascular invasion, lymph node metastasis, and perineural invasion (Fig. 18.15b).
- *Papillary adenocarcinoma* is only included in the WHO carcinoma classification of the stomach. It is characterized by an exophytic growth pattern with elongated finger-like projections that have fibrovascular cores. Tumor cells may be cuboidal or columnar in shape. These tumors are also thought to carry an unfavorable prognosis with frequent liver metastasis.
- *Spindle cell carcinoma* (sarcomatoid carcinoma or carcinoma with sarcomatoid components) shows biphasic morphology featuring admixed spindle cell and gland-forming areas. The spindle cell component is usually of high grade and may contain pleomorphic giant cells and rhabdoid cells but typically shows at least focal immunoreactivity for keratins to support the diagnosis. Recent studies have shown that the aggressive rhabdoid phenotype is associated with loss

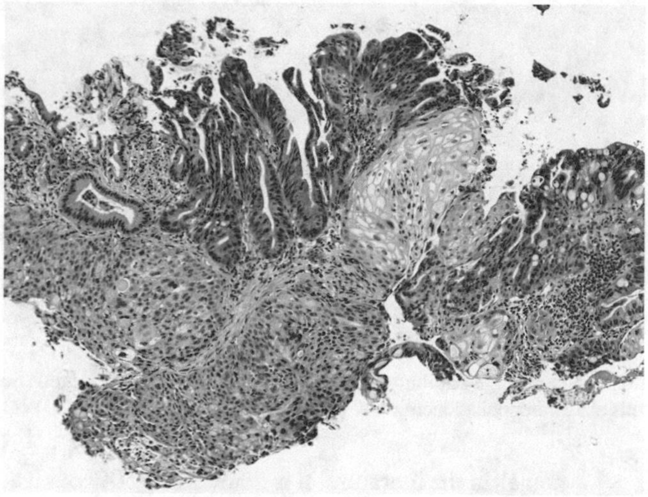

Fig. 18.14 A biopsy of an anorectal lesion showing a neoplasm consisting of both glandular and squamous components, suggesting the possibility of adenosquamous carcinoma

of nuclear expression in one or more of the switch/sucrose-nonfermenting (SWI/SNF) complex subunits including the core subunit SMARCB1 (INI1). Spindle cell carcinoma seen the esophagus typically arises from squamous cell carcinoma (Fig. 18.15c).

- *Hepatoid adenocarcinoma* (adenocarcinoma with hepatoid differentiation) is included in the WHO carcinoma classification of the stomach but can occur in the esophagus, ampulla of Vater, and colon. It is composed of large polygonal tumor cells with abundant eosinophilic cytoplasm which may contain pink globules (positive on PAS with diastase). The tumor may partially or entirely recapitulate a hepatocellular carcinoma (Fig. 18.15d). These tumors can cause elevation of serum alpha-fetoprotein (AFP) levels. Tumor cells may also express hepatocellular markers such as HepPar-1 and arginase and show canalicular pCEA and CD10 immunostaining pattern. This may

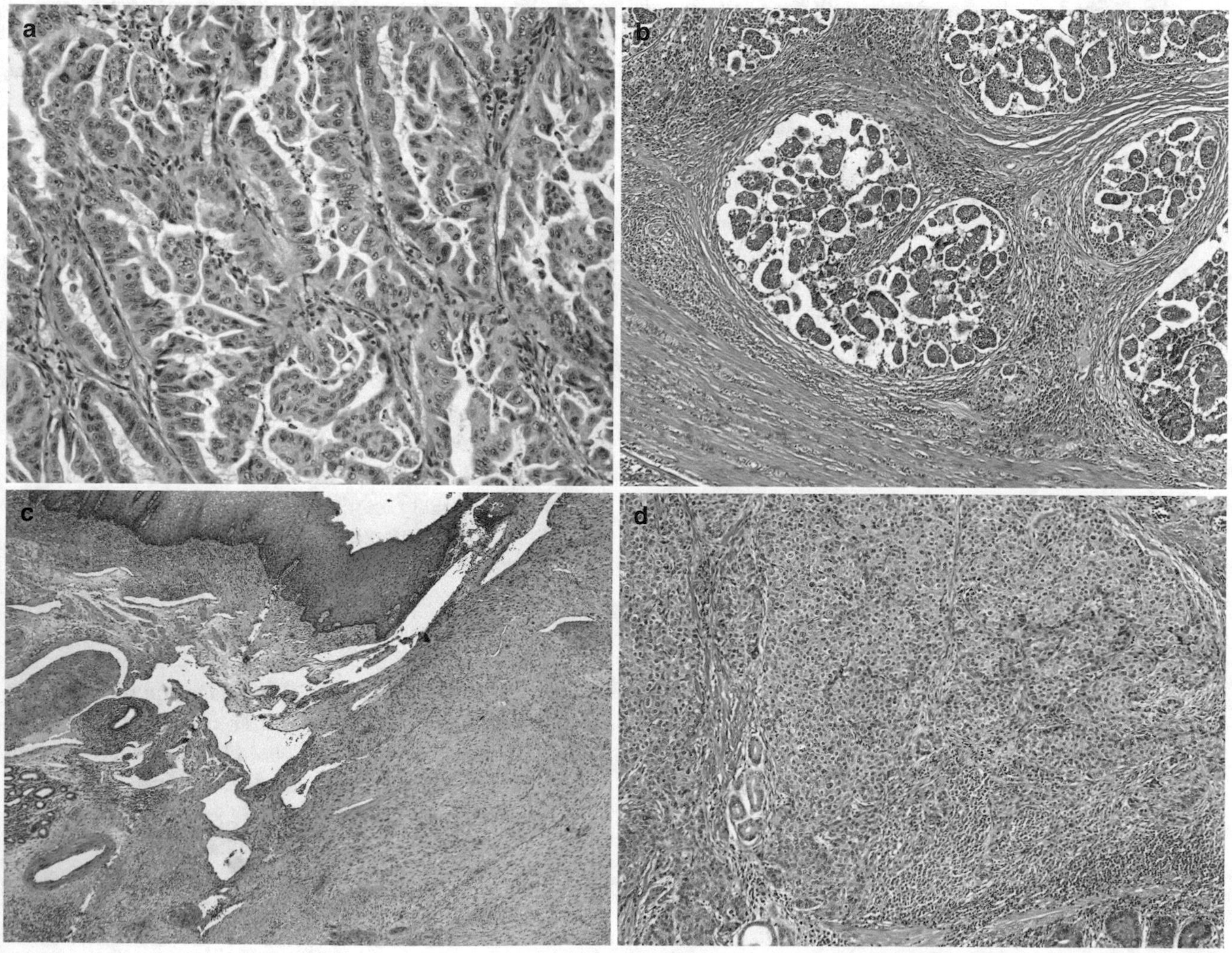

Fig. 18.15 (**a**) Serrated adenocarcinoma of the colon showing serrated architecture with tufted fronds. (**b**) Micropapillary adenocarcinoma showing small nests of tumor cells protruding into clear spaces in fibrous stroma. (**c**) Squamous cell carcinoma of the esophagus with admixed spindle cell component. (**d**) Hepatoid adenocarcinoma of the stomach

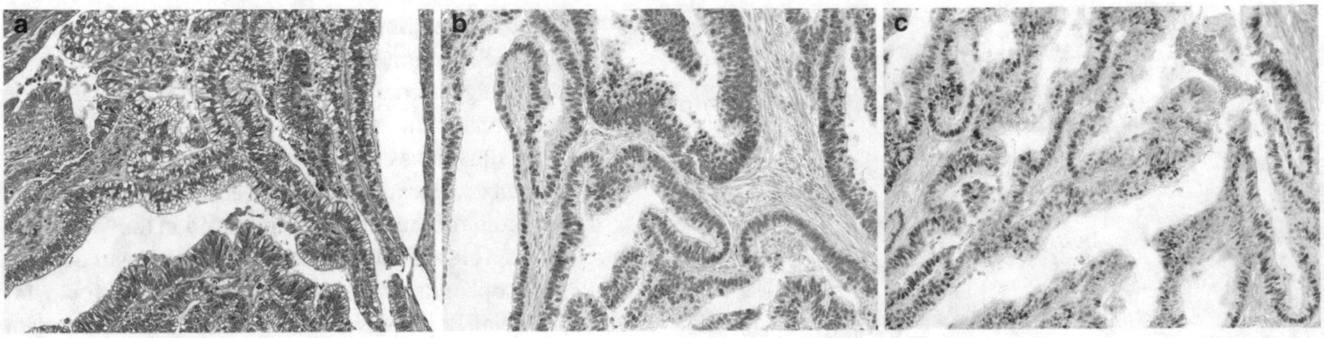

Fig. 18.16 (**a**) Adenocarcinoma with enteroblastic differentiation of the stomach showing a papillary architecture lined by columnar neoplastic cells with cleared out cytoplasm, resembling fetal gut epithelium. Tumor cells are immunohistochemically positive for CDX2 (**b**) and SALL4 (**c**)

cause confusion during workup of metastatic disease, especially in the presence of liver lesions.

- *Adenocarcinoma with enteroblastic differentiation* belongs to a category of well-differentiated papillary or tubular-type adenocarcinoma. It has been also described as adenocarcinoma with clear cells or yolk sac tumor-like carcinoma. This tumor resembles primitive gut histologically, forming papillary and tubular structures lined by cuboidal or columnar cells with clear cytoplasm and "piano-key" appearance. This tumor type has been described most frequently in the stomach but can occur in other parts of the gut. These tumors can also cause elevation of serum AFP levels and show positivity for oncofetal immunomarkers such as SALL4, glypican3, and AFP, in addition to variable immunoreactivity to keratins and CDX2 (Fig. 18.16a–c).
- *Adenocarcinoma of fundic gland type* is included in the WHO carcinoma classification of the stomach, but it is a controversial entity currently. It is assumed to develop from an oxyntic gland adenoma predominantly seen in the upper third of the stomach (see Chap. 14, Question 6). The vast majority of reported cases (~99%) are chief cell-predominant, but parietal cell-predominant or mixed variants may rarely occur. The distinction between adenocarcinoma of fundic-type gland and oxyntic gland adenoma appears to entirely rely on the presence or absence of submucosal extension. It remains debatable, however, whether the presence of fundic-type glands in the submucosa represents prolapse-type change or true submucosal invasion. Nevertheless, all reported cases in the literature are small (typically <1 cm), lack desmoplastic reaction, and show no recurrence or metastasis following endoscopic excision.
- *Adenoma-like adenocarcinoma* is a new entity included in the WHO carcinoma classification of the colon and rectum, which has been termed "villous adenocarcinoma" and "invasive papillary adenocarcinoma" in the literature. It is defined as ≥50% of invasive component having an adenoma-like histology with a villous architecture (Fig. 18.17a, b). These tumors are believed to have a low rate of metastasis with a good prognosis. This variant can be difficult to diagnose on a biopsy because of low-grade histology and lack of overt desmoplasia.
- *Undifferentiated carcinoma* is a malignant epithelial tumor that lacks histologic, immunohistochemical, and molecular evidence of glandular, squamous, or neuroendocrine differentiation. It usually forms variably sized nests or sheets by anaplastic, primitive epithelioid cells.
  - It is a diagnosis of exclusion, requiring clinical and radiographic correlation in order to exclude metastasis. Extensive sampling may also prove helpful in the search for a precursor lesion or areas of histologic differentiation.
  - Focal immunohistochemical evidence of epithelial differentiation is typically present. EMA immunostaining may be helpful for keratin-negative tumors.
  - It does not exhibit typical histologic features of medullary carcinoma, such as pushing borders and prominent tumor-infiltrating lymphocytes, and only rarely shows MSI.
  - Undifferentiated carcinoma with osteoclast-like giant cells, typically seen in the pancreas, may rarely occur in the GI tract, particularly at the ampullary region. Direct extension or metastasis from the pancreas should be excluded.
  - Areas showing a rhabdoid histology may be present. These tumors may be associated with loss of nuclear expression in one or more of the SWI/SNF complex subunits such as SMARCB1 (INI1) as described above.
- *Gastroblastoma* is a rare tumor of the stomach typically centered in the muscularis propria, but transmural or limited serosal involvement may occur. Both male and female patients have been reported, and they range in age from 9 to 74 years (majority under

30 years). Histologically, these tumors feature a biphasic pattern with varying proportions of spindled and epithelial elements. The spindle cells are relative uniform with blunt-ended nuclei. There may be variation in cell density in different areas. The epithelial cells usually form variable-sized clusters or tubular structures dispersed in the spindle cell background (Fig. 18.18a, b). They have round nuclei, inconspicuous nucleoli, and variable mitotic activity.

- Epithelial cells are positive for pankeratin and low molecular weight cytokeratins and variably positive for CD56 and CD10.
- Spindle cells are keratin negative and CD10 and CD56 positive.
- The biologic behavior of gastroblastoma is uncertain because there are <15 cases reported in the literature, but it is considered to be a low-grade malignancy because liver metastasis and local recurrence do occur.
- There is only one case of presumed duodenoblastoma reported in the English literature, which is also described as an epitheliomesenchymal biphasic tumor.

• *Choriocarcinoma of GI primary* can occur anywhere in the GI tract. It is composed of a mixture of syncytiotrophoblastic and cytotrophoblastic cells, typically with a hemorrhagic and necrotic appearance (Fig. 18.19a, b). Pure choriocarcinoma is exceed-

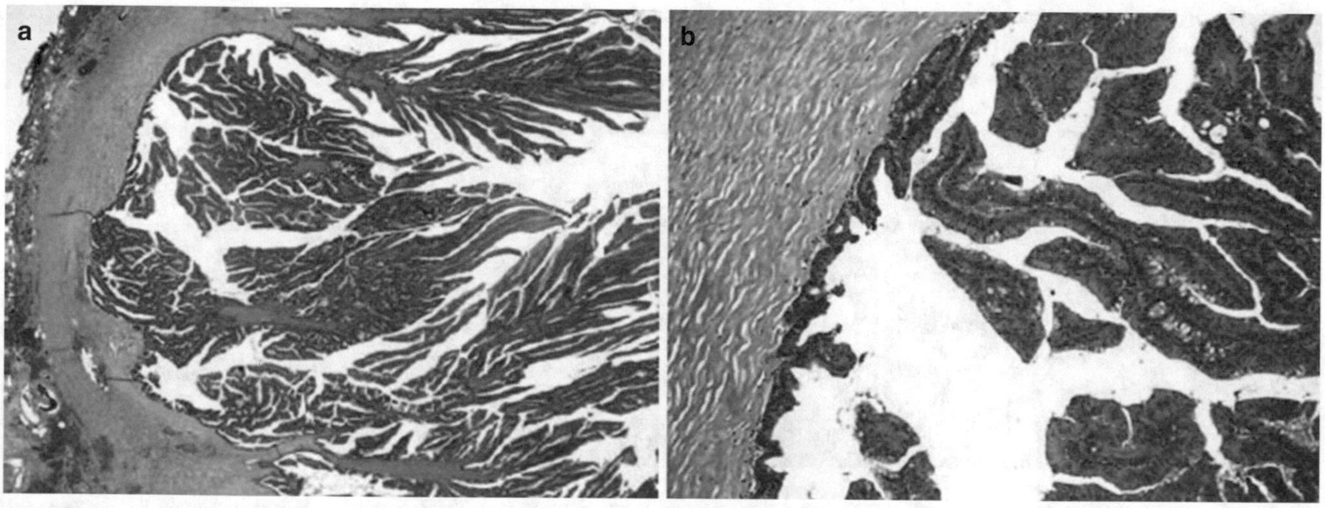

Fig. 18.17 (**a**) Typical appearance of an adenoma-like colorectal carcinoma, with a pushing border and villiform architecture. These tumors demonstrate low-grade nuclear features and often lack stromal desmoplasia. (**b**) True invasion is indicated by the absence of surrounding lamina propria. (From Gonzalez et al. [26], with permission)

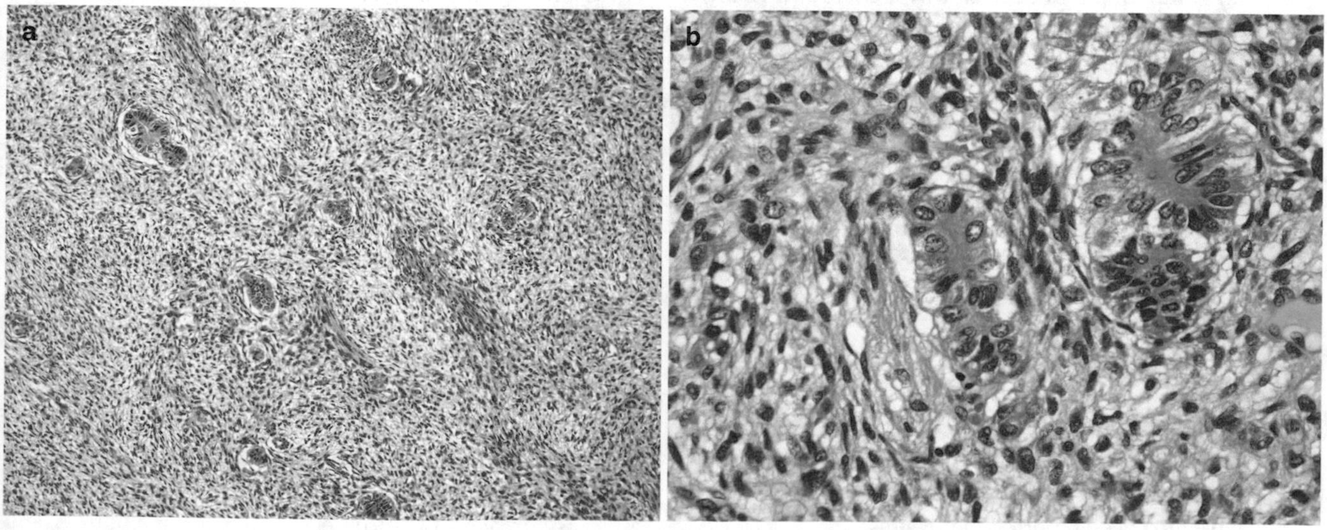

Fig. 18.18 (**a**) Gastroblastoma showing spindled and epithelial components. (**b**) Higher power view

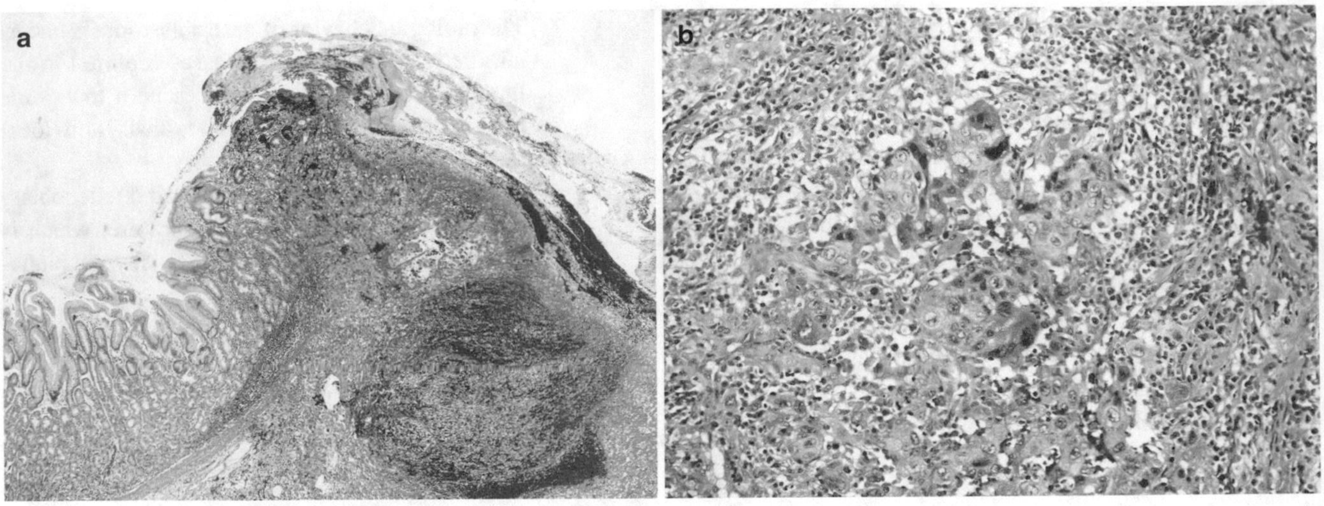

Fig. 18.19 (**a**) Choriocarcinoma of the gastric primary showing marked hemorrhage on low power view. (**b**) Higher power view showing syncytiotrophoblastic and cytotrophoblastic cells

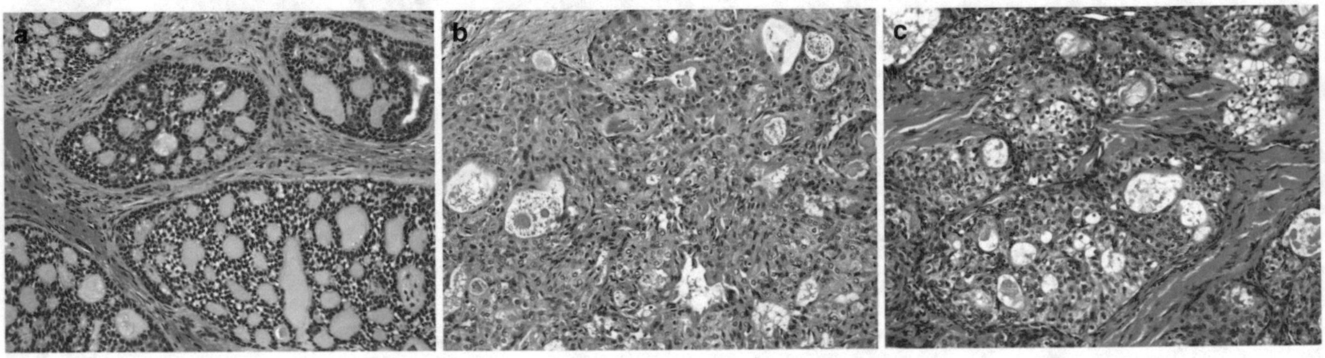

Fig. 18.20 (**a**) Adenoid cystic carcinoma showing a cribriform pattern with luminal basophilic glycosaminoglycans and basal lamina material. (**b**) Mucoepidermoid carcinoma showing admixed squamoid and mucin-producing cells. (**c**) Mucoepidermoid carcinoma showing intermediate cells with clusters of clear cells

ingly rare in the GI tract, however. Most cases show a combination with variable components of conventional adenocarcinoma, hepatoid carcinoma, yolk sac tumor, or even squamous cell carcinoma (in the esophagus). Immunohistochemically, trophoblastic cells are positive for human chorionic gonadotropin (HCG).

  - Hematogenous and lymphatic dissemination is common, with a poor prognosis.
  - Metastasis must be excluded before GI primary is diagnosed.

  References: [1, 26–43]

13. **Do salivary gland tumors occur in the GI tract?**
    - Salivary gland carcinomas can rarely occur in the gastrointestinal tract, especially in the esophagus, but have also been reported in the anus.
    - Among these, adenoid cystic carcinoma has been described most frequently in the esophagus, accounting for 0.1% of all esophageal malignancies. This tumor may show cribriform, tubular, and/or solid growth patterns and is composed of a mixture of epithelial and myoepithelial cells. Characteristically, the luminal spaces contain either hyalinized basal lamina material or basophilic glycosaminoglycans (Fig. 18.20a).
    - Rare cases of esophageal and anal mucoepidermoid carcinoma have been reported. This needs to be differentiated from the more common adenosquamous carcinoma in these regions. Like its salivary gland counterpart, mucoepidermoid carcinoma is composed of malignant squamoid (epidermoid), mucous, and intermediate cells (Fig. 18.20b, c). Glycogen-rich clear cells can be prominent.

    References: [44–46]

14. What should be considered when diagnosing diffuse-type adenocarcinoma of the stomach?

- Gastric adenocarcinoma can be divided into intestinal and diffuse types (Lauren classification). Diffuse-type adenocarcinoma, also referred to as poorly cohesive carcinoma, is comprised of malignant cells without conspicuous gland formation. Tumor cells can be single and mucin-poor (Fig. 18.11b) or form signet-ring cells (Fig. 18.11a).
- A significant consideration in the setting of a young patient with diffuse-type adenocarcinoma is the possibility of an underlying cancer susceptibility syndrome, including hereditary diffuse gastric cancer. It is caused by inactivating germline mutations of the *CDH1* gene that encodes a transmembrane protein E-cadherin, a cell-cell adhesion molecule. These autosomal dominant mutations predispose patients to a high risk of developing diffuse-type gastric cancer (signet-ring cell carcinoma) and lobular carcinoma of the breast. The affected patients range in age from 14 to 85 years. Early lesions in gastric cancer development include signet-ring cell carcinoma in situ and intramucosal signet-ring cell carcinoma typically seen in the superficial mucosa. There is usually no association with intestinal metaplasia, *H. pylori* infection, or atrophic gastritis. Pagetoid spread of signet-ring cells within normal gastric glands (beneath epithelial cell nuclei but within the basement membrane) may be seen (Fig. 18.21a–c). Complete loss or marked reduction of E-cadherin expression can be demonstrated in tumor cells by immunohistochemistry. However, E-cadherin immunostaining is not required for the diagnosis of hereditary diffuse gastric cancer because loss of E-cadherin expression can also occur in sporadic diffuse gastric cancer (Fig. 18.22a, b).
- Genetic counseling may be helpful for family members of patients with hereditary diffuse gastric cancer.
- If prophylactic total gastrectomy specimens from patients with *CDH1* mutation do not show gross lesions, extensive sampling or entire submission of the gastric mucosa for histologic examination should be performed to look for occult foci of carcinoma, which may show focal or multifocal in situ or invasive signet-ring cell carcinoma. Periodic acid-Schiff (PAS) stain may be performed instead of H&E stain to decrease the amount of time required to screen the slides. On scanning magnification, signet-ring cells are visible as PAS-positive cells that disrupt the normal packed glandular architecture of the gastric mucosa (Fig. 18.23).
- An important consideration in women with diffuse-type adenocarcinoma of the stomach is to exclude the possibility of an occult metastatic lobular breast adenocarcinoma. Immunostains for breast markers such as GATA3 and estrogen receptor can be helpful to evaluate for this possibility.

  References: [47–51]

15. Does the staging system for carcinomas differ depending on the gastrointestinal site?

- Staging protocols are similar but not identical across various parts of the GI tract (Tables 18.3 and 18.4).
- pT1 colorectal cancer implies submucosal invasion, whereas for small bowel, esophagus, or stomach, pT1 adenocarcinoma can either represent cancer with mucosal or submucosal invasion.
- Current pT staging protocols for most GI malignancies are primarily based on the depth of invasion through the wall, invasion of the visceral peritoneum, and direct involvement of adjacent organs. However, this approach differs for ampullary carcinomas, which are staged with more emphasis on involvement of surrounding structures, and for anal carcinomas, which are staged with an emphasis on tumor size.
- Low-grade appendiceal mucinous neoplasm (LAMN) has a unique pT staging system, which is described in detail in Chap. 8, Question 19.

  Reference: [7]

16. How is tumor involvement of the serosal surface (pT4a) evaluated?

- Invasion of tumor through the serosa (visceral peritoneum) is characterized by tumor cells present on the serosal surface (Fig. 18.24).
- Gross perforation of the viscera through tumor also qualifies as involvement of the serosa.
- Free-floating tumor cells present on the serosal surface with underlying erosion/ulceration of mesothelial lining, mesothelial hyperplasia, and/or inflammatory reaction also constitute serosal involvement.
- If tumor is present <1 mm from the serosal surface with mesothelial hyperplasia and/or inflammatory reaction, multiple deeper levels should be examined to determine if tumor involves the serosal surface.
  - If deeper levels do not demonstrate involvement of the serosal surface, the tumor should be staged as pT3.
  - The use of elastic stain (Verhoeff-Van Gieson stain) to help demonstrate tumor invasion of the peritoneal elastic lamina has been recommended for pT3 colorectal carcinomas by some studies. Peritoneal elastic lamina is present in close proximity to the serosal surface. Its involvement has been shown to be an adverse prognostic factor for pT3N0M0 colorectal carcinomas, with an overall survival worse than pT3 without peritoneal elastic lamina involvement but better than or equivalent to pT4a. However, this stain is not currently con-

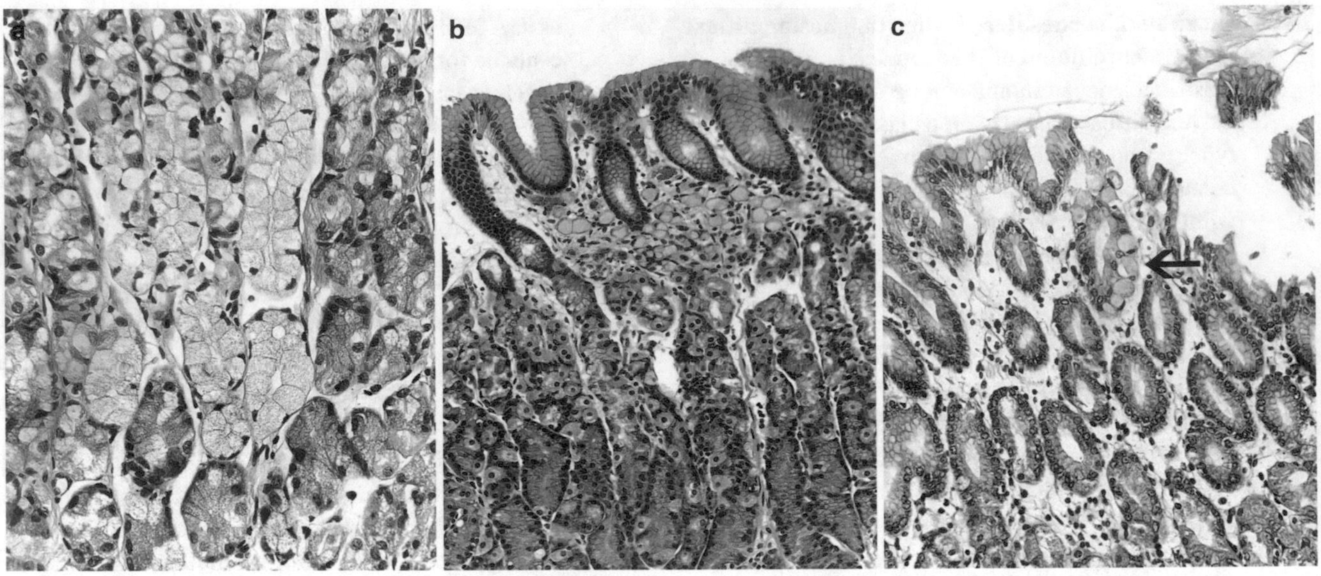

Fig. 18.21 Hereditary diffuse gastric cancer showing (**a**) signet-ring cell carcinoma in situ, (**b**) intramucosal signet-ring cell carcinoma in the superficial lamina propria, and (**c**) pagetoid spread of signet-ring cells (arrow). (Courtesy of Dr. Wei Zheng of Emory University)

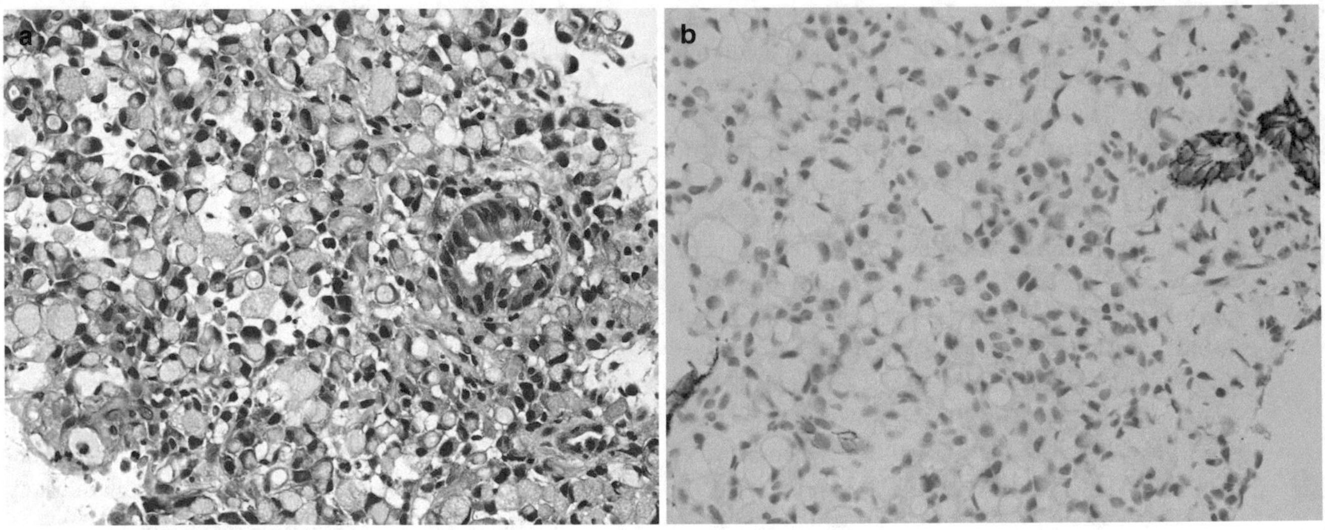

Fig. 18.22 A sporadic case of diffuse gastric cancer (signet-ring cell carcinoma) (**a**) showing complete loss of E-cadherin expression in tumor cells as demonstrated by immunohistochemistry (**b**)

sidered standard practice because the stain can be difficult to interpret and the elastic lamina is not uniformly present in the normal colon.

– Immunostains for mesothelial cells (such as calretinin and CK5/6) to highlight mesothelial lining may help in difficult cases.

References: [52–55]

17. **What should be considered as a radial margin at different sites of the GI tract for resection specimens?**
   - The serosal surface of the bowel is not a margin, while surfaces that are dissected/transected by the surgeon are true margins.
   - Esophagus – the entire adventitial surface.
   - Stomach – the lesser and greater omentum resection margins.
   - Small bowel – the mesenteric resection margin.
   - Colon – dependent on the anatomic location of tumor.
     – The cecum is entirely covered by peritoneum but does not have its own mesentery. The closest mesenteric margin of the terminal ileum or retroperitoneal surface of the ascending colon should be evaluated.
     – The ascending colon and descending colon are retroperitoneal. The posterior surface, which lacks peritoneal covering, is the radial margin.

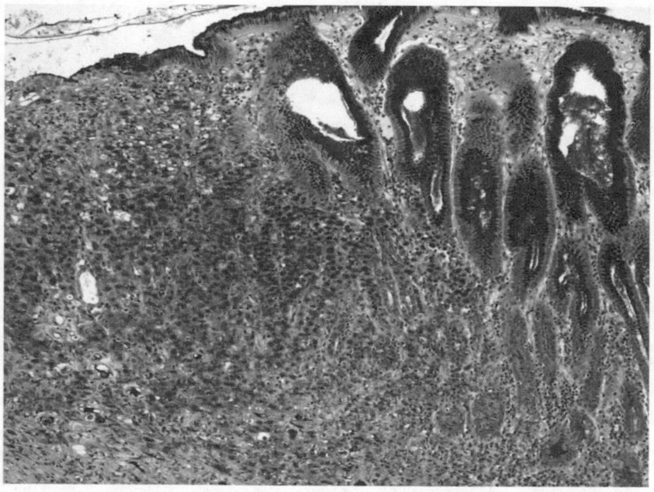

Fig. 18.23 PAS stained section from a prophylactic gastrectomy specimen highlighting poorly cohesive tumor cells with abundant intracytoplasmic mucin that disrupt the normal packed glandular architecture of the gastric mucosa

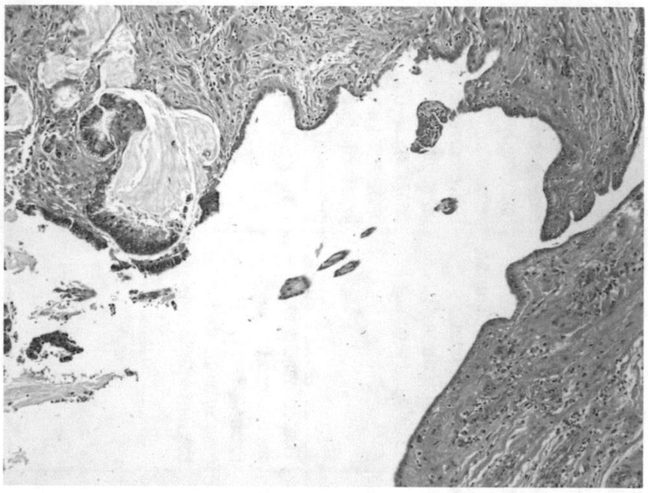

Fig. 18.24 Carcinoma invading through the serosal surface with adjacent reactive mesothelial cells

- The transverse colon, sigmoid colon, and appendix are intraperitoneal and have mesentery. The mesenteric margin is the radial margin for these locations.
- Rectum – depending on anatomic locations of tumor.
  - The upper third is covered by peritoneum on the anterior and lateral surfaces. The posterior retroperitoneal surface is the radial margin.
  - The middle third is covered by peritoneum only on the anterior surface. The posterior and lateral retroperitoneal surfaces are radial margins.
  - The lower third has no peritoneal covering. The entire circumference of the mesorectal surface is the radial margin.
- There is no pT4a tumor in the distal third of the rectum, as well as in the retroperitoneal surfaces of the colorectum.

18. What is the significance of mesorectal envelop evaluation and how is it evaluated?

- Gross assessment of completeness of the mesorectal envelop in surgical specimens (such as low anterior resection and abdominoperineal resection) for rectal cancer provides useful information about the adequacy of surgery and probability of tumor recurrence. Studies have shown that patients with incomplete excision of the mesorectal envelop have a higher risk of recurrence than those with complete excision.
- The specimen should be inspected circumferentially before the radial margin is inked and margin sections are taken. The completeness of the mesorectal envelop is evaluated using the criteria outlined in Table 18.5 based on the worst area in the specimen.
- The mesorectal tissue may become fragmented during surgical dissection. This should not be interpreted as incomplete if bulky tissue is present with no coning toward the distal margin. A discussion with the surgeon should help if there is question.

References: [56–59]

19. What distance from margin to tumor is adequate to achieve a negative margin?

- In the esophagus, tumor present at inked radial (circumferential) margin is considered positive by the College of American Pathologists (CAP); however, the Royal College of Pathologists considers tumor within 1 mm of the margin as positive.
- Proximal and distal colon/rectal margins of ≥5 cm are typically considered adequate with low risk of local recurrence.
  - For low anterior resections, distal margins of 2 cm are typically considered adequate. For pT1 and pT2 carcinomas, a distal margin of 1 cm may be adequate.
- In the colorectum, the radial margin is considered negative if tumor is >1 mm from inked nonperitonealized surface.
  - Tumor present ≤1 mm from inked nonperitonealized surface is considered positive. The local recurrence rates are similar for tumors with a microscopic clearance of 0 to 1 mm.
- Data for the presence of intravascular or intranodal tumor at the radial margin or <1 mm from radial margin are limited; however, they suggest outcomes similar to those with negative radial margins. Therefore, the radial margin should be considered negative, but

Table 18.3 pT staging systems for GI carcinomas[a]

pT stage	Esophagus and GEJ	Stomach	Small intestine	Ampulla of Vater	Appendix[b]	Colon and rectum	Anus
pTis	High-grade dysplasia, defined as malignant cells confined to the epithelium by basement membrane	Carcinoma in situ: intraepithelial tumor without invasion of the lamina propria, high-grade dysplasia	High-grade dysplasia/ carcinoma in situ	Carcinoma in situ	Carcinoma in situ (intramucosal carcinoma; invasion of the lamina propria or extension into but not through the muscularis mucosae)	Carcinoma in situ, intramucosal carcinoma (involvement of lamina propria with no extension through muscularis mucosae)	High-grade squamous intraepithelial lesion (previously termed carcinoma in situ, Bowen disease, anal intraepithelial neoplasia II–III, high-grade anal intraepithelial neoplasia)
pT1	Tumor invades the lamina propria, muscularis mucosae, or submucosa	Tumor invades the lamina propria, muscularis mucosae, or submucosa	Tumor invades the lamina propria or submucosa	Tumor limited to ampulla of Vater or sphincter of Oddi or tumor invades beyond the sphincter of Oddi (perisphincteric invasion) and/or into the duodenal submucosa	Tumor invades the submucosa (through the muscularis mucosae but not into the muscularis propria)	Tumor invades the submucosa (through the muscularis mucosae but not into the muscularis propria)	Tumor ≤2 cm
pT1a	Tumor invades the lamina propria or muscularis mucosae	Tumor invades the lamina propria or muscularis mucosae	Tumor invades the lamina propria	Tumor limited to ampulla of Vater or sphincter of Oddi			
pT1b	Tumor invades the submucosa	Tumor invades the submucosa	Tumor invades the submucosa	Tumor invades beyond the sphincter of Oddi (perisphincteric invasion) and/or into the duodenal submucosa			
pT2	Tumor invades the muscularis propria	Tumor invades the muscularis propria	Tumor invades the muscularis propria	Tumor invades into the muscularis propria of the duodenum	Tumor invades the muscularis propria	Tumor invades the muscularis propria	Tumor >2 cm but ≤5 cm
pT3	Tumor invades adventitia	Tumor penetrates the subserosal connective tissue without invasion of the visceral peritoneum or adjacent structures	Tumor invades through the muscularis propria into the subserosa or extends into the nonperitonealized perimuscular tissue (mesentery or retroperitoneum) without serosal penetration	Tumor directly invades the pancreas (up to 0.5 cm) or tumor extends more than 0.5 cm into the pancreas, or extends into peripancreatic or periduodenal tissue or duodenal serosa without involvement of the celiac axis or superior mesenteric artery	Tumor invades through the muscularis propria into the subserosa or mesoappendix	Tumor invades through the muscularis propria into pericolorectal tissues	Tumor >5 cm

pT3a				Tumor directly invades the pancreas (up to 0.5 cm)			
pT3b				Tumor extends more than 0.5 cm into the pancreas, or extends into peripancreatic tissue or periduodenal tissue or duodenal serosa without involvement of the celiac axis or superior mesenteric artery			
pT4	Tumor invades adjacent structures	Tumor invades the serosa (visceral peritoneum) or adjacent structures	Tumor perforates the visceral peritoneum or directly invades other organs or structures (e.g., other loops of small intestine, mesentery of adjacent loops of bowel, and abdominal wall by way of serosa; for duodenum only, invasion of pancreas or bile duct)	Tumor involves the celiac axis, superior mesenteric artery, and/or common hepatic artery, irrespective of size	Tumor invades the visceral peritoneum, including the acellular mucin or mucinous epithelium involving the serosa of the appendix or mesoappendix, and/or directly invades adjacent organs or structures	Tumor invades the visceral peritoneum or invades or adheres to adjacent organs or structures	Tumor of any size invading adjacent organ(s) such as the vagina, urethra, or bladder
pT4a	Tumor invades the pleura, pericardium, azygos vein, diaphragm, or peritoneum	Tumor invades the serosa (visceral peritoneum)			Tumor invades through the visceral peritoneum, including the acellular mucin or mucinous epithelium involving the serosa of the appendix or serosa of the mesoappendix	Tumor invades through the visceral peritoneum (including gross perforation of the bowel through tumor and continuous invasion of tumor through areas of inflammation to the surface of the visceral peritoneum)	
pT4b	Tumor invades other adjacent structures, such as aorta, vertebral body, or airway	Tumor invades adjacent structures/organs			Tumor directly invades (or adheres to) adjacent organs or structures[c]	Tumor directly invades or adheres to adjacent organs or structures[c]	

GEJ gastroesophageal junction

[a]The staging systems do not apply to well differentiated neuroendocrine tumor of the GI tract

[b]The staging system for appendix is also used for goblet cell adenocarcinoma and high-grade appendiceal mucinous neoplasm

[c]Tumor that is adherent to other organs or structures grossly but no tumor is found in the adhesion microscopically; the tumor should be staged as pT1-4a according on the depth of wall invasion, rather than pT4b

Table 18.4 pN and pM staging systems for GI carcinomas

	Esophagus and GEJ	Stomach[a]	Small intestine	Ampulla of Vater	Appendix	Colon and rectum	Anus
pN0	No regional lymph node metastasis	No regional lymph node metastasis	No regional lymph node metastasis	No regional lymph node metastasis	No regional lymph node metastasis	No regional lymph node metastasis	No regional lymph node metastasis
pN1	Metastasis in one or two regional lymph nodes	Metastasis in one or two regional lymph nodes	Metastasis in one or two regional lymph nodes	Metastasis to one to three regional lymph nodes	One to three regional lymph nodes are positive (tumor in lymph nodes measuring ≥0.2 mm), or any number of tumor deposits is present, and all identifiable lymph nodes are negative	One to three regional lymph nodes are positive (tumor in lymph nodes measuring ≥0.2 mm), or any number of tumor deposits are present and all identifiable lymph nodes are negative	Metastasis in inguinal, mesorectal, internal iliac, or external iliac nodes
pN1a					One regional lymph node is positive	One regional lymph node is positive	Metastasis in inguinal, mesorectal, or internal iliac lymph nodes
pN1b					Two or three regional lymph nodes are positive	Two or three regional lymph nodes are positive	Metastasis in external iliac lymph nodes
pN1c					No regional lymph nodes are positive, but there are tumor deposits in the subserosa or mesentery	No regional lymph nodes are positive, but there are tumor deposits in the subserosa, mesentery, or nonperitonealized pericolic, or perirectal/mesorectal tissues[b]	Metastasis in external iliac with any N1a nodes
pN2	Metastasis in three to six regional lymph nodes	Metastasis in three to six regional lymph nodes	Metastasis in three or more regional lymph nodes	Metastasis to four or more regional lymph nodes	Four or more regional lymph nodes are positive	Four or more regional lymph nodes are positive	
pN2a						Four to six regional lymph nodes are positive	
pN2b						Seven or more regional lymph nodes are positive	
pN3	Metastasis in seven or more regional lymph nodes	Metastasis in seven or more regional lymph nodes					

pN3a		Metastasis in 7 to 15 regional lymph nodes					
pN3b		Metastasis in 16 or more regional lymph nodes					
pM1	Distant metastasis	Distant metastasis	Distant metastasis	Distant metastasis	Distant metastasis	Metastasis to one or more distant sites or organs or peritoneal metastasis is identified	Distant metastasis
pM1a					Intraperitoneal acellular mucin, without identifiable tumor cells in the disseminated peritoneal mucinous deposits	Metastasis to one site or organ is identified without peritoneal metastasis	
pM1b					Intraperitoneal metastasis only, including peritoneal mucinous deposits containing tumor cells	Metastasis to two or more sites or organs is identified without peritoneal metastasis	
pM1c					Metastasis to sites other than peritoneum	Metastasis to the peritoneal surface is identified alone or with other site or organ metastases	

GEJ gastroesophageal junction

[a]Tumor deposits in the subserosal fat adjacent to a gastric carcinoma are considered regional lymph node metastasis for pN staging (see Question 21)

[b]The number of tumor deposits should be recorded for colorectal carcinomas. If lymph node metastasis (including micrometastasis) is also present, the pN stage should be determined by the number of positive lymph nodes. The presence of tumor deposits does not affect pN in that case (see Question 21)

Table 18.5 Gross assessment of the completeness of the mesorectal envelop

Complete	Intact bulky mesorectum with a smooth surface Only minor irregularities of the mesorectal surface No surface defects deeper than 5 mm No coning toward the distal margin of the specimen After transverse sectioning, the circumferential margin is smooth
Nearly complete	Moderate bulk to the mesorectum Irregular mesorectal surface with defects deeper than 5 mm, but none extending to the muscularis propria No areas of visibility of the muscularis propria except at the insertion site of the levator ani muscles
Incomplete	Little bulk to the mesorectum Defects in the mesorectum down to the muscularis propria After transverse sectioning, the circumferential margin is very irregular

the presence of intravascular or intranodal tumor within 1 mm of the margin should be documented in pathology reports.

References: [60, 61]

20. What are the minimal numbers of regional lymph nodes at different sites of the GI tract required for adequate pN staging?

- In general, all lymph nodes should be harvested and examined histologically to accurately stage carcinomas.
- For esophageal cancer, the minimum number of lymph nodes has not been determined. Some data suggest that the optimal lymph node harvest ranges from 10 to 30 lymph nodes.
  - Others suggest that the number varies by pT stage.
    pT1: 10 nodes.
    pT2: 20 nodes.
    pT3 and pT4: 30 nodes.
    Some suggest that more nodes are necessary for earlier pT stage carcinomas to adequately stage the carcinoma.
  - For esophagectomy or esophagogastrectomy, the regional lymph nodes may be separately submitted by surgeons. There usually is minimal periesophageal (adventitial) soft tissue present in the specimens, which does not contain an adequate number of lymph nodes. In cases that have received preoperative treatment, lymph nodes may become atrophic and difficult to identify. Therefore, the entire periesophageal soft tissue may need to be submitted to maximize lymph node retrieval.
- For gastrectomy, at least 16 nodes are suggested, with >30 being optimal for staging.
- For small bowel carcinoma, the minimum number of lymph nodes has not been well defined. There are limited data to suggest five to nine, and at least eight have been suggested as optimal.
- For colorectal carcinoma, at least 12 lymph nodes are recommended.

21. How to diagnose tumor deposits?

- A tumor deposit is defined as a discrete tumor focus, irrespective of size and shape, separate from the primary tumor but within its lymph drainage area (Fig. 18.25a). It is present within the subserosal fat, pericolorectal soft tissue, or the adjacent mesentery. It lacks evidence of lymphovascular invasion or perineural invasion and lacks recognizable lymph node architecture (Fig. 18.25b, c). If the vessel wall or neural structure or their remnants are recognizable on H&E or other stains (such as elastic stain), the lesion should be classified as vascular (venous) or perineural invasion.
- For colorectal and appendiceal carcinomas, the presence of tumor deposits in the absence of lymph node metastasis is staged as pN1c (Table 18.4). Patients with pN1c will often receive adjuvant therapy regardless of pT stage. The presence of tumor deposits only changes pN0 to pN1c but does not affect pN if there is any number of positive lymph nodes. The number of tumor deposits should be separately recorded and

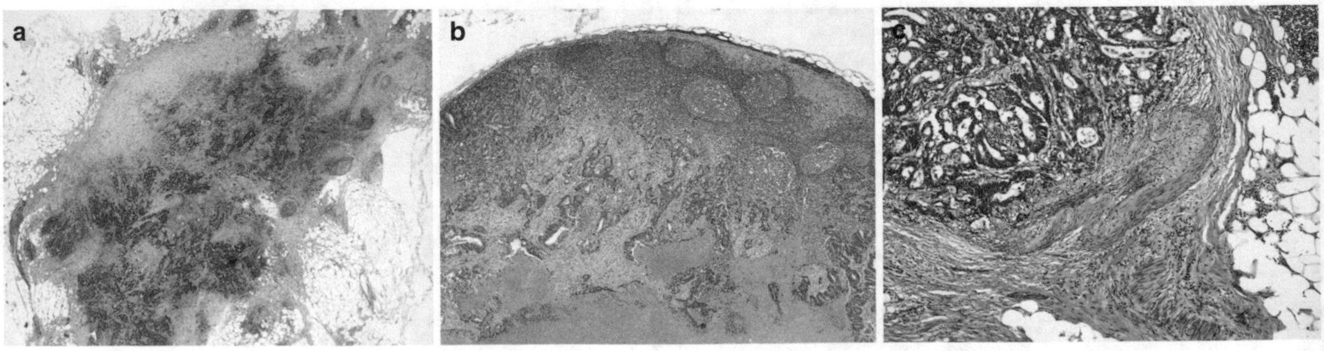

Fig. 18.25 (**a**) A tumor deposit in the mesenteric fat showing an irregular contour. No residual nodal structures or evidence of vascular or neural invasion are seen. (**b**) Nodal metastasis showing near-complete replacement by tumor but residual nodal structures are recognized. (**c**) A discrete cluster of tumor cells in the subserosal fat showing evidence of vascular invasion

should not be added to the total number of positive lymph nodes.

- For gastric carcinoma, tumor deposits are considered regional lymph node metastases. In the gastric location, the number of tumor deposits is added to the total number of positive lymph nodes.
- For small bowel carcinoma, tumor deposits should be documented in pathology reports as potential metastatic disease but are not counted as positive regional lymph nodes.
- Reporting of tumor deposit should be done with caution in the setting of neoadjuvant therapy where findings may represent incompletely regressed tumor rather than a true tumor deposit.

References: [7, 62–64]

22. What is the significance of isolated tumor cells in a lymph node?

- Isolated tumor cells are defined as single tumor cells or small tumor clusters measuring <0.2 mm (Fig. 18.26), identified either on H&E or by immunostains. They are usually detected in the subcapsular sinus and may be present as a single focus in a single lymph node or multiple foci in one or more nodes.
- The significance of isolated tumor cells in the lymph node evaluation performed for gastrointestinal cancer is currently uncertain. Some studies failed to demonstrate worse prognosis in cases only showing isolated tumor cells within the lymph nodes; therefore, these cases are currently staged as pN0 disease.
- However, others suggest worse disease-free survival in early cancers with isolated tumor cells as the only manifestation of lymphatic spread.

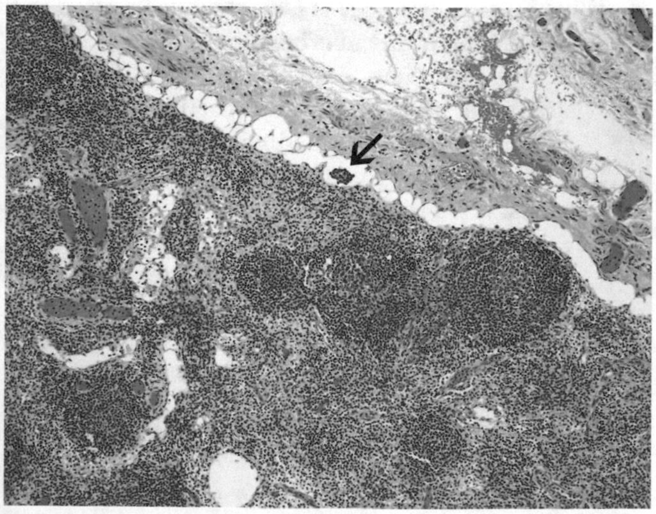

Fig. 18.26 A single tumor cell cluster of <0.2 mm (arrow) present in the subcapsular sinus of a lymph node, recognized on H&E stain

- Tumor clusters of 0.2–2.0 mm have been traditionally defined as micrometastasis. Lymph nodes with micrometastasis should be counted as positive.
- In practice, the 0.2 mm rule does not appear to be strictly followed. Many pathologists count lymph nodes positive if tumor cells are readily recognized on routine H&E stain, no matter if the tumor cluster is greater or smaller than 0.2 mm. Ancillary techniques such as immunohistochemistry to help identify tumor cells are not recommended for H&E-negative lymph nodes.

References: [7, 65–68]

23. What is the significance of acellular mucin in pTNM staging or present at surgical margin?

- With the exception of appendix, acellular mucin should not be used for pTNM staging for GI carcinomas. Instead, the presence of tumor cells is required.
- For the appendix, acellular mucin and tumor cells are considered equally important for pT staging (Table 18.3), although the pure presence of acellular mucin on the serosal surface (pT4a) carries a much lower risk of recurrence than the presence of cellular mucin. Acellular mucin is also used for pM staging but is not used for pN staging for appendiceal carcinomas (Table 18.4). As in other sites of the GI tract, the presence of acellular mucin within lymph nodes or subserosal/mesenteric deposits is categorized as pN0 (Fig. 18.27a).
- In treated tumors, the presence of acellular mucin in viscera or within nodal tissue is considered complete treatment response and is not considered when assigning pT, pN, or pM categories.
- The presence of acellular mucin at the surgical margin does not appear to increase the likelihood of local recurrence or metastasis (Fig. 18.27b). Technically, the margin should not be considered positive, but the finding should be documented and conveyed to the surgeon. Multiple deeper sections should be examined to ensure the absence of tumor cells at the margin.

References: [69–71]

24. What is tumor budding and its significance?

- High tumor budding in colorectal adenocarcinoma is considered to be high-risk feature, which predicts an increased likelihood of nodal metastasis, similar to the presence of lymphovascular invasion. Studies have suggested it to be most useful as a risk factor for malignant polyps as well as stage I and II colorectal adenocarcinomas.

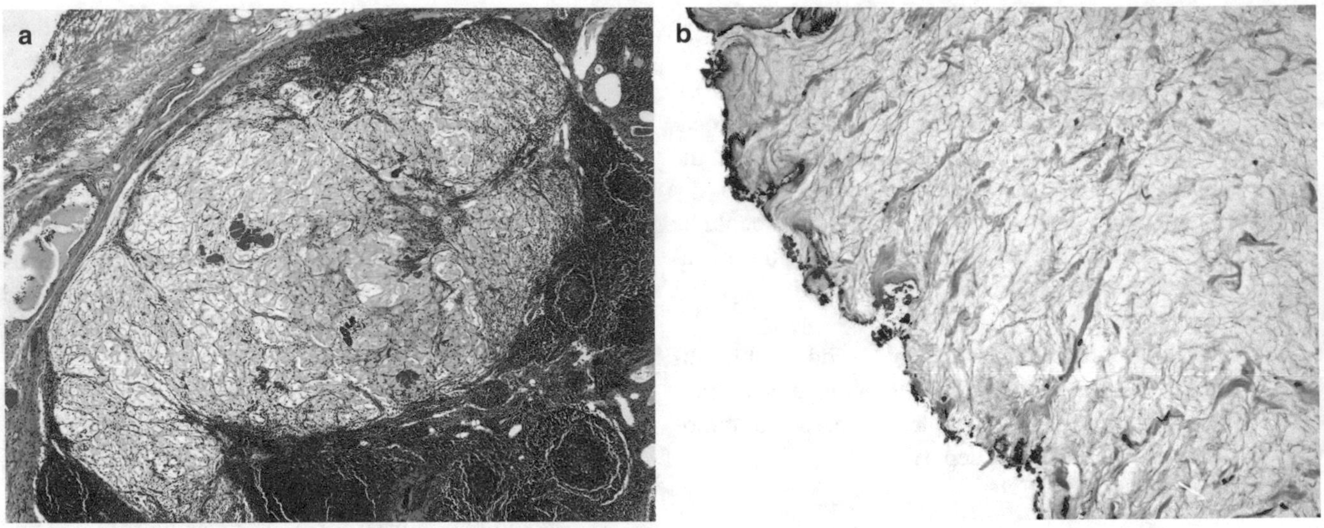

Fig. 18.27 (**a**) An acellular mucin pool present in a lymph node retrieved from a partial gastrectomy specimen. The patient received neoadjuvant chemotherapy for gastric adenocarcinoma. (**b**) Acellular mucin dissecting the rectal wall and extending to inked radial margin

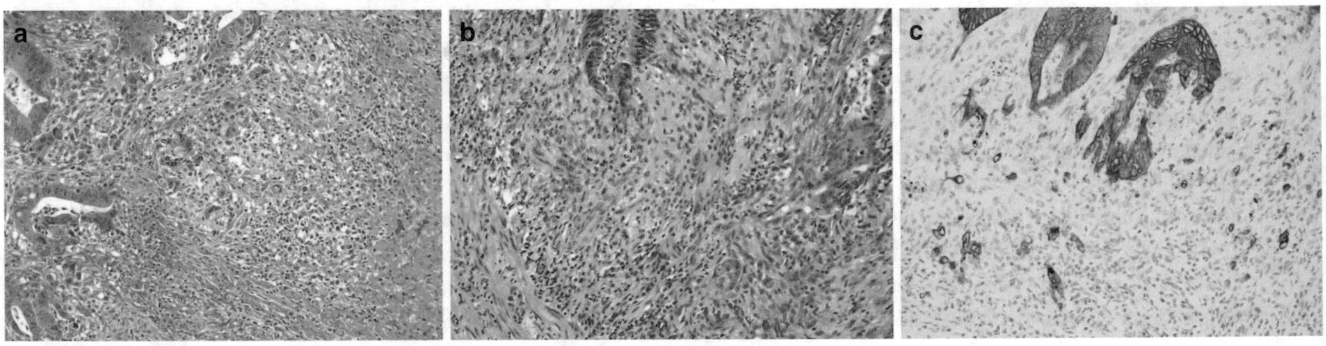

Fig. 18.28 (**a**) Adenocarcinoma with high tumor budding characterized by single cells or small clusters of tumor cells (up to four cells) at the advancing front of the tumor. (**b**) Tumor budding is difficult to assess in this area due to presence of inflammation but much easier to appreciate on immunostaining for cytokeratin (**c**)

- Tumor buds are defined as single cells or small clusters composed of <5 tumor cells present at the advancing front of the tumor (Fig. 18.28a).
- Tumor budding is assessed in a "hot spot" area after reviewing all available tumor sections. Tumor buds are counted within an area of 0.785 mm^2 that corresponds to a 20x field in a standard microscope.
- A keratin immunostain can be used to aid microscopic assessment in difficult cases where tumor buds may be obscured by inflammation (Fig. 18.28b, c), but the count should be performed on routine H&E-stained sections.
- A three-tiered scoring system is used to report tumor budding: low (0–4 buds), intermediate (5–9 buds), and high (10 or more buds).

References: [72–75]

25. What is the significance of large venous invasion versus small lymphovascular invasion?

- Small vessels are endothelium-lined, thin-walled spaces that include lymphatics, capillaries, and postcapillary venules. They differ from large venous vessels by lacking smooth muscle layer and elastic lamina in the walls.
- Tumors with small lymphovascular invasion (Fig. 18.29a) have more frequent regional nodal metastases, whereas tumors with extramural (beyond the muscularis propria) large venous invasion (Fig. 18.29b) are associated with metastasis to more distant sites such as the liver. The significance of intramural (submucosa and muscularis propria) venous invasion is less clear.

- Tissue evaluation with D2–40 or CD31 immunostain can help in highlighting small lymphovascular invasion (Fig. 18.29c).
- Large venous invasion often appears histologically as a circumscribed tumor nodule surrounded by fibromuscular tissue, often adjacent to an uninvolved artery (orphan artery sign).
- Elastic stain can aid in interpretation of large venous invasion by highlighting the residual elastic lamina of the venous wall (Fig. 18.29d). Residual muscle layer can be highlighted by immunostains for muscle markers such as desmin or caldesmon.

References: [76–79]

26. What is the significance of perineural invasion?

- Invasion of nerves by tumor cells has been shown to be a negative prognostic factor for GI carcinomas. It is characterized by tumor cells invading around or into the nerve fibers (Fig. 18.30). It is usually readily recognizable on H&E stain.

27. How is tumor regression in response to neoadjuvant therapies assessed in a resection specimen?

- Failure of tumor to respond to neoadjuvant treatment is an adverse prognostic indicator. Several tumor regression grading systems have been proposed. The widely used modified Ryan scheme for tumor regression score has been shown to be reproducible and has prognostic significance (Table 18.6).
- The specimen should be examined thoroughly for treatment effect at the tumor site, lymph nodes, and peritumoral deposits. However, tumor regression score is only assessed in the main tumor and not in lymph node metastasis.
- Acellular mucin pools are considered to represent completely treated tumor and are not considered in pT and pN assessment.

References: [80, 81]

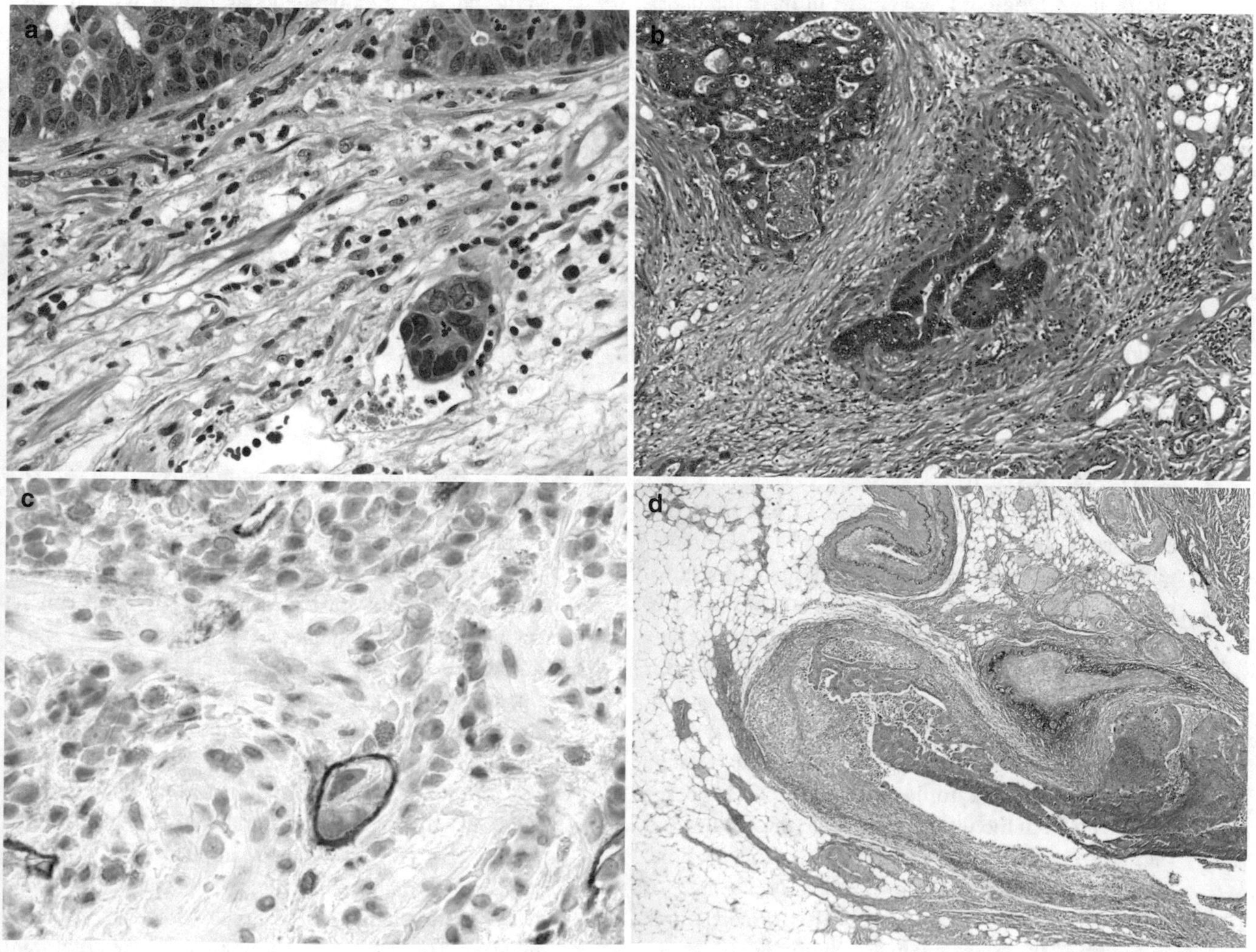

Fig. 18.29 (**a**) Small vessel (lymphovascular) invasion. (**b**) Large vessel (venous) invasion. (**c**) Small vessel invasion highlighted by D2–40 immunostaining. (**d**) Large extramural venous invasion highlighted by elastic stain, which is commonly found next to an artery

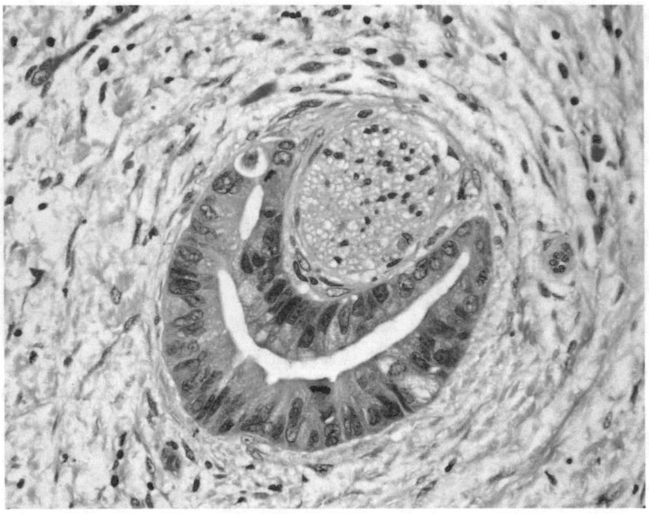

Fig. 18.30 Perineural invasion

28. What is lymphoglandular complex and how to distinguish it from invasive adenocarcinoma?

- Benign colorectal crypts can occasionally be present within large lymphoid aggregates in the submucosa where the muscularis mucosae are discontinuous. These structures are referred to as lymphoglandular complexes (Fig. 18.31a). In the rectum, lymphoglandular complexes may occur in localized/nodular reactive proliferation of lymphoid tissue, which is sometimes referred to as "rectal tonsil."
- The epithelium may be involved by adenoma/dysplasia. Misplacement of the adenomatous/dysplastic epithelium deep into these areas may simulate invasive adenocarcinoma (Fig. 18.31b).
- Single infiltrating cells or small clusters of cells; poorly formed, fused, and irregular glands; solid nests; desmoplastic stromal reaction; and lymphovascular invasion are features of invasive adenocarcinoma (Fig. 18.31c, d).
- There are a handful reported cases of so-called gut-associated lymphoid tissue (GALT) carcinoma, which can be confused with lymphoglandular complexes with misplaced adenomatous/dysplastic epithelium. This peculiar adenocarcinoma is characterized by submucosal localization, prominent lymphoid tissue with germinal center formation, tumor-infiltrating lymphocytes, lack of desmoplasia, and dilated glands with bland nuclear features and eosinophilic cytoplasm. The reported cases were seen from the ileocecal valve to the rectum and ranged from 0.5 to 3 cm in size. Interestingly, none of reported cases developed local recurrence or metastasis during follow-up. It is also termed "dome carcinoma" by some given its characteristic endoscopic appearance. It is postulated that GALT carcinoma originates from M-cells of GALT. Associated adenomatous component is identified in only half of the cases.
- This topic is also discussed in Chap. 14, Question 28.

Reference: [82–84]

Table 18.6 Modified Ryan schema for tumor regression score

Score	Description
0	No viable tumor cells (complete response)
1	Single cells or rare small groups of tumor cells (near-complete response)
2	Residual cancer with evident tumor regression, but more than single cells or rare small groups of cancer cells (partial response)
3	Extensive residual cancer with no evidence of tumor regression (poor or no response)

29. What is a colorectal-type adenocarcinoma of the appendix?

- This type of adenocarcinoma arises within the appendix which morphologically resembles a conventional colorectal adenocarcinoma without significant mucin production (Fig. 18.32). These tumors display an infiltrating growth pattern, desmoplasia, and variable necrosis, similar to their colorectal counterpart. Cribriform and angulated glands may be present depending on the degree of differentiation.
- As in other sites of the GI tract, tumors consisting of >50% of extracellular mucin are designated as mucinous adenocarcinoma.
- Nodal and distant metastases are more common with nonmucinous adenocarcinomas as compared to mucinous carcinomas of the appendix.

References: [85, 86]

30. What is the definition of adenocarcinoma of the ampulla of Vater?

- Adenocarcinoma of the ampulla of Vater is defined as a tumor in which the epicenter is grossly located at the ampulla of Vater. Based on its cell origin, it can be divided into intra-ampullary type arising from intra-ampullary papillary-tubular neoplasm or ampullary ducts, peri-ampullary type arising from duodenal mucosa of the papilla, and mixed intra- and peri-ampullary type.
- Histologically, ampullary adenocarcinoma can be generally divided into intestinal and pancreatobiliary types, which have prognostic implications. Intestinal type has been shown to have a better prognosis compared with pancreatobiliary type. However, approximately 40% of cases show mixed intestinal and pancreatobiliary histology.

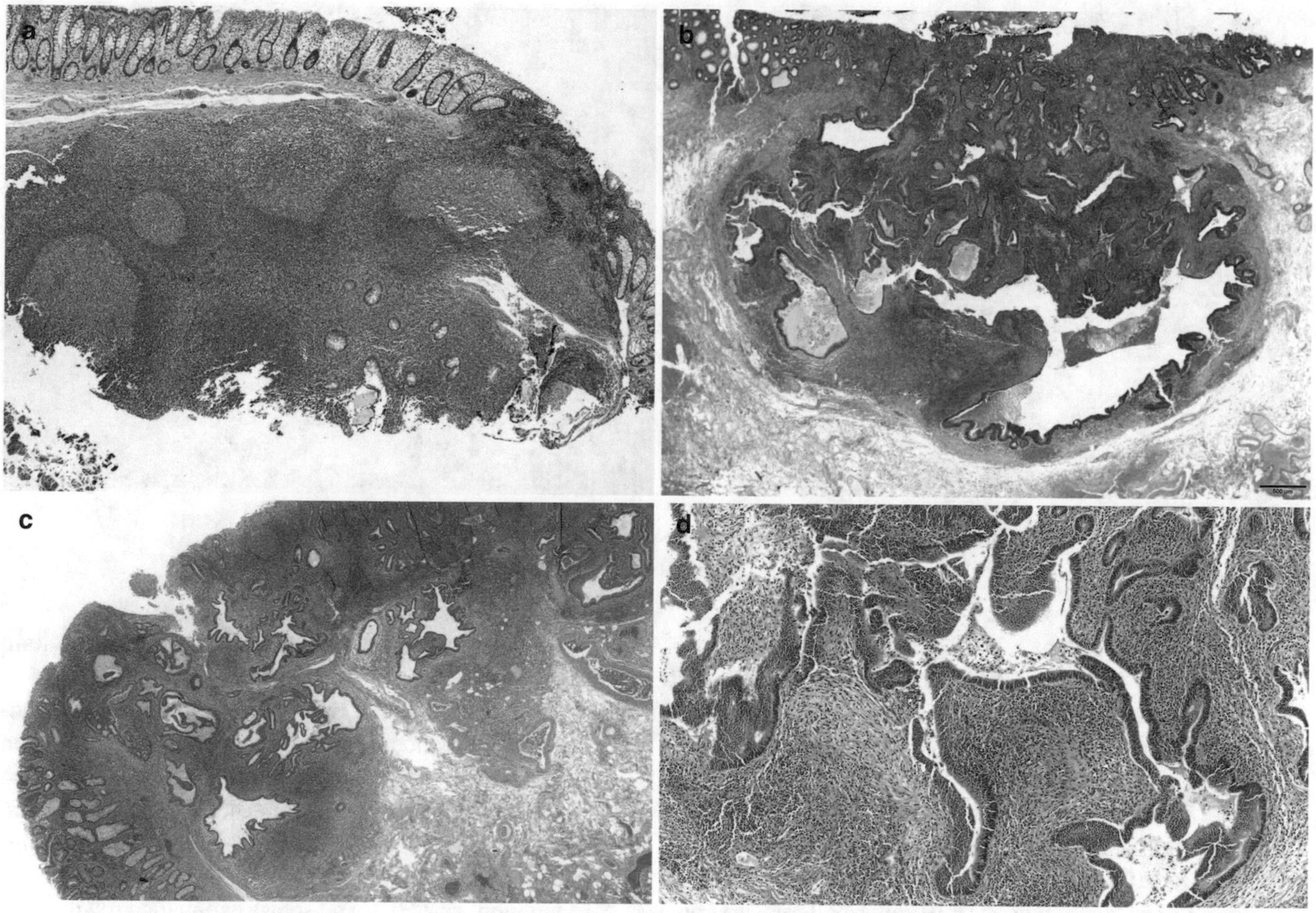

Fig. 18.31 (**a**) A lymphoglandular complex of the rectum showing nonneoplastic crypts in a large submucosal lymphoid nodule ("rectal tonsil"). (**b**) A rectal adenoma involving a submucosal lymphoglandular complex. The rounded contour, retained lamina propria, and lack of desmoplastic stroma favor a benign process. (**c**) A polypoid rectal lesion showing prominent lymphoid tissue with markedly irregular neoplastic glands extending to the submucosa. A component of tubular adenoma is noted in the left lower corner. (**d**) Focal desmoplasia is noted, which along with marked glandular irregularity supports a diagnosis of invasive adenocarcinoma. This case shares some of the histologic features described for "gut-associated lymphoid tissue carcinoma"

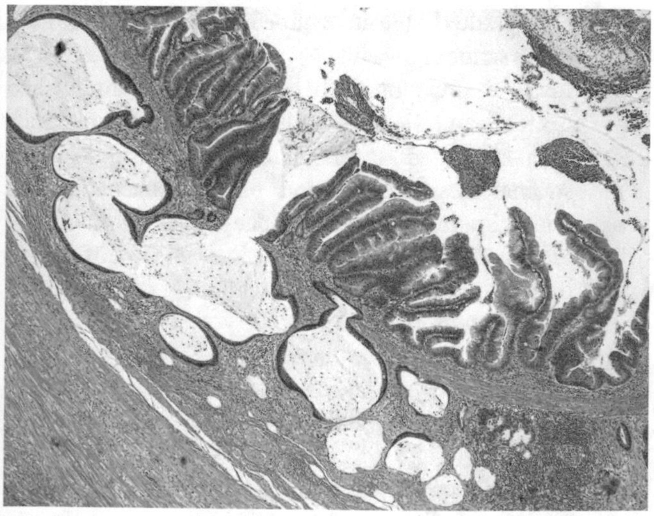

Fig. 18.32 Colorectal-type adenocarcinoma of the appendix arising from an adenoma

- Intestinal type resembles colorectal adenocarcinoma (Fig. 18.33a). Tumor glands are lined by tall columnar cells with elongated pseudostratified nuclei. Luminal necrosis and mucin production are common. Scattered goblet cells and Paneth cells may be present.
- Pancreatobiliary type resembles pancreatic ductal carcinoma or cholangiocarcinoma (Fig. 18.33b). Tumor glands are usually small, widely separated by desmoplastic stroma, and lined by a single layer of cuboidal or low columnar cells. There is no significant nuclear pseudostratification. In comparison to intestinal type, nuclear pleomorphism is more prominent.
- Differentiating these histologic types is based on resection specimens and is typically considered a morphologic diagnosis. In tumors with equivocal histologic features, immunostains for CK20, CDX2, MUC1, and MUC2 can be helpful.

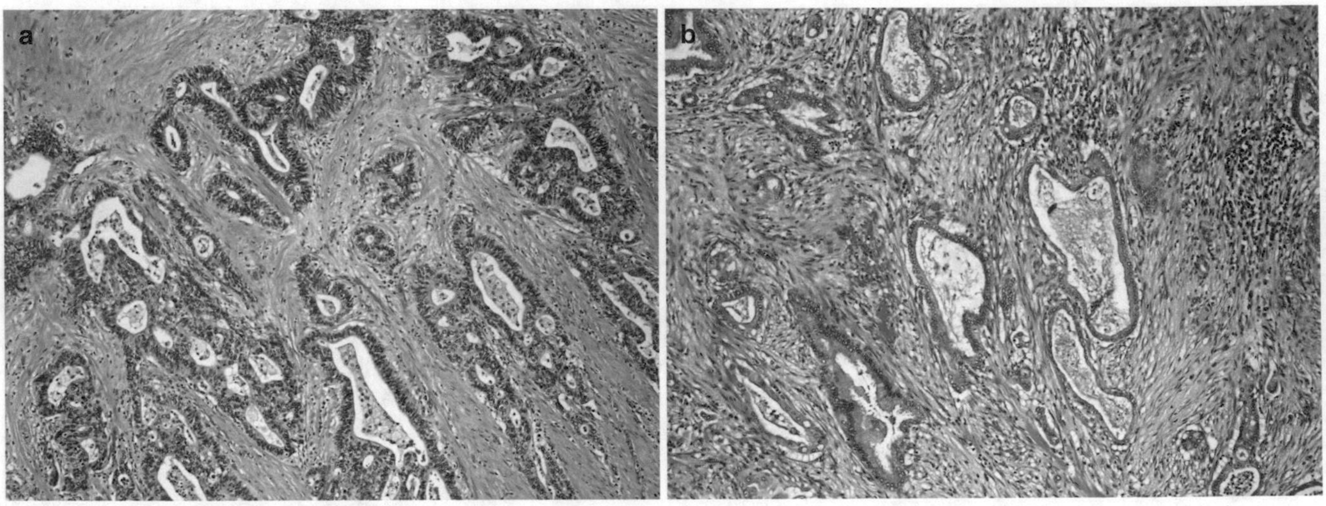

Fig. 18.33 Ampullary adenocarcinoma, (**a**) intestinal type, (**b**) pancreatobiliary type

- Intestinal type:
  Positive for CK20 or CDX2 or MUC2 and negative for MUC1
  Positive for CK20, CDX2, and MUC2, irrespective of MUC1
- Pancreatobiliary type:
  Positive for MUC1 and negative for CDX2 and MUC2, irrespective of CK20
- Other combinations of staining patterns are considered ambiguous.

Reference: [87]

31. **What are the histologic features of conventional squamous cell carcinoma versus verrucous carcinoma of the anus?**
    - Conventional squamous cell carcinoma of the anus can show basaloid features or demonstrate frank keratinization. The tumor typically shows infiltrative growth of rounded to jagged nests of tumor cells with mild to marked cytologic atypia (Fig. 18.34a).
    - Verrucous carcinoma is a squamoproliferative lesion characterized by a large gross tumor size. The tumor is predominantly exophytic, with papillomatous growth and acanthosis of the epithelial layer. Broad, blunt downward projections of the epithelium represent pushing-type invasion. Cytologically, tumor cells are bland with some mild atypia and mitotic activity at the base with maturation toward the surface (Fig. 18.34b, c). Foci of conventional squamous cell carcinoma may arise within the large tumor, and thus extensive sampling of the tumor base is advised to rule this out.
    - Verrucous carcinoma is locally destructive and typically treated with surgical debulking, if possible. The lesions may recur but do not metastasize unless a conventional squamous cell carcinoma arises within the lesion.
    - Giant condyloma of Buschke-Lowenstein was considered synonymous with verrucous carcinoma; however, they are now thought to represent different entities. Importantly, verrucous carcinoma is not associated with HPV and shows exophytic growth and pushing-type invasion, whereas giant condyloma is associated with low-risk HPV and shows exophytic growth only.
    - Please see Chap. 9 for additional discussion on this topic.

    Reference: [1]

32. **How to distinguish in situ from invasive squamous cell carcinoma?**
    - Squamous cell carcinoma in situ implies that there is high-grade dysplasia confined to the basement membrane without invasion.
    - Invasive squamous cell carcinoma is distinguished from in situ lesions by infiltrative nests of tumor cells with angulated or irregular contours, single cells, stromal desmoplasia, and paradoxical maturation with keratinization in the deep component of the tumor. Early superficial invasion can be difficult to diagnose and may only show blurring of the smooth epithelial-stromal interface.
    - In basaloid tumors without overt keratinization, nests of tumor cells in the submucosa that do not connect to the overlying epithelium can be clues to invasion.

33. **What is the significance of p16 positivity in squamous lesions of the anus?**
    - Squamous intraepithelial neoplasia or lesion (AIN) and squamous cell carcinoma of the anus are frequently related to HPV infection. Overexpression of

p16 is a surrogate marker for high-risk HPV infection, indicating viral-related expression of E6 and E7 and inactivation of the Rb protein. In high-grade AIN, diffuse block-like nuclear and cytoplasmic staining of p16 is characteristic.

- Invasive tumors with strong and diffuse p16 positivity may suggest HPV involvement in tumorigenesis (Fig. 18.35a, b), but the staining is not entirely specific for HPV effect.
- Please see Chap. 9 for additional discussion on this topic.

References: [88, 89]

34. How is anorectal squamous cell carcinoma treated compared with adenocarcinoma?

- Invasive anorectal squamous cell carcinoma is typically treated with chemotherapy and radiation, with surgery reserved for cases that do not respond well to the initial therapy.
- Anorectal adenocarcinoma is usually treated with neoadjuvant chemotherapy and radiation, typically followed by surgical resection.
- Given the treatment difference, it is imperative that the diagnosis be accurate. In a poorly differentiated malignancy with no overt gland formation or mucin production to indicate adenocarcinoma, or keratinization to indicate squamous cell carcinoma, immunostains for p40, CK5/6, CK20, CDX2, and SATB2 can be helpful to confirming the tumor type.
- Treated squamous cell carcinoma (including that of the esophagus) may show degenerative changes with space formation within tumor nests, which should not be confused with adenocarcinoma (Fig. 18.36).

References: [90, 91]

35. What is anal canal adenocarcinoma?

- Adenocarcinomas arising from the anal canal including the mucosal surface, fistula, and anal glands are all called anal canal adenocarcinomas. Some are associated with Crohn disease and perianal fistula.
- Most cases appear histologically identical to rectal adenocarcinoma, but primary rectal adenocarcinoma extending into the anus is far more common.

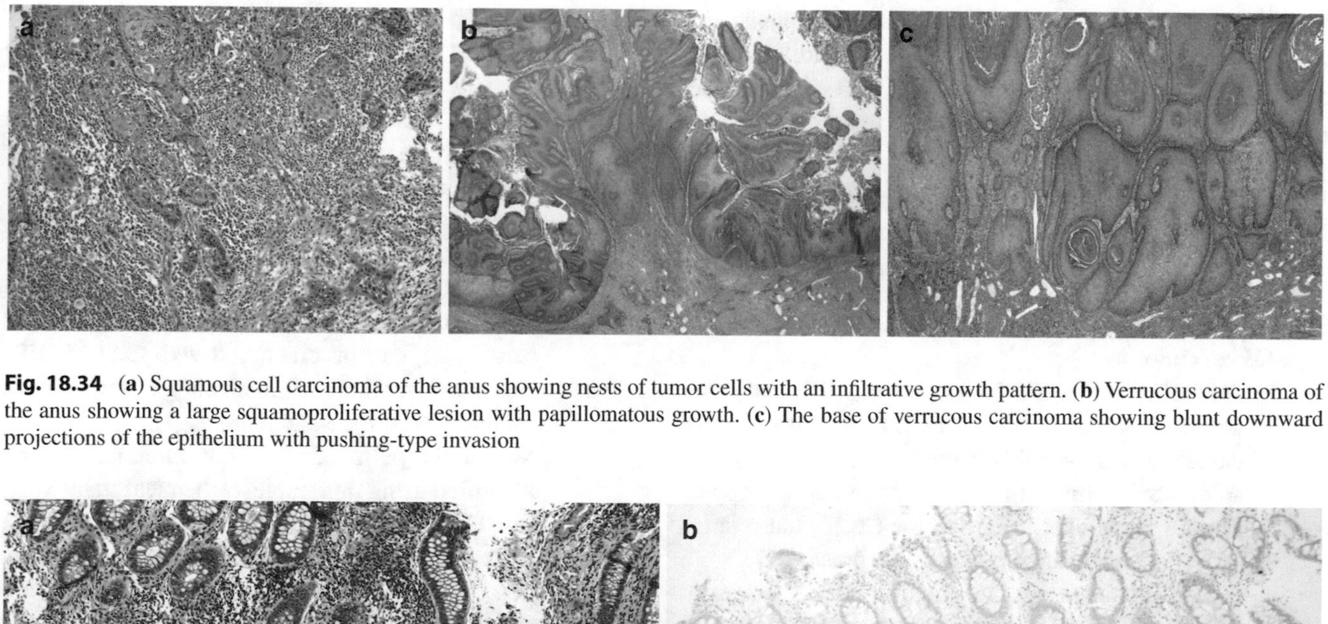

Fig. 18.34 (**a**) Squamous cell carcinoma of the anus showing nests of tumor cells with an infiltrative growth pattern. (**b**) Verrucous carcinoma of the anus showing a large squamoproliferative lesion with papillomatous growth. (**c**) The base of verrucous carcinoma showing blunt downward projections of the epithelium with pushing-type invasion

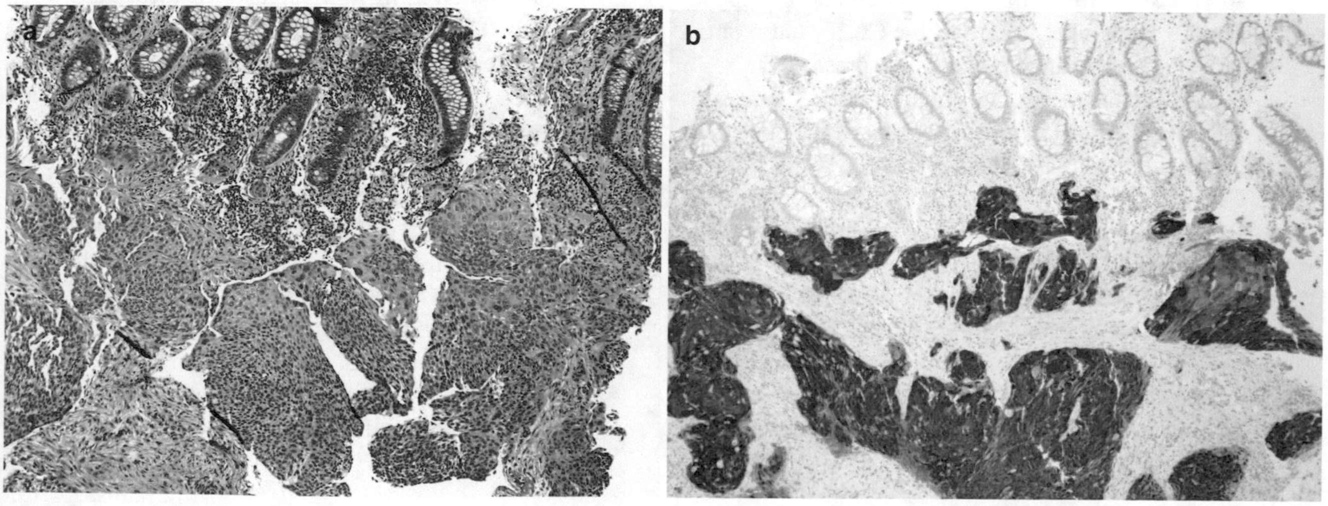

Fig. 18.35 (**a**) A case of invasive squamous cell carcinoma of the anus showing no overt keratinization. (**b**) Immunostaining for p16 shows strong positivity indicating a high probability of HPV involvement in tumorigenesis

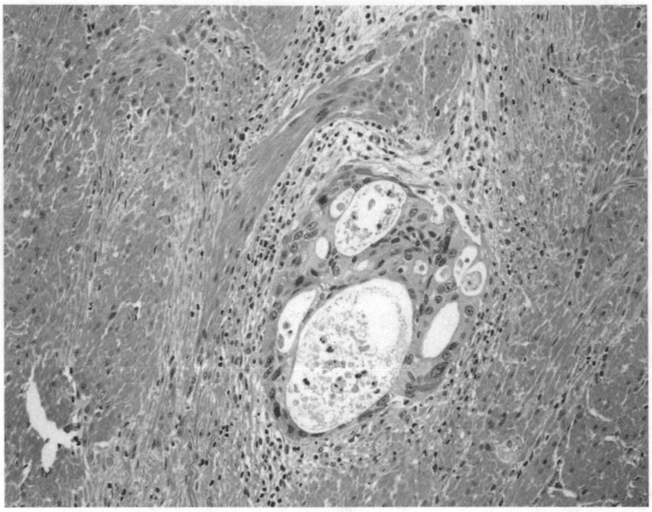

Fig. 18.36 Treated squamous cell carcinoma of the esophagus showing a residual tumor nest with spaces containing necrotic debris, mimicking adenocarcinoma

- The majority of anal canal adenocarcinomas are mucinous tumors immunoreactive for CDX2 and CK20 while being CK7 negative.
- Anal gland carcinoma is a special type of anal canal tumor originating from anal gland epithelium and composed of ductal architecture with scant production of mucin. Tumor cells are immunoreactive for CK7 while being negative for CDX2 and CK20.
- Please see Chap. 9 for additional discussion on this topic.

  References: [92, 93]

36. What are useful immunohistochemical markers for GI carcinomas?

- Adenocarcinomas of the esophagus, GEJ, and stomach are typically positive for CK7. A small subset of cases may also variably express CK20.
- Adenocarcinomas of the colorectum and the appendix are more likely positive for CK20, but a small subset of cases can also variably express CK7.
- Adenocarcinoma of the small intestine expresses CK7 and CK20 at similar frequencies. It can be CK7 positive only, CK20 positive only, or both CK7 and CK20 positive.
- Other markers of intestinal differentiation include CDX2, SATB2, CDH17, and villin. While these markers are more commonly expressed in colorectal and appendiceal adenocarcinomas, they may also be expressed in esophageal, GEJ, gastric, small bowel, and pancreatobiliary adenocarcinomas at lower frequencies. In addition, mucinous lung tumors, ovarian mucinous tumors arising in teratomas, and bladder adenocarcinomas may show expression of these markers.
- Poorly differentiated or undifferentiated adenocarcinomas as well as medullary carcinomas may completely lose the expression of CK7, CK20, and CDX2, but they may remain positive for SATB2 and CDH17.
- Markers of squamous differentiation include high molecular weight CK such as CK5/6. p40 and p63 commonly show positive nuclear staining in squamous cell carcinoma. These markers can be helpful in the distinction between basaloid squamous cell carcinoma and neuroendocrine carcinoma, the latter of which also expresses neuroendocrine markers chromogranin and synaptophysin.

  References: [94–96]

37. What are the common metastatic lesions encountered in the GI tract, and how do you diagnose them?

- Metastatic lesions that can be encountered in the GI tract are wide ranging and can include epithelial malignancies, sarcomas, and melanoma. A detailed patient history is critical to investigating the possibility of metastasis.
- In general, the presence of an in situ or precursor component is histologic evidence that the lesion is primary to that organ. In some cases, metastatic lesions or those with direct spread from an adjacent organ may colonize the nonneoplastic mucosa leading to confusion with a primary in situ lesion.
- Immunohistochemical workup can be helpful in many cases.
  - Metastatic breast carcinoma, including lobular carcinoma, can be diagnosed with GATA3, ER, and other markers of mammary differentiation such as GCDFP-15 and mammaglobin.
  - Metastatic pulmonary adenocarcinoma can be identified using immunohistochemical stains such as TTF-1 and napsin-A.
  - Metastatic gynecologic carcinomas can be identified using PAX8 and ER, while metastatic renal and thyroid tumors will also stain for PAX8.
  - Metastatic prostatic carcinoma can be diagnosed with NKX3.1, PSA, and PAP.
  - Involvement of the GI tract by mesothelioma can be demonstrated by positive stains for calretinin, WT1, CK5/6, and D2–40.
- Benign lesions such as endometriosis may also mimic primary or metastatic carcinoma to the GI tract. The infiltrative-appearing pattern of involvement can closely mimic invasive adenocarcinoma. When

mucosa is involved, it may mimic dysplasia or adenoma on an endoscopic biopsy (Fig. 18.37). Clues to the presence of endometriosis include hemosiderin-laden macrophages and endometrial stroma. Immunostain for CD10 can help highlight the endometrial stroma. PAX8 and ER can help highlight the glandular epithelium in challenging cases.

- Malignant transformation of GI endometriosis into endometrioid adenocarcinoma has been well documented, which can be confused with primary GI adenocarcinomas. In contrast to GI primaries, these tumors mainly involve the serosa and subserosa and invade the visceral wall from the outside. Involvement of the mucosal surface is uncommon. Microscopically, squamous differentiation is more common than primary GI adenocarcinomas. Immunomarkers such as CK7, CK20, CDX2, SATB2, PAX8, ER, PR, and CD10 can help in difficult cases. Rarely, endometrial stromal sarcoma may develop from GI endometriosis.

  References: [94, 97, 98]

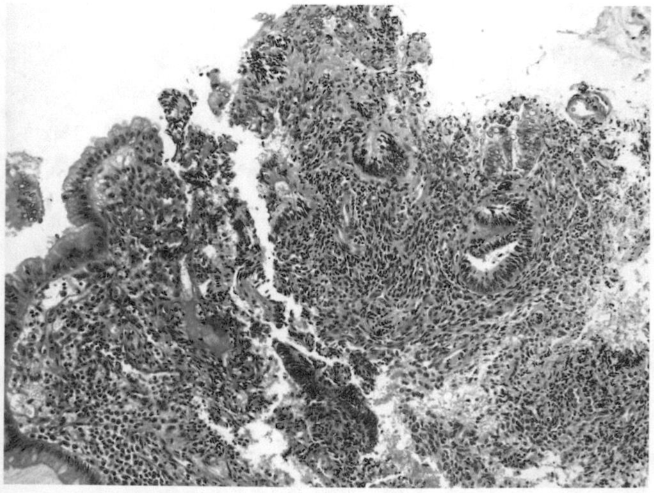

Fig. 18.37 Colonic mucosa involved by endometriosis mimicking adenoma on endoscopic biopsy

38. When to perform and how to report Her2 testing on gastric and GEJ adenocarcinomas?

- In accordance with results of the TOGA trial in 2010, which demonstrated a survival benefit with trastuzumab (Herceptin) compared with chemotherapy alone, reporting of the biomarker Her2/neu status is recommended for certain patients with gastric or GEJ adenocarcinoma. In the setting of locally advanced tumors not amenable to surgical resection, recurrent, or metastatic adenocarcinoma, assessment of the tumor by immunohistochemistry for Her2 protein overexpression and/or fluorescence in situ hybridization (FISH) for *Her2* gene amplification is indicated.
- Many centers perform universal Her2 immunohistochemistry testing on all newly diagnosed gastric and GEJ adenocarcinomas on biopsy specimens. Testing will be performed on a resection specimen if not done so on a prior biopsy.
- The Her2 scoring system is different in this setting than for breast carcinoma and is also different between biopsy and resection specimens (Table 18.7).
- Tumors that show immunohistochemical scores of 0 and 1+ are considered negative for Her2 overexpression, while 3+ is considered positive for overexpression. A tumor with a score of 2+ is considered equivocal and should undergo further testing by FISH for *Her2* gene amplification.
- Her2 is amplified and/or overexpressed in 9–27% of gastric and GEJ adenocarcinomas. It is more commonly detected in intestinal-type than in diffuse-type tumors and is more frequent in well- and moderately differentiated than in poorly differentiated tumors, but exceptions do occur (Fig. 18.38a, b).

  References: [94, 99, 100]

39. What is the current recommendation for MMR deficiency testing and what is the significance of MMR deficiency?

- Universal MMR testing is recommended on all newly diagnosed colorectal adenocarcinomas regardless of patients' age or tumor histology. Patients with evidence of MMR deficiency may have an underlying germline genetic defect (Lynch syndrome).
- Tumors that are MMR deficient have a better stage-adjusted prognosis than those that are MMR proficient. For example, poorly differentiated (including signet-ring cell type) and undifferentiated carcinomas are generally considered to have an aggressive clinical course. However, tumors with MMR deficiency may behave less aggressively. MMR-deficient mucinous carcinoma may also behave less aggressively than its proficient counterpart.
- MMR-deficient tumors may have a poor response to 5-fluorouracil (5-FU)-based chemotherapeutic treatments.
- MMR testing is also performed on adenocarcinomas of the esophagus, GEJ, and stomach as well as any other locations for patients who are selected for possible immune checkpoint inhibitor therapies. Tumors that are MMR deficient have been reported to have increased sensitivity to treatments with immunotherapies such as programmed death receptor-1 (PD-1) blockage.

  References: [4, 94, 101–106]

40. What are the common tests used to evaluate for MMR deficiency?

- Immunohistochemistry for the expression of MMR proteins MLH1, MSH2, MSH6, and PMS2 is most widely used. Loss of nuclear staining for one or more of these proteins is a good marker for MMR deficiency. It has the following advantages: easy performance on small biopsy specimens, fast turnaround time, and identification of a MMR gene that may need to be further sequenced based on the staining pattern.
- Polymerase chain reaction (PCR) assay for MSI is another method. Changes in the length of microsatellites (short tandem nucleotide repeats) with a PCR result of MSI-high are indication of MMR deficiency.
- Next-generation sequencing (NGS) assays can evaluate numerous microsatellite repeats and provide an excellent determination of MSI. NGS can also measure the overall tumor mutation burden, which is usually elevated in tumors with MMR deficiency. Tumor mutation burden may also be elevated in tumors with polymerase epsilon or delta mutations.
- Studies have shown that immunohistochemistry and PCR results correlate well in detecting MMR deficiency, but each technique may miss a small number (5–10%) of cases and may show discordant results. The current recommendation is to use immunohistochemistry and/or PCR analysis as screening tests for Lynch syndrome.
  References: [107–111]

Table 18.7 Interpretation of Her2 immunohistochemistry on gastric and GEJ adenocarcinomas

Score	Biopsy	Resection	Interpretation
0	No reactivity or no membranous reactivity in any cancer cell	No reactivity or membranous reactivity in <10% of cancer cells	Negative
1+	Cancer cell cluster (≥5 neoplastic cells) with a faint or barely perceptible membranous reactivity irrespective of percentage of cancer cells positive	Faint or barely perceptible membranous reactivity in ≥10% of cancer cells; cells are reactive only in part of their membrane	Negative
2+	Cancer cell cluster (≥5 neoplastic cells) with a weak to moderate complete, basolateral, or lateral membranous reactivity irrespective of percentage of cancer cells positive	Weak to moderate complete, basolateral, or lateral membranous reactivity in ≥10% of tumor cells	Equivocal Her2 FISH to be performed
3+	Cancer cell cluster (≥5 neoplastic cells) with a strong complete, basolateral, or lateral membranous reactivity irrespective of percentage of cancer cells positive	Strong complete, basolateral, or lateral membranous reactivity in ≥10% of cancer cells	Positive

41. How are MMR immunostains interpreted?

- Functionally, MMR proteins act as heterodimers, with MLH1 pairing with PMS2 and MSH2 pairing with MSH6. MLH1 and MSH2 are obligate binding partners, such that abnormalities in either one of these proteins will result in loss of its respective secondary partner. As a result, loss of MLH1 protein is almost always accompanied by loss of PMS2; loss of MSH2 protein is almost always accompanied by loss of MSH6. In contrast, loss of PMS2 or MSH6 protein alone usually results from isolated mutations of the

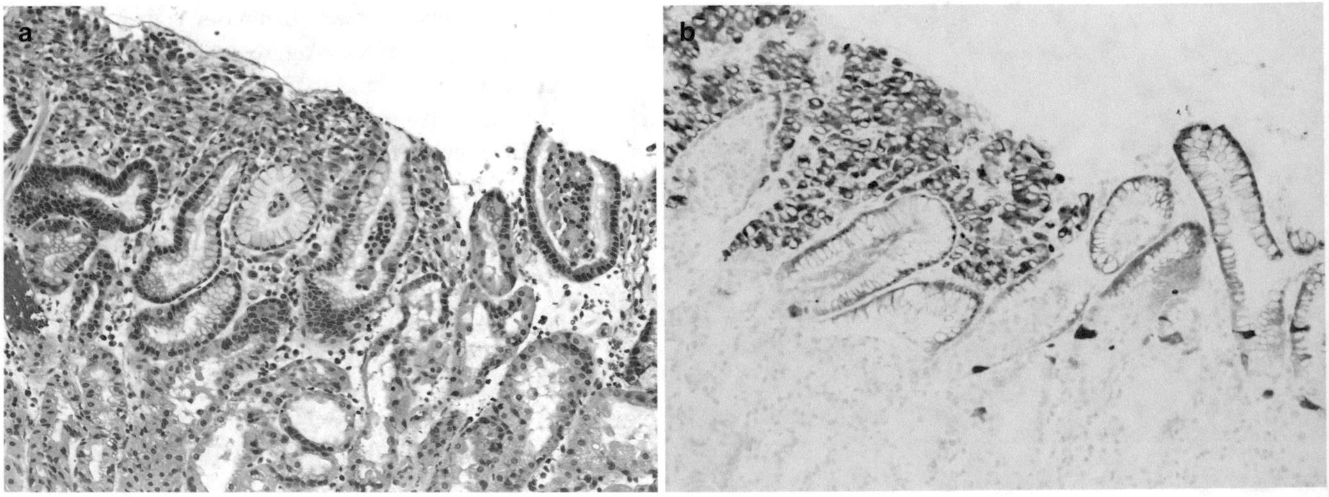

Fig. 18.38 An example of poorly cohesive (signet-ring cell) carcinoma of the stomach (**a**) showing Her2 overexpression (score 3+) by immunohistochemistry (**b**)

PMS2 or *MSH6* gene, which does not affect MLH1 or MSH2 protein expression.

- When MMR proteins are examined by immunohistochemistry, background inflammatory cells, stromal cells, and nonneoplastic epithelial cells should show positive nuclear staining, which serves as an internal control.
- Current understanding is that any positive staining in the nuclei of tumor cells should be considered intact (normal) expression. Patchy distribution of positive nuclear staining is not an uncommon finding, and thus patchy loss of nuclear expression in tumor cells is still considered intact expression. An interpretation of loss of expression should be made only if no nuclear staining is seen in all tumor cells and a positive reaction is present in internal control cells.
  - A recent study used 10% as a cutoff and considered staining in <10% of tumor cells as indeterminate. The authors found that 16 of 479 (3.3%) of their cancer cases showed an indeterminate pattern and that 8 of 13 (61.5%) tested indeterminate cases had MMR germline mutations. Therefore, an indeterminate staining result may need further investigation for possible Lynch syndrome.
- Detailed assessment of MMR immunohistochemical patterns and recommendations for further investigation are summarized in Table 18.8.

  References: [94, 107, 112]

42. What are some pitfalls in the interpretation of MMR protein immunohistochemical testing?

- False-negative testing, in which the nuclear expression of MMR proteins is intact but an underlying MMR mutation is present, can occur. If the clinical index of suspicion for Lynch syndrome or acquired MMR deficiency is high enough, alternative testing, such as PCR for MSI or germline testing, may be considered. In fact, if the patient is younger than 50 years, genetic evaluation is recommended regardless of test results.
- Technical problems with the immunohistochemical staining procedure, or a lack of maintained antigenicity within the tissue, may lead to the incorrect interpretation of loss of expression. It is important to evaluate the staining of tumor cell nuclei in areas with intact internal control staining of nonneoplastic cells.
- Although staining variation within a tumor is common, positively and negatively stained tumor cells are usually intermingled. If completely negative staining is seen in a large area of tumor cells sharply demarcated from surrounding heterogeneous areas, MSI PCR should be performed, which may demonstrate MSI-high.
- Altered MMR protein expression results may be seen after neoadjuvant chemotherapy and/or radiation therapy, especially loss of MSH6 immunoreactivity (Fig. 18.39a–c). In those situations, evaluation of pretreatment biopsy specimens should be helpful before proceeding to further genetic workup. MSI PCR is another helpful option. A nucleolar-only staining pattern can also be observed, particularly for MLH1 and MSH6. This should be interpreted as loss of expression. Nucleolar pattern can also be occasionally seen in untreated colorectal adenocarcinoma in our experience (Fig. 18.40a–c).
- Immunohistochemistry may be performed on colorectal adenomas if cancer tissue is not available. However, negative results should not be used to exclude the possibility of Lynch syndrome because of lower sensitivity comparing to cancer tissue samples.
- Data have shown that the results derived from primary tumors match those of metastatic diseases. Thus, metastatic lesions can be used for analysis if primary tumors are not available.

  References: [107, 113, 114]

43. When an abnormal MMR protein test result is seen, what are the next steps taken to determine the significance of the findings?

- General recommendations following immunohistochemical testing of MMR proteins are summarized in Table 18.8.
- Loss of nuclear expression of MLH1 and PMS2 is the most common abnormal staining pattern observed in tumors. This may be due to an underlying germline mutation of the *MLH1* gene, but more commonly it is a sporadic event due to acquired hypermethylation of the *MLH1* promoter that silences its expression. *MLH1* promoter methylation assay and/or *BRAF* mutation analysis should be performed for those cases. If either is positive, the tumor is likely sporadic rather than the result of an inherited condition. Negative results indicate likely Lynch syndrome. Genetic testing may be undertaken to assess for germline *MLH1* mutations.
- *BRAF* mutation testing is chosen over methylation analysis in most centers because of its availability. Tumor DNA used for *BRAF* testing can also be further used for mutation analysis of other genes such as *KRAS*, *NRAS*, *PIK3CA*, and *AKT1*. In many centers, *BRAF* is one of the molecular panel members that include all these genes for colorectal carcinomas.
- Immunohistochemistry using a specific antibody (VE1) to detect *BRAF* V600E mutant is available, but its reliability in clinical practice has been contro-

Table 18.8 Immunostaining patterns of MMR proteins, interpretation, and recommendations

Pattern				Interpretation	Recommendations
MHL1	MSH2	MSH6	PMS2		
+	+	+	+	1. Sporadic cancer 2. Non-LS hereditary CRC	1. None 2. MSI PCR or other genetic testing if indicated by clinical and/or family history
–	+	+	–	1. Sporadic CRC with *MLH1* promoter hypermethylation 2. LS with *MLH1* germline mutation 3. Rarely, LS with *PMS2* germline mutation	1. *BRAF* mutation and/or *MLH1* methylation testing 2. Germline testing for *MLH1* and/or *PMS2* if the above tests are negative 3. Consider somatic MMR genetic testing if above tests are negative
+	–	–	+	1. LS with *MSH2* germline mutation 2. LS with *EPCAM* germline mutation[a] 3. Rarely, LS with *MSH6* germline mutation 4. Sporadic CRC	1. Germline testing for *MSH2* 2. Germline testing for *EPCAM* if the above test is negative 3. Germline testing for *MSH6* if the above tests are negative 4. Consider somatic MMR genetic testing if germline tests are negative
+	+	+	–	1. LS with *PMS2* germline mutation 2. Rarely, LS with *MLH1* germline mutation 3. Sporadic CRC	1. Germline testing for *PMS2* 2. Germline testing for *MLH1* if the above test is negative 3. Consider somatic MMR genetic testing if germline tests are negative
+	–	+	+	1. LS with *MSH2* germline mutation 2. LS with *EPCAM* germline mutation 3. Sporadic CRC	1. Germline testing for *MSH2* 2. Germline testing for *EPCAM* if the above test is negative 3. Consider somatic MMR genetic testing if germline tests are negative
+	+	–	+	1. LS with *MSH6* germline mutation 2. Rarely, LS with *MSH2* germline mutation 3. Sporadic CRC 4. Treatment effect	1. Repeat IHC in nontreated tumor if possible 2. Germline testing for *MSH6* 3. Germline testing for *MSH2* if the above test is negative 4. MSI PCR 5. Consider somatic MMR genetic testing if germline tests are negative
–	+	+	+	1. Sporadic CRC 2. LS with *MLH1* germline mutation 3. Rarely, LS with *PMS2* germline mutation	1. *BRAF* mutation and/or *MLH1* methylation 2. Germline testing for *MLH1* if the above tests are negative 3. Germline testing for *PMS2* if the above tests are negative 4. Consider somatic MMR genetic testing if germline tests are negative
–	–	–	–	1. Germline mutation in any MMR gene 2. *MSH2* germline mutation with concurrent *MLH1* promoter hypermethylation 3. Sporadic CRC	1. Germline testing for all four MMR genes 2. *BRAF* mutation and/or *MLH1* methylation if germline test for *MLH1* gene is negative 3. Consider somatic MMR genetic testing if germline tests are negative

CRC colorectal cancer, *LS* lynch syndrome, *MSI* microsatellite instability, *IHC* immunohistochemistry, + intact nuclear expression, – loss of nuclear expression

[a]*EPCAM* (epithelial cell adhesion molecule) is a gene located just upstream from the *MSH2* gene. Deletions of the terminal codon of the *EPCAM* gene result in silencing of the *MSH2* gene, leading to a phenotype very similar to Lynch syndrome

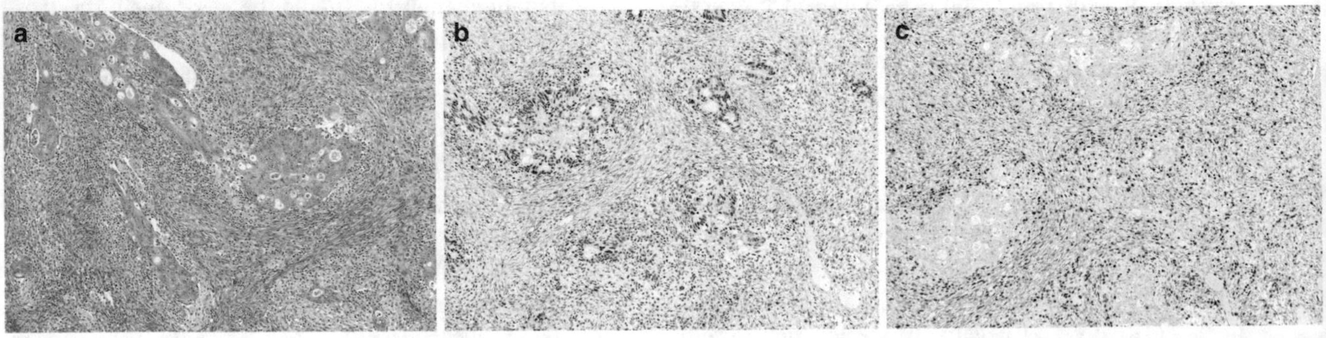

Fig. 18.39 This rectal adenocarcinoma was treated with neoadjuvant chemoradiation therapy prior to resection. Immunostains performed on the residual carcinoma (**a**) show intact nuclear expression of MLH1, PMS2, and MSH2 (**b**), with isolated loss of MSH6 (**c**). The tumor had the same markers performed on the original biopsy specimen which showed intact nuclear expression of all of these proteins, leading to the conclusion that the loss of MSH6 was related to therapeutic effect

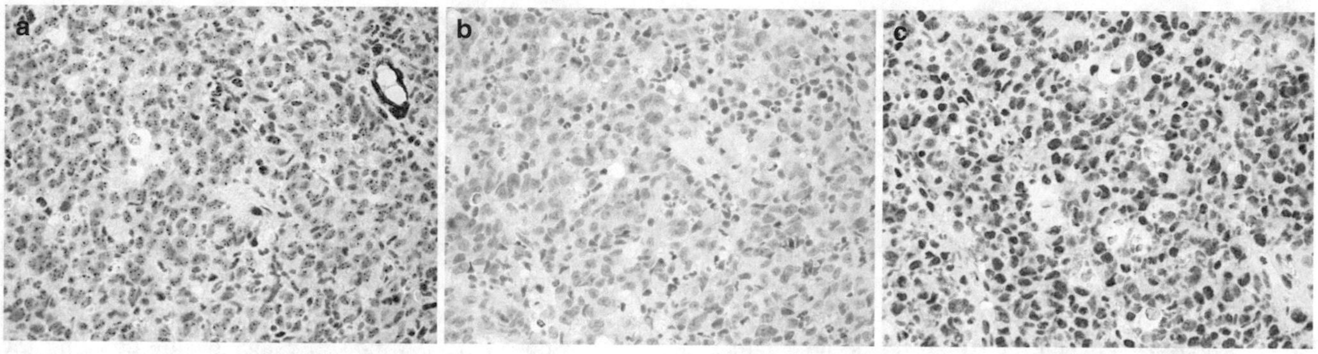

Fig. 18.40 An untreated ascending colon adenocarcinoma biopsied from a 47-year-old man showing a speckled nucleolar staining pattern for MLH1 (**a**), loss of PMS2 expression (**b**), and intact MSH2 and MSH6 nuclear expression (**c**). No mutations were detected in the *BRAF* gene. The patient was diagnosed with Lynch syndrome as confirmed by demonstration of germline mutation in the *MLH1* gene

versial. It is not currently recommended to replace DNA testing due to low sensitivity and discordant results. However, it may be an option in situation where there is not enough tumor tissue for DNA testing.

- Loss of nuclear expression of both MSH2 and MSH6, isolated loss of MSH6, and isolated loss of PMS2 are suggestive of underlying germline mutations (Lynch syndrome), and genetic testing is likely indicated.
References: [94, 107, 115]

44. What colorectal tumor morphologic subtypes are likely to be associated with MMR deficiency?

- MMR deficiency may be associated with signet-ring cell carcinoma, mucinous carcinoma, and medullary carcinoma. Medullary carcinoma is almost invariably MMR deficient, whereas only a subset of signet-ring cell and mucinous cancers are MMR deficient.
- The morphologic appearance of MMR-deficient tumors is highly variable. These tumors may have a heterogeneous appearance, poor differentiation, and/or prominent lymphoid infiltration along the periphery of the tumor (Crohn-like lymphoid reaction) and within the tumor including tumor-infiltrating lymphocytes (Fig. 18.41).
- As discussed in Question 39, most laboratories now screen all colorectal tumors (and endometrial cancers) for MMR deficiency, regardless of patient demographics or morphologic features. If clinically required, such as for potential immunotherapy, MMR testing may also be performed on tumors arising from other GI and extra-GI sites.
References: [13, 116, 117]

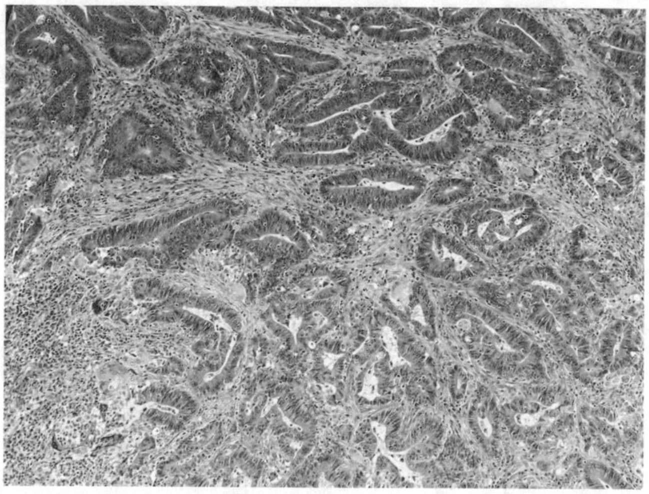

Fig. 18.41 Tumor-infiltrating lymphocytes is a histologic feature that can be associated with MMR deficiency

45. What molecular tests may be performed on metastatic (stage IV) colorectal adenocarcinoma?

- Molecular testing may be indicated in patients with metastatic colorectal adenocarcinoma to identify appropriate chemotherapeutic regimens.
- Treatments involving epidermal growth factor receptor (EGFR)-targeted therapies may not be indicated in patients with mutations in *KRAS* or *NRAS*. Detection of mutations in codons 12, 13, 59, 61, 117, and 146 of both genes (extended RAS testing) has been associated with a lack of responsiveness to the drugs as these mutations activate signaling pathways downstream of EGFR.
- *BRAF* V600E mutations in MMR-proficient tumors have been associated with a poor prognosis regardless of whether or not anti-EGFR therapy is employed.
- In many centers, *KRAS* mutations are universally tested for all stage IV colorectal adenocarcinomas. If it is wild type, reflex testing for mutations of the *NRAS*, *BRAF*, *PIK3CA*, and *AKT1* genes will be performed.
References: [118–121]

46. What is the role of Her2 testing in colorectal adenocarcinoma?

- The Her2 pathway has been identified as important in some colorectal adenocarcinomas that develop resistance to EGFR-targeted therapies.
- Tumors that have wild-type *BRAF* and *RAS* genes may show enhancement in amplification of the *Her2* gene.
- Early studies have shown a role for anti-Her2 therapy in patients with *Her2*-amplified tumors, but further studies are needed before Her2 is routinely tested as a biomarker and potential therapeutic target in colorectal adenocarcinoma.
- By IHC, intense (3+) circumferential, basolateral or lateral membrane staining in ≥50% of tumor cells is considered positive. Intense staining in >10% but <50% of tumor cells is also considered positive, but FISH for Her2 amplification is recommended. Moderate (2+) staining in ≥50% of tumor cells is considered equivocal, which should be followed by FISH test. No staining, faint staining (1+) in any cellularity, moderate staining in <50% of tumor cells and intense staining in ≤10% of tumor cells are all considered negative.
  References: [122, 123, 124]

47. What is the significance of PIK3CA mutations in colorectal adenocarcinoma?

- *PIK3CA* mutations can lead to activation of the AKT pathway and may play a role in colorectal carcinogenesis. Mutations have also been shown to be associated with poor survival and resistance to anti-EGFR therapy in some studies. *PIK3CA* mutations can co-occur with *KRAS* or *BRAF* mutations, but the adverse effect appears to be limited to tumors with wild-type *KRAS*.
  Reference: [125, 126]

48. What is the significance of PTEN expression in colorectal adenocarcinoma?

- Loss of PTEN expression by immunohistochemistry has been associated with lack of benefit from EGFR-targeted therapies in metastatic colorectal cancer. It is also associated with decreased progression-free and overall survival rates in patients with colorectal adenocarcinoma. Loss of PTEN has been found to co-occur with *KRAS*, *BRAF*, and *PIK3CA* mutations.
- PTEN expression by immunohistochemistry as a clinical biomarker is not standardized and is not commonly utilized at this point in time.
  References: [126, 127]

49. How to report programmed death-ligand 1 (PD-L1) immunostaining results?

- PD-L1 is a biomarker that by immunohistochemistry can aid in identifying tumors that are likely to respond to anti-PD-1 and anti-PD-L1 therapies.
- Assays and interpretation of results vary based on the tumor type and by the inhibitor being considered for treatment.
- For gastric and GEJ adenocarcinomas, an FDA-approved PD-L1 immunohistochemical assay using the 22C3 antibody (PD-L1 IHC 22C3 pharmDx) is utilized to help identify patients who may benefit from treatment with Keytruda (pembrolizumab), a humanized monoclonal PD-1 blocking antibody. The staining results are reported using Combined Positive Score (CPS), which is calculated by counting the total number of PD-L1 stained tumor cells and mononuclear inflammatory cells (lymphocytes and macrophages) divided by the total number of viable tumor cells (stained and non-stained), multiplied by 100.
  - CPS <1: No PD-L1 expression
  - CPS ≥1: PD-L1 expression
- For specimen to be considered adequate for PD-L1 evaluation, a minimum of 100 viable tumor cells must be present in PD-L1 stained slide.
- For viable tumor cells, any convincing partial or complete linear membranous staining at any intensity (≥weak) that is perceived as distinct from cytoplasmic staining is considered positive and should be included for CPS (Fig. 18.42). Tumor cells with cytoplasmic staining only are considered negative. Adenoma, dysplasia, or carcinoma in situ should not be evaluated.
- For mononuclear inflammatory cells, only the cells within tumor nests and/or in adjacent supporting stroma (directly associated with the response against tumor) are evaluated. These also include lymphoid aggregates. Any convincing membranous and/or

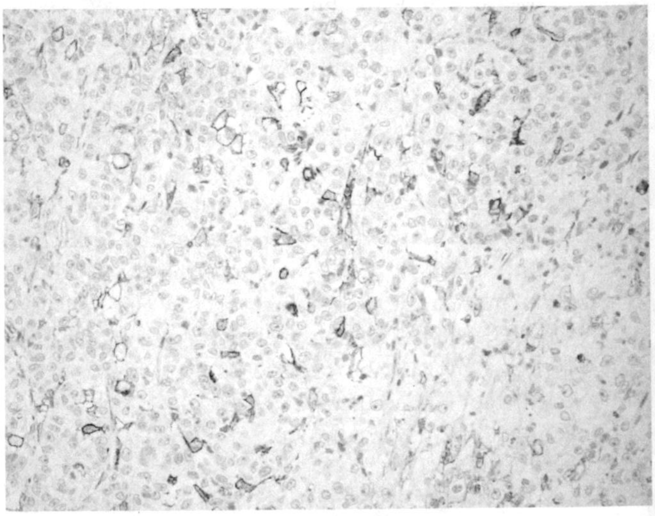

Fig. 18.42 PD-L1 immunostaining using the 22C3 antibody performed on a poorly differentiated gastric adenocarcinoma showing convincing membranous staining in tumor cells and occasional mononuclear inflammatory cells, with a CPS of ~25 (>1)

cytoplasmic staining at any intensity in these cells is considered positive and should be included for CPS.
- PD-L1 protein expression in some non-GI tumors (such as non-small cell lung cancer) is reported using Tumor Proportion Score (TPS), which is the percentage of viable tumor cells that show partial or complete membranous staining at any intensity. PD-L1 is considered expressed if TPS ≥1% and high expression if ≥50%.

Case Presentation

Case 1

Learning Objectives

1. To learn to evaluate the histologic features of gastric adenocarcinoma
2. To refine diagnosis with consideration of differential diagnosis
3. To recognize clinical implications of the diagnosis and to recommend appropriate testing

Case History

A 33-year-old female, status post renal transplantation, presented with a 4-month history of abdominal pain.

Endoscopy

Gastritis with a focal area of abnormal mucosa. A biopsy was performed.

Histologic Findings

The biopsy consisted of oxyntic mucosa that showed a superficial area of architectural disruption by neoplastic cells (Fig. 18.43a). The cells had expanded mucinous cytoplasm with a "signet-ring cell" morphology (Fig. 18.43b).

Differential Diagnosis

- Adenocarcinoma of gastric primary, diffuse type
- Metastatic adenocarcinoma

Immunohistochemistry

- CK7 positive.
- GATA3 and ER negative.

Final Diagnosis

Adenocarcinoma of gastric primary, diffuse type with signet-ring cells.

Take-Home Messages

- Adenocarcinoma of the stomach may be primary or represent metastatic disease.
- Differentials for a poorly differentiated adenocarcinoma in a female patient should always include lobular carcinoma from the breast.
- In a young patient, diffuse-type adenocarcinoma raises the possibility of hereditary diffuse gastric cancer, and genetic counseling should be advised. This patient had a germline mutation in *CDH1* gene and a strong family history of gastric cancer.

References: [47–50]

Case 2

Learning Objectives

1. To learn to evaluate histologic features of carcinoma in the stomach
2. To utilize histologic and immunohistochemical features to generate differential diagnosis
3. To understand the differing treatment considerations in a patient with a tumor of the stomach

Case History

A 47-year-old female with no significant past medical history presented with upper abdominal pain of recent onset. The patient had lost weight and was anemic.

Endoscopy

A 1.5 cm ulcer with oozing was seen in the body of the stomach. A biopsy was performed.

Histologic Findings

The biopsy showed neoplastic proliferation with small clusters of or single discohesive tumor cells infiltrating the gastric mucosa (Fig. 18.44a).

Differential Diagnosis

- Diffuse-type adenocarcinoma of gastric primary, hereditary or sporadic
- Metastatic carcinoma

Immunohistochemistry

- CK7 positive.
- GATA3 and ER positive (Fig. 18.44b).

Final Diagnosis

Metastatic adenocarcinoma of breast origin.

Take-Home Messages

- When diffuse-type adenocarcinoma is found in the stomach of a young person, consideration should be given to the possibility of hereditary diffuse-type gastric cancer resulting from germline *CDH1* mutations.
- Diffuse-type gastric adenocarcinoma in a female should also raise the possibility of an occult metastatic breast carcinoma. Immunohistochemical studies may need to be performed to rule out that possibility.

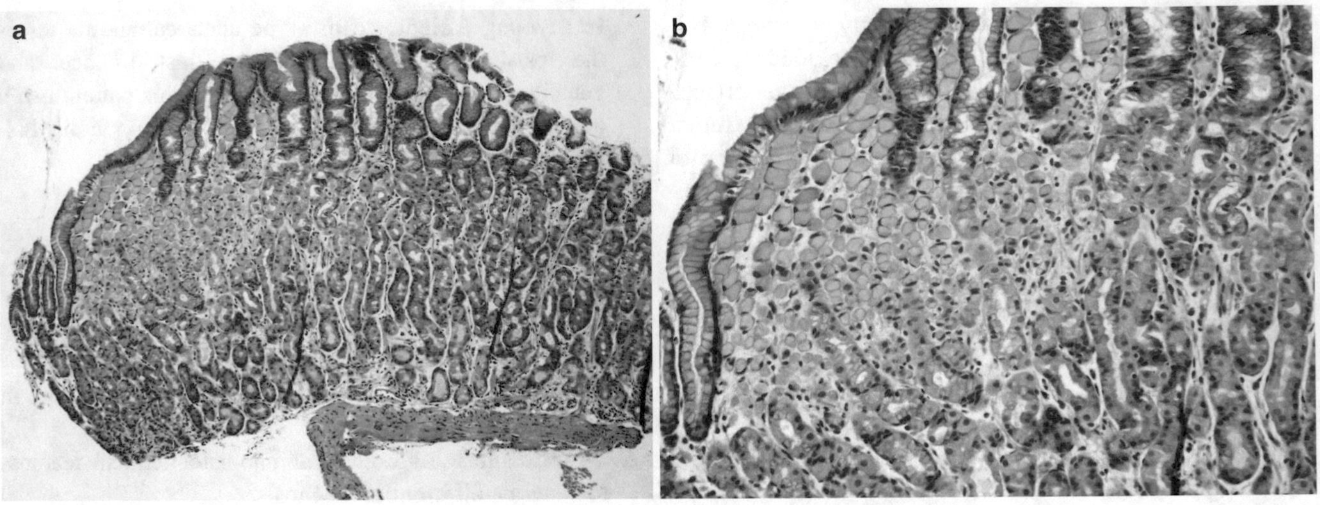

Fig. 18.43 (Case 1) Oxyntic mucosa with focal disruption by a cluster of neoplastic cells (**a**) showing a "signet-ring cell" morphology (**b**)

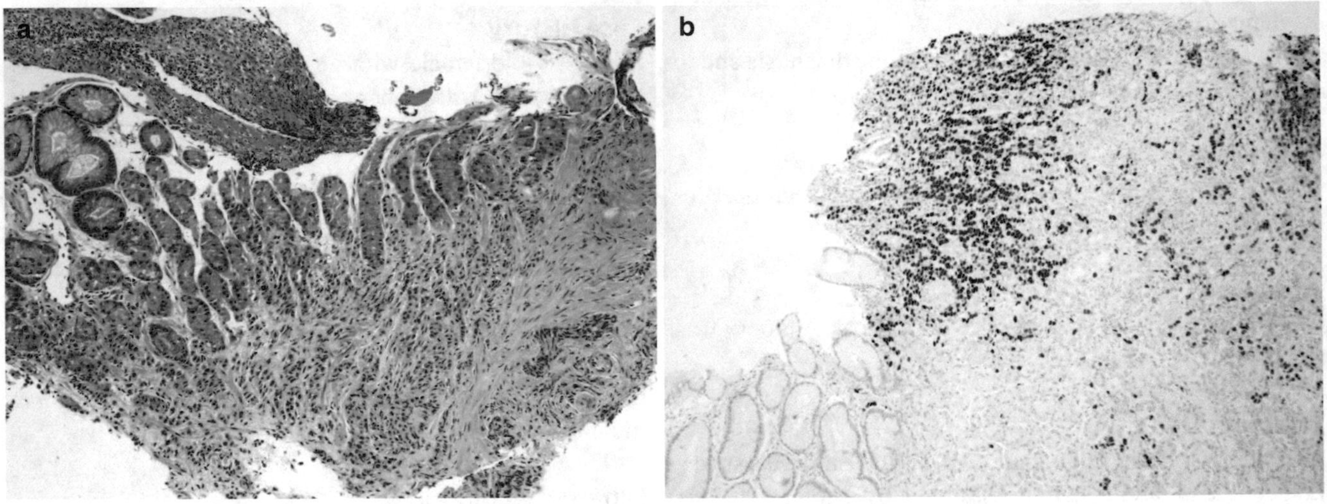

Fig. 18.44 (Case 2) (**a**) Ulcerated gastric mucosa showing involvement by a poorly differentiated malignant process. No definitive gland formation or mucin production was evident. (**b**) ER immunostain was strongly positive in the tumor cells, supportive of metastatic breast carcinoma

- Markers for confirmation of a gastric primary tumor are not specific, but GATA3, ER, GCDFP15, and mammaglobin can be helpful to evaluate for the possibility of metastatic breast carcinoma.
  References: [49, 50]

Case 3

Learning Objectives

1. To become familiar with features suggestive of metastasis to the GI tract
2. To learn about metastatic disease workup in a GI biopsy

Case History

A 63-year-old female presented with duodenal obstruction.

Endoscopy

A large fungating and ulcerated mass with no bleeding was found in the duodenum.

Histologic Findings

The biopsy showed large sheets of poorly differentiated epithelioid neoplasm. Tumor cells had large round nuclei, prominent nucleoli, and modest amounts of amphophilic cytoplasm (Fig. 18.45a, b). Poorly formed glandular structures and hemorrhage were focally seen (Fig. 18.45c).

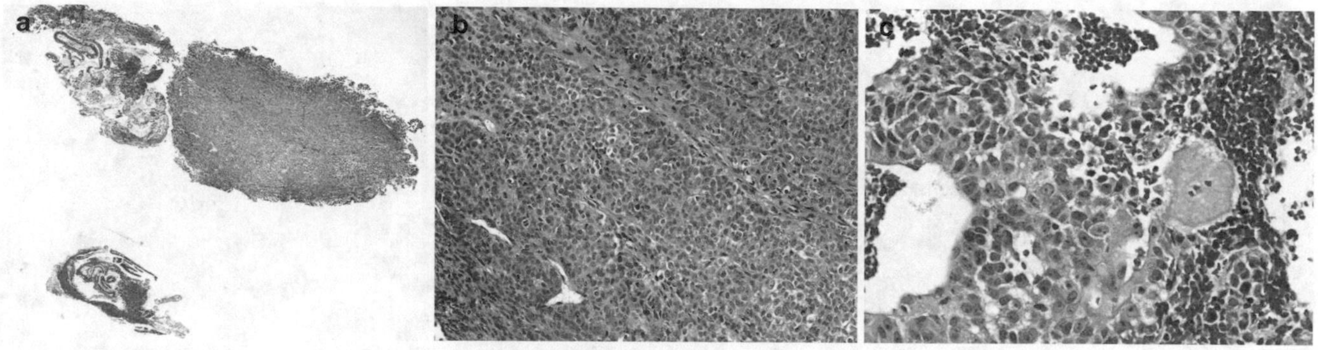

Fig. 18.45 (Case 3) (**a**) Duodenal biopsy at low magnification showing sheets of poorly differentiated tumor replacing duodenal mucosa. (**b**) Tumor cells had large round nuclei, prominent nucleoli, and modest amounts of amphophilic cytoplasm. Mitotic figures were readily identified. (**c**) Focal gland formation and background hemorrhage were seen

Differential Diagnosis

- Poorly differentiated carcinoma, primary vs. metastatic
- Lymphoma
- Metastatic melanoma

IHC and Other Ancillary Studies

- AE1/3, CK7, and PAX8 positive.
- CK20, CDX2, GATA3, S100, and CD45 negative.
- Loss of nuclear expression for MLH1 and PMS2 with intact nuclear expression of MSH2 and MSH6.
- Positive for *MLH1* promotor hypermethylation.

Additional Clinical Information

History of high-grade endometrioid carcinoma, status post hysterectomy, and bilateral salpingo-oophorectomy.

Final Diagnosis

Metastatic endometrial carcinoma.

Take-Home Messages

- Metastasis is very likely given the small intestinal location because primary adenocarcinoma of the small intestine is rare.
- Absence of precursor adenomatous change in non-ulcerated surface mucosa should raise the suspicion for metastasis.
- Endometrial carcinomas can show glandular formation and MMR deficiency, similarly to intestinal adenocarcinomas.
- Clinical history and immunohistochemistry can be helpful in difficult cases.
- Endometrial cancers can also arise within foci of endometriosis involving the GI tract.

  References: [98, 128–130]

Case 4

Learning Objectives

1. To become familiar with screening biopsies performed during surveillance colonoscopy for inflammatory bowel disease patient
2. To learn how to recognize features worrisome for carcinoma

Case History

A 36-year-old female with a clinical history of ulcerative colitis and primary sclerosing cholangitis, status post liver transplant.

Colonoscopy

Altered vascular, erythematous, and granular mucosa in the entire examined colon. One 20 mm polyp was found at 60 cm proximal to the anal verge, which was biopsied.

Histologic Findings

The biopsy from the 20 mm colonic polyp showed glandular structures with irregular contours and a haphazard arrangement. The epithelial cells lining the glandular structures were tall columnar and exhibited only mild cytologic atypia. There was a lack of maturation from bottom to top of the biopsy. The intervening stroma had prominent inflammatory cell infiltrates but no definitive desmoplasia (Fig. 18.46a, b).

Differential Diagnosis

- Inflammatory polyp with reactive changes
- Polypoid dysplasia or tubular adenoma
- Invasive well-differentiated adenocarcinoma

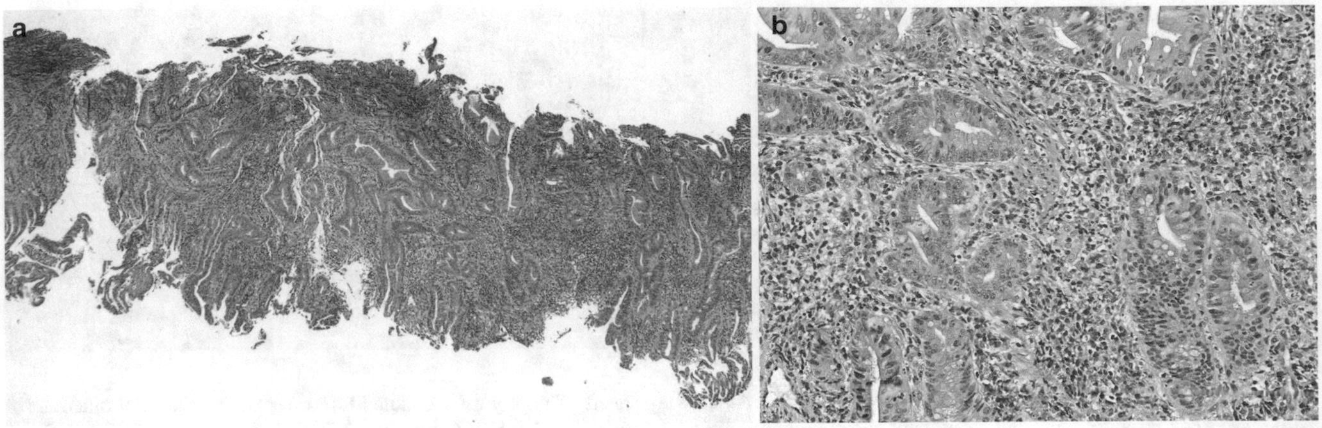

Fig. 18.46 (Case 4) (**a**) At low magnification, the biopsy of colonic polyp showed irregular glandular structures arranged in a haphazard fashion without maturation toward the surface. (**b**) The intervening stroma contained numerous inflammatory cells and twigs of smooth muscle but showed no definitive desmoplasia. The proliferating glands exhibited only mild cytologic atypia

Ancillary Studies

- Deeper sections were examined, which showed similar findings.

Follow-Up

Given the glandular complexity and irregularity, a concern for invasive adenocarcinoma was raised, and rebiopsy was recommended. The patient underwent another colonoscopy, but repeat biopsy was also not definitive. Subsequent total colectomy revealed invasive well-differentiated adenocarcinoma invading through the muscularis propria and into pericolic fibroadipose tissue.

Final Diagnosis

Invasive well-differentiated adenocarcinoma.

Take-Home Messages

- Glandular proliferation without maturation arranged in a haphazard fashion should raise concern for a neoplastic process.
- Well-differentiated adenocarcinoma (such as low-grade tubuloglandular adenocarcinoma in the setting of inflammatory bowel disease) may show very little cytologic atypia and lack obvious desmoplasia, which can be very difficult to diagnose on a biopsy.
  References: [3, 131]

References

1. WHO Classification of Tumours Editorial Board. Digestive system tumours. 5th ed. Lyon, France: International Agency for Research on Cancer; 2019.
2. Ushiku T, Arnason T, Ban S, Hishima T, Shimizu M, Fukayama M, Lauwers GY. Very well-differentiated gastric carcinoma of intestinal type: analysis of diagnostic criteria. Mod Pathol. 2013;26(12):1620–31.
3. Levi GS, Harpaz N. Intestinal low-grade tubuloglandular adenocarcinoma in inflammatory bowel disease. Am J Surg Pathol. 2006;30(8):1022–9.
4. Leopoldo S, Lorena B, Cinzia A, Gabriella DC, Angela Luciana B, Renato C, Antonio M, Carlo S, Cristina P, Stefano C, Maurizio T, Luigi R, Cesare B. Two subtypes of mucinous adenocarcinoma of the colorectum: clinicopathological and genetic features. Ann Surg Oncol. 2008;15(5):1429–39.
5. Andrici J, Farzin M, Sioson L, Clarkson A, Watson N, Toon CW, Gill AJ. Mismatch repair deficiency as a prognostic factor in mucinous colorectal cancer. Mod Pathol. 2016;29(3):266–74.
6. Asare EA, Compton CC, Hanna NN, Kosinski LA, Washington MK, Kakar S, Weiser MR, Overman MJ. The impact of stage, grade, and mucinous histology on the efficacy of systemic chemotherapy in adenocarcinomas of the appendix: analysis of the National Cancer Data Base. Cancer. 2016;122(2):213–21.
7. Amin MB, editor. AJCC Cancer staging manual. 8th ed. Switzerland: Springer International Publishing, American Joint Commission on Cancer; 2017.
8. Wang HB, Liao XF, Zhang J. Clinicopathological factors associated with HER2-positive gastric cancer: a meta-analysis. Medicine (Baltimore). 2017;96(44):e8437.
9. Ahn JY, Jung HY, Choi KD, Choi JY, Kim MY, Lee JH, Choi KS, Kim DH, Song HJ, Lee GH, Kim JH, Park YS. Endoscopic and oncologic outcomes after endoscopic resection for early gastric cancer: 1370 cases of absolute and extended indications. Gastrointest Endosc. 2011;74(3):485–93.
10. Soetikno R, Kaltenbach T, Yeh R, Gotoda T. Endoscopic mucosal resection for early cancers of the upper gastrointestinal tract. J Clin Oncol. 2005;23(20):4490–8.
11. Lewin MR, Fenton H, Burkart AL, Sheridan T, Abu-Alfa AK, Montgomery EA. Poorly differentiated colorectal carcinoma with invasion restricted to lamina propria (intramucosal carcinoma): a follow-up study of 15 cases. Am J Surg Pathol. 2007;31(12):1882–6.
12. Schlemper RJ, Riddell RH, Kato Y, Borchard F, Cooper HS, Dawsey SM, Dixon MF, Fenoglio-Preiser CM, Fléjou JF, Geboes K, Hattori T, Hirota T, Itabashi M, Iwafuchi M, Iwashita A, Kim YI, Kirchner T, Klimpfinger M, Koike M, Lauwers GY, Lewin KJ, Oberhuber G, Offner F, Price AB, Rubio CA, Shimizu M, Shimoda T, Sipponen P, Solcia E, Stolte M, Watanabe H, Yamabe H. The Vienna classification of gastrointestinal epithelial neoplasia. Gut. 2000;47(2):251–5.
13. Fleming M, Ravula S, Tatishchev SF, Wang HL. Colorectal carcinoma: pathologic aspects. J Gastrointest Oncol. 2012;3(3):153–73.

14. Loughrey MB, Shepherd NA. Problematic colorectal polyps: is it cancer and what do I need to do about it? Surg Pathol Clin. 2017;10(4):947–60.
15. Littler ER, Gleibermann E. Gastritis cystica polyposa (gastric mucosal prolapse at gastroenterostomy site, with cystic and infiltrative epithelial hyperplasia). Cancer. 1972;29(1):205–9.
16. Kitajima K, Fujimori T, Fujii S, Takeda J, Ohkura Y, Kawamata H, Kumamoto T, Ishiguro S, Kato Y, Shimoda T, Iwashita A, Ajioka Y, Watanabe H, Watanabe T, Muto T, Nagasako K. Correlations between lymph node metastasis and depth of submucosal invasion in submucosal invasive colorectal carcinoma: a Japanese collaborative study. J Gastroenterol. 2004;39(6):534–43.
17. Aarons CB, Shanmugan S, Bleier JI. Management of malignant colon polyps: current status and controversies. World J Gastroenterol. 2014;20(43):16178–83.
18. Wick MR, Vitsky JL, Ritter JH, Swanson PE, Mills SE. Sporadic medullary carcinoma of the colon: a clinicopathologic comparison with nonhereditary poorly differentiated enteric-type adenocarcinoma and neuroendocrine colorectal carcinoma. Am J Clin Pathol. 2005;123(1):56–65.
19. Cunningham J, Kantekure K, Saif MW. Medullary carcinoma of the colon: a case series and review of the literature. In Vivo. 2014;28(3):311–4.
20. Kang DB, Oh JT, Jo HJ, Park WC. Primary adenosquamous carcinoma of the colon. J Korean Surg Soc. 2011;80(Suppl 1):S31–5.
21. Iizasa H, Nanbo A, Nishikawa J, Jinushi M, Yoshiyama H. Epstein-Barr virus (EBV)-associated gastric carcinoma. Viruses. 2012;4(12):3420–39.
22. Cancer Genome Atlas Research Network. Comprehensive molecular characterization of gastric adenocarcinoma. Nature. 2014;513(7517):202–9.
23. Lim H, Park YS, Lee JH, Son DH, Ahn JY, Choi KS, Kim DH, Choi KD, Song HJ, Lee GH, Jung HY, Kim JH, Yook JH, Kim BS. Features of gastric carcinoma with lymphoid stroma associated with Epstein-Barr virus. Clin Gastroenterol Hepatol. 2015;13(10):1738–1744.e2.
24. Lino-Silva LS, Salcedo-Hernández RA, Herrera-Gómez A, Padilla-Rosciano A, Ramírez-Jaramillo M, Herrera-Goepfert RE, Meneses-García A. Colonic cribriform carcinoma, a morphologic pattern associated with low survival. Int J Surg Pathol. 2015;23(1):13–9.
25. Fukayama M, Abe H, Kunita A, Shinozaki-Ushiku A, Matsusaka K, Ushiku T, Kaneda A. Thirty years of Epstein-Barr virus-associated gastric carcinoma. Virchows Arch. 2020;476(3):353–65.
26. Gonzalez RS, Cates JM, Washington MK, Beauchamp RD, Coffey RJ, Shi C. Adenoma-like adenocarcinoma: a subtype of colorectal carcinoma with good prognosis, deceptive appearance on biopsy and frequent KRAS mutation. Histopathology. 2016;68(2):183–90.
27. Mäkinen MJ. Colorectal serrated adenocarcinoma. Histopathology. 2007;50(1):131–50.
28. Shida Y, Fujimori T, Tanaka H, Fujimori Y, Kimura R, Ueda H, Ichikawa K, Tomita S, Nagata H, Kubota K, Tsubaki M, Kato H, Yao T, Sugai T, Sugihara K, Ohkura Y, Imura J. Clinicopathological features of serrated adenocarcinoma defined by Mäkinen in dukes' B colorectal carcinoma. Pathobiology. 2012;79(4):169–74.
29. Guzińska-Ustymowicz K, Niewiarowska K, Pryczynicz A. Invasive micropapillary carcinoma: a distinct type of adenocarcinomas in the gastrointestinal tract. World J Gastroenterol. 2014;20(16):4597–606.
30. Choi YY, Jeen YM, Kim YJ. Sarcomatoid carcinoma of colon: extremely poor prognosis. J Korean Surg Soc. 2011;80(Suppl 1):S26–30.
31. Murakami T, Yao T, Mitomi H, Morimoto T, Ueyama H, Matsumoto K, Saito T, Osada T, Nagahara A, Watanabe S. Clinicopathologic and immunohistochemical characteristics of gastric adenocarcinoma with enteroblastic differentiation: a study of 29 cases. Gastric Cancer. 2016;19(2):498–507.
32. Akazawa Y, Saito T, Hayashi T, Yanai Y, Tsuyama S, Akaike K, Suehara Y, Takahashi F, Takamochi K, Ueyama H, Murakami T, Watanabe S, Nagahara A, Yao T. Next-generation sequencing analysis for gastric adenocarcinoma with enteroblastic differentiation: emphasis on the relationship with hepatoid adenocarcinoma. Hum Pathol. 2018;78:79–88.
33. Kumashiro Y, Yao T, Aishima S, Hirahashi M, Nishiyama K, Yamada T, Takayanagi R, Tsuneyoshi M. Hepatoid adenocarcinoma of the stomach: histogenesis and progression in association with intestinal phenotype. Hum Pathol. 2007;38(6):857–63.
34. Agaimy A, Daum O, Märkl B, Lichtmannegger I, Michal M, Hartmann A. SWI/SNF complex-deficient undifferentiated/rhabdoid carcinomas of the gastrointestinal tract: a series of 13 cases highlighting mutually exclusive loss of SMARCA4 and SMARCA2 and frequent co-inactivation of SMARCB1 and SMARCA2. Am J Surg Pathol. 2016;40(4):544–53.
35. Ushiku T, Uozaki H, Shinozaki A, Ota S, Matsuzaka K, Nomura S, Kaminishi M, Aburatani H, Kodama T, Fukayama M. Glypican 3-expressing gastric carcinoma: distinct subgroup unifying hepatoid, clear-cell, and alpha-fetoprotein-producing gastric carcinomas. Cancer Sci. 2009;100(4):626–32.
36. Ushiku T, Shinozaki A, Shibahara J, Iwasaki Y, Tateishi Y, Funata N, Fukayama M. SALL4 represents fetal gut differentiation of gastric cancer, and is diagnostically useful in distinguishing hepatoid gastric carcinoma from hepatocellular carcinoma. Am J Surg Pathol. 2010;34(4):533–40.
37. Winn B, Tavares R, Fanion J, Noble L, Gao J, Sabo E, Resnick MB. Differentiating the undifferentiated: immunohistochemical profile of medullary carcinoma of the colon with an emphasis on intestinal differentiation. Hum Pathol. 2009;40(3):398–404.
38. Lin F, Shi J, Zhu S, Chen Z, Li A, Chen T, Wang HL, Liu H. Cadherin-17 and SATB2 are sensitive and specific immunomarkers for medullary carcinoma of the large intestine. Arch Pathol Lab Med. 2014;138(8):1015–26.
39. Singhi AD, Lazenby AJ, Montgomery EA. Gastric adenocarcinoma with chief cell differentiation: a proposal for reclassification as oxyntic gland polyp/adenoma. Am J Surg Pathol. 2012;36(7):1030–5.
40. Chan K, Brown IS, Kyle T, Lauwers GY, Kumarasinghe MP. Chief cell-predominant gastric polyps: a series of 12 cases with literature review. Histopathology. 2016;68(6):825–33.
41. Castri F, Ravegnini G, Lodoli C, Fiorentino V, Abatini C, Giustiniani MC, Angelini S, Ricci R. Gastroblastoma in old age. Histopathology. 2019;75(5):778–82.
42. Centonze G, Mangogna A, Salviato T, Belmonte B, Cattaneo L, Monica MAT, Garzone G, Brambilla C, Pellegrinelli A, Melotti F, Testi A, Monti V, Kankava K, Gasparini P, Dagrada G, Mazzaferro V, Cotsoglou C, Collini P, Pruneri G, Milione M. Gastroblastoma in adulthood: a rarity among rare cancers – a case report and review of the literature. Case Rep Pathol. 2019;2019:4084196.
43. Poizat F, de Chaisemartin C, Bories E, Delpero JR, Xerri L, Flejou JF, Monges G. A distinctive epitheliomesenchymal biphasic tumor in the duodenum: the first case of duodenoblastoma? Virchows Arch. 2012;461(4):379–83.
44. Na YJ, Shim KN, Kang MJ, Jung JM, Ha CY, Jung HS, Baik SJ, Kim SE, Jung SA, Yoo K, Moon IH, Cho MS. Primary esophageal adenoid cystic carcinoma. Gut Liver. 2007;1(2):178–81.
45. Batoon SB, Banzuela M, Angeles HG, Zoneraich S, Maniego W, Co J. Primary mucoepidermoid carcinoma of the esophagus misclassified as adenocarcinoma on endoscopic biopsy. Am J Gastroenterol. 2000;95(10):2998–9.
46. Yamamoto M, Hirata K, Tuneyoshi M, Yoshida Y, Matsuda H, Gion T, Tominaga Y. Mucoepidermoid carcinoma of the anal

canal: a case report and review of the literature. Mol Clin Oncol. 2018;9(5):504–6.
47. Shenoy S. CDH1 (E-Cadherin) mutation and gastric cancer: genetics, molecular mechanisms and guidelines for management. Cancer Manag Res. 2019;11:10477–86.
48. Rocha JP, Gullo I, Wen X, Devezas V, Baptista M, Oliveira C, Carneiro F. Pathological features of total gastrectomy specimens from asymptomatic hereditary diffuse gastric cancer patients and implications for clinical management. Histopathology. 2018;73(6):878–86.
49. El-Hage A, Ruel C, Afif W, Wissanji H, Hogue JC, Desbiens C, Leblanc G, Poirier É. Metastatic pattern of invasive lobular carcinoma of the breast: emphasis on gastric metastases. J Surg Oncol. 2016;114(5):543–7.
50. Hui Y, Wang Y, Nam G, Fanion J, Sturtevant A, Lombardo KA, Resnick MB. Differentiating breast carcinoma with signet ring features from gastrointestinal signet ring carcinoma: assessment of immunohistochemical markers. Hum Pathol. 2018;77:11–9.
51. Lee AF, Rees H, Owen DA, Huntsman DG. Periodic acid-Schiff is superior to hematoxylin and eosin for screening prophylactic gastrectomies from CDH1 mutation carriers. Am J Surg Pathol. 2010;34(7):1007–13.
52. Liang WY, Chang WC, Hsu CY, Arnason T, Berger D, Hawkins AT, Sylla P, Lauwers GY. Retrospective evaluation of elastic stain in the assessment of serosal invasion of pT3N0 colorectal cancers. Am J Surg Pathol. 2013;37(10):1565–70.
53. Nakanishi Y, LeVea C, Dibaj S, Habib F, Cheney R, Kanehira K. Reappraisal of serosal invasion in patients with T3 colorectal cancer by elastic stain: clinicopathologic study of 139 surgical cases with special reference to peritoneal elastic lamina invasion. Arch Pathol Lab Med. 2016;140(1):81–5.
54. Odate T, Vuong HG, Mochizuki K, Oishi N, Kondo T. Assessment of peritoneal elastic laminal invasion improves survival stratification of pT3 and pT4a colorectal cancer: a meta-analysis. J Clin Pathol. 2019;72(11):736–40.
55. Liang WY, Wang YC, Hsu CY, Yang SH. Staging of colorectal cancers based on elastic lamina invasion. Hum Pathol. 2019;85:44–9.
56. Compton CC. Colorectal carcinoma: diagnostic, prognostic, and molecular features. Mod Pathol. 2003;16(4):376–88.
57. Nagtegaal ID, van de Velde CJ, van der Worp E, Kapiteijn E, Quirke P, van Krieken JH, Cooperative Clinical Investigators of the Dutch Colorectal Cancer Group. Macroscopic evaluation of rectal cancer resection specimen: clinical significance of the pathologist in quality control. J Clin Oncol. 2002;20(7):1729–934.
58. Tzardi M. Role of total mesorectal excision and of circumferential resection margin in local recurrence and survival of patients with rectal carcinoma. Dig Dis. 2007;25(1):51–5.
59. Bosch SL, Nagtegaal ID. The importance of the pathologist's role in assessment of the quality of the mesorectum. Curr Colorectal Cancer Rep. 2012;8(2):90–8.
60. Birbeck KF, Macklin CP, Tiffin NJ, Parsons W, Dixon MF, Mapstone NP, Abbott CR, Scott N, Finan PJ, Johnston D, Quirke P. Rates of circumferential resection margin involvement vary between surgeons and predict outcomes in rectal cancer surgery. Ann Surg. 2002;235(4):449–57.
61. Nagtegaal ID, Marijnen CA, Kranenbarg EK, van de Velde CJ, van Krieken JH, Pathology Review Committee, Cooperative Clinical Investigators. Circumferential margin involvement is still an important predictor of local recurrence in rectal carcinoma: not one millimeter but two millimeters is the limit. Am J Surg Pathol. 2002;26(3):350–7.
62. Li J, Yang S, Hu J, Liu H, Du F, Yin J, Liu S, Li C, Xing S, Yuan J, Lv B, Fan J, Leng S, Zhang X, Wang B. Tumor deposits counted as positive lymph nodes in TNM staging for advanced colorectal cancer: a retrospective multicenter study. Oncotarget. 2016;7(14):18269–79.
63. Jin M, Roth R, Rock JB, Washington MK, Lehman A, Frankel WL. The impact of tumor deposits on colonic adenocarcinoma AJCC TNM staging and outcome. Am J Surg Pathol. 2015;39(1):109–15.
64. Belt EJ, van Stijn MF, Bril H, de Lange-de Klerk ES, Meijer GA, Meijer S, Stockmann HB. Lymph node negative colorectal cancers with isolated tumor deposits should be classified and treated as stage III. Ann Surg Oncol. 2010;17(12):3203–11.
65. Weixler B, Warschkow R, Güller U, Zettl A, von Holzen U, Schmied BM, Zuber M. Isolated tumor cells in stage I & II colon cancer patients are associated with significantly worse disease-free and overall survival. BMC Cancer. 2016;16:106.
66. Faerden AE, Sjo OH, Bukholm IR, Andersen SN, Svindland A, Nesbakken A, Bakka A. Lymph node micrometastases and isolated tumor cells influence survival in stage I and II colon cancer. Dis Colon Rectum. 2011;54(2):200–6.
67. Lee MR, Hong CW, Yoon SN, Lim SB, Park KJ, Lee MJ, Kim WH, Park JG. Isolated tumor cells in lymph nodes are not a prognostic marker for patients with stage I and stage II colorectal cancer. J Surg Oncol. 2006;93(1):13–8.
68. Protic M, Stojadinovic A, Nissan A, Wainberg Z, Steele SR, Chen DC, Avital I, Bilchik AJ. Prognostic effect of ultra-staging node-negative colon cancer without adjuvant chemotherapy: a prospective National Cancer Institute-sponsored clinical trial. J Am Coll Surg. 2015;221(3):643–51.
69. Bhatti AB, Akbar A, Khattak S, Kazmi AS, Jamshed A, Syed AA. Impact of acellular mucin pools on survival in patients with complete pathological response to neoadjuvant treatment in rectal cancer. Int J Surg. 2014;12(10):1123–6.
70. Ingle P, Bal M, Engineer R, Ostwal V, Desouza A, Saklani A. Do acellular mucin pools in resection margins for rectal cancer influence outcomes? Indian J Surg Oncol. 2019;10(3):515–9.
71. Hornick JL, Farraye FA, Odze RD. Prevalence and significance of prominent mucin pools in the esophagus post neoadjuvant chemoradiotherapy for Barrett's-associated adenocarcinoma. Am J Surg Pathol. 2006;30(1):28–35.
72. Dawson H, Lugli A. Molecular and pathogenetic aspects of tumor budding in colorectal cancer. Front Med (Lausanne). 2015;2:11.
73. Mitrovic B, Schaeffer DF, Riddell RH, Kirsch R. Tumor budding in colorectal carcinoma: time to take notice. Mod Pathol. 2012;25(10):1315–25.
74. Cho SJ, Kakar S. Tumor budding in colorectal carcinoma: translating a morphologic score into clinically meaningful results. Arch Pathol Lab Med. 2018;142(8):952–7.
75. Lugli A, Kirsch R, Ajioka Y, Bosman F, Cathomas G, Dawson H, El Zimaity H, Fléjou JF, Hansen TP, Hartmann A, Kakar S, Langner C, Nagtegaal I, Puppa G, Riddell R, Ristimäki A, Sheahan K, Smyrk T, Sugihara K, Terris B, Ueno H, Vieth M, Zlobec I, Quirke P. Recommendations for reporting tumor budding in colorectal cancer based on the International Tumor Budding Consensus Conference (ITBCC) 2016. Mod Pathol. 2017;30(9):1299–311.
76. Dawson H, Kirsch R, Driman DK, Messenger DE, Assarzadegan N, Riddell RH. Optimizing the detection of venous invasion in colorectal cancer: the Ontario, Canada, experience and beyond. Front Oncol. 2015;4:354.
77. Messenger DE, Driman DK, Kirsch R. Developments in the assessment of venous invasion in colorectal cancer: implications for future practice and patient outcome. Hum Pathol. 2012;43(7):965–73.
78. Liang P, Nakada I, Hong JW, Tabuchi T, Motohashi G, Takemura A, Nakachi T, Kasuga T, Tabuchi T. Prognostic significance of immunohistochemically detected blood and lymphatic vessel

invasion in colorectal carcinoma: its impact on prognosis. Ann Surg Oncol. 2007;14(2):470–7.
79. Sternberg A, Amar M, Alfici R, Groisman G. Conclusions from a study of venous invasion in stage IV colorectal adenocarcinoma. J Clin Pathol. 2002;55(1):17–21.
80. Ryan R, Gibbons D, Hyland JMP, Treanor D, White A, Mulcahy HE, O'Donoghue DP, Moriarty M, Fennelly D, Sheahan K. Pathological response following long-course neoadjuvant chemoradiotherapy for locally advanced rectal cancer. Histopathology. 2005;47(2):141–6.
81. Kim SH, Chang HJ, Kim DY, Park JW, Baek JY, Kim SY, Park SC, Oh JH, Yu A, Nam BH. What is the ideal tumor regression grading system in rectal cancer patients after preoperative chemoradiotherapy? Cancer Res Treat. 2016;48(3):998–1009.
82. Lee HE, Wu TT, Chandan VS, Torbenson MS, Mounajjed T. Colonic adenomatous polyps involving submucosal lymphoglandular complexes: a diagnostic pitfall. Am J Surg Pathol. 2018;42(8):1083–9.
83. Farris AB, Lauwers GY, Ferry JA, Zukerberg LR. The rectal tonsil: a reactive lymphoid proliferation that may mimic lymphoma. Am J Surg Pathol. 2008;32(7):1075–9.
84. McCarthy AJ, Chetty R. Gut-associated lymphoid tissue or so-called "dome" carcinoma of the colon: review. World J Gastrointest Oncol. 2019;11(1):59–70.
85. Leonards LM, Pahwa A, Patel MK, Petersen J, Nguyen MJ, Jude CM. Neoplasms of the appendix: pictorial review with clinical and pathologic correlation. Radiographics. 2017;37(4):1059–83.
86. Connor SJ, Hanna GB, Frizelle FA. Appendiceal tumors: retrospective clinicopathologic analysis of appendiceal tumors from 7,970 appendectomies. Dis Colon Rectum. 1998;41(1):75–80.
87. Ang DC, Shia J, Tang LH, Katabi N, Klimstra DS. The utility of immunohistochemistry in subtyping adenocarcinoma of the ampulla of Vater. Am J Surg Pathol. 2014;38(10):1371–9.
88. Serup-Hansen E, Linnemann D, Skovrider-Ruminski W, Høgdall E, Geertsen PF, Havsteen H. Human papillomavirus genotyping and p16 expression as prognostic factors for patients with American Joint Committee on Cancer stages I to III carcinoma of the anal canal. J Clin Oncol. 2014;32(17):1812–7.
89. Graham RP, Arnold CA, Naini BV, Lam-Himlin DM. Basaloid squamous cell carcinoma of the anus revisited. Am J Surg Pathol. 2016;40(3):354–60.
90. National Comprehensive Cancer Network. Anal carcinoma (version 1.2020 – December 19, 2019). https://www.nccn.org/professionals/physician_gls/pdf/anal.pdf. Accessed 4 Jan 2020.
91. National Comprehensive Cancer Network. Rectal cancer (version 1.2020 – December 19, 2019). https://www.nccn.org/professionals/physician_gls/pdf/rectal.pdf. Accessed 4 Jan 2020.
92. Lisovsky M, Patel K, Cymes K, Chase D, Bhuiya T, Morgenstern N. Immunophenotypic characterization of anal gland carcinoma: loss of p63 and cytokeratin 5/6. Arch Pathol Lab Med. 2007;131(8):1304–11.
93. Shia J. An update on tumors of the anal canal. Arch Pathol Lab Med. 2010;134(11):1601–11.
94. Wang HL, Kim CJ, Koo J, Zhou W, Choi EK, Arcega R, Chen ZE, Wang H, Zhang L, Lin F. Practical immunohistochemistry in neoplastic pathology of the gastrointestinal tract, liver, biliary tract, and pancreas. Arch Pathol Lab Med. 2017;141(9):1155–80.
95. Ma C, Lowenthal BM, Pai RK. SATB2 is superior to CDX2 in distinguishing signet ring cell carcinoma of the upper gastrointestinal tract and lower gastrointestinal tract. Am J Surg Pathol. 2018;42(12):1715–22.
96. Magnusson K, de Wit M, Brennan DJ, Johnson LB, McGee SF, Lundberg E, Naicker K, Klinger R, Kampf C, Asplund A, Wester K, Gry M, Bjartell A, Gallagher WM, Rexhepaj E, Kilpinen S, Kallioniemi OP, Belt E, Goos J, Meijer G, Birgisson H, Glimelius B, Borrebaeck CA, Navani S, Uhlén M, O'Connor DP, Jirström K, Pontén F. SATB2 in combination with cytokeratin 20 identifies over 95% of all colorectal carcinomas. Am J Surg Pathol. 2011;35(7):937–48.
97. Selves J, Long-Mira E, Mathieu MC, Rochaix P, Ilié M. Immunohistochemistry for diagnosis of metastatic carcinomas of unknown primary site. Cancers (Basel). 2018;10(4): pii:E108.
98. Palla VV, Karaolanis G, Bliona T, Katafigiotis I, Anastasiou I, Hassiakos D. Endometrioid adenocarcinoma arising from colon endometriosis. SAGE Open Med Case Rep. 2017;5:2050313X17745204.
99. Bang YJ, Van Cutsem E, Feyereislova A, Chung HC, Shen L, Sawaki A, Lordick F, Ohtsu A, Omuro Y, Satoh T, Aprile G, Kulikov E, Hill J, Lehle M, Rüschoff J, Kang YK, ToGA Trial Investigators. Trastuzumab in combination with chemotherapy versus chemotherapy alone for treatment of HER2-positive advanced gastric or gastro-oesophageal junction cancer (ToGA): a phase 3, open-label, randomized controlled trial. Lancet. 2010;376(9742):687–97.
100. Bartley AN, Washington MK, Ventura CB, Ismaila N, Colasacco C, Benson AB 3rd, Carrato A, Gulley ML, Jain D, Kakar S, Mackay HJ, Streutker C, Tang L, Troxell M, Ajani JA. HER2 testing and clinical decision making in gastroesophageal adenocarcinoma: guideline from the College of American Pathologists, American Society for Clinical Pathology, and American Society of Clinical Oncology. Arch Pathol Lab Med. 2016;140(12):1345–63.
101. Le DT, Durham JN, Smith KN, Wang H, Bartlett BR, Aulakh LK, Lu S, Kemberling H, Wilt C, Luber BS, Wong F, Azad NS, Rucki AA, Laheru D, Donehower R, Zaheer A, Fisher GA, Crocenzi TS, Lee JJ, Greten TF, Duffy AG, Ciombor KK, Eyring AD, Lam BH, Joe A, Kang SP, Holdhoff M, Danilova L, Cope L, Meyer C, Zhou S, Goldberg RM, Armstrong DK, Bever KM, Fader AN, Taube J, Housseau F, Spetzler D, Xiao N, Pardoll DM, Papadopoulos N, Kinzler KW, Eshleman JR, Vogelstein B, Anders RA, Diaz LA Jr. Mismatch repair deficiency predicts response of solid tumors to PD-1 blockade. Science. 2017;357(6349):409–13.
102. Schneider NI, Langner C. Prognostic stratification of colorectal cancer patients: current perspectives. Cancer Manag Res. 2014;6:291–300.
103. Yoon YS, Kim J, Hong SM, Lee JL, Kim CW, Park IJ, Lim SB, Yu CS, Kim JC. Clinical implications of mucinous components correlated with microsatellite instability in patients with colorectal cancer. Colorectal Dis. 2015;17(8):O161–7.
104. Zhang X, Li J. Era of universal testing of microsatellite instability in colorectal cancer. World J Gastrointest Oncol. 2013;5(2):12–9.
105. Guinney J, Dienstmann R, Wang X, de Reyniès A, Schlicker A, Soneson C, Marisa L, Roepman P, Nyamundanda G, Angelino P, Bot BM, Morris JS, Simon IM, Gerster S, Fessler E, De Sousa E, Melo F, Missiaglia E, Ramay H, Barras D, Homicsko K, Maru D, Manyam GC, Broom B, Boige V, Perez-Villamil B, Laderas T, Salazar R, Gray JW, Hanahan D, Tabernero J, Bernards R, Friend SH, Laurent-Puig P, Medema JP, Sadanandam A, Wessels L, Delorenzi M, Kopetz S, Vermeulen L, Tejpar S. The consensus molecular subtypes of colorectal cancer. Nat Med. 2015;21(11):1350–6.
106. Le DT, Uram JN, Wang H, Bartlett BR, Kemberling H, Eyring AD, Skora AD, Luber BS, Azad NS, Laheru D, Biedrzycki B, Donehower RC, Zaheer A, Fisher GA, Crocenzi TS, Lee JJ, Duffy SM, Goldberg RM, de la Chapelle A, Koshiji M, Bhaijee F, Huebner T, Hruban RH, Wood LD, Cuka N, Pardoll DM, Papadopoulos N, Kinzler KW, Zhou S, Cornish TC, Taube JM, Anders RA, Eshleman JR, Vogelstein B, Diaz LA Jr. PD-1 blockade in tumors with mismatch-repair deficiency. N Engl J Med. 2015;372(26):2509–20.
107. National Comprehensive Cancer Network. Genetic/familial high-risk assessment: colorectal (version 3.2019 – December 13, 2019). https://www.nccn.org/professionals/physician_gls/pdf/genetics_colon.pdf. Accessed 4 Jan 2020.

108. Stadler ZK, Battaglin F, Middha S, Hechtman JF, Tran C, Cercek A, Yaeger R, Segal NH, Varghese AM, Reidy-Lagunes DL, Kemeny NE, Salo-Mullen EE, Ashraf A, Weiser MR, Garcia-Aguilar J, Robson ME, Offit K, Arcila ME, Berger MF, Shia J, Solit DB, Saltz LB. Reliable detection of mismatch repair deficiency in colorectal cancers using mutational load in next-generation sequencing panels. J Clin Oncol. 2016;34(18):2141–7.
109. Zehir A, Benayed R, Shah RH, Syed A, Middha S, Kim HR, Srinivasan P, Gao J, Chakravarty D, Devlin SM, Hellmann MD, Barron DA, Schram AM, Hameed M, Dogan S, Ross DS, Hechtman JF, DF DL, Yao J, Mandelker DL, Cheng DT, Chandramohan R, Mohanty AS, Ptashkin RN, Jayakumaran G, Prasad M, Syed MH, Rema AB, Liu ZY, Nafa K, Borsu L, Sadowska J, Casanova J, Bacares R, Kiecka IJ, Razumova A, Son JB, Stewart L, Baldi T, Mullaney KA, Al-Ahmadie H, Vakiani E, Abeshouse AA, Penson AV, Jonsson P, Camacho N, Chang MT, Won HH, Gross BE, Kundra R, Heins ZJ, Chen HW, Phillips S, Zhang H, Wang J, Ochoa A, Wills J, Eubank M, Thomas SB, Gardos SM, Reales DN, Galle J, Durany R, Cambria R, Abida W, Cercek A, Feldman DR, Gounder MM, Hakimi AA, Harding JJ, Iyer G, Janjigian YY, Jordan EJ, Kelly CM, Lowery MA, LGT M, Omuro AM, Raj N, Razavi P, Shoushtari AN, Shukla N, Soumerai TE, Varghese AM, Yaeger R, Coleman J, Bochner B, Riely GJ, Saltz LB, Scher HI, Sabbatini PJ, Robson ME, Klimstra DS, Taylor BS, Baselga J, Schultz N, Hyman DM, Arcila ME, Solit DB, Ladanyi M, Berger MF. Mutational landscape of metastatic cancer revealed from prospective clinical sequencing of 10,000 patients. Nat Med. 2017;23(6):703–13.
110. Cheng DT, Prasad M, Chekaluk Y, Benayed R, Sadowska J, Zehir A, Syed A, Wang YE, Somar J, Li Y, Yelskaya Z, Wong D, Robson ME, Offit K, Berger MF, Nafa K, Ladanyi M, Zhang L. Comprehensive detection of germline variants by MSK-IMPACT, a clinical diagnostic platform for solid tumor molecular oncology and concurrent cancer predisposition testing. BMC Med Genet. 2017;10(1):33.
111. Hampel H, Pearlman R, Beightol M, Zhao W, Jones D, Frankel WL, Goodfellow PJ, Yilmaz A, Miller K, Bacher J, Jacobson A, Paskett E, Shields PG, Goldberg RM, de la Chapelle A, Shirts BH, Pritchard CC, Ohio Colorectal Cancer Prevention Initiative Study Group. Assessment of tumor sequencing as a replacement for Lynch syndrome screening and current molecular tests for patients with colorectal cancer. JAMA Oncol. 2018;4(6):806–13.
112. Sarode VR, Robinson L. Screening for Lynch syndrome by immunohistochemistry of mismatch repair proteins: significance of indeterminate result and correlation with mutational studies. Arch Pathol Lab Med. 2019;143(10):1225–33.
113. Bao F, Panarelli NC, Rennert H, Sherr DL, Yantiss RK. Neoadjuvant therapy induces loss of MSH6 expression in colorectal carcinoma. Am J Surg Pathol. 2010;34(12):1798–804.
114. Radu OM, Nikiforova MN, Farkas LM, Krasinskas AM. Challenging cases encountered in colorectal cancer screening for Lynch syndrome reveal novel findings: nucleolar MSH6 staining and impact of prior chemoradiation therapy. Hum Pathol. 2011;42(9):1247–58.
115. Gould-Suarez M, El-Serag HB, Musher B, Franco LM, Chen GJ. Cost-effectiveness and diagnostic effectiveness analyses of multiple algorithms for the diagnosis of Lynch syndrome. Dig Dis Sci. 2014;59(12):2913–26.
116. Smyrk TC, Watson P, Kaul K, Lynch HT. Tumor-infiltrating lymphocytes are a marker for microsatellite instability in colorectal carcinoma. Cancer. 2001;91(12):2417–22.
117. Xiao H, Yoon YS, Hong SM, Roh SA, Cho DH, Yu CS, Kim JC. Poorly differentiated colorectal cancers: correlation of microsatellite instability with clinicopathologic features and survival. Am J Clin Pathol. 2013;140(3):341–7.
118. Lièvre A, Bachet JB, Le Corre D, Boige V, Landi B, Emile JF, Côté JF, Tomasic G, Penna C, Ducreux M, Rougier P, Penault-Llorca F, Laurent-Puig P. KRAS mutation status is predictive of response to cetuximab therapy in colorectal cancer. Cancer Res. 2006;66(8):3992–5.
119. Amado RG, Wolf M, Peeters M, Van Cutsem E, Siena S, Freeman DJ, Juan T, Sikorski R, Suggs S, Radinsky R, Patterson SD, Chang DD. Wild-type KRAS is required for panitumumab efficacy in patients with metastatic colorectal cancer. J Clin Oncol. 2008;26(10):1626–34.
120. Allegra CJ, Jessup JM, Somerfield MR, Hamilton SR, Hammond EH, Hayes DF, McAllister PK, Morton RF, Schilsky RL. American Society of Clinical Oncology provisional clinical opinion: testing for KRAS gene mutations in patients with metastatic colorectal carcinoma to predict response to anti-epidermal growth factor receptor monoclonal antibody therapy. J Clin Oncol. 2009;27(12):2091–6.
121. Douillard JY, Oliner KS, Siena S, Tabernero J, Burkes R, Barugel M, Humblet Y, Bodoky G, Cunningham D, Jassem J, Rivera F, Kocákova I, Ruff P, Błasińska-Morawiec M, Šmakal M, Canon JL, Rother M, Williams R, Rong A, Wiezorek J, Sidhu R, Patterson SD. Panitumumab-FOLFOX4 treatment and RAS mutations in colorectal cancer. N Engl J Med. 2013;369(11):1023–34.
122. Valtorta E, Martino C, Sartore-Bianchi A, Penaullt-Llorca F, Viale G, Risio M, Rugge M, Grigioni W, Bencardino K, Lonardi S, Zagonel V, Leone F, Noe J, Ciardiello F, Pinto C, Labianca R, Mosconi S, Graiff C, Aprile G, Frau B, Garufi C, Loupakis F, Racca P, Tonini G, Lauricella C, Veronese S, Truini M, Siena S, Marsoni S, Gambacorta M. Assessment of a HER2 scoring system for colorectal cancer: results from a validation study. Mod Pathol. 2015;28(11):1481–91. https://doi.org/10.1038/modpathol.2015.98. Epub 2015 Oct 9. PMID: 26449765.
123. Ross JS, Fakih M, Ali SM, Elvin JA, Schrock AB, Suh J, Vergilio JA, Ramkissoon S, Severson E, Daniel S, Fabrizio D, Frampton G, Sun J, Miller VA, Stephens PJ, Gay LM. Targeting HER2 in colorectal cancer: the landscape of amplification and short variant mutations in ERBB2 and ERBB3. Cancer. 2018;124(7):1358–73.
124. Greally M, Kelly CM, Cercek A. HER2: an emerging target in colorectal cancer. Curr Probl Cancer. 2018;42(6):560–71.
125. Mei ZB, Duan CY, Li CB, Cui L, Ogino S. Prognostic role of tumor PIK3CA mutation in colorectal cancer: a systematic review and meta-analysis. Ann Oncol. 2016;27(10):1836–48.
126. De Roock W, De Vriendt V, Normanno N, Ciardiello F, Tejpar S. KRAS, BRAF, PIK3CA, and PTEN mutations: implications for targeted therapies in metastatic colorectal cancer. Lancet Oncol. 2011;12(6):594–603.
127. Hocking C, Hardingham JE, Broadbridge V, Wrin J, Townsend AR, Tebbutt N, Cooper J, Ruszkiewicz A, Lee C, Price TJ. Can we accurately report PTEN status in advanced colorectal cancer? BMC Cancer. 2014;14:128.
128. Kurra V, Krajewski KM, Jagannathan J, Giardino A, Berlin S, Ramaiya N. Typical and atypical metastatic sites of recurrent endometrial carcinoma. Cancer Imaging. 2013;13(1):113–22.
129. Petersen VC, Underwood JC, Wells M, Shepherd NA. Primary endometrioid adenocarcinoma of the large intestine arising in colorectal endometriosis. Histopathology. 2002;40(2):171–6.
130. Hubers JA, Soni A. A rare case of endometrial cancer metastatic to the sigmoid colon and small bowel. Case Rep Gastrointest Med. 2017;2017:9382486.
131. Yamamoto T, Hiroi A, Itagaki H, Kato Y, Iizuka B, Itabashi M, Shibata N, Nagashima Y. Well-differentiated adenocarcinoma associated with ulcerative colitis. SAGE Open Med Case Rep. 2017;5:2050313X17692902.

Gastrointestinal Stromal Tumor

19

Karen E. Matsukuma and Zongming Eric Chen

List of Frequently Asked Questions

1. What is GIST, and what are some characteristic features?
2. What is the histologic differential diagnosis of GIST?
3. What immunostains should be used to evaluate for GIST? What if they are negative, but GIST is still a serious consideration?
4. What is the significance of dot-like or membranous CD117 staining?
5. What is the immunoprofile of epithelioid GIST? What pitfalls should one be aware of?
6. What histologic features meet criteria for a "mixed" type GIST? Is there any prognostic significance to this term?
7. What is a syndromic GIST? What morphologic features are indicative of syndromic GISTs?
8. What is the definition of pediatric GIST? How is it different from classical GIST in morphology and molecular mechanism?
9. What tumor characteristics are important for assessing malignant potential (risk stratification)?
10. What criteria should be used to diagnose and grade extra-gastrointestinal GISTs? Is the immunoprofile similar to typical GISTs?
11. What histologic criteria should be used to identify mitotic figures in GIST?
12. Where and how many high-power fields should I count for the mitotic index?
13. What are the histologic features of treatment effect? How do you estimate % viable tumor?
14. What is the significance of tumor necrosis in GIST?
15. To confirm a GIST diagnosis at the primary site, why is endoscopic ultrasound-guided fine needle aspiration preferred over percutaneous biopsy? What information should be reported from such tissue samples for clinical management purposes?
16. Should the terms "malignant GIST" and "benign GIST" be used? Are there other terms I should be aware of?
17. What are the most common sites of metastasis for sporadic GISTs?
18. If no lymph nodes are found or submitted with the tumor resection, should pN0 or pNX be used for AJCC tumor staging?
19. Should all GISTs be staged according to the AJCC staging manual?
20. Should grading and risk assessment be performed on post-therapy resections?
21. What is the significance of multifocal GIST? How does one differentiate multifocal disease from intraperitoneal metastasis?
22. What risk assessment category should be used if the primary site of GIST is an anatomic site other than stomach or small intestine?
23. Should all GISTs be tested for KIT and PDGFRα mutation? Can the type of mutation predict prognosis?
24. How can specific mutation profiles help guide therapy?
25. When should the possibility of germline KIT or PDGFRα syndrome be considered?
26. In the absence of KIT and PDGFRA mutations, would a GIST still be responsive to imatinib therapy?
27. When is it appropriate to order SDHB immunohistochemistry?
28. When is BRAF V6000E mutation testing appropriate, and what is the clinical significance of this mutation?

K. E. Matsukuma (✉)
University of California at Davis School of Medicine, Sacramento, CA, USA
e-mail: kmatsukuma@ucdavis.edu

Z. E. Chen
Mayo Clinic, Rochester, MN, USA

H. L. Wang, Z. E. Chen (eds.), *Practical Gastrointestinal Pathology*, Practical Anatomic Pathology,
https://doi.org/10.1007/978-3-030-51268-2_19

Frequently Asked Questions

1. **What is GIST, and what are some characteristic features?**
   - Gastrointestinal stromal tumor (GIST) is a neoplasm derived from the interstitial cells of Cajal. These cells are normally present in the myenteric plexus and function as neuronal pacemaker cells (e.g., responsible for initiating and propagating contractions along the gut).
   - Proliferation of interstitial cells of Cajal (ICC) leads to formation of mass lesions that are centered in the muscularis propria.
   - Histologically, GISTs are characterized by elongate spindle cells with eosinophilic cytoplasm, arranged in loose interweaving fascicles. In more hypercellular areas, cells are typically packed closely together (e.g., nuclei almost contact one another or are one nucleus length away) (Fig. 19.1a).
   - The neoplastic cells may also demonstrate an "epithelioid" appearance in which individual tumor cells have more abundant cytoplasm and a rounded (rather than spindled) morphology. Epithelioid cells may demonstrate prominent cytoplasmic borders (Fig. 19.1b).
   - Gastric GISTs may demonstrate perinuclear vacuoles (Fig. 19.1c), and small bowel and colon GISTs may demonstrate skeinoid fibers (short, thick collagen bands scattered within the tumor) (Fig. 19.1d). There is no prognostic significance to perinuclear vacuoles. However, skeinoid fibers are associated with favorable prognosis.
   - A number of variant histologic patterns of gastric GIST have been described. These include sclerosing, palisading-vacuolated, hypercellular, and sarcomatous spindle cell and sclerosing epithelioid, dyscohesive epithelioid, hypercellular epithelioid, and sarcomatous epithelioid cell. These are descriptive designations that may aid in identification of GIST but have not been established as independent prognostic factors.
   - GISTs can be derived from all organs of the tubular gastrointestinal tract as well as from extra-gastrointestinal sites.
   - The majority of GISTs harbor mutations in the *KIT* gene (75%), a tyrosine kinase. A smaller subset (10%) harbor mutations in *PDGFRA*, an evolutionarily

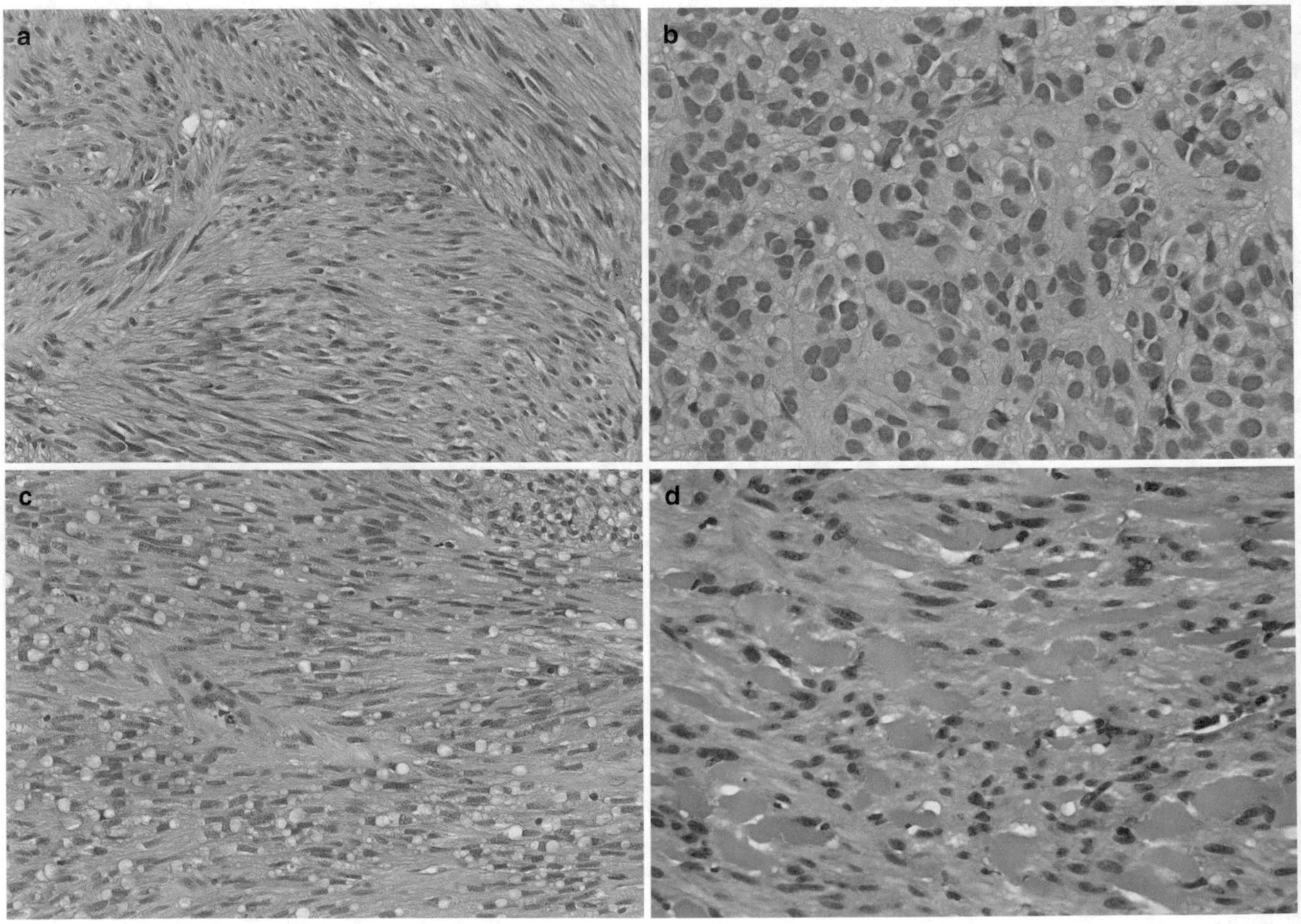

Fig. 19.1 (**a**–**d**) Classic morphology of GIST

related tyrosine kinase. The remainder of the GISTs harbor mutations in (or demonstrate functional inactivation of) one of the four succinate dehydrogenase genes (*SDHA*, *SDHB*, *SDHC*, *SDHD*), *BRAF*, *NF1*, or other driver genes. The specific genetic alterations in many cases correlate with morphology, biologic behavior, and response to therapy.
References: [8, 10, 34, 35, 54]

2. **What is the histologic differential diagnosis of GIST?**
The histologic differential diagnosis of GIST is long and can be broadly divided into two categories: (1) spindle cell lesions and (2) epithelioid/epithelial tumors. See Table 19.1.
   - In most cases, utilization of a panel of immunostains will help distinguish GIST from other entities listed in Table 19.1.
   - Attention to the relationship of the GIST to the layers of the bowel wall can help pare down the list of diagnostic possibilities. Specifically, GISTs are centered in the muscularis propria of the bowel, and thus primary tumors centered in the mucosa (e.g., neuroendocrine tumors, carcinoma) or submucosa (e.g., inflammatory fibroid polyp, granular cell tumor, glomus tumor, paraganglioma) are less likely if no involvement of the superficial layers is identified.

   References: [7, 10, 27]

Table 19.1 Histologic differential diagnosis of GIST

Spindle cell	Epithelioid
Leiomyoma	Glomus tumor
Schwannoma	Paraganglioma
Neurofibroma	Granular cell tumor
Perineurioma	Carcinoma
Inflammatory fibroid polyp	Melanoma
Plexiform fibromyxoma	Perivascular epithelioid cell tumor
Sarcomatoid carcinoma	Neuroendocrine neoplasm
Mesenteric fibromatosis	Solid pseudopapillary neoplasm
Leiomyosarcoma	Granulosa cell tumor
Malignant peripheral nerve sheath tumor	Epithelioid leiomyosarcoma
Inflammatory myofibroblastic tumor	Epithelioid angiosarcoma
Dedifferentiated/cellular liposarcoma	Lymphoma/myeloid sarcoma
Low-grade fibromyxoid sarcoma	Other small round blue cell tumors
Low-grade myofibroblastic sarcoma	
Solitary fibrous tumor	
Endometrial stromal sarcoma	
Angiosarcoma	

3. **What immunostains should be used to evaluate for GIST? What if they are negative, but GIST is still a serious consideration?**
The vast majority of GISTs are positive for both CD117 and DOG1 with a sensitivity of approximately 95% for each marker. Since many of those that are CD117 negative are DOG1 positive, to test for both immunomarkers in daily practice should not be regarded as redundancy. CD34 is positive in approximately two-thirds of GISTs. Because CD34 is frequently positive in vascular and other mesenchymal lesions as well as some hematolymphoid tumors, it should be used as a second-line stain and should not be the primary justification for the diagnosis of GIST.
If one or more of the above immunostains is negative but GIST is still a serious consideration, other morphologic and clinical features of the tumor are important to consider. In particular, *PDGFRA*-mutated GISTs can be CD117 and CD34 negative. Thus, in addition to excluding other entities in the differential diagnosis, immunohistochemistry for PKCθ (protein kinase C theta) can be useful, as it is relatively specific for GIST. Additionally, molecular testing for *KIT* (because it is the most commonly mutated gene in GIST) and *PDGFRA* mutations may be appropriate if a GIST is suspected but not confirmed by the pattern of CD117, DOG1, and CD34 expression.
   - *Pitfall* #1: Some tumors in the differential diagnosis of GIST may be CD117 positive, including melanoma, angiosarcoma, perivascular epithelioid cell tumor (PEComa), fibromatosis, and lymphoma/myeloid sarcoma. Thus, if the histologic features and location of the tumor are not classic, additional stains both to support GIST (specifically DOG1) and to exclude other entities are prudent.
   - *Pitfall* #2: Smooth muscle actin (SMA) can be positive in approximately one-half of GISTs (as well as smooth muscle and glomus tumors). In contrast, 10% or less of GISTs are positive for desmin. As such, desmin is more useful for distinguishing between GIST and a smooth muscle neoplasm.
   - *Pitfall* #3: Leiomyomas may on occasion have a number of mast cells or may demonstrate the presence of prominent interstitial cells of Cajal. Both of these situations result in CD117-positive elements within a spindle cell neoplasm with otherwise diffuse desmin or smooth muscle actin positivity. These should not be confused with GIST.
   - *Pitfall* #4: Although DOG1 is relatively specific in the realm of mesenchymal neoplasms, it can also stain epithelial neoplasms. Thus, if the differential diagnosis includes an epithelial malignancy, cytokeratin stains are useful. Of note, DOG1 also stains

colonized interstitial cells of Cajal in leiomyomas, like CD117.

- *Pitfall #5*: Cytokeratin may be expressed in epithelioid GISTs. Typically, it is weak and focal, but in some cases, it may be more diffuse. Correlation with location within the bowel wall and CD117, DOG1, and CD34 stains is useful for excluding carcinoma.

  References: [1–8]

4. **What is the significance of dot-like or membranous CD117 staining?**
   - The CD117 immunostain typically demonstrates diffuse cytoplasmic staining of GISTs.
   - In some cases, the CD117 pattern may show cytoplasmic staining along with dot-like perinuclear staining. This pattern should be regarded as positive and is not associated with mutation type or a specific response to therapy.
   - Some GISTs may demonstrate predominantly membranous CD117 staining. This pattern should also be regarded as positive and does not correlate with mutation type or response to therapy.

   References: [8, 9]

5. **What is the immunoprofile of epithelioid GIST? What pitfalls should one be aware of?**
   - Most epithelioid GISTs have the same immunoprofile as spindle cell GISTs.
   - However, they may demonstrate focal, weak expression of CD117.
   - They may also be cytokeratin positive. Cytokeratin expression is typically focal and weak but on occasion can be moderate and diffuse (Fig. 19.2a–c).
   - DOG1 is useful when CD117 is weak or when cytokeratin expression is present.

   Reference: Miettinen and Lasota [10]

6. **What histologic features meet criteria for a "mixed"-type GIST? Is there any prognostic significance to this term?**
   - GISTs are classified into three categories based on cytomorphology (Fig. 19.3a–c):
     - Spindle cell type – which is entirely spindled
     - Epithelioid type – which is entirely epithelioid
     - Mixed – which has both spindled and epithelioid morphologies
   - No declared minimum proportion of epithelioid (or spindled) morphology is necessary to be considered a mixed GIST, and even focal epithelioid cytology is recognized.

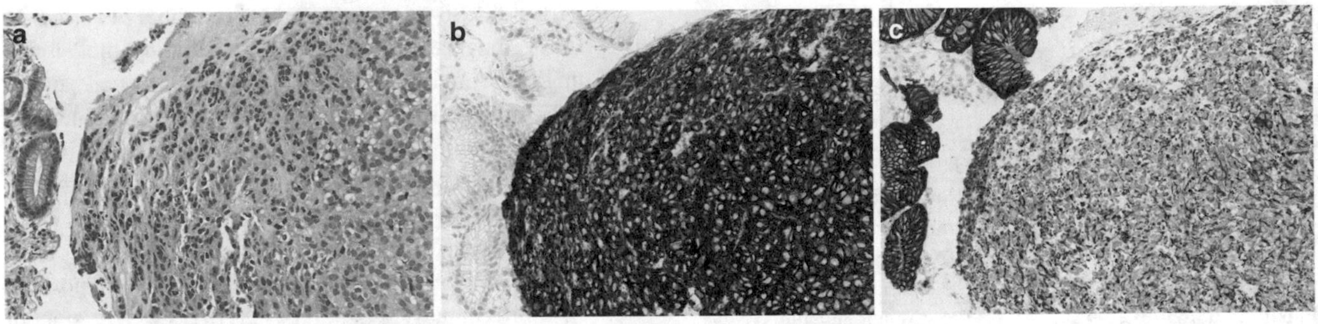

Fig. 19.2 Epithelioid GIST. (**a**) H&E. (**b**) CD117. (**c**) CK AE1/3. This tumor was confirmed to have a *KIT* mutation and responded to imatinib therapy with marked therapy-related changes noted on subsequent resection

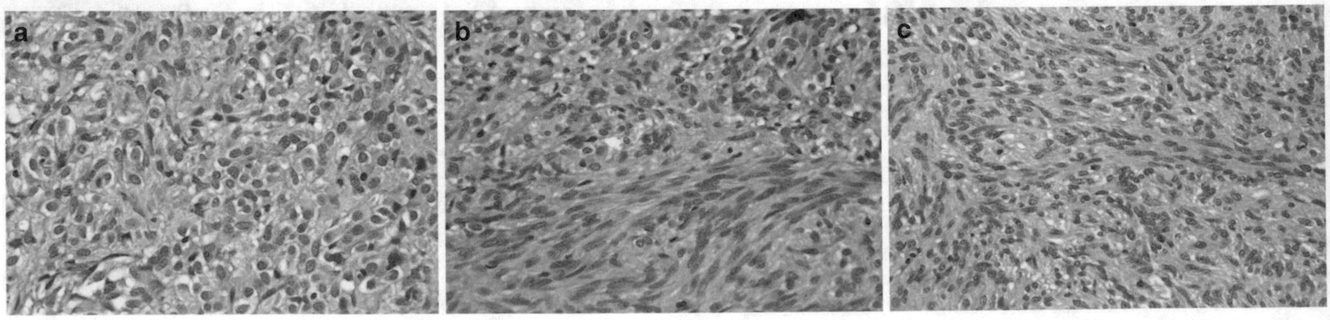

Fig. 19.3 Mixed-type GIST. (**a**) Epithelioid area. (**b**) Transition from epithelioid to spindled morphology. (**c**) Spindled area

- Mixed GISTs can have either distinct areas showing spindled and epithelioid morphologies or intermixed spindle and epithelioid cells. They may even have an "intermediate" ovoid appearance when the two cell morphologies are intimately commingled.
- Because there may be an abrupt transition from spindle cell morphology to epithelioid morphology, adequate tumor sampling (e.g., a minimum of one section per centimeter of tumor) is recommended.
- Although in some cases epithelioid or mixed-type GISTs are associated with more aggressive behavior, no official prognostic significance is currently attributed to these morphologic subtypes. However, the presence of epithelioid morphology in a tumor should prompt review of the clinical history in order to evaluate for the possibility of a *PDGFRA*-mutated or SDHB-deficient GIST (either of which may have consequences for treatment).

References: [9–11]

7. **What is a syndromic GIST? What morphologic features are indicative of syndromic GISTs?**

The term "syndromic GIST" refers to those tumors arising in association with a germline mutation or somatic DNA alteration (e.g., methylation) that predisposes to GISTs and is associated with other clinical signs and symptoms. Multiplicity with or without diffuse or confluent ICC hyperplasia is an important morphologic clue for pathologists to consider the diagnosis of syndromic GIST (more in question #25). The largest group is the Carney triad/Carney-Stratakis group (which accounts for almost all SDHB-deficient GISTs) and is estimated to represent approximately 5% of all GISTs. See Table 19.2.

References: [12–17]

8. **What is the definition of pediatric GIST? How is it different from classical GIST in morphology and molecular mechanism?**
   - The term "pediatric GIST" was originally defined as GIST occurring in a patient 18 years or younger and was coined to describe the unique features of GISTs occurring in this age group.
   - It is now clear that the vast majority of these tumors are SDHB-deficient GISTs. SDHB-deficient GISTs comprise virtually all GISTs in patients less than 20 years old and half of those aged 20–30 years.
   - SDHB-deficient GISTs are characterized by mutation in one of the four subunits of the succinate dehydrogenase complex. Mutation in any one of these genes (*SDHA*, *SDHB*, *SDHC*, *SDHD*) results in a defective SDH complex and destabilization of the SDHB protein. Alternatively, *SDHC* gene inactivation via promoter methylation has been described (and has the same impact on SDHB protein stability).
   - Loss or attenuation of SDHB protein expression serves as a marker of a defective succinate dehydrogenase complex. Thus, these tumors are collectively known as SDHB-deficient GISTs.
   - SDHB-deficient GISTs are associated with unique clinicopathologic features and biologic behavior compared to sporadic GISTs (summarized in Table 19.3).

   References: [5, 10, 18–20]

Table 19.2 Clinicopathologic features of GIST syndromes

Syndrome	Gene defect	Incidence	GIST phenotype	Tumor behavior	Associated features
Familial *KIT*	Germline *KIT* mutation	35 families identified to date	Spindle cell GISTs, multifocal, anywhere in GI tract, ICC hyperplasia	Thought to be similar to sporadic *KIT*-mutated GIST	Achalasia, melanoma, lentigines, urticaria pigmentosa
Familial *PDGFRA*	Germline *PDGFRA* mutation	5 families identified to date	Epithelioid GISTs, stomach	Appear to be low risk, but too few cases	Female predominance, inflammatory fibroid polyp, lipoma, large hands
Carney triad	*SDHC* promoter methylation	7.5% of all gastric GIST (estimated)	Epithelioid or mixed; plexiform/nodular architecture, multifocal, stomach	Can present with metastasis, but can have paradoxically indolent behavior	Pulmonary chondroma, paraganglioma; not heritable
Carney-Stratakis	*SDHA, SDHB, SDHC*, or *SDHD* mutation				Overlaps with Carney triad, renal cell carcinoma; heritable
Neurofibromatosis-1	*NF1*	1:5000 with germline mutation; only 7% develop GIST	Spindle cell GISTs, multifocal, small bowel, ICC hyperplasia	Generally low risk, but unclear if they respond to imatinib	Neurofibroma, ganglioneuroma, café au lait spots, pheochromocytoma, neuroendocrine tumors

ICC interstitial cells of Cajal

Table 19.3 Comparison of clinicopathologic features between sporadic and SDHB-deficient GISTs

Characteristic	Sporadic	SDHB-deficient
Age at presentation	>50 years	~20 years
Site	Anywhere in the abdomen	Stomach
Lymph node metastasis	Uncommon	Common
Focality	Unifocal	Often multifocal
Architecture	Well-circumscribed	Plexiform/nodular
Morphology	Spindle cell (most common)	Epithelioid or mixed
Molecular mechanism	*KIT* or *PDGFRA* mutation (most often)	Defect in one of the SDH genes
Prognosis	Variable by size, mitotic activity, metastasis	Can be indolent despite metastasis

9. **What tumor characteristics are important for assessing malignant potential (risk stratification)?**
   - Although GISTs are sarcomas, their behavior is distinct compared to other types of sarcoma. In particular, aggressive behavior is seen at lower mitotic counts than that seen in other sarcomas.
   - As such, it is recognized that the established French Federation of Comprehensive Cancer Centers (FNCLCC) system, used to classify other soft tissue sarcomas, is not optimal for classification for GISTs.
   - Based on the work of Miettinen and colleagues, three features have been found to be independent prognostic indicators: tumor size, tumor site, and mitotic activity. These were combined to develop a disease progression table (Tables 19.4a and 19.4b), endorsed by the American Joint Committee on Cancer (AJCC), the National Comprehensive Cancer Network (NCCN), and the College of American Pathologists (CAP) (see CAP protocol for corresponding risk assessment table, Laurini et al. [8]).
   - This disease progression table was developed after clinicopathologic evaluation of a large number of GISTs of various sites and has since been validated by others. Importantly, the risk stratification table is appropriate for treatment-naïve tumors only, and it is primarily used to determine whether systemic therapy should be considered (either before or following resection).
   - Additional features, in particular intra-abdominal tumor rupture, have shown some association with biological aggressiveness but are currently not considered in the disease progression table or risk assessment.

   References: [10, 18, 21–25]

Table 19.4a Disease progression table for gastric GISTs

Stage	Tumor size (cm)	Mitotic rate (mitoses/5 mm^2)	Rate of aggressive disease
IA	≤5	≤5	0–2%
IB	>5–10	≤5	3–4%
II	≤2	>5	Insufficient data
	>2–5	>5	16%
	>10	≤5	12%
IIIA	>5–10	>5	55%
IIIB	>10	>5	86%

Modified from AJCC Cancer Staging Manual 8th edition

Table 19.4b Disease progression table for small intestinal GISTs

Stage	Tumor size (cm)	Mitotic rate (mitoses/5 mm^2)	Rate of aggressive disease
IA	≤5	≤5	0–4%
II	>5–10	≤5	24%
IIIA	≤2	>5	50%
	>10	≤5	52%
IIIB	>2–5	>5	73%
	>5–10	>5	85%
	>10	>5	90%

Modified from AJCC Cancer Staging Manual 8th edition

10. **What criteria should be used to diagnose and grade extra-gastrointestinal GISTs? Is the immunoprofile similar to typical GISTs?**
    - Extra-gastrointestinal GISTs (E-GIST) are uncommon (<1% of all GISTs).
    - Aside from mesenteric and omental locations, E-GISTs have been reported (rarely) to arise in other organs such as the gallbladder, pancreas, liver, urinary bladder, and vagina.
    - The same histologic and immunophenotypic criteria should be used to diagnose E-GIST as that used for conventional gastrointestinal GIST. Specifically, E-GISTs display the same spindle cell, epithelioid, or mixed morphology as GISTs, express differentiation markers compatible with interstitial cells of Cajal (e.g., CD117, DOG1, CD34), and frequently harbor *KIT* or *PDGFRA* mutations.
    - Risk assessment is based on the criteria developed by Miettinen and Lasota in 2006, with omental E-GISTs included in the same site category as the stomach (as their behavior appears to be similar and they may in fact represent detached gastric primaries). All other E-GISTs are included in the same risk category as small intestinal tumors.
    - Careful intraoperative and/or gross examination of the tumor is imperative, as seemingly focal attachment or apparent adhesion of tumor to the bowel may in fact demonstrate origin within the bowel wall on microscopic evaluation (and thus exclude the diagnosis of E-GIST).

- Similarly, careful histologic examination of the tumor pseudocapsule to identify possible residual muscularis propria is important when an intra-abdominal tumor is large and its precise relationship to the gastric or bowel wall is not evident. This finding would also exclude a diagnosis of E-GIST.
- Finally, it is essential to rule out the possibility of metastatic GIST before rendering the diagnosis of E-GIST.

  References: [9, 10, 26–28]

11. What histologic criteria should be used to identify mitotic figures in GIST?

- Mitotic counts can be overestimated in the assessment of GIST.
- It is necessary to apply stringent criteria when counting mitotic figures. In particular, pyknotic, karyorrhectic, and apoptotic nuclei must be distinguished from true mitoses (Fig. 19.4a–c).
  - Pyknotic – chromatin tightly condensed, often in a single dark globule. Cytoplasm (if visible) is typically eosinophilic and glassy, and the cell appears shrunken.
  - Karyorrhectic – irregularly fragmented and hyperchromatic chromatin associated with necrosis.
  - Apoptotic – small, generally smooth contoured chromatin particles, in intact tissue.
- Normal mitoses demonstrate "hairy" extensions of nuclear membrane material present as either:
  - A single plane or ring (metaphase/early anaphase)
  - Two separate bands (late anaphase/telophase)
- Atypical forms should also be included in the mitotic count, in particular those with tripolar or multipolar mitotic spindles.
- Fortunately, most GISTs have either very low or high mitotic activity. Thus, in practice a single equivocal mitotic figure will rarely impact treatment or management.

  References: [8, 24, 29–31]

12. Where and how many high-power fields should I count for the mitotic index?

To perform a mitotic count, it is important to first scan all tumor sections using the 10× objective in order to find a mitotic figure or, if easily identified, to find the area with the highest density of mitotic figures. Once this area has been identified, switch the objective to 40× (high-power field (HPF)), and count mitotic figures in consecutive fields until a surface area of 5 mm^2 has been viewed. The standard cutoff for low mitotic rate category is 5. Tumors with greater than 5 mitotic figures are classified as having a high mitotic rate. Note: It is not necessary to count mitotic figures separately in areas with epithelioid or spindled morphology; it is only the area of highest mitotic activity that determines the mitotic count.

To determine the number of HPFs equivalent to 5 mm^2, you must know the field number (FN) of the microscope eyepiece. This number is typically displayed on the barrel of the eyepiece. Once the FN is identified, use the chart below to obtain the number of HPFs required for 5 mm^2. See Table 19.5.

13. What are the histologic features of treatment effect? How do you estimate % viable tumor?

- Histologic features attributed to treatment effect include tumor with:
  - Paucicellular hyalinized and/or myxoid stroma
  - Fibrosis
  - Calcification
  - Necrosis
- These histologic features can also be seen in treatment-naïve GISTs. Thus, it is important not to classify changes as treatment effect if incompatible with the clinical setting.
- At least some residual viable tumor nests (morphologically recognizable as GIST) are present in most treated GISTs. Complete pathologic response is uncommon.

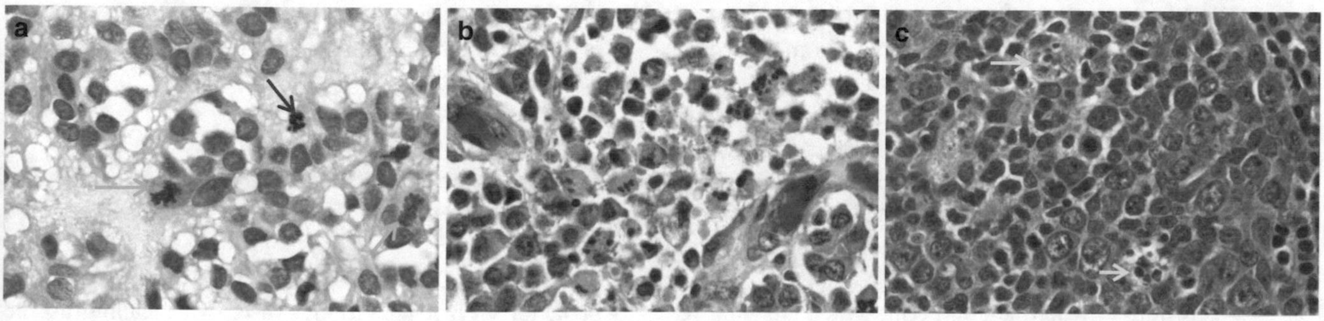

Fig. 19.4 Mitotic figures and mimics. (**a**) True mitotic figures (green arrows) and a pyknotic nucleus (red arrow). (**b**) Karyorrhexis: numerous tumor nuclei with irregularly fragmented chromatin within necrotic debris. (**c**) Apoptotic nuclei (yellow arrows)

Table 19.5 Conversion of 5 mm^2 to high-power fields

40× objective	Eyepiece field number (FN)								
	18	19	20	21	22	23	24	25	26
No. of HPFs for 5 mm^2	31.4	28.2	25.5	23.1	21.0	19.3	17.7	16.3	15.1

- In some cases, it may be difficult to distinguish non-neoplastic stromal cells in the paucicellular matrix from tumor cells. Immunostaining for markers of GIST can be useful, but it is important to note that CD117 and CD34 expression can be lost after targeted therapy (and desmin expression can be gained).
- The histologic features of treatment effect in metastases to lymph nodes and other distant sites are similar to those seen in the primary tumor.
- No specific procedure for estimation of percent viable tumor has been established, but in practice, it is performed by visually assessing percentage of viable tumor volume over all tumor sections at scanning power (4× or 10× objective).

References: [8, 32, 33]

14. What is the significance of tumor necrosis in GIST?

In the seminal papers by Miettinen and colleagues (Gastric GIST, 2005, and SB GIST, 2006), two types of tumor necrosis were described in GISTs: (1) coagulative and (2) liquefactive. A third type of necrosis, hyaline necrosis, is also worth mentioning, as discussed below (Fig. 19.5):

- Coagulative necrosis is characterized histologically by an abrupt transition from viable tumor cells to necrotic tissue. At the interface, discernible cell outlines ("ghost" cells) and hyperchromatic nuclear fragments are frequently present. Viable tumor cells may be clustered around intact intratumoral vessels.
- Liquefactive necrosis in GISTs is characterized by the presence of paucicellular fluid-filled spaces (necrosis) that in some cases may be rimmed or interspersed with a homogeneous, pale, glassy matrix. "Ghost" cells are not seen. Scattered plasma cells and lymphocytes may be seen within the spaces.
- Hyaline necrosis is characterized by the presence of paucicellular collagenous matrix (homogeneous, pale) separating areas of necrosis from viable tumor cells. Areas of necrosis may demonstrate intact, uniformly pale cell outlines, with similar changes in adjacent intratumoral vessels. These findings are thought to reflect prior infarction with reparative fibrosis. This type of necrosis is best characterized in uterine smooth muscle tumors.

According to Miettinen and colleagues, coagulative necrosis correlated with adverse prognosis. However, it is worth noting that ischemia can cause tumor necrosis in a "histologically benign" tumor. Although hyaline necrosis may be more frequently observed, in practice, it is difficult to distinguished it from coagulative necrosis. Presence of liquefactive necrosis had no prognostic value.

Because the original description of tumor necrosis only distinguishes coagulative and liquefactive necrosis, at this time, both coagulative necrosis and hyaline-type necrosis (if observed) should be reported. However, if the necrosis is exclusively hyaline type, it may be useful to mention it.

References: [30, 34, 35]

15. To confirm a GIST diagnosis at the primary site, why is endoscopic ultrasound-guided fine needle aspiration preferred over percutaneous biopsy? What information should be reported from such tissue samples for clinical management purposes?

Endoscopic ultrasound-guided fine needle aspiration (EUS-FNA) is preferred over percutaneous biopsy because it is associated with decreased risk of hemorrhage and tumor rupture (both of which can occur with large GISTs). Tumor rupture into the abdominal cavity is associated with peritoneal dissemination. Percutaneous biopsy may be suitable for evaluation of metastatic disease (e.g., liver, lymph nodes).

Information that should be reported with biopsies revealing a newly diagnosed GIST includes:

- Method of tissue procurement (e.g., EUS-FNA, computed tomography-guided percutaneous biopsy, etc.)
- Organ/site biopsied
- Morphologic subtype (spindle cell, epithelioid, mixed)
- Mitotic count per 5 mm^2
- Radiologically determined size of the tumor

This information is necessary for risk assessment and is used to determine the need for (or the benefit of) neoadjuvant therapy.

References: [6, 25]

16. Should the terms "malignant GIST" and "benign GIST" be used? Are there other terms I should be aware of?

Although the concept of benign and malignant behavior with regard to GISTs is still meaningful, the terms "malignant GIST" and "benign GIST" are no lon-

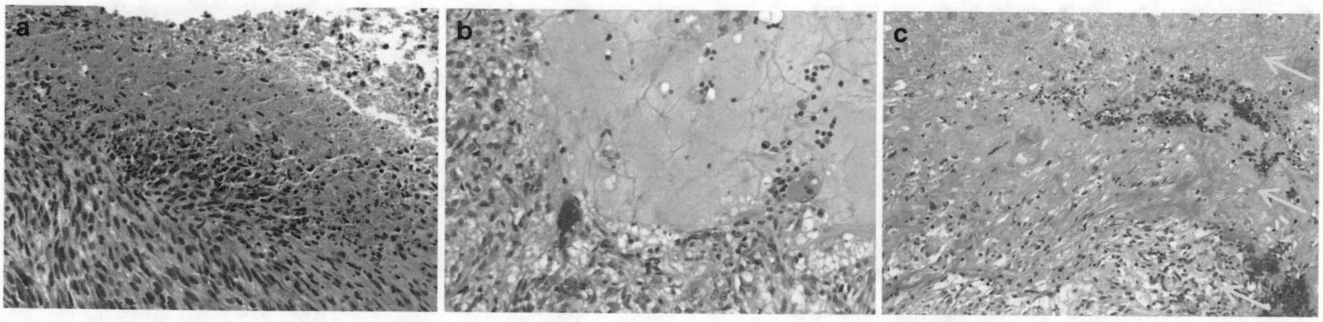

Fig. 19.5 Coagulative, liquefactive, and hyaline necrosis. (**a**) Coagulative (tumor-type) necrosis. (**b**) Liquefactive necrosis. (**c**) Hyaline (infarct-type) necrosis (top arrow, necrotic debris; middle arrow, hyaline interface; bottom arrow, GIST)

ger used because this dichotomous classification does not accurately capture the spectrum of biologic behavior observed in these tumors.

The currently accepted method for describing GIST behavior, endorsed by the AJCC, NCCN, and CAP is based on the risk stratification scheme developed by Miettinen and Lasota. In particular, all GISTs measuring less than 2 cm and having less than 5 mitotic figures per 5 mm^2 are considered to have no risk of progression (e.g., benign). All other categories of GISTs are considered to have malignant potential, with risk being divided into very low, low, moderate, and high categories, depending on tumor site, size, and mitotic activity.

Other Terms Used in Relation to GIST

Advanced GIST

- Metastatic or unresectable GIST

Mini-GIST

- GISTs measuring 1–2 cm, also referred to as "subclinical"
- Term not officially endorsed by AJCC, NCCN, or CAP

Microscopic GIST (Micro-GIST)

- GISTs measuring 1 cm or less; usually reserved for incidental lesions of the stomach and gastroesophageal junction
- Also described as "seedling mesenchymal tumors," if <0.5 cm; characterized in the gastroesophageal junction and proximal stomach
- Term not officially endorsed by AJCC, NCCN, or CAP

GIST Tumorlet

- 0.5–1.0 cm, grossly visible or palpable, in the proximal stomach
- Term not officially endorsed by AJCC, NCCN, or CAP

ICC Hyperplasia: Diffuse

- Microscopic expansion of interstitial cells of Cajal between layers of muscularis propria (not grossly identifiable); can be nodular or diffuse, presumably less than 0.5 cm if nodular
- Term not officially endorsed by AJCC, NCCN, or CAP

References: [9, 10, 36–39]

17. **What are the most common sites of metastasis for sporadic GISTs?**
    - The most common sites of metastasis both at presentation and following surgical resection are the liver (Fig. 19.6a) and peritoneum. Multiple microscopic tumor nodules of various sizes in the vicinity of a primary tumor demonstrating infiltrative growth pattern are characteristic of intraperitoneal spreading (Fig. 19.6b, c).
    - Less common sites of metastasis include the lymph node, lung, and bone.
    - When metastasis to the lung occurs, it is typically associated with a rectal primary (due to drainage of the lymphatic system) or with widely metastatic disease.

    References: [11, 34, 35, 40–43]

18. **If no lymph nodes are found or submitted with the tumor resection, should pN0 or pNX be used for AJCC tumor staging?**

    Because sporadic GISTs rarely metastasize to lymph nodes, the AJCC recommends lymph node sampling at the time of resection *only if* abnormal or suspicious lymph nodes are identified. In the absence of information on regional lymph node involvement, AJCC recommends using "cN0" (clinically no lymph node metastasis) instead of "NX" for purposes of clinical staging (e.g., TNM classification). According to the 2019 College of American Pathologists (CAP) GIST reporting template, for those resections without lymph nodes, the pathological "N" category is not assigned and should not be reported.

    References: [8, 24]

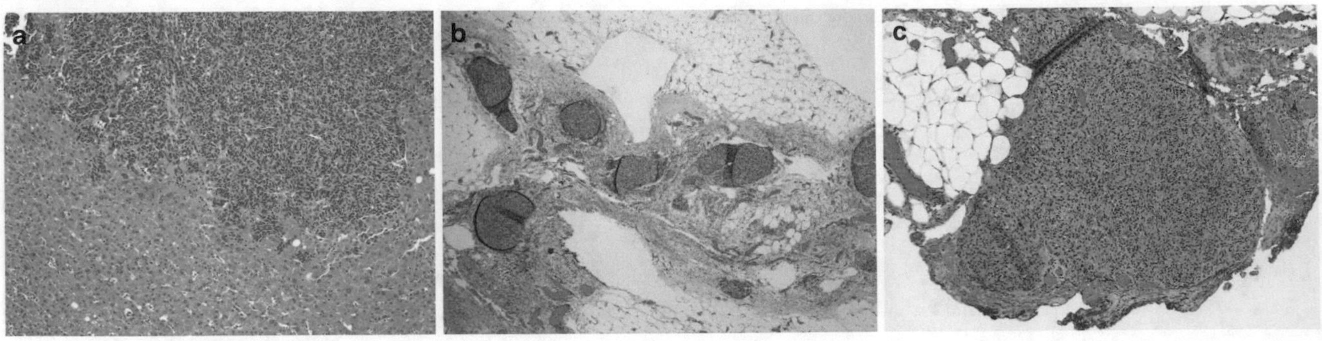

Fig. 19.6 Characteristic pattern of intraperitoneal spreading. (**a**) Metastatic epithelioid GIST in the liver. (**b**) Multiple tumor nodules in the mesentery. (**c**) Isolated nodule in the omentum. (Courtesy of Dr. Michael Torbenson, Mayo Clinic)

19. **Should all GISTs be staged according to the AJCC staging manual?**
    - Only sporadic GISTs should be given a TNM classification.
    - TNM classification is not appropriate for GISTs associated with germline *KIT* mutation, germline *PDGFRA* mutation, Carney triad, Carney-Stratakis syndrome, or neurofibromatosis type 1. This recommendation reflects the unique biologic behavior of each of the GISTs associated with these syndromes.
    - If a tumor is suspected to be associated with a syndrome based on pathologic findings or other clinical information (e.g., young patient age, gastric GIST with epithelioid and multinodular/plexiform features), it may be useful to suspend TNM classification until further information is available. However, reporting the elements needed for TNM classification (tumor size, lymph node involvement, evidence of metastasis) is important for completeness and in the event that TNM staging is needed.

    References: [8, 24]

20. **Should grading and risk assessment be performed on post-therapy resections?**

    Both grading and risk assessment criteria were developed for treatment-naïve GISTs. As such, they do not provide clinically meaningful information for post-therapy specimens and thus should be avoided.

    References: [10]

21. **What is the significance of multifocal GIST? How does one differentiate multifocal disease from intraperitoneal metastasis?**
    - Multifocal GIST mostly occurs in GIST-associated syndromes (i.e., Carney triad, Carney-Stratakis syndrome, neurofibromatosis type 1, germline *KIT* and germline *PDGFRA* syndromes) and may be the first clue to the presence of a syndromic GIST.
    - However, multifocal GISTs are also occasionally seen in the sporadic setting.
    - The gold standard for distinction of syndromic and sporadic GISTs is mutational analysis of all (or at least a subset of) the patient's GISTs. Syndromic GISTs will all bear the same driver mutation, whereas sporadic multifocal GISTs will possess mutational profiles that are distinct from one another.
    - Distinction of multifocal disease from intraperitoneal metastasis is important because metastatic lesions may not be subjected to genotyping.
    - The following morphologic features favor metastasis over multifocal disease:
      - High-risk morphology (e.g., high mitotic activity, coagulative necrosis)
      - Infiltrative growth (e.g., invasion into fat)
      - Poor circumscription of tumor
      - No clear association with muscularis propria
      - Presence of tumor at other sites where GIST is known to metastasize (liver, lung, bone)

      References: [44, 45]

22. **What risk assessment category should be used if the primary site of GIST is an anatomic site other than stomach, duodenum, jejunum/ileum, or rectum?**
    - GISTs arising in locations not specified in the risk assessment scheme (e.g., esophagus, colon, peritoneum- with the exception for omentum) are placed in the corresponding jejunum/ileum GIST risk category. This is due to the fact that too few documented examples exist to derive an independent risk category for these sites.
    - In some categories of the risk assessment table, there is "insufficient data" to assign a risk category (such as for duodenal GISTs less than or equal to 2 cm with greater than 5 mitotic figures per 5 mm^2). It is also recommended that the corresponding jejunum/ileum-risk category be used in these cases.

- One potential source of confusion is that clinical staging (stages I–IV) of GISTs is divided into two systems, one for gastric and one for small intestine. In this clinical classification, omental GISTs are included in the gastric staging system, whereas all other anatomic sites are recommended to follow the small intestinal group staging scheme.
  References: [8, 10, 24]

23. Should all GISTs be tested for KIT and PDGFRA mutation? Can the type of mutation predict prognosis?

- The current NCCN recommendation is to test all GISTs for *KIT* and *PDGFRA* mutations, without regard to whether or not systemic therapy is planned.
- The primary rationale for *KIT* and *PDGFRA* mutation testing is to determine susceptibility to imatinib (which, depending on clinical and pathologic findings, may or may not be indicated).
- This recommendation also allows for identification of the subset of GISTs without *KIT* or *PDGFRA* mutation. This is important since the majority of the non-*KIT*- and non-*PDGFRA*-mutated GISTs are SDHB-deficient tumors which have a markedly different biologic behavior and warrant consideration of an alternative management approach.
- With regard to *KIT*- and *PDGFRA*-mutated GISTs, the specific type of mutation (e.g., *KIT* exon 11 mutation versus *KIT* exon 9 mutation) may be associated with more or less aggressive behavior (see next question). If systemic therapy is indicated, the specific mutation in *KIT* or *PDGFRA* predicts tumor response to imatinib and will in turn determine selection of tyrosine kinase inhibitor and overall prognosis.
  References: [18, 25]

24. How can specific mutation profiles help guide therapy?

***KIT* Mutations**

KIT mutations cluster in four exons: 11, 9, 13, and 17.

- Mutations in exon 11 are the most common (65–70%). Although GISTs with mutations in this exon have been noted to be more aggressive than those with mutations in other *KIT* exons, the vast majority of the *KIT* exon 11-mutated GISTs (90%) respond to standard imatinib therapy.
- Mutations in exon 9 account for 13% of *KIT*-mutated GISTs. Studies have shown that they are relatively less sensitive to imatinib (50% response). However, at increased imatinib dose (800 mg vs 400 mg), response rates approach those seen with the exon 11-mutant GISTs.
- Mutations in exon 13 account for approximately 1% of *KIT*-mutated GISTs. Some evidence suggests that they are sensitive to imatinib therapy.
- Mutations in exon 17 are present in 0.6% of GISTs. Although in theory they may be less sensitive to imatinib (based on in vitro studies), they have been documented to respond to imatinib.

***PDGFRA* Mutations**

PDGFRA mutations mainly occur in three exons: 18, 12, and 14. Studies have shown that they are less likely to recur compared to *KIT*-mutated GISTs.

- Mutations in exon 18 cluster around amino acid 842. The most common mutation, D842V, representing 70% of *PDGFRA*-mutated GISTs, is resistant to imatinib. However, the second most common mutation in exon 18, deletion of amino acids 842–845, is imatinib-sensitive.
- Mutations in exon 12 are thought to be imatinib-sensitive.
- Mutations in exon 14 are thought to have a favorable prognosis; however, sensitivity to imatinib therapy is not known.
- Other tyrosine kinase inhibitors crenolanib and regorafenib appear to have activity against the *PDGFRA*-mutated, imatinib-resistant GISTs.
  References: [7, 46]

25. When should the possibility of germline KIT or PDGFRα syndrome be considered?

Both germline *KIT* syndrome and germline *PDGFRA* syndrome are rare, with only 40 affected kindreds identified to date. Yet knowledge of the clinical and pathologic features of these two syndromes is important, as they have significant consequences for both the patients (e.g., risk of other tumors) and their families (inherited disease).

Germline *KIT* Syndrome

- Described in 35 kindreds to date.
- Multiple synchronous or metachronous GISTs in the stomach and/or small bowel.
- Most GISTs have spindled morphology.
- Background Cajal cell hyperplasia present (can also be seen in patients with neurofibromatosis type 1).
- Variable presentation in terms of number of GISTs and other clinical features.
- Other diseases include melanoma; hyperpigmentation/lentigines of mucocutaneous sites, trunk and

face; urticaria pigmentosa/systemic mastocytosis; and achalasia.

Germline *PDGFRA* Syndrome

- Described in five families to date.
- Most GISTs are gastric and some in the small bowel and colon.
- Most GISTs have epithelioid or mixed morphology.
- No Cajal cell hyperplasia.
- Other diseases include multiple inflammatory fibroid polyps (frequently outnumbering the GISTs), other mesenchymal fibrous tumors of the GI tract, lipomas, and large hands.
- One expert recommends consideration of *PDGFRA* syndrome when two or greater inflammatory fibroid polyps and/or gastric GISTs are identified in a single patient or in a single family.

References: [13, 15, 47, 48]

26. In the absence of KIT and PDGFRA mutations, would a GIST still be responsive to imatinib therapy?

Generally speaking, *KIT*- and *PDGFRA*-negative GISTs do not respond to imatinib. GISTs that are negative for both *KIT* and *PDGFRA* mutations were originally termed "wildtype GISTs." They account for approximately 10–15% of all GISTs. Approximately 5% of these GISTs contain defects in the succinate dehydrogenase complex, most of which are due to germline mutation in one of the four SDH genes (*SDHA*, *SDHB*, *SDHC*, *SDHD*). Among the SDHB-defective GISTs, germline mutation in *SDHA* is the most common. The rest of the SDHB-defective tumors (a small minority) have normal *SDH* genes and are instead characterized by hypermethylation of the *SDHC* promoter. The hypermethylation is a somatic change and non-heritable, which explains the non-heritability of the Carney triad. The remaining non-*KIT*- and *non-PDGFRA*-mutated GISTs are *NF1*- or *BRAF*-mutated (each accounting for approximately 3% of all GISTs) or have other rare mutations or as yet unclassified molecular defects.

Because non-*KIT*- and non-*PDGFRA*-mutated GISTs are relatively uncommon and as a group consist of a genetically heterogeneous mix of tumors (e.g., SDHB-deficient, *NF1*-mutated, *BRAF*-mutated, and others), there is currently insufficient data to support a specific treatment paradigm for all or any subset of them. However, clinical trials, both recent and ongoing, as well as case reports do point to a role for different tyrosine kinase inhibitors in clinical management and also offer other treatment opportunities to those who would otherwise have no validated chemotherapeutic options.

- For SDHB-deficient tumors, sunitinib and regorafenib have demonstrated some beneficial effects. As of August 2020, two clinical trials were recently completed for SDH-deficient tumors: one testing the glutaminase inhibitor CB-839, and the other testing the DNA methyltransferase inhibitor guadecitabine. Results are still pending for both studies.
- For all advanced GISTs regardless of driver mutation, the antibody-conjugated drug DS-6157a, targeting GPR20, is currently being tested for activity against GIST. GPR20 is a G-protein coupled receptor highly expressed in GIST (clinical trial currently recruiting).
- For *BRAF*-mutated tumors, dabrafenib, a BRAF inhibitor, showed clinical activity in one *BRAF*-mutated GIST. Dabrafenib and trametinib are currently being tested for *BRAF*-mutated GISTs (clinical trial open, no longer recruiting as of August 2020).

References: [19, 49–54]

27. When is it appropriate to order SDHB immunohistochemistry?

- Because of their frequently multifocal and metastatic presentation yet indolent behavior, SDHB-deficient tumors may not undergo surgical resection. As such, identification of this subset is critical for appropriate clinical management.
- Clinical and morphologic features suggesting the possibility of a SDHB-deficient GIST include:
  - Young patient age (<40 years)
  - Gastric primary with histology that is epithelioid or mixed type and/or plexiform/nodular
  - Multiple synchronous GISTs
  - Lymph node metastasis
  - Concurrent or prior tumors such as paraganglioma, pulmonary chondroma, and renal cell carcinoma
- The most commonly mutated gene in SDHB-deficient GISTs is *SDHA*. Because expression of both SDHA and SDHB is lost in *SDHA*-mutated tumors, SDHB immunohistochemistry can be a useful screen.
- Immunohistochemistry for both SDHB and SDHA is recommended when an epithelioid gastric GIST with multinodular architecture is identified at resection or when a small biopsy of gastric GIST demonstrates epithelioid morphology, particularly those occurring in young patients.

– The current version of the CAP GIST reporting template (published in August 2019) recommends that all gastric GISTs be screened for SDH deficiency by SDHB immunohistochemistry.
  References: [12, 19, 55]

28. When is BRAF V600E mutation testing appropriate, and what is the clinical significance of this mutation?

The NCCN Sarcoma Guidelines (version 2.2020) recommends that tumors lacking *KIT* or *PDGFRA* mutations undergo further evaluation, including SDHB immunohistochemistry for gastric GISTs and next generation sequencing (including BRAF, NF1, and other genes) for non-gastric GISTs and gastric GISTs with intact SDHB expression. The rationale is that if systemic therapy is indicated, identification of a *BRAF*-mutated GIST (or other targetable gene abnormality) would allow for the possibility of targeted therapy.

The following molecular testing algorithm has been proposed for GISTs, based on the relative incidence of the various gene defects (which are mutually exclusive, except in rare cases):

(a) *KIT* mutation testing, with reflex to *PDGFRA* mutation testing
(b) If negative for (a), then SDHB immunohistochemistry; if abnormal, germline testing for mutation in one of the four *SDH* genes
(c) If SDHB expression is intact, *BRAF* and *NF1* gene mutation testing

This algorithm is based on the rationale that unique therapeutic options and responses are available for each type of gene defect. Additionally, for genetic alterations that are indicative of syndromes (e.g., neurofibromatosis type 1, Carney-Stratakis syndrome), genetic counseling and/or surveillance for additional tumors may be indicated.

References: [7, 28, 46]

Case Presentation

Case 1

Learning Objectives

1. To learn the histologic features of classic spindle cell GIST
2. To learn the histologic features of treatment effect
3. To learn the pathologic assessment of treated tumors

Case History

A 47-year-old female presented to the local emergency department with constipation, urinary retention, and a 2-week history of abdominal pain.

Imaging

By magnetic resonance imaging, a well-circumscribed 15 cm heterogeneously enhancing mass was identified between the vaginal wall and rectum. A needle core biopsy was performed.

Histologic Findings (Fig. 19.7a, b)

- Dense proliferation of spindle cells.
- Hyperchromatic nuclei.
- Abundant eosinophilic cytoplasm.
- Short, overlapping fascicles.

Differential Diagnosis

- Mullerian leiomyosarcoma
- Melanoma
- Gastrointestinal stromal tumor
- Malignant peripheral nerve sheath tumor

IHC and Other Ancillary Findings

- CD117 and DOG1 positive (Fig. 19.7c, d).
- Negative for S100, desmin, and cytokeratin AE1/3.
- Molecular testing revealed a *KIT* exon 11 mutation.

Final Diagnosis

KIT-mutated gastrointestinal stromal tumor.

Follow-Up

The patient was treated with 400 mg imatinib daily, resulting in marked diminution of the tumor over a period of 18 months. En bloc resection including the rectum, uterus, and posterior vaginal wall was subsequently performed, revealing a 6 cm nodular mass partially surfaced by bowel mucosa on one side and by vaginal wall on the opposite side. On sectioning, the tumor was predominantly solid with areas of cystic degeneration (Fig. 19.8).

Histologic Findings in Resection Specimen (Fig. 19.9a–d)

- Tumor present in association with the muscular layer of the rectum (confirming GI origin).
- Paucicellular, pale matrix with small intact vessels and scattered (non-neoplastic) stromal cells.
- Foci of calcification.
- Rare focus of residual tumor.
- ypT3.
- No "risk assessment" reported.

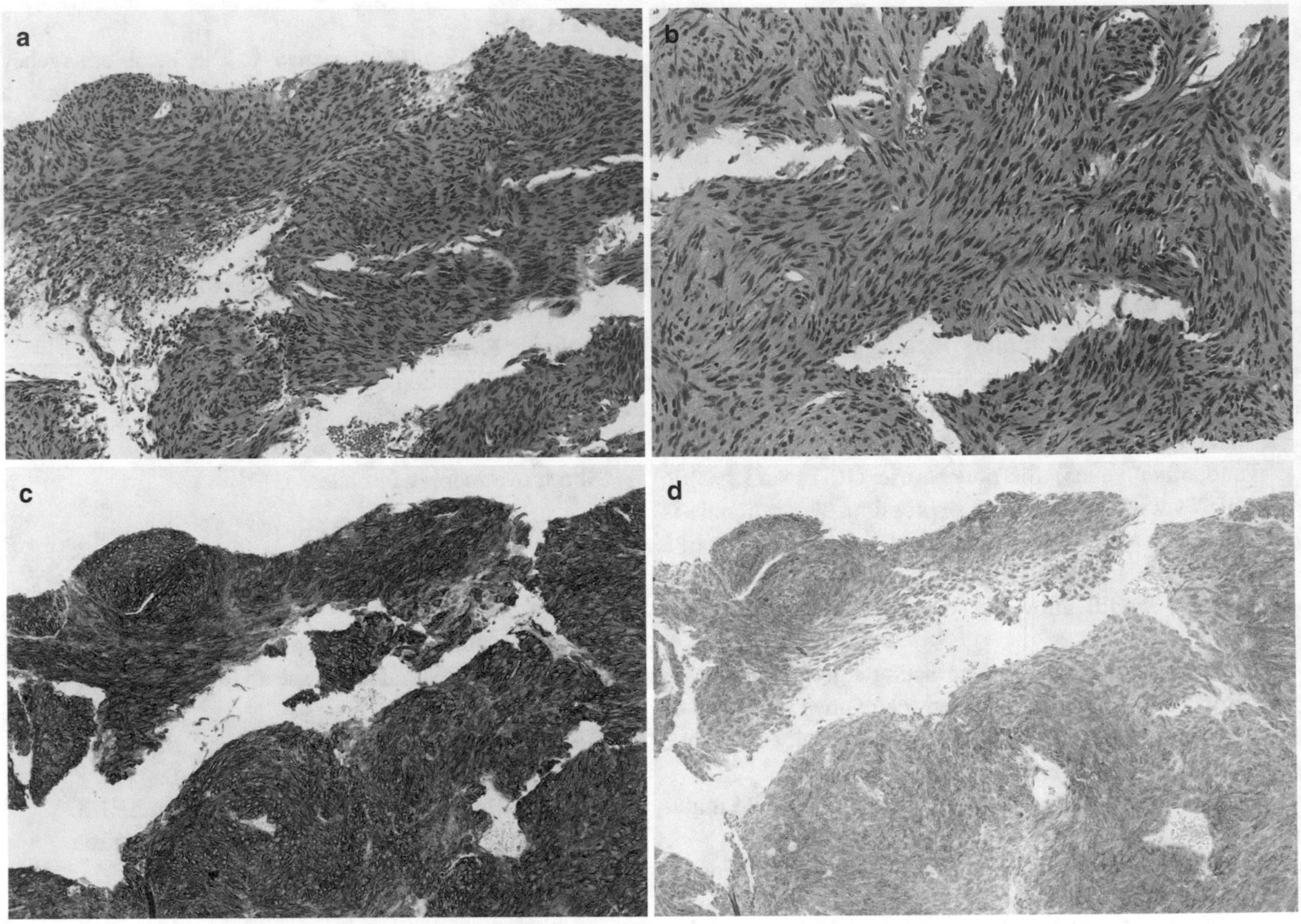

Fig. 19.7 Core biopsy of large pelvic mass. (**a**) H&E low-power view. (**b**) H&E high-power view showing hyperchromatic spindle cells in loose fascicles. (**c**) CD117 immunostain. (**d**) DOG1 immunostain

Take-Home Messages

- Demonstration of tumor relation to bowel wall is important to establish the diagnosis of GIST when other organs are involved.
- Even GISTs that show marked response to therapy usually demonstrate some residual viable tumor on histologic sections.
- If no lymph nodes are retrieved, no pathologic "N" category is assigned. Per CAP reporting guidelines, the designation "pNX" should not be used for GIST.
- Tumor size (for TNM purposes) is based on gross measurement (even if only a fraction of the tumor is viable).
- Risk assessment is not applicable in the post-treatment setting.

Case 2

Learning Objectives

1. To learn the morphologic and immunophenotypic features of *PDGFRA*-mutated GISTs
2. To learn the therapeutic consequences of the *PDGFRA* D842V mutation in GIST
3. To learn how to distinguish between tumor adhesion and tumor invasion

Case History

A 68-year-old female with a remote history of colon cancer (status post resection) and multiple episodes of small bowel obstruction presented to the emergency department for intermittent abdominal pain.

Imaging

On computed tomography, a large well-circumscribed heterogeneous mass arising between the stomach and liver was identified (Fig. 19.10).

Gross Findings

A 9 cm soft tissue mass associated with gastric wall and a small portion of the liver was received. On cut surface, the tumor demonstrated fleshy pink-tan and hemorrhagic cut

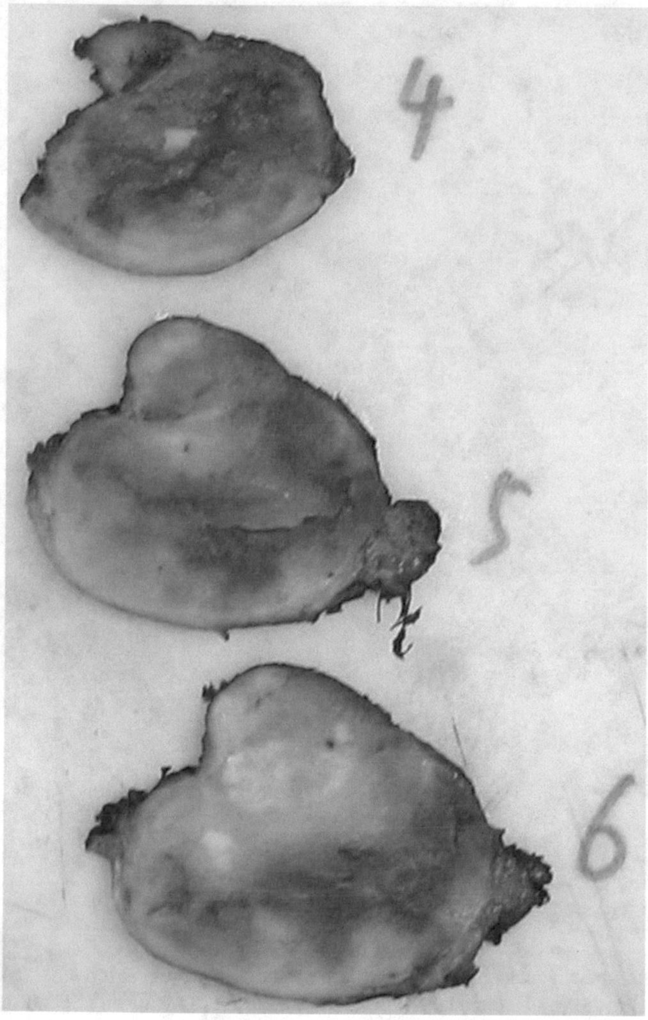

Fig. 19.8 Gross findings of treated GIST. This tumor is predominantly solid with central cystic degeneration (slice 4) as well as areas of fibrosis (solid white areas) and hemorrhage (dark areas)

surfaces with multiple small irregularly shaped cystic spaces (Fig. 19.11).

Histologic Findings (Figs. 19.12a–d and 19.13)

- Round to ovoid nuclei.
- Abundant eosinophilic cytoplasm.
- More prominent cytoplasmic borders, accentuating spherical shape of cells.
- 5 mitotic figures per 5 mm^2.
- Tumor abutting the liver but without evidence of parenchymal invasion.

Differential Diagnosis

- Glomus tumor
- Gastrointestinal stromal tumor
- Paraganglioma
- Carcinoma
- Melanoma

IHC and Other Ancillary Findings

- CD117, DOG1, and CD34 positive.
- Negative for S100, desmin, and cytokeratin AE1/3.
- Negative for *KIT* mutation in exons 9, 11, 13, 17, and 18.
- Positive for *PDGFRA* D842V mutation.

Final Diagnosis

Epithelioid gastrointestinal stromal tumor, intermediate risk, with *PDGFRA* D842V mutation.

Follow-Up

Given the risk of recurrence, adjuvant therapy was discussed with the patient. As *PDGFRA*-mutated GISTs with D842V mutation have been shown to be resistant to imatinib, alternative tyrosine kinase inhibitors were considered.

Take-Home Messages

- *PDGFRA*-mutated gastric GISTs are more frequently epithelioid than *KIT*-mutated gastric GISTs.
- Certain *PDGFRA*-mutated GISTs have been shown to be resistant to imatinib therapy, including those with *PDGFRA* D842V mutation (the most common *PDGFRA* mutation in GISTs).
- Large GISTs can impinge on neighboring organs and form adhesions. Invasion of another organ requires histologic evidence of infiltration beyond the tumor capsule into parenchyma.

Case 3

Learning Objectives

1. To recognize clinical and pathologic features of SDHB-deficient GISTs
2. To become familiar with interpretation of the SDHB immunostain
3. To learn the unique prognostic and therapeutic considerations of SDHB-deficient GISTs

Case History

A 15-year-old male presented with a 2-day history of acute periumbilical abdominal pain and was subsequently found to have a large gastric mass.

Imaging

On computed tomography, a 5 cm hemorrhagic and centrally necrotic mass arising from the gastric antrum was identified. In addition to the gastric mass, a hypermetabolic right com-

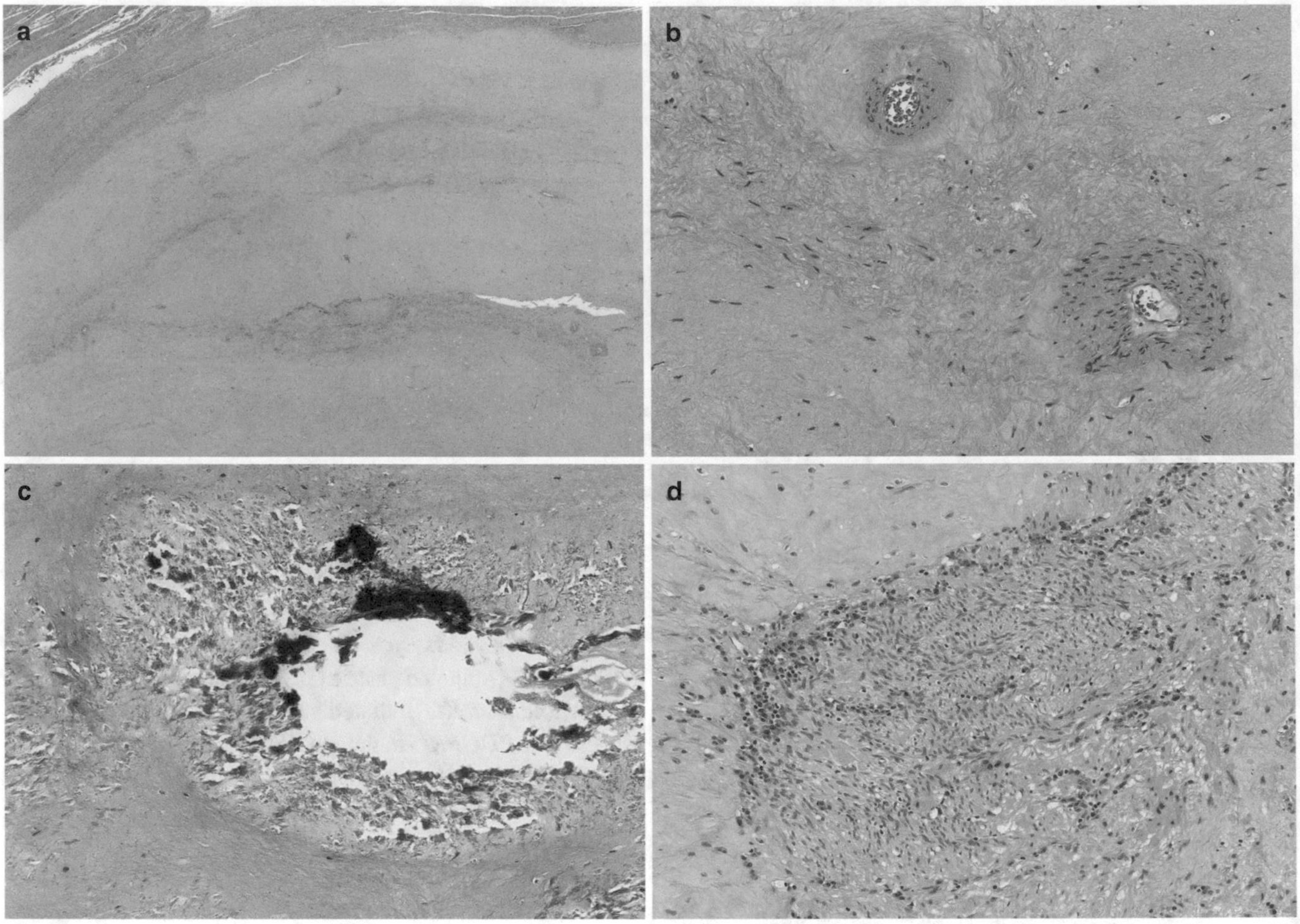

Fig. 19.9 Histologic features of treated GIST. (**a**) Low-power view showing pale, paucicellular matrix (note muscularis propria at top left). (**b**) High-power view showing residual small vessels and stromal cells. (**c**) Calcifications. (**d**) Residual tumor (center) adjacent to treatment effect (top left of image)

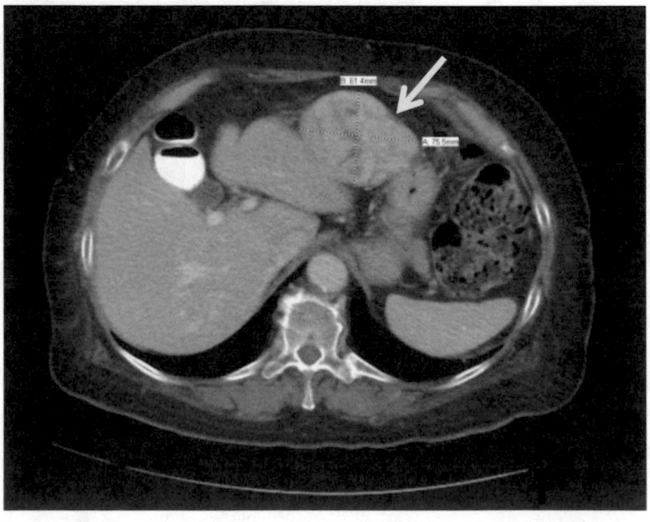

Fig. 19.10 Large abdominal mass. The large heterogeneous tumor (arrow) is situated between the liver (left) and stomach (right)

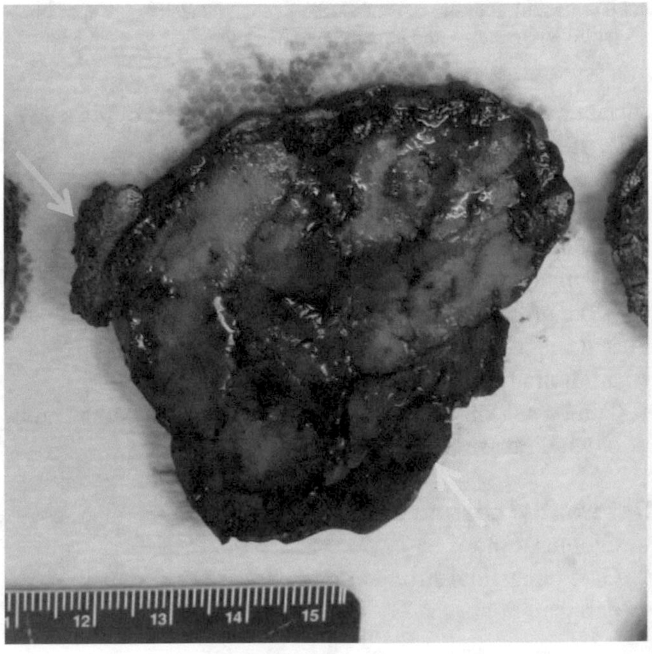

Fig. 19.11 Gross findings. The tumor is well-circumscribed and predominantly solid with areas of degeneration and fresh hemorrhage. The tumor is associated with gastric wall (orange arrow) and abuts the liver (yellow arrow)

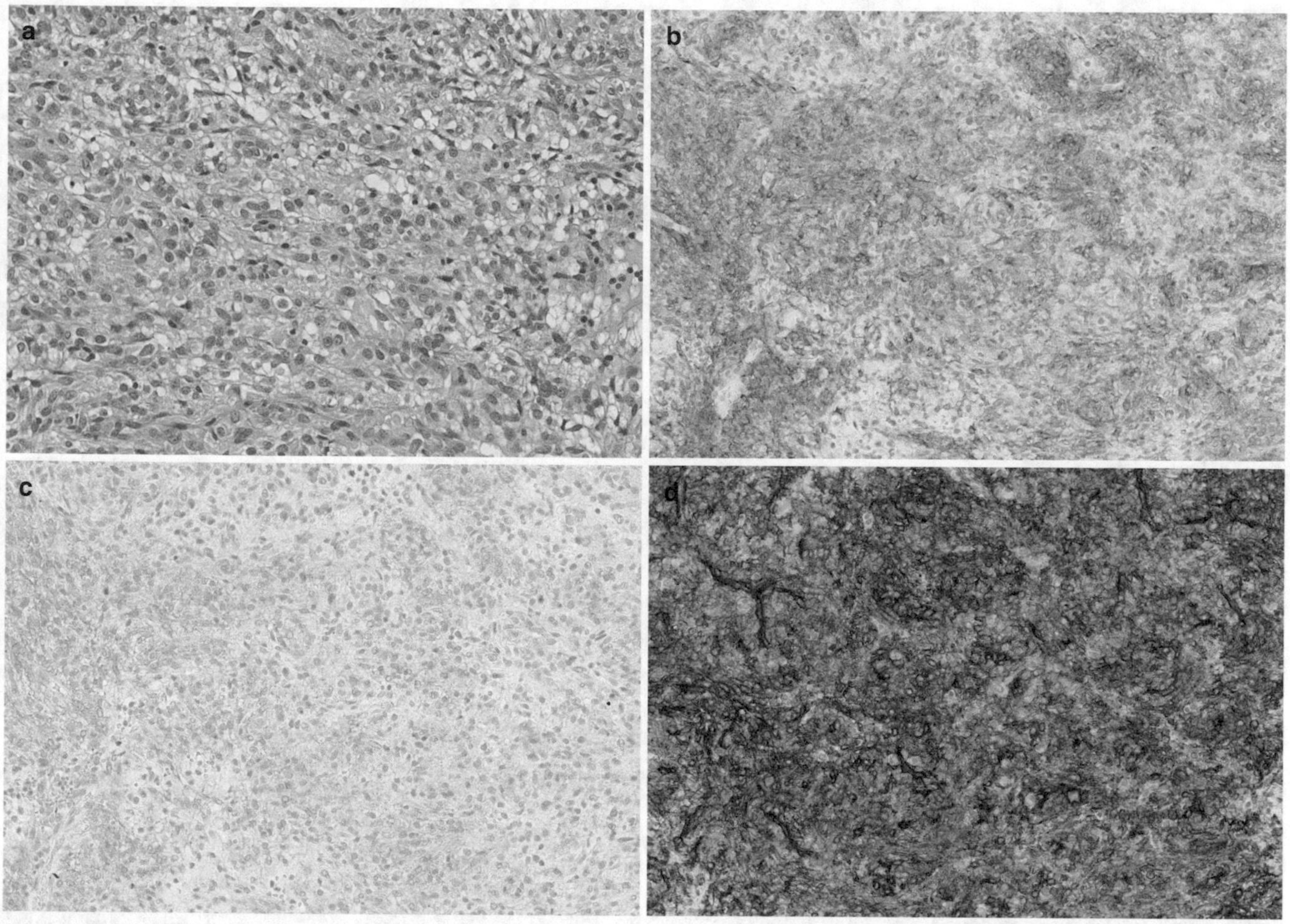

Fig. 19.12 Epithelioid GIST. (**a**) Tumor cells are round to ovoid with abundant eosinophilic cytoplasm and distinct cytoplasmic borders. (**b**) CD117 stain. (**c**) DOG1 stain. (**d**) CD34 stain

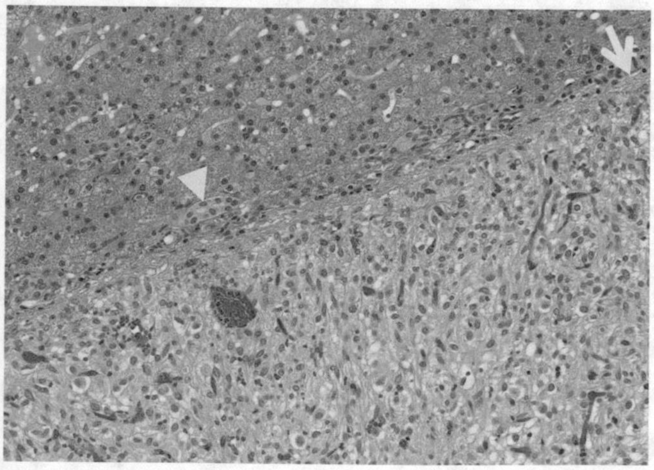

Fig. 19.13 GIST abutting the liver. Note the thin fibrous band separating the GIST and liver parenchyma (arrow). Also note the small biliary ducts (arrowhead) at the liver edge, a normal histologic finding near the liver capsule

mon iliac lymph node highly suspicious for metastatic disease was noted by positron emission tomography. Laparoscopy was initially performed with the intent of resection, but given the extent of disease, only biopsy was performed.

Histologic Findings (Figs. 19.14a, d and 19.15a).

- Round to ovoid nuclei.
- Abundant eosinophilic cytoplasm.
- Some areas with more spindled morphology.

Differential Diagnosis

- Melanoma
- Pancreatic solid pseudopapillary neoplasm (possibly impinging on the stomach)
- Neuroendocrine tumor
- Gastrointestinal stromal tumor

IHC and Other Ancillary Findings

- CD117 and DOG1 positive (Fig. 19.14b, c).
- Negative for synaptophysin.
- No *KIT* or *PDGFRA* mutation identified.
- Reduced SDHB expression in tumor cells by immunohistochemistry (Fig. 19.15b).

Final Diagnosis

SDHB-deficient gastrointestinal stromal tumor.

Follow-Up

The patient was started sunitinib therapy. Repeat imaging is planned to assess response to therapy in 6 weeks' time.

Take-Home Messages

- A SDHB-deficient tumor should be considered in a young patient who presents with a GIST, particularly when arising in the stomach, presenting with metastasis, and demonstrating epithelioid morphology.
- Immunohistochemistry for SDHB is useful for identification of SDHB-deficient tumors. Decreased or complete loss of expression of SDHB protein is consistent with SDH deficiency and merits follow-up molecular testing for a *SDH* mutation. SDHB-deficient GISTs also indicate a high risk of Carney-Stratakis syndrome, and genetic counseling may be useful.
- The risk assessment algorithm for GISTs does not apply to non-sporadic tumors, such as SDHB-deficient GISTs, as their biologic behavior is distinct. Additionally, TNM classification is not appropriate for non-sporadic GISTs.
- SDHB-deficient tumors do not respond to imatinib but have been shown to respond to sunitinib and regorafenib.
- Because SDHB-deficient tumors are frequently multifocal, present with metastasis, and yet are typically indolent, the risks and benefits of radical surgical resection for reasons other than symptomatic relief must be weighed carefully (particularly in a young patient).

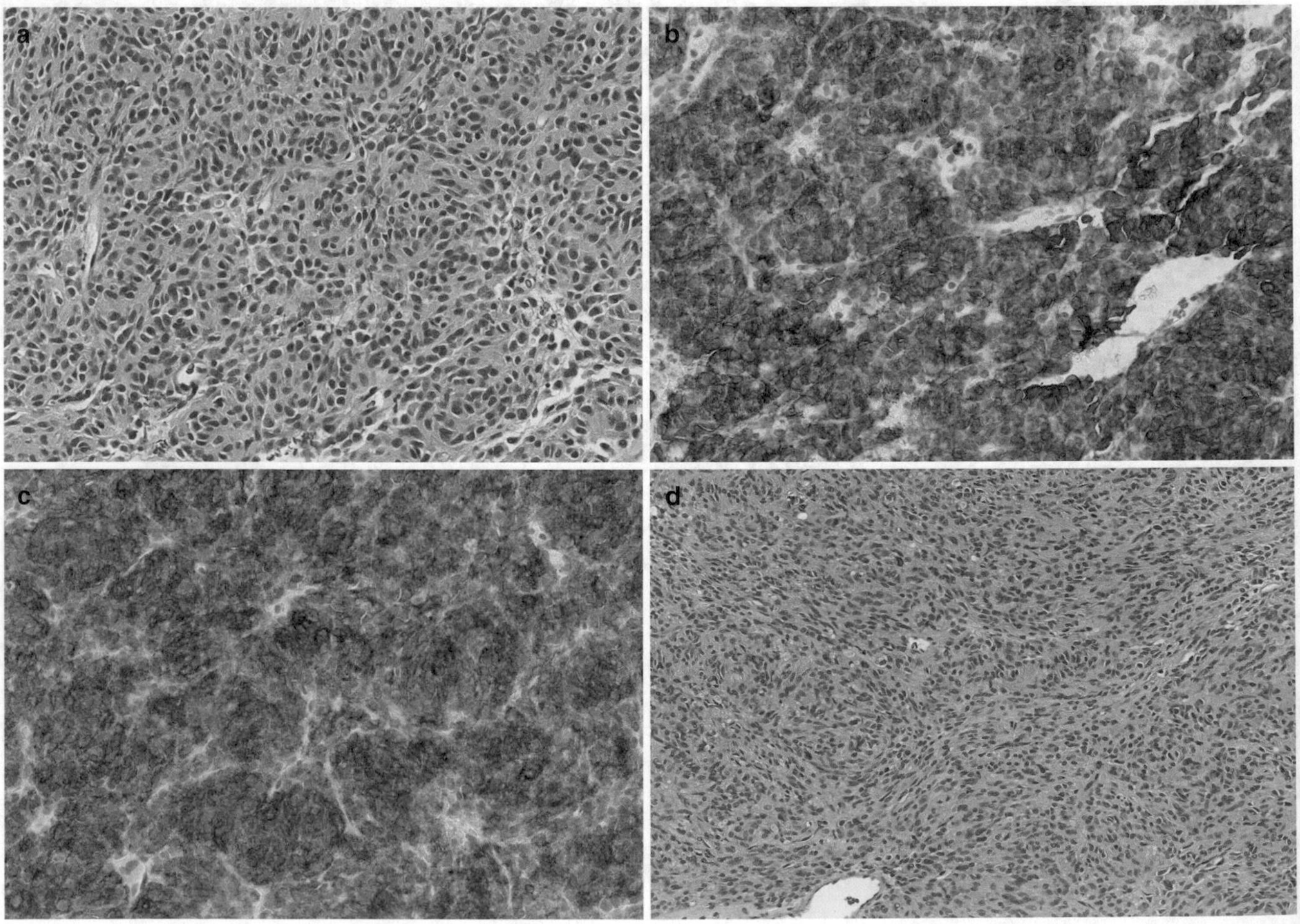

Fig. 19.14 Biopsy of gastric mass. (**a**) Tumor cells are round to ovoid with abundant eosinophilic cytoplasm. (**b**) CD117 stain. (**c**) DOG1 stain. (**d**) Focally, the tumor demonstrated more spindled morphology

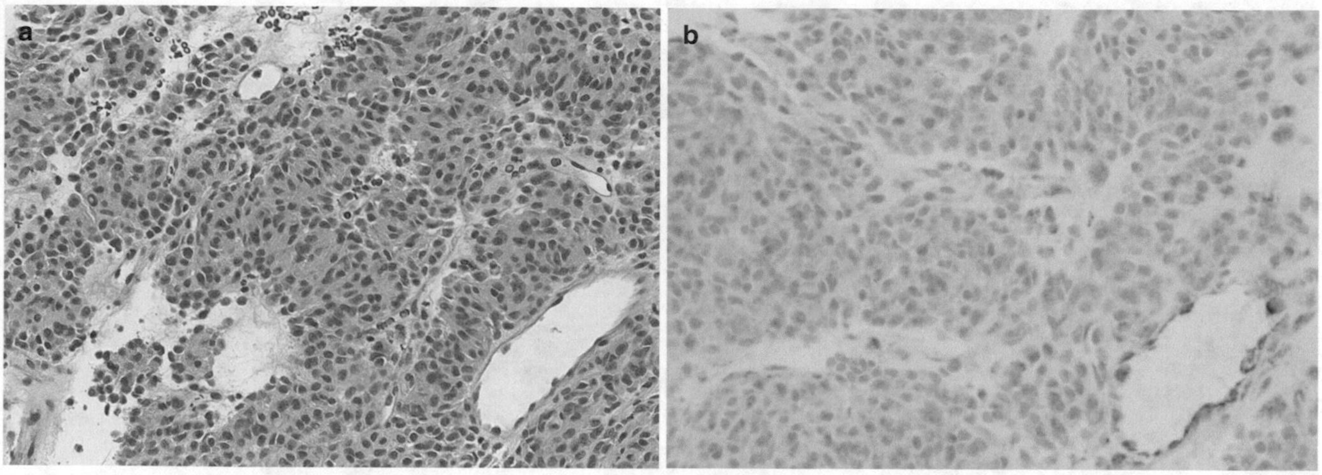

Fig. 19.15 SDHB immunostain. (**a**) H&E-stained section. (**b**) SDHB immunostain. Staining in the tumor is decreased compared to that seen in the small vein (bottom right of image) which serves as an internal positive control. Decreased or absent staining supports a diagnosis of SDHB-deficient GIST. (SDHB image courtesy of ARUP Laboratories in Salt Lake City, Utah)

Case 4

Learning Objectives

1. To recognize clinical and pathologic features of extra-intestinal and metastatic GISTs
2. To be aware of the commonly aberrant immunostaining profile of epithelioid GISTs
3. To avoid common pitfalls that lead to misdiagnosis of GISTs

Case History

A 55-year-old female presented with acute bowel obstruction and was subsequently found to have multiple mesenteric and abdominal wall masses.

Histologic Findings Including Initial IHC Results (Fig. 19.15a–e)

- Epithelioid tumor cells forming nests and cords.
- Scant to moderate eosinophilic cytoplasm with abundant mitotic figures.
- Stroma with distinct myxoid hyaline matrix.
- Tumor cells positive for pancytokeratin (AE1/3), CD56, calretinin, and CD34.

Differential Diagnosis

- Poorly differentiated carcinoma with neuroendocrine features
- Epithelioid hemangioendothelioma
- Mesothelioma
- Gastrointestinal stromal tumor

Additional IHC and Other Ancillary Findings

- CD117 and DOG1 positive (Fig. 19.16f).
- Negative for CD31, WT-1, and synaptophysin.
- *PDGFRA* mutation identified.

Final Diagnosis

Epithelioid gastrointestinal stromal tumor of the mesentery with intraperitoneal metastasis.

Follow-Up

The patient was treated with imatinib therapy and showed partial response at 6 weeks' clinical follow-up.

Take-Home Messages

- Extra-intestinal GISTs and metastatic GISTs are relatively uncommon and may present a significant diagnostic challenge. To include them in the differential is the key to an accurate diagnosis.
- Uniformity of tumor cells with myxoid hyaline stroma, sometimes with mixed spindle cells and skeinoid fibers, is a morphological clue to consider a diagnosis of GIST. To apply immunostains of CD117 and DOG1 in such lesions is necessary to confirm or exclude a probable diagnosis of GIST.
- Immunohistochemistry for epithelioid GISTs may show unexpected results such as immunoreactivity to cytokeratin and other markers that are not commonly associated with GIST. Aberrant immunostaining profile is a common pitfall leading to misdiagnosis of GIST as poorly differentiated carcinoma or other entities. Conversely, melanoma may be misdiagnosed as GIST because of its immunoreactivity to CD117. To be aware of these common pitfalls is critical to ensure diagnostic accuracy.

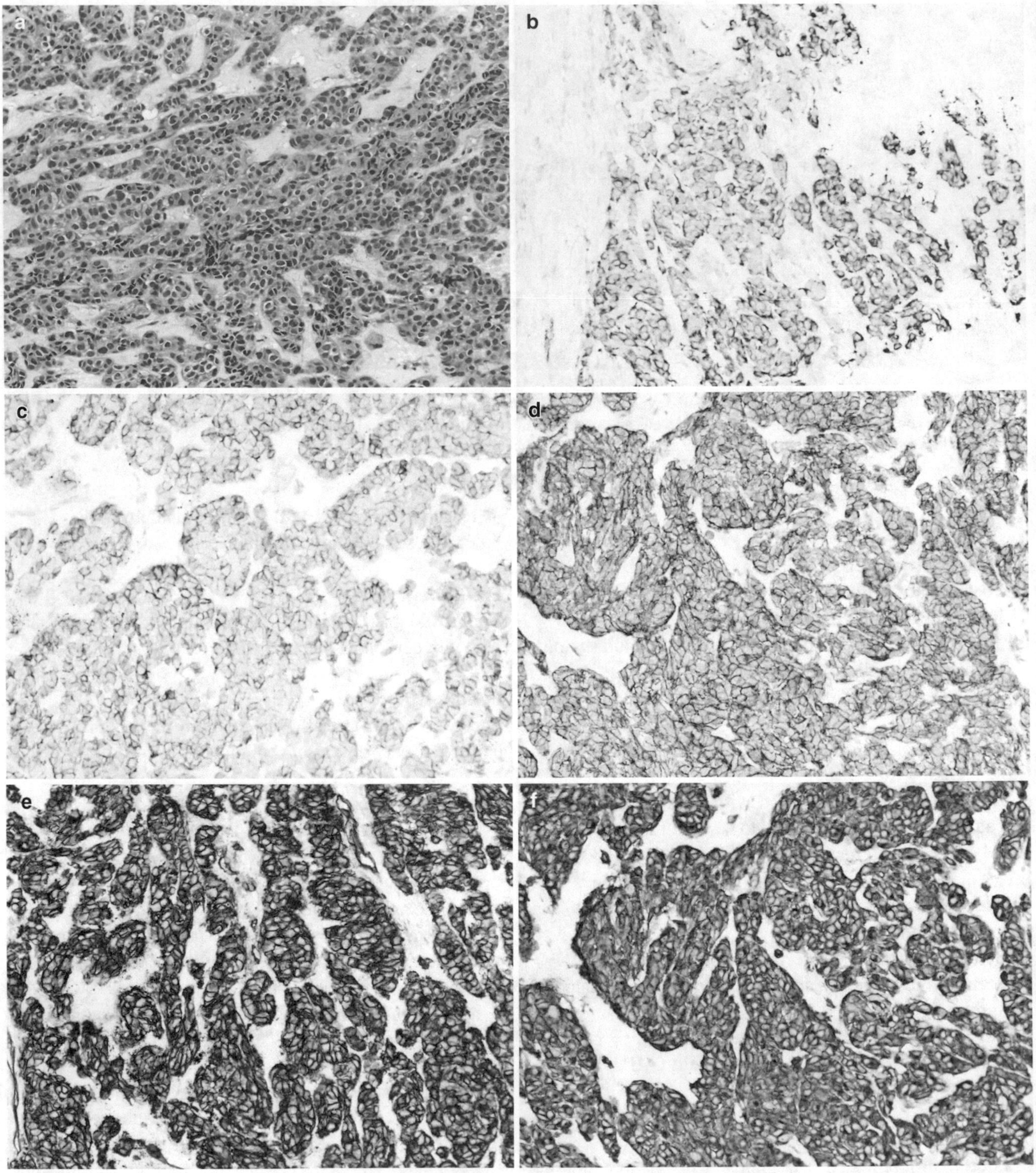

Fig. 19.16 (**a**) H&E-stained section. (**b**) Pancytokeratin (AE1/3) immunostain. (**c**) CD56 immunostain. (**d**) Calretinin immunostain. (**e**) CD34 immunostain. (**f**) CD117 immunostain

References

1. Miettinen M, Sobin LH, Sarlomo-Rikala M. Immunohistochemical spectrum of GISTs at different sites and their differential diagnosis with a reference to CD117 (KIT). Mod Pathol. 2000;13(10):1134–42.
2. Blay P, Astudillo A, Buesa JM, Campo E, Abad M, Garcia-Garcia J, Miquel R, Marco V, Sierra M, Losa R, Lacave A, Brana A, Balbin M, Freije JM. Protein kinase C theta is highly expressed in gastrointestinal stromal tumors but not in other mesenchymal neoplasias. Clin Cancer Res. 2004;10(12 Pt 1):4089–95.
3. Duensing A, Joseph NE, Medeiros F, Smith F, Hornick JL, Heinrich MC, Corless CL, Demetri GD, Fletcher CD, Fletcher JA. Protein Kinase C theta (PKCtheta) expression and constitutive activation in gastrointestinal stromal tumors (GISTs). Cancer Res. 2004;64(15):5127–31.
4. Motegi A, Sakurai S, Nakayama H, Sano T, Oyama T, Nakajima T. PKC theta, a novel immunohistochemical marker for gastrointestinal stromal tumors (GIST), especially useful for identifying KIT-negative tumors. Pathol Int. 2005;55(3):106–12.
5. Miettinen M, Wang ZF, Lasota J. DOG1 antibody in the differential diagnosis of gastrointestinal stromal tumors: a study of 1840 cases. Am J Surg Pathol. 2009;33(9):1401–8.
6. Joensuu H, Hohenberger P, Corless CL. Gastrointestinal stromal tumour. Lancet. 2013;382(9896):973–83.
7. Charville GW, Longacre TA. Surgical pathology of gastrointestinal stromal tumors: practical implications of morphologic and molecular heterogeneity for precision medicine. Adv Anat Pathol. 2017;24(6):336–53.
8. Laurini JA, Blanke CD, Kumarasen C, Demetri GD, Dematteo RP, Fletcher CDM, Goldblum JR, Krausz T, Lasota J, Lazar A, Maki RG, Miettinen M, Noffsinger A, Olson JE, Rubin BP, Washington MK. Protocol for the examination of specimens from patients with gastrointestinal stromal tumor. GIST 4.1.0.0; 2019.
9. Fletcher CD, Berman JJ, Corless C, Gorstein F, Lasota J, Longley BJ, Miettinen M, O'Leary TJ, Remotti H, Rubin BP, Shmookler B, Sobin LH, Weiss SW. Diagnosis of gastrointestinal stromal tumors: a consensus approach. Int J Surg Pathol. 2002;10(2):81–9.
10. Miettinen M, Lasota J. Gastrointestinal stromal tumors: pathology and prognosis at different sites. Semin Diagn Pathol. 2006;23(2):70–83.
11. Miettinen M, Kopczynski J, Makhlouf HR, Sarlomo-Rikala M, Gyorffy H, Burke A, Sobin LH, Lasota J. Gastrointestinal stromal tumors, intramural leiomyomas, and leiomyosarcomas in the duodenum: a clinicopathologic, immunohistochemical, and molecular genetic study of 167 cases. Am J Surg Pathol. 2003;27(5):625–41.
12. Miettinen M, Wang ZF, Sarlomo-Rikala M, Osuch C, Rutkowski P, Lasota J. Succinate dehydrogenase-deficient GISTs: a clinicopathologic, immunohistochemical, and molecular genetic study of 66 gastric GISTs with predilection to young age. Am J Surg Pathol. 2011;35(11):1712–21.
13. Ricci R, Martini M, Cenci T, Carbone A, Lanza P, Biondi A, Rindi G, Cassano A, Larghi A, Persiani R, Larocca LM. PDGFRA-mutant syndrome. Mod Pathol. 2015;28(7):954–64.
14. Ricci R. Syndromic gastrointestinal stromal tumors. Hered Cancer Clin Pract. 2016;14:15.
15. Manley PN, Abu-Abed S, Kirsch R, Hawrysh A, Perrier N, Feilotter H, Pollett A, Riddell RH, Hookey L, Walia JS. Familial PDGFRA-mutation syndrome: somatic and gastrointestinal phenotype. Hum Pathol. 2018;76:52–7.
16. Mei L, Smith SC, Faber AC, Trent J, Grossman SR, Stratakis CA, Boikos SA. Gastrointestinal stromal tumors: the GIST of precision medicine. Trends Cancer. 2018;4(1):74–91.
17. Gopie P, Mei L, Faber AC, Grossman SR, Smith SC, Boikos SA. Classification of gastrointestinal stromal tumor syndromes. Endocr Relat Cancer. 2018;25(2):R49–58.
18. Janeway KA, Weldon CB. Pediatric gastrointestinal stromal tumor. Semin Pediatr Surg. 2012;21(1):31–43.
19. Boikos SA, Pappo AS, Killian JK, LaQuaglia MP, Weldon CB, George S, Trent JC, von Mehren M, Wright JA, Schiffman JD, Raygada M, Pacak K, Meltzer PS, Miettinen MM, Stratakis C, Janeway KA, Helman LJ. Molecular subtypes of KIT/PDGFRA wild-type gastrointestinal stromal tumors: a report from the National Institutes of Health Gastrointestinal Stromal Tumor Clinic. JAMA Oncol. 2016;2(7):922–8.
20. Mullassery D, Weldon CB. Pediatric/"Wildtype" gastrointestinal stromal tumors. Semin Pediatr Surg. 2016;25(5):305–10.
21. Takahashi T, Nakajima K, Nishitani A, Souma Y, Hirota S, Sawa Y, Nishida T. An enhanced risk-group stratification system for more practical prognostication of clinically malignant gastrointestinal stromal tumors. Int J Clin Oncol. 2007;12(5):369–74.
22. Goh BK, Chow PK, Yap WM, Kesavan SM, Song IC, Paul PG, Ooi BS, Chung YF, Wong WK. Which is the optimal risk stratification system for surgically treated localized primary GIST? Comparison of three contemporary prognostic criteria in 171 tumors and a proposal for a modified Armed Forces Institute of Pathology risk criteria. Ann Surg Oncol. 2008;15(8):2153–63.
23. Reece-Smith AM, MacGoey P, Shah MA, Leeder P, Andrew DR, McCulloch T, Parsons SL. A multi-centre analysis of the impact of updated risk stratification on follow-up of gastric gastro-intestinal stromal tumours in the post-imatinib era. Eur J Surg Oncol. 2012;38(6):484–9.
24. Amin M, editor. AJCC cancer staging manual. Cham: Springer International Publishing AG; 2017.
25. NCCN. "Soft tissue sarcoma." NCCN clinical practice guidelines in oncology, Version 2.2020. 28 May 2020. From https://www.nccn.org/store/login/login.aspx?ReturnURL=https://www.nccn.org/professionals/physician_gls/pdf/sarcoma.pdf.
26. Miettinen M, Sobin LH, Lasota J. Gastrointestinal stromal tumors presenting as omental masses--a clinicopathologic analysis of 95 cases. Am J Surg Pathol. 2009;33(9):1267–75.
27. Miettinen M, Felisiak-Golabek A, Wang Z, Inaguma S, Lasota J. GIST manifesting as a retroperitoneal tumor: clinicopathologic immunohistochemical, and molecular genetic study of 112 cases. Am J Surg Pathol. 2017;41(5):577–85.
28. Sawaki A. Rare gastrointestinal stromal tumors (GIST): omentum and retroperitoneum. Transl Gastroenterol Hepatol. 2017;2:116.
29. van Diest PJ, Baak JP, Matze-Cok P, Wisse-Brekelmans EC, van Galen CM, Kurver PH, Bellot SM, Fijnheer J, van Gorp LH, Kwee WS, et al. Reproducibility of mitosis counting in 2,469 breast cancer specimens: results from the Multicenter Morphometric Mammary Carcinoma Project. Hum Pathol. 1992;23(6):603–7.
30. Bell SW, Kempson RL, Hendrickson MR. Problematic uterine smooth muscle neoplasms. A clinicopathologic study of 213 cases. Am J Surg Pathol. 1994;18(6):535–58.
31. Agaimy A. Gastrointestinal stromal tumors (GIST) from risk stratification systems to the new TNM proposal: more questions than answers? A review emphasizing the need for a standardized GIST reporting. Int J Clin Exp Pathol. 2010;3(5):461–71.
32. Pauwels P, Debiec-Rychter M, Stul M, De Wever I, Van Oosterom AT, Sciot R. Changing phenotype of gastrointestinal stromal tumours under imatinib mesylate treatment: a potential diagnostic pitfall. Histopathology. 2005;47(1):41–7.
33. Dennis KL, Damjanov I. Evaluating and reporting gastrointestinal stromal tumors after imatinib mesylate treatment. Open Pathol J. 2009;3:53–7.

34. Miettinen M, Sobin LH, Lasota J. Gastrointestinal stromal tumors of the stomach: a clinicopathologic, immunohistochemical, and molecular genetic study of 1765 cases with long-term follow-up. Am J Surg Pathol. 2005;29(1):52–68.
35. Miettinen M, Makhlouf H, Sobin LH, Lasota J. Gastrointestinal stromal tumors of the jejunum and ileum: a clinicopathologic, immunohistochemical, and molecular genetic study of 906 cases before imatinib with long-term follow-up. Am J Surg Pathol. 2006;30(4):477–89.
36. Abraham SC, Krasinskas AM, Hofstetter WL, Swisher SG, Wu TT. “Seedling” mesenchymal tumors (gastrointestinal stromal tumors and leiomyomas) are common incidental tumors of the esophagogastric junction. Am J Surg Pathol. 2007;31(11):1629–35.
37. Demitri GD, Benjamin R, Blanke CD, Blay J-Y, Casali P, Choi H, Corless CL, Debiec-Rychter M, DeMatteo RP, Ettinger DS, Fisher GA, Fletcher CDM, Gronchi A, Hohenberger P, Hughes M, Joensuu H, Judson I, Le Cesne L, Make RG, Morse M, Pappo AS, Pisters PWT, Raut CP, Reichardt P, Tyler DS, Van de Abbeele AD, von Mehren M, Wayne JD, Zalcberg J. NCCN: task force report: optimal management of patients with gastrointestinal stromal tumor (GIST) - update of the NCCN clinical practice guidelines. J Natl Compr Canc Netw. 2007;5(Supplement 2):40.
38. Agaimy A, Markl B, Arnholdt H, Hartmann A, Schneider-Stock R, Chetty R. Sporadic segmental Interstitial cell of cajal hyperplasia (microscopic GIST) with unusual diffuse longitudinal growth replacing the muscularis propria: differential diagnosis to hereditary GIST syndromes. Int J Clin Exp Pathol. 2010;3(5):549–56.
39. Nishida T, Goto O, Raut CP, Yahagi N. Diagnostic and treatment strategy for small gastrointestinal stromal tumors. Cancer. 2016;122(20):3110–8.
40. DeMatteo RP, Lewis JJ, Leung D, Mudan SS, Woodruff JM, Brennan MF. Two hundred gastrointestinal stromal tumors: recurrence patterns and prognostic factors for survival. Ann Surg. 2000;231(1):51–8.
41. Miettinen M, Sarlomo-Rikala M, Sobin LH, Lasota J. Esophageal stromal tumors: a clinicopathologic, immunohistochemical, and molecular genetic study of 17 cases and comparison with esophageal leiomyomas and leiomyosarcomas. Am J Surg Pathol. 2000;24(2):211–22.
42. Miettinen M, Furlong M, Sarlomo-Rikala M, Burke A, Sobin LH, Lasota J. Gastrointestinal stromal tumors, intramural leiomyomas, and leiomyosarcomas in the rectum and anus: a clinicopathologic, immunohistochemical, and molecular genetic study of 144 cases. Am J Surg Pathol. 2001;25(9):1121–33.
43. Burkill GJ, Badran M, Al-Muderis O, Meirion Thomas J, Judson IR, Fisher C, Moskovic EC. Malignant gastrointestinal stromal tumor: distribution, imaging features, and pattern of metastatic spread. Radiology. 2003;226(2):527–32.
44. Haller F, Schulten HJ, Armbrust T, Langer C, Gunawan B, Fuzesi L. Multicentric sporadic gastrointestinal stromal tumors (GISTs) of the stomach with distinct clonal origin: differential diagnosis to familial and syndromal GIST variants and peritoneal metastasis. Am J Surg Pathol. 2007;31(6):933–7.
45. Agaimy A, Markl B, Arnholdt H, Wunsch PH, Terracciano LM, Dirnhofer S, Hartmann A, Tornillo L, Bihl MP. Multiple sporadic gastrointestinal stromal tumours arising at different gastrointestinal sites: pattern of involvement of the muscularis propria as a clue to independent primary GISTs. Virchows Arch. 2009;455(2):101–8.
46. Mei L, Du W, Idowu M, von Mehren M, Boikos SA. Advances and challenges on management of gastrointestinal stromal tumors. Front Oncol. 2018;8:135.
47. Neuhann TM, Mansmann V, Merkelbach-Bruse S, Klink B, Hellinger A, Hoffkes HG, Wardelmann E, Schildhaus HU, Tinschert S. A novel germline KIT mutation (p.L576P) in a family presenting with juvenile onset of multiple gastrointestinal stromal tumors, skin hyperpigmentations, and esophageal stenosis. Am J Surg Pathol. 2013;37(6):898–905.
48. Jones DH, Caracciolo JT, Hodul PJ, Strosberg JR, Coppola D, Bui MM. Familial gastrointestinal stromal tumor syndrome: report of 2 cases with KIT exon 11 mutation. Cancer Control. 2015;22(1):102–8.
49. NCT02034110. Efficacy and safety of the combination therapy of dabrafenib and trametinib in subjects with BRAF V600E- mutated rare cancers. Retrieved August 2020, from https://clinicaltrials.gov/ct2/show/NCT02034110?term=NCT02034110&rank=1.
50. NCT02071862. Study of the glutaminase inhibitor CB-839 in solid tumors. Retrieved August 2020, from https://clinicaltrials.gov/ct2/show/study/NCT02071862.
51. NCT04276415. DS-6157a in participants with advance gastrointestinal stromal tumor (GIST). Retrieved August 2020, https://clinicaltrials.gov/ct2/show/NCT04276415.
52. NCT03165721. A phase II trial of the DNA methyl transferase inhibitor, guadecitabine (SGI-110), in children and adults with wild type GIST, pheochromocytoma and paraganglioma associated with succinate dehydrogenase deficiency and HLRCC-associated kidney cancer. Retrieved August 2020, from https://clinicaltrials.gov/ct2/show/NCT03165721.
53. Falchook GS, Trent JC, Heinrich MC, Beadling C, Patterson J, Bastida CC, Blackman SC, Kurzrock R. BRAF mutant gastrointestinal stromal tumor: first report of regression with BRAF inhibitor dabrafenib (GSK2118436) and whole exomic sequencing for analysis of acquired resistance. Oncotarget. 2013;4(2):310–5.
54. Ben-Ami E, Barysauskas CM, von Mehren M, Heinrich MC, Corless CL, Butrynski JE, Morgan JA, Wagner AJ, Choy E, Yap JT, Van den Abbeele AD, Solomon SM, Fletcher JA, Demetri GD, George S. Long-term follow-up results of the multicenter phase II trial of regorafenib in patients with metastatic and/or unresectable GI stromal tumor after failure of standard tyrosine kinase inhibitor therapy. Ann Oncol. 2016;27(9):1794–9.
55. Hameed M, Corless C, George S, Hornick JL, Kakar S, Lazar A, Tang L. Template for reporting results of biomarker testing of specimens from patients with gastrointestinal stromal Tumors. Feb 2015. Retrieved July 2018, 2018, from http://www.cap.org/web/oracle/webcenter/portalapp/pagehierarchy/cancer_protocol_templates.jspx?_adf.ctrl-state=fdh0vui9d_9&_afrLoop=29330867362706#!%40%40%3F_afrLoop%3D29330867362706%26_adf.ctrl-state%3D3ql6t7wta_4.

Non-GIST Primary Mesenchymal Tumors of the GI Tract

20

Katy Lawson, David Borzik, Aaron W. James, and Sarah M. Dry

List of Frequently Asked Questions

1. What mesenchymal tumors characteristically involve the esophagus?
2. What mesenchymal tumors characteristically involve the stomach?
3. What mesenchymal tumors characteristically involve the small bowel?
4. What mesenchymal tumors characteristically involve the colon and rectum?
5. How are schwannomas distinguished from neurofibromas of the GI tract?
6. How are neurofibromas differentiated from malignant peripheral nerve sheath tumor?
7. What are the characteristic location and features of a plexiform fibromyxoma?
8. What are the molecular abnormalities of inflammatory myofibroblastic tumor (IMT)?
9. What tumors fall within the differential diagnosis of IMT?
10. What are the immunohistochemical findings in IMT?
11. What are the histologic patterns of IMT?
12. What are the typical histologic findings in gastrointestinal neuroectodermal tumor (GNET)?
13. What are the common immunohistochemical and molecular features of GNET?
14. What are the similarities and differences between GNET and clear cell sarcoma (CCS) of soft tissue?
15. What are common S100-positive GI tumors and how may they be distinguished?
16. What demographic populations commonly are affected by fibromatosis?
17. What are the growth patterns of intra-abdominal fibromatosis?
18. How can intra-abdominal fibromatosis be distinguished from other spindle cell neoplasms of the GI tract?
19. What genetic syndromes are associated with fibromatosis?
20. What are the characteristic histologic findings of leiomyosarcoma?
21. What patient populations are affected by EBV-associated smooth muscle tumors?
22. What are the characteristic histologic and immunohistochemical features of EBV-associated smooth muscle tumors?
23. What is the differential diagnosis for EBV-associated smooth muscle tumors?
24. What vascular neoplasms affect the GI tract?
25. What patient populations are affected by angiosarcoma of the GI tract?
26. What differentiates angiosarcoma from hemangioma?
27. What differentiates hemangioma from glomus tumor?
28. What are the distinguishing features of angiosarcoma from other malignant tumors of the GI tract?
29. What are the immunohistochemical features of angiosarcoma?
30. What tumors of adipose tissue may involve the GI tract, and how to distinguish lipoma from well-differentiated liposarcoma?
31. What immunohistochemical or molecular tests may help in the diagnosis of liposarcoma?
32. How does well-differentiated liposarcoma differ from dedifferentiated liposarcoma?
33. May dedifferentiated liposarcoma be diagnosed in the absence of a well-differentiated component?
34. How does liposarcoma of the retroperitoneum differ from atypical lipomatous tumor of the deep soft tissue?
35. How is angiomyolipoma distinguished from liposarcoma?
36. What are the histological variants of angiomyolipoma?
37. What are the immunohistochemical features of angiomyolipoma?
38. What are histologic features predicting a malignant angiomyolipoma?

K. Lawson · S. M. Dry (✉)
University of California at Los Angeles, Los Angeles, CA, USA
e-mail: kllawson@mednet.ucla.edu

D. Borzik · A. W. James
Johns Hopkins University, Baltimore, MD, USA

H. L. Wang, Z. E. Chen (eds.), *Practical Gastrointestinal Pathology*, Practical Anatomic Pathology,
https://doi.org/10.1007/978-3-030-51268-2_20

Frequently Asked Questions

1. **What mesenchymal tumors characteristically involve the esophagus?**
   - Leiomyoma is the most common mesenchymal tumor of the esophagus, accounting for approximately two-thirds of benign tumors of the esophagus. It is most commonly seen in patients aged 20–50 years with a 2:1 male-to-female ratio. The distal esophagus is the most common location (79%), followed by mid-esophagus (18%). It is often detected incidentally at routine chest radiograph but can present with dysphagia and chest pain or in association with an esophageal ulcer.
   - Gastrointestinal stromal tumor (GIST) of the esophagus accounts for <1% of all GIST cases of the gastrointestinal (GI) tract. Unique features of esophageal GISTs include more frequently seen in men and patients under 60 years of age, more likely to have a larger tumor size that confers a higher risk stratification and a less favorable prognosis, and a higher frequency of KIT wild-type tumors.
   - Fibrovascular polyp is a rare benign intraluminal lesion arising in the proximal esophagus, with synonyms including fibroma, fibrolipoma, pedunculated lipoma, and fibroepithelial polyp. Most are diagnosed only after the lesion becomes symptomatic or grossly visible. Histologically, these lesions show loose fibrovascular tissue with varying degrees of myxomatous and fatty change.
   - Leiomyosarcoma (LMS) is rare, accounting for <1% of all malignant esophageal tumors. Features suggesting malignancy in an esophageal smooth muscle tumor on a biopsy include mitotic rate >5/50 HPF, cytologic atypia, and/or necrosis.

   References: [1–5]

2. **What mesenchymal tumors characteristically involve the stomach?**
   - GIST (see Chap. 19 for more details) is common in the stomach, accounting for the vast majority of gastric mesenchymal tumors. It is driven by *KIT* or *PDGFRA* mutations and is generally CD117 (c-kit) and DOG1 positive by immunohistochemistry (IHC). The succinate dehydrogenase (SDH)-deficient variant typically occurs in the stomach, particularly in children. Approximately 20–25% of gastric GISTs are malignant.
   - Lipoma accounts for <1% of all tumors of the stomach. It typically occurs in the fifth or sixth decade of life, with no sex predisposition. It is a submucosal fatty tumor composed of mature adipocytes surrounded by a fibrous capsule, most commonly arising from the submucosa of the antrum. GI bleeding secondary to mucosal ulceration is seen in 50–60% of cases.
   - Leiomyoma accounts for 2% of all resected neoplasms of the stomach, most commonly seen in the body (40%) and antrum (25%). Patients with gastric leiomyoma are typically asymptomatic but may present with anemia secondary to mucosal ulceration.
   - Schwannoma and neurofibroma account for 4% of all benign neoplasms of the stomach. Patients with these tumors commonly present with bleeding (40%) and/or obstructive symptoms.
   - Glomus tumor occurs in adults of all ages, with a significant female preponderance. Virtually all glomus tumors of the GI tract arise in the stomach. Patients often present with epigastric pain, GI bleeding, and gastric ulceration. Nuclear atypia and vascular invasion may be seen in gastric glomus tumors, but these findings do not necessarily represent malignant behavior.
   - Plexiform fibromyxoma is rare. The vast majority arise in the antrum of the stomach; some may extend into the duodenum. This tumor has previously been described as "plexiform angiomyxoid myofibroblastic tumor" or "myxoma." It is seen in a wide age range (children to elderly), with most cases occurring in young to middle-aged adults. There is no sex predisposition. Clinically, it often clinically mimics GIST. Symptoms include anemia and hematemesis. Large tumors may lead to gastric outlet obstruction

   References: [6–11]

3. **What mesenchymal tumors characteristically involve the small bowel?**
   - GIST is more likely to cause perforation at this location compared to other sites of the GI tract. Large GISTs (>4 cm) of the small bowel may present as abdominal emergencies.
   - Lipoma of the small bowel most commonly arises from the submucosa in the terminal ileum. Large tumors may cause intussusception in adults.
   - Gastrointestinal neuroectodermal tumor (GNET) arises from the submucosa and muscularis propria, with 66% of cases showing ulceration. Histologically it is characterized by sheets or nests of primitive epithelioid-to-spindled cells, with osteoclast-like giant cells seen in approximately 50% of cases. Immunohistochemically, these tumors display markers suggestive of primitive neural phenotype without expression of specific melanocytic markers. Specifically, tumor cells are positive for S100 and SOX10 (100%), CD56 (70%), and synaptophysin (56%). Molecular alterations include translocations involving the EWSR1, ATF1, or CREB1 genes.

   References: [12–15]

4. What mesenchymal tumors characteristically involve the colon and rectum?

- Lipoma and GIST also occur in the colon and rectum.
- Leiomyoma is commonly seen in the colorectum. It is usually small, arising from the muscularis mucosae, and found as an incidental polyp on screening colonoscopy.
- Angioma, including hemangioma and lymphangioma, also occurs in the colorectum.

5. How are schwannomas distinguished from neurofibromas of the GI tract?

- Schwannomas are composed exclusively of Schwann cells, while neurofibromas are composed of all the cells normally present in the nerve sheath, including Schwann cells and perineural fibroblasts.
- GI schwannomas show plump, dense nuclei and often display some pleomorphism, as well as a distinctive peritumoral lymphoplasmacytic cuff. They typically show more uniform cellularity and lack the classic features of schwannomas of soft tissue, such as encapsulation, alternating hypercellular ("Antoni A") and hypocellular ("Antoni B") areas, nuclear palisading around cell process ("Verocay bodies"), and thick hyalinized vessel walls (Fig. 20.1a, b).
- The microcystic/reticular variant of schwannoma, first described in 2008, predominantly affects the GI tract and shows a microcystic and reticular growth pattern with anastomosing and intersecting spindle cells in a background of myxoid or collagenous, hyalinizing stromal islands. This variant is seen in a wide age range (11–93 years), with a median age of 63 years. There is no association with NF1 nor NF2. IHC show diffuse and strong nuclear and cytoplasmic S100 expression, patchy GFAP positivity, and negative stains for keratins, EMA, CD117, and smooth muscle markers.
- Neurofibromas are typically more uniformly cellular, with cells present in sheets or vague whirling patterns in a collagenous or myxoid matrix. Collagen fibers are often broad and have a so-called "shredded carrots" appearance (Fig. 20.2).
- Immunohistochemically, Schwann cells express S100, while fibroblasts stain for CD34. Thus, Schwann cells show diffuse and strong nuclear and cytoplasmic S100 positivity and are negative for CD34, while neurofibromas show a mixture of S100- and CD34-positive cells.
- Both schwannomas and neurofibromas are negative for DOG1 and CD117, which rules out GIST, and negative for STAT6, which rules out solitary fibrous tumor (SFT). Desmoid fibromatosis is negative for S100 and typically shows longer fascicles of spindle cells.
- Schwannomas most commonly arise in the submucosa or muscularis propria of the stomach and small bowel. This differs from mucosal proliferation of Schwann cells, known as Schwann cell hamartoma, which forms a small polypoid lesion and almost always arises in the colorectum (see Chap. 16 for more details).

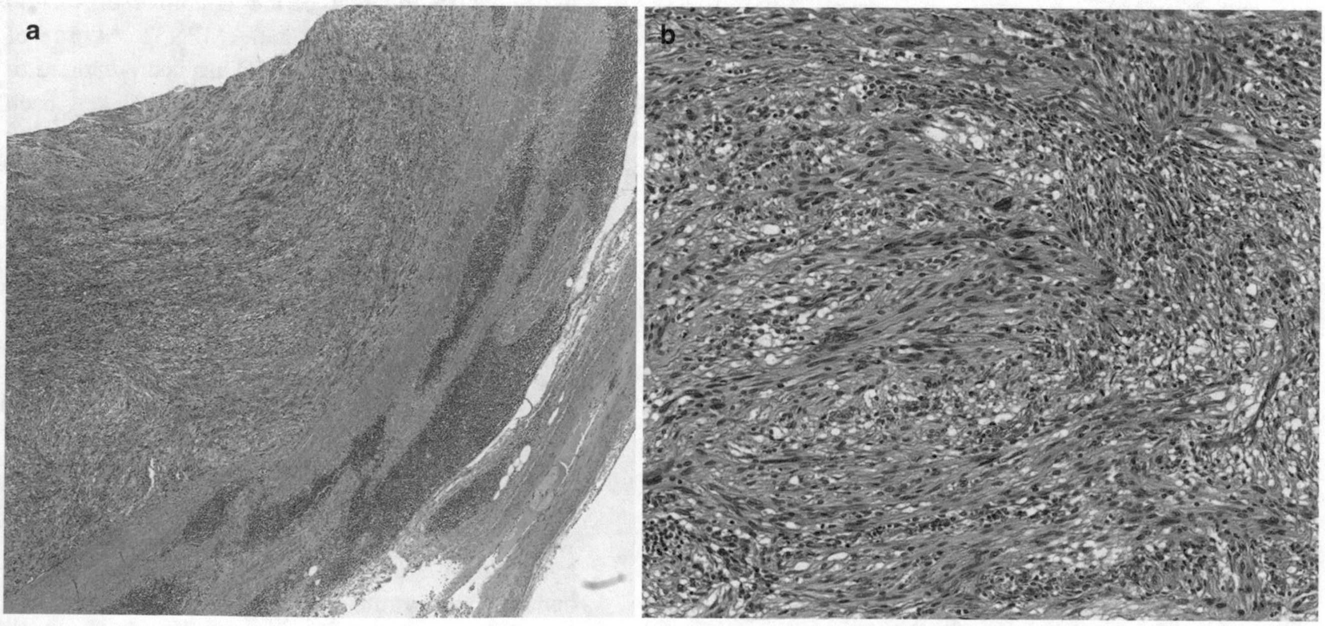

Fig. 20.1 (**a**) Gastric schwannoma showing spindled cells with relatively uniform cellularity and a prominent peritumoral lymphoid cuff. (**b**) Higher-power view showing interlacing fascicles of bland spindle cells with plump, dense nuclei and mild nuclear pleomorphism (degenerative-type atypia)

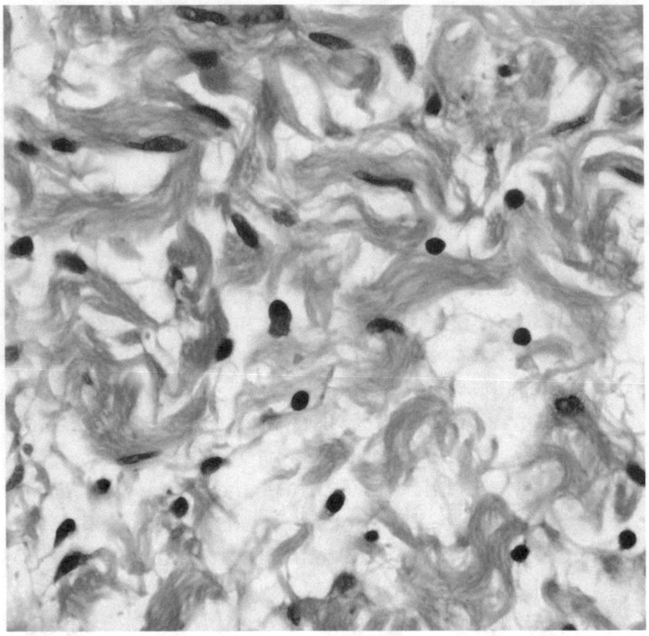

Fig. 20.2 High-power view of a neurofibroma showing low cellularity composed of small, uniform, elongated spindle cells arranged loosely in a vague whirling pattern in coarse collagen bundles, the so-called "shredded carrot" or myxoid background

- GI schwannomas typically show patchy prominent peritumoral lymphocytic aggregates or cuff (Fig. 20.1a) that help distinguish from GISTs.
- The majority of neurofibromas and schwannomas are sporadic, but they may arise in the context of well-described clinical syndromes, NF1 and NF2, respectively.
  - NF1 occurs as the result of mutations in the *NF1* gene and is the most common sporadic human mutation, occurring in 1/300 births. The clinical presentation of NF1 is extremely variable, and patients may not be diagnosed with NF1 until a diagnosis of a plexiform or visceral neurofibroma is made. Manifestations of NF1 include café au lait spots, cutaneous neurofibromas, plexiform neurofibromas, and Lisch nodules of the iris.
  - GI manifestations of NF1 are common, occurring in an estimated 25% of affected individuals. These include hyperplasia of submucosal and myenteric nerve plexuses; GISTs, often multiple, which tend to arise in the small bowel; diffuse ganglioneuromatosis; and somatostatinoma of the ampulla of Vater.
  - The majority, but not all, of visceral neurofibromas occur in the setting of NF1, and thus clinicians should be alerted to this possibility when a diagnosis of a GI neurofibroma is rendered.
  - NF2 occurs as a result of mutation in the *NF2* gene that encodes protein merlin. It may be sporadic (50% of cases) or inherited in an autosomal dominant manner. It is far less common than NF1 with an incidence of 1/25,000.
  - NF2 is clinically characterized by bilateral vestibular schwannomas, meningiomas, ependymomas, and cataracts. GI manifestations in NF2 are very rare.

References: [16–22]

6. **How are neurofibromas differentiated from malignant peripheral nerve sheath tumor?**
   - Malignant peripheral nerve sheath tumors (MPNSTs) most commonly arise from neurofibromas and rarely from schwannomas. Transformation to MPNST occurs in both sporadic and NF1-associated neurofibromas and also in about 10% of irradiated neurofibromas. Patients with NF1 develop MPNSTs at an earlier age (20s–40s) than those with sporadic neurofibromas. Clinically worrisome features for transformation to MPNST include rapid growth or pain in a preexisting neurofibroma.
   - To make a diagnosis of MPNST, one should see malignant transformation of a neurofibroma, a malignant tumor arising in a nerve trunk, or a malignant tumor in a patient with NF1. For the latter two situations, judicious use of IHC and molecular studies to exclude other tumors in the differential diagnosis is required, as up to 20% of "sporadic" MPNSTs have been reclassified as other tumors on re-review.
   - There are no immunohistochemical features or molecular testing that permit definitive distinction between neurofibroma and MPNST. Loss of H3K27me3 expression by IHC has been reported in about 50% of MPNSTs, while loss has not been reported in neurofibromas. While loss of this marker can help support the diagnosis of MPNST, loss (complete or partial) has also been reported in a number of other tumors in the differential diagnosis of MPNST including spindle cell sarcoma NOS, synovial sarcoma, and dedifferentiated dermatofibrosarcoma protuberans.
   - High-grade MPNSTs are easy to identify as malignant tumors, as they show highly cellular fascicles and sheets of spindled cells with scattered cells showing marked pleomorphism and readily identifiable mitoses (including atypical mitoses) and necrosis (Fig. 20.3). Perivascular accentuation and hyper- and hypocellular areas are often seen. Staghorn or hemangiopericytoma-like vessels may be seen and may cause confusion with malignant SFT or synovial sarcoma. Ancillary testing can help diagnose tumors

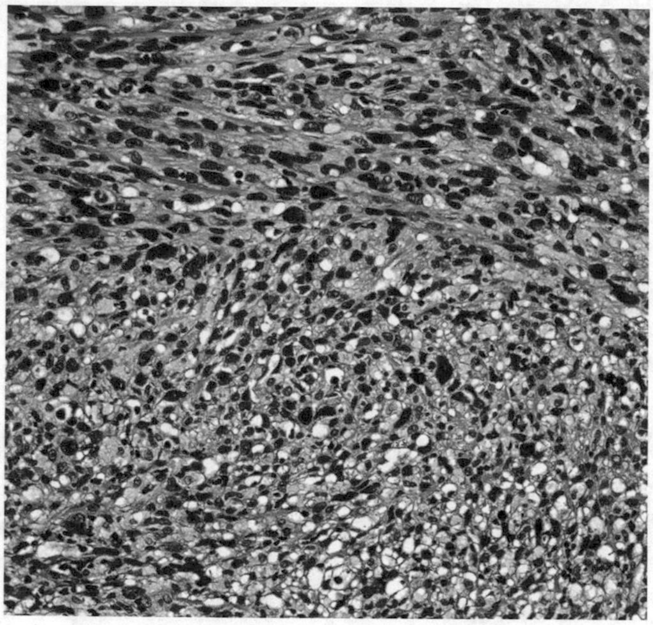

Fig. 20.3 High-grade malignant peripheral nerve sheath tumor showing highly cellular fascicles and sheets of hyperchromatic spindled cells with scattered cells exhibiting marked nuclear pleomorphism

in the differential diagnosis of MPNST, including malignant SFT (STAT6 positive), synovial sarcoma (*SYT* gene rearrangement), or dedifferentiated liposarcoma (*MDM2* gene amplification).

- Low-grade MPNSTs show scattered atypical cells with pleomorphic, hyperchromatic nuclei and low levels of mitoses. Low-grade MPNSTs can be very difficult to distinguish from neurofibromas with atypical features and are best reviewed by pathologists with subspecialty expertise in soft tissue sarcomas.
- Heterologous differentiation is seen in 10% of MPNSTs, including rhabdomyosarcoma ("triton" tumors), osteosarcoma, angiosarcoma, or chondrosarcoma.

References: [16, 23, 24]

7. **What are the characteristic location and features of a plexiform fibromyxoma?**
   - Most plexiform fibromyxomas arise in the antrum of the stomach, rarely in the body, and may extend into the duodenum. It is a benign tumor, previously described as "plexiform angiomyxoid myofibroblastic tumor" or "myxoma," which often clinically mimics GISTs. It occurs in a wide age range (children to elderly), but most cases are seen in young to middle-aged adults. There is no sex predisposition. Symptoms include anemia and hematemesis. Large tumors may lead to gastric outlet obstruction.
   - Plexiform fibromyxomas are typically multinodular, ranging in size from 2 to 15 cm (mean 4–5 cm). They arise in the muscularis propria and may extend into the subserosa or adjacent soft tissues or extend toward the lumen to involve the submucosa or mucosa with associated mucosal ulceration. Tumors may also extend into lymphovascular spaces, including muscular-walled large veins, which does NOT confer a different prognosis.
   - Histologically, these are plexiform and multinodular lesions, with nodules well-demarcated from surrounding tissues (Fig. 20.4a). Lesional cells show relatively uniform delicate spindled morphology with small nuclei without prominent nucleoli and scant eosinophilic cytoplasm (Fig. 20.4b). Clear cell features may be seen. Mitoses are low, usually <1/10 HPF. Prominent small capillary network may be present, sometimes with plexiform features. The matrix is typically myxoid, though some have a collagenous matrix.
   - Lesional cells typically express SMA (may be patchy or absent), desmin, and CD10 (variable). They are negative for DOG1, CD117, keratins, S100, and CD34.
   - A recent study showed 20% to have *MALAT1-GLI1* gene fusions, t(11;12)(q11;q13), and an additional 10% have polysomy of *GLI1*; both of these resulted in upregulation of the GLI1 protein. Cases with these fusions did not differ in histology or clinical features. Interestingly, a *MALAT1-GLI1* gene fusion with an identical structure as that reported in plexiform fibromyxoma was reported in four cases of gastroblastoma. It is unclear currently how or if these are related, particularly since plexiform fibromyxoma is clinically benign, while gastroblastoma has a high rate of metastases and is potentially fatal.

   References: [25–29]

8. **What are the molecular abnormalities of inflammatory myofibroblastic tumor (IMT)?**
   - IMT is predominantly a tumor of children and adolescents, which only rarely appears after the age of 50. The retroperitoneum, lung, and abdominal cavity are the most common locations, although it is reported at a wide variety of anatomic sites. It is associated with clinical symptoms in up to one-third of patients, mainly pediatric, including weight loss, fever, elevated erythrocyte sedimentation rate (ESR), hypergammaglobulinemia, and anemia. These symptoms usually disappear after tumor resection.
   - *ALK* gene rearrangements (with various partner genes) are seen overall in 50% of cases. Most pediatric cases (80%) have an *ALK* gene rearrangement, while few are seen in adult cases (20%). These are identified by tumor cell positivity for ALK1 by immu-

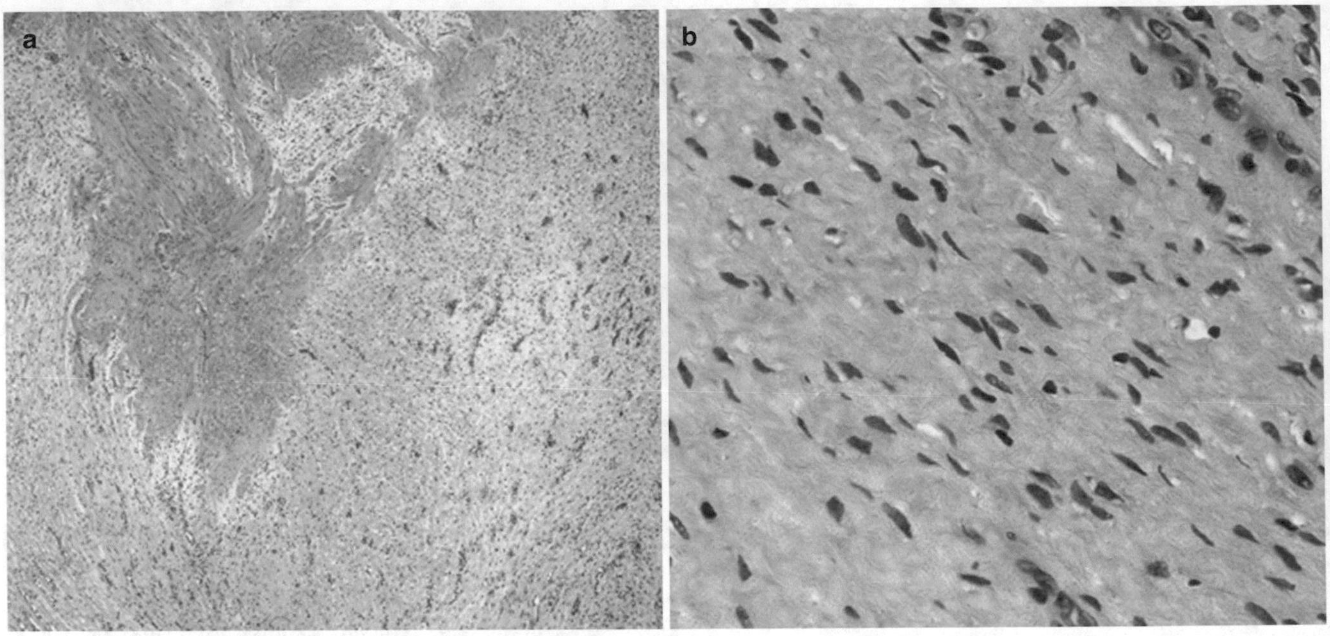

Fig. 20.4 (**a**) Plexiform fibromyxoma in the antrum of the stomach, which clinically mimics GISTs, showing characteristic infiltration of the muscularis propria by a multinodular, plexiform growth pattern within an abundant fibromyxoid stroma with prominent vasculature. (**b**) Higher-power view showing small, bland spindled cells and eosinophilic cytoplasm with indistinct borders

nohistochemical staining (Fig. 20.24). An ALK-RANBP2 fusion was recently identified to occur in the epithelioid variant of IMT and is thought to result in the characteristic ALK membrane staining seen in this variant.

9. **What tumors fall within the differential diagnosis of IMT?**
   - Both sarcomas and hematolymphoid neoplasms are in the differential diagnosis of IMT. In the GI tract, GISTs always should be considered. GISTs typically do not show fascicles like those in IMT and only rarely show the presence of plasma cells. By IHC, GISTs are positive for CD117 and DOG1 and negative for ALK1, while IMTs are negative for CD117 and DOG1, and about half are positive for ALK1.
   - Follicular dendritic cell (FDC) sarcomas also show an admixture of spindled cells and inflammatory cells, as is seen in IMT. FDC sarcomas tend to show a more whorling or storiform pattern than is typically present in IMTs, which typically show fascicles of spindle cells. In FDC sarcoma, the inflammatory cells are lymphocytes, whereas IMT usually shows a mixture of lymphocytes and plasma cells, with neutrophils and eosinophils more rarely present. FDC sarcomas are positive for CD21, CD23, and CD35, which are all negative in IMTs.
   - Desmoid fibromatosis typically shows more slender spindled cells, is less cellular, does not have a significant inflammatory cell component, and is not positive for ALK1.
   - For the epithelioid variant of IMT, anaplastic large cell lymphoma (ALCL) may enter the differential diagnosis. IMTs and ALCLs are both positive for ALK1 and may additionally share CD30 positivity; but importantly, IMTs express SMA (80%) and desmin (60%), which are both typically negative in ALCL.
   - Dedifferentiated or cellular well-differentiated liposarcoma may be in the differential diagnosis of both classic and epithelioid IMTs. It can be distinguished from IMT by MDM2 gene amplification and the presence of areas of classic well-differentiated liposarcoma.
   - It is important to remember that IMT classically shows very uniform cells. Any significant nuclear atypia should prompt consideration of a different tumor.

10. **What are the immunohistochemical findings in IMT?**
    - Lesional cells in IMTs are positive for SMA (80%), desmin (60%), keratins (1/3 of cases), and CD30 (epithelioid variant). ALK1 is positive in 50% of cases, which shows cytoplasmic staining in spindled cells and membranous staining in epithelioid variants.

11. **What are the histologic patterns of IMT?**
    - Typical spindled cell tumors show uniform, plump spindled cells with ill-defined cell borders present in

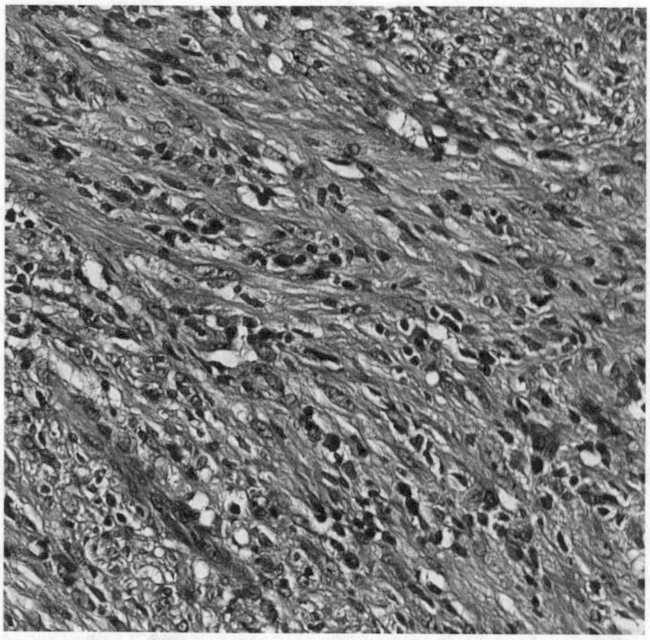

Fig. 20.5 Inflammatory myofibroblastic tumor with typical spindled morphology composed of relatively uniform, plump, spindled cells present in variably cellular fascicles among scattered lymphocytes and plasma cells

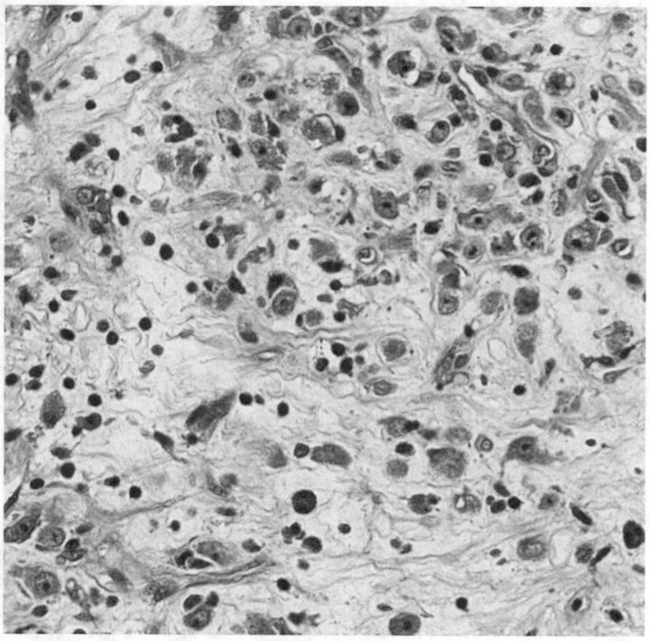

Fig. 20.6 Inflammatory myofibroblastic tumor, epithelioid variant, with vesicular nuclei and prominent nucleoli in loose sheets set in a myxoid stroma among scattered mixed inflammatory cells including neutrophils

variably cellular fascicles (Fig. 20.5). Nuclei are ovoid with small nucleoli. Scattered lymphocytes and plasma cells are typically present. Neutrophils and eosinophils are less common. A myxoid or collagenous stroma is often present. Ganglion-like cells with eccentric nuclei and eosinophilic cytoplasm are present in about half of cases. Significant nuclear atypia is not seen and should prompt consideration of a different tumor.

- Epithelioid variant (Fig. 20.6) is almost exclusively seen in the omentum or mesentery, with a marked male predominance. Lesional cells show vesicular nuclear chromatin and prominent large nucleoli and are arranged in loose sheets set in a myxoid stroma. Mitoses may be readily seen. There are abundant mixed inflammatory cells, and a prominent neutrophilic infiltrate may be present.

References: [30–32]

12. **What are the typical histologic findings in gastrointestinal neuroectodermal tumor (GNET)?**
    - GNET is characterized by sheets and nests of predominantly epithelioid cells with infrequent spindling (Fig. 20.7a). Tumor cells have moderate amounts of clear to pale eosinophilic cytoplasm. Nuclei are vesicular and centrally placed and have small nucleoli (Fig. 20.7b). Osteoclast-like multinucleated giant cells are common, which are distributed unevenly throughout tumor: some fields may show frequent giant cells, while others may not have any. There is a highly variable mitotic activity, ranging from 0 to 20 mitoses per 10 HPF, with a mean of 6 mitoses per 10 HPF. Necrosis is common.
    - A variety of architectural patterns have been described, including pseudoalveolar, pseudopapillary, microcystic, fascicular, or trabecular patterns (Fig. 20.7c, d).

13. **What are the common immunohistochemical and molecular features of GNET?**
    - Tumor cells are positive for S100 (100%), SOX10 (100%), CD56 (70%), and synaptophysin (56%) and negative for HMB45, melan-A, MiTF, and tyrosinase.
    - *EWSR1* gene (22q12) rearrangement with *CREB1* (2q34) or *ATF1* (12q13) occurs in 25% and 50% of the tumors, respectively.

14. **What are the similarities and differences between GNET and clear cell sarcoma (CCS) of soft tissue?**
    - Both GNET and CCS may have an indistinguishable appearance on H&E staining, and both are S100 immunoreactive. *EWSR1* gene rearrangement with *CREB1* or *ATF1* may occur in both tumors. Both CCS and GNET carry an overall poor prognosis, with a tumor size >5 cm in CCS being associated with a worse prognosis than smaller lesions.

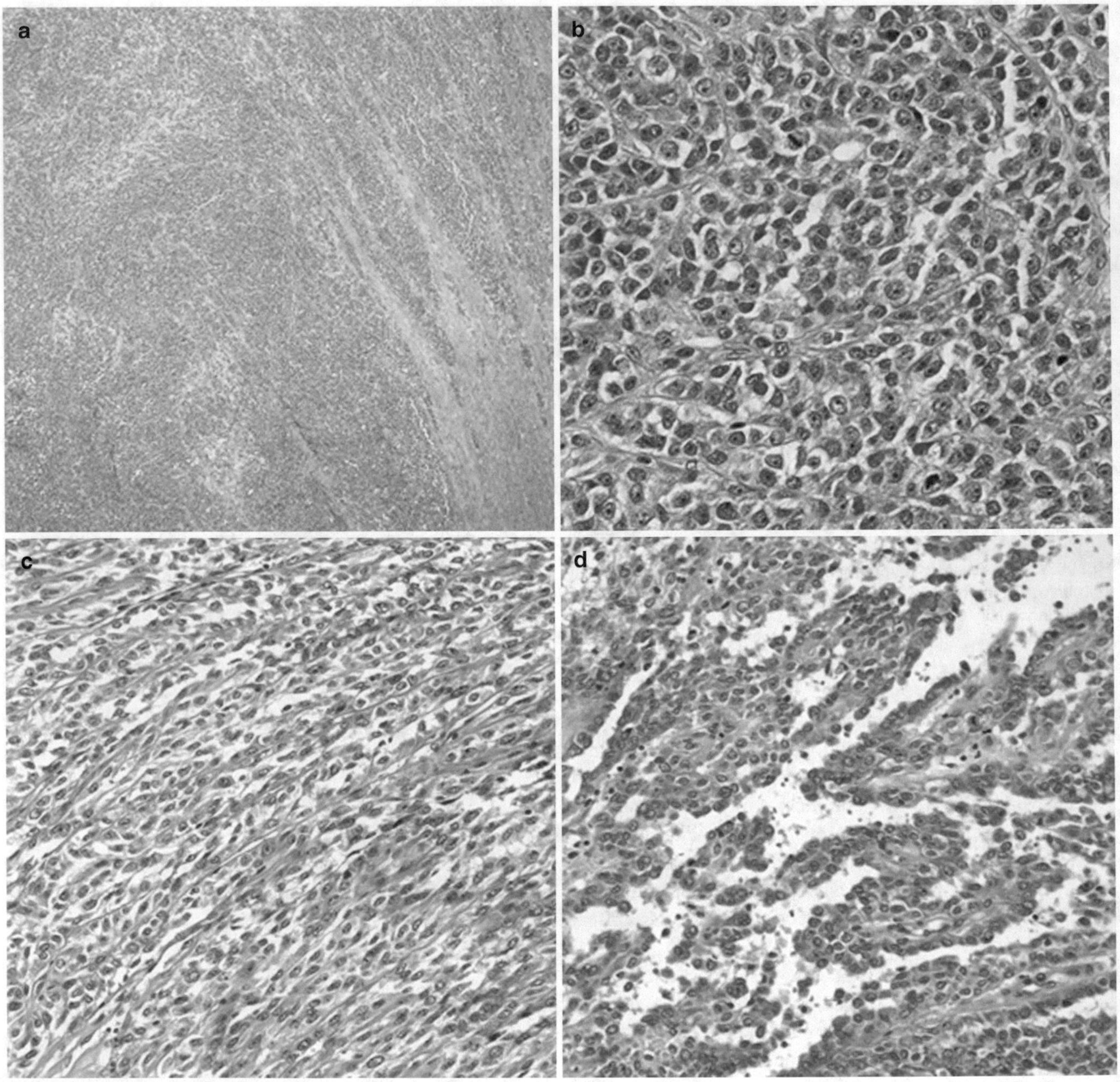

Fig. 20.7 (**a**) Gastrointestinal neuroectodermal tumor (GNET) showing sheets and nests of predominantly epithelioid cells with infrequent spindling. (**b**) Higher-power view reveals polygonal cells with vesicular nuclei; small, centrally located nucleoli; and moderate amounts of clear to pale eosinophilic cytoplasm. (**c**, **d**) GNETs display a variety of architectural patterns, including pseudoalveolar, pseudopapillary, microcystic, fascicular, or trabecular patterns

- However, CCS typically occurs in the dermis and soft tissues, while GNET occurs exclusively in the GI tract. CCS expresses melanocytic markers (such as HMB45, melan-A, MiTF, and tyrosinase), while GNET does not. Therefore, the presence of melanoma-like features suggests CCS. In addition, CCS demonstrates macronucleoli, while GNET primarily does not.

References: [14, 33–37]

15. **What are common S100-positive GI tumors and how may they be distinguished?**
    - See Tables 20.1 and 20.2 for benign and malignant S100-positive GI tumors.

16. **What demographic populations commonly are affected by fibromatosis?**
    - Desmoid fibromatosis presents in superficial and deep forms. Superficial forms arise in the superficial

Table 20.1 Benign S100-positive GI tumors

	Location	Histology	IHC/special stains
Schwannoma	90% in the stomach	Intramural tumor, spindled cells with relatively uniform cellularity, degenerative-type atypia, lymphoid cuff Microcystic/reticular variant shows microcystic and reticular growth pattern with anastomosing and intersecting spindle cells in a background of myxoid or collagenous, hyalinizing stromal islands	Strong diffuse S100 +, SOX10 + CD34 may be + near capsule
Schwann cell hamartoma	Virtually all in colorectum	Spindled cells with no ganglion cells, no lymphoid cuff, no nuclear pleomorphism. Confined to lamina propria	Strong diffuse S100+, CD34–
Ganglioneuroma	Three clinical presentations, described in Chap. 16	Ganglion cells and spindled cells with no axons, no epithelial component. No atypia	S100+ in spindle component, synaptophysin+ in ganglion cell component
Gangliocytic paraganglioma	Virtually all in ampulla of Vater	Can be distinguished by characteristic triphasic morphology, consisting of epithelial cells, ganglion cells, and spindled cells.	S100+, SOX10+
Granular cell tumor	Esophagus most common, followed by the colon	Dense granular cytoplasm, pseudoepitheliomatous hyperplasia	S100+, CD68+

Table 20.2 Malignant S100-positive GI tumors

	Location	Histology	IHC/special stains
Malignant granular cell tumor	Commonly the esophagus	Dense granular cytoplasm, necrosis, spindling, pleomorphism, increased mitoses, high N/C ratio	S100+, CD68+, Ki-67 > 10%, strong p53 expression
GNET	Small bowel most common	Sheets and nests of epithelioid or spindled cells, inconspicuous nucleoli. Osteoclast-like giant cells common	S100+, SOX10+, HMB45-, melan-A-
Melanoma	GI primary melanomas usually occur in the anus or esophagus, but majority of lesions in the GI tract are metastatic	Sheets and nests of epithelioid or spindled cells, with prominent nucleoli and increased mitotic activity	S100+, HMB45+, melan-A+, SOX10+. Staining for all these may be patchy or lost in metastatic tumors

soft tissues of the hand (palmar fibromatosis, aka "Dupuytren's contracture"), foot (plantar fibromatosis, aka "Ledderhose disease"), and penis (penile fibromatosis, aka "Peyronie disease").

- Classically, deep desmoid fibromatosis has been divided into three clinical presentations: abdominal wall, intra-abdominal/pelvis, and extra-abdominal.
  - Abdominal wall desmoids typically arise in young women during pregnancy or within their first year of childbirth, are associated with Cesarean sections, and arise in the rectus muscles and associated aponeurosis.
  - Intra-abdominal/pelvis most often affect adults between the ages of 20 and 40 years old and occur in the mesentery, pelvis, or retroperitoneum, with the mesentery being the most common site. Due to location, these tumors often grow to very large sizes before they become symptomatic. Overall, more than 50% of patients have a history of surgery. Mesenteric lesions often show myxoid features and arise either in association with Gardner syndrome (often following colectomy) or sporadically.
  - Extra-abdominal desmoid fibromatosis affects a similar population as intra-abdominal/pelvis cases (adults between the age of 20 and 50 years) and arises in the deep soft tissue, involving muscles and associated aponeuroses, particularly of the limb girdles, proximal extremities, and head and neck regions.
- Mutations in the *APC* and *CTNNB1* genes are seen in deep fibromatosis, while frequently observed molecular aberrations in superficial fibromatosis include trisomies 7 and 8 and loss of the Y chromosome. *APC* mutations usually occur in the setting of familial cases, while *CTNNB1* mutations arise in sporadic tumors.

17. **What are the growth patterns of intra-abdominal fibromatosis?**
    - In all sites, desmoid fibromatosis shows extensive infiltration into adjacent structures, with entrapped and atrophic skeletal muscles and adipose tissue (depending on location).
    - Overall, the histologic appearance is deceptively benign, with relatively uniform, spindled to stellate

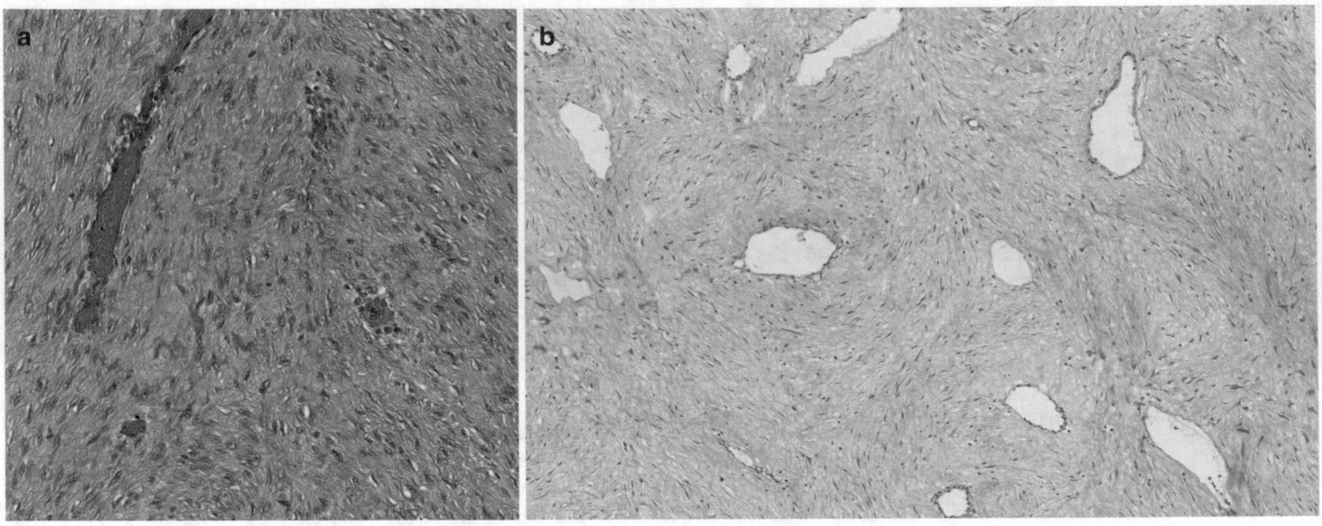

Fig. 20.8 (**a**) Intra-abdominal fibromatosis showing relatively uniform, spindled to stellate cells with vesicular nuclei, fine chromatin, one or more nucleoli, and moderate amounts of eosinophilic cytoplasm. (**b**) Medium-sized blood vessels with thin muscular walls are frequently seen

cells with vesicular nuclei, fine chromatin, one or more nucleoli, and moderate amounts of eosinophilic cytoplasm (Fig. 20.8a). Mitoses (typical) usually are scant, though often are seen easily in cellular forms. Cells are arranged in long, sweeping fascicles, while storiform patterns may be seen, which usually are focal. Superficial fibromatosis can be quite cellular, and the cellularity of deep fibromatosis can vary.

- The background matrix may be collagenous or show marked keloidal hyalinization and myxoid change (particularly in mesenteric tumors). Ossification or chondroid metaplasia may be present and should not be mistaken for malignancy.
- A characteristic feature, which can allow distinction from other (myo)fibroblastic process or scar tissue, is the presence of medium-sized vessels with thin muscular walls which are slightly gaping (Fig. 20.8b); this feature is especially helpful on a small needle core biopsy.
- The radiographic features of deep desmoid fibromatosis are strongly suggestive of this entity (particularly with abdominal wall desmoids), due to poor circumscription.
- Desmoid fibromatosis is associated with a high rate of local recurrence, even in cases with apparently negative surgical resection margins. Many different therapies have been tried, including surgery, antiestrogen therapy, chemotherapy (thalidomide), and radiation, but none has proven to offer a significantly lower rate of local recurrence. However, spontaneous regression is seen in about one-third of cases. Collectively, clinical experience to date has resulted in a more conservative clinical approach to therapy for desmoid fibromatosis, including observation only. Distant metastases do not occur.

18. How can intra-abdominal fibromatosis be distinguished from other spindle cell neoplasms of the GI tract?

- The histologic features of fibromatosis, in resections, are quite typical and do not frequently cause confusion. Cases with more myxoid areas, particularly in small biopsies, may mimic nodular fasciitis; however, the clinical features are different, as nodular fasciitis tends to arise in the subcutaneous tissues and has a history of rapid growth.
- In difficult cases, beta-catenin IHC may be helpful. Beta-catenin nuclear positivity is seen in about 75% of cases of fibromatosis. However, a significant percentage of other (myo)fibroblastic tumors and reactive myofibroblastic processes may show beta-catenin nuclear staining, and thus this must be just one factor of many that contributes to the diagnosis.
- Other immunohistochemical stains that are often positive in desmoid fibromatosis include SMA, MSA, and calponin. Scattered desmin-positive cells may be seen. CD34, S100, CD117, and DOG1 are negative, which help in difficult cases to distinguish desmoid fibromatosis from neurofibroma (CD34 and S100 positive), schwannoma (S100 positive), and GIST (CD117 and DOG1 positive). Keratins, particularly low molecular weight keratins, may sometimes be positive in desmoid fibromatosis and may lead to erroneous consideration of mesothelioma or carcinoma.

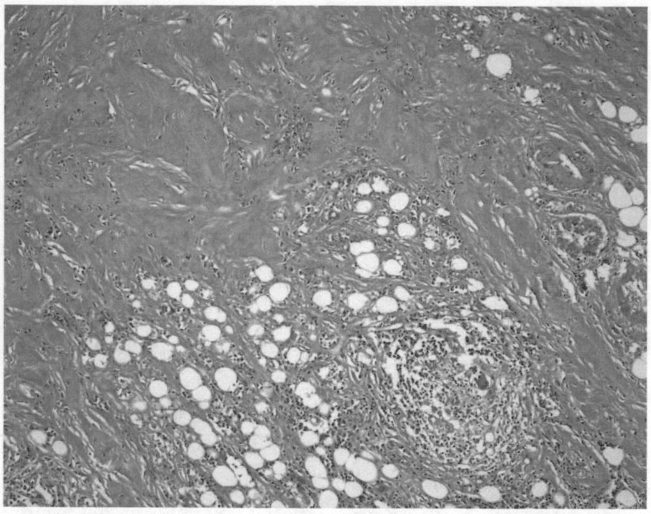

Fig. 20.9 Sclerosing mesenteritis showing dense fibrosis involving the mesentery. Areas of fat necrosis and inflammatory cell infiltrates consisting mostly of lymphocytes are seen

- Low-grade fibromyxosarcomas most often arise in the proximal extremities and limb girdles and typically show a whorling pattern, with alternating myxoid and collagenous areas. These are positive for MUC4 by IHC and for *FUS* rearrangement by fluorescence in situ hybridization (FISH), both of which are negative in desmoid fibromatosis.
- Sclerosing mesenteritis (aka retractile mesenteritis, mesenteric panniculitis, mesenteric lipodystrophy, and Weber-Christian disease in the literature) may present as diffuse mesenteric thickening or a single or multiple discrete mass lesions involving the mesenteric root. Histologically, it shows mesenteric fibrosis with dense collagen but also shows fat necrosis and chronic inflammation particularly around blood vessels (Fig. 20.9). Focal calcifications, lymphoid follicles, multinucleated giant cells, and obliterated vessels may be seen. However, these features may be absent in a small needle core biopsy. It appears that some cases previously described as sclerosing mesenteritis may represent manifestations of IgG4-related disease. Imaging findings may be helpful.
- Reactive myofibroblastic proliferation is often more cellular and inflamed. The clinical history can be very helpful, particularly if the lesion has appeared recently and rapidly. Scar tissue, especially in small biopsies, can look identical to desmoid.
- The clinical presentation, the radiographic findings, and the presence of medium-sized, muscular, slightly gaping vessels help favor desmoid fibromatosis.

19. What genetic syndromes are associated with fibromatosis?

- Most (90%) cases of deep desmoid fibromatosis are sporadic. Non-sporadic cases occur in the setting of a germline mutations of the *APC* or *CTNNB1* genes, which leads to activation of the Wnt pathway and to nuclear accumulation of beta-catenin.
- Inherited forms (*APC* mutations) usually arise in the setting of Gardner syndrome (familial adenomatous polyposis, osteomas, desmoid fibromatosis, and cutaneous epidermoid cysts, which are seen synchronously or metachronously).

References: [21, 38–45]

20. What are the characteristic histologic findings of leiomyosarcoma?

- Only reliable data on LMS of the GI tract are from cases reported after 2000. Prior to this, most cases reported as LMS are actually GISTs. Fewer than 100 cases are reported since 2000.
- LMS is associated with a local recurrence rate of 40–80% and a metastatic rate of 55–70%. Death from the disease ranges from 25% to 50%.
  - Tumors >5 cm appear to be associated with a worse prognosis.
  - Mitotic rate and degree of nuclear atypia do not correlate with prognosis.
  - Several studies have reported that gene expression patterns correlate with prognosis and thus have proposed different LMS classes; however, these currently are not used clinically.
- LMS is most commonly seen in the small intestine and colorectum (40% each) with no gender preference. The stomach and esophagus (10% each; about 2.5 more common in males) are less common locations. The median age of presentation is about 60 years old, except gastric tumors (median age 37). Clinical signs and symptoms may include weight loss, GI bleeding, anemia, abdominal pain, dysphagia, gastroesophageal reflux, and intestinal obstruction. On endoscopy, LMS is seen most commonly as a lobulated intraluminal or polypoid lesion. It may also present as an ulcerating, sessile, solid, or cystic mass.
- LMS is an infiltrative tumor composed of long intersecting fascicles of spindle cells with ample eosinophilic cytoplasm (Fig. 20.10), often oriented parallel and perpendicular to the plane of section. Tumor cell nuclei have blunt ends (so-called "cigar"-shaped nuclei). Severe nuclear pleomorphism is often present, but some tumors show more relatively uniform vesicular nuclei. Mitoses are typically high in GI LMS (50–100/50 HPF), but there are reports of rare

tumors with a low mitotic rate. Necrosis may be seen, but is not required for the diagnosis.
- Tumor cells are positive for SMA by IHC; most are also desmin positive. Muscle-specific actin, calponin, and caldesmon are usually positive. Rare cases are positive for keratins and CD34.

References: [2, 46–52]

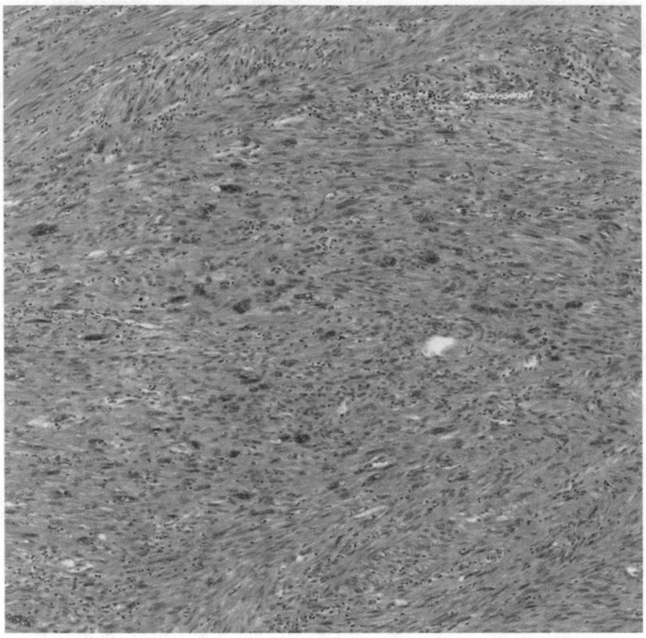

Fig. 20.10 Leiomyosarcoma showing spindled to stellate cells with moderate amounts of eosinophilic cytoplasm. Scattered cells show marked nuclear pleomorphism

21. **What patient populations are affected by EBV-associated smooth muscle tumors?**
    - EBV-associated smooth muscle tumors arise in immunosuppressed patients such as solid organ transplant recipients, bone marrow transplant patients, and AIDS patients.
    - Prognosis is variable and is closely related to the patient's immune status. Persistent disease is common; one large study reported 58% of patients having persistent disease up to 5 years after diagnosis. Death from disease is rare but has been reported.

22. **What are the characteristic histologic and immunohistochemical features of EBV-associated smooth muscle tumors?**
    - Patients with EBV-associated smooth muscle tumors often present with multifocal lesions, which can be easily mistaken for metastatic disease clinically. They have been reported at numerous visceral sites and soft tissue.
    - Different tumors in the same patient usually represent multiple different clones. Histology thus can be quite variable, within the same tumor and between tumors within the same patient. These range from primitive small ovoid blue cells, to spindled cells, to cells showing histologic and immunohistochemical features of mature smooth muscle/leiomyoma (Fig. 20.11a). Some tumors show a combination of these features.
    - In general, tumor cell nuclei are relatively uniform with minimal pleomorphism within a histologic type, i.e., small ovoid cells all relatively uniform

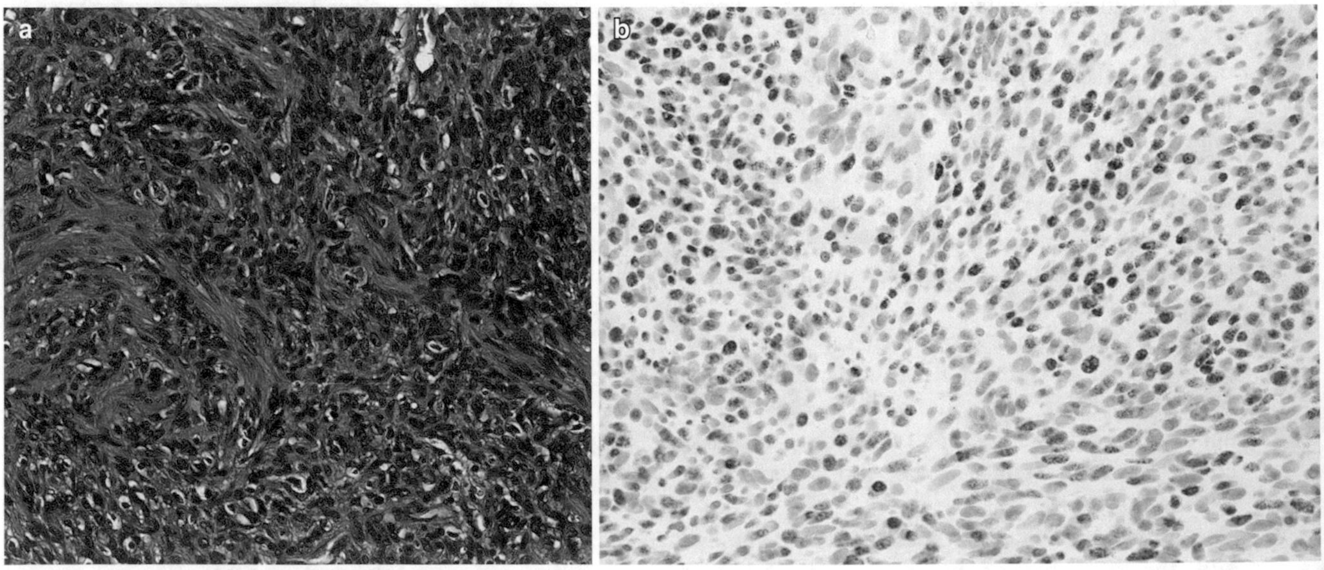

Fig. 20.11 (**a**) EBV-associated smooth muscle tumor featuring a mixture of primitive small ovoid blue cells and spindled cells with blunt-ended nuclei and moderate amounts of eosinophilic cytoplasm set in fascicles. (**b**) Tumor cells are positive for EBV by in situ hybridization (EBER)

Table 20.3 Differential diagnosis for EBV-associated smooth muscle tumors

Tumor	Features that distinguish from EBV-associated smooth muscle tumor	Association with immunosuppression
Leiomyoma	Mature smooth muscle cells only Solitary lesion Colorectum (as polyp) or esophagus (as mural mass) most common	No
Leiomyosarcoma	Moderate/marked nuclear pleomorphism Mitoses abundant (1–2/HPF) Necrosis often present	No
Rhabdomyosarcoma (spindle cell variant)	Spindle cells only No areas of primitive ovoid cells or mature-appearing smooth muscle cells MyoD1 and myogenin positive	No
Kaposi sarcoma	Gaping vessels in early-stage lesions Extravasated red blood cells, hemosiderins, and hyaline globules No areas of primitive ovoid cells or mature-appearing smooth muscle cells HHV8 positive EBV EBER negative	Yes

compared to each other, spindled cells also all relatively uniform compared to each other, etc. Primitive areas are often hypercellular, with overlapping nuclei. Lymphocytes often infiltrate the tumor(s), as seen in other EBV-associated tumors. Mitoses are often difficult to identify.

- SMA is positive by IHC in all histologic types. Desmin is often positive in the more mature-appearing areas and overall more variable in expression. In situ hybridization for EBV (EBER) is strongly and diffusely positive and is diagnostic (Fig. 20.11b).

References: [53–56]

23. What is the differential diagnosis for EBV-associated smooth muscle tumors?

- The diagnosis of EBV-associated smooth muscle tumors can be difficult, especially on small biopsies. In immunosuppressed patients, this should always be a diagnostic consideration. Multiple tumors with different histologic features, ranging from primitive ovoid to spindled cells, are characteristic and help make the diagnosis. EBV EBER in situ hybridization is diagnostic. Differential diagnosis is summarized in Table 20.3.

24. What vascular neoplasms affect the GI tract?

- Vascular neoplasms involving the GI tract are summarized in Table 20.4.
- Angiodysplasia is also included in this table but it is not a neoplastic process. Unlike true arteriovenous malformation, which is a congenital disorder, angiodysplasia is an acquired vascular lesion that may cause GI bleeding. Endoscopically, angiodysplasia appears as small (usually 0.5–1.0 cm), flat, cherry-red lesions, which can be solitary or multiple. It does not form a polyp or mass lesion.

References: [57–63]

25. What patient populations are affected by angiosarcoma of the GI tract?

- Based on studies on hepatic angiosarcoma, it is most commonly associated with carcinogen exposure, such as arsenic, vinyl chloride, radium, and anabolic steroids.
- Thorotrast (thorium dioxide), a radiocontrast dye used in the USA until the 1950s, was also implicated.

26. What differentiates angiosarcoma from hemangioma?

- Morphologic features favoring hemangioma include lack of cytologic atypia or mitotic activity. Cavernous hemangioma is characterized by large, cystically dilated thin-walled vessels, commonly seen with intravascular thrombi or mineralization. Capillary hemangioma features densely packed spindled cells with vascular spaces containing few RBCs, scant fibrous stroma, and hemosiderin-laden macrophages. Thrombi may be present.
- Morphologic features favoring angiosarcoma include infiltrative growth pattern and variable mitotic activity ranging from <5 to 30+ mitoses per 10 HPF. Most angiosarcomas have an epithelioid morphology with nuclear atypia, consisting of sheets or vascular networks of pleomorphic epithelioid cells with amphophilic cytoplasm, hyperchromatic nuclei, and prominent nucleoli.
- Histologic appearance alone should be the main determiner for malignancy in vascular tumors. However, IHC favoring angiosarcoma includes high Ki-67 proliferation index, diffuse and strong p53+, and diffuse MYC+.

References: [63–65]

27. What differentiates hemangioma from glomus tumor?

- The growth pattern may be similar in both tumors; both can grow in a solid pattern and may show

Table 20.4 Vascular neoplasms of the GI tract

	Location	Morphology	IHC
Hemangioma	Most common in small bowel, followed by rectosigmoid colon	Well-circumscribed, vasculogenic tumor without atypical endothelial cells. Secondary changes such as calcification and thrombosis may be seen	CD31+, CD34+, ERG+, factor VIII+. Epithelioid hemangioma may be CK+
Lymphangioma	Most common in small bowel	Anastomosing dilated vascular spaces with lymphatic lining, at least partially involving smooth muscle	D2-40+, VEGFR-3+, and LYVE-1+
Angiosarcoma	Most common in the colon and rectum	Pleomorphic, atypical, and infiltrative endothelial cells. Can be epithelioid. Vasculogenic nature may be obvious or inconspicuous (Fig. 20.12a, b)	CD31+, CD34+, ERG+, factor VIII+. Epithelioid angiosarcoma may be CK+
Glomus tumor	Most common in the stomach	Round to ovoid, monomorphic cells (Fig. 20.13). Can have prominent nucleolus	Diffuse SMA+ (99%), MSA+ (95%), and focal to diffuse CD34+ (32%), type IVcollagen+,CD31−,ERG−
Kaposi sarcoma	Can arise throughout the GI tract, most frequently in the stomach and intestine	Whorls of mucosal and submucosal vascular spindled cells with small vessel proliferation, extravasated RBCs, and hemosiderins (Fig. 20.14a–c)	HHV8+, CD31+, CD34+, ERG+, factor VIII+
Epithelioid hemangioendothelioma	Most common in the liver though may arise in a variety of sites	Abundant cytoplasm with round or oval nuclei. Central necrosis, hyalinization, or mineralization can be seen. Low-level atypical mitoses are tolerated	CD31+, ERG+, Fli-1+
Angiodysplasia	Most common in the right colon but can be seen anywhere in the large and small intestines. Typically seen in elderly	Small cluster of dilated and tortuous submucosal veins, mucosal venules, and capillaries (Fig. 20.15). Ecstatic vessels lined by endothelium only with scant or no smooth muscle. Dilated vessels passing through the muscularis mucosae may be seen	Not needed

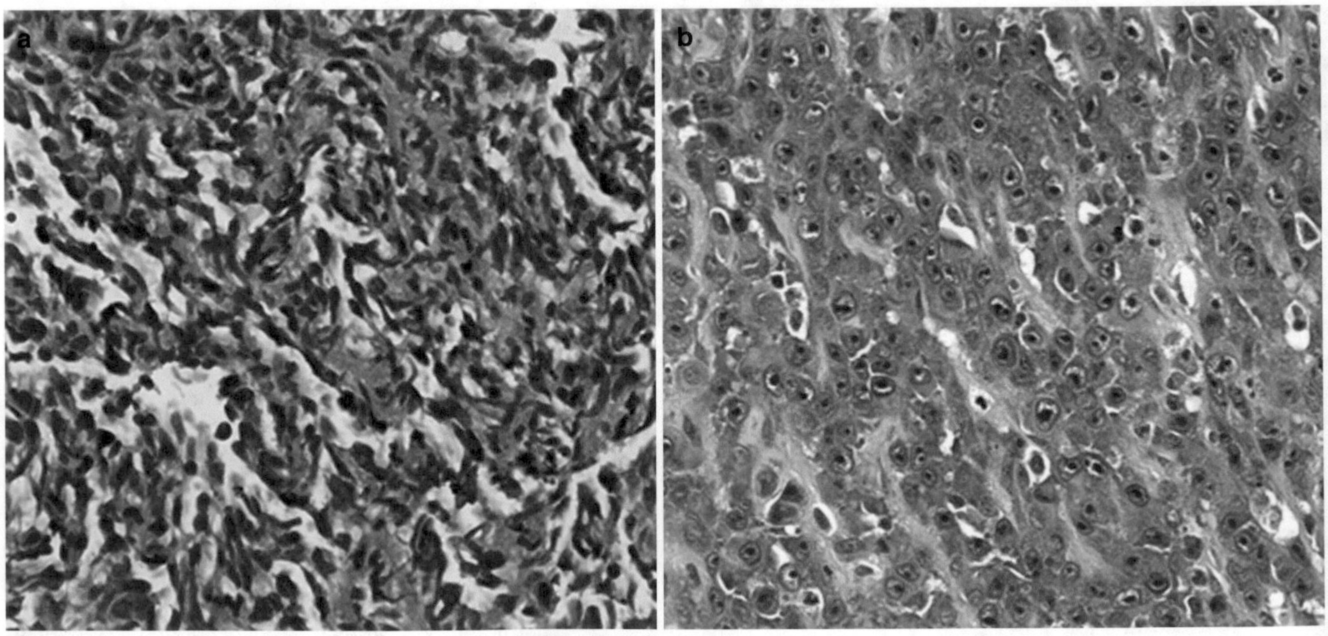

Fig. 20.12 (**a**) Angiosarcoma showing poorly formed slit-like vessels lined by pleomorphic endothelial cells. (**b**) Epithelioid angiosarcoma showing plump epithelioid cells with vesicular nuclei and prominent nucleoli, which may be confused on H&E for carcinoma or melanoma

dilated vascular spaces. However, glomus tumors have characteristic nuclei that are small, round, and monomorphic with a single "punched-out" nucleolus. The presence of characteristic glomus cells lining dilated vasculature is diagnostic.

- Immunohistochemical features are distinct: CD31, CD34, and ERG are positive in tumor cells of vascular neoplasms. Glomus tumors are rich in vasculature, but tumor cells are negative for endothelial markers. Instead, they are positive for SMA, type IV collagen, and CD34 (minority). Synaptophysin can be weakly positive in glomus tumor cells.

- Deep-seated glomus tumors have an increased risk of aggressive behavior, whereas deep-seated hemangiomas have no risk of malignancy. Glomus tumors can further be placed into categories of malignant, symplastic, or uncertain malignant potential.
  - Malignant glomus tumor: deep location and size >2 cm, or atypical mitotic figures, or moderate to high nuclear grade and ≥5 mitotic figures per 50 HPF
  - Symplastic glomus tumor: high nuclear grade without other malignant features described above
  - Glomus tumor of uncertain malignant potential: high mitotic rate and superficial location only, or large size only, or deep location only

References: [61, 66–69]

28. What are the distinguishing features of angiosarcoma from other malignant tumors of the GI tract?

- Angiosarcomas of the GI tract are frequently epithelioid and may express cytokeratins, representing a diagnostic pitfall. Positive vascular markers (CD31, CD34, FVIII, ERG) are useful in distinguishing vascular neoplasms from carcinomas. Angiosarcomas are uniformly negative for CK20, which is helpful in distinguishing it from carcinomas of the bowel.
- Epithelioid hemangioendothelioma (EHE) has indolent behavior and multifocal involvement. EHE shows a lobular architecture with cords/strands of primitive epithelioid cells with intracytoplasmic lumina set in a myxoid or hyaline matrix. In contrast, angiosarcoma grows in diffuse sheets with large, pleomorphic cells and prominent nucleoli. In challenging cases, FISH for CAMTA1 can be performed and should be positive in EHE.

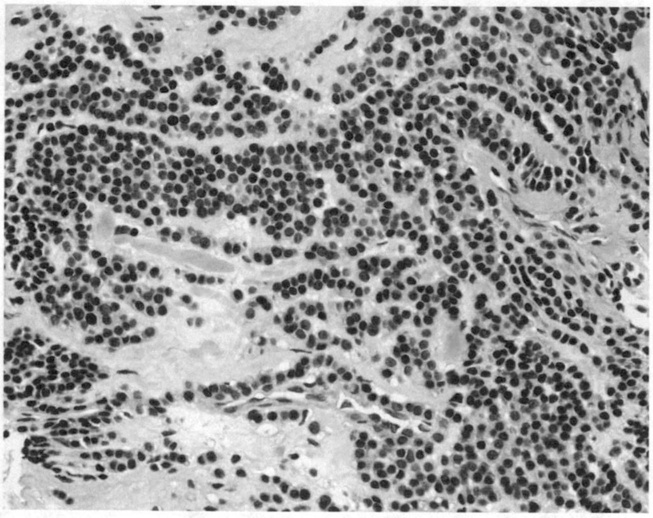

Fig. 20.13 Glomus tumor showing small round, monomorphic cells in a vascular and hyalinized background

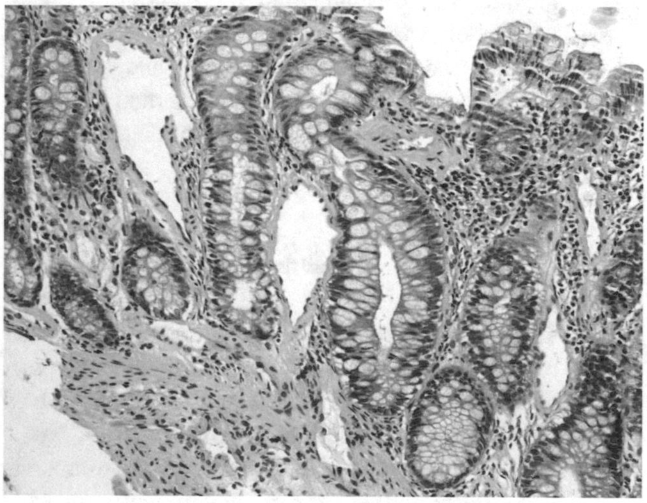

Fig. 20.15 Angiodysplasia seen in a colonic biopsy showing dilated veins, venules, and capillaries in the mucosa and the muscularis mucosae

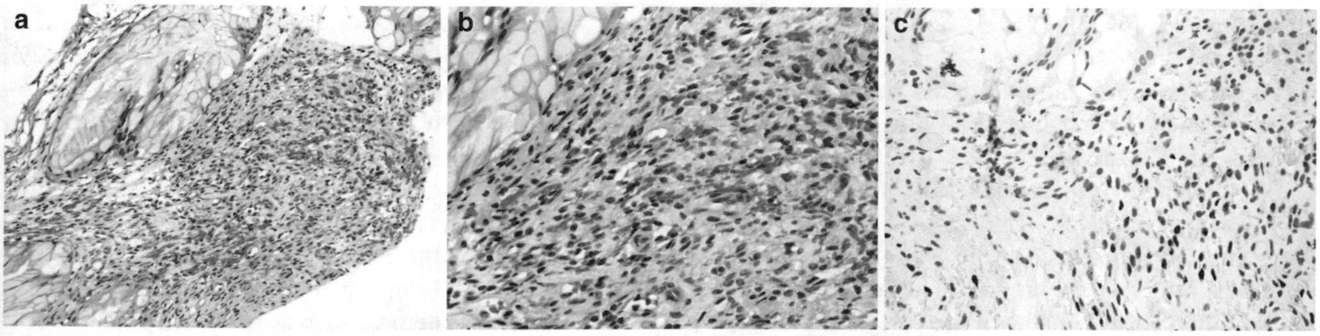

Fig. 20.14 (**a**) Kaposi sarcoma seen in a gastric biopsy showing destruction of the gastric mucosa by a short spindled cell proliferation in a vascular and hemorrhagic background. (**b**) The spindled cells exhibiting minimal to mild nuclear pleomorphism. Mitoses are difficult to find. Hemosiderin granules are noted. (**c**) Many spindled cells are positive for HHV8 by immunohistochemistry

Table 20.5 Distinction between lipoma and well-differentiated liposarcoma involving the GI tract

	Location	Size	Morphology
Lipoma	Usually the right colon, arising from the submucosa	Usually <10 cm, though there are rare cases reaching sizes up to 55 cm	Mature, uniformly sized adipocytes that lack cytologic atypia. No enlarged, hyperchromatic nuclei. Fat necrosis or histologic preparation artifact may mimic liposarcoma
Well-differentiated liposarcoma	Retroperitoneum, secondarily encasing GI tract	Usually >10 cm	Enlarged, hyperchromatic stromal cells with smudgy chromatin, commonly located within thick fibrous septa, which are visible at low magnification (Fig. 20.16). Lipoblasts are not required for the diagnosis

- Pronounced nuclear atypia is a helpful clue in distinguishing angiosarcoma from benign vascular lesions such as arteriovenous malformation or angiodysplasia. In addition, an association with mucosal prolapse or intussusception favors a benign process.
- Angiosarcoma can be categorized as low, intermediate, or high grade, with high grade correlating with the presence of epithelioid morphology, necrosis, degree of vasoformative architecture, and high nuclear grade. However, consensus guidelines from AJCC does not recommend grading angiosarcomas as conventional schemes do not correlate well with prognosis.

References: [64, 70]

29. What are the immunohistochemical features of angiosarcoma?

- Tumor cells are positive for cytoplasmic vascular markers (CD31, CD34, factor VIII) and show positive nuclear staining for transcription factors involved in vascular differentiation (Fli-1 and ERG).
- Keratins are often positive in angiosarcoma. Particularly, epithelioid variants can show strong and diffuse positivity for pancytokeratins AE1/AE3, CAM5.2, and CK19. Notably, CK20 is negative. Other cytokeratin-positive sarcomas, including epithelioid sarcoma and synovial sarcoma, do not characteristically affect the GI tract.

References: [64, 71–75]

30. What tumors of adipose tissue may involve the GI tract, and how to distinguish lipoma from well-differentiated liposarcoma?

- Tumors of adipose tissue that may involve the GI tract include lipoma, liposarcoma, and angiomyolipoma.
- Features that can help distinguish lipoma from well-differentiated liposarcoma are summarized in Table 20.5.

References: [76–86]

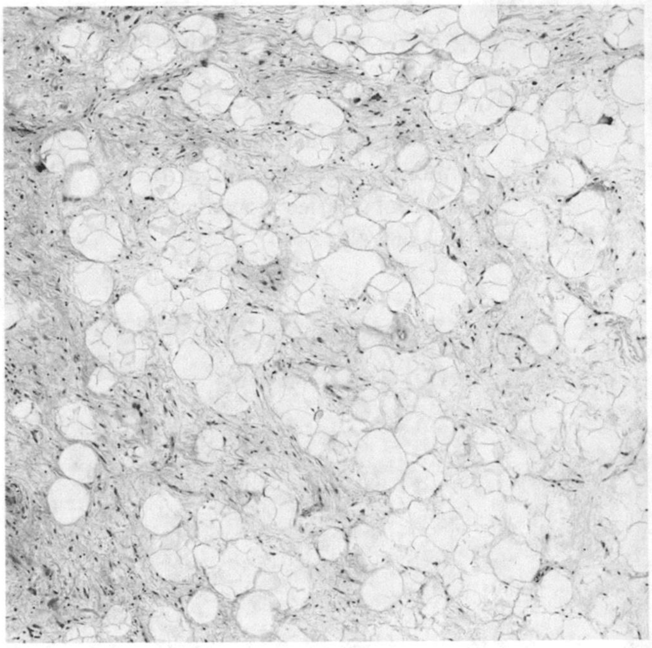

Fig. 20.16 Well-differentiated liposarcoma showing hyperchromatic stromal cells with smudgy chromatin. Lipoblasts are not required for the diagnosis

31. What immunohistochemical or molecular tests may help in the diagnosis of liposarcoma?

- To distinguish between well-differentiated liposarcoma (WDLPS) and lipoma, IHC can be helpful. MDM2 and CDK4 should be strongly positive in atypical stromal cells of WDLPS in 97% and 92% of the cases, respectively, and should be essentially negative in lipoma (5% and 2%, respectively).
  - MDM2/CDK4 IHC may have background or nonspecific staining and may be difficult to interpret.
  - Similar staining pattern is seen in atypical lipomatous tumor (ALT) of soft tissue.
  - MDM2 staining may occasionally be seen in other sarcomas such as low-grade osteosarcoma or non-sarcomatous malignancies such as non-small cell lung cancers.

- *MDM2* gene amplification by FISH is present in ALT/WDLPS and absent in lipomas. FISH shows a higher specificity in comparison to IHC. Specifically, IHC shows a sensitivity of 65–100% and a specificity of 59–96%, while FISH shows a sensitivity and a specificity approaching 100%. FISH can be especially helpful in the following situations:
  - Lipomatous tumor with questionable cytologic atypia
  - Recurrent lipomas
  - Large lipomatous tumors (>15 cm) without cytologic atypia
- Retroperitoneal WDLPS can usually be distinguished from other fat-containing neoplasms by H&E alone. With small biopsies, particularly of cellular well-differentiated or dedifferentiated liposarcoma (both of which may show large areas without adipocytes), analysis of *MDM2* amplification may be diagnostically useful. Other fat-containing neoplasms of the GI tract include lipoma, angiomyolipoma, and myxoid liposarcoma.
- Epithelial malignancies with signet ring cells may focally mimic lipoblasts. Lipoblasts are uncommonly seen in WDLPS, and abundant lipoblast-like cells should prompt consideration of alternate diagnoses.

32. How does well-differentiated liposarcoma differ from dedifferentiated liposarcoma?

- Dedifferentiated liposarcoma (DDLPS) is a biphasic tumor that demonstrates areas of WDLPS as well as a high-grade sarcomatous component. The dedifferentiated component is usually cellular and nonlipomatous. The morphological rangc is likewise broad, including fascicular and spindled, storiform, meningothelial, epithelioid, myxoid, pleomorphic, and rhabdomyomatous, among others.
- There exists some controversy in the cutoff between WDLPS and DDLPS. In authors' practice, we adhere to the guidelines as set forth by Evans et al. to distinguish these entities based on mitotic activity. The diagnosis of DDLPS requires at least 5 mitoses/10 HPF. For those cases that do not meet this criterion, the diagnosis of "cellular WDLPS" is used, which behaves in a more indolent fashion similar to WDLPS.
- Approximately 80% of patients with a dedifferentiated histology will recur locally, and ~30% will metastasize to distant sites within 3 years of diagnosis. Patients may present with either WDLPS or DDLPS, and recurrences may switch between WDLPS and DDLPS.

33. May dedifferentiated liposarcoma be diagnosed in the absence of a well-differentiated component?

- In a patient with known WDLPS, a local recurrent tumor may appear as DDLPS only.
- In the absence of a personal history of liposarcoma, the diagnosis of DDLPS in the context of a high-grade sarcoma with evidence of MDM2 overexpression (by IHC or FISH) is controversial. In the appropriate clinical context (e.g., large retroperitoneal mass), many practicing soft tissue pathologists would regard this as a presumptive DDLPS. However, other sarcomas, such as MPNST, have been shown to overexpress MDM2 in a minority of cases; thus, clinical and radiographic correlation is required.

34. How does liposarcoma of the retroperitoneum differ from atypical lipomatous tumor of the deep soft tissue?

- The histologic appearances of WDLPS and ALT are essentially identical. MDM2 overexpression is seen in both WDLPS and ALT. The biological behavior and overall prognosis for ALT differ greatly than WDLPS, which gives rise to the distinction in nomenclature. ALT has a high rate of local recurrence (up to 50%) but with very little to no metastatic potential in the absence of a dedifferentiated component. WDLPS has a higher rate of local recurrence (91%), and secondary involvement of the visceral organs confers a poorer prognosis. The estimated 10-year survival for ALT is 100%, while for WDLPS of the retroperitoneum, the 10-year survival is 82%

References: [75–83, 87, 88]

35. How is angiomyolipoma distinguished from liposarcoma?

- Features that can help distinguish between angiomyolipoma and liposarcoma are summarized in Table 20.6.

Reference: [80]

36. What are the histological variants of angiomyolipoma?

- Angiomyolipoma (AML) is a member of the perivascular epithelioid cell tumor family, otherwise called PEComa.
  - Typical AML shows a classic triphasic pattern with adipocytes, smooth muscle, and thick-walled vessels (Fig. 20.17a). Rarely, large retroperitoneal masses with abundant fat may be mistaken for a lipoma or liposarcoma. Likewise, AML with a scant fatty component may be confused for a LMS.

Table 20.6 Distinction between angiomyolipoma and liposarcoma involving the GI tract

	Histology	IHC	Molecular
Angiomyolipoma	Triphasic pattern consisting of abundant mature adipose tissue and smooth muscle surrounding convoluted, thick-walled, medium-sized vessels	Positive for HMB45 (100%), melan-A (87%), and SMA (73%)	Not routinely used
Liposarcoma	Enlarged, hyperchromatic stromal cells with smudgy chromatin, commonly located within thick fibrous septa, which are visible at low magnification. Lipoblasts are not required for the diagnosis	MDM2/CDK4 positive in atypical stromal cells	*MDM2* amplification by FISH

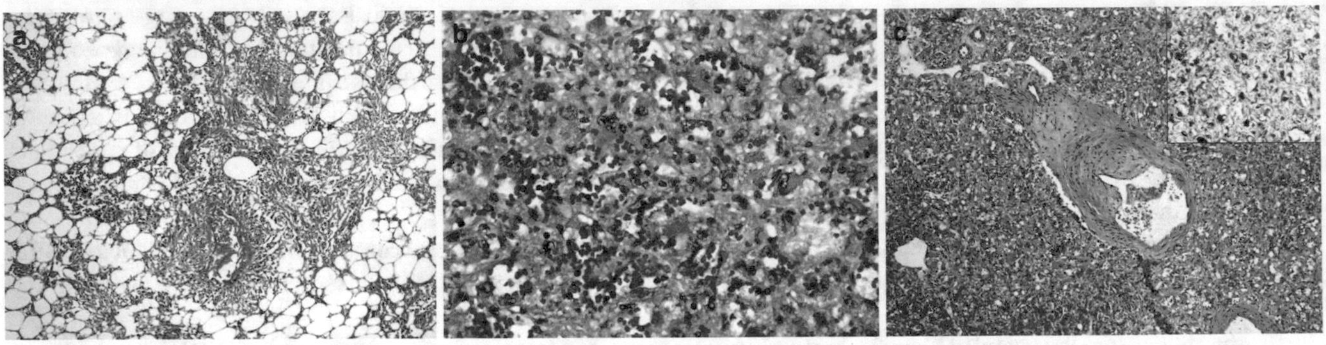

Fig. 20.17 (**a**) Typical angiomyolipoma showing a triphasic pattern with adipocytes, thick-walled vessels, and smooth muscle bundles around the vessels. (**b**) Epithelioid angiomyolipoma (PEComa) showing sheets of polygonal cells with abundant eosinophilic cytoplasm and indistinct cell borders. (**c**) A medium-sized, thick-walled blood vessel is shown, but no adipose tissue is present. Tumor cells are diffusely positive for melan-A (inset)

In each case, HMB45 or melan-A positivity will confer the diagnosis of AML.

- Spindle cell AML consists predominantly of spindled cells with no or sparse adipose-like tissue. Differentials include other spindle cell tumors, including leiomyoma, LMS, spindle cell melanoma, and GNET.
- Epithelioid AML consists predominantly of epithelioid cells with no or inconspicuous adipose tissue (Fig. 20.17b, c). Tumor cells are polygonal with clear or densely eosinophilic cytoplasm. Multinucleation and/or multilobation, hemorrhage, and necrosis can be seen. This variant generally has a more aggressive clinical behavior. Differentials include melanoma, carcinoma, CCS, and GNET.

37. What are the immunohistochemical features of angiomyolipoma?

- IHC can confirm a dual myoid-melanocytic differentiation.
  - Positive for melanocytic markers (HMB45, melan-A) and myoid markers (SMA).
  - Negative for epithelial markers.
  - IHC is usually not required for classic triphasic tumors, which can be diagnosed with confidence on morphology alone.
- Both melanoma and CCS are SMA negative and S100 positive.

References: [80, 89–93]

38. What are histologic features predicting a malignant angiomyolipoma?

- AML, as well as other PEComas, may be classified into categories of benign, uncertain malignant potential, or malignant. Lesions with two or more of the following features should be considered malignant:
  - Size >5 cm
  - Mitotic figures >1/50 HPF, or atypical mitosis
  - Nuclear pleomorphism or multinucleated giant cells
  - Necrosis
  - Infiltrative growth
  - Vascular invasion
- Based on a study on PEComas of the kidney, clinicopathologic parameters associated with disease progression (recurrence, metastasis, or death due to disease) include association with tuberous sclerosis complex or concurrent AML, necrosis, large tumor size (>7 cm), extrarenal extension and/or renal vein involvement, and carcinoma-like growth pattern (characterized by large cells arranged as cohesive nests, broad alveoli, and compartmentalized sheets separated by thin vascular-rich septa).
- Other features that indicate a poor prognosis may include a higher percentage of epithelioid component, p53 immunoreactivity, and decreased membranous E-cadherin.

References: [94–96]

Case Presentation

Case 1

Learning Objectives

1. To become familiar with the histologic features of the tumor
2. To become familiar with the immunohistochemical features of the tumor
3. To generate the differential diagnosis

Case History

A 49-year-old male underwent endoscopy for abdominal pain with biopsies showing two tumors – one in the duodenum and one in the stomach. At surgery, multiple distinct tumors were identified in the stomach, small bowel, and large bowel. Representative tumors from each site were excised.

Gross

A gastric wedge, partial small bowel resection, and partial colectomy were received, each showing a well-circumscribed mass with white-tan fleshy cut surface.

Histologic Findings

- The gastric tumor was composed entirely of primitive appearing ovoid blue cells (Fig. 20.18).
- The small bowel tumor showed only spindled cells with ample amounts of eosinophilic cytoplasm and cigar-shaped nuclei (Fig. 20.19).
- The colonic tumor showed a biphasic appearance, with primitive ovoid blue cells and scattered foci of spindled cells with eosinophilic cytoplasm.

Differential Diagnosis

- Multiple discrete tumors, including a leiomyoma of the small bowel and malignant granular cell tumors of the stomach and colon (unclear which is primary)
- EBV-associated smooth muscle tumors

IHC and Other Ancillary Studies

- SMA is positive in all tumors, in both primitive and more mature-appearing spindled cells.
- Desmin is positive predominantly in more mature-appearing spindled cells.
- EBV EBER shows strong and diffuse nuclear positivity in all tumors (Fig. 20.20).

Additional Clinical Information

After reviewing the initial H&E slides, the attending physician was contacted and asked if the patient was immunosuppressed. Indeed, the patient was a renal transplant patient.

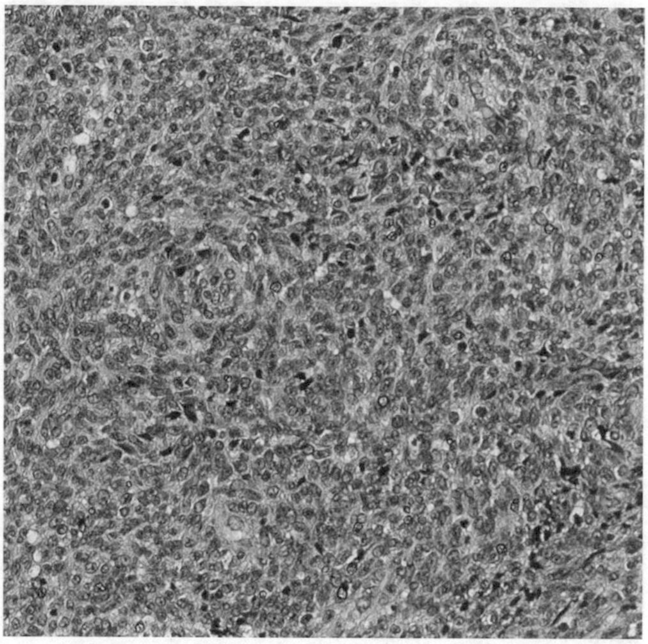

Fig. 20.18 (Case 1). EBV-associated smooth muscle tumor of the stomach composed entirely of primitive-appearing ovoid blue cells

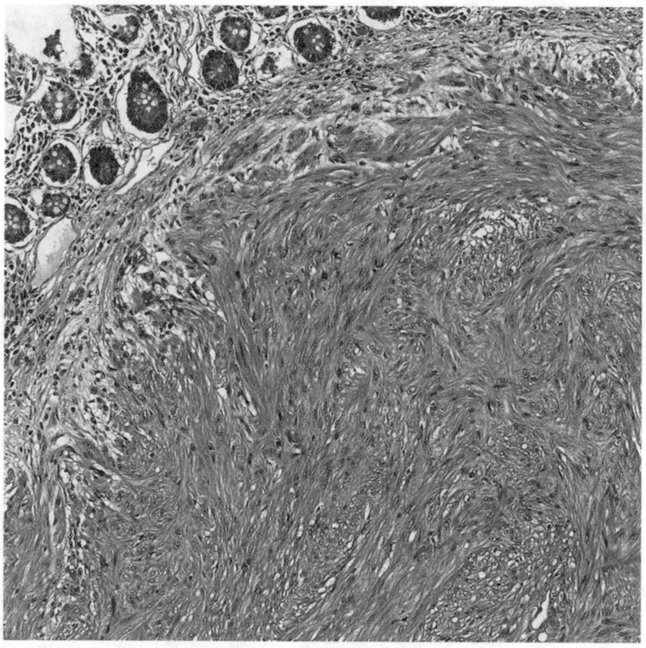

Fig. 20.19 (Case 1). EBV-associated smooth muscle tumor of the small bowel showing spindled cells with ample amounts of eosinophilic cytoplasm and cigar-shaped nuclei

Final Diagnosis

EBV-associated smooth muscle neoplasm.

Take-Home Messages

- EBV-associated smooth muscle neoplasm arises in immunosuppressed patients.
- Classically presents as multifocal tumors, which represent individual EBV clones rather than metastases.

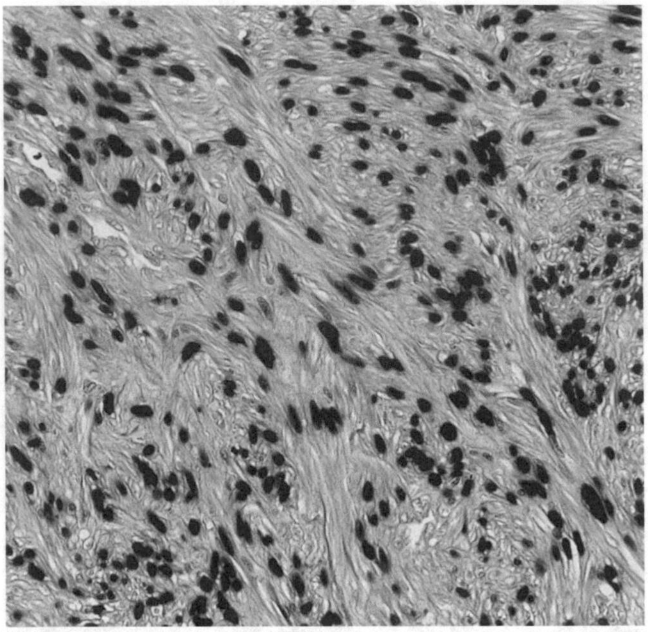

Fig. 20.20 (Case 1). EBV-associated smooth muscle tumors showing strong and diffuse positivity for EBV (EBER)

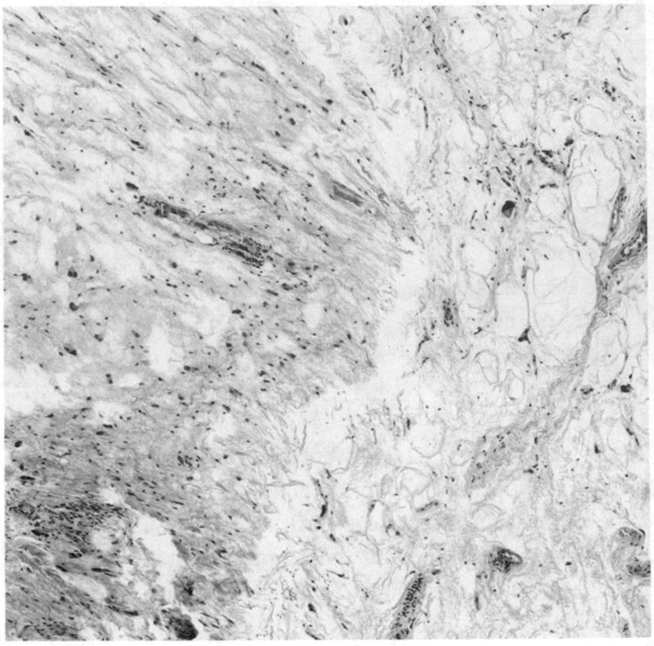

Fig. 20.21 (Case 2). Well-differentiated liposarcoma showing adipose tissue with fibrous septa of increased thickness and scattered enlarged, hyperchromatic, and pleomorphic cells in the fibrous septa and adipose tissue

- It shows diverse histologic features ranging from primitive ovoid blue cells to more mature spindled cells with the appearance of smooth muscle cells.
- EBV EBER is diffusely positive and is diagnostic.
- SMA is usually positive in all cells; and desmin shows more patchy positivity, usually staining more mature-appearing smooth muscle cells.
  References: [53–56]

Case 2

Learning Objectives

1. To become familiar with the gross and histologic features of the tumor
2. To become familiar with the immunohistochemical features of the tumor
3. To generate the differential diagnosis

Case History

A large (25 cm) abdominal/retroperitoneal mass was identified in a 65-year-old female on imaging studies following a motor vehicle accident. CT images showed two distinct areas, one appearing more solid. The tumor was located in the right retroperitoneum, surrounding the right kidney, with extension to the pericolic tissue of the ascending colon.

Gross

A radical resection of the tumor was performed and showed a tumor with distinct areas showing varying appearances, ranging from creamy yellow to tan/white and firm.

Histologic Findings

- Areas that were creamy yellow on gross examination showed adipose tissue with fibrous septa of increased thickness and scattered enlarged, hyperchromatic, and pleomorphic cells in fibrous septa and adipose tissue (Fig. 20.21).
- Areas that were tan-white and firm on gross exam showed non-adipogenic areas with varying appearances (Fig. 20.22), including highly cellular areas with scattered hyperchromatic/pleomorphic cells, spindled cells, floret-type giant cells, and readily identifiable mitoses (>5 mitoses/10 HPF) to less cellular areas composed of less pleomorphic cells and inconspicuous mitoses (1–4/10 HPF).

Differential Diagnosis

- Well-differentiated/dedifferentiated liposarcoma
- High-grade spindled and pleomorphic sarcoma, not otherwise specified

IHC and Other Ancillary Studies

- *MDM2* amplification present by FISH.
- Scattered positive cells for SMA in non-adipogenic areas; S100, keratins, and vascular markers are negative.

Final Diagnosis

Well-differentiated/dedifferentiated liposarcoma.

Take-Home Messages

- Most common sarcoma of the retroperitoneum, which may extend into or primarily occur within the abdomen/pelvis.

- Varying histologic appearances, from low to high grade, which are common in non-adipogenic areas.
- Definitive diagnosis requires identification of areas of WDLPS, a prior history of WDLPS, or *MDM2* amplification within a tumor with histologic and clinical features consistent with liposarcoma (*MDM2* amplification not exclusive to well-differentiated/dedifferentiated liposarcoma).
- Clinically characterized by a prolonged course (often decades) comprised of multiple recurrences as both well-differentiated and dedifferentiated tumors.

References: [77, 97–99]

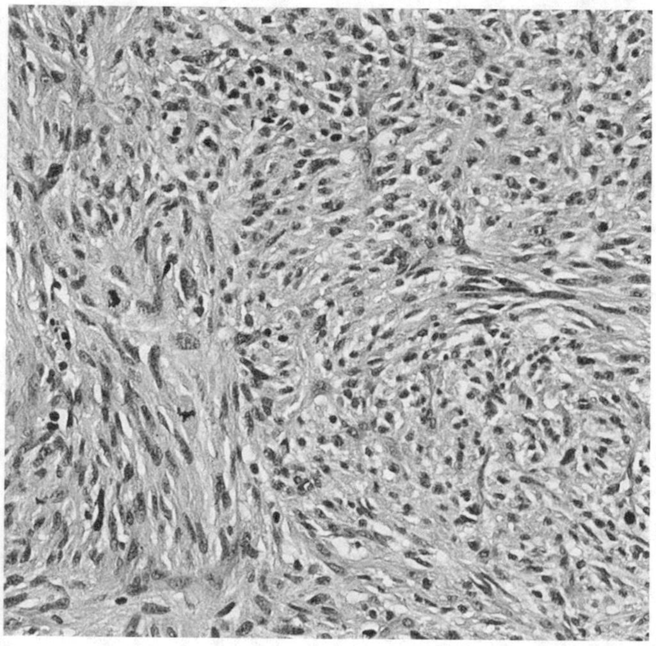

Fig. 20.22 (Case 2). Dedifferentiated liposarcoma showing highly cellular areas with scattered hyperchromatic and pleomorphic cells, spindled cells, and readily identifiable mitoses (>5 mitoses/10 HPF)

Case 3

Learning Objectives

1. To become familiar with the gross and histologic features of the tumor
2. To become familiar with the immunohistochemical features of the tumor
3. To generate the differential diagnosis

Case History

A 62-year-old male presented with symptoms of intestinal obstruction and an unintentional 25 pound weight loss over the preceding 6 months. Imaging showed an 8.5 cm mass of the jejunum, which was excised. The clinical diagnosis was GIST.

Gross

The tumor appeared to be arising from the muscularis propria. Cut surface showed a white, fleshy tumor with areas of necrosis and hemorrhage.

Histologic Findings

- Fascicles of spindled cells with ample eosinophilic cytoplasm and scattered marked pleomorphism (Fig. 20.23a).
- Mitoses, including atypical mitoses, were readily identified and numbered up to 20/10 HPF (Fig. 20.23b).

Differential Diagnosis

- Leiomyosarcoma
- GIST

IHC and Other Ancillary Studies

- Tumor cells strongly positive for SMA and desmin (Fig. 20.23c).
- Tumor cells negative for DOG-1 and CD117.

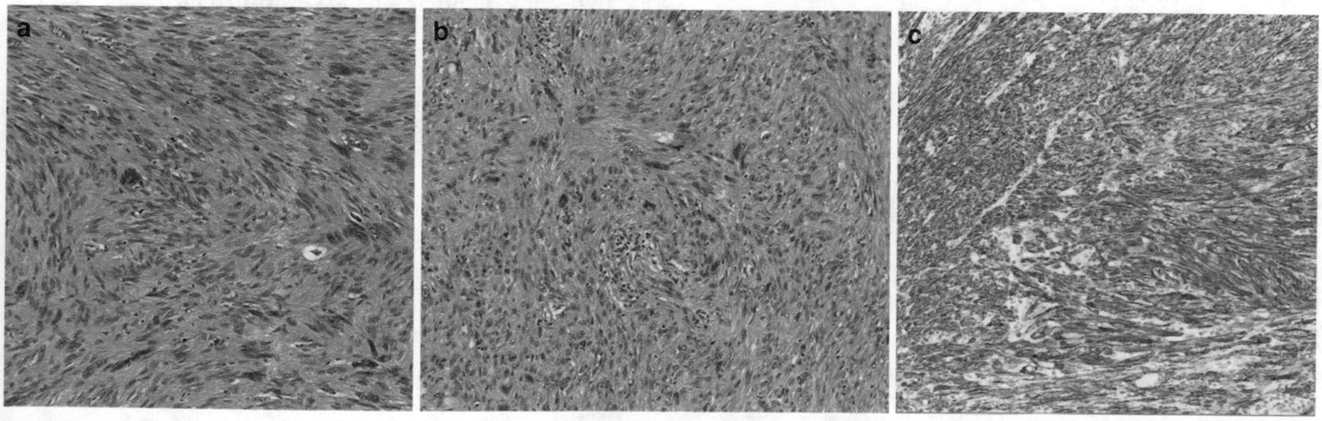

Fig. 20.23 (Case 3). (**a**) Leiomyosarcoma showing fascicles of spindled cells with ample eosinophilic cytoplasm and scattered cells exhibiting marked pleomorphism. (**b**) Mitoses, including atypical ones, are readily identified, which numbers up to 20/10 HPF. (**c**) Tumor cells showing strong positive staining for desmin

Final Diagnosis

Leiomyosarcoma, high grade.

Take-Home Messages

- Rare tumor in the GI tract in comparison to GIST.
- Most commonly seen in the small and large intestines.
- Most cases of "leiomyosarcoma" reported prior to 2000 actually represent GISTs.
- Malignant tumor, with a high rate of local recurrence, metastasis, and death from disease.
  References: [2, 46–52, 100]

Case 4

Learning Objectives

4. To become familiar with the gross and histologic features of the tumor
5. To become familiar with the immunohistochemical features of the tumor
6. To generate the differential diagnosis

Case History

A 7-year-old male had been experiencing 2 months of weight loss and 4 weeks of persistent fevers when he developed postprandial periumbilical abdominal pain and early satiety. An abdominal CT was performed, which showed a 5.5 cm abdominal mass.

Gross

The tumor was well-circumscribed and attached to the small intestine. Cut section showed a white, fleshy tumor with areas of necrosis and hemorrhage.

Histologic Findings

- Plump spindled cells present in variably cellular fascicles with admixed lymphocytes and plasma cells (Fig. 20.5).

Differential Diagnosis

- Inflammatory myofibroblastic tumor
- Spindle cell rhabdomyosarcoma

IHC and Other Ancillary Studies

- Tumor cells strongly positive for ALK1 (Fig. 20.24).
- Tumor cells negative for desmin, MyoD1, and myogenin.

Final Diagnosis

Inflammatory myofibroblastic tumor.

Take-Home Messages

- About one-third of patients, usually pediatric, have associated symptoms including fever, weight loss, elevated ESR, hypergammaglobulinemia, and anemia, which usually disappear after tumor resection.
- Positive ALK1 immunostaining is seen overall only in 50% of cases.
- The spindled variant does not show significant nuclear atypia, and the presence of atypia should prompt consideration of a different tumor.
  References: [30–32]

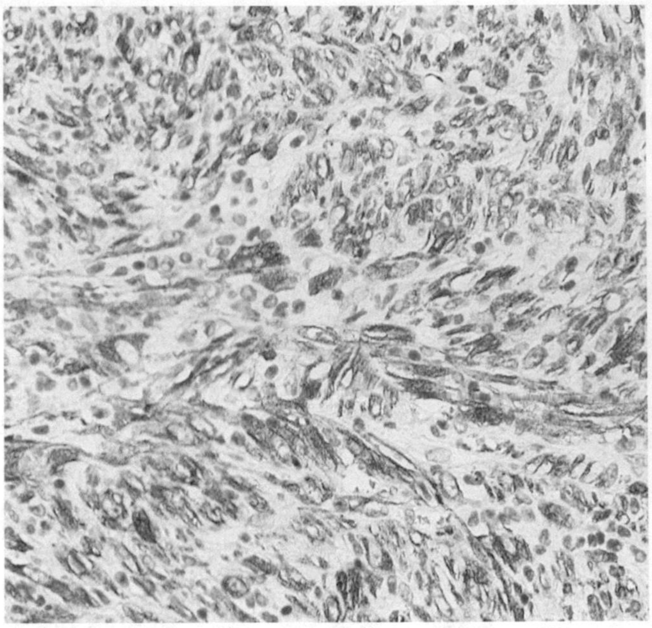

Fig. 20.24 (Case 4). Inflammatory myofibroblastic tumor showing strongly positive staining for ALK1 in tumor cells

Case 5

Learning Objectives

1. To become familiar with the gross and histologic features of the tumor
2. To become familiar with the immunohistochemical features of the tumor
3. To generate the differential diagnosis

Case History

A 37-year-old female with familial adenomatous polyposis and a history of prior total colectomy presented with abdominal pain. Imaging studies showed an 8 cm mass in the small bowel mesentery.

Gross

The tumor was centered in the mesentery with indistinct borders. Cut surface showed a firm white mass lesion.

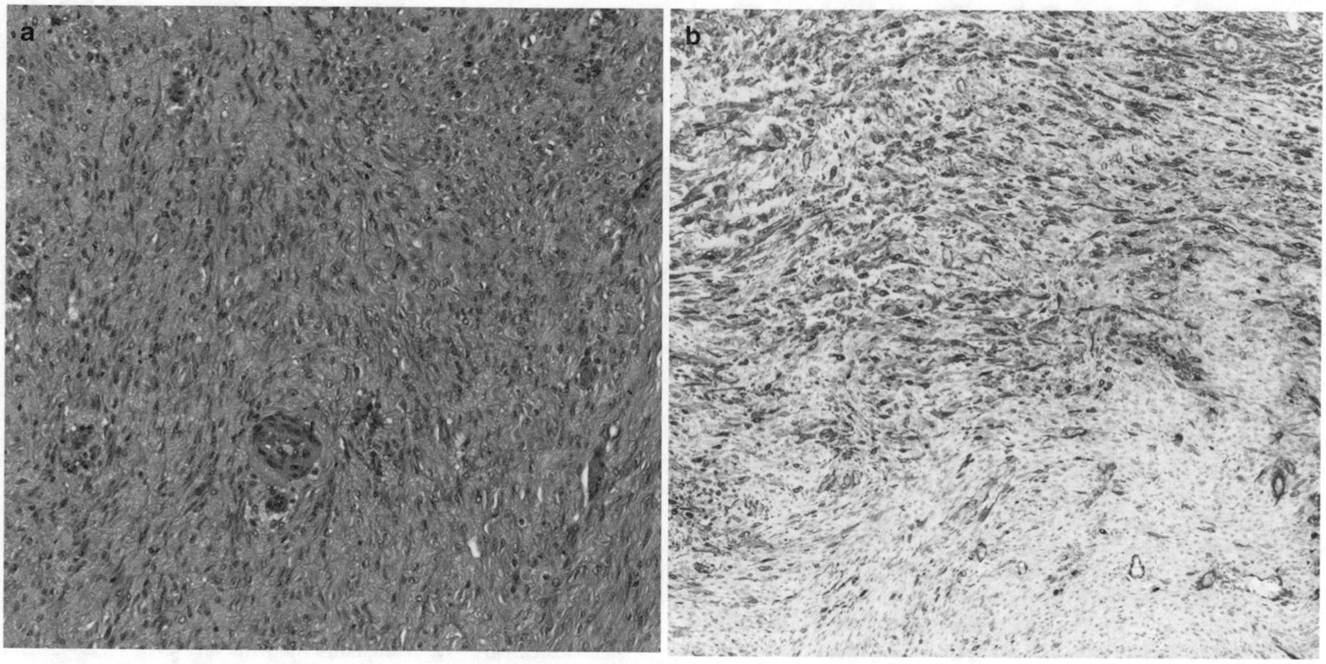

Fig. 20.25 (Case 5). (**a**) Desmoid fibromatosis showing long sweeping fascicles of spindled cells with ample eosinophilic cytoplasm and relatively uniform vesicular nuclei. Mitoses are inconspicuous. (**b**) Tumor cells are patchy positive for SMA

Histologic Findings

- Long sweeping fascicles of spindled cells with ample eosinophilic cytoplasm and relatively uniform vesicular nuclei; mitoses were inconspicuous (Fig. 20.25a).
- Scattered small- to medium-sized vessels with thin muscular walls that were slightly gaping were present.
- The lesion showed infiltrative borders with invasion into the small bowel wall.

Differential Diagnosis

- Desmoid fibromatosis
- Inflammatory myofibroblastic tumor
- GIST
- Sclerosing mesenteritis

IHC and Other Ancillary Studies

- Tumor cells show nuclear beta-catenin staining.
- Tumor cells are patchy positive for SMA (Fig. 20.25b) and rare cells positive for desmin.
- Tumor cells are negative for CD117 and DOG1.

Final Diagnosis

Desmoid fibromatosis.

Take-Home Messages

- Desmoid fibromatosis occurs both as sporadic forms and in Gardner syndrome.
- Beta-catenin staining may be seen in tumors other than desmoid fibromatosis, and not all cases of desmoid are positive.
- The clinical course is highly variable and cannot be predicted by histologic features. While a third of cases regress spontaneously, the rate of local recurrence (even with apparently negative surgical resection margins) is high. Many different therapies have been tried without consistent success. The current clinical approach is more conservative, including observation only.

  References: [39–43]

References

1. Lee LS, Singhal S, Brinster CJ, Marshall B, Kochman ML, Kaiser LR, Kucharzuk JC. Current management of esophageal leiomyoma. J Am Coll Surg. 2004;198(1):136–46.
2. Miettinen M, Sarlomo-Rikala M, Sobin LH, Lasota J. Esophageal stromal tumors: a clinicopathologic, immunohistochemical, and molecular genetic study of 17 cases and comparison with esophageal leiomyomas and leiomyosarcomas. Am J Surg Pathol. 2000;24(2):211–22.
3. Lott S, Schmieder M, Mayer B, Henne-Bruns D, Knippschild U, Agaimy A, Schwab M, Kramer K. Gastrointestinal stromal tumors of the esophagus: evaluation of a pooled case series regarding clinicopathological features and clinical outcome. Am J Cancer Res. 2014;5(1):333–43.
4. Levine MS, Buck JL, Pantongrag-Brown L, Buetow PC, Lowry MA, Sobin LH. Esophageal leiomyomatosis. Radiology. 1996;199(2):533–6.
5. Levine MS, Buck JL, Pantonngrag-Brown L, Buetow PC, Hallman JR, Sobin LH. Leiomyosarcoma of the esophagus: radiographic findings in 10 patients. AJR Am J Roentgemol. 1996;167(1):27–32.
6. Tran T, Davila JA, El-Serag HB. The epidemiology of malignant gastrointestinal stromal tumors: an analysis of 1,458 cases from 1992 to 2000. Am J Gastroentrol. 2005;100(1):162–8.

7. Miettinen M, Wang ZF, Sarlomo-Rikala M, Osuch C, Ruthkowski P, Lasota J. Succinate dehydrogenase-deficient GISTs: a clinicopathologic, immunohistochemical, and molecular genetic study of 66 gastric GISTs with predilection to young age. Am J Surg Pathol. 2011;35(11):1712–21.
8. Miettinen M, Majidi M, Lasota J. Pathology and diagnostic criteria of gastrointestinal stromal tumors (GISTS): a review. Eur J Cancer. 2002;38 Suppl 5:S39–51.
9. Miettinen M, El-Rifai W, Sobin HL, Lasota J. Evaluation of malignancy and prognosis of gastrointestinal stromal tumors: a review. Hum Pathol. 2002;33(5):478–83.
10. Kang HC, Menias CO, Gaballah AH, Shroff S, Taggart MW, Garg N, Elsayes KM. Beyond the GIST: mesenchymal tumors of the stomach. Radio Graphics. 2013;33(6):1673.
11. Fernandez MJH, Davis RP, Nora PF. Gastrointestinal lipomas. Arch Surg. 1983;118(9):1081–3.
12. Skipworth JR, Fanshawe AE, West MJ, Al-Bahrani A. Perforation as a rare presentation of gastric gastrointestinal stromal tumors: a case report and review of the literature. Ann R Coll Surg Engl. 2014;96(1):96E–100E.
13. Vagholkar K, Chavan R, Mahadik A, Maurya I. Lipoma of the small intestine: a cause for intussusception in adults. Case Rep Surg. 2015;2015:856030.
14. Stockman DL, Miettinen M, Suster S, Spagnolo D, Dominguez-Malagon H, Hornick JL, Adsay V, Chou PM, Amanuel B, Vantuine P, Zambrano EV. Malignant gastrointestinal neuroectodermal tumor: clinicopathologic, immunohistochemical, ultrastructural, and molecular analysis of 16 cases with a reappraisal of clear cell sarcoma-like tumors of the gastrointestinal tract. Am J Surg Pathol. 2012;36(6):857–68.
15. Khuri S, Gilshtein H, Darawshy AA, Bahouth H, Kluger Y. Primary small bowel GIST presenting as a life-threatening emergency: a report of two cases. Case Rep Surg. 2017;2017:1814254.
16. Antonescu CR, Scheithauer BW, Woodruff JD. Tumors of the peripheral nervous system. Silver Spring: American Registry Pathology; 2013. Fourth Series.
17. Hou YY, Tan YS, Xu JF, Wang XN, Lu SH, Ji Y, Wang J, Zhu XZ. Schwannoma of the gastrointestinal tract: a clinicopathological, immunohistochemical and ultrastructural study of 33 cases. Histopathology. 2006;48(5):536–45.
18. Kudose S, Kyriakos M, Awad MM. Gastric plexiform schwannoma in association with neurofibromatosis type 2. Clin J Gastroenterol. 2016;9(6):352–7.
19. Mekras A, Krenn V, Perrakis A, Croner RS, Kalles V, Atamer C, Grutzmann R, Vassos N. Gastrointestinal schwannomas: a rare but important differential diagnosis of mesenchymal tumors of gastrointestinal tract. BMC Surg. 2018;18(1):47.
20. Miettinin M, Shekitka KM, Sobin LH. Schwannomas in the colon and rectum: a clinicopathologic immunohistochemical study of 20 cases. Am J Surg Pathol. 2001;25(7):846–55.
21. Liegl B, Bennet MW, Fletcher CDM. Microcystic/reticular schwannoma: a distinct variant with predilection for visceral locations. Am J Surg Pathol. 2008;32(7):1080–7.
22. Asthagiri AR, Parry DM, Butman JA, Kim HJ, Tsilou ET, Zhuang Z, Lonser RR. Neurofibromatosis type 2. Lancet. 2009;373(9679):1974–86.
23. Fuller CE, Williams GT. Gastrointestinal manifestations of type 1 neurofibromatosis (von Recklinghausen's disease). Histopathology. 1991;19(1):1–11.
24. Le Guellec S, Decouvelaere AV, Filleron T, Valo I, Charon-Barra C, Robin YM, Terrier P, Chevreau C, Coindre JM. Malignant peripheral nerve sheath tumor is a challenging diagnosis: a systematic pathology review, immunohistochemistry, and molecular analysis in 160 patients from the French Sarcoma Group Database. Am J Surg Pathol. 2016;40(7):896–908.
25. Spans L, Fletcher CD, Antonescu CR, Rouqutte A, Coindre JM, Sciot R, Debiec-Rychter M. Recurrent MALAT1-GLI1 oncogenic fusion and GLI1 up-regulation define a subset of plexiform fibromyxoma. J Pathol. 2016;3:335–43.
26. Miettinen M, Makhlouf HR, Sobin LH, Lasota J. Plexiform fibromyxoma: a distinctive benign gastric antral neoplasm not to be confused with a myxoid GIST. Am J Surg Pathol. 2009;33(11):1624–32.
27. Graham RP, Nair AA, Davila JI, Jin L, Jen J, Sukov WR, Wu TT, Appleman HD, Torres-Mora J, Perry KD, Zhang L, Kloft-Nelson SM, Knudsen RA, Greipp PT, Folpe AL. Gastroblastoma harbors a recurrent somatic MALAT1-GLI1 fusion gene. Mod Pathol. 2017;30(10):1443–52.
28. Takahashi Y, Shimizu S, Ishida T, Aita K, Toida S, Fukusato T, Mori S. Plexiform angiomyxoid myofibroblastic tumor of the stomach. Am J Surg Pathol. 2007;31(5):724–8.
29. Lai J, Kresak JL, Cao D, Zhang D, Zhang S, Leon ME, Shenoy A, Liu W, Trevino J, Starostik P, Gonzalo DH, Wang H, Liu X, Fan X. Gastric plexiform fibromyxoma: a great mimic of gastrointestinal stromal tumor (GIST) and diagnostic pitfalls. J Surg Res. 2019;239:76–82.
30. Coffin CM, Hornick JL, Fletcher CD. Inflammatory myofibroblastic tumor: comparison of clinicopathologic, histologic, and immunohistochemical features including ALK expression in atypical and aggressive cases. Am J Surg Pathol. 2007;31(4):509–20.
31. Coffin CM, Watterson J, Priest JR, Dehner LP. Extrapulmonary inflammatory myofibroblastic tumor (inflammatory pseudotumor). A clinicopathologic and immunohistochemical study of 84 cases. Am J Surg Pathol. 1995;19(8):859–72.
32. Marino-Enriquez A, Wang WL, Roy A, Lopez-Terrada D, Lazar AJ, Fletcher CD, Coffin CM, Hornick JL. Epithelioid inflammatory myofibroblastic sarcoma: an aggressive intra-abdominal variant of inflammatory myofibroblastic tumor with nuclear membrane or perinuclear ALK. Am J Surg Pathol. 2011;35(1):135–44.
33. Antonescu CR, Nafa K, Segal NH, Dal Cin P, Ladanyl M. EWS-CREB1: a recurrent variant fusion in clear cell sarcoma--association with gastrointestinal location and absence of melanocytic differentiation. Clin Cancer Res. 2006;12(18):5356–62.
34. Kosemehmetoglu K, Folpe AL. Clear cell sarcoma of tendons and aponeuroses, and osteoclast-rich tumour of the gastrointestinal tract with features resembling clear cell sarcoma of soft parts: a review and update. J Clin Pathol. 2010;63(5):416–23.
35. Lyle PL, Amato CM, Fitspatrick JE, Robinson WA. Gastrointestinal melanoma or clear cell sarcoma? Molecular evaluation of 7 cases previously diagnosed as malignant melanoma. Am J Surg Pathol. 2008;32(6):858–66.
36. Rosai J. Editorial: clear cell sarcoma and osteoclast-rich clear cell sarcoma-like tumór of the gastrointestinal tract: one tumor type or two? Melanoma or sarcoma? Int J Surg Pathol. 2005;13(4):309–11.
37. Zambrano E, Reyes-Mugica M, Franchi A, Rosai J. An osteoclast-rich tumor of the gastrointestinal tract with features resembling clear cell sarcoma of soft parts: reports of 6 cases of a GIST simulator. Int J Surg Pathol. 2003;11(2):75–81.
38. Carlson JW, Fletcher CD. Immunohistochemistry for beta-catenin in the differential diagnosis of spindle cell lesions: analysis of a series and review of the literature. Histopathology. 2007;51(4):509–14.
39. Fiore M, MacNeill A, Gronchi A, Colombo C. Desmoid-type fibromatosis: evolving treatment standards. Surg Oncol Clin N Am. 2016;25(4):803–26.
40. Kasper B, Baumgarten C, Bonvalot S, Haas R, Haller F, Hohenberger P, Moreau G, van der Graaf WT, Gronchi A, Desmoid Working Group. Management of sporadic desmoid-type fibromatosis: a European consensus approach based on patients' and professionals' expertise - a sarcoma patients EuroNet and

European Organisation for Research and Treatment of Cancer/Soft Tissue and Bone Sarcoma Group initiative. Eur J Cancer. 2015;51(2):127–36.
41. Penel N, Le Cesne A, Bonvalot S, Giraud A, Bompas E, Rios M, Salas S, Isambert N, Boudou-Rouquette P, Honore C, Italiano A, Ray-Coquard I, Piperno-Neumann S, Gouolin F, Bertucci F, Ryckewaert T, Kurtz JE, Ducimetiere F, Coindre JM, Blay JY. Surgical versus non-surgical approach in primary desmoid-type fibromatosis patients: a nationwide prospective cohort from the French Sarcoma Group. Eur J Cancer. 2017;83:125–31.
42. Skubitz KM. Biology and treatment of aggressive fibromatosis or desmoid tumor. Mayo Clin Proc. 2017;92(6):947–64.
43. Thway K, Abou Sherif S, Riddell AM, Mudan S. Fibromatosis of the sigmoid colon with CTNNB1 (β-Catenin) gene mutation, arising at the site of ileocolic anastomosis for resection of gastrointestinal stromal tumor. Int J Surg Pathol. 2016;24(3):264.
44. Chen TA, Montgomery EA. Are tumefactive lesions classified as sclerosing mesenteritis a subset of IgG4-related sclerosing disorders? J Clin Pathol. 2008;61(10):1093–7.
45. Minato H, Shimizu J, Arano Y, Saito K, Masunaga T, Sakashita T, Nojima T. IgG4-related sclerosing mesenteritis: a rare mesenteric disease of unknown etiology. Pathol Int. 2012;62(4):281–6.
46. Guo X, Jo VY, Mills AM, Zhu SX, Lee CH, Espinosa I, Nucci MR, Varma S, Forgo E, Hastie T, Anderson S, Ganjoo K, Bck AH, West RB, Fletcher CD, van de Rijn M. Clinically relevant molecular subtypes in leiomyosarcoma. Clin Cancer Res. 2015;21(15):3501–11.
47. Hilal L, Barada K, Mukherji D, Temraz S, Shamseddine A. Gastrointestinal (GI) leiomyosarcoma (LMS) case series and review on diagnosis, management, and prognosis. Med Oncol. 2016;33(2):20.
48. Italiano A, Lagarde P, Brulard C, Terrier P, Lae M, Marques B, Ranchere-Vince D, Michels JJ, Trassard M, Cioffi A, Piperno-Neumann S, Chevreau C, Blay JY, Delcambre C, Isambert N, Penel N, Bay JO, Bonvalot S, Le Cesne A, Chibon F. Genetic profiling identifies two classes of soft-tissue leiomyosarcomas with distinct clinical characteristics. Clin Cancer Res. 2013;19(5):1190–6.
49. Miettinen M, Sarlomo-Rikala M, Sobion LH, Lasota J. Gastrointestinal stromal tumors and leiomyosarcomas in the colon: a clinicopathologic, immunohistochemical, and molecular genetic study of 44 cases. Am J Surg Pathol. 2000;24(10):1339–52.
50. Miettinen M, Furlong M, Sarlomo-Rikala M, Burke A, Sobin LH, Lasota J. Gastrointestinal stromal tumors, intramural leiomyomas, and leiomyosarcomas in the rectum and anus: a clinicopathologic, immunohistochemical, and molecular genetic study of 144 cases. Am J Surg Pathol. 2001;25(9):1121–33.
51. Miettinen M, Sobin LH, Lasota J. True smooth muscle tumors of the small intestine: a clinicopathologic, immunohistochemical, and molecular genetic study of 25 cases. Am J Surg Pathol. 2009;33(3):430–6.
52. Yamamoto H, Handa M, Tobo T, Setsu N, Fujita K, Oshiro Y, Mihara Y, Yoshikawa Y, Oda Y. Clinicopathological features of primary leiomyosarcoma of the gastrointestinal tract following recognition of gastrointestinal stromal tumours. Histopathology. 2013 Aug;63(2):194–207.
53. Deyrup T, Lee VK, Hill CE, Cheuk W, Toh HC, Kesavan S, Chan EW, Weiss SW. Epstein-Barr virus-associated smooth muscle tumors are distinctive mesenchymal tumors reflecting multiple infection events: a clinicopathologic and molecular analysis of 29 tumors from 19 patients. Am J Surg Pathol. 2006;30(1):75–82.
54. Deyrup AT. Epstein-Barr virus-associated epithelial and mesenchymal neoplasms. Hum Pathol. 2008;39(4):473–83.
55. Jonigk D, Laenger F, Maegel L, Izykowski N, Rische J, Tiede C, Klein C, Maecker-Kolhoff B, Kreipe H, Hussein K. Molecular and clinicopathological analysis of Epstein-Barr virus-associated posttransplant smooth muscle tumors. Am J Transplant. 2012;12(7):1908–17.
56. Stubbins RJ, Alami Laroussi N, Peters AC, Urschel S, Dicke F, Lai RL, Zhu J, Mabilangan C, Preiksaitis JK. Epstein-Barr virus associated smooth muscle tumors in solid organ transplant recipients: incidence over 31 years at a single institution and review of the literature. Transpl Infect Dis. 2018;9:e13010.
57. Becq A, Rahmi G, Perrod G, Cellier C. Hemorrhagic angiodysplasia of the digestive tract: pathogenesis, diagnosis, and management. Gastrointest Endoc. 2017;86(5):792–806.
58. Sardaro A, Bardoscia L, Petruzzelli MF, Nikolaou A, Detti B, Angelelli G. Pulmonary epithelioid hemangioendothelioma presenting with vertebral metastases: a case report. J Med Case Reports. 2014;8:201.
59. Lau K, Massad M, Pollack C, Rubin C, Yeh J, Wang J, Edelman G, Yeh J, Prasad S, Weinberg G. Clinical patterns and outcome in epithelioid hemangioendothelioma with or without pulmonary involvement: insights from an internet registry in the study of rare cancer. Chest. 2011;140(5):1312–8.
60. Lee AJ, Brenner L, Mourad B, Monteiro C, Vega KJ, Munoz JC. Gastrointestinal Kaposi's sarcoma: case report and review of the literature. World J Gastrointest Pharmacol Ther. 2015;6(3):89–95.
61. Mravic M, LaChaud G, Nguyen A, Scott MA, Dry SM, James AW. Clinical and histopathological diagnosis of glomus tumor: an institutional experience of 138 cases. Int J Surg Pathol. 2015;23(3):181–8.
62. Lawless ME, Lloyd KA, Swanson PE, Upton MP, Yeh MM. Lymphangiomatous lesions of the gastrointestinal tract: a clinicopathologic study and comparison between adult and children. Am J Clin Pathol. 2015;144(4):563–9.
63. Han EC, Kim SH, Kim HY, Jung SE, Park KW. Gastrointestinal hemangioma in childhood: a rare cause of gastrointestinal bleeding. Korean J Pediatr. 2014;57(5):245–9.
64. Allison KH, Yoder BJ, Bronner MP, Goldblum JR, Rubin BP. Angiosarcoma involving the gastrointestinal tract: a series of primary and metastatic cases. Am J Surg Pathol. 2004;28(3):298–307.
65. Lin J, Bigge J, Ulbright TM, Montgomery E. Anastomosing hemangioma of the liver and gastrointestinal tract: an unusual variant histologically mimicking angiosarcoma. Am J Surg Pathol. 2013;37(11):1761–5.
66. Folpe AL, Fanburg-Smith JC, Miettinen M, Weiss SW. Atypical and malignant glomus tumors: analysis of 52 cases, with a proposal for the reclassification of glomus tumors. Am J Surg Pathol. 2001;25(1):1–12.
67. Fan C, Liu Y, Lin X, Han Y, He A, Wang E. Epithelioid angiosarcoma at chest wall which needs to be carefully distinguished from malignant mesothelioma: report of a rare case. Int J Clin Exp Pathol. 2014;17(12):9056–60.
68. Gombos Z, Zhang PJ. Glomus tumor. Arch Pathol Lab Med. 2008;132(9):1448–52.
69. Miettinen M, Paal E, Lasota J, Sobin LH. Gastrointestinal glomus tumors: a clinicopathologic, immunohistochemical, and molecular genetic study of 32 cases. Am J Surg Pathol. 2002;26(3):301–11.
70. Buehler D, Rice SR, Moody JS, Ruch P, Hafez GR, Attia S, Longley BJ, Kozak KR. Angiosarcoma outcomes and prognostic factors: a 25-year single institution experience. Am J Clin Oncol. 2014;37(5):473–9.
71. Sullivan HC, Edgar MA, Cohen C, Kovach CK, Hookim K, Reid MD. The utility of ERG, CD31 and CD34 in the cytological diagnosis of angiosarcoma: an analysis of 25 cases. J Clin Pathol. 2015;68(1):44–50.
72. McKay KM, Doyle LA, Lazar AJ, Hornick JL. Expression of ERG, an Ets family transcription factor, distinguishes cutaneous

angiosarcoma from histological mimics. Histopathology. 2012;61(5):989–91.
73. Folpe AL, Chand EM, Goldblum JR, Weiss SW. Expression of Fli-1, a nuclear transcription factor, distinguishes vascular neoplasms from potential mimics. Am J Surg Pathol. 2001;25(8):1061–6.
74. Rao P, Lahat G, Arnold C, Gavino AC, Lahat S, Hornick JL, Lev D, Lazar AJ. Angiosarcoma: a tissue microarray study with diagnostic implications. Am J Dermatopathol. 2013;35(4):432–7.
75. Gray MH, Rosenberg AE, Dickerson GR, Bhan AK. Cytokeratin expression in epithelioid vascular neoplasms. Hum Pathol. 1990;21(2):212–7.
76. Knebel C, Lenze U, Pohlig F, Lenze F, Harrasser N, Suren C, Breitenbach J, Rechl H, von Eisenhart-Rothe R, Muhlhofer HML. Prognostic factors and outcome of Liposarcoma patients: a retrospective evaluation over 15 years. BMC Cancer. 2017;17(1):410.
77. Evans HL. Atypical lipomatous tumor, its variants, and its combined forms: a study of 61 cases, with a minimum follow-up of 10 years. Am J Surg Pathol. 2007;31(1):1–14.
78. Wallander ML, Tripp S, Layfield LJ. MDM2 amplification in malignant peripheral nerve sheath tumors correlates with p53 protein expression. Arch Pathol Lab Med. 2012;136(1):95–9.
79. Singer S, Antonescu CR, Riedel E, Brennan MF. Histologic subtype and margin of resection predict pattern of recurrence and survival for retroperitoneal liposarcoma. Ann Surg. 2003;238(3):358–70.
80. Park JH, Lee C, Suh JH, Kim G, Song B, Moon KC. Renal epithelioid angiomyolipoma: histopathologic review, immunohistochemical evaluation and prognostic significance. Pathol Int. 2016;66(10):571–7.
81. Kimura H, Dobashi Y, Nojima T, Nakamura H, Yamamoto N, Tsuchiya H, Ikeda H, Sawada-Kitamura S, Oyama T, Ooi A. Utility of fluorescence in situ hybridization to detect MDM2 amplification in liposarcomas and their morphological mimics. Int J Clin Exp Pathol. 2013;6(7):1306–16.
82. Dworakowska D, Jassem E, Jassem J, Peters B, Dziadziuszko R, Zylicz M, Jakobkiewicz-Banecka J, Kobierska-Gulida G, Szymanowski A, Roessner A, Schneider-Stock R. MDM2 gene amplification: a new independent factor of adverse prognosis in non-small cell lung cancer (NSCLC). Lung Cancer. 2004;43(3):285–95.
83. Dujardin F, Binh MB, Bouvier C, Gomez-Brouchet A, Larousserie F, Muret AD, Louis-Brennetot C, Aurias A, Coindre JM, Guillou L, Pedeutour F, Duval H, Collin C, de Pinieux G. MDM2 and CDK4 immunohistochemistry is a valuable tool in the differential diagnosis of low-grade osteosarcoma and other primary fibro-osseous lesions of the bone. Mod Pathol. 2011;24(5):624–37.
84. Binh MB, Sastre-Garau X, Guillou L, de Pinieux G, Terrier P, Lagace R, Aurias A, Hostein I, Coindre JM. MDM2 and CDK4 immunostainings are useful adjuncts in diagnosing well-differentiated and dedifferentiated liposarcoma subtypes: a comparative analysis of 559 soft tissue neoplasms with genetic data. Am J Surg Pathol. 2005;29(10):1340–7.
85. Fisher C. The diversity of soft tissue tumours with EWSR1 gene rearrangements: a review. Histopathology. 2014;64(1):134–50.
86. Durr HR, Rauh J, Bauer-Melnyk A, Knosel T, Lindner L, Roeder F, Jansson V, Klein A. Myxoid liposarcoma: local relapse and metastatic pattern in 43 patients. BMC Cancer. 2018;18(1):304.
87. Weniger M, D'Haese JG, Kunz W, Pratschke S, Guba M, Werner J, Angele MK. En-bloc resection of a giant retroperitoneal lipoma: a case report and review of the literature. BMC Res Notes. 2015;8:75.
88. Nagano S, Yokouchi M, Setoguchi T, Ishidou Y, Sasaki H, Shimada H, Komiya S. Differentiation of lipoma and atypical lipomatous tumor by a scoring system: implication of increased vascularity on pathogenesis of liposarcoma. BMC Muculoskelet Disord. 2015;16:36.
89. Libertini M, Thway K, Noujaim J, Puls F, Messiou C, Fisher C, Jones RL. Clear cell sarcoma-like tumor of the gastrointestinal tract: clinical outcome and pathologic features of a molecularly characterized tertiary center case series. Anticancer Res. 2018;38(3):1479–83.
90. Alyousef MJ, Alratroot JA, El Sharkawy T, Shawarby MA, Al Hamad MA, Hashem TM, Alsayyah A. Malignant gastrointestinal neuroectodermal tumor: a case report and review of the literature. Diagn Pathol. 2017;12(1):29. Published 2017 Mar 20.
91. Hoon V, Thung SN, Kaneko M, Unger PD. HMB-45 reactivity in renal angiomyolipoma and lymphangioleiomyomatosis. Arch Pathol Lab Med. 1994;118(7):732–4.
92. Fetsch PA, Fetsch JF, Marincola FM, Travis W, Batts KP, Abati A. Comparison of melanoma antigen recognized by T cells (MART-1) to HMB-45: additional evidence to support a common lineage for angiomyolipoma, lymphangiomyomatosis, and clear cell sugar tumor. Mod Pathol. 1998;11(8):699–703.
93. Zavala-Pompa A, Folpe AL, Jimenez RE, Lim SD, Cohen C, Eble JN, Amin MB. Immunohistochemical study of microphthalmia transcription factor and tyrosinase in angiomyolipoma of the kidney, renal cell carcinoma, and renal and retroperitoneal sarcomas: comparative evaluation with traditional diagnostic markers. Am J Surg Pathol. 2001;25(1):65–70.
94. Brimo F, Robinson B, Guo C, Zhou M, Latour M, Epstein JI. Renal epithelioid angiomyolipoma with atypia: a series of 40 cases with emphasis on clinicopathologic prognostic indicators of malignancy. Am J Surg Pathol. 2010;34(5):715–22.
95. D'Andrea D, Hanspeter E, D'Elia C, Martini T, Pycha A. Malignant perivascular epithelioid cell neoplasm (PEComa) of the pelvis: a case report. Urol Case Rep. 2016;6:36–8.
96. Nese N, Martignoni G, Fletcher CD, Gupta R, Pan CC, Kim H, Ro JY, Hwang IS, Sato K, Bonetti F, Pea M, Amin MB, Hes O, Svec A, Kida M, Vankalakunti M, Berel D, Rogatko A, Gown AM, Amin MB. Pure epithelioid PEComas (so-called epithelioid angiomyolipoma) of the kidney: a clinicopathologic study of 41 cases: detailed assessment of morphology and risk stratification. Am J Surg Pathol. 2011;35(2):161–76.
97. Evans HL, Soule EH, Winkelmann RK. Atypical lipoma, atypical intramuscular lipoma, and well differentiated retroperitoneal liposarcoma: a reappraisal of 30 cases formerly classified as well differentiated liposarcoma. Cancer. 1979;43(2):574–84.
98. Hasegawa T, Seki K, Hasegawa F, Matsuno Y, Shimodo T, Hirose T, Sano T, Hirohashi S. Dedifferentiated liposarcoma of retroperitoneum and mesentery: varied growth patterns and histological grades--a clinicopathologic study of 32 cases. Hum Pathol. 2000;31(6):717–27.
99. Huang HY, Brennan MF, Singer S, Antonescu CR. Distant metastasis in retroperitoneal dedifferentiated liposarcoma is rare and rapidly fatal: a clinicopathological study with emphasis on the low-grade myxofibrosarcoma-like pattern as an early sign of dedifferentiation. Mod Pathol. 2005;18(7):976–84.
100. Deshpande A, Nelson D, Corless CL, Deshpande V, O'Brien MJ. Leiomyoma of the gastrointestinal tract with interstitial cells of Cajal: a mimic of gastrointestinal stromal tumor. Am J Surg Pathol. 2014;38(1):72–7.

Lymphomas of the Gastrointestinal Tract

21

Robert S. Ohgami and Ryan M. Gill

List of Frequently Asked Questions

1. How does one distinguish among common low-grade or small B-cell lymphomas of the stomach on mucosal biopsy?
2. How does one distinguish extranodal marginal zone lymphoma with increased large cells from extranodal marginal zone lymphoma transformed to diffuse large B-cell lymphoma?
3. How does one differentiate between an extranodal marginal zone lymphoma and reactive marginal zone hyperplasia in the gastrointestinal tract?
4. What prognostic testing is needed for gastrointestinal diffuse large B-cell lymphoma?
5. How does one distinguish between duodenal-type follicular lymphoma and systemic usual adult-type follicular lymphoma?
6. How does one distinguish between enteropathy associated T-cell lymphoma (EATL) and monomorphic epitheliotropic intestinal T-cell lymphoma (MEITL)?
7. How are EATL and MEITL distinguished from other systemic T-cell lymphomas?
8. How does one diagnose refractory celiac disease type 1 and type 2?
9. How does one make a diagnosis of systemic mastocytosis in the gastrointestinal tract?
10. Which hematopoietic neoplasms are associated with a preceding gastrointestinal disease?
11. Which lymphomas can present as multiple mucosal polyps?
12. What are indolent NK- and T-cell neoplasms that may involve the gastrointestinal tract?
13. What is a rectal tonsil and how does it mimic lymphoma?
14. What is immunoproliferative small intestinal disease and is it a plasma cell neoplasm?
15. What is the differential diagnosis and workup for a plasma cell-rich lesion in the gastrointestinal tract?
16. How does one diagnose a high-grade B-cell lymphoma in the gastrointestinal tract?
17. How does acute leukemia present in the gastrointestinal tract?
18. When do mucosal eosinophils indicate a hematolymphoid neoplasm?
19. Are there gastrointestinal lymphomas to watch for in patients with primary immunodeficiencies?
20. I performed an EBV in situ hybridization and all the lymphoma cells are positive; what are my next steps?
21. What types of lymphoma occur in the appendix?
22. How does one distinguish between histiocytic and dendritic neoplasms of the gastrointestinal tract?

Frequently Asked Questions

1. How does one distinguish among common low-grade or small B-cell lymphomas of the stomach on mucosal biopsy?

Gastric low-grade or small B-cell lymphomas include (in order of frequency) (1) extranodal marginal zone lymphoma (ENMZL) of mucosa-associated lymphoid tissue (MALT) and then (2) mantle cell lymphoma (MCL), followed by rarely follicular lymphoma (FL) and chronic lymphocytic leukemia/small lymphocytic lymphoma (CLL/SLL). While MCL is a consideration for any B-cell lymphoma in the gastrointestinal (GI) tract with small-medium-sized lymphoid cells, it should be noted that MCL is not truly a low-grade lymphoma, as it typically proliferates more aggressively.

A simplified algorithm for how to immunophenotypically distinguish among low-grade or small B-cell lymphomas of the stomach is outlined in Fig. 21.1. Staining patterns of

R. S. Ohgami (✉) · R. M. Gill
University of California, San Francisco, San Francisco, CA, USA
e-mail: Robert.ohgami@ucsf.edu

H. L. Wang, Z. E. Chen (eds.), *Practical Gastrointestinal Pathology*, Practical Anatomic Pathology,
https://doi.org/10.1007/978-3-030-51268-2_21

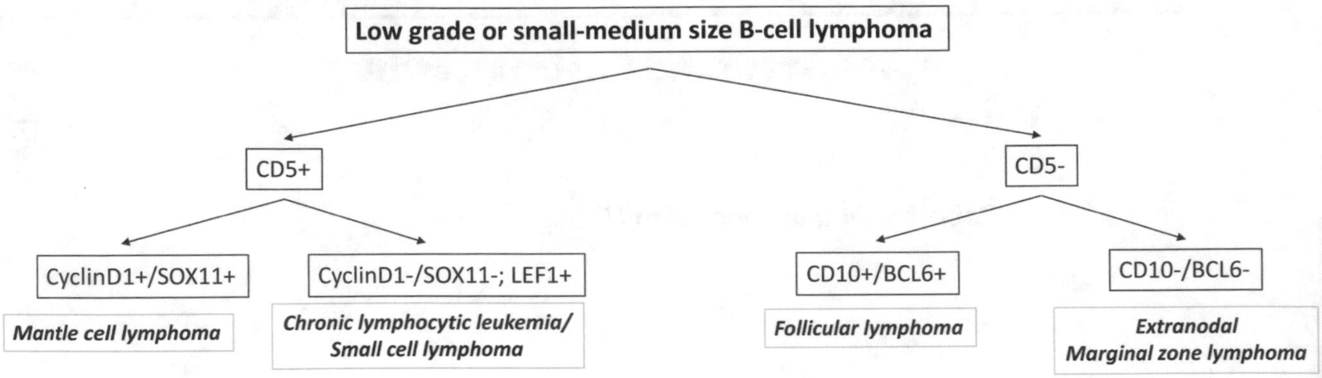

Fig. 21.1 Algorithmic approach to the diagnosis of a low-grade or small-medium-sized B-cell lymphoma

CD5, CD10, BCL6, and cyclin D1 form a basis for differentiating among these lymphomas. Table 21.1 contains relevant detailed information on how to distinguish different types of low-grade or small B-cell lymphomas using morphology, immunophenotyping, and genetics.

- *Extranodal marginal zone lymphoma*: A significant proportion of ENMZL are associated with *H. pylori* infections (30–90% of cases depending on different studies), and the organisms may be readily seen on H&E-stained slides or may benefit from special stains or immunohistochemistry for ease of visualization. By morphology, the cells of ENMZL tend to have a monocytoid appearance, with cleared cytoplasm, and encroach on glands with lymphoepithelial lesions (invasion of B cells into glands with destruction of the epithelium) (Fig. 21.2a–h). A subset of cases will demonstrate amyloid deposition. The immunophenotype is typically that of mature B cells (i.e., CD20 and PAX5 positive), with the absence of CD5 and CD10 staining, though rarer cases may be positive for either or both CD5 and CD10. Cyclin D1 is always negative, and MNDA (myeloid cell nuclear differentiation antigen) and CD43 may be positive in a subset of cases. Both MNDA and CD43 may be particularly useful for differentiating between FL and ENMZL: FL is nearly always negative for CD43 and MNDA, but ENMZL is frequently positive. A subset of cases may be positive for t(11;18)(q21;q21), which may be more resistant to *H. pylori* eradication therapy, or show trisomies of chromosome 3 or 18. Coexpression of CD43 can aid in determining that the infiltrate is neoplastic.
- *Mantle cell lymphoma*: Diffuse effacement, or a nodular appearance, may be present in cases of MCL in the stomach. Typically, if MCL involves the stomach, it is high stage, though cases primary to the stomach exist (very rare), and therefore an early mantle zone pattern is almost never seen. The cells are small-medium in size with irregular notched or slightly indented nuclei. The immunophenotype is CD5 positive without expression of germinal center markers CD10 and BCL6. Importantly,

Table 21.1 Low-grade or small B-cell lymphomas of the stomach

Entity	Morphology	Immunophenotype	Genetics
ENMZL	Monotonous infiltrate of small cells with cleared cytoplasm or monocytoid appearance, may show plasmacytic differentiation	CD20+, CD5−, CD10−, BCL6−, cyclin D1−, CD43+/−, MNDA+/−	May show t(11;18)(q21;q21);*BIRC3/MALT1*, trisomy 3 or 18
CLL/SLL	Monotonous infiltrate of small cells with blocky chromatin. Proliferation centers may be seen	CD20+, CD5+, CD10−, BCL6−, cyclin D1−, CD43+/−, MNDA+/−, LEF1+	May show deletions of 11q, 13q, 17p, and trisomy 12
FL	Back-to-back follicles without polarization and no tingible body macrophages. Centrocytic cells and centroblastic cells in varying proportions depending on grading (1–3A/B)	CD20+, CD5−, CD10+, BCL6+, cyclin D1−, CD43−, MNDA−	t(14;18)(q32;q21);*IGH/BCL2* or less frequently t(3;14)(q27;q32);*IGH/BCL6*. The presence of either of these translocations in the setting of small B cells is diagnostic for FL
MCL	Vague nodules or diffuse effacement by monotonous small-medium-sized cells with irregular indented nuclei	CD20+, CD5+, cyclin D1+, SOX11+, CD10−, BCL6−	t(11;14)(q13;q32);*IGH/CCND1*. The presence of this translocation is diagnostic for MCL

ENMZL extranodal marginal zone lymphoma, *CLL/SLL* chronic lymphocytic leukemia/small lymphocytic lymphoma, *FL* follicular lymphoma, *MCL* mantle cell lymphoma

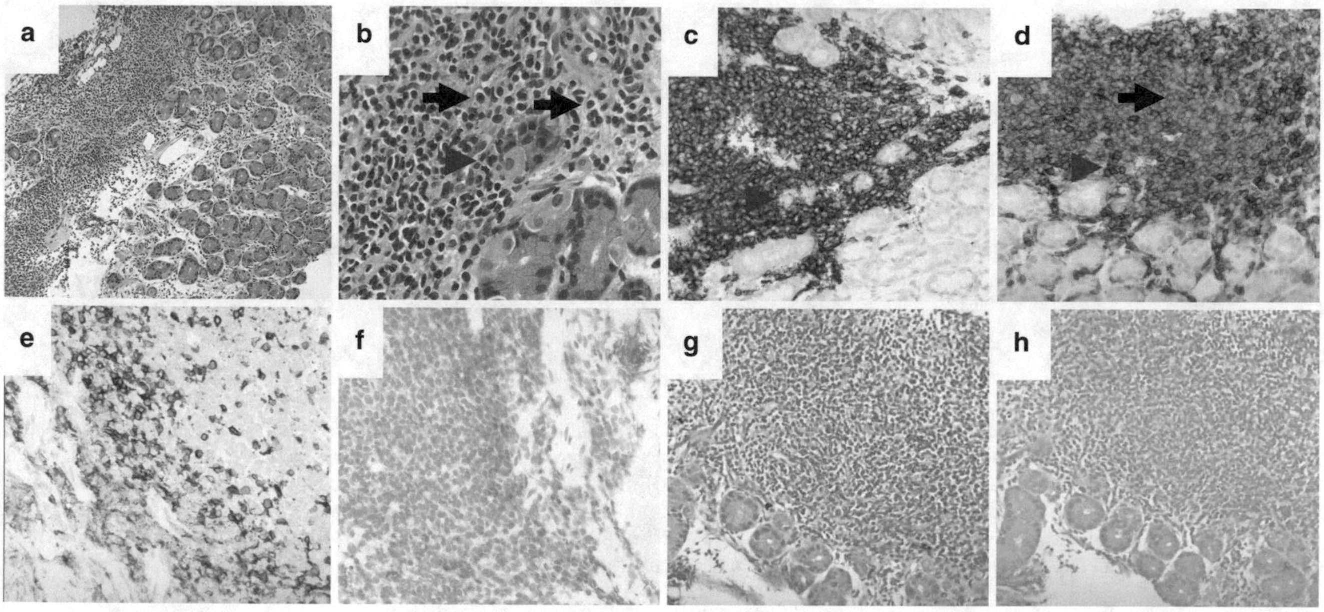

Fig. 21.2 Extranodal marginal zone lymphoma in the stomach. (**a**) A low-power view shows stomach mucosa with an infiltrate of small lymphocytes. (**b**) High-power magnification shows atypical lymphocytes, some with a monocytoid or cleared cytoplasm appearance (black arrows); a lymphoepithelial lesion is seen with several atypical small lymphocytes invading into glands (red arrowhead). (**c**) A CD20 immunostain highlights the small lymphocytes, some invading into glands resulting in lymphoepithelial lesions (red arrowhead). (**d**) A CD43 immunostain highlights B cells (black arrow) where the staining intensity is slightly dimmer than that in T cells, which show stronger staining (red arrowhead). (**e**) A CD5 immunostain highlights rarer small T cells, but is negative in B cells. (**f**) A CD10 immunostain is negative in B cells. (**g**) An in situ hybridization for kappa light chain shows faint staining in B cells. (**h**) In situ hybridization for lambda light chain is negative

cyclin D1 and SOX11 stains will be positive. A Ki67 stain should be performed to determine the proliferative index, as a MCL with a proliferative index of >30% will behave more aggressively. Finally, t(11;14)(q13;q32);*IGH/CCND1* is diagnostic of MCL. Two variants of MCL are now recognized based on SOX11 staining. The SOX11-positive classic variant involves lymph nodes or extranodal sites and can become blastoid or pleomorphic (and has unmutated or minimally mutated *IGHV*). The SOX11-negative variant presents as an indolent leukemic form without tissue involvement, but secondary mutations result in aggressive disease (and this variant has mutated *IGHV)*.

- *Follicular lymphoma*: In the stomach, as in other sites, FL will appear as dense collections of nodules of lymphoid cells, which lack tingible body macrophages and lack polarization. As in other sites, FL is graded based on the number of centroblasts per high-power field (HPF): grade 1, 0–5 centroblasts/HPF; grade 2, 6–15; grade 3A, >15; and grade 3B, solid sheets of centroblasts. However, one important point is that frequently stomach biopsies are scant and only one or a few follicles may be present. In these cases, definitive grading of the FL may not be possible, but one can convey the predominant pattern seen (low grade or high grade 3A or 3B) with a caveat that the biopsy is scant. Immunostains will highlight the B cells as CD20 and PAX5 positive, with coexpression of germinal center markers, such as CD10 and BCL6. FL cases will typically lack expression of MNDA and CD43; expression of either of these would argue against FL and can help when one is attempting to differentiate between FL and ENMZL. Expression of BCL2 is common and can aid in determining that the infiltrate is neoplastic. FL in the stomach routinely shows translocation of the *BCL2* gene with *IGH*, t(14;18)(q32;q21);*IGH/*BCL2, or less frequently shows a *BCL6* gene translocation; and identification of either of these translocations in the setting of small neoplastic B cells would be diagnostic for FL.
- *Chronic lymphocytic leukemia/small lymphocytic lymphoma*: While a CLL/SLL is an overall common leukemia/lymphoma, it is a most unusual finding in the stomach. When it does involve the stomach, as in other anatomic sites, it effaces the normal glandular structures. Proliferation centers, or vague pseudo-follicles, may be seen. The typical cytologic appearance of the lymphoid cells is expected (i.e., blocky nuclear chromatin), though the proliferation centers will have an increased number of prolymphocytes with characteristic prominent single nucleoli and mitotic figures. The immunophenotype is characteristically CD20 dimly positive, CD79a-positive, and CD5-positive B cells with expression of LEF1 and absence of CD10, absence of BCL6, and absence of cyclin D1 expression.

References: [1–5]

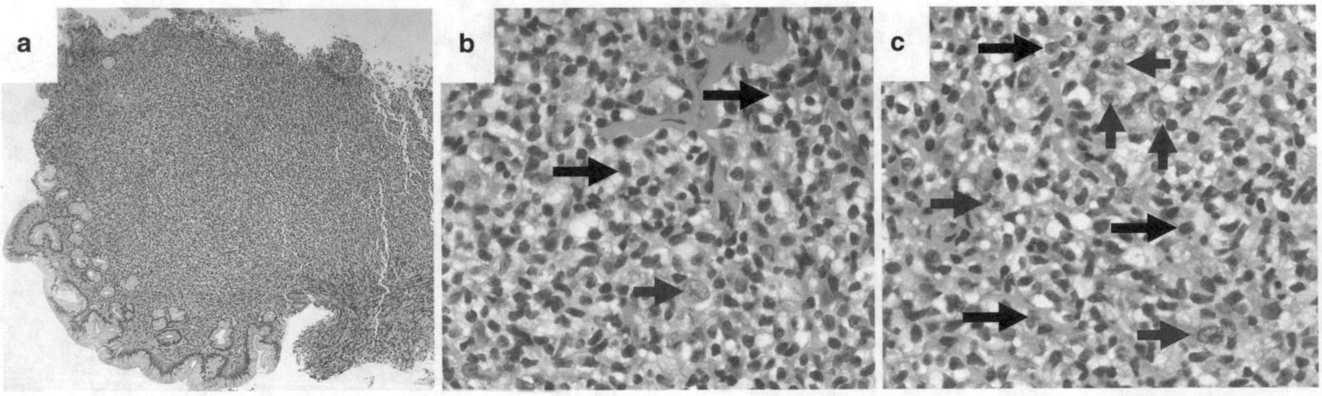

Fig. 21.3 Extranodal marginal zone lymphoma with increased large cells. (**a**) A dense infiltrate of atypical lymphoid cells with cleared cytoplasm is apparent at low-power magnification of this stomach biopsy. (**b**) High-power magnification shows the infiltrate to be composed mostly of small- or medium-sized cells with irregular nuclear contours and cleared cytoplasm/monocytoid appearance (black arrows). Scattered atypical larger lymphoid cells with vesicular chromatin and prominent nucleoli are seen (red arrow). (**c**) In another field of view, numerous small-medium-sized atypical lymphocytes with a monocytoid appearance are seen (black arrows). In addition, numerous atypical large lymphoid cells with immature chromatin and prominent nucleoli (red arrows) are noted (5–10% of the infiltrate); however, no sheets of atypical large cells are seen

2. **How does one distinguish extranodal marginal zone lymphoma with increased large cells from extranodal marginal zone lymphoma transformed to diffuse large B-cell lymphoma?**

A subset of ENMZL cases of the GI tract may have a significant number of large cells, which raises concern for transformation to diffuse large B-cell lymphoma (DLBCL). Criteria for determining if a case simply has increased large cells or it is truly transformed to DLBCL are not well defined, but a simple rule of thumb is that DLBCL can be diagnosed if there are sheets of large B cells (Fig. 21.3a–c). Of course, while cases where sheets of large B cells are seen are generally not difficult to diagnose, there is one exception when large reactive secondary follicles are disrupted. In these instances, small sheets of large B cells, which are actually disrupted reactive germinal center B cells, may be confusing on histology. In this situation, immunohistochemistry will be helpful. A germinal center marker, BCL6 (preferably) or CD10 (less preferred due to background stromal cell staining), along with CD21 to highlight follicular dendritic cells, will reveal that the large B cells are in fact reactive germinal center B cells associated with the follicular dendritic cell meshworks in a disrupted germinal center.

Returning to our original question, cases with fewer than 20% large cells should not be diagnosed as large cell transformation, but in the range of 20–50% large cells, there is no general standard as to whether these cases should be diagnosed as transformed DLBCL or not. In these instances, a description of ENMZL with increased large cells concerning for transformation may be an appropriate diagnosis. In such cases, it is important to convey to the clinical team that, regardless of whether the final diagnostic line outright states transformation to DLBCL or there is concern for transformation, the literature supports that cases of ENMZL with increased large cells (in the range of 20 to >50%) tend to clinically behave more aggressively than typical ENMZL.

Finally, while a Ki67 immunostain may be useful in highlighting the nuclei of larger cells and draws attention to regions with a higher proliferative index, we note that there is no standard for using Ki67 to diagnose large cell transformation in ENMZL.

References: [6–12]

3. **How does one differentiate between an extranodal marginal zone lymphoma and reactive marginal zone hyperplasia in the gastrointestinal tract?**

Distinguishing ENMZL from reactive marginal zone hyperplasia (rMZH) in mucosa-associated lymphoid tissue may be difficult, even with ancillary studies. B cells may appear to be monotypic by immunostains for lambda and kappa (or by flow cytometric evaluation) in rMZH, in certain anatomic sites particularly the appendix where they may appear to be lambda restricted. CD43 is not specific for a malignant B-cell population in this setting. However, the pattern of lymphoid involvement (diffuse or marginal zone localized), presence of prominent lymphoepithelial lesions, follicular colonization, and clonality as demonstrated by DNA sequencing studies for IgH and/or light-chain genes will allow one to render a correct diagnosis.

A diffuse pattern is not seen in rMZH; lymphoepithelial lesions and follicular colonization favor ENMZL.

rMZH may be monotypic by immunostains (kappa and lambda), possibly with anomalous CD43 coexpression on B cells, but clonality will not be present by DNA sequencing studies of IgH or light-chain genes.

We note that positive expression of BCL2 does not help to distinguish ENMZL from rMZH as reactive marginal zone B

Table 21.2 Comparison of features between extranodal marginal zone lymphoma and reactive marginal zone hyperplasia

	ENMZL	rMZH
Morphology	Small-medium-sized lymphocytes with cleared cytoplasm/ monocytoid in a diffuse or marginal zone pattern. Lymphoepithelial lesions and/or follicular colonization may be present	Small-medium-sized lymphocytes with cleared cytoplasm/ monocytoid in a marginal zone pattern. Lymphoepithelial lesions and/or follicular colonization is rare
Immunophenotype	CD20+, CD43+/–, MNDA+/–,BCL2+/–	CD20+, CD43+/–, MNDA+/–, BCL2+
B-cell light-chain restriction (by immunostains)	Restricted light-chain expression expected	May show restricted light-chain expression
B-cell clonality (by DNA sequencing)	Clonal	Non-clonal

ENMZL extranodal marginal zone lymphoma, *rMZH* reactive marginal zone hyperplasia

cells express BCL2. However, BCL2, along with germinal center markers and CD21 for follicular meshworks, may help evaluate the architecture and establish follicular colonization in ENMZL.

rMZH would typically demonstrate a higher proliferative index than ENMZL, and thus Ki-67 immunostain can aid in diagnosis.

Table 21.2 summarizes the differences and similarities between ENMZL and rMZH to allow for a correct diagnosis.

References: [13, 14]

4. What prognostic testing is needed for gastrointestinal diffuse large B-cell lymphoma?

As in other sites, DLBCLs of the GI tract should be phenotyped to determine if they are germinal center B-cell-like (GCB) versus activated B-cell-like (ABC) and analyzed for double-expressor status (c-Myc and BCL2 protein expression). While determination of GCB versus ABC, and/or double-expressor status, has not been definitively shown to be important in the prognosis of DLBCL of the GI tract, the studies to date have mostly been retrospective and limited in scope and data; as such, DLBCLs of the GI tract should be prognostically worked up similarly to nodal DLBCL (Table 21.3).

Testing and analysis required are:

- Determination of GCB vs ABC
- Ki67 index (higher value may indicate poor prognosis)
- CD5 expression (expression may be associated with poor prognosis)
- *MYC* gene rearrangement (*MYC* translocation may be associated with poor prognosis)
- EBV infection as demonstrated by in situ hybridization (EBV-positive cases may be associated with poor prognosis and would warrant classification as "EBV-positive DLBCL, NOS")

Table 21.3 Prognostic testing for diffuse large B-cell lymphoma and Paris staging system for primary gastrointestinal lymphomas

Classification	Comment
GCB vs ABC (Hans' algorithm)	Use CD10, BCL6, and MUM1 expression to phenotype GCB: CD10+ (BCL6 and MUM1 + or –) or CD10–/BCL6+/MUM1– ABC: all non-GCB combinations of CD10, BCL6, and MUM1 expression
Double expressor	c-Myc protein expression ≥40% and BCL2 protein expression ≥50%
Paris staging system	TX – lymphoma extent not specified T0 – no evidence of lymphoma T1 – lymphoma confined to the mucosa/ submucosa T1m – confined to mucosa T1sm – confined to submucosa T2 – infiltration of muscularis propria or subserosa T3 – penetration of serosa (visceral peritoneum) without invasion of adjacent structure T4 – invasion of adjacent structures/organs
	NX – lymph nodes not assessed N0 – no lymph nodal involvement N1 – involvement of regional lymph nodes N2 – involvement of intraabdominal nodes beyond the regional area N3 – spread to extraabdominal nodes (at least 6 lymph nodes are typically assessed)
	MX – dissemination not assessed M0 – no extranodal dissemination M1 – non-continuous involvement of other GI sites M2 – non-continuous involvement of other tissues outside of GI tract
	BX – bone marrow involvement not assessed B0 – no bone marrow involvement B1 – bone marrow involvement

GCB germinal center B-cell-like, *ABC* activated B-cell-like

One nuance to DLBCL in the GI tract is that several studies have demonstrated that the depth of tissue invasion may correlate with outcome. Indeed, a histopathologic Tumor (T), Nodes (N), Metastases (M) TNM classification, the Paris staging system, exists which captures these data (Table 21.3).

Here we are not including "double-hit" large B-cell lymphomas. In the 2016 revised World Health Organization (WHO) classification of lymphomas, "double-hit" lymphomas are an entirely separate entity. Genetic analysis by fluorescence in situ hybridization for the *MYC* gene rearrangement is important in excluding this diagnosis.

References: [15–21]

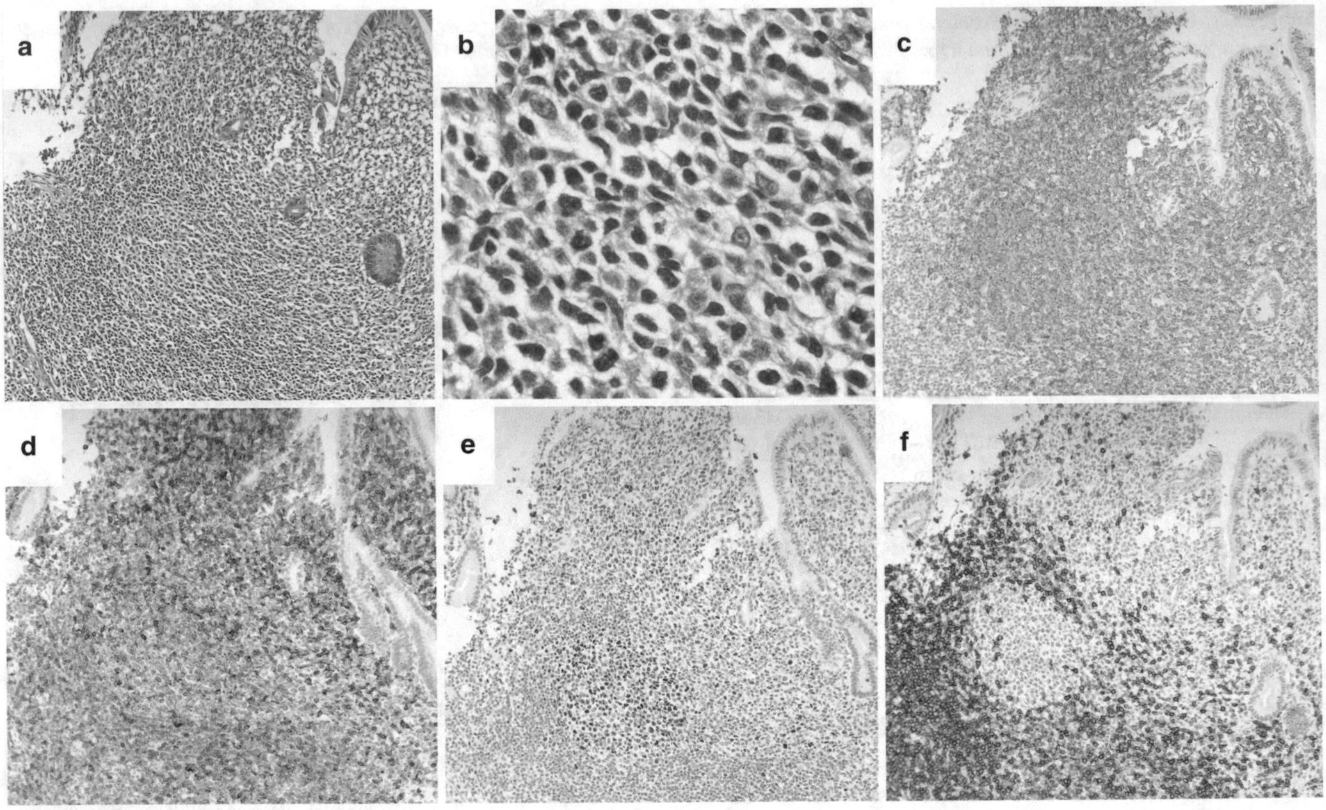

Fig. 21.4 Duodenal-type follicular lymphoma. (**a**) A low-power view shows a nodule of atypical lymphocytes in the duodenum. No tingible body macrophages are present. (**b**) A high-power view shows atypical lymphocytes with cleaved and angulated nuclei. (**c**) A CD20 immunostain highlights the atypical lymphocytes in the nodule and outside the nodule. Invasion into the surface epithelium is seen. (**d**) A BCL2 immunostain highlights the nodule, as well as neoplastic lymphocytes outside the follicle. (**e**) A BCL6 immunostain highlights the nodule and B cells outside the nodule. (**f**) A CD3 immunostain highlights T cells mostly outside the nodule

5. **How does one distinguish between duodenal-type follicular lymphoma and systemic usual adult-type follicular lymphoma?**

The distinction between duodenal-type follicular lymphoma (d-FL) and systemic usual adult-type follicular lymphoma (u-FL) is based largely on clinical features, though some histopathologic findings are also contributory. d-FL in its classic form is localized to the small intestine, though multiple localized polyps may be seen. d-FL has an excellent prognosis as it behaves indolently without dissemination. Therefore, a patient with disseminated nodal involvement by FL (typically involving mesenteric lymph nodes) should not be classified as d-FL but u-FL. Histologically aggressive features such as extensive infiltration into the muscularis propria or high-grade classification (grade 3) are findings not typically seen in d-FL. Immunophenotypically and cytogenetically, cases of d-FL and u-FL are identical with expression of germinal center markers (CD10 and BCL6) and gene rearrangements of *BCL2* in the majority of cases (>90%) (Fig. 21.4a–f). It is important to note that involvement of the ampulla of Vater and head of the pancreas (i.e., typically in the setting of u-FL) can present with jaundice and may clinically mimic pancreatic carcinoma.

References: [22–24]

6. **How does one distinguish between enteropathy associated T-cell lymphoma (EATL) and monomorphic epitheliotropic intestinal T-cell lymphoma (MEITL)?**

There are two main types of primary GI T-cell lymphomas: enteropathy-associated T-cell lymphoma (EATL) and monomorphic epitheliotropic intestinal T-cell lymphoma (MEITL) (Fig. 21.5a–f). Table 21.4 contains critical details for distinguishing between these two.

The diagnosis of EATL versus MEITL begins with morphology. As the name suggests, cases of MEITL show a monomorphic infiltrate of generally small-medium-sized lymphoid cells with condensed nuclear chromatin, whereas in EATL, the cells are medium-large in size and more pleomorphic in appearance and often associated with eosinophils. Cases of MEITL frequently express CD8 and CD56, which is the opposite of EATL, though both lymphomas demonstrate expression of proteins associated with a cyto-

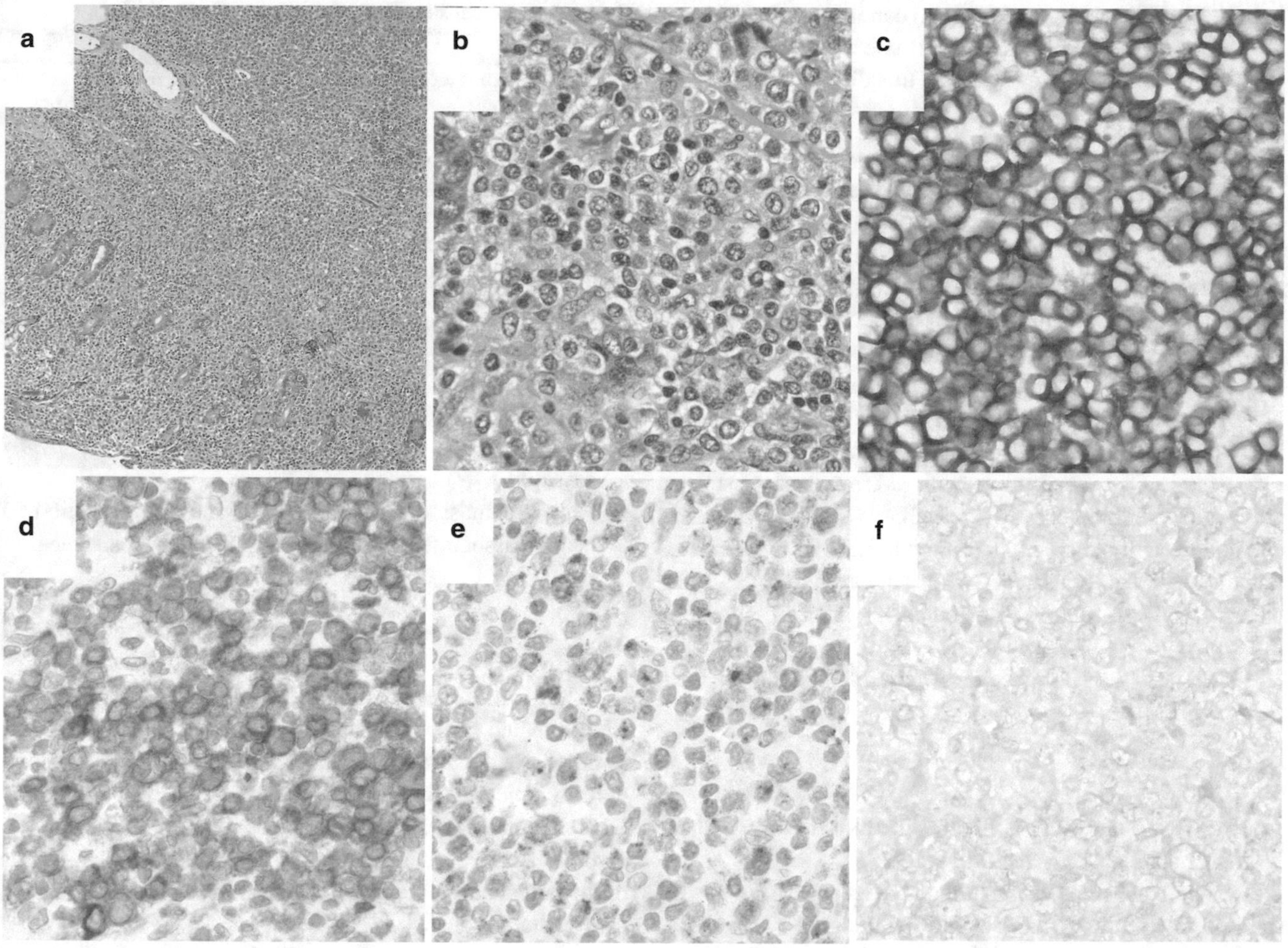

Fig. 21.5 Monomorphic epitheliotropic intestinal T-cell lymphoma. (**a**) A diffuse infiltrate of atypical lymphocytes is seen in the colon at low-power magnification. (**b**) These lymphocytes are medium-large in size with immature/fine chromatin and visible nucleoli. (**c**) A CD3 immunostain highlights these cells. A TCR-gamma immunostain is positive in these lymphoma cells (**d**), as is a granzyme stain (**e**). (**f**) An EBV in situ hybridization is negative

Table 21.4 Distinction between enteropathy-associated T-cell lymphoma and monomorphic epitheliotropic intestinal T-cell lymphoma

	EATL	MEITL
Associated disease	Celiac disease	None
Ethnicity	European	Hispanic, Asian
Morphology	Polymorphic	Monomorphic
Immunophenotype	CD3+, cytotoxic marker+, CD5−, CD4−, CD8−, CD56−, EBV−, CD30+/−	CD3+, cytotoxic marker+, CD5−, CD4−, CD8+, CD56+, EBV−, CD30−
TCR	Alpha/beta > gamma/delta	Gamma/delta > alpha/beta

EATL enteropathy-associated T-cell lymphoma, *MEITL* monomorphic epitheliotropic intestinal T-cell lymphoma

toxic phenotype. Clinically, the two are quite different with EATL cases being associated with celiac disease and those of Northern European descent, whereas MEITL is very infrequently seen with concurrent celiac disease and is more prevalent in Asian and Hispanic populations.

References: [25–28]

7. **How are EATL and MEITL distinguished from other systemic T-cell lymphomas?**

Other T-cell lymphomas can occur in the GI tract and need to be distinguished from EATL and MEITL. Specifically, peripheral T-cell lymphoma not otherwise specified (PTCL NOS) and angioimmunoblastic T-cell lymphoma (AITL) may be considerations, but these lymphomas tend to be CD4 positive and typically lack cytotoxic markers, which would be expressed by both EATL and MEITL. Another consideration may be anaplastic large cell lymphoma (ALCL). However, ALCL is positive for CD30 in essentially all of neoplastic cells, which is unlike EATL that may show partial CD30 expression but not in all cells. Finally, extranodal NK/T-cell lymphoma (ENKTL) can involve the GI tract, but expression of Epstein-Barr virus-encoded small RNA (EBER) in ENKTL helps establish this diagnosis.

References: [29, 30]

8. **How does one diagnose refractory celiac disease type 1 and type 2?**

Refractory celiac disease is defined by malabsorptive symptoms, despite a gluten-free diet for at least 6–12 months along with villous atrophy. It is divided into two types: type 1 with increased but phenotypically normal intraepithelial lymphocytes (IELs) and type 2 with immunophenotypically abnormal IELs (i.e., with downregulation of CD8 in >50% of IELs compared with CD3 immunostaining which detects cytoplasmic CD3 epsilon) or with aberrant loss of surface CD3 and CD8 in at least 20–25% T cells by flow cytometric evaluation, if fresh tissue is available. IELs in type 2 cases are also frequently clonal (with demonstration of TCR-gamma or TCR-delta rearrangement), whereas clonality is not typical of type 1.

Please see Chap. 5, question 10, for additional discussion on this topic.

References: [31]

9. **How does one make a diagnosis of systemic mastocytosis in the gastrointestinal tract?**

Systemic mastocytosis is diagnosed similarly in the GI tract as in the bone marrow and other tissue sites. Major and/or minor criteria must be met: either one major and one minor or three minor criteria (Table 21.5 and Fig. 21.6a–d).

In GI biopsies where there is suspicion for systemic mastocytosis, immunostaining for CD117 or mast cell tryptase to highlight mast cells, along with CD25 immunostaining, is sufficient to help identify mast cell aggregates and to help evaluate for aberrant CD25 coexpression. Minor criteria also include atypical morphology (usually spindled and enlarged, resembling fibroblasts or histiocytes), *KIT* mutation, and elevated serum tryptase level. One note about *KIT* mutational analysis is that mast cells may be sparse in a mucosal biopsy, and thus the method used for molecular testing must have a high sensitivity.

Please see Chap. 12, questions 9–13, for further discussion on this topic.

References: [32–35]

10. **Which hematopoietic neoplasms are associated with a preceding gastrointestinal disease?**

Three neoplasms are associated with a preceding GI disease.

- Enteropathy-associated T-cell lymphoma (discussed above in questions 6 and 7) is associated with celiac disease.

Table 21.5 Diagnostic criteria for systemic mastocytosis[a]

Criteria	
Major	Tumor mass/aggregate of mast cells (15 mast cells or more)
Minor	1. *KIT* D816V mutation 2. Morphologically atypical/spindled mast cells, at least 25% atypical 3. Elevated serum tryptase (>20 ng/mL)[b] 4. Expression of CD25 and/or CD2 by mast cells

[a]Diagnosis requires either one major and one minor or three minor criteria

[b]Cannot use elevated serum tryptase as a criterion if there is an unrelated myeloid neoplasm

- Extranodal marginal zone lymphoma (discussed above in question 1) is frequently associated with *H. pylori* gastritis.
- Systemic mastocytosis (discussed above in question 9) may be associated with malabsorption due to diarrhea.

11. **Which lymphomas can present as multiple mucosal polyps?**

While MCL can present with multiple mucosal polyps (the so-called lymphomatous polyposis), which is a top differential diagnosis in a patient with intestinal polyposis and clinical concern for lymphoma, FL, ENMZL, and even DLBCL can all present as mucosal polyps. MCL most often involves the ileocecal region but can involve large stretches of the bowel and often demonstrates mesenteric lymph node involvement.

In a retrospective study by Kodama et al., however, of patients with multiple mucosal polyps and a diagnosis of lymphoma, the majority of lymphomas were found to be cases of FL, followed closely by MCL and then ENMZL. Intestinal polyposis is very rarely due to DLBCL.

References: [36, 37]

12. **What are indolent NK- and T-cell neoplasms that may involve the gastrointestinal tract?**

Two entities to bear in mind are:

- NK-cell enteropathy is a clinically indolent proliferation of immunophenotypically normal NK cells (CD56+/TIA1+/cytoplasmic CD3+) that are EBER negative. This condition can involve the stomach, small bowel, and large bowel. Hemorrhage, ulceration, and edema can be seen. Morphologic findings can be alarming because it is composed of medium- to large-sized lymphoid cells. T-cell receptor (TCR) clonality testing will be negative. A clinical watch-and-wait approach can be adopted.
- Indolent T-cell lymphoproliferative disorder of the GI tract is characterized by an indolent dense proliferation of small lymphocytes with an immunophenotype identical to normal small cytotoxic T cells (CD8+, TIA1+,

CD56−). It is EBER negative and shows a low Ki67 proliferative index (<10%). However, these cases show clonal rearrangements of T-cell receptor genes. Patients may present with diarrhea and abdominal pain. A clinical watch-and-wait approach can be adopted, though a subset of patients may progress to aggressive T-cell lymphoma.

References: [38–40]

13. What is a rectal tonsil and how does it mimic lymphoma?

A rectal tonsil is an exuberant proliferation of reactive lymphoid follicles that often expands into the submucosa in the rectum. The irregular follicular shape, large size, and infiltration into the submucosa may result in a morphologic picture mimicking lymphoma. However, immunostains for CD20, CD3, and CD21 will show normal B- and T-cell distributions with variable follicular meshworks, usually asso-

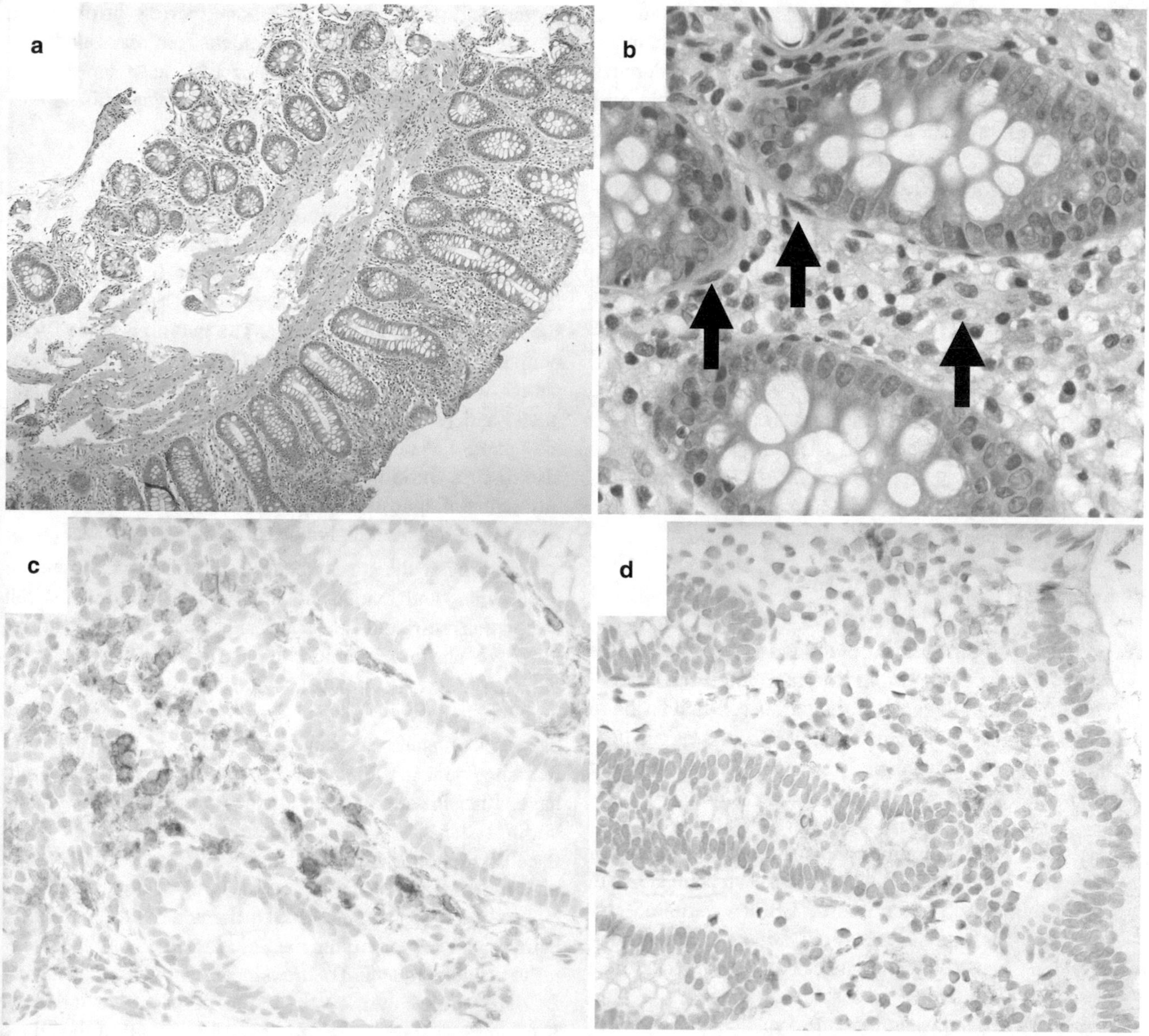

Fig. 21.6 Systemic mastocytosis in the colon. (**a**) Low-power magnification shows colonic mucosa with subtle changes in surface epithelium. (**b**) High-power magnification shows intact crypts with a subtle infiltrate of spindled to larger oval-shaped cells (arrows). (**c**) A CD117 immunostain highlights an infiltrate of atypical mast cells, which are enlarged in size and occasionally spindled. (**d**) A CD25 immunostain is positive in many of the CD117-positive mast cells

ciated with B cells. Light-chain analysis is polytypic, and there is no evidence of B-cell clonality. Prominent rectal tonsils may be encountered with *Treponema pallidum* or *Chlamydia trachomatis* infection.

References: [41]

14. What is immunoproliferative small intestinal disease and is it a plasma cell neoplasm?

Immunoproliferative small intestinal disease (IPSID) is a variant of ENMZL and also known as alpha heavy-chain disease. It is not a plasma cell neoplasm, but a neoplasm of B cells. It is most common in geographical regions bordering the Mediterranean Sea. The patients tend to be younger males with poor hygiene, who present with diarrhea and abdominal pain, along with malabsorption, wasting, hypocalcemia, fever, and steatorrhea. The disease may be associated with *Campylobacter jejuni* infection and tends to involve the small intestine and mesenteric lymph nodes. Histologically, the disease shows dense plasma cells and B cells expanding the lamina propria along the length of the small intestine. Infiltration into glands with lymphoepithelial lesions is seen. The cells express monoclonal cytoplasmic alpha heavy chains but lack light-chain expression. Thus, serum protein electrophoresis may be normal; immunofixation would be required to identify the abnormal alpha heavy chain in such cases. Progression to DLBCL may occur. As seen in other ENMZL cases, IPSID cells are CD5 and CD10 negative. They also lack the t(11;18)(q21;q21);*BIRC3/MALT1* translocation, which can be seen in other ENMZL cases. If detected early, IPSID may respond to antibiotic therapy.

References: [42, 43]

15. What is the differential diagnosis and workup for a plasma cell-rich lesion in the gastrointestinal tract?

The differential diagnosis for a plasma cell-rich lesion in the GI tract is generally limited to ENMZL, plasma cell neoplasm (PCN), posttransplant lymphoproliferative disorder (PTLD), and syphilis.

- Cases will require immunostains and a focused panel of markers to include CD20, CD3, kappa and lambda in situ hybridization or immunostains, EBER, Warthin-Starry silver stain, or immunostain for *T. pallidum*. PTLD is discussed in Chap. 22. If spirochete organisms are identified, then GI syphilis should be considered, which can be confirmed by immunostaining. GI syphilis, discussed in detail in Chaps. 9 and 10, is usually seen in the anorectum and stomach. Clinically, it can mimic carcinoma.
- Differentiating ENMZL from a PCN can be more complex, as cases of ENMZL with extreme plasmacytic differentiation can be seen. In difficult cases, CD117, CD56, CD45, CD19, and CD20 stains are useful. Expression of CD19, CD20, and CD45 on the plasmacytoid and plasma cells would support ENMZL, while expression of CD117 and CD56 would support a PCN. Regardless of the final classification, presence of prominent plasma cells allows for utilization of in situ hybridization (which has less background staining than immunostains for kappa and lambda) for the detection of a monotypic kappa or lambda population, which can aid in diagnosis of a neoplasm, especially in limited samples. Lymphoplasmacytic lymphoma (LPL), although very rare in the GI tract, is another consideration with a monotonous lymphoplasmacytic infiltrate. LPL may be associated with an IgM paraprotein, and such patients, with bone marrow involvement, will be considered to have Waldenstrom macroglobulinemia. The majority of cases of LPL have the *MYD88 L265P* mutation, which can assist with diagnosis.

References: [44, 45]

16. How does one diagnose a high-grade B-cell lymphoma in the gastrointestinal tract?

High-grade B-cell lymphomas must be distinguished from DLBCL, not otherwise specified (NOS), as they have a significantly different prognosis. The two high-grade B-cell lymphomas bearing that name are (1) high-grade B-cell lymphoma with *MYC* and *BCL2* and/or *BCL6* gene rearrangements and (2) high-grade B-cell lymphoma, NOS, which may present as destructive/ulcerative colorectal masses. We also discuss Burkitt lymphoma here as this would be in the differential diagnosis, though this is almost always encountered in the ileocecal region, usually in young males.

Reaching a diagnosis requires morphologic, immunophenotypic, and cytogenetic analysis. High-grade B-cell lymphomas show either a "starry sky" appearance ("Burkitt-like"), or blastoid cytomorphology, or relatively pleomorphic large B cells ("DLBCL-like," usually with a GCB immunophenotype), or can be diagnosed as such if they have a *MYC* gene rearrangement and/or at least a second rearrangement in either *BCL2* or *BCL6*. Cases that do not have either the morphology or the appropriate cytogenetic findings should not be considered as either a high-grade B-cell lymphoma with *MYC* and *BCL2* and/or *BCL6* gene rearrangements or high-grade B-cell lymphoma, NOS. Burkitt lymphoma shows a characteristic "starry sky" pattern with monomorphic medium-large cells, without significant nucleoli, and *MYC* translocation without concurrent *BCL2* or *BCL6* translocation. The proliferative index by Ki67 immunostain is typically over 90% in all of the above considerations. DLBCL should also be evaluated for EBV to exclude EBV-positive DLBCL. Table 21.6 shows the morphologic, immunophenotypic, and genetic differences among these groups.

References: [46–48]

Table 21.6 Comparison of high-grade B-cell lymphomas

Entity	Morphology	Immunophenotype	Genetics
High-grade B-cell lymphoma with *MYC* and *BCL2* and/or *BCL6* gene rearrangements	Variable: may include Burkitt-like, blastoid, and DLBCL-like morphology (i.e., large B cells with pleomorphism and visible nucleoli)	CD20+, CD10+/−, BCL2+/−	*MYC* and *BCL2* and/or *BCL6* gene rearrangement (i.e., double- or triple-hit lymphomas; excluding cases demonstrated to arise from follicular lymphoma or from established B lymphoblastic lymphoma)
High-grade B-cell lymphoma, NOS	Starry sky pattern present and/or large lymphoid cells with blastoid chromatin	CD20+, CD10+/−, BCL2+/−	No translocations in both *MYC* and *BCL2* and/or *BCL6*
Burkitt lymphoma	Starry sky pattern	CD20+, CD10+, BCL2−, EBV+/−	*MYC* translocation present; *TCF3* or *ID3* mutations detected in 70% of sporadic and endemic cases and 40% of immunodeficiency-associated cases
Diffuse large B-cell lymphoma, NOS	Sheets of pleomorphic large B cells	CD20+, CD10+/−, BCL2+/−, EBV−	No translocations in both *MYC* and *BCL2* and/or *BCL6*

17. How does acute leukemia present in the gastrointestinal tract?

Acute leukemias presenting in the GI tract can be T-cell, B-cell, myeloid, or of ambiguous lineage. The most common presenting feature of acute leukemia in the GI tract is that of abdominal pain, which may be due to leukemic infiltrates, most commonly in the stomach, ileum, and proximal colon. Gingival hyperplasia in the mouth is a well-known presentation of acute myeloid leukemia and particularly in cases with monocytic differentiation. Destructive involvement (i.e., effacement of mucosa) of the GI tract by a myeloid neoplasm (without bone marrow involvement) may occur and would be considered diagnostic of a myeloid sarcoma. Myelodysplasia may also rarely present with GI involvement. For example, a case of oral Sweet syndrome has been reported with the same cytogenetic abnormality detected in clonal neutrophils, within oral tissue, as was identified in a bone marrow specimen. Isolated involvement of the GI tract by lymphoblasts (without bone marrow involvement) would be considered diagnostic of B or T lymphoblastic lymphoma. The most helpful immunohistochemical stains for assessing an immature hematopoietic neoplasm are CD34 (immature blast marker), CD117 (immature myeloid blast marker), TdT (immature lymphoid blast marker), MPO (myeloid marker), PAX5 (labeling most B lymphoblasts), and CD3 (labeling most T lymphoblasts). If fresh tissue is available, the tissue should be sent for both flow cytometric and cytogenetic analyses. Cytogenetic analysis in particular can be critical for appropriate classification and treatment of immature hematopoietic neoplasms.

References: [49–51]

18. When do mucosal eosinophils indicate a hematolymphoid neoplasm?

Eosinophils may be significantly increased in the mucosa of the small and large intestines without relation to a malignancy (discussed in more detail in Chap. 12). However, in association with other clinical sequelae and particular morphologic findings, increased eosinophils may be a marker of a neoplasm. This may be true in patients presenting with diarrhea, urticaria, and increased eosinophils in the intestinal mucosa. In that case, careful evaluation for mast cell infiltrates can be undertaken using immunostains for CD117, mast cell tryptase, CD25, and CD2. Other instances to be aware of are acute myeloid leukemias/myeloid sarcoma, which may have increased eosinophils and eosinophilic myelocytes, and chronic eosinophilic leukemia, which will have increased circulating eosinophils. Eosinophils may also be elevated in the instances of peripheral T-cell lymphoma and EATL. Finally, eosinophils may be prominent in classical Hodgkin lymphoma. Although this is very rare in the GI tract, both nodular sclerosing and mixed cellularity variants have been described. There is perhaps an association with development of disease in inflamed areas of the bowel in Crohn disease.

- Systemic mastocytosis may present with increased mucosal eosinophils as well as CD117-positive mast cells with CD25 and CD2 coexpression. These mast cells may form dense clusters. *KIT* D816V mutation is present in nearly all cases.
- Langerhans cell histiocytosis (LCH) would demonstrate a characteristic infiltrate of Langerhans cells, which may be identified on S100, CD1a, and langerin (CD207) immunostains.
- Myeloid sarcomas, as described in question 17, in the GI tract may have increased eosinophils and eosinophilic myelocytes.
- EATL may show numerous eosinophils associated with the neoplastic T cells, which typically are medium-large in size with variable nuclear pleomorphism.
- Chronic eosinophilic leukemia is a myeloproliferative neoplasm with clonal eosinophils, which circulate at high levels and may also infiltrate and damage tissue.

- Classical Hodgkin lymphoma can be considered if Reed-Sternberg cells are identified, in which a typical immunophenotype (e.g., CD30+, CD15+, PAX5 weakly positive, CD20−, CD45−) is expected.
  – A consideration in this differential diagnosis is a rare type of acute T-cell lymphoma/leukemia (ATLL), which may demonstrate Hodgkin-like morphology and may involve the GI tract. The disease is usually systemic, however, and is associated with HTLV-1 infection. The neoplastic cells express T-cell markers (e.g., CD2, CD3, CD5, and CD4).

References: [33, 52–55]

19. Are there gastrointestinal lymphomas to watch for in patients with primary immunodeficiencies?

Patients with primary immunodeficiencies are prone to developing lymphomas of T-cell and B-cell origins. The primary immunodeficiency that we typically consider in the context of GI lymphomas is common variable immunodeficiency (CVID). In patients with CVID, the most frequent lymphomas are ENMZL and EBV-associated DLBCL, though other types are possible as well. A pitfall in the diagnosis is that patients with CVID may demonstrate evidence of B- or T-cell clonality on PCR testing, without morphologic evidence of lymphoma.

References: [56–59]

20. I performed an EBV in situ hybridization and all the lymphoma cells are positive; what are my next steps?

EBV-positive hematopoietic neoplasms occurring in the GI tract include extranasal NK/T-cell lymphoma; peripheral T-cell lymphoma, NOS; DLBCL; Burkitt lymphoma; classic Hodgkin lymphoma; plasmablastic lymphoma; primary effusion lymphoma; and PTLD. To distinguish among these entities, immunostains are necessary and should first focus on determining the lineage of neoplastic cells (T, NK, B, or plasmablastic) as well as if there is another concomitant viral infection (e.g., HHV8). Morphology is also important, but immunophenotyping is critical in establishing the diagnosis. Each entity is outlined in Table 21.7.

- Initial immunostains should include CD3, CD20, and CD138. If the neoplastic cells are strongly CD20 positive, then the findings would argue for consideration of an EBV-positive DLBCL or Burkitt lymphoma. A starry sky pattern with monotonous medium-large-sized cells would lead one to the diagnosis of Burkitt lymphoma. On the other hand, more pleomorphic large cells with geographic necrosis and expression of BCL2 would steer one toward EBV-positive DLBCL. If the neoplastic cells are CD3 positive, then one would consider either an extranodal NK/T-cell lymphomas or EBV-positive peripheral T-cell lymphoma, NOS. CD56 expression and absence of TCR ßF1 expression would favor an extranodal NK/T-cell lymphoma. Identification of necrosis centered around vessels would further support this consideration. Absence of CD56 expression would lead to the diagnosis of an EBV-positive peripheral T-cell lymphoma, NOS. Absence of concurrent HHV8 infection by immunostain, along with expression of CD138, without CD20 or CD3, in the morphologic setting of large plasmablastic-appearing cells, would result in a diagnosis of plasmablastic lymphoma (Fig. 21.7a–h). Alternatively, if HHV8 immunostaining is positive, then this finding would lead one to the diagnosis of primary effusion lymphoma, which is rare to occur as a solid tumor mass (i.e., an extracavitary variant) in the GI tract. This entity is more commonly seen in peritoneal fluid.

References: [60–66]

21. What types of lymphoma occur in the appendix?

Appendiceal lymphomas are rare, or rather, the diagnosis of lymphoma based on an appendectomy or appendiceal orifice biopsy is unusual. Any B-cell or T-cell lymphoma can occur in the appendix, but B-cell lymphomas are much more frequently diagnosed compared to T-cell lymphomas. B-cell lymphomas that occur in the appendix, in order of relative frequency, are DLBCL, MCL, Burkitt lymphoma, FL, CLL/SLL, and rarely ENMZL.

References: [67–70]

Table 21.7 Comparison of EBV-positive lymphomas in the gastrointestinal tract

Entity	Morphology	Immunophenotype
Extranodal NK/T-cell lymphoma	Medium-large-sized cells with mature chromatin, necrosis centered around vessels	EBV+, HHV8−, CD3+ (typically cytoplasmic), CD20−, CD56+, TCR ßF1−
Peripheral T-cell lymphoma, NOS	Medium-large-sized cells, often with increased eosinophils	EBV+, HHV8−, CD3+, CD20−, CD56−/+, TCR ßF1+
Diffuse large B-cell lymphoma	Large lymphoid cells with vesicular chromatin and visible nucleoli; geographic necrosis may be present	EBV+, HHV8−, BCL2−, CD20+, CD3−
Plasmablastic lymphoma	Sheets of large plasmablastic-appearing cells	EBV+, HHV8−, CD3−, CD20−, CD138+, CD38+, c-Myc+/−
Primary effusion lymphoma	Plasmablastic or anaplastic large cells typically with a less cohesive appearance	EBV+, HHV8+, CD3−, CD20+/−, CD38+/−
Burkitt lymphoma	"Starry sky" pattern; monotonous proliferation of medium-large-sized cells without pleomorphism	EBV+, CD3−, CD20+, CD10+, c-Myc+, BCL2-

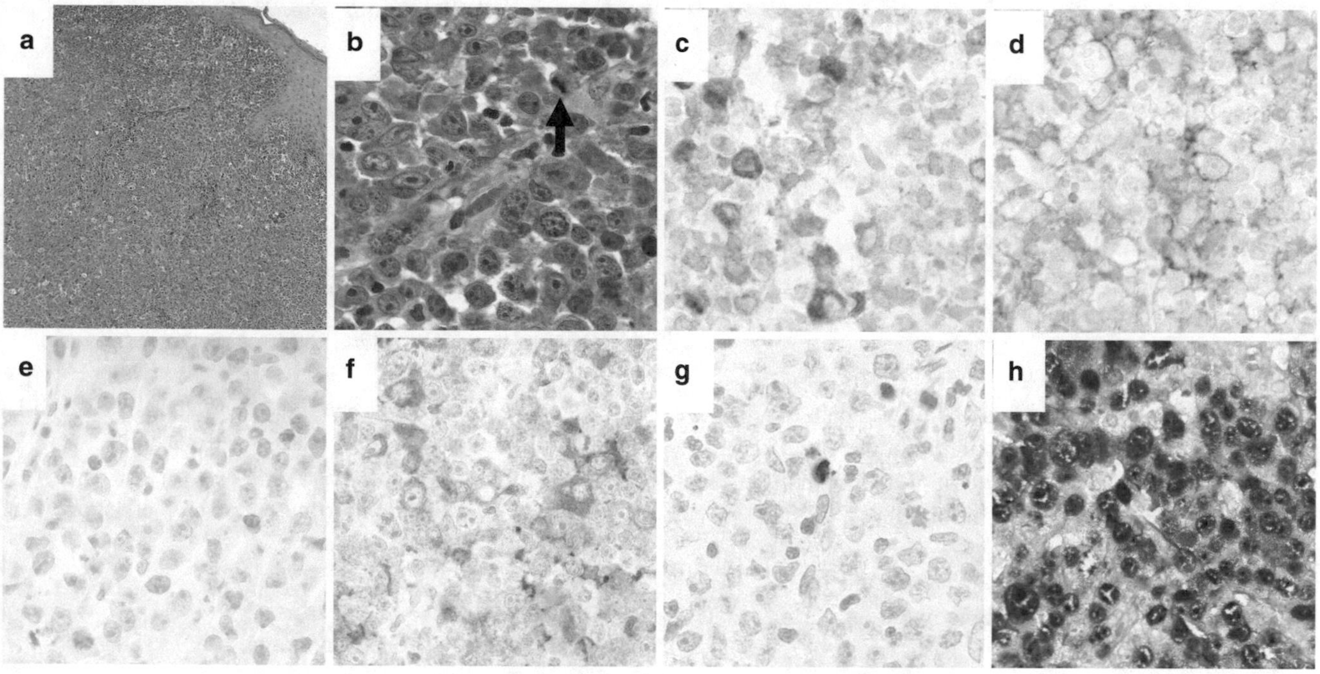

Fig. 21.7 Plasmablastic lymphoma involving the anorectal junction. (**a**) A diffuse infiltrate of atypical large cells is seen. (**b**) At higher-power magnification, these cells are large in size, many with eccentric nuclei and prominent nucleoli and the appearance of plasmablasts. Mitotic figures are seen (arrow). (**c**) A CD79a immunostain highlights the infiltrate. (**d**) A CD38 immunostain is positive. (**e**) A CD20 immunostain is negative. (**f**) Immunostain for kappa light chain is positive. (**g**) Immunostain for lambda light chain is negative. (**h**) An EBV in situ hybridization is positive in plasmablasts

22. How does one distinguish between histiocytic and dendritic neoplasms of the gastrointestinal tract?

While not a lymphoma, histiocytic and dendritic neoplasms are an important diagnostic consideration in the GI tract, though presentation in this location is quite rare. In addition to LCH (discussed in question 18), those to consider include histiocytic sarcomas, Erdheim-Chester disease, interdigitating dendritic cell sarcoma, indeterminate dendritic cell tumor, Rosai-Dorfman disease, follicular dendritic cell sarcomas, and Langerhans cell sarcoma. Below is a summary of key points that can be used to distinguish among these entities:

- Histiocytic sarcoma – An anaplastic cell population with expression of several histiocytic markers (e.g., CD68, CD163, PU.1), but absence of staining with S100, markers of Langerhans cells (CD1a, langerin), markers of follicular dendritic cells (CD21, CD23, CD35), or other lymphoid markers (e.g., CD20, CD3).
- Langerhans cell sarcoma (LCS) – Pleomorphic cells with expression of langerin, S100, CD68, and CD1a. LCS has a high proliferative index by Ki67.
- Erdheim-Chester disease – Lipid-laden histiocytes intermingled with fibrosis and Touton giant cells may be seen. The histiocytes are positive for CD68, CD163, and PU.1, but negative for CD21, CD23, CD1a, and langerin. Radiographically symmetric diaphyseal and metaphyseal osteosclerosis of the legs is present in most cases, with a subset showing perinephric fat infiltration.
- Interdigitating dendritic cell sarcoma – Cells are typically spindled but show variable pleomorphism throughout the tumor, with bizarre multinucleated cells as a common finding. The neoplastic cells are positive for S100 but lack expression of CD21, CD23, langerin, CD1a, CD68, CD163, and lysozyme.
- Indeterminate dendritic cell tumor – Cells show reniform vesicular nuclei with inconspicuous nucleoli and are positive for CD1a and S100, but negative for langerin and lack Birbeck granules on ultrastructural examination.
- Follicular dendritic cell sarcoma – Another neoplasm of spindled cells with some bilobed nuclei that is positive for at least two specific follicular dendritic cell markers (i.e., CD21, CD23, CD35) and negative on CD1a and langerin.
- Rosai-Dorfman disease – Conglomerates of histiocytes with abundant cytoplasm and round to oval large nuclei with visible nucleoli. Emperipolesis is typical, and a background of increased plasma cells may be seen. Cells are positive for S100 but lack expression of markers of Langerhans cells (CD1a, langerin) and markers of follicular dendritic cells (CD21, CD23).

Case Presentation

Case 1

Learning Objectives

1. To become familiar with the histologic and immunophenotypic features of the lymphoma
2. To become familiar with the genetics associated with the lymphoma
3. To generate a differential diagnosis

Case History

A 65-year-old man complained of stomach pain that was not well resolved with proton pump inhibitor therapy. The patient underwent endoscopic examination of his stomach, and several ulcers were identified and biopsied.

Histologic Findings

- Monotonous infiltrate of monocytoid-appearing small B cells (Fig. 21.8a, b).
- Lymphoepithelial lesions (Fig. 21.8a, b).

Differential Diagnosis

- Reactive lymphoid infiltrate
- Extranodal marginal zone lymphoma
- Follicular lymphoma
- Mantle cell lymphoma

Immunohistochemistry and Other Ancillary Studies (Fig. 21.8c–f)

- *H. pylori* organisms identified (not shown).
- CD20 positive.
- CD5 and CD10 negative (arguing against CLL/SLL, MCL, or FL).
- t(11;18)(q21;q21) positive.
- Clonal by B-cell gene rearrangement studies (supporting a neoplastic process).

Final Diagnosis

Extranodal marginal zone lymphoma.

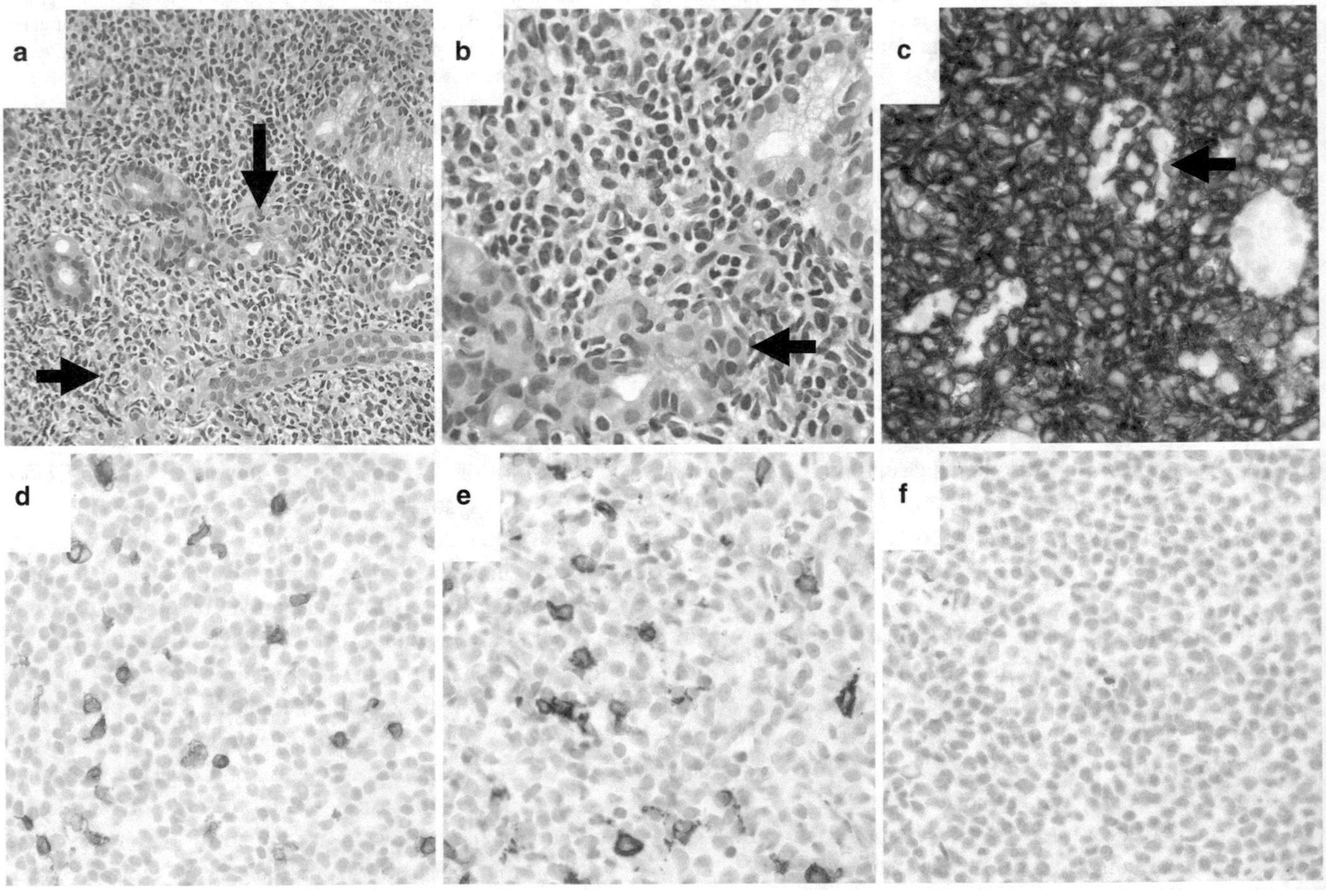

Fig. 21.8 (Case 1). Extranodal marginal zone lymphoma of the stomach. (**a**) Atypical small lymphocytes are seen diffusely infiltrating around and into gastric pits. Lymphoepithelial lesions (lymphocytes invading into and destroying epithelium) are seen (arrows). (**b**) At high-power magnification, these lymphocytes have a monocytoid appearance with cleared cytoplasm. Again, lymphoepithelial lesions are clearly seen (arrow). (**c**) A CD20 immunostain is positive in lymphoma cells, which also invade into gastric pits (arrow). (**d**) Small scattered CD3-positive T cells are present. (**e**) A CD5 immunostain only highlights T cells. (**f**) A CD10 immunostain is negative

Take-Home Messages

- ENMZL in the stomach is frequently associated with *H. pylori* infection (30–90% of cases in the stomach).
- The classic immunophenotype is CD20-positive B cells which are CD5 and CD10 negative.
- CD43 immunostain can be helpful if coexpressed in B cells.

References: [5, 56]

Case 2

Learning Objectives

1. To become familiar with the histologic and immunophenotypic features of the lymphoma
2. To become familiar with the prognosis and staging associated with the lymphoma

Case History

A healthy 55-year-old man had several endoscopic biopsies of his GI tract. Several small sub-centimeter polyps were identified in the second portion of the duodenum. No lymphadenopathy was identified during physical exam.

Histologic Findings

- Large lymphoid nodules comprised of small centrocytes with angulated nuclei and rare larger centroblasts (Fig. 21.9a, b).
- No polarization and absence of tingible body macrophages (Fig. 21.9a, b).

Differential Diagnosis

- Reactive lymphoid aggregates
- Extranodal marginal zone lymphoma
- Follicular lymphoma
- Mantle cell lymphoma

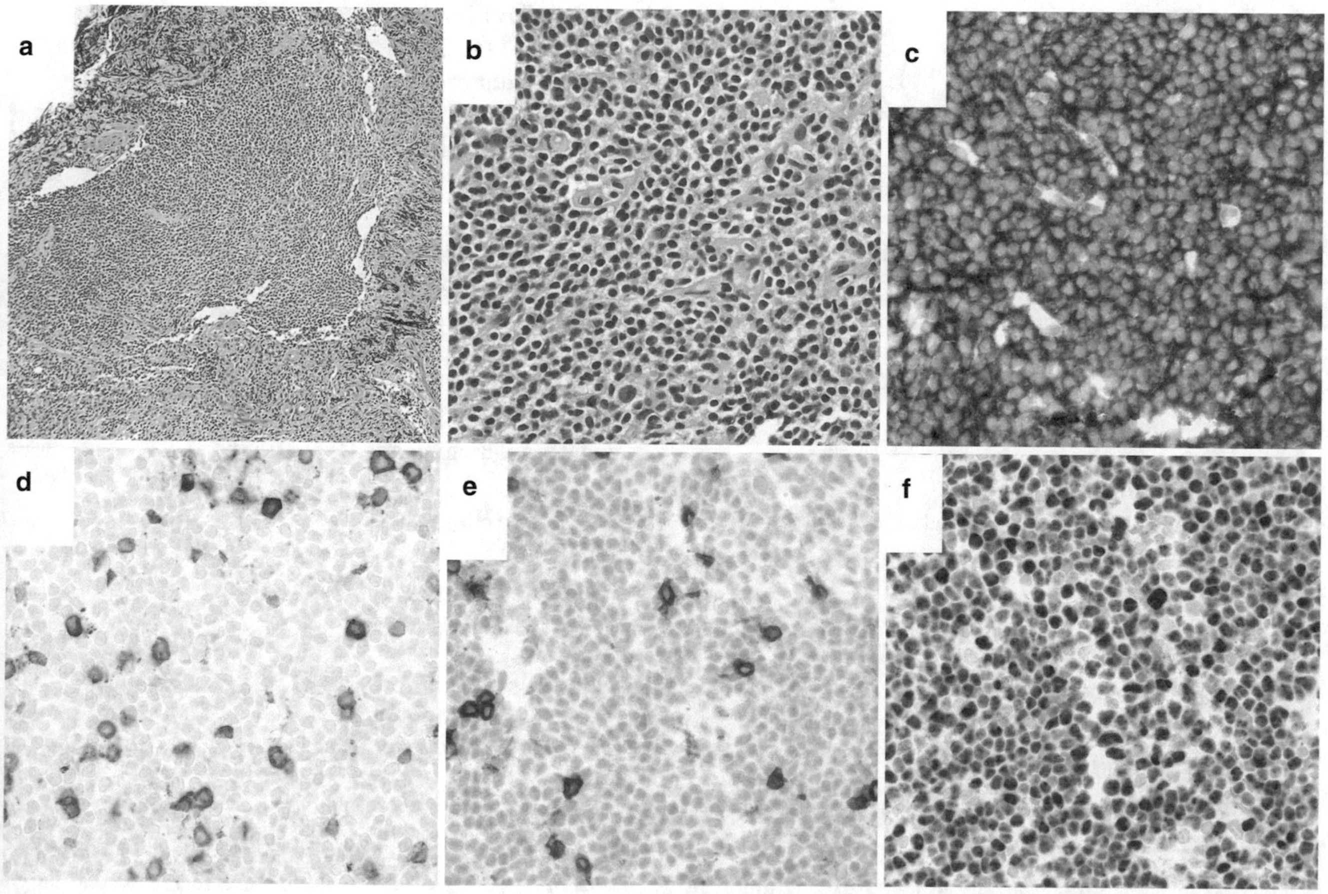

Fig. 21.9 (Case 2). Duodenal-type follicular lymphoma. (**a**) A low-power view shows a nodule of atypical lymphocytes in the duodenum. No tingible body macrophages are seen. (**b**) A high-power view shows predominantly small atypical lymphocytes with cleaved and angulated nuclei. The lymphoma cells also show a slightly monocytoid appearance. (**c**) A CD20 immunostain is positive. (**d**) A CD3 immunostain is negative in lymphoma cells. (**e**) A CD5 immunostain is negative. (**f**) A BCL6 immunostain is positive

Immunohistochemistry and Other Ancillary Studies (Fig. 21.9c–f)

- CD20 and BCL6 positive (supporting B-cell and germinal center phenotype).
- CD5 negative (arguing against MCL).
- t(14;18)(q32;q21) identified (*IGH* and *BCL2* translocation).

Final Diagnosis

Duodenal-type follicular lymphoma.

Staging and Prognosis

- Typically low grade and isolated to the duodenum.
- Good prognosis of 70% survival at 10 years.
- Appropriate treatment may be a watch-and-wait approach.

Take-Home Messages

- Duodenal-type FL is typically clinically low stage with a good prognosis.
- The immunophenotype is that of germinal center B cells (CD10, BCL6 positive).

References: [1, 22]

Case 3

Learning Objectives

1. To become familiar with the histologic and immunophenotypic features of the lymphoma
2. To understand the genetic abnormality associated with the lymphoma
3. To understand the prognostic workup

Case History

A 69-year-old man with a gastric nodule.

Histologic Findings

- A monotonous infiltrate of small-medium-sized lymphoid cells with slightly indented, irregular nuclei (Fig. 21.10a, b).

Differential Diagnosis

- Extranodal marginal zone lymphoma
- Follicular lymphoma
- Mantle cell lymphoma

Immunohistochemistry and Other Ancillary Studies (Fig. 21.10c–f)

- CD20, CD5, cyclin D1, and SOX11 positive (supporting MCL).
- CD10 negative (arguing against FL).
- t(11;14)(q13;q32) identified by fluorescence in situ hybridization (supporting MCL).
- Ki67 index of 80% (poor prognosis due to high Ki67 index >40%).

Final Diagnosis

Mantle cell lymphoma (SOX11-positive classic variant).

Take-Home Messages

- MCL may present anywhere in the GI tract. In the colon, MCL may present as an intestinal polyposis, as can FL or ENMZL.
- Cyclin D1 protein expression and the identification of t(11;14)(q13;q32) are diagnostic of this entity.
- A Ki67 index must be evaluated to assess for prognosis.
- MCL can be separated into two variants based on SOX11 staining.

References: [4, 36]

Case 4

Learning Objectives

1. To become familiar with the histologic and immunophenotypic features of the lymphoma
2. To become familiar with the prognostic workup
3. To generate a differential diagnosis

Case History

A 78-year-old woman with a 6-month history of dull abdominal pain, and a computed tomography scan of the abdomen demonstrated a mass along the ascending colon.

Histologic Findings

- Sheets of large lymphoid cells with prominent nucleoli and vesicular chromatin (Fig. 21.11a).

Differential Diagnosis

- Carcinoma
- Diffuse large B-cell lymphoma
- T-cell lymphoma

Immunohistochemistry and Other Ancillary Studies (Fig. 21.11b–h)

- CD20+/CD10−/BCL6+/MUM1+ (non-germinal center/activated B-cell-like).
- CD30 negative.
- Both c-Myc and BCL2 proteins expressed above 40% and 50%, respectively, (i.e., a double-expressor diffuse large B-cell lymphoma).

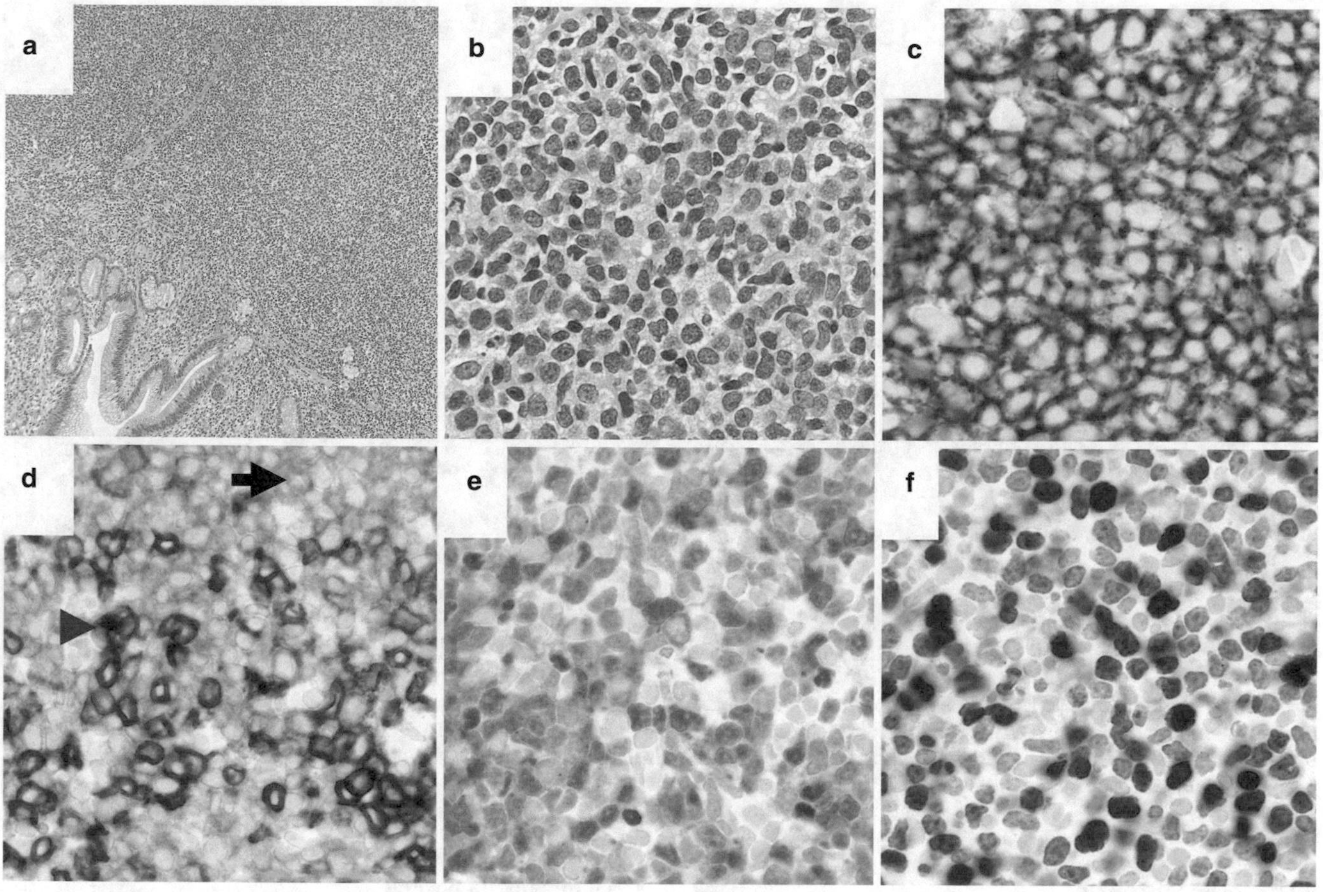

Fig. 21.10 (Case 3). Mantle cell lymphoma in the stomach. (**a**) Low-power magnification shows a lymphoid infiltrate within the stomach forming a vaguely nodular and diffuse pattern of involvement. (**b**) High-power magnification shows these lymphoid cells to be small-medium in size with irregular, slightly indented nuclei. (**c**) A CD20 immunostain is positive. (**d**) A CD5 immunostain strongly highlights T cells (red arrowhead) and dimly stains B cells (black arrow). (**e**) A cyclin D1 immunostain is positive in the atypical B cells. (**f**) A KI67 immunostain shows a high proliferative index of ~80%

Final Diagnosis

Diffuse large B-cell lymphoma.

Take-Home Messages

- A battery of immunohistochemistry and ancillary studies must be performed to determine (a) germinal center versus activated B-cell type, (b) c-Myc and BCL2 protein expression, (c) CD30 expression (for therapeutic interventions), and (d) *MYC*, *BCL2*, and *BCL6* gene rearrangement status.
- The prognostic workup of DLBCL in the GI tract is similar to DLBCL in other sites.

References: [18, 46]

Case 5

Learning Objectives

1. To become familiar with the histologic and immunophenotypic features of the lymphoma
2. To understand the clinical associations
3. To generate a differential diagnosis

Case History

A 69-year-old man with a small intestinal mass and no history of celiac disease.

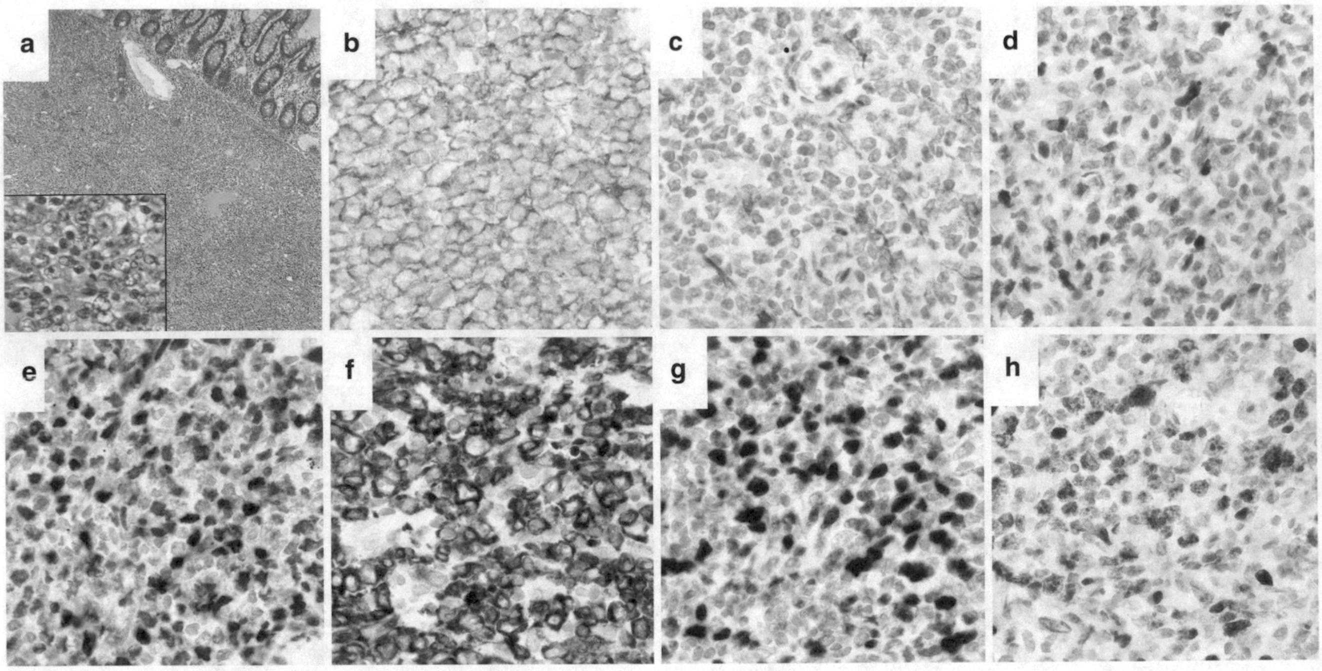

Fig. 21.11 (Case 4). Diffuse large B-cell lymphoma in the colon. (**a**) Atypical lymphocytes show a diffuse pattern of infiltration. High-power magnification (inset) shows large lymphoid cells with vesicular nuclei and prominent nucleoli. (**b**) A CD20 immunostain is positive. (**c**) A CD10 immunostain is negative. (**d**) A BCL6 immunostain is positive. (**e**) A MUM1 immunostain is positive. (**f**) A BCL2 immunostain is positive. (**g**) A c-Myc immunostain is positive (>40%). (**h**) A KI67 immunostain shows a proliferative index of ~50%

Histologic Findings

- An infiltrate of small-medium-sized lymphoid cells with cleared cytoplasm, effacing small intestinal mucosal architecture (Fig. 21.12a).

Differential Diagnosis

- Monomorphic epitheliotropic intestinal T-cell lymphoma
- Enteropathy-associated T-cell lymphoma
- Mantle cell lymphoma
- Diffuse large B-cell lymphoma

Immunohistochemistry and Other Ancillary Studies (Fig. 21.12b–f)

- CD3, CD8, and granzyme positive (supporting cytotoxic T-cell phenotype).
- CD56 negative.
- Gamma/delta positive.
- T-cell receptor gamma (TRG) gene and T-cell receptor beta (TRB) clonally rearranged.

Final Diagnosis

Monomorphic epitheliotropic intestinal T-cell lymphoma.

Take-Home Messages

- MEITL is not associated with celiac disease, but EATL is.
- T cells in MEITL are monomorphic and more monotonous than in EATL.
- MEITL cells are CD3+ with frequent expression of CD8, CD56, and TCR gamma/delta.
- Both EATL and MEITL can occur in the colon.

References: [27]

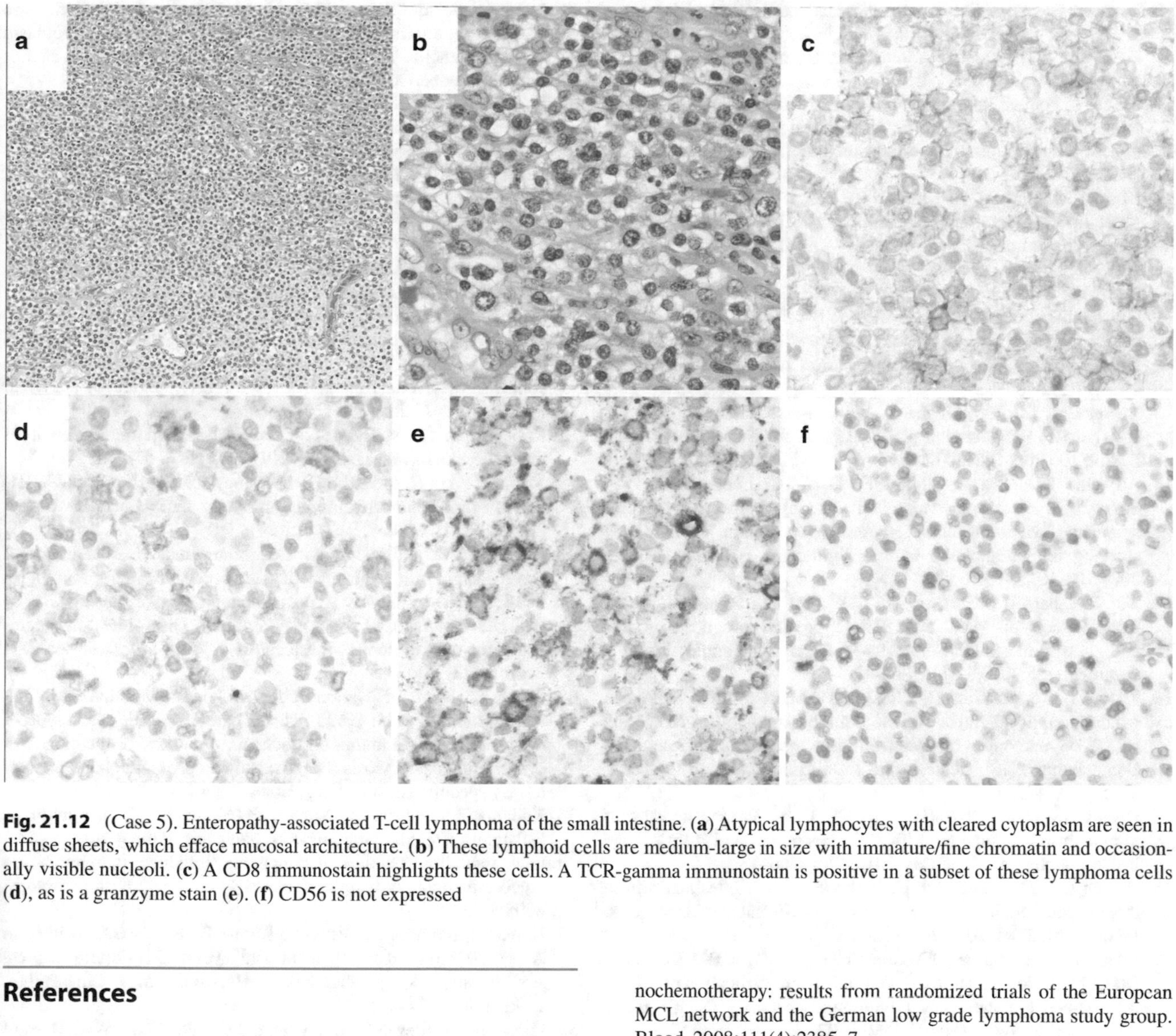

Fig. 21.12 (Case 5). Enteropathy-associated T-cell lymphoma of the small intestine. (**a**) Atypical lymphocytes with cleared cytoplasm are seen in diffuse sheets, which efface mucosal architecture. (**b**) These lymphoid cells are medium-large in size with immature/fine chromatin and occasionally visible nucleoli. (**c**) A CD8 immunostain highlights these cells. A TCR-gamma immunostain is positive in a subset of these lymphoma cells (**d**), as is a granzyme stain (**e**). (**f**) CD56 is not expressed

References

1. Nakamura S, Matsumoto T, Nakamura S, Kusano Y, Esaki M, Kurahara K, et al. Duodenal mucosa-associated lymphoid tissue lymphoma treated by eradication of helicobacter pylori: report of 2 cases including EUS findings. Gastrointest Endosc. 2001;54(6):772–5.
2. Luminari S, Cesaretti M, Marcheselli L, Rashid I, Madrigali S, Maiorana A, et al. Decreasing incidence of gastric MALT lymphomas in the era of anti-helicobacter pylori interventions: results from a population-based study on extranodal marginal zone lymphomas. Ann Oncol. 2010;21(4):855–9.
3. Swerdlow SH, Campo E, Pileri SA, Harris NL, Stein H, Siebert R, et al. The 2016 revision of the World Health Organization (WHO) classification of lymphoid neoplasms. Blood. 2016;127(20):2375–90.
4. Determann O, Hoster E, Ott G, Wolfram Bernd H, Loddenkemper C, Leo Hansmann M, et al. Ki-67 predicts outcome in advanced-stage mantle cell lymphoma patients treated with anti-CD20 immunochemotherapy: results from randomized trials of the European MCL network and the German low grade lymphoma study group. Blood. 2008;111(4):2385–7.
5. Bautista-Quach MA, Ake CD, Chen M, Wang J. Gastrointestinal lymphomas: morphology, immunophenotype and molecular features. J Gastrointest Oncol. 2012;3(3):209–25.
6. Petit B, Chaury MP, Le Clorennec C, Jaccard A, Gachard N, Moalic-Judge S, et al. Indolent lymphoplasmacytic and marginal zone B-cell lymphomas: absence of both IRF4 and Ki67 expression identifies a better prognosis subgroup. Haematologica. 2005;90(2):200–6.
7. Camacho FI, Algara P, Mollejo M, Garcia JF, Montalban C, Martinez N, et al. Nodal marginal zone lymphoma: a heterogeneous tumor: a comprehensive analysis of a series of 27 cases. Am J Surg Pathol. 2003;27(6):762–71.
8. Camacho FI, Mollejo M, Mateo MS, Algara P, Navas C, Hernandez JM, et al. Progression to large B-cell lymphoma in splenic marginal zone lymphoma: a description of a series of 12 cases. Am J Surg Pathol. 2001;25(10):1268–76.

9. Traverse-Glehen A, Felman P, Callet-Bauchu E, Gazzo S, Baseggio L, Bryon PA, et al. A clinicopathological study of nodal marginal zone B-cell lymphoma. A report on 21 cases. Histopathology. 2006;48(2):162–73.
10. Berger F, Felman P, Thieblemont C, Pradier T, Baseggio L, Bryon PA, et al. Non-MALT marginal zone B-cell lymphomas: a description of clinical presentation and outcome in 124 patients. Blood. 2000;95(6):1950–6.
11. Kojima M, Inagaki H, Motoori T, Itoh H, Shimizu K, Tamaki Y, et al. Clinical implications of nodal marginal zone B-cell lymphoma among Japanese: study of 65 cases. Cancer Sci. 2007;98(1):44–9.
12. Nathwani BN, Anderson JR, Armitage JO, Cavalli F, Diebold J, Drachenberg MR, et al. Marginal zone B-cell lymphoma: a clinical comparison of nodal and mucosa-associated lymphoid tissue types. Non-Hodgkin's lymphoma classification project. J Clin Oncol. 1999;17(8):2486–92.
13. Bacon CM, Du MQ, Dogan A. Mucosa-associated lymphoid tissue (MALT) lymphoma: a practical guide for pathologists. J Clin Pathol. 2007;60(4):361–72.
14. Attygalle AD, Liu H, Shirali S, Diss TC, Loddenkemper C, Stein H, et al. Atypical marginal zone hyperplasia of mucosa-associated lymphoid tissue: a reactive condition of childhood showing immunoglobulin lambda light-chain restriction. Blood. 2004;104(10):3343–8.
15. Xia B, Zhang L, Guo SQ, Li XW, Qu FL, Zhao HF, et al. Coexpression of MYC and BCL-2 predicts prognosis in primary gastrointestinal diffuse large B-cell lymphoma. World J Gastroenterol. 2015;21(8):2433–42.
16. Kawajiri A, Maruyama D, Maeshima AM, Nomoto J, Makita S, Kitahara H, et al. Impact of the double expression of MYC and BCL2 on outcomes of localized primary gastric diffuse large B-cell lymphoma patients in the rituximab era. Blood Cancer J. 2016;6(9):e477.
17. Hwang HS, Yoon DH, Suh C, Park CS, Huh J. Prognostic value of immunohistochemical algorithms in gastrointestinal diffuse large B-cell lymphoma. Blood Res. 2013;48(4):266–73.
18. Hwang HS, Yoon DH, Suh C, Park CS, Huh J. Intestinal diffuse large B-cell lymphoma: an evaluation of different staging systems. J Korean Med Sci. 2014;29(1):53–60.
19. Hans CP, Weisenburger DD, Greiner TC, Gascoyne RD, Delabie J, Ott G, et al. Confirmation of the molecular classification of diffuse large B-cell lymphoma by immunohistochemistry using a tissue microarray. Blood. 2004;103(1):275–82.
20. Alizadeh AA, Eisen MB, Davis RE, Ma C, Lossos IS, Rosenwald A, et al. Distinct types of diffuse large B-cell lymphoma identified by gene expression profiling. Nature. 2000;403(6769):503–11.
21. Ruskone-Fourmestraux A, Dragosics B, Morgner A, Wotherspoon A, De Jong D. Paris staging system for primary gastrointestinal lymphomas. Gut. 2003;52(6):912–3.
22. Marks E, Shi Y. Duodenal-type follicular lymphoma: a clinicopathologic review. Arch Pathol Lab Med. 2018;142(4):542–7.
23. Bende RJ, Smit LA, Bossenbroek JG, Aarts WM, Spaargaren M, de Leval L, et al. Primary follicular lymphoma of the small intestine: alpha4beta7 expression and immunoglobulin configuration suggest an origin from local antigen-experienced B cells. Am J Pathol. 2003;162(1):105–13.
24. Misdraji J, del Castillo CF, Ferry JA. Follicle center lymphoma of the ampulla of Vater presenting with jaundice: report of a case. Am J Surg Pathol. 1997;21(4):484–8.
25. Gentille C, Qin Q, Barbieri A, Ravi PS, Iyer S. Use of PEG-asparaginase in monomorphic epitheliotropic intestinal T-cell lymphoma, a disease with diagnostic and therapeutic challenges. Ecancermedicalscience. 2017;11:771.
26. Tan SY, Chuang SS, Tang T, Tan L, Ko YH, Chuah KL, et al. Type II EATL (epitheliotropic intestinal T-cell lymphoma): a neoplasm of intra-epithelial T-cells with predominant CD8alphaalpha phenotype. Leukemia. 2013;27(8):1688–96.
27. Delabie J, Holte H, Vose JM, Ullrich F, Jaffe ES, Savage KJ, et al. Enteropathy-associated T-cell lymphoma: clinical and histological findings from the international peripheral T-cell lymphoma project. Blood. 2011;118(1):148–55.
28. Zettl A, Deleeuw R, Haralambieva E, Mueller-Hermelink HK. Enteropathy-type T-cell lymphoma. Am J Clin Pathol. 2007;127(5):701–6.
29. Kim SJ, Jung HA, Chuang SS, Hong H, Guo CC, Cao J, et al. Extranodal natural killer/T-cell lymphoma involving the gastrointestinal tract: analysis of clinical features and outcomes from the Asia lymphoma study group. J Hematol Oncol. 2013;6:86–8722.
30. Carey MJ, Medeiros LJ, Roepke JE, Kjeldsberg CR, Elenitoba-Johnson KS. Primary anaplastic large cell lymphoma of the small intestine. Am J Clin Pathol. 1999;112(5):696–701.
31. Rubio-Tapia A, Murray JA. Classification and management of refractory coeliac disease. Gut. 2010;59(4):547–57.
32. Valent P, Akin C, Metcalfe DD. Mastocytosis: 2016 updated WHO classification and novel emerging treatment concepts. Blood. 2017;129(11):1420–7.
33. Nanagas VC, Kovalszki A. Gastrointestinal manifestations of Hypereosinophilic syndromes and mast cell disorders: a comprehensive review. Clin Rev Allergy Immunol. 2019;57:194–212.
34. Lee JK, Whittaker SJ, Enns RA, Zetler P. Gastrointestinal manifestations of systemic mastocytosis. World J Gastroenterol. 2008;14(45):7005–8.
35. Sotlar K, Horny HP, Simonitsch I, Krokowski M, Aichberger KJ, Mayerhofer M, et al. CD25 indicates the neoplastic phenotype of mast cells: a novel immunohistochemical marker for the diagnosis of systemic mastocytosis (SM) in routinely processed bone marrow biopsy specimens. Am J Surg Pathol. 2004;28(10):1319–25.
36. Kodama T, Ohshima K, Nomura K, Taniwaki M, Nakamura N, Nakamura S, et al. Lymphomatous polyposis of the gastrointestinal tract, including mantle cell lymphoma, follicular lymphoma and mucosa-associated lymphoid tissue lymphoma. Histopathology. 2005;47(5):467–78.
37. Kumar S, Krenacs L, Otsuki T, Kumar D, Harris CA, Wellmann A, et al. bc1-1 rearrangement and cyclin D1 protein expression in multiple lymphomatous polyposis. Am J Clin Pathol. 1996;105(6):737–43.
38. Perry AM, Bailey NG, Bonnett M, Jaffe ES, Chan WC. Disease progression in a patient with indolent T-cell lymphoproliferative disease of the gastrointestinal tract. Int J Surg Pathol. 2019;27(1):102–7.
39. Perry AM, Warnke RA, Hu Q, Gaulard P, Copie-Bergman C, Alkan S, et al. Indolent T-cell lymphoproliferative disease of the gastrointestinal tract. Blood. 2013;122(22):3599–606.
40. Mansoor A, Pittaluga S, Beck PL, Wilson WH, Ferry JA, Jaffe ES. NK-cell enteropathy: a benign NK-cell lymphoproliferative disease mimicking intestinal lymphoma: clinicopathologic features and follow-up in a unique case series. Blood. 2011;117(5):1447–52.
41. Farris AB, Lauwers GY, Ferry JA, Zukerberg LR. The rectal tonsil: a reactive lymphoid proliferation that may mimic lymphoma. Am J Surg Pathol. 2008;32(7):1075–9.
42. Al-Saleem T, Al-Mondhiry H. Immunoproliferative small intestinal disease (IPSID): a model for mature B-cell neoplasms. Blood. 2005;105(6):2274–80.
43. Lecuit M, Abachin E, Martin A, Poyart C, Pochart P, Suarez F, et al. Immunoproliferative small intestinal disease associated with campylobacter jejuni. N Engl J Med. 2004;350(3):239–48.

44. Cha JM, Choi SI, Lee JI. Rectal syphilis mimicking rectal cancer. Yonsei Med J. 2010;51(2):276–8.
45. Seegmiller AC, Xu Y, McKenna RW, Karandikar NJ. Immunophenotypic differentiation between neoplastic plasma cells in mature B-cell lymphoma vs plasma cell myeloma. Am J Clin Pathol. 2007;127(2):176–81.
46. Rimsza L, Pittaluga S, Dirnhofer S, Copie-Bergman C, de Leval L, Facchetti F, et al. The clinicopathologic spectrum of mature aggressive B cell lymphomas. Virchows Arch. 2017;471(4):453–66.
47. Staiger AM, Ziepert M, Horn H, Scott DW, Barth TFE, Bernd HW, et al. Clinical impact of the cell-of-origin classification and the MYC/ BCL2 dual expresser status in diffuse large B-cell lymphoma treated within prospective clinical trials of the German high-grade non-Hodgkin's lymphoma study group. J Clin Oncol. 2017;35(22):2515–26.
48. Sesques P, Johnson NA. Approach to the diagnosis and treatment of high-grade B-cell lymphomas with MYC and BCL2 and/or BCL6 rearrangements. Blood. 2017;129(3):280–8.
49. Van Loon K, Gill RM, McMahon P, Chigurupati R, Siddiqi I, Fox L, et al. 20q- Clonality in a case of Oral sweet syndrome and myelodysplasia. Am J Clin Pathol. 2012;137(2):310–5.
50. Robazzi TC, Silva LR, Mendonca N, Barreto JH. Gastrointestinal manifestations as initial presentation of acute leukemias in children and adolescents. Acta Gastroenterol Latinoam. 2008;38(2):126–32.
51. Ebert EC, Hagspiel KD. Gastrointestinal manifestations of leukemia. J Gastroenterol Hepatol. 2012;27(3):458–63.
52. Hovenga S, de Graaf H, Joosten P, Van den Berg GA, Storm H, Langerak AW, et al. Enteropathy-associated T-cell lymphoma presenting with eosinophilia. Neth J Med. 2003;61(1):25–7.
53. Avni B, Koren-Michowitz M. Myeloid sarcoma: current approach and therapeutic options. Ther Adv Hematol. 2011;2(5):309–16.
54. Sokol H, Georgin-Lavialle S, Grandpeix-Guyodo C, Canioni D, Barete S, Dubreuil P, et al. Gastrointestinal involvement and manifestations in systemic mastocytosis. Inflamm Bowel Dis. 2010;16(7):1247–53.
55. Zuo L, Rothenberg ME. Gastrointestinal eosinophilia. Immunol Allergy Clin North Am. 2007;27(3):443–55.
56. Desar IM, Keuter M, Raemaekers JM, Jansen JB, van Krieken JH, Van der Meer JW. Extranodal marginal zone (MALT) lymphoma in common variable immunodeficiency. Neth J Med. 2006;64(5):136–40.
57. Al-Muhsen SZ. Gastrointestinal and hepatic manifestations of primary immune deficiency diseases. Saudi J Gastroenterol. 2010;16(2):66–74.
58. Chua I, Quinti I, Grimbacher B. Lymphoma in common variable immunodeficiency: interplay between immune dysregulation, infection and genetics. Curr Opin Hematol. 2008;15(4):368–74.
59. Williams SA, Moench LE, Khan F, Vercellotti G, Linden MA. Clonal lymphoproliferations in a patient with common variable immunodeficiency. Lab Med. 2016;47(4):318–25.
60. Castillo JJ, Bibas M, Miranda RN. The biology and treatment of plasmablastic lymphoma. Blood. 2015;125(15):2323–30.
61. Shimada K, Hayakawa F, Kiyoi H. Biology and management of primary effusion lymphoma. Blood. 2018;132(18):1879–88.
62. Castillo JJ, Beltran BE, Miranda RN, Young KH, Chavez JC, Sotomayor EM. EBV-positive diffuse large B-cell lymphoma of the elderly: 2016 update on diagnosis, risk-stratification, and management. Am J Hematol. 2016;91(5):529–37.
63. Ok CY, Papathomas TG, Medeiros LJ, Young KH. EBV-positive diffuse large B-cell lymphoma of the elderly. Blood. 2013;122(3):328–40.
64. Ha SY, Sung J, Ju H, Karube K, Kim SJ, Kim WS, et al. Epstein-Barr virus-positive nodal peripheral T cell lymphomas: clinicopathologic and gene expression profiling study. Pathol Res Pract. 2013;209(7):448–54.
65. Chen CL, Sadler RH, Walling DM, Su IJ, Hsieh HC, Raab-Traub N. Epstein-Barr virus (EBV) gene expression in EBV-positive peripheral T-cell lymphomas. J Virol. 1993;67(10):6303–8.
66. Tse E, Kwong YL. Diagnosis and management of extranodal NK/T cell lymphoma nasal type. Expert Rev Hematol. 2016;9(9):861–71.
67. Weledji EP, Ngowe MN, Abba JS. Burkitt's lymphoma masquerading as appendicitis--two case reports and review of the literature. World J Surg Oncol. 2014;12:187–7819.
68. Guo J, Wu G, Chen X, Li X. Primary appendiceal lymphoma presenting as suspected perforated acute appendicitis: clinical, sonography and CT findings with pathologic correlation. Int J Clin Exp Pathol. 2014;7(10):7068–71.
69. Pickhardt PJ, Levy AD, Rohrmann CA, Kende AI. Primary neoplasms of the appendix: radiologic spectrum of disease with pathologic correlation. Radiographics. 2003;23(3):645–62.
70. Pickhardt PJ, Levy AD, Rohrmann CA, Abbondanzo SL, Kende AI. Non-Hodgkin's lymphoma of the appendix: clinical and CT findings with pathologic correlation. AJR Am J Roentgenol. 2002;178(5):1123–7.

Transplant-Related Issues in the Gastrointestinal Tract

22

Jamie Koo and Hanlin L. Wang

List of Frequently Asked Questions

1. What are the indications and the types of small bowel transplantation?
2. What are the most common posttransplant complications?
3. What are the clinical and endoscopic features suggesting acute or chronic rejection?
4. What are the histologic features of acute cellular rejection?
5. How is acute cellular rejection graded?
6. How do you distinguish a crypt apoptotic body from an intraepithelial lymphocyte, an isolated fragment of nuclear chromatin or a cytoplasmic mucin granule?
7. Do apoptotic bodies seen in surface lining epithelium have any value in the diagnosis of acute rejection?
8. What is the differential diagnosis for increased crypt apoptotic activity in the setting of small bowel transplant?
9. How can comparison to a biopsy from native bowel be helpful in establishing the diagnosis of acute cellular rejection?
10. Can acute cellular rejection coexist with other processes such as infection?
11. What are the histologic features of chronic rejection?
12. Can chronic rejection be diagnosed on a mucosal biopsy?
13. Does antibody-mediated rejection occur in small bowel transplant?
14. In cases where colon and/or stomach are also transplanted, how do you evaluate for acute cellular rejection of transplanted colon and stomach?
15. What are the most common infections seen in the setting of small bowel transplantation?
16. In addition to the presence of infectious organisms, what other histologic features may be seen in the setting of infection?
17. What special and immunohistochemical stains can be used to help identify infectious organisms?
18. In addition to bone marrow or stem cell transplant, can solid organ transplants cause GVHD?
19. What are the histologic features of acute GVHD in the esophagus and stomach?
20. What are the histologic features of acute GVHD in the small bowel and colon?
21. What is the differential diagnosis for increased apoptotic activity in the GI tract?
22. How is acute GVHD of the GI tract graded?
23. What is the distinction between acute and chronic GVHD?
24. What are the clinical features of PTLD occurring after small bowel transplant? What sites does it involve?
25. What are the general types of PTLD?
26. What are some basic morphologic features that can be used to distinguish benign lymphoid aggregates from possible PTLD?
27. What basic immunostains and special studies can help establish a diagnosis of PTLD?

J. Koo
ProPath, Dallas, TX, USA

H. L. Wang (✉)
University of California at Los Angeles David Geffen School of Medicine, Los Angeles, CA, USA

Frequently Asked Questions

1. What are the indications and the types of small bowel transplantation?

Small bowel transplant has shown an increasing success for treatment of irreversible intestinal failure in both pediatric and adult patients, which may result from a variety of conditions such as gastroschisis, necrotizing enterocolitis, volvulus, microvillus inclusion disease, tufting enteropathy, and Hirschsprung disease in children or mesenteric venous thrombosis, trauma, and extensive bowel resection for a mass lesion or Crohn disease in

H. L. Wang, Z. E. Chen (eds.), *Practical Gastrointestinal Pathology*, Practical Anatomic Pathology,
https://doi.org/10.1007/978-3-030-51268-2_22

adults. Retransplantation is performed for patients with graft failure or dysfunction due to rejection or other complications. There are four different types of intestinal grafts, including (1) isolated intestinal transplants (with or without the colon), (2) combined intestinal-liver transplants, (3) multivisceral transplants (including the small intestine with the duodenum, liver, pancreas, and stomach, with or without the colon), and (4) modified multivisceral transplants (multivisceral transplants without the liver and with or without the stomach).

References: [1–3]

2. **What are the most common posttransplant complications?**

Posttransplant complications are similar to those seen in other solid organ transplants and mainly include rejection, infection, medication effect, and posttransplant lymphoproliferative disorder (PTLD). Because of the unique and complex immunologic environment of the small bowel, maintenance of immunosuppression after bowel transplantation is challenging, thus leading to higher rates of acute cellular rejection (ACR) and infection as compared to other solid organ transplants. ACR is relatively common, occurring in 39% of patients in the first year and 44% in the 2 years following transplant. Infrequently, recurrent intestinal diseases, such as Crohn disease, can occur.

References: [1–3]

3. **What are the clinical and endoscopic features suggesting acute or chronic rejection?**

Clinical symptoms of ACR are relatively non-specific and may include increased stoma output, fever, nausea, vomiting, abdominal pain, and diarrhea. Endoscopic findings are likewise non-specific and can range from mucosal edema, erythema, friability, focal to diffuse ulcerations, and frank mucosal sloughing when severe. Chronic rejection is difficult to diagnose clinically but may be suspected in cases of persistent diarrhea, ulcers unresponsive to increased immunosuppression, dysmotility, and poor nutritional status. Endoscopic findings may include loss of regular mucosal folds, extensive ulceration, the appearance of firm and fibrotic bowel wall, and stricture. Treatment of ACR requires increased immunosuppression to prevent graft loss.

References: [1–3]

4. **What are the histologic features of acute cellular rejection?**

The main histologic features of ACR include:

- Increased apoptotic activity in the crypt epithelium (Fig. 22.1a), which is a hallmark of ACR.
- Varying degrees of lamina propria mixed inflammatory infiltrates composed predominantly of small and activated lymphocytes with admixed eosinophils and neutrophils. The lamina propria may be edematous or congested.
- Varying degrees of epithelial injury that range from focal, minimal, and reactive, including loss of mucin, nuclear enlargement and hyperchromasia, and villous blunting; to focal crypt destruction, withering, and dropout; to complete crypt dropout, extensive erosion, and ulceration when severe. In cases with crypt dropout, empty crypt contours can be recognized, but without epithelial cells, which can be mistaken for lamina

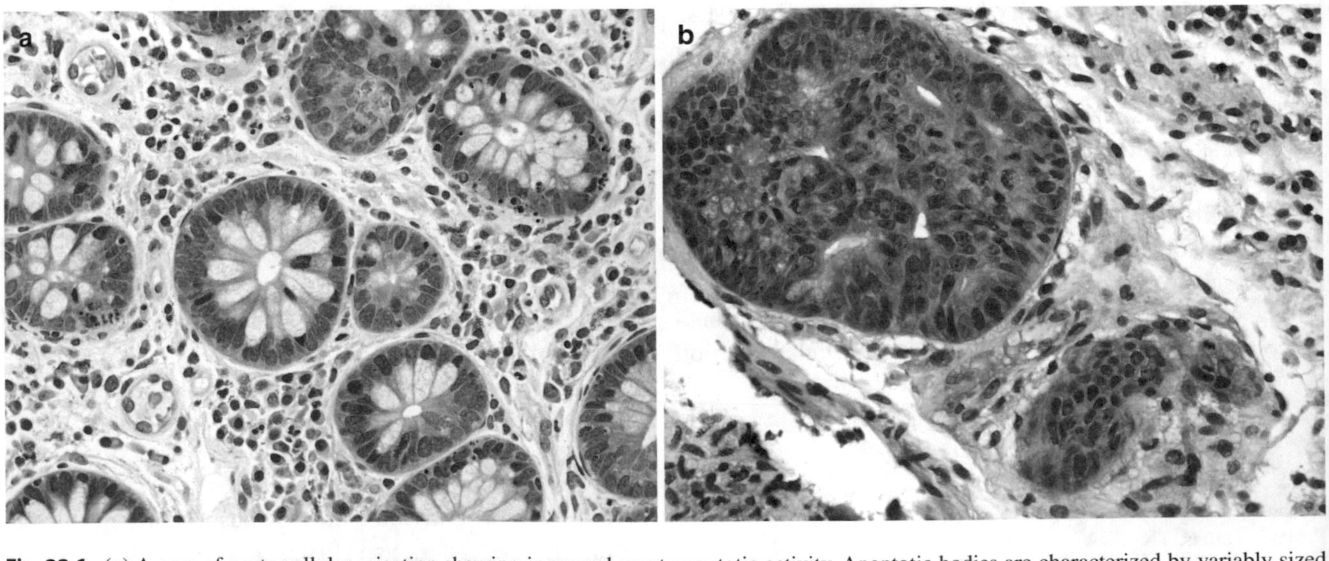

Fig. 22.1 (**a**) A case of acute cellular rejection showing increased crypt apoptotic activity. Apoptotic bodies are characterized by variably sized fragments of pyknotic nuclei within eosinophilic cytoplasm or with a rim of clear cytoplasm. They are typically located at the base of crypts beneath or between non-apoptotic epithelial cells. (**b**) Regenerating crypts can be seen in the setting of severe rejection, characterized by increased mitoses, hyperchromatic nuclei, and distorted crypt architecture

propria capillaries/lymphatics. In treated rejection, regenerating crypts may be seen, which typically show increased mitoses, hyperchromatic nuclei, and distorted crypt architecture (Fig. 22.1b). Apoptotic activity is not prominent in regenerating crypts, in contrast to those that are still undergoing rejection.
References: [4–6]

5. **How is acute cellular rejection graded?**
Based on the evaluation of the criteria above, ACR can be graded as mild, moderate, or severe as shown in Table 22.1. An additional diagnostic category includes indeterminate for ACR, which may be used in the presence of minimal increased crypt apoptotic bodies that does not reach the threshold for mild ACR.

- Apoptotic bodies are counted per ten consecutive crypts in a selected area with the most active apoptotic activity. This should ideally be assessed in well-oriented, longitudinally arranged crypts (Fig. 22.2a). If a biopsy is tangentially sectioned, resulting in multiple donut-shaped cross sections from each crypt, one should not count each "donut" as an individual crypt (Fig. 22.2b). For biopsies that are superficially sectioned, which show only villi or less than ten crypts, deeper sections should be examined.
- If no crypt dropout0 is appreciated on low-power view, the possibility of moderate and severe ACR is essentially ruled out. Higher-power view to search for apoptotic bodies then becomes important for the diagnosis of mild or indeterminate ACR.
- One exception is the finding of confluent apoptosis involving all or the vast majority of the epithelial cells forming a crypt. This would qualify for moderate ACR in the absence of crypt dropout or erosion (Fig. 22.3a–c).
- Biopsies from or near the stoma or anastomosis may show non-specific inflammation, villous architectural change, and epithelial injury, which should not be used to evaluate for rejection.

References: [4, 5]

6. **How do you distinguish a crypt apoptotic body from an intraepithelial lymphocyte, an isolated fragment of nuclear chromatin, or a cytoplasmic mucin granule?**
   - An apoptotic body is the result of programed cell death, consisting of variably sized fragments of pyknotic nuclei with condensed nuclear dust and debris within

Table 22.1 Histologic grading of acute cellular rejection in small bowel allograft biopsies

Grade	Apoptotic bodies per 10 consecutive crypts	Degree of epithelial injury	Degree of lamina propria inflammation
No ACR	≤2	None	Normal components
Indeterminate	3–5	Minimal, usually focal	Minimal, usually localized
Mild	≥6	Mild, usually focal with intact mucosa	Mild, usually localized
Moderate[a]	≥6 or confluent	Focal crypt dropout, focal mucosal erosion	Moderate, usually extensive
Severe[a]	Variable in residual crypts	Extensive crypt dropout, extensive erosion, and/or ulceration	Moderate to severe, extensive

[a]A varying degree of arteritis may be present in the setting of moderate and severe ACR, but this feature is not evident in superficial mucosal biopsies

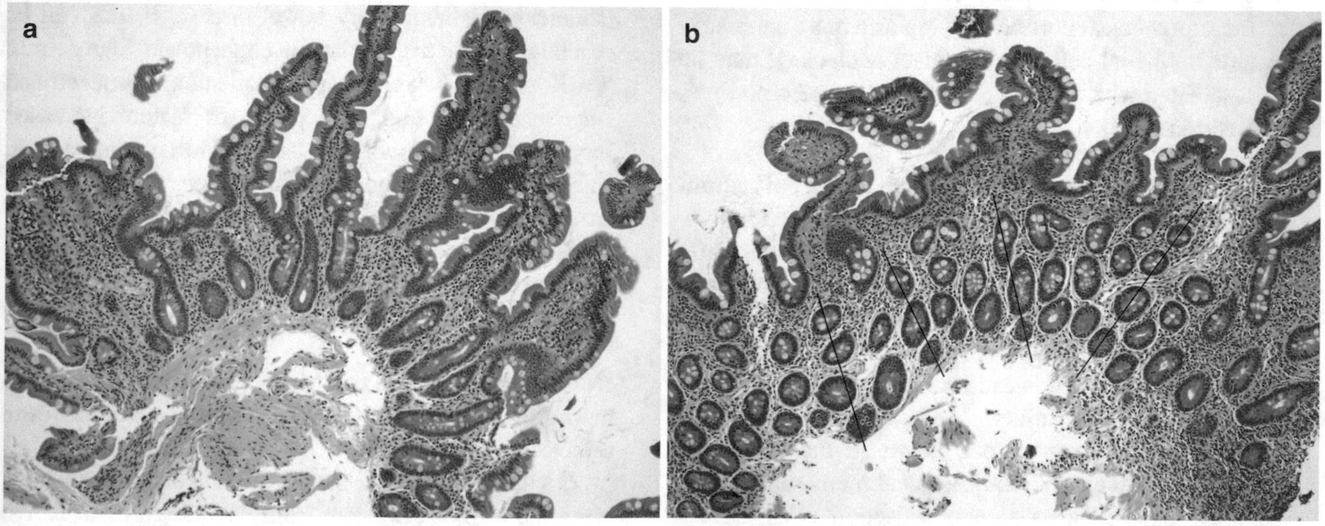

Fig. 22.2 (a) Well-oriented, longitudinally arranged crypts are the best areas to assess crypt apoptosis. (**b**) In tangentially sectioned specimens, multiple linear arranged donut-shaped cross sections may be counted as one crypt as highlighted by black lines

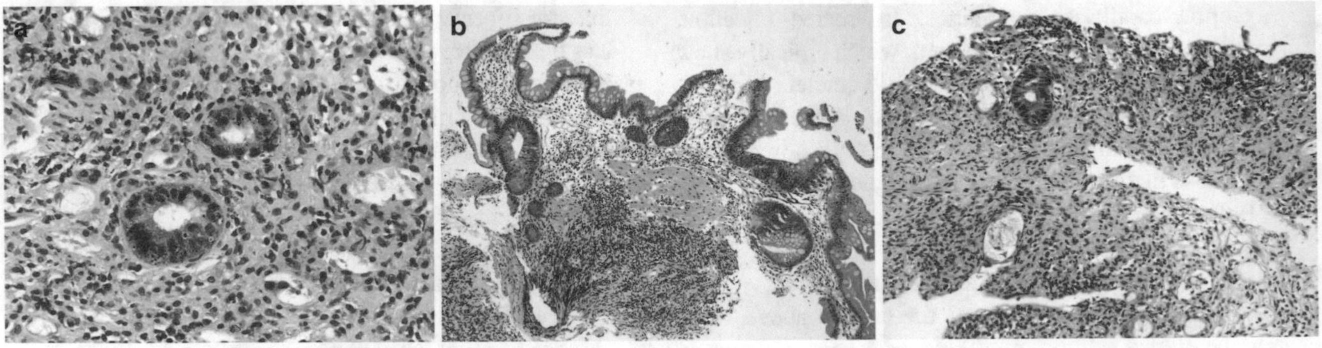

Fig. 22.3 (**a**) Two residual crypts showing confluent apoptosis. The adjacent crypts are dropped out, leaving empty contours. (**b**) This biopsy shows focal/partial crypt dropout, qualifying for moderate acute cellular rejection. (**c**) This biopsy shows more severe rejection with more significant crypt destruction and more extensive crypt dropout

eosinophilic cytoplasm or with a rim of clear cytoplasm (Figs. 22.1a and 22.3a). Occasionally they can be subtle, consisting of only small, pinpoint basophilic fragments of nuclear debris. In the setting of ACR, they are typically located at the base of crypts beneath or between other non-apoptotic epithelial cells.

- Intraepithelial lymphocytes can also show condensed nuclei with a clear halo but can be distinguished by its uniform size of about 10 microns and lack of nuclear fragmentation.
- In contrast to an apoptotic body, an isolated fragment of nuclear chromatin is tiny, single, usually round and dark, and typically found free-floating within the supranuclear portion of cytoplasm in an unremarkable epithelial cell with an intact nucleus. It does not cluster with other nuclear fragments as an apoptotic body would do and usually does not show an associated rim of clear cytoplasm (Fig. 22.4a).
- A cytoplasmic mucin granule is also tiny, single, usually dot-like, and basophilic. It is also present within the supranuclear portion of cytoplasm in an unremarkable epithelial cell with an intact nucleus. It may be associated with a rim of clear halo (Fig. 22.4b).

Reference: [1]

7. **Do apoptotic bodies seen in surface lining epithelium have any value in the diagnosis of acute rejection?**

Epithelial apoptosis associated with ACR typically involves the crypt bases, as this represents the regenerative zone in the small bowel. Apoptosis involving the surface lining epithelium is not considered a diagnostic feature of ACR, as this can be seen in association with infections, drug injury, and bowel preparation (Fig. 22.5a). Also, apoptotic debris in the superficial lamina propria beneath the basement membrane should not be regarded as a sign of rejection (Fig. 22.5b). However, in cases of severe ACR with ulceration, areas adjacent to an ulcer or of healing mucosa may show only scant surface epithelium overlying an area of crypt dropout. Apoptotic bodies may be seen in these residual cells as part of the ongoing process of ACR.

8. **What is the differential diagnosis for increased crypt apoptotic activity in the setting of small bowel transplant?**

While an increased crypt apoptotic body count is a key histologic feature of ACR, it is not specific for ACR as it may also be seen in the setting of infection and medication effect. Medications, and mycophenolate mofetil (CellCept) in particular, are known to cause increased apoptotic activity in crypts (see Chap. 11). Mycophenolate is an immunosuppressant commonly used in transplant patients that in high doses may cause GI toxicity, typically manifesting as diarrhea. A wide spectrum of histologic changes associated with mycophenolate toxicity has been described, which includes increased crypt apoptotic activity resembling graft-versus-host disease (GVHD-like pattern), ischemia-type injury, and mucosal damage mimicking inflammatory bowel disease. It thus can be challenging to distinguish mycophenolate injury from ACR, as small bowel transplant patients are frequently on mycophenolate, and both processes feature increased crypt apoptotic activity. In addition to correlation with medication history, comparison of biopsy findings from native bowel can be helpful (see question 9 below). Treatment of mycophenolate toxicity requires dose reduction or cessation, with quick clinical improvement.

References: [2, 7–10]

9. **How can comparison to a biopsy from native bowel be helpful in establishing the diagnosis of acute cellular rejection?**

As discussed above, the distribution of apoptotic bodies seen in biopsies taken from the allograft and native bowel (small bowel or colon) can potentially help distinguish between ACR and medication effect from myco-

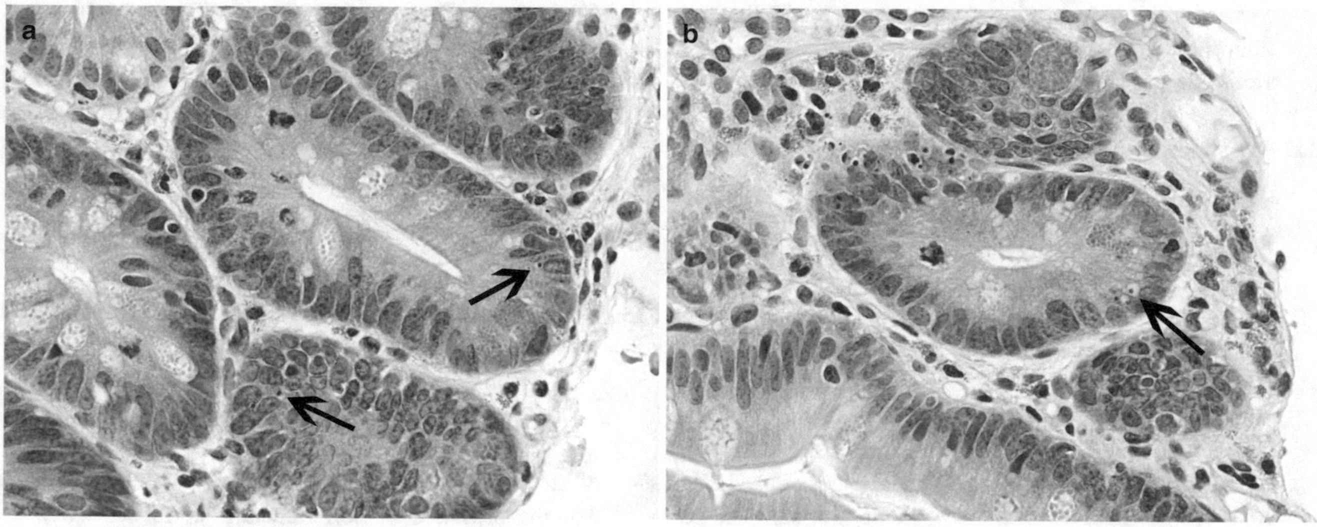

Fig. 22.4 (**a**) An isolated fragment of nuclear chromatin (arrows) is tiny, single, and typically free-floating within the supranuclear portion of cytoplasm in an unremarkable epithelial cell with an intact nucleus. This should not be counted as an apoptotic body for the diagnosis of acute rejection. (**b**) A cytoplasmic mucin granule (arrow) is also tiny, single, usually dot-like, basophilic, and with a rim of clear halo. It is also present within the supranuclear portion of cytoplasm in an unremarkable epithelial cell with an intact nucleus. This should not be counted as an apoptotic body

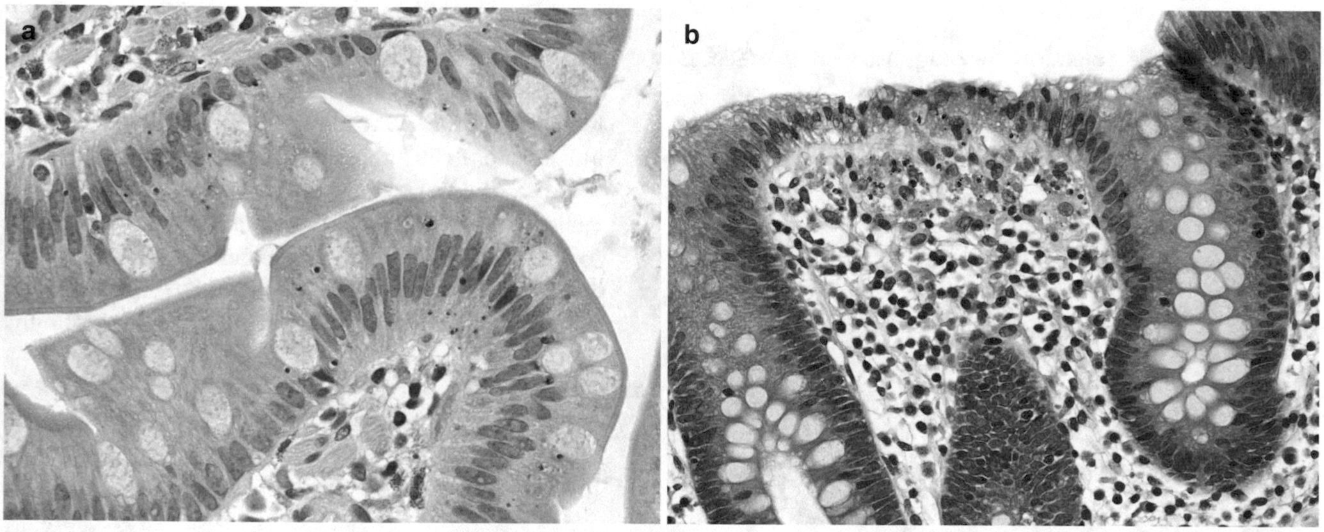

Fig. 22.5 Apoptotic debris within the surface lining epithelial cells (**a**) or in the superficial lamina propria beneath the basement membrane (**b**) should not be counted for the diagnosis of acute rejection

phenolate. Features of ACR including apoptotic bodies, while known to be patchy in distribution in the allograft, would not be expected in the patient's native bowel; in contrast, medication effect would be expected to have a more diffuse distribution involving both allograft and native bowel. Thus, attention to the distribution of apoptotic bodies can help one favor either ACR or medication effect. In our experience, a concurrent native bowel biopsy has been helpful in about 25% of these cases.
References: [1, 2]

10. **Can acute cellular rejection coexist with other processes such as infection?**

Yes. However, because the histologic features of ACR overlap with those of infection and medication effect, it can be difficult to definitely diagnose both concurrently. If infection can be verified based on identification of microorganisms on biopsy or positive results of stool or blood studies but the possibility of ACR also remains, it may be prudent to discuss with the clinical team for the necessity of treatment for ACR. Close fol-

low-up with repeat biopsies to reassess for ACR appears appropriate once the infection has resolved.
References: [11–16]

11. **What are the histologic features of chronic rejection?**
    The defining histologic finding in chronic rejection is obliterative arteriopathy (Fig. 22.6a, b), characterized by intimal hyperplasia and luminal narrowing, which may involve blood vessels of the mesentery, subserosa, muscularis propria, and submucosa. This finding is much more likely to be seen on a resected allograft specimen, which may also show fibrosis and thickening of the bowel wall and serosal adhesions with possible encasement of bowel loops, among other changes (Fig. 22.7a, b). Because these vessels are typically not sampled on an endoscopic mucosal biopsy, full-thickness biopsies have been suggested to allow for better sampling and identification of arterial changes. However, in our experience, even full-thickness biopsies fail to show diagnostic lesions of chronic rejection.
    References: [17–19]

12. **Can chronic rejection be diagnosed on a mucosal biopsy?**
    Due to the difficulty in identifying obliterative arteriopathy in both mucosal and full-thickness biopsies, some studies have attempted to identify mucosal changes that may be associated with chronic rejection. These findings include pyloric metaplasia, lamina propria fibrosis, submucosal fibrosis, widespread loss of crypts, ulceration with granulation tissue, and villous blunting (Fig. 22.7c). However, many of these features are non-specific, and consensus criteria for the diagnosis of chronic rejection on biopsy specimens have not been established. Thus, while the presence of these histologic findings may raise the possibility of chronic rejection in the appropriate clinical setting and should be noted, it is not possible to definitively make this diagnosis on biopsy alone.
    References: [1, 2, 17–19]

13. **Does antibody-mediated rejection occur in small bowel transplant?**
    Although well established as a cause of graft failure in kidney and heart transplants, antibody-mediated rejection (AMR) remains poorly characterized in the setting of small bowel transplant. Several studies have shown that the presence of donor-specific antibodies (DSAs) after small bowel transplant is associated with worse outcome and higher rates of rejection. However, only a few studies have examined C4d immunohistochemical staining as an indicator of AMR in small bowel allografts, and most have found C4d positivity to be relatively equally present in patients with or without concurrent positive DSAs and/or biopsies with or without ACR. Other histologic findings indicative of AMR have also not been established. Although Rabant and colleagues recently found the histologic features of capillaritis (presence of inflammatory cells in lumens of lamina propria capillaries), mucosal erosion/ulceration, lamina propria inflammation, and edema to be associated with C4d positivity and thus AMR in their study cohort, there was a high incidence of positive DSAs in their pediatric study cohort, which may have affected the results. Interestingly,

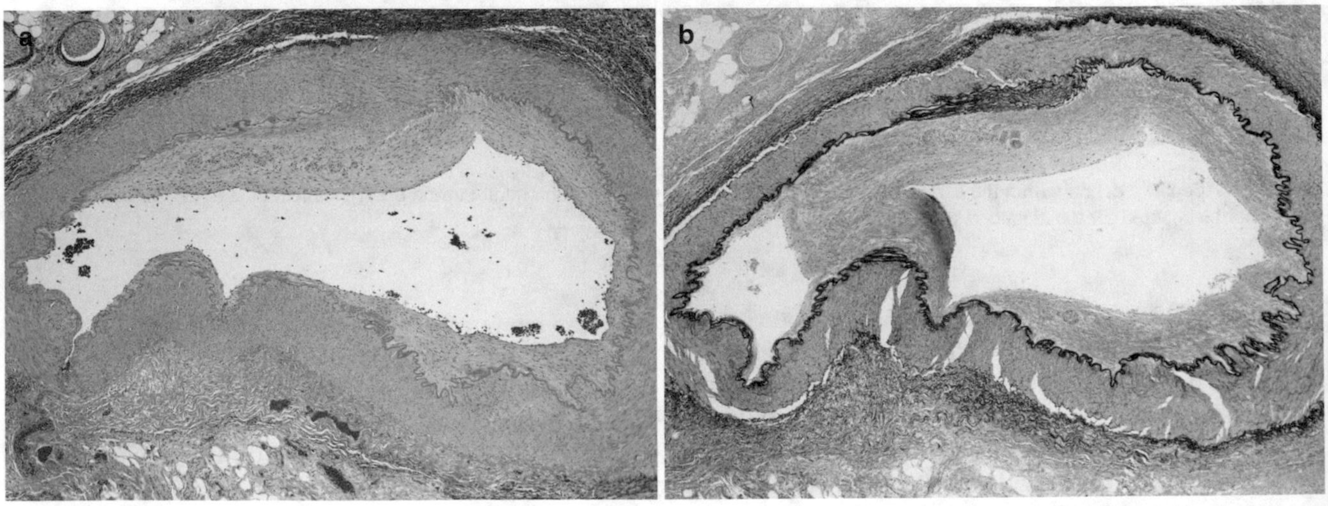

Fig. 22.6 Obliterative arteriopathy characterized by intimal hyperplasia and luminal narrowing (**a**), which is better evaluated by EVG (Verhoeff-van Gieson) stain (**b**). (From Ref. [1] with permission)

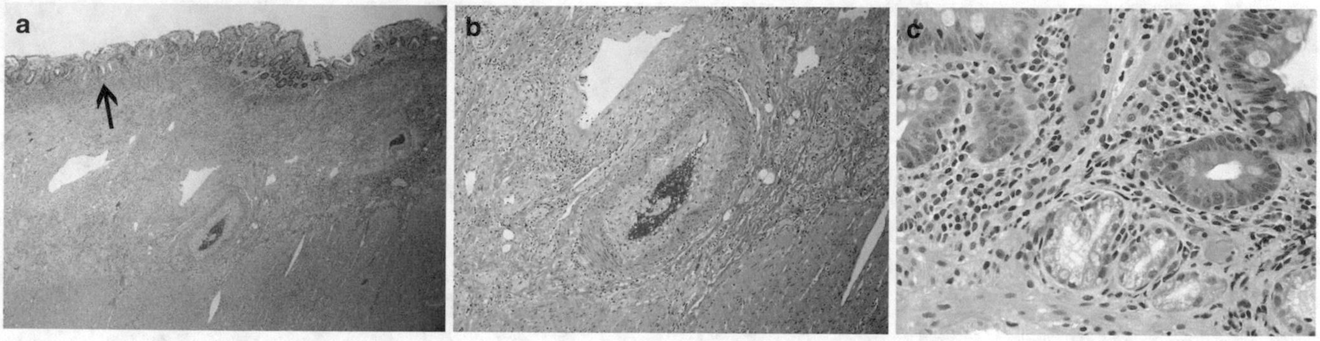

Fig. 22.7 (**a** and **b**) A resected small bowel graft showing submucosal fibrosis and features of obliterative arteriopathy in submucosal vessels. Pyloric metaplasia (arrow) is noted in the mucosa (**a**). The findings are consistent with chronic rejection. (From Ref. [1] with permission). (**c**) Focal pyloric metaplasia is seen in a biopsy from transplanted small bowel, which is an indication of chronic mucosal injury including chronic rejection

C4d positivity was found in both patients with and without DSAs in this study as well. Overall, the utility of C4d immunohistochemical staining or specific histologic features to identify AMR is not well established and is an area that requires further investigation (Fig. 22.8a, b).
References: [2, 20–22]

14. **In cases where colon and/or stomach is also transplanted, how do you evaluate for acute cellular rejection of transplanted colon and stomach?**

The diagnostic and grading criteria of ACR in transplanted colon are similar to those used for small bowel transplants, primarily based on apoptotic activity in crypts and the degree of epithelial injury (Fig. 22.9a). Similar criteria are also used for histologic evaluation of transplanted stomach (Fig. 22.9b). In 2004, Garcia and colleagues proposed a grading schema specifically for gastric ACR, which are somewhat different than that used for small bowel transplants. It is summarized below:

- Grade 0 (no rejection) – Absent or very minimal inflammatory cell infiltrates in the lamina propria, normal glandular architecture, and no increased apoptotic activity
- Grade 1 (indeterminate for ACR) – Scattered mixed inflammatory cell infiltrates in the lamina propria, edema or focal congestion, normal glandular architecture, and no increased apoptotic activity
- Grade 2 (mild ACR) – Increased lamina propria inflammatory cell infiltrates, increased apoptotic bodies in glands, mild glandular architectural distortion, and mild cytologic atypia
- Grade 3 (moderate ACR) – Prominent mixed inflammatory cell infiltrates in lamina propria, increased or confluent apoptotic bodies in glands, increased cytologic atypia, vacuolization of parietal cells, erosion or ulceration of the surface epithelium, and glandular architectural disarray
- Grade 4 (severe ACR) – Significant distortion of the glandular architecture with subtotal destruction of the glands and gastric pits, accompanied by ulceration.

Reference: [23]

15. **What are the most common infections seen in the setting of small bowel transplantation?**

Infections after small bowel transplant can be bacterial, viral, fungal, and rarely protozoal. Bacterial infections are the most common and tend to occur in the first month after transplantation due to postsurgical complications. Viral infections due to immunosuppression typically occur a few months post transplantation and can include viral enteritis involving the allograft from organisms such as rotavirus, adenovirus, and CMV. Fungal infections occur less frequently and may cause peritonitis, fungemia, or pneumonia. Protozoal infections such as cryptosporidiosis have been reported rarely.
References: [11–16]

16. **In addition to the presence of infectious organisms, what other histologic features may be seen in the setting of infection?**

Histologic features of infectious enteritis may show increased lamina propria inflammatory cells including neutrophils, neutrophil infiltration of the crypts and surface epithelium, increased intraepithelial lymphocytes, mild to moderate villous blunting, and a varying degree of crypt dropout, and sometimes erosion and ulceration. Apoptotic activity may be increased in both the surface epithelium and in the crypt bases, particularly in adenovirus and CMV infections. In infectious enteritis, the degree of neutrophilic inflammation and epithelial injury may be disproportionate to the degree of apoptotic activity as compared to ACR. Correlation with microbiology studies (serologies, cultures, PCR) may be helpful in confirming an infectious etiology.

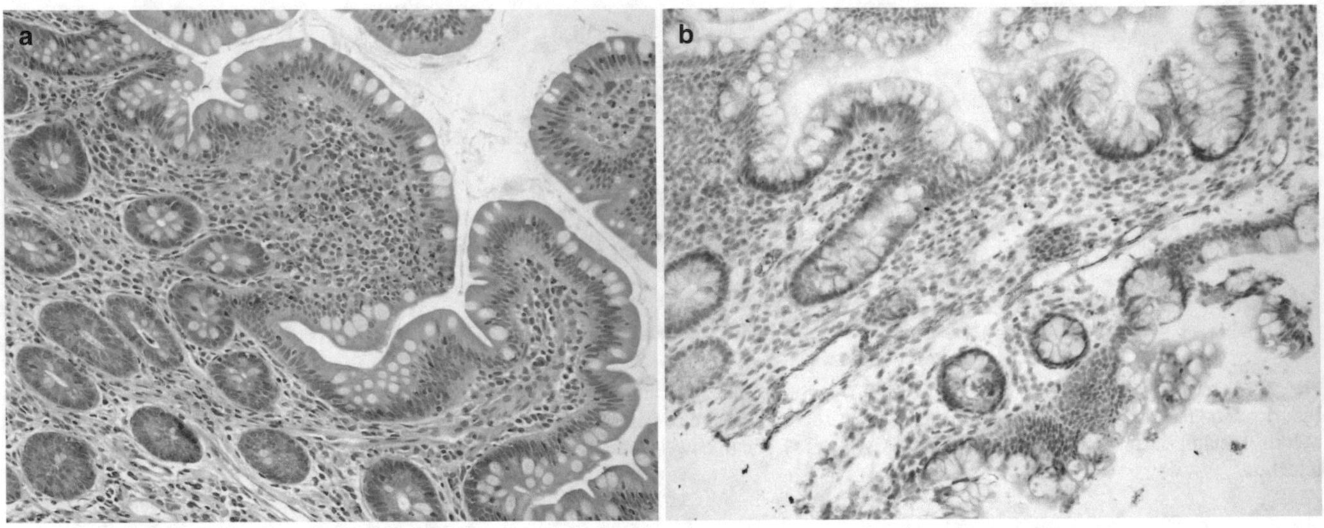

Fig. 22.8 (**a**) A biopsy from transplanted small bowel showing focal minimally active inflammation with neutrophils seen in the lamina propria and within the epithelium. No features of capillaritis or increased crypt apoptotic activity are seen in this biopsy. (**b**) Positive C4d immunoreactivity is observed in endothelial cells lining the lamina propria capillaries. This case is considered antibody-medicated rejection because the patient also has positive donor-specific antibodies against HLA DQ7 and DQ9

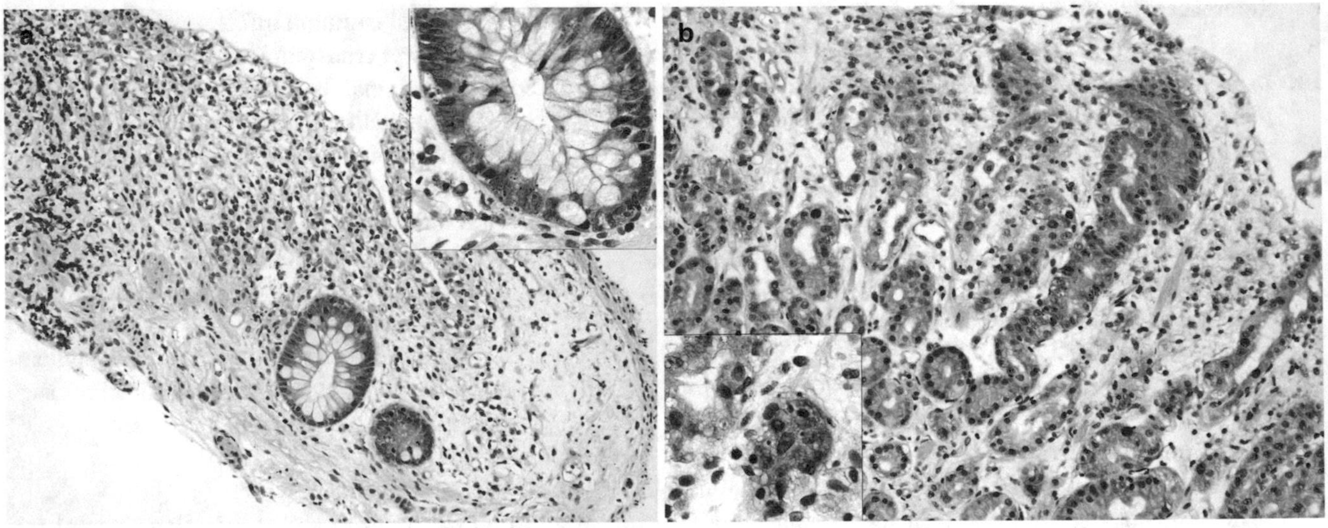

Fig. 22.9 (**a**) Moderate acute cellular rejection seen in transplanted colon showing partial crypt dropout. Some of the remaining crypts show increased apoptotic activity (inset). (**b**) Acute cellular rejection seen in transplanted stomach showing partial glandular injury and increased apoptotic activity in glands (inset)

Adenovirus infection typically involves surface enterocytes, which often show layering or "piling up" of nuclei. Characteristic smudged or glassy nuclear chromatin can be seen (Fig. 22.10a). CMV shows characteristic nuclear and cytoplasmic eosinophilic viral inclusions accompanied by cytomegaly, which typically involve endothelial and stromal cells, but can also be seen in epithelial and inflammatory cells. Cryptosporidium enteritis occurs rarely and shows characteristic, spherical, regular, 3–5 micron basophilic organisms present on the surface of luminal enterocytes.

References: [1, 11–16]

17. **What special and immunohistochemical stains can be used to help identify infectious organisms?**

Immunostains for adenovirus are helpful in highlighting infected enterocytes, which can be overlooked on H&E sections when only a few cells are affected

(Fig. 22.10b). Routine immunostaining for adenovirus is performed at some institutions. CMV inclusions can usually be identified on H&E, but immunostaining can be helpful in confirming the diagnosis in ulcerated areas where residual ganglion cells and reactive or degenerating stromal cells can mimic CMV.
References: [1, 11–16]

18. In addition to bone marrow or stem cell transplant, can solid organ transplants cause GVHD?

GVHD is a T-cell-mediated process in which donor T lymphocytes attack host tissues. It is most commonly seen in patients after stem cell transplant (SCT) but may also be seen after solid organ transplantation or even blood transfusions. GVHD occurs in approximately 5% of patients receiving small bowel transplant and in 0.1–2% of those with liver transplant. A similar clinical syndrome has been described after autologous SCT, and while its pathogenesis is not well understood, it is thought to be due to a failure of self-tolerance. Fortunately, it tends to be mild and responds well to corticosteroids.
References: [24–26]

19. What are the histologic features of acute GVHD in the esophagus and stomach?

The key histologic feature of GVHD in the tubular GI tract includes epithelial apoptosis leading to mucosal injury and denudation as the degree of severity increases. In the esophagus, in addition to individual apoptotic bodies or dyskeratotic keratinocytes, other non-specific features may include increased intraepithelial lymphocytes or a lichenoid interface inflammatory infiltrate (Fig. 22.11a). When severe, ulceration or bullous disease with sloughing of the mucosa may occur. In the stomach, increased apoptotic bodies are found in the neck area of gastric mucosa with a sparse associated inflammatory cell infiltrate. Dilated and degenerating glands with luminal eosinophilic debris as well as gland dropout may be seen (Fig. 22.11b).
References: [24, 25, 27, 28]

20. What are the histologic features of acute GVHD in the small bowel and colon?

Acute GVHD in the small bowel and colon resembles ACR, which also features increased apoptotic bodies in the crypts. This may be the only finding in mild cases. There is typically a sparse associated inflammatory infiltrate. With increasing severity, crypts may become attenuated and dilated with luminal debris, which may progress to larger areas of crypt dropout that can eventually become completely replaced by ulceration and loose granulation tissue (Fig. 22.12a–c).

- Apoptotic activity in the surface epithelium should not be used to diagnose GVHD, as these may occur as the result of bowel preparation regimens, drug injury, or infections.
- The exact threshold of minimum number of crypt apoptotic bodies needed for a diagnosis of mild acute GVHD is not well established. While not specific for GVHD, at least one apoptotic body per biopsy tissue fragment has been recommended.
- Multiple serial sections should be examined to avoid missing focal, infrequent apoptotic bodies.
- Paneth cells and neuroendocrine cells at the crypt bases usually survive longer than epithelial cells,

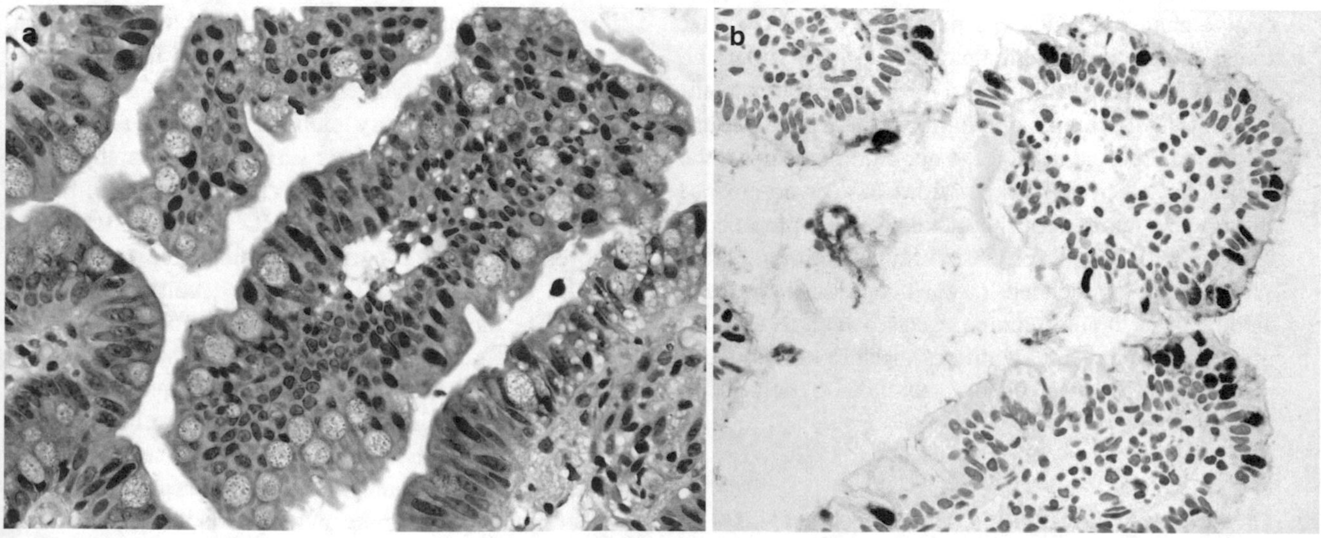

Fig. 22.10 Adenovirus enteritis showing smudged nuclear chromatin in surface lining epithelial cells (**a**), which is confirmed by immunostain (**b**)

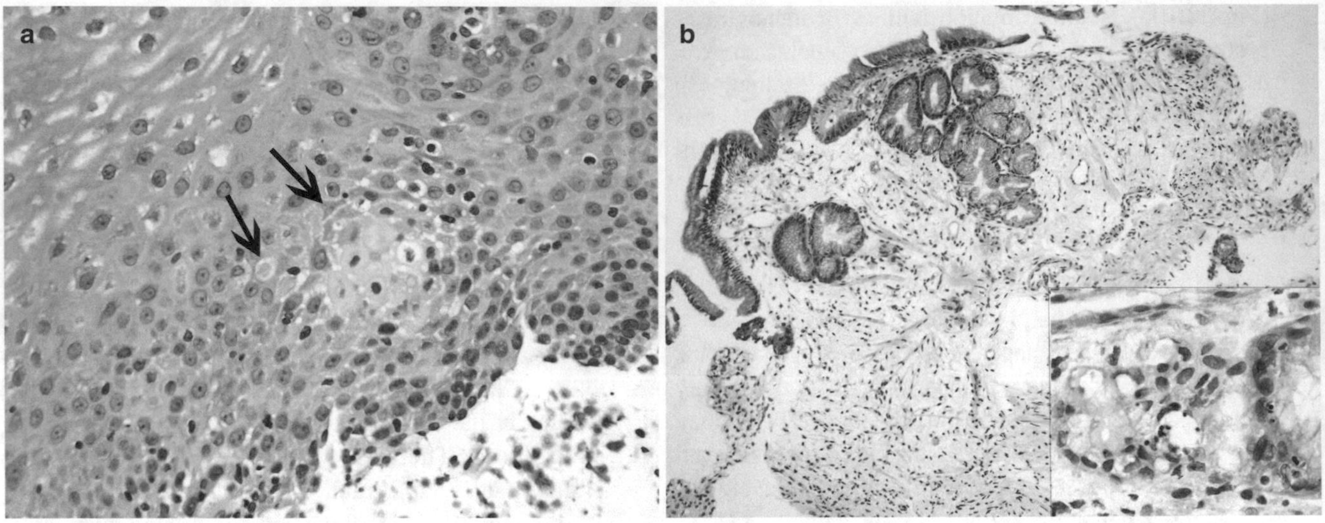

Fig. 22.11 (**a**) Acute graft-versus-host disease seen in an esophageal biopsy showing focal damage with dyskeratotic keratinocytes (arrows). A mild increase in intraepithelial lymphocytes is also seen. (**b**) Acute graft-versus-host disease seen in a gastric biopsy showing glandular dropout. Increased apoptotic activity is seen in some of the remaining glands (inset)

which should not be confused with viral inclusions (Fig. 22.12d).

References: [24, 25, 27–29]

21. **What is the differential diagnosis for increased apoptotic activity in the GI tract?**

    Increased apoptotic bodies may be seen in other conditions such as drug-related injury and infection, making clinical correlation invaluable. As discussed above, mycophenolate-induced injury in particular can histologically show increased crypt apoptotic bodies with crypt damage, ulceration, and a mixed inflammatory infiltrate. Cytoreductive conditioning regimens in patients recently undergoing stem cell transplant can also cause increased apoptotic bodies and regenerative changes, which can persist up to day 20 after transplantation; thus, a diagnosis of GVHD should be made with caution in this early period post transplantation. Use of proton pump inhibitors and NSAIDs has also been reported to increase apoptotic activity in the GI tract. Infections such as with CMV or cryptosporidium also commonly show increased apoptotic bodies. A low threshold for CMV immunostaining in this setting is recommended. Crypt apoptotic bodies can also be seen in autoimmune diseases such as autoimmune enteropathy and common variable immunodeficiency, but clinical history should be helpful in separating these from GVHD.

    References: [25, 27–30]

22. **How is acute GVHD of the GI tract graded?**

    While severe injury from GVHD (grade 4) has been associated with poor survival, the other less severe grades do not necessarily correlate with clinical symptoms or outcomes. Thus, histologic grading of GVHD is not universally performed at all centers. However, when used, the Lerner grading system for colonic GVHD is the most common. The most severe grade should be provided if there is variability across different biopsy sites.

    - Grade 1 – Increase in apoptotic cells only, without crypt damage
    - Grade 2 – Loss or damage of individual crypts
    - Grade 3 – Loss of two or more contiguous crypts
    - Grade 4 – Complete crypt loss/mucosal ulceration.

    References: [28, 31]

23. **What is the distinction between acute and chronic GVHD?**

    Acute and chronic GVHD were historically defined based on timing of presentation post transplantation, with acute GVHD occurring within the first 100 days. However, due to changes in conditioning regimens used clinically, this arbitrary temporal distinction is no longer applied, and characteristic skin, GI tract, or liver findings are classified as acute GVHD regardless of timing after transplant. Chronic GVHD of the GI tract may develop after prolonged or incompletely treated episodes of acute GVHD, leading to architectural distortion. The most commonly affected part of the GI tract is the esophagus, which may show esophageal webs by endoscopy or imaging and ulceration and submucosal fibrosis histologically. In the small bowel and colon, changes of chronicity are similar to those seen in inflammatory bowel disease and include crypt architectural distortion, crypt atrophy, pyloric metaplasia, Paneth cell metaplasia in the distal colon, and fibrosis of the lamina propria or even submucosal fibrosis (uncommon).

    References: [25–28]

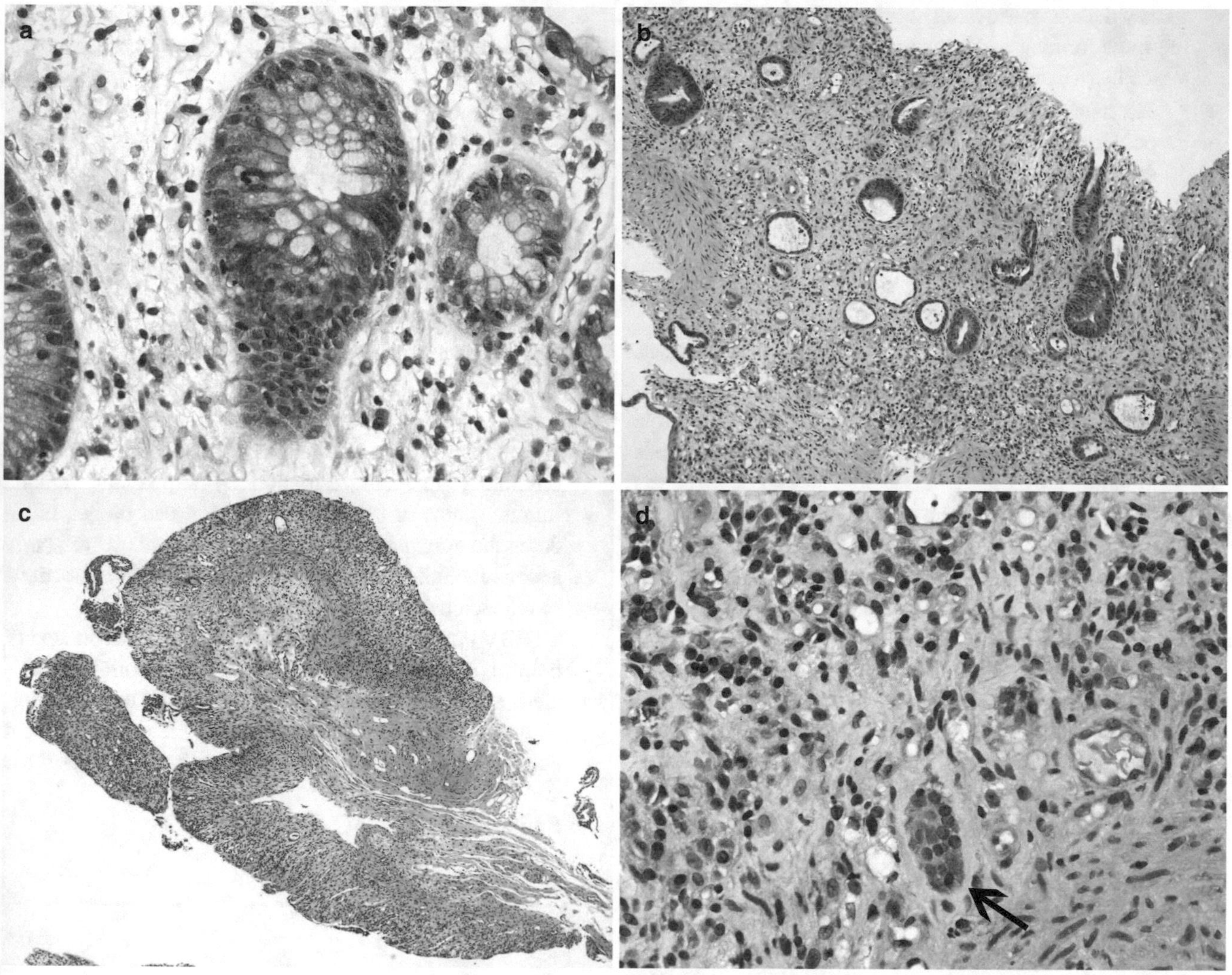

Fig. 22.12 Acute graft-versus-host disease seen in colonic biopsies showing increased crypt apoptotic activity (**a**), crypt damage with attenuated and dilated crypts and partial crypt dropout (**b**), or complete crypt dropout (**c**). Paneth cells and neuroendocrine cells (arrow) may survive longer (**d**)

24. What are the clinical features of PTLD occurring after small bowel transplant? What sites does it involve?

Posttransplant lymphoproliferative disorders (PTLDs) occurring as a result of immunosuppression have been reported in up to 21% of patients after small bowel transplant and are seen more frequently in pediatric patients. While type of immunosuppression can influence the incidence of PTLD development, there is no significant relationship between PTLD and type of intestinal graft received. Patients may be asymptomatic or can show variable symptoms, including fever, lymphadenopathy, shock, and GI bleeding. The diagnosis of PTLD can be made anywhere from a month to several years after transplantation. In addition to involving the intestinal graft, other sites including the lymph nodes, thymus, bone marrow, liver, and native bowel may be involved. EBV infection is associated with PTLD in the majority of cases, over 90% in most studies. Treatment of PTLD includes reduction of immunosuppression, which may be effective in some early lesions, but therapy with rituximab and chemotherapy is required in some cases to achieve durable remission.

References: [1, 2, 32–36]

25. What are the general types of PTLD?

The 2016 WHO classification identifies the following types of PTLD:

- Plasmacytic hyperplasia PTLD
- Infectious mononucleosis PTLD
- Florid follicular hyperplasia PTLD
- Polymorphic PTLD
- Monomorphic PTLD (B- and T-/NK-cell types)
- Classical Hodgkin lymphoma PTLD

A detailed discussion of the classification of PTLD is beyond the scope of this chapter, but briefly, plasmacytic hyperplasia, infectious mononucleosis, and florid follicular hyperplasia PTLDs are considered non-destructive lesions as they demonstrate overall intact architecture. They usually are mass-forming and/or show significant EBV positivity, which helps distinguish them from reactive processes.

- Plasmacytic hyperplasia PTLD shows a mixture of polyclonal plasma cells and small B and T lymphocytes with a few immunoblasts, and is typically EBV associated.
- Infectious mononucleosis PTLD shows variably hyperplastic follicles with expanded paracortical areas containing numerous immunoblasts in a background of small T cells and plasma cells.
- Florid follicular hyperplasia PTLD is a newly included entity, which forms a mass lesion with follicular hyperplasia (including the presence of tingible body macrophages) that does not suggest infectious mononucleosis.
- Polymorphic PTLD shows effaced architecture with a mixture of cells including small and medium B lymphocytes, immunoblasts, plasma cells, and T lymphocytes, often associated with EBV. Areas of necrosis may be present.
- Monomorphic PTLD is the most common, can be B-cell or T-cell lymphoma, and is classified according to the WHO criteria for the lymphoma type it resembles (however, indolent B-cell lymphomas are excluded as they are not considered PTLD). Most commonly these are diffuse large B-cell lymphomas but may also be Burkitt lymphoma, plasma cell neoplasm, or T-cell lymphomas such as peripheral T-cell lymphoma or hepatosplenic lymphoma (Fig. 22.13a–f). The monomorphic PTLDs are usually clonal proliferations and show variable association with EBV.
- Classical Hodgkin lymphoma PTLD is the least common, fulfills the WHO criteria for classical Hodgkin lymphoma, and is usually associated with EBV.

  References: [35, 36]

26. **What are some basic morphologic features that can be used to distinguish benign lymphoid aggregates from possible PTLD?**

    Lymphoid aggregates are common findings in small bowel allograft biopsies, particularly those from the terminal ileum. Features suggestive of a benign, reactive process include retention of underlying architecture, presence of germinal centers, tingible body macrophages, and a polymorphic population of lymphoid cells of varying sizes. Rare EBV-positive small lymphocytes may be detected on in situ hybridization. Large confluent lymphoid aggregates may be difficult to distinguish from the newly included florid follicular hyperplasia PTLD in some cases. Immunohistochemical work-up and EBV in situ hybridization (see question 27 below) as well as hematopathogy consultation may be necessary in difficult cases. Plasmacytic hyperplasia PTLD also shows retention of architecture but will show sheets of plasma cells and small lymphocytes. Polymorphic PTLD shows effacement of architecture by a proliferation of various cell types (small lymphocytes, plasma cells, immunoblasts, histiocytes) with varying degrees of cytologic atypia and some areas of necrosis.

    References: [35, 36]

27. **What basic immunostains and special studies can help establish a diagnosis of PTLD?**

    A general panel of immunostains may include CD20, PAX5, CD3, CD5, CD10, BCL2, BCL6, BCL1, CD21, CD30, CD15, CD138, kappa light chain, lambda light chain, and Ki-67, among others, and will depend on the morphology of the infiltrate in question. Assessment of possible light-chain restriction by kappa and lambda immunostains or in situ hybridization can be helpful in cases showing plasmacytic differentiation; however, early lesions including plasmacytic hyperplasia and infectious mononucleosis PTLDs are typically polyclonal.

    EBV detection by EBER in situ hybridization is very helpful, as most subtypes of PTLD are strongly associated with EBV infection. EBV-positive cells are typically numerous. Immunoglobulin gene rearrangement studies can also establish monoclonality in polymorphic and monomorphic PTLDs.

    References: [1–2, 36]

Case Presentation

Case 1

Learning Objectives

1. To become familiar with the diagnostic criteria of the disease
2. To generate the differential diagnosis

Case History

A 16-year-old male had a history of jejunal atresia and is status post isolated small bowel transplant 13 years ago. His posttransplant course was complicated by episodes of ACR, atypical mycobacterial infection, and Hodgkin lymphoma PTLD treated with chemotherapy. He underwent combined small bowel, liver, and pancreas transplants 6 months ago. Following ileostomy takedown a few months ago, the patient had experienced fecal urgency. Endoscopy was performed for assessment of bowel graft rejection, which showed normal-appearing transplanted small bowel and native colon. Multiple surveillance biopsies were performed. The patient had been on mycophenolate.

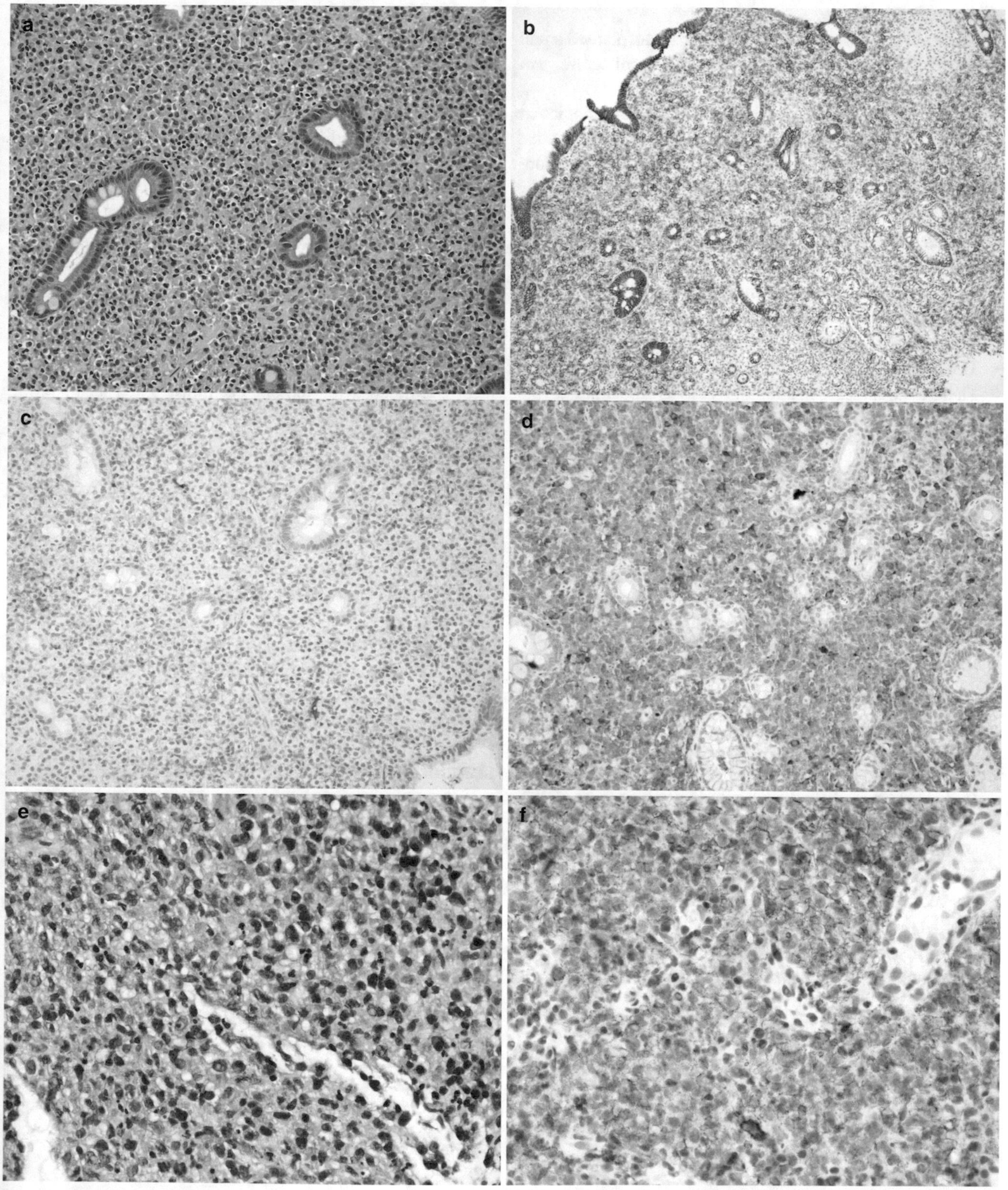

Fig. 22.13 Posttransplant lymphoproliferative disorders. (**a**) A biopsy from abnormally thickened and bumpy duodenal mucosa showing diffuse, predominantly plasmacytic proliferation that expands the lamina propria. Similar findings are also seen in the biopsies from the bumpy ileal mucosa and polypoid colonic mucosa. (**b**) Immunostain for CD138 highlights numerous plasma cells. (**c** and **d**) Immunostains for lambda and kappa show lambda light-chain restriction, consistent with plasma cell neoplasm. (**e**) A biopsy from a rectal mass from the same patient showing diffuse large B-cell lymphoma, which is diffusely positive for CD20 (**f**). The patient has a history of two liver transplants 32 and 18 years ago

Histologic Findings

- Low-power view of the biopsies from transplanted small bowel shows well-preserved normal architecture. No crypt dropout is appreciated (Fig. 22.14a).
- Higher-power view shows increased apoptotic bodies in crypts (Fig. 22.14b, arrows), up to 13 per 10 consecutive crypts in a concentrated area. This is seen in multiple biopsies from different locations of transplanted small bowel.
- The number of lamina propria inflammatory cells is not significantly increased. No features of erosion or ulceration are seen.
- No infectious agents are identified.
- A few benign-appearing lymphoid aggregates are present, but no features of PTLD are seen.
- The biopsies from the native colon are unremarkable. There is no increase in apoptotic activity in colonic crypts (Fig. 22.14c).

Differential Diagnosis

- Normal (no histopathologic abnormality)
- Mild acute cellular rejection
- Mycophenolate-induced injury
- Moderate acute cellular rejection

Immunohistochemistry and Ancillary Studies

- Routine immunostain is negative for adenovirus.

Final Diagnosis

Mild acute cellular rejection.

Take-Home Messages

- Increased crypt apoptotic activity is a hallmark of ACR.
- Mild ACR is defined by ≥6 apoptotic bodies per 10 consecutive crypts.
- Lack of crypt dropout or confluent crypt apoptosis rules out moderate ACR.
- Medication effect, particularly that of mycophenolate, can mimic ACR by causing crypt cell apoptosis. Histologic assessment of both graft and native bowel biopsies can be helpful.

  References: [1, 2, 4–6]

Case 2

Learning Objectives

1. To become familiar with the diagnostic criteria of the disease
2. To generate the differential diagnosis

Case History

A 31-year-old woman with a history of intestinal failure secondary to chronic intestinal pseudo-obstruction is status post multivisceral transplant 4 years ago. Her posttransplant complications included episodes of mild and moderate rejection and CMV and adenovirus enteritis treated with foscarnet and cidofovir. She now presents with abdominal pain and hematemesis. Endoscopy showed erythematous, friable, and ulcerated mucosa throughout the transplanted small bowel and colon.

Histologic Findings

- Multiple biopsies from transplanted small bowel and colon show complete crypt dropout (Fig. 22.15a).
- The remaining lamina propria shows an increased number of inflammatory cells. Empty crypt contours without epithelial cells are seen (Fig. 22.15b).

Differential Diagnosis

- Severe acute cellular rejection
- Severe drug-induced injury
- Severe graft-versus-host disease

Immunohistochemistry and Ancillary Studies

- Immunostains are negative for adenovirus and CMV.

Final Diagnosis

Severe acute cellular rejection.

Take-Home Messages

- Severe ACR is characterized by extensive or complete crypt dropout.

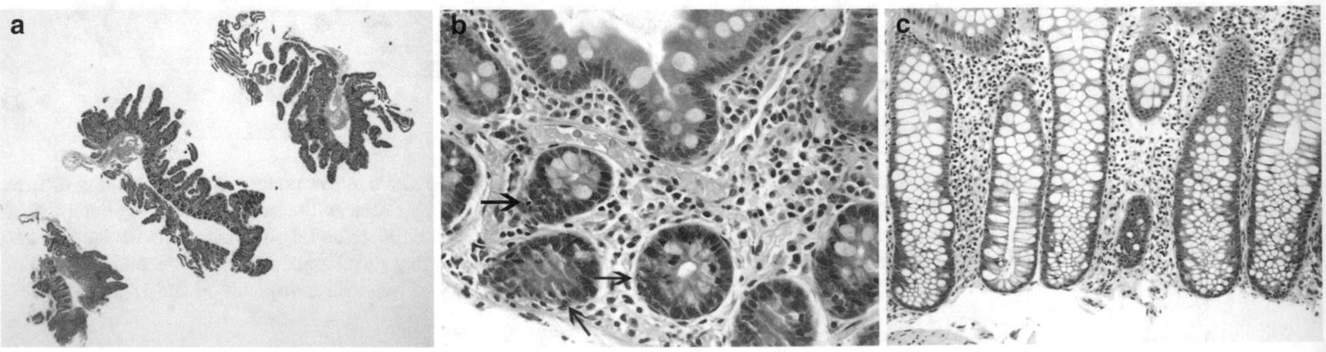

Fig. 22.14 (case 1). (**a**) Lower-power view showing well-preserved normal architecture with no crypt dropout. (**b**) Higher-power view showing increased crypt apoptotic activity (arrows). (**c**) Unremarkable colonic mucosa

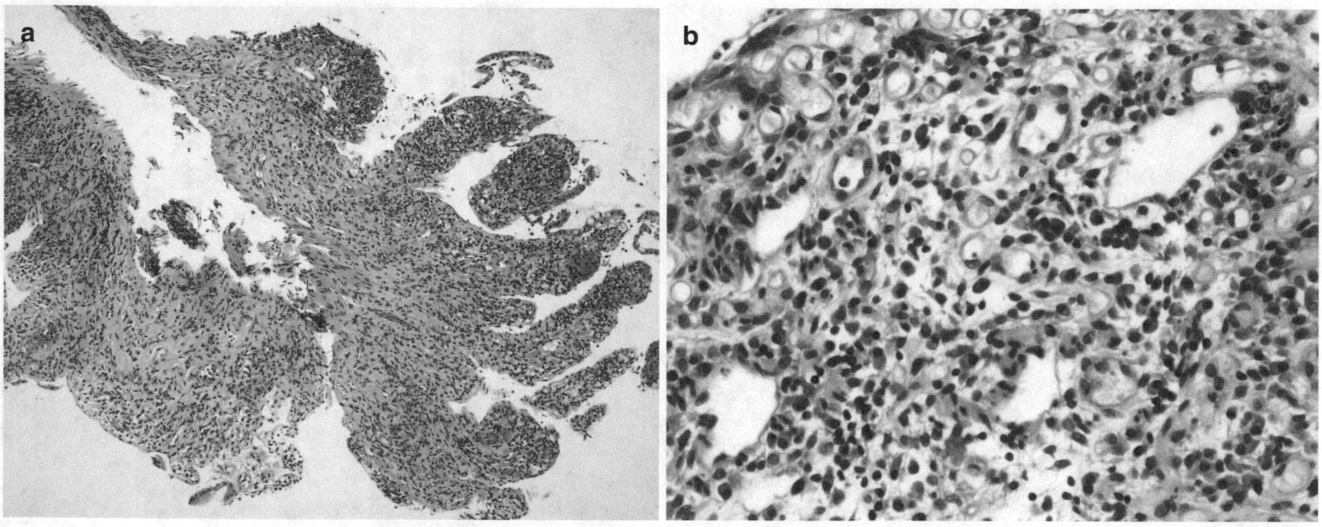

Fig. 22.15 (case 2). (**a**) Low-power view showing complete crypt dropout. (**b**) Empty crypt contours without epithelial cells are seen

- Drug-induced injury (such as that by mycophenolate) usually does not cause this degree of diffuse crypt damage.
- GVHD can occur in the setting of solid organ transplantation, which would occur early post transplantation and should not injure the transplanted organs.

  References: [1, 2, 4–6, 23, 24]

Case 3

Learning Objectives

1. To become familiar with the histologic features of the disease
2. To become familiar with the special staining findings of the disease
3. To generate the differential diagnosis

Case History

A 9-year-old girl with a history of intestinal failure due to necrotizing enterocolitis as a neonate and advanced intestinal failure-associated liver disease underwent multivisceral transplant including the liver, pancreas, duodenum, spleen, jejunoileum, and transverse colon 33 days ago. Her posttransplant course was complicated by stool leakage from an incision site, status post repair, debridement of necrotic fascia, peritoneal lavage, and abdominal closure. An endoscopic exam via stoma showed erythematous mucosa at 25 cm.

Histologic Findings

- The biopsy from 25 cm shows ulceration and complete crypt dropout. Abundant fungal hyphae are noted, which are either free-floating, admixed with necrotic debris, or embedded within fibrotic tissue (Fig. 22.16a, b).
- The hyphae appear wide ribbonlike with branches.
- The biopsies from endoscopically unremarkable locations of transplanted small bowel show 1–2 apoptotic bodies per 10 consecutive crypts. No fungal or other infectious organisms are identified.

Differential Diagnosis

- Fungal infection
- Severe acute cellular rejection

Immunohistochemistry and Ancillary Studies

- GMS and PASD stains highlight fungal organisms (Fig. 22.16c, d).

Additional Clinical Information

- Negative blood and peritoneal fluid cultures.
- Positive detection of *Rhizopus oryzae* in blood by next-generation sequencing.

Final Diagnosis

Fungal infection, consistent with mucormycosis.

Take-Home Messages

- Transplant recipients are prone to infections.
- The most common infections are bacterial and viral, but fungal and protozoal infections can occur.
- Special stains, IHC, and molecular tests can be very useful.

  References: [2, 13, 14]

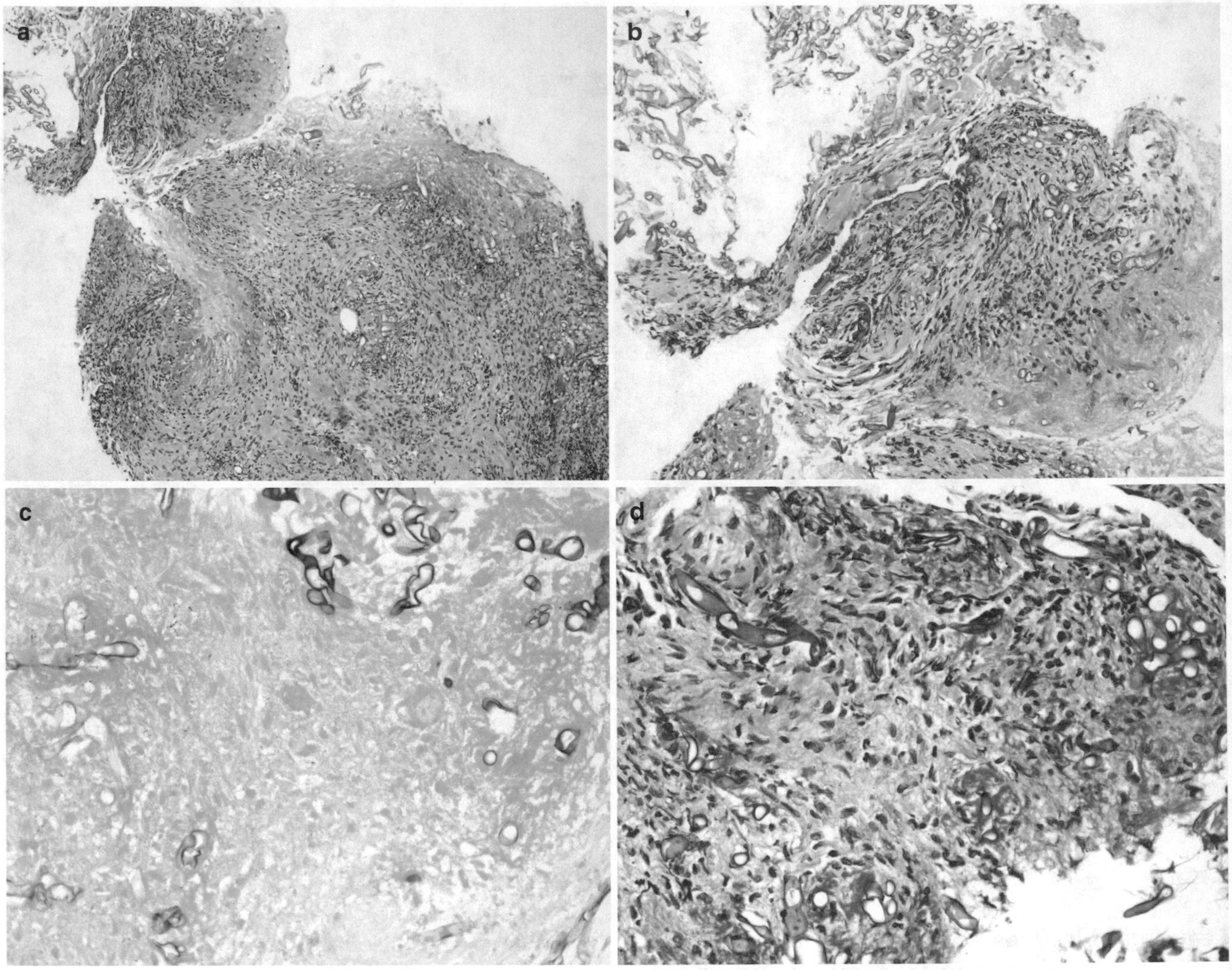

Fig. 22.16 (case 3). (**a** and **b**) Ulceration with complete crypt dropout and abundant fungal hyphae. (**c**) Grocott methenamine silver (GMS) stain. (**d**) Periodic acid–Schiff with diastase (PASD) stain

Case 4

Learning Objectives

1. To become familiar with the histologic features of the lesion
2. To become familiar with the immunohistochemical features of the lesion
3. To generate the differential diagnosis

Case History

A 56-year-old man underwent isolated small bowel transplant 3 months ago for short bowel syndrome secondary to mesenteric venous thrombosis. He had an unremarkable postoperative course and was eligible for ileostomy takedown.

Gross

Received was an ileostomy specimen consisting of a 17.0 cm segment of edematous small bowel with a diffusely roughened peritonealized surface. The bowel lumen was patent and averaged 4.0 cm in circumference. In the mid-portion of the specimen, there were two tan-red, focally ulcerated, and raised lesions measuring 2.0 × 1.0 cm and 2.5 × 2.0 cm. The surrounding mucosa was edematous with normal folds.

Histologic Findings

- Sections of ulcerated and raised lesions show dense, band-like, vaguely nodular, and well-demarcated lymphoplasmacytic proliferation, primarily involving the submucosa (Fig. 22.17a). Extension into the mucosa with areas of superficial ulceration is seen.

- Higher-power view shows numerous plasma cells (Fig. 22.17b).

Differential Diagnosis

- Peyer patches of the terminal ileum
- Posttransplant lymphoproliferative disorder

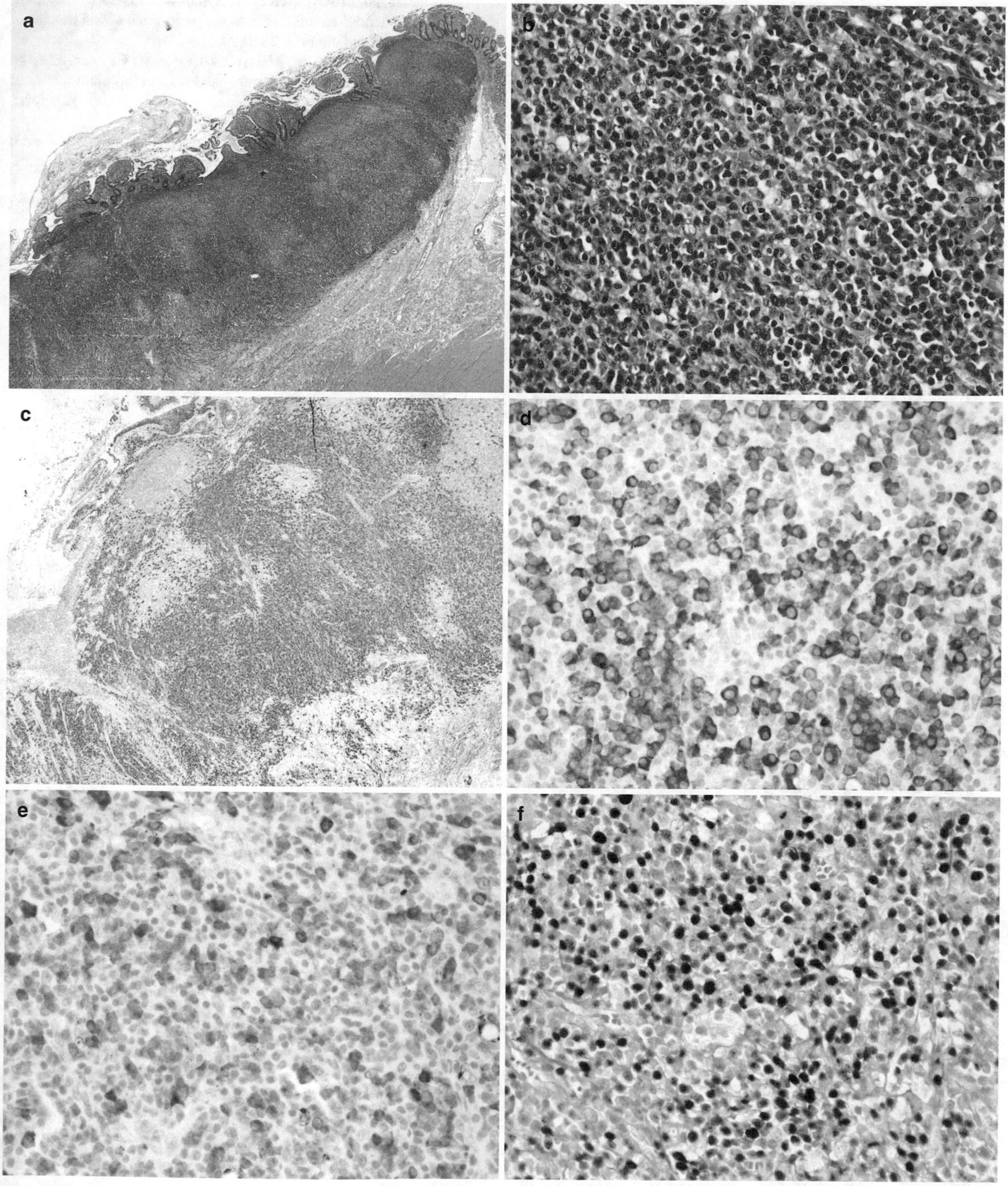

Fig. 22.17 (case 4). (**a**) Dense, band-like lymphoplasmacytic proliferation. (**b**) Numerous plasma cells. (**c**) CD138 immunostain. (**d**) Kappa immunostain. (**e**) Lambda immunostain. (**f**) In situ hybridization for EBV

Immunohistochemistry and Ancillary Studies

- CD138 immunostain highlights numerous plasma cells (Fig. 22.17c).
- Kappa and lambda immunostains show no light-chain restriction (Fig. 22.17d, e).
- In situ hybridization for EBV (EBER) shows numerous positive cells (Fig. 22.17f).

Final Diagnosis

Posttransplant lymphoproliferative disorder, plasmacytic hyperplasia type.

Take-Home Messages

- PTLD is one of the three major posttransplant complications, the others being rejection and infection.
- It is a spectrum of diseases ranging from non-destructive lesions (plasmacytic hyperplasia, infectious mononucleosis, florid follicular hyperplasia), to polymorphic lymphocytic proliferation, to full-blown lymphomas (monomorphic).
- Even non-destructive lesions are usually mass-forming.
- There is a strong association with EBV, but EBV can be negative in minority of cases.

References: [35, 36]

References

1. Koo J, Wang HL. Small bowel. In: Wallace WD, Naini BV, editors. Practical atlas of transplant pathology. Cham: Springer; 2016. p. 133–51.
2. Koo J, Dawson DW, Dry S, French SW, Naini BV, Wang HL. Allograft biopsy findings in patients with small bowel transplantation. Clin Transpl. 2016;30:1433–9.
3. Remotti H, Subramanian S, Martinez M, Kato T, Magid MS. Small-bowel allograft biopsies in the management of small-intestinal and multivisceral transplant recipients: histopathologic review and clinical correlations. Arch Pathol Lab Med. 2012;136:761–71.
4. Wu T, Abu-Elmagd K, Bond G, Nalesnik MA, Randhawa P, Demetris AJ. A schema for histologic grading of small intestine allograft acute rejection. Transplantation. 2003;75:1241–8.
5. Ruiz P, Bagni A, Brown R, Cortina G, Harpaz N, Magid MS, et al. Histological criteria for the identification of acute cellular rejection in human small bowel allografts: results of the pathology workshop at the VIII International Small Bowel Transplant Symposium. Transplant Proc. 2004;36:335–7.
6. Lee RG, Nakamura K, Tsamandas AC, Abu-Elmagd K, Furukawa H, Hutson WR, et al. Pathology of human intestinal transplantation. Gastroenterology. 1996;110:1820–34.
7. Delacruz V, Weppler D, Island E, Gonzalez M, Tryphonopoulos P, Moon J, et al. Mycophenolate mofetil-related gastrointestinal mucosal injury in multivisceral transplantation. Transplant Proc. 2010;42:82–4.
8. Nguyen T, Park JY, Scudiere JR, Montgomery E. Mycophenolic acid (CellCept and Myofortic) induced injury of the upper GI tract. Am J Surg Pathol. 2009;33:1355–63.
9. Parfitt JR, Jayakumar S, Driman DK. Mycophenolate mofetil-related gastrointestinal mucosal injury: variable injury patterns, including graft-versus-host disease-like changes. Am J Surg Pathol. 2008;32:1367–72.
10. Selbst MK, Ahrens WA, Robert ME, Friedman A, Proctor DD, Jain D. Spectrum of histologic changes in colonic biopsies in patients treated with mycophenolate mofetil. Mod Pathol. 2009;22:737–43.
11. Florescu DF, Islam MK, Mercer DF, Grant W, Langnas AN, Freifeld AG, et al. Adenovirus infections in pediatric small bowel transplant recipients. Transplantation. 2010;90:198–204.
12. Adeyi OA, Randhawa PA, Nalesnik MA, Ochoa ER, Abu-Elmagd KM, Demetris AJ, et al. Posttransplant adenoviral enteropathy in patients with small bowel transplantation. Arch Pathol Lab Med. 2008;132:703–5.
13. Ziring D, Tran R, Edelstein S, McDiarmid SV, Gajjar N, Cortina G, et al. Infectious enteritis after intestinal transplantation: incidence, timing, and outcome. Transplantation. 2005;79:702–9.
14. Guaraldi G, Cocchi S, Codeluppi M, Di Benedetto F, De Ruvo N, Masetti M, et al. Outcome, incidence, and timing of infectious complications in small bowel and multivisceral organ transplantation patients. Transplantation. 2005;80:1742–8.
15. Talmon GA. Histologic features of cytomegalovirus enteritis in small bowel allografts. Transplant Proc. 2010;42:2671–5.
16. Adeyi OA, Costa G, Abu-Elmagd KM, Wu T. Rotavirus infection in adult small intestine allografts: a clinicopathological study of a cohort of 23 patients. Am J Transplant. 2010;10(12):2683–9.
17. Parizhskaya M, Redondo C, Demetris A, Jaffe R, Reyes J, Ruppert K, et al. Chronic rejection of small bowel grafts: pediatric and adult study of risk factors and morphologic progression. Pediatr Dev Pathol. 2003;6:240–50.
18. White FV, Ranganathan S. Small intestine. In: Liapis H, Wang HL, editors. Pathology of solid organ transplantation. Heidelberg: Springer; 2011. p. 347–70.
19. Swanson BJ, Talmon GA, Wisecarver JW, Grant WJ, Radio SJ. Histologic analysis of chronic rejection in small bowel transplantation: mucosal and vascular alterations. Transplantation. 2013;95:378–82.
20. de Serre NP, Canioni D, Lacaille F, Talbotec C, Dion D, Brousse N, et al. Evaluation of c4d deposition and circulating antibody in small bowel transplantation. Am J Transplant. 2008;8:1290–6.
21. Troxell ML, Higgins JP, Kambham N. Evaluation of C4d staining in liver and small intestine allografts. Arch Pathol Lab Med. 2006;130:1489–96.
22. Rabant M, Racapé M, Petit LM, et al. Antibody-mediated rejection in pediatric small bowel transplantation: capillaritis is a major determinant of C4d positivity in intestinal transplant biopsies. Am J Transplant. 2018;18:2250–60.
23. Garcia M, Delacruz V, Ortiz R, Bagni A, Weppler D, Kato T, Tzakis A, Ruiz P. Acute cellular rejection grading scheme for human gastric allografts. Hum Pathol. 2004;35:343–9.
24. Salomao M, Dorritie K, Mapara MY, Sepulveda A. Histopathology of graft-vs-host disease of gastrointestinal tract and liver: an update. Am J Clin Pathol. 2016;145(5):591–603.
25. Washington K, Jagasia M. Pathology of graft-versus-host disease in the gastrointestinal tract. Hum Pathol. 2009;40(7):909–17.
26. Cogbill CH, Drobyski WR, Komorowski RA. Gastrointestinal pathology of autologous graft-versus-host disease following hematopoietic stem cell transplantation: a clinicopathological study of 17 cases. Mod Pathol. 2011;24(1):117–25.
27. Shulman HM, Kleiner D, Lee SJ, et al. Histopathologic diagnosis of chronic graft-versus-host disease: National Institutes of Health Consensus Development Project on Criteria for Clinical Trials in Chronic Graft-versus-Host Disease: II. Pathology Working Group Report. Biol Blood Marrow Transplant. 2006;12(1):31–47.
28. Shulman HM, Cardona DM, Greenson JK, et al. NIH Consensus development project on criteria for clinical trials in chronic graft-

versus-host disease: II. The 2014 Pathology Working Group Report. Biol Blood Marrow Transplant. 2015;21(4):589–603.
29. Epstein RJ, McDonald GB, Sale GE, Shulman HM, Thomas ED. The diagnostic accuracy of the rectal biopsy in acute graft-versus-host disease: a prospective study of thirteen patients. Gastroenterology. 1980;78(4):764–71.
30. Snover DC. Mucosal damage simulating acute graft-versus-host reaction in cytomegalovirus colitis. Transplantation. 1985;39(6):669–70.
31. Lerner KG, Kao GF, Storb R, Buckner CD, Clift RA, Thomas ED. Histopathology of graft-vs.-host reaction (GvHR) in human recipients of marrow from HL-A-matched sibling donors. Transplant Proc. 1974;6(4):367–71.
32. Selvaggi G, Gaynor JJ, Moon J, Kato T, Thompson J, Nishida S, et al. Analysis of acute cellular rejection episodes in recipients of primary intestinal transplantation: a single center, 11-year experience. Am J Transplant. 2007;7:1249–57.
33. Abu-Elmagd KM, Mazariegos G, Costa G, Soltys K, Bond G, Sindhi R, et al. Lymphoproliferative disorders and de novo malignancies in intestinal and multivisceral recipients: improved outcomes with new outlooks. Transplantation. 2009;88:926–34.
34. Nassif S, Kaufman S, Vahdat S, Yazigi N, Kallakury B, Island E, et al. Clinicopathologic features of post-transplant lymphoproliferative disorders arising after pediatric small bowel transplant. Pediatr Transplant. 2013;17:765–73.
35. Said J. Post-transplantation lymphoproliferative disorders. In: Wallace WD, Naini BV, editors. Practical atlas of transplant pathology. Cham: Springer; 2016. p. 173–85.
36. Swerdlow SH, Webber SA, Chadburn A, Ferry JA. Post-transplant lymphoproliferative disorders. In: Swerdlow SH, et al., editors. WHO classification of tumours of haematopoietic and lymphoid tissues. Lyon: IARC; 2017. p. 453–62.

Index

A

Achalasia
 histopathologic findings in, 319, 320
 motility disorder, 333, 335
Acquired appendiceal diverticula, 171
Acute appendicitis
 causes of, 168
 histologic features of, 167, 168
Acute cellular rejection (ACR), 544
Acute gastritis, 67, 68
 histological findings of, 68
 phlegmonous gastritis, 68
Acute graft-versus-host disease, 551–553
Acute ischemic injury, 153
Acute leukemias, 531
Adenocarcinoma, 215, 428, 432, 440, 452
 anal gland adenocarcinoma, 205
 extramucosal anal canal adenocarcinoma, non-anal gland-type and non-fistula-associated, 206, 207
 fistula-associated adenocarcinoma, 206
 mucosal type adenocarcinoma, 206
Adenoid cystic carcinoma, 442
Adenoma-like adenocarcinoma, 440
Adenoma-like colorectal carcinoma, 441
Adenosquamous carcinoma, 438
Adenovirus, 230, 232
Advanced ECL cell hyperplasia, 79
Aeromonas colitis, 225
Aganglionic appendix, 13
Aganglionosis, 11
AIDS, 232, 233
Alcian blue, 57
Allied disorders of HSCR, 329
Alpha-methylacyl-CoA racemase (AMACR) overexpression, 130
Amanita phalloides, 323
Amastigotes, 252
Amebic colitis, 119
Amoebae, 249
Amoebiasis, 250
Ampulla of Vater, 454–456
Ampullary adenocarcinoma, 456
Ampullary adenomas, 348
Amyloidosis, 318
Anal adenocarcinoma, 215
Anal canal adenocarcinoma, 457, 458
Anal canal extramucosal lesion, 215
Anal cancer, 200
Anal condyloma, 220
Anal diseases, 195
 adenocarcinoma, 205
  anal gland adenocarcinoma, 205
  extramucosal anal canal adenocarcinoma, non-anal gland-type and non-fistula-associated, 206, 207
  fistula-associated adenocarcinoma, 206
  mucosal type adenocarcinoma, 206
 anatomical anal canal, 196
 atypical squamous cells of undetermined significance, 219–221
 basal cell carcinoma, 208, 209
 Bowen disease, 201
  diagnosis, recommendations for, 203
  giant condyloma of Buschke-Lowenstein, 202, 203
  lower anogenital squamous terminology, 201, 202
  verrucous carcinoma, 202
 cloacogenic carcinoma, 203, 205
 epithelioid sarcomas, 209
 high grade/high grade-appearing cellular neoplasms, differential diagnosis of, 207
 histologic anal canal, 195
 IBD/malignancy, 214–216
 inflammatory bowel disease, 199
  Crohn disease, 199
  syphilis and lymphogranuloma venereum, 199
  ulcerative colitis, 199
 lymphoma, 209
 medical conditions, 197
  anal fistula, 197
  hemorrhoids, varices, and Dieulafoy lesion, 198
  hypertrophied papillae, 197, 198
  inflammatory cloacogenic polyp, 198
 neuroendocrine neoplasms, 209
 perianal skin, 196
 poorly differentiated squamous cell carcinoma, 208
 pruritus, 216, 217
 skin adnexal tumors, 200
  hidradenoma papilliferum, 200
  trichoepithelioma, 200
 squamous cell carcinoma, 203–205
 stage of anal tumors, 200
  AJCC definition, 201
  clinical definition, 200, 201
 surgical anal canal, 195
 WHO classification for anal tumors, 199, 200
Anal duct, 197
Anal fistula, 197
Anal fistula-associated adenocarcinoma, 208
Anal gland adenocarcinoma, 206, 208
Anal hemorrhoid, 211, 213
Anal herpes simplex virus, 231
Anal hidradenoma papilliferum, 201
Anal intraepithleial neoplasia, 234
Anal malignant neoplasms, 211
Anal margin, 196

H. L. Wang, Z. E. Chen (eds.), *Practical Gastrointestinal Pathology*, Practical Anatomic Pathology,
https://doi.org/10.1007/978-3-030-51268-2

Anal nodular lesion, 219
Anal Paget disease, 200, 206, 207
Anal pruritus, 216, 217
Anal squamous cell carcinoma, 206, 212
Anal squamous intraepithelial neoplasia (AIN), 219, 233
Anal syphilis, 199
Anal transition zone (ATZ), 195, 196
Anal tumors
  fifth edition WHO classification of, 200
  fourth edition WHO classification of, 200
  pitfalls in immunohistochemistry of, 211
Angiodysplasia, 507, 509
Angioma, 497
Angiomyolipoma (AML)
  distinguished from liposarcoma, 511, 512
  histologic features of, 512
  immunohistochemical features of, 512
Angiosarcoma, 508
  distinguishing features of, 509, 510
  from hemangioma, 507
  immunohistochemical features of, 510
Angiotensin II receptor antagonist olmesartan, 275, 276
Anorectal adenocarcinoma, 457
Anorectal junction, 533
Anorectal malformation, 4
Anorectal syphilis, 259
Antibody-mediated rejection (AMR), 548
Antitumor necrosis factor (anti-TNF), 120
Antrum
  autoimmune pangastritis, 83
  eosinophilic gastritis, 82
Anus, 196
  high-risk HPV infection in, 233–235
Aphthous ulcer, 115
Apoptotic debris, 547
Appendiceal adenoma, 182
Appendiceal carcinoid, 20
Appendiceal diseases
  acute appendicitis
    causes of, 168
    histologic features of, 167, 168
  appendiceal adenoma, serrated lesions and retention cyst, 182, 183
  appendiceal diverticulosis, 171
  appendiceal epithelial tumors, classification of, 173
  appendiceal mucinous neoplasms, staging, 178, 180
  appendiceal neuroendocrine neoplasms, WHO classification of, 171, 172
  appendix
    mucinous adenocarcinoma of, 183
    parasitic infections in, 170, 171
  eosinophilic appendicitis, 170
  goblet cell adenocarcinoma, 173, 174
    clinical features, 174
    grading systems and prognostic significance, 174, 177
    gross and histologic features of, 174
    immunohistochemical features of, 177
    molecular alterations, 177
  granulomatous appendicitis, 169, 170
  high-grade appendiceal mucinous neoplasm, 178
  low-grade appendiceal mucinous neoplasm, 177, 178
  periappendicitis, 169
  pseudomyxoma peritonei, 180
  rectal bleeding, 187, 188
  ruptured diverticulum, endometriosis, 182, 183
  symptoms and signs, 184
  tubular neuroendocrine tumor, 172, 173
Appendiceal diverticulosis, 171
Appendiceal diverticulum, 172
Appendiceal epithelial tumors, classification of, 173
Appendiceal lymphomas, 532
Appendiceal mucinous neoplasms, 178, 180
Appendiceal neuroendocrine neoplasms, 172, 418
Appendiceal polyps, 359
Appendiceal sessile serrated lesion, 189
Appendix
  acute inflammation, 168
  distorted serrated crypts, 190
  fibrotic submucosa, 191
  infiltrating neoplasm, 186
  mucinous adenocarcinoma of, 183, 184
  parasitic infections in, 170, 171
  PSOGI classification, noncarcinoid epithelial neoplasia, 173
  three-tier grading system, mucinous adenocarcinoma, 183
  villous adenoma of, 182
  WHO classification, epithelial tumors of, 173
Apple-peel atresia, 4
Architectural disarray, 115
Arteriovenous malformation (AVM), 152
Artifactual cytoplasmic vacuolation, 323
Ascaris lumbricoides, 256
Aspergillus species, 235–237
Atezolizumab, 121
Atrophic gastritis, 421
  in CTLA-4 deficiency, 29
Atrophic microcrypts, 270
Atrophy of outer muscle layer, 321
Attenuated familial adenomatous polyposis (AFAP), 370, 380
Atypical squamous cells of undetermined significance (ASC-US), 219–221
Auerbach plexus, 318
Autoimmune atrophic pangastritis, 83, 84
Autoimmune enteropathy (AIE), 23, 97, 103, 123
  clinical features, 96
  histologic features of, 97
Autoimmune gastritis, 80, 84
  body pyloric metaplasia, 78
  ECL cell hyperplasia, 79
  ECL hyperplasia and neuroendocrine tumors, 79
  histological findings, 77, 78
  neuroendocrine tumor, 79
Autoimmune pangastritis, 83, 84

B

Bacterial overgrowth, 100
Balantidium coli, 248, 249
Band-like lymphoplasmacytic proliferation, 559
Barrett esophagus, 433
Barrett esophagus (BE), 56, 433
  ancillary testing, 61
  basal crypt atypia, significance of, 57, 58
  diagnostic criteria, 56
  duplicated muscularis mucosae, 60
  endoscopic findings, 56
  high-grade dysplasia, 59, 60
  histologic features and progression, 59
  immunostains, 57
  indefinite for dysplasia, 58
  intramucosal adenocarcinoma, 60

low-grade dysplasia, 59
non-conventional dysplasia, types and identification, 61
pseudo-goblet cells, 57
reactive atypia versus dysplasia, 58
reflux symptoms, 62–64
risk of progression, 61
screening and surveillance, 57
submucosally invasive adenocarcinoma, 60, 61
treatment modalities, 61, 62
Basal cell carcinoma, 200
Basal crypt epithelium, 58
Basal lymphoplasmacytosis, 115, 135
Basidiobolomycosis, 236
Basidiobolus ranarum, 236, 237
Basophilic inclusion, 261
Basophils, 289
Behçet disease, 161
clinicopathologic features of, 159
Bile acid sequestrants (BAS), 41, 278, 279
Billroth II gastrojejunostomy, 341
Bland spindle cells, 417
Blisters, esophagitis, 50, 51
Body pyloric metaplasia, autoimmune gastritis, 78
Botox injection, 360
Bowen disease, 201
BRAF mutation testing, 461
Bronchogenic cyst, 2, 3
Brown bowel syndrome, 331
Brunner gland cyst, 346
Brunner gland hyperplasia, 345
Brunner glands, 345
Budding yeasts, 236
Bullous disease, 50, 51
Bullous pemphigoid (BP), 43
Burkitt lymphoma, 15, 17, 554

C
C. difficile, 227, 228
infections of gastrointestinal tract, 246–248
pseudomembranous colitis, 159, 247
Calcifying fibrous pseudotumor/reactive nodular fibrous pseudotumor (CFPT/RNFP), 391, 392
Calpain 14 (CAPN14), 293
Calretinin immunohistochemistry, 9
Calretinin positive mucosal neurites, 9
Campylobacter spp., 225, 227
C.jejuni infection, 530
C.pyloridis, 239
Candida spp., 238
C. albicans, 235
C. esophagitis, 38, 45, 232
infections of gastrointestinal tract, 236
Carcinoid tumor, 387
Carcinomas, 132
abnormal MMR protein test, 461, 463
adenocarcinoma, 428, 433
adenoma-like adenocarcinoma, 440
adenosquamous carcinoma, 438
AJCC tumor staging system, 443
ampulla of Vater, 454–456
anal canal adenocarcinoma, 457, 458
anorectal adenocarcinoma, 457
choriocarcinoma, 441
clear cells or yolk sac tumor-like carcinoma, 440
colorectal-type adenocarcinoma, 454
conventional adenocarcinomas, 436
conventional squamous cell carcinoma, 456
E-cadherin expression, 443
gastroblastoma, 440, 441
gastroesophageal junction, 432
giant condyloma of Buschke-Lowenstein, 456
hepatoid adenocarcinoma, 439
Her2 immunohistochemistry, 460
Her2 pathway, 464
Her2 testing, 459
high tumor budding, 451
high-grade dysplasia, 433, 434
immunohistochemical markers for, 458
intramucosal adenocarcinoma, 434
invasive adenocarcinoma, 434
invasive squamous cell carcinoma, 456, 457
isolated tumor cells, 451
large venous invasion versus small lymphovascular invasion, 452
low-grade tubuloglandular adenocarcinoma, 428
lymphoglandular complex, 454
malignant polyps, 436
medullary carcinoma, 437
mesorectal envelop, 445, 450
metastatic lesions, 458
micropapillary adenocarcinoma, 438
MMR
deficiency testing, 459, 460
immunostains, 460, 461
interpretation and recommendations, 462
molecular testing, 463
mucinous carcinoma, 437
neoadjuvant treatment, 453
neuroendocrine carcinomas, 428
MMR deficiency, colorectal tumor morphologic subtypes, 463
nonmucinous adenocarcinoma, 430
oxyntic gland adenoma, 440
papillary adenocarcinoma, 438
PD-L1, 464
perineural invasion, 453
PIK3CA mutations, 464
poorly cohesive carcinoma, 443
proximal and distal colon/rectal margins, 445
pseudoinvasion and true submucosal invasion, 435
PTEN expression, 464
radial margin, 444, 445
rectal tonsil, 455
regional lymph nodes, 450
salivary gland carcinomas, 442
serrated adenocarcinoma, 438
signet-ring cell carcinoma, 436, 443
spindle cell carcinoma, 438
squamous cell carcinoma, 432
submucosal invasion, 434
submucosal misplacement (pseudoinvasion), 434
TNM staging, 451
tumor buds, 452
tumor deposit, 450, 451
tumor regression score, 454
undifferentiated carcinoma, 440
verrucous carcinoma, 456
Cardia, 55, 56
Cavernous hemangioma, 507

CD138 immunostain, 559
Celiac disease, 27–29, 80, 93, 224, 433
  complications of, 94, 95
  drugs cause changes, 98, 99
  environmental and genetic risk factors for, 92
  features of, 96
  gastrointestinal tract, infections, 227
  modified marsh score system for, 93
  serologic markers in, 92
  specific histologic features of, 92, 93
Cervical cancer, 234
Cervical intraepithelial neoplasia (CIN), 233
Chemical gastritis, 269, 270
Chemical gastropathy, 74
Chlamydia, 243
Chlamydia proctitis, 120
Chlamydia trachomatis, 244
Cholestyramine, 278
Choriocarcinoma, 441, 442
Chromogranin A, 416, 420, 422, 423
Chromosomal instability pathway (CIN), 381
Chronic active colitis, 27
Chronic constipation, 330, 331
Chronic eosinophilic leukemia, 531
Chronic gastritis
  Crohn disease, 85
  idiopathic, 85
Chronic granulomatous disease (CGD), 23, 24
Chronic idiopathic constipation, 322, 323
Chronic idiopathic inflammatory bowel disease, 224
Chronic ingestion of laxatives, 323
Chronic ischemic injury, diagnosis of, 154
Chronic kidney disease, 45–48
Chronic lymphocytic leukemia/small lymphocytic lymphoma, 523
Chronic NSAID-associated enteropathy, 120
Chronic rejection, 544
Chronic ulcerative colitis, characteristic pathologic features of, 109–111
CK7, 130
Classical Hodgkin lymphoma, 532, 554
Clear cell sarcoma of soft tissue, 501, 502
Cloacogenic carcinoma, 203–205
Clostridium perfringens, 246
Coagulative necrosis, 480
Coccidial infection, 252
Colchicine, 42, 275
Colectomy, 136
  ulcerative colitis, 110
Collagenous colitis, 123, 146, 148, 162
Collagenous gastritis, 80, 81
  cause, 81
  treatment, 81
Collagenous sprue, 95
Colon, 290, 294
  arteriovenous malformation of, 158
  cancer, 305
  diffuse large B-cell lymphoma in, 538
  non-IBD noninfectious colitis, 148, 149
  non-GIST primary mesenchymal tumors of, 497
  systemic mastocytosis in, 529
Colonic Crohn disease, 112
Colonic diverticulosis, 331
Colonic inflammatory polyp, 349
Colonic malakoplakia, 301
Colonic mucosa, 283, 459
Colorectal carcinoma, 132, 134
Colorectal neurofibroma, 389
Colorectal-type adenocarcinoma, 454, 455
Common variable immunodeficiency (CVID), 23, 104, 124
  clinical features, 97
  histologic features, 97
Composite intestinal villous adenoma-microcarcinoid, 362
Condyloma, 213
Condyloma acuminatum, 219
Congenital diverticulosis, 171
Constipation, motility disorder, 327–329
Conventional adenocarcinomas, 436
Conventional adenomas, 355
Conventional squamous cell carcinoma, 456
Corrosive ingestion, 40
Corrosive injury, 39, 40
Cowden/PTEN hamartoma syndrome, 341, 377, 382
Crohn-associated granulomas, 117
Crohn colitis
  histological features, 116, 117
  pathologic features of, 111, 112
  superficial, 113
Crohn disease, 27, 38, 50, 81, 85, 103, 161, 163, 164, 226, 351, 543
  Behçet disease, 161
  characteristic histologic features of, 116
  esophagitis, 49, 50
  infections of gastrointestinal tract, 261
  malabsorption disorders, 96
  with massive inflammatory thickening and stricture of the transverse colon, 111
  pouchitis, 125
  upper GI manifestations, 124, 125
Crohn gastritis, 124
Crohn ileitis, 115
Cronkhite–Canada syndrome, 20, 377, 381, 382
Crypt abscess, 114, 117, 147, 243
Crypt cell dysplasia, 127, 128, 138
Crypt inflammation, 115, 116
Cryptococcus spp., 115, 235
Cryptolytic granulomas, 116, 117
Cryptosporidia, 102
Cryptosporidium, 253
Crystal-storing histiocytosis, 302
CTLA-4 deficiency, 28, 29
Cuffitis, 125
Cyclospora, 253
Cyclospora cayetanensis, 253
Cystoisospora, 254
Cytomegalovirus (CMV) infection, 42, 45, 228, 230, 232, 285
  colitis, 230
  esophagitis, 261
  inclusion, 104
  PCR, 229
Cytoplasmic hyaline inclusions, 333
Cytotoxic T-lymphocyte antigen-4 (CTLA-4), 42

D

Dedifferentiated liposarcoma (DDLPS), 511, 515
Dense lymphocytic inflammation, 322
Dentate line, 8
Desmin, 507
Desmoglein 1, 43
Desmoid fibromatosis, 500, 503, 504, 517
Desmoplastic small round cell tumor, 21
Developmental anomalies
  anorectal malformation repair specimens, 4, 5

cyst, 5
disorder with ileocolonic and colonic atresia, 4
intestinal perforation, 7, 8
intestinal stenoses and atresias common location and pathologic features, 3, 4
mutation with familial multiple intestinal atresias, 3, 4
omphalomesenteric remnant, gastrointestinal duplication, bronchogenic cyst, and neurenteric cyst, 2, 3
pediatric gastrointestinal tract, 2
Diabetes type II, 331, 333
Diaphragm disease, 272
Diarrhea, 103–105, 324
Dieulafoy lesion, 152, 198
Diffuse ganglioneuromatosis, 403
Diffuse infiltration of the lamina propria, 27
Diffuse large B-cell lymphoma (DLBCL), 523, 525, 537
in the colon, 538
malabsorption disorders, 106
Paris staging system, 525
Dilated stomach, 334
"Diminutive" polyps, 358
Diphyllobothrium, 256
Direct immunofluorescence (DIF), 38, 43
Dirty necrosis, 436
Discontinuous inflammation, 112
Diversion colitis, 155, 159, 164
diagnosis of, 155
histologic features, 154
Diverticular-disease-associated colitis, 152
diagnosis of, 150
features of, 150
histologic and endoscopic features of, 151
Diverticulosis, 307
Donor-specific antibodies (DSAs), 548
Drug-induced gastrointestinal tract injury, 267, 284, 285
angiotensin II receptor antagonist olmesartan, 275, 276
encountered medication-induced injury patterns, 268
gastric mucosal calcinosis, 273, 274
gout, 283, 284
immunotherapy agents, 279, 280
idelalisib, 281
ipilimumab, 280
programmed cell death protein 1 (PD-1) inhibitors, 280, 281
melanosis coli, 278, 279
mitotic arrest-related changes, 275
mucosal changes associated with iron therapy, 272, 273
mucosal injury patterns and associated offending agents, 268
mycophenolate mofetil, 276–278
non-specific drug-induced gastrointestinal tract injury patterns, 268
chemical gastritis/ reactive gastropathy, 269, 270
focal active colitis, 271
increased epithelial apoptosis, 271
ischemic colitis, 270, 271
microscopic colitis, 270
pill esophagitis, 268, 269
sloughing esophagitis, 269
non-steroidal anti-inflammatory drugs (NSAIDs)-related GI tract mucosal injury, 271, 272
proton pump inhibitors, 274, 275
renal failure, hemodialysis for, 281, 282
resins, 278
bile acid sequestrants, 278
sevelamer, 278
sodium polystyrene sulfonate, 278
Yttrium-90 microspheres, 275
Duodenal and rectal NETs, 412
Duodenal biopsy, 23, 94, 467
Duodenal injury, 106
Duodenal somatostatinoma, 416
Duodenal-type follicular lymphoma (d-FL), 526, 535, 536
Duodenum, 416, 417
Duplicated muscularis mucosae, 60
Duplication cyst of the ileum, 2
Dysmotility, 333
Dysphagia, 47, 48
Dysplasia
diagnosis of, 131, 132
IBD, 125, 126
reactive atypia versus, 58
types of Barrett dysplasia, 61
Dysplastic epithelium, 129, 213

E

E. coli-associated colitis, 227
EBV-associated gastric carcinoma, 438
EBV-associated smooth muscle tumors, 506, 513, 514
characteristic histologic and immunohistochemical features, 506, 507
differential diagnosis, 507
patient populations, 506
EBV in situ hybridization, 532
EBV-positive lymphomas, 532
ECL cell hyperplasia, 79
Edema, 227
Electron microscopy (EM), 316
Embolic beads in stomach, 68
Encountered viral infections, 230
Endometrial carcinomas, 467
Endometriosis, 182
Endoscopic mucosal resection, 64
Endoscopic ultrasound-guided fine needle aspiration (EUS-FNA), 480
End-stage renal disease, 105, 106
Entamoeba histolytica, 248–250
Enteric coccidians, 252
Enterobiasis, 257
Enterobius vermicularis, 170, 171
Enterocolic lymphocytic phlebitis, 156
Enterocytes, 105, 106
Enteroendocrine dysgenesis, 25
Enteropathy-associated T-cell lymphoma (EATL 1), 94, 95, 527
and monomorphic epitheliotropic intestinal T-cell lymphoma, 526, 527
small intestine, 539
Environmental metaplastic atrophic gastritis, 70
Eosinophilic appendicitis, 170
Eosinophilic esophagitis(EoE), 21, 35, 292, 308
clinicopathologic findings in, 34, 35
criteria, diagnosis of, 292, 293
esophagus, intraepithelial eosinophils in, 37
pathogenesis of, 293
Eosinophilic gastroenteritis (EGE), 22, 82, 295, 308, 322
antrum, 82
causes, 82
diagnosis of, 82
small bowel biopsy samples, 97, 98
Eosinophilic gastrointestinal disease (EGID), 22
Eosinophilic myenteric ganglionitis, 322
Eosinophils, 289
distribution of, 22
gastroesophageal reflux disease, 37
in inflammatory bowel disease, 294

Epidermolysis bullosa, 43
Epigastric pain, 49, 50
Epithelial adenomatous polyposis, 369
Epithelial apoptosis, 106, 546
Epithelioid gastrointestinal stromal tumor (GIST), 476, 487, 489, 491
Epithelioid granuloma, 124, 241, 302
Epithelioid hemangioendothelioma, 491
Epithelioid sarcomas, 209
Epithelium overlying lymphoid follicles, 90
Erdheim–Chester disease (ECD), 304, 533
Esophageal candidiasis, 291
Esophageal squamous papilloma, 340
Esophageal ulcer, cause of, 44, 45
Esophagitis, 33, 267
  corrosive injury, causes and long-term implications, 39, 40
  dysphagia and hepatitis B infection, 47, 48
  eosinophilic esophagitis, 34, 35
  epigastric pain and Crohn disease, 49, 50
  esophageal ulcer, cause of, 44, 45
  gastroesophageal reflux disease, 33, 34, 37
  GERD and EoE, 36, 37
  immunosuppression and chronic kidney disease, 45–48
  intraepithelial eosinophils, 36, 37
  lichenoid esophagitis, clinicopathologic characteristics of, 38–39
  lymphocytic and lichenoid esophagitis patterns, 39
  lymphocytic esophagitis pattern, clinical and histologic characteristics of, 37, 38
  medications, cause morphologic change, 42
  odynophagia, bullae, blisters and erosions of oral mucosa, 50, 51
  pemphigus vulgaris, 43, 44
  pill fragments, types of, 40, 41
  PPI, 36, 37
  sloughing esophagitis/esophagitis dissecans, 42, 43
Esophagitis dissecans superficialis, 40, 42, 44, 269, 270
Esophagus, 290
  intraepithelial eosinophils in, 37
  non-GIST primary mesenchymal tumors, GI tract, 496
Exophytic adenocarcinoma, 430
External hemorrhoids, 198
Extra-abdominal desmoid fibromatosis, 503
Extra-gastrointestinal GISTs (E-GIST), 478
Extra-intestinal GISTs, 491
Extramucosal adenocarcinomas, 216
Extramucosal anal canal adenocarcinoma, 206, 207
Extranodal marginal zone lymphoma (ENMZL), 522, 524, 534
  and reactive marginal zone hyperplasia, 524, 525
  stomach, 534
Extranodal Rosai–Dorfman disease, 304

F

Familial adenomatous polyposis (FAP), 342, 367, 380, 516
Familial visceral myopathy, 320
Fibrin thrombi, 76
Fibromatosis, 502, 505
Fibromuscular dysplasia, 153, 154
Fibrovascular polyps (FVPs), 387, 496
Filamentous fungi, 236
Filiform polyps, 350
Fish tapeworm, 256
Fistula-associated adenocarcinoma, 206, 215
Florid follicular hyperplasia PTLD, 554
Fluke infection, 255
Fluorescent treponemal antibody absorbed test (FTA-ABS), 244
Focal active colitis, 271
Focal colitis, 117
Focal inflammation, 116
Follicular dendritic cell (FDC) sarcomas, 500, 533
Follicular lymphoma, 523
Foveolar hyperplasia, 75
Foveolar-type gastric adenoma, 343
Full thickness/seromuscular biopsy, 314
Fulminant colitis, 110, 112, 113
Fundic gland polyps, 342
Fungal infection, 557
Fungi, 235, 236, 238, 239
Fusarium, 236

G

Galactomannan, 239
Gangliocytic paraganglioma, 417
Ganglion cells, 328, 333
  Auerbach plexus, 318
  Hirschsprung disease, 9, 10
  within myenteric plexus, 10
Ganglioneuroma, 403
Ganglioneuromatosis, 403
Ganglioneuromatous lesions, 403
Ganglioneuromatous polyps, 20, 392, 403
Gardner syndrome, 369, 503
Gas-filled cysts, 156
Gastric adenocarcinoma, 344, 433, 443
Gastric adenocarcinoma and proximal polyposis of the stomach (GAPPS), 342, 379, 382
Gastric adenomas, 342
Gastric anisakiasis, 258
Gastric antral vascular ectasia (GAVE) syndrome, 76, 77
Gastric corpus mucosa, 421
Gastric duplication cyst, 5
Gastric foveolar dysplasia, 61
Gastric heterotopia, 24
Gastric hyperplastic polyp, 341, 342
Gastric mucosal calcinosis, 273, 274
Gastric poorly cohesive carcinoma, 437
Gastric rugal folds, 308
Gastric schwannoma, 497
Gastric siderosis, 272, 273
Gastric xanthoma, 301, 388
Gastrin cell neoplasms, 416
Gastritis, 84, 261
Gastritis cystica profunda/polyposa, 345
Gastroblastoma, 440, 441
Gastroenteric infections, 119
Gastroesophageal junction (GEJ), 55, 56
Gastroesophageal reflux disease (GERD), 340
  clinicopathologic features, 33, 34
  eosinophils, 37
  esophagus, intraepithelial eosinophils in, 37
Gastrointestinal anisakiasis, 258
Gastrointestinal disorders, pediatric
  developmental anomalies
    anorectal malformation repair specimens, 4, 5
    cyst, 5
    disorder with ileocolonic and colonic atresia, 4
    ileum segment, 6, 7
    intestinal perforation, 7, 8
    intestinal stenoses and atresias, 3, 4
    mutation with familial multiple intestinal atresias, 3, 4

omphalomesenteric remnant, gastrointestinal duplication, bronchogenic cyst and neurenteric cyst, 2, 3
pediatric gastrointestinal tract, 2
Hirschsprung disease
biopsy, 9, 10
dentate line, 8
dilated bowel and rectosigmoid, 12
ganglion cells, 8–10
Hirschsprung-associated enterocolitis, 11
ileocecal obstruction, loop ileostomy for, 12, 13
intestinal neuronal dysplasia, hypoganglionosis, hyperganglionosis and ultrashort HD, 11
lamina propria, calretinin positive neurites in, 9
suction rectal biopsies, 13, 14
suction rectal biopsy, 8, 9
transition zone, feature of, 10, 11
ileocecal intussusception, 16, 17
inflammatory disorders
celiac disease, 27–29
congenital onset diarrhea and non-inflammatory enteropathy, 25
eosinophilic esophageal disease, pathologic features of, 21
eosinophilic gastrointestinal disease, differential of, 22
granulomatous appendicitis, differentials of, 27
inflammatory bowel disease, early onset of, 25, 26
inflammatory enteropathy, differential for, 22, 23
non-infectious lamina propria histiocytic infiltrate, differentials for, 27
plasma cells, in gastrointestinal tract, 22
necrotizing enterocolitis, 15, 16
pediatric intussusceptions
malignancy associated with, 15
pathologic lead points, 15
pediatric volvulus
vs. adult volvulus, 14
and intussusception, 14
tumors and polyps
abdomen and pelvis, intraabdominal mass filling, 20, 21
appendiceal carcinoid, pathologic characteristics and clinical behavior of, 20
gastrointestinal stromal tumor, 17, 18
hamartomatous polyp, 19, 20
juvenile polyp, 18, 19
malignant gastrointestinal neuroectodermal tumor, 18
Gastrointestinal graft *versus* host disease (GVHD), 99, 100
Gastrointestinal mucosae, 296
Gastrointestinal neuroectodermal tumor (GNET), 496, 502
and clear cell sarcoma of soft tissue, 501, 502
histologic findings, 501
immunohistochemical and molecular features, 501
Gastrointestinal stromal tumor (GIST), 17, 18, 392, 485, 487, 489, 491
advanced GIST, 481
AJCC staging manual, 482
benign GIST, 480
BRAF V6000E mutation testing, 485
BRAF-mutated tumors, 484
CD117 immunostain, 476
clinical staging, 483
coagulative necrosis, 480
common sites of metastasis, 481
definition, 474
E-GISTs, 478, 479
of esophagus, 496
EUS-FNA approach for diagnosis, 480
germline KIT syndrome, 483
germline PDGFRA syndrome, 484
grading and risk assessment criteria, 482
histologic features, 474–477, 479
hyaline necrosis, 480
ICC hyperplasia, 481
immunostains, 475, 476
KIT and PDGFRA mutations, 483
KIT gene, 474
liquefactive necrosis, 480
malignant GIST, 480
microscopic GIST, 481
mini-GIST, 481
mitotic count, 479
multifocal GISTs, 482
neoplastic cells, 474
PDGFR mutations, 483
pediatric GIST, 477
risk assessment scheme, 478, 482
SDHB immunostain, 484, 491
sporadic and SDHB-deficient GISTs, 478
syndromic GIST, 477
tubular gastrointestinal tract, 474
tumorlet, 481
tyrosine kinase, 475
Gastrointestinal tract
angiosarcoma of, 507
endoscopic and histologic, systemic mastocytosis in, 298, 299
eosinophil count, 290
eosinophils, distribution of, 22
granulomas, differential diagnosis for, 300
histiocytic disorders, 303–305
histiocytic infiltrate, differential diagnosis for, 299, 300
lymphomas of
acute leukemia, 531
appendix, lymphoma types, 532
diffuse large B-cell lymphoma, prognostic testing, 525
duodenal-type follicular lymphoma and systemic usual adult type follicular lymphoma, 526
EATL and MEITL, 527, 528
EBV in situ hybridization, 532
enteropathy-associated T-cell lymphoma, 526, 527
extranodal marginal zone lymphoma, 524
gastric nodule, 536
hematopoietic neoplasms, 528
high grade B-cell lymphoma, diagnose, 530
histiocytic and dendritic neoplasms, 533
immunoproliferative small intestinal disease and plasma cell neoplasm, 530
monomorphic epitheliotropic intestinal T-cell lymphoma, 526, 527
mucosal eosinophils, 531, 532
multiple mucosal polyps, 528
NK-cell enteropathy, 528, 529
plasma cell-rich lesion, differential diagnosis and workup for, 530
primary immunodeficiencies, 532
reactive marginal zone hyperplasia, 524, 525
rectal tonsil and mimics of lymphoma, 529, 530
refractory celiac disease type 1 and type 2, 528
stomach, low-grade/small B-cell lymphomas of, 521–523
systemic mastocytosis, diagnosis of, 528
mast cell counts in, 295
motility disorders of (*see* Motility disorders)
neurofibroma, 390
plasma cells, 22

Gastrointestinal tract, infections
aeromonas, 225
AIDS, 232, 233
antibiotic-associated injury, 246
C. difficile, 227
laboratory methodologies, diagnosis, 246–248
Campylobacter species, 225
chronic idiopathic inflammatory bowel disease, celiac disease, and ischemic colitis, 224
clinical significance with stool PCR assay, 245, 246
Crohn disease, 261
E.coli, 227
fungi, 235, 236, 238, 239
Helicobacter pylori and drug resistant organisms, 239, 240
helminths/worms, 254
ascaris lumbricoides, 256
diphyllobothrium, 256
fluke infection, 255
gastrointestinal anisakiasis, 258
hookworms, 256
hymenolepsis nana, 256
pinworms, 256, 257, 259
schistosomiasis, 255
strongyloides stercoralis, 257, 258
T. saginata, 256
tapeworms, 255
whipworm, 256
high-risk HPV infection in anus and clinical implications, 233–235
idiopathic inflammatory bowel disease and clinical significance, 228, 229
intestinal spirochetosis and clinical significance, 244, 245
lung adenocarcinoma, 260, 261
M. tuberculosis, 228
mimic celiac disease, 227
mimic chronic idiopathic inflammatory bowel disease, 224
mimic ischemia, 226, 227
mycobacterium avium-intracellulare complex, 242, 243
mycobacterium tuberculosis, 241, 242
PCR, 223, 224
plasma CMV PCR, 229
protozoa, 248
amoebic trophozoites, 249
balantidium coli, 248
coccidial infection, 252
cryptosporidium, 253
cyclospora cayetanensis, 253
cystoisospora spp., 253
entamoeba histolytica, 248–250
giardia lamblia, 251
leishmania, 252
leishmaniasis, 251, 252
microsporidia spp., 253
toxoplasma gondii, 254
rectal bleeding, 259
salmonella, 225
sexually transmitted infectious, chronic idiopathic inflammatory bowel disease from, 243, 244
upper GI bleeding, 260
viruses, 229–232
Whipple disease, 240, 241
yersinia, 225, 226
Gastroparesis, 333
causes of, 335
Gastrospirillum hominis, 240
GEJ biopsies, Barrett esophagus, 57
Generalized juvenile polyposis (GJP), 377
Germline KIT syndrome, 483
Germline PDGFRA syndrome, 484
GI tract, non-GIST primary mesenchymal tumors of
abdominal/retroperitoneal mass, 514, 515
adipose tissue, tumors of, 510
angiomyolipoma
histologic features of, 512
histological variants of, 511, 512
immunohistochemical features of, 512
angiosarcoma
distinguishing features of, 509, 510
from hemangioma, 507
immunohistochemical features of, 510
patient populations, 507
colon and rectum involvement, 497
dedifferentiated liposarcoma
absence of well-differentiated component, 511
liposarcoma differ from, 511
EBV-associated smooth muscle tumors
characteristic histologic and immunohistochemical features, 506, 507
differential diagnosis, 507
patient populations, 506
esophagus, 496
familial adenomatous polyposis, 516, 517
fibromatosis, demographic populations, 502, 503
gastrointestinal neuroectodermal tumor
and clear cell sarcoma of soft tissue, 501, 502
histologic findings, 501
immunohistochemical and molecular features, 501
genetic syndromes, 505
glomus tumor, hemangioma from, 508, 509
inflammatory myofibroblastic tumor
differential diagnosis, 500
histologic patterns, 500, 501
immunohistochemical findings, 500
molecular abnormalities, 499, 500
intestinal obstruction, 515, 516
intra-abdominal fibromatosis
spindle cell neoplasms, 504, 505
growth patterns of, 503, 504
leiomyosarcoma, characteristic histologic findings of, 505, 506
liposarcoma
angiomyolipoma distinguished from, 511, 512
immunohistochemical or molecular tests, 510, 511
malignant peripheral nerve sheath tumor, neurofibromas differentiated from, 498, 499
mesenchymal tumors, 496
neurofibromas, schwannomas from, 497, 498
plexiform fibromyxoma, characteristic location and features of, 499
retroperitoneum, liposarcoma of, 511
S100-positive GI tumors, 503
small bowel involvement, 496
stomach, characteristically involvement, 496
vascular neoplasms, 507, 508
Giant condyloma of Buschke-Lowenstein (GCBL), 202–204, 456
Giant inflammatory polyposis, 113
Giardia lamblia, infections of gastrointestinal tract, 251
Giardiasis, 251
Glomus, 496
Glomus tumor, 397, 487, 509
hemangioma from, 508, 509
stain, 397
Glutamate dehydrogenase (GDH), 248
Glycogenic acanthosis, 340, 378

Goblet cell adenocarcinoma (GCA), 173–176
  clinical features, 174
  grading system for, 177
  grading systems and prognostic significance, 174, 177
  gross and histologic features of, 174
  immunohistochemical features of, 177
  molecular alterations, 177
Goblet cell-rich hyperplastic polyp (GCHP), 352
Goblet-cell-deficient dysplasia, 127
Goblet-cell-deficient epithelium, 140
Goblets cells, 56
Gout, drug-induced gastrointestinal tract injury, 283, 284
Grading B-cell lymphomas, 531
Grading neuroendocrine tumors (NETs), 411
Graft-*vs.*-host disease (GVHD), 42, 99, 123, 277, 546
  malabsorption disorders, 106
Granular cell tumor, 387, 390, 391
Granulomas, 116, 241, 303
  differential diagnosis for, 300, 303
  IBD, 115
  in UC and CD, 113
Granulomatous appendicitis, 169, 170
  differentials of, 27
Granulomatous gastritis, 81, 82
Gut-associated lymphoid tissue (GALT) carcinoma, 454

H
H. Heilmanni gastritis, 74
H. pylori gastritis, 70, 239
  active inflammation, 71
  immunostain, 70
  lymphoid aggregate, 71
  residual chronic inflammation, 72
  superficial predominant pattern, 71
  treatment, 70
Hamartomatous Peutz-Jeghers type polyp, 19
Hamartomatous polyp
  gastrointestinal disorders, 19, 20
Hamazaki-Wesenberg bodies, 299
Helicobacter heilmanni, 73, 74, 240
  clinical significance, 74
Helicobacter organisms, 421
Helicobacter pylori gastritis
  and *Helicobacter heilmanni*, 73, 74
  biopsy, 70
  chronic infection, 69
  environmental metaplastic atrophic gastritis, 70
  infections of gastrointestinal tract, 239, 240
  histochemical/immunostains for, 71, 72
  histological findings in, 70, 71
  infection with, 69
  laboratory tests, 69
  metaplasia, significance of, 72, 73
  mucosal atrophy, significance of, 72
Helminths/worms, 255
  infections of gastrointestinal tract, 254
    ascaris lumbricoides, 256
    diphyllobothrium, 256
    fluke infection, 255
    gastrointestinal anisakiasis, 258
    hookworms, 256
    hymenolepsis nana, 256
    pinworms, 256, 257, 259
    schistosomiasis, 255
    strongyloides stercoralis, 257, 258
    T. saginata, 256
    tapeworms, 255
    whipworm, 256
Hemangioma, 387
  angiosarcoma from, 507
  from glomus tumor, 508, 509
Hematopoietic neoplasms, 528
Hemorrhoids, 198
Hepatitis B infection
  esophagitis, 47, 48
Hepatoid adenocarcinoma, 439
Hereditary diffuse gastric cancer, 444
Hereditary hemorrhagic telangiectasia (HHT), 152
Herpes esophagitis, 47
Herpes simplex virus (HSV), 40
Heterotopic gastric mucosa, 24, 346, 347
Heterotopic pancreatic tissue, 347
Hidradenoma papilliferum, 200
High grade-appearing cellular neoplasms, differential
    diagnosis of, 207
High-grade appendiceal mucinous neoplasm (HAMN), 178, 180
High grade B-cell lymphoma, diagnose, 530
High grade squamous intraepithelial neoplasia (HSIL), 233
High-grade appendiceal mucinous neoplasm (HAMN), 178, 180
High-grade dysplasia, 60, 127, 433
  from intramucosal adenocarcinoma, 59, 60
  histologic features of, 59
High-grade malignant peripheral nerve sheath tumor, 499
High-risk HPV infection, in anus, 233–235
Hindgut NETs, 412
Hirschsprung associated enterocolitis, 11
Hirschsprung disease (HD), 4, 13, 313, 324, 325, 329, 330
  allied disorders of, 329
  biopsies evaluation and special stains, 324, 325
  biopsy, 9, 10
  dentate line, 8
  dilated bowel and rectosigmoid, 12
  ganglion cells, 9, 10
  ganglion cells, absence of, 8, 9
  hirschsprung-associated enterocolitis, 11
  ileocecal obstruction, loop ileostomy for, 12, 13
  intestinal neuronal dysplasia, hypoganglionosis, hyperganglionosis
    and ultrashort HD, 11
  lamina propria, calretinin positive neurites in, 9
  pull-through surgery, intraoperative consultation during, 325
  resection, evaluation, 326
  suction rectal biopsies, 8, 9, 13, 14
  symptoms frequent persistence and implications, 326
  transition zone, feature of, 10, 11
  triage biopsy tissues, 324
Histiocytic disorders, 303–305
Histiocytic infiltrate, differential diagnosis for, 299, 300
Histiocytic sarcoma, 304, 305, 533
Histochemical stains, motility disorder, stains, workup, 314
Histoplasma, 236, 238, 239
Histoplasma capsulatum var. capsulatum, 235
Histoplasmosis, 237
Hodgkin lymphoma PTLD, 554
Hookworms, infections of gastrointestinal tract, 256
Human chorionic gonadotropin (HCG), 442
Human papillomavirus (HPV), 340, 432
Hyaline necrosis, 480
Hymenolepsis nana
  infections of gastrointestinal tract, 256
Hyperchromatic nuclei, 485
Hyperemia, 109

Hyperganglionosis
  Hirschsprung disease, 11
Hyperinfective, 257
Hypermucinous (villous) dysplasia, 129
Hypermucinous dysplasia, 128
Hyperplastic polyp with iron deposition, 361
Hyperplastic polyps, 341, 342, 344, 352, 433
Hypertension, 305, 306
Hypertrophied muscle, 319
Hypertrophied papillae, 197, 198
Hypobetalipoproteinemia, 25
Hypoganglionosis, 329
  and ganglia number evaluation, 327
  Hirschsprung disease, 11
Hypoproteinemia, 349
Hypothyroidism, 318

I

Idelalisib, 99
  drug-induced gastrointestinal tract injury, 281
Idelalisib-associated injury, 282
Idiopathic eosinophilic gastroenteritis, 308
Idiopathic inflammatory bowel disease, 224, 225
  infections of gastrointestinal tract, 228, 229, 243, 244
IHC stains, motility disorder, stains, workup, 315, 316
Iischemic colitis, 152, 153
Ileal pouch-anal anastomosis (IPAA), 125
Ileocecal and jejuno-ileal segments, 241
Ileocecal intussusception, gastrointestinal disorders, 16, 17
Ileocecal obstruction, loop ileostomy for, 12, 13
Ileoanal pouch surgery
  complications of, 125
    CD of pouch, 125
    cuffitis, 125
    pouchitis, 125
  with Crohn disease, 126
Ileocolonic and colonic atresia, developmental anomalies, 4
Ileum, 417, 418
Ileum segment, developmental anomalies, 6, 7
Immune checkpoint inhibitors, 98, 121, 279
Immunohistochemistry, 403
Immunoproliferative small intestinal disease (IPSID), 530
Immunostains, Barrett esophagus, 57
In situ hybridization for EBV (EBER), 507
Inactive chronic colitis, 138
Increased crypt apoptosis, 27
Increased epithelial apoptosis, 271
Indeterminate colitis, diagnosis and clinical implications, 113, 114
Indeterminate dendritic cell tumor, 533
Indolent SM, 297
Indolent T-cell lymphoproliferative disorder of the GI tract, 528
Induction chemotherapy, 99
Infections of gastrointestinal tract
  aeromonas, 225
  AIDS, 232, 233
  antibiotic-associated injury, 246
  Campylobacter species, 225
  C. difficile, 227
    laboratory methodologies, diagnosis, 246–248
  chronic idiopathic inflammatory bowel disease, celiac disease, and ischemic colitis, 224
  clinical significance with stool PCR assay, 245, 246
  Crohn disease, 261
  Cryptosporidia, 102
  E.coli, 227
  fungi, 235, 236, 238, 239
  Helicobacter pylori and drug resistant organisms, 239, 240
  helminths/worms, 254
    ascaris lumbricoides, 256
    diphyllobothrium, 256
    fluke infection, 255
    gastrointestinal anisakiasis, 258
    hookworms, 256
    hymenolepsis nana, 256
    pinworms, 256, 257, 259
    schistosomiasis, 255
    strongyloides stercoralis, 257, 258
    T. saginata, 256
    tapeworms, 255
    whipworm, 256
  high-risk HPV infection in anus and clinical implications, 233–235
  idiopathic inflammatory bowel disease and clinical significance, 228, 229
  intestinal spirochetosis and clinical significance, 244, 245
  lung adenocarcinoma, 260, 261
  M. tuberculosis, 228
  mimic celiac disease, 227
  mimic chronic idiopathic inflammatory bowel disease, 224
  mimic ischemia, 226, 227
  mycobacterium avium-intracellulare complex, 242, 243
  mycobacterium tuberculosis, 241, 242
  PCR, 223, 224
  plasma CMV PCR, 229
  protozoa, 248
    amoebic trophozoites, 249
    Balantidium coli, 248
    coccidial infection, 252
    cryptosporidium, 253
    cyclospora cayetanensis, 253
    cystoisospora spp., 253
    entamoeba histolytica, 248–250
    giardia lamblia, 251
    leishmania, 252
    leishmaniasis, 251, 252
    microsporidia spp., 253
    toxoplasma gondii, 254
  rectal bleeding, 259
  Salmonella, 225
  sexually transmitted infectious, chronic idiopathic inflammatory bowel disease from, 243, 244
  viruses, 229–232
  Whipple disease, 240, 241
  Yersinia, 225, 226
Infectious colitis, 117–119, 135
Infectious mononucleosis PTLD, 554
Infiltrative disorders, intestinal pseudo-obstruction, 321, 322
Inflammatory bowel disease (IBD), 150, 152
  acute and chronic infectious colitis, 118
  adjunctive markers, distinguishing dysplasia, 129, 130
  anal diseases, 199, 214–216
    Crohn disease, 199
    syphilis and lymphogranuloma venereum, 199
    ulcerative colitis, 199
  CD, characteristic histologic features of, 116
  characteristic histological features, 114–115
    architectural disarray, 115
    basal lymphoplasmacytosis, 115
    crypt and surface inflammation, 115
    granulomas, 115
    mucin depletion, 115
    paneth cell metaplasia, 115, 116
    pyloric gland metaplasia, 116

chronic ulcerative colitis, characteristic pathologic features of, 109–111
colorectal carcinoma, pathological features, 132, 134
Crohn-associated and cryptolytic granulomas, 117
Crohn colitis
characteristic pathologic features of, 111, 112
histological features, 116, 117
Crohn disease, upper GI manifestations, 124
cryptolytic granulomas in, 116
differential diagnoses of, 122, 123
drugs and toxic agents, 120–122
dysplasia
diagnosis of, 131, 132
histological characteristics of, 125, 126
early onset of, 26
fulminant colitis, 112, 113
giant inflammatory polyposis, 113
IBD-associated dysplasia, sporadic adenomas distinguished from, 130, 131
ileoanal pouch surgery, complications of, 125
CD of pouch, 125
cuffitis, 125
pouchitis, 125
indeterminate colitis, diagnosis and clinical implications, 113, 114
infectious colitis, 117–119, 135
LGD, 136
long-standing well-controlled UC, 135
low-grade dysplasia, 138, 139
non-adenomatous dysplasia, spectrum of, 126–128
pathology of, 122, 123
reactive and dysplastic epithelium, 129
reactive epithelial changes, dysplasia distinguished from, 128, 129
superficial Crohn colitis, 113
ulcerative colitis
anti-inflammatory therapy with mesalamine, 139
backwash ileitis in, 113
characteristic histologic features of, 116
discontinuous inflammation in, 112
granulomas in, 113
histological features, 116, 117
rectal sparing in, 112
transmural inflammation in, 113
upper GI manifestations, 124
ulcerative pancolitis, 139–141
villous dysplasia, 136
well-controlled Crohn colitis, 137
Inflammatory cap polyps, 349
Inflammatory cloacogenic polyp, 198, 351
Inflammatory disorders
celiac disease, 27–29
congenital onset diarrhea and non-inflammatory enteropathy, 25
eosinophilic esophageal disease, pathologic features of, 21
eosinophilic gastrointestinal disease, differential of, 22
eosinophils, clinical differential diagnosis of, 21
esophageal biopsy, heterotopic gastric mucosa in, 24
gastrointestinal tract, eosinophils distribution, 22
granulomatous appendicitis, differentials of, 27
inflammatory bowel disease, early onset of, 25, 26
inflammatory enteropathy, differential for, 22, 23
non-infectious lamina propria histiocytic infiltrate, differentials for, 27
plasma cells, in gastrointestinal tract, 22
small intestinal biopsies, pathologic features in, 22, 23
Inflammatory enteropathy, differential for, 22, 23
Inflammatory fibroid polyp (IFP), 388, 395–397, 406
Inflammatory myofibroblastic tumor (IMT), 391, 405, 501, 516
differential diagnosis, 500
molecular abnormalities, 499, 500
Inflammatory myoglandular polyp, 351, 352
Inflammatory polyps, 139, 348, 349, 467
Inflammtory fibroid polyp, 405
Internal sphincter achalasia, 329
Intestinal atresias, developmental anomalies, 3, 4
Intestinal dysmotility, 323
Intestinal heterotopia, in pyloric region of stomach, 24
Intestinal lymphangiectasia, 401
Intestinal metaplasia
complete type, 72, 73
incomplete type, 73
Intestinal mucosa, 101
umbilical polyp with, 7
Intestinal muscularis propria, segmental absence of, 8
Intestinal neuronal dysplasia (IND), 326, 327
Hirschsprung disease, 11
Intestinal perforation, developmental anomalies, 7, 8
Intestinal pseudo-obstruction, 321–323
Intestinal spirochetosis, 244, 245
Intestinal type adenocarcinoma, 207
Intestinal-type gastric adenomas, 343
Intestines, tissue eosinophils, differential diagnosis of, 293
Intra-abdominal (desmoid) fibromatosis, 391
Intra-abdominal fibromatosis, 504
growth patterns of, 503, 504
spindle cell neoplasms, 504, 505
Intra-abdominal/pelvis, 503
Intraepithelial eosinophils, 37, 48, 290
esophagitis, 36
esophagus, 37
Intraepithelial lymphocytes (IELs), 146
immunohistochemistry, 94
Intraepithelial lymphocytosis, 90, 91, 93, 94, 100, 285
infection cause, 101
malabsorption disorders, 104
Intramucosal adenocarcinoma, 60, 63
high-grade dysplasia from, 60
Intussusception, 14
Invasive adenocarcinoma, 358
Invasive moderately differentiated adenocarcinoma, 362
Invasive squamous cell carcinoma, 456, 457
Invasive strongyloidiasis, 261
Invasive well differentiated adenocarcinoma, 467, 468
Inverted inflammatory polyp, 216
"Invisible" dysplasia, 132
Ion-exchange resins, 278
Ipilimumab, 42, 121
drug-induced gastrointestinal tract injury, 280
Ipilimumab-associated colitis, 121
Ipilimumab-associated injury, 281
Iron pill esophagitis, 41
Iron pill gastritis, 272
Iron pills, 40
Iron therapy, drug-induced gastrointestinal tract, 272, 273
Irritable bowel syndrome (IBS)
histologic characteristics of, 161
mast cells in, 296
Ischemic bowel injury, etiologies for, 152, 155
Ischemic colitis, 123, 158, 159, 163, 224, 270, 271, 282
gross and histologic features of, 153
histologic features of, 157
Ischemic enterocolitis, 155
Ischemic injury, 282
Isolated granulomatous appendicitis, 28
Isolated tumor cells, 451

J
Jejunal atresia, 4
Juvenile polyposis, 18, 19, 376, 381
  gastrointestinal disorders, 19
Juvenile polyposis coli (JPC), 377
Juvenile polyposis of infancy (JPI), 377
Juvenile xanthogranuloma (JXG), 304

K
K. oxytoca, 246
K. oxytoca toxin, 246
Kaposi sarcoma, 509
Kappa immunostain, 559
Karyosome, 249
Kayexalate, 40, 42, 278, 279
Kayexalate crystals, 41, 282
Keratin immunostain, 452
Keratins, 510
Ki-67 proliferative index, 410–412
KIT-mutated gastrointestinal stromal tumor, 485
Klebsiella oxytoca, 246

L
L cell neuroendocrine tumor, 419
Lambda immunostain, 559
Lamina propria, 104
  calretinin positive neurites, 9
  fibrosis, 293
  hyalinization, 154
Langerhans cell histiocytosis (LCH), 27, 28, 303, 304, 531
Langerhans cell sarcoma (LCS), 533
Lanthanum deposition in duodenal mucosa, 274
Large cell neuroendocrine carcinoma (LCNEC), 410
Laxatives, 323
Leiomyoma, 18, 387, 398, 399, 403, 404, 496, 497
Leiomyosarcoma (LMS), 496
  characteristic histologic findings of, 505, 506
  high grade, 516
Leishmaniasis, 252
  infections of gastrointestinal tract, 251, 252
Lerner grading system, 552
LGV proctitis, 244
Lichen planus, 38
Lichenoid esophagitis, 47
  clinicopathologic characteristics of, 38, 39
Lichenoid esophagitis pattern, 39, 49
Lipid transport defects, 25
Lipomas, 400, 496, 497
Liposarcoma, 400, 401
  angiomyolipoma distinguished from, 511, 512
  diagnosis of, 510, 511
  retroperitoneum, 511
Loop ileostomy, ileocecal obstruction, 12, 13
Low grade AIN (AIN1), 219
Low grade squamous intraepithelial neoplasia (LSIL), 233
Low grade/small B-cell lymphomas, stomach, 521
Lower anogenital squamous terminology (LAST), 201, 202
Low-grade appendiceal mucinous neoplasm (LAMN), 177–179, 181, 192, 443
  unique T definition for, 180
Low-grade dysplasia, 59, 62, 127
  IBD, 138, 139
  histologic features of, 59
Low-grade fibromyxosarcomas, 505
Low-grade/small B-cell lymphomas
  of stomach, 522
Low-grade tubuloglandular adenocarcinoma, 141
Luminal GI tract, eosinophil count in, 290, 292
Lung adenocarcinoma, infections of gastrointestinal tract, 260, 261
Lymphadenopathy, 243
Lymphangiectasia, 25
Lymphangiomas, 401
Lymphocytic colitis, 146, 148, 161
  histologic features of, 147
Lymphocytic esophagitis, 125
Lymphocytic esophagitis pattern, 37
  clinical and histologic characteristics of, 37, 38
Lymphocytic gastritis, 80
  causes, 80
  clinical significance of, 80
Lymphocytic inflammation, 322
Lymphocytic leiomyositis, 322
Lymphoglandular complex, 358
Lymphogranuloma venereum (LGV), 199
Lymphoid aggregate, 71
Lymphoid hyperplasia, 24
Lymphomas
  gastrointestinal tract
    acute leukemia, 531
    appendix, lymphoma types, 532
    diffuse large B-cell lymphoma, prognostic testing, 525
    dull abdominal pain, 536, 537
    duodenal-type follicular lymphoma and systemic usual adult type follicular lymphoma, 526
    EATL and MEITL, 527, 528
    EBV in situ hybridization, 532
    endoscopic biopsies, 535, 536
    enteropathy-associated T-cell lymphoma, 526, 527
    extranodal marginal zone lymphoma, 524
    gastric nodule, 536
    hematopoietic neoplasms, 528
    high grade B-cell lymphoma, diagnose, 530
    histiocytic and dendritic neoplasms, 533
    immunoproliferative small intestinal disease and plasma cell neoplasm, 530
    monomorphic epitheliotropic intestinal T-cell lymphoma, 526, 527
    multiple mucosal polyps, 528
    NK-cell enteropathy, 528, 529
    plasma cell-rich lesion, differential diagnosis and workup for, 530
    primary immunodeficiencies, 532
    reactive marginal zone hyperplasia, 524, 525
    refractory celiac disease type 1 and type 2, 528
    small intestinal mass, 537, 538
    stomach, low-grade/small B-cell lymphomas of, 521–523
    systemic mastocytosis, diagnosis of, 528
Lymphoplasmacytic lymphoma (LPL), 530
Lynch syndrome, 371, 380, 381, 433

M
Malabsorption disorders
  adequate tissue sample with malabsorptive symptoms, 89, 90
  autoimmune enteropathy
    clinical features, 96
    histologic features of, 97
  bacterial overgrowth, 100

biopsy samples, artifacts simulate chronic enteritis in, 90
celiac disease
complications of, 94, 95
drugs cause changes, 98, 99
environmental and genetic risk factors for, 92
evaluation, serologic markers in, 92
specific histologic features of, 92, 93
collagenous sprue, differential diagnosis of, 95
common variable immunodeficiency
clinical features, 97
histologic features, 97
Crohn disease, 96
diarrhea, 103–105
diffuse large B-cell lymphoma, 106
duodenal injury, 106
end-stage renal disease, malnutrition, and failure to thrive, 105, 106
eosinophilic gastroenteritis, small bowel biopsy samples, 97, 98
epithelial cell apoptosis, 106
GVHD and mycophenolate mofetil, 106
intraepithelial lymphocytosis
immunohistochemistry, 94
infection cause, 101
intraepithelial lymphocytosis and villous blunting, 104
malabsorptive pattern of small bowel injury, differential diagnosis for, 91
medication-related injury, gastrointestinal graft *versus* host disease, 99–100
small bowel injury, malabsorptive pattern of, 91
tropical sprue, features, 100
Malabsorptive pattern of small bowel injury
differential diagnosis for, 91
Malakoplakia, 307
Malignant gastrointestinal neuroectodermal tumor, 18
Malignant peripheral nerve sheath tumors (MPNSTs), 485, 498, 499
Malignant polyps, 436
Malnutrition, malabsorption disorders, 105, 106
Mantle cell lymphoma, 522, 536
in stomach, 537
Massive inflammatory polyposis, 139
Masson trichrome stain, 148
Mast cells disorders, 289, 325, 328
classification of, 298
gastrointestinal mucosae, 296
irritable bowel syndrome, 296
Mastocytic colitis, 296
Mastocytic enterocolitis, 296
Mastocytosis, 299
classification of, 297, 298
diagnosis of, 297
Maturation, 126
Maturation gradient, 128
M-bodies, 333
Meckel diverticulum, 6, 7
Meconium peritonitis, 15
Medication-related injury, gastrointestinal graft *vs.* host disease, 99, 100
Medullary carcinoma, 437, 438
Meissner plexus ganglion cells, 330
Melanosis, 278
Melanosis coli, 279, 283, 331
drug-induced gastrointestinal tract injury, 278, 279
Menetrier disease, 85, 86
Mesenchymal entities, 200
Mesenchymal lesions
admixture of Schwann cells and ganglion cells, 392
CFPT/RNFP, 391, 392
diagnosis of granular cell tumor, 397
FVPs, 387, 388
ganglioneuroma, 392
ganglioneuromatous polyposis, 392
GIST, IMT and mucosal perineurioma *vs.* IFP, 396
glomus tumors stain, 397
granular cell tumor, 390, 391
IFP, 395–397
leiomyoma, 398, 399
leiomyosarcoma, histologic features, 399
lipomas, 400
liposarcomas, 400, 401
lymphangiomas, 401
mucosal perineurioma, 393, 394
Schwann cell hamartomas, 389, 390
Schwannomas *vs.* Schwann cell hamartomas, 389, 390
smooth muscle neoplasm, 398
solitary polypoid gangliomas, 392
solitary polypoid ganglioneuroma, 392
xanthoma
diagnosis of, 388
differential diagnosis for, 388, 389
endoscopic appearance of, 388
Mesentery, 21
Metaplasia, significance of, 72, 73
Metastatic adenocarcinoma, 465
Metastatic breast carcinoma, 458
Metastatic calcification, 273
Metastatic carcinoma, 465
Metastatic endometrial carcinoma, 467
Metastatic gynecologic carcinomas, 458
Metastatic melanoma, 467
Metastatic prostatic carcinoma, 458
Metastatic pulmonary adenocarcinoma, 458
Michaelis–Guttmann bodies, 307
Micropapillary adenocarcinoma, 438
Microsatellite instability pathway (MSI), 381
Microscopic colitis, 150, 270
diagnosis of, 146
histologic characteristics of, 146
Microsporidia spp., 254
infections of gastrointestinal tract, 253
Microvesicular hyperplastic polyp (MVHP), 352
Microvillus inclusion disease, 25, 26, 106
Midgut neuroendocrine tumor (NET), 418
Mild acute cellular rejection, 556
Mild villous blunting, 230
Mimic ischemia, 226, 227
Misplaced adenomatous glands, 435
Mitotic arrest-related changes in
drug-induced gastrointestinal tract injury, 275
Mixed adenoneuroendocrine carcinomas (MANECs), 413, 414
Mixed neuroendocrine-nonneuroendocrine neoplasm (MiNEN), 172, 413, 424
Mixed-type GIST, 476
Moderate acute cellular rejection, 550
Moderately differentiated adenocarcinoma, 428
Modified Marsh score system for celiac disease, 93
Monomorphic epitheliotropic intestinal T-cell lymphoma, 527, 538
enteropathy-associated T-cell lymphoma and, 526, 527

Monomorphic PTLD, 554
Motility disorder
abnormalities, neurohormonal apparatus, 327
achalasia, 333, 335
achalasia cardia, histopathologic findings in, 319, 320
chronic constipation and intestinal pseudo-obstruction, 330, 331
chronic idiopathic constipation and intestinal pseudo-obstruction, 322, 323
classification and distinctive pathologic features, 318
clinical information, 316
constipation, 327–329
diabetes type II, 331, 333
distended abdomen, 329, 330
electron microscopy, evaluation, 316
Hirschsprung disease
biopsies evaluation and special stains, 324, 325
biopsy type, 324
pull-through surgery, intraoperative consultation during, 325
resection, evaluation, 326
symptoms frequent persistence and implications, 326
triage biopsy tissues, 324
hypoganglionosis and ganglia number evaluation, 327
infiltrative disorders, intestinal pseudo-obstruction, 321, 322
intestinal neuronal dysplasia, 326, 327
medications, 323, 324
neurological disorders, 318
postinfectious intestinal pseudo-obstruction, 320, 321
scleroderma, histopathologic features of, 319
stains, workup
histochemical stains, 314
IHC stains, 315, 316
systemic disorders, 318
tissue specimens, 313
full thickness/seromuscular biopsy, 314
resection specimens, 314
studies, triage tissues for, 314
suction mucosal biopsies, 313
Mucin depletion, IBD, 115
Mucin poor hyperplastic polyp (MCHP), 352
Mucinous adenocarcinoma, 437
appendix, 183, 184
three-tier grading system for, 183
Mucinous carcinoma, 437
Mucinous cystadenoma of ovary, 182
Mucinous dysplasia, 128
Muciphages, 301
Mucopolysaccharidoses, 27
Mucor, 236
Mucormycosis, 235, 260
Mucosal architecture, 110
Mucosal atrophy, significance of, 72
Mucosal changes, drug-induced gastrointestinal tract, 272, 273
drug-induced gastrointestinal tract, 272, 273
Mucosal eosinophils, 531, 532
Mucosal immunity, eosinophils, mast cells, and basophils in, 289
Mucosal injury patterns, 268
drug-induced gastrointestinal tract injury, 268
Mucosal perineurioma, 393, 394, 396, 397, 402, 404, 405
Mucosal prolapse, 350, 351
Mucosal Schwann cell hamartoma, 402–404
Mucosal type adenocarcinoma anal diseases, 205
Mullerian leiomyosarcoma, 485
Multifocal GIST, 482
Multiple mucosal polyps (MCL), 528
Muscularis mucosae
calretinin positive neurite in, 14
multiple calretinin positive neurites in, 14
Muscularis propria, 332
smooth muscle cells of, 333
MUTYH associated polyposis (MAP), 377
Mycobacteria, 243
Mycobacterium avium-intracellulare, 233
Mycobacterium avium-intracellulare colitis, 233
Mycobacterium avium-intracellulare complex (MAI)
gastrointestinal tract, infections, 242, 243
Mycobacterium tuberculosis, 228
infections of gastrointestinal tract, 241, 242
Mycophenolate, 42, 43
Mycophenolate mofetil, 106
drug-induced gastrointestinal tract injury, 276–278
Mycophenolate mofetil (MMF), 120
Mycophenolate-associated injury, 106, 277
Myeloid sarcomas, 531
Myenteric ganglia, 322
Myenteric plexus, ganglion cells within, 10
Myenteric plexuses, 315
Myocytes, 323

N

Necrotizing enterocolitis, 16, 161
etiologies/risk factors for, 159
histopathologic features, 15, 16
pathologic features of, 159
Neoplastic glands, 434
Neurenteric cyst, 6
gastrointestinal disorders, developmental anomalies, 2, 3
Neurenteric remnant, 6
Neuroendocrine carcinomas, 428
Neuroendocrine cell hyperplasia, 414
Neuroendocrine neoplasms, 209, 409
Neuroendocrine tumors (NETs), 409, 489
abdominoperineal resection, 424
AJCC staging manual, 423
appendiceal NETs, 418
autoimmune gastritis, 79
characteristic molecular features of, 419
Chromogranin A, 409
definition, 409
differential diagnostic of, 412
duodenum, 416, 417, 422
gangliocytic paragangliomas, 422
grading of, 411
grading schemes, 411, 412
histological features of, 410
ileum, 417, 418
immunohistochemical markers, 412
immunohistochemical staining and serum measurements, 412
L cell rectal NETs, 419
LCNECs, 410, 423
MANECs, 413, 414
MiNEN, 425
vs. NECs, 410
neuroendocrine cell hyperplasia, 414
neuroendocrine markers, 424
neuroendocrine neoplasms, 409
neuroendocrine tumors, synaptophysin, 409
small cell carcinoma, 410
staging of, 412, 413
synaptophysin immunostains, 423
type 1 gastric NETs, 415
type 2 gastric NETs, 415

type 3 gastric NETs, 415
type 4 gastric NET, 415
Neurofibromas, 496–498
from malignant peripheral nerve sheath tumor, 498, 499
Neurofibromatosis, 20
Neurological disorders, 318
Neuromuscular apparatus, 331
Neuropathy, 320
Neutrophilic cryptitis, 226, 243
Neutrophils, 34
acute esophagitis with, 21
Next generation sequencing (NGS) assays, 460
Nivolumab, 121, 280, 323
Nivolumab associated colitis, 285
Nivolumab-associated injury, 282
NK-cell enteropathy, 528, 529
Non-adenomatous dysplasia, 126–128
Non-anal gland-type and non-fistula-associated adenocarcinoma, 206, 207
Noncarcinoid epithelial neoplasia, PSOGI classification of, 173
Non-conventional dysplasia, types and identification, 61
Non-distorted biopsy, non-IBD noninfectious colitis, 149
Non-GIST primary mesenchymal tumors, GI tract
abdominal pain with biopsies, 513, 514
abdominal/retroperitoneal mass, 514, 515
angiomyolipoma
histologic features of, 512
histological variants of, 511, 512
immunohistochemical features of, 512
angiosarcoma
adipose tissue, tumors of, 510
distinguishing features of, 509, 510
from hemangioma, 507
immunohistochemical features of, 510
angiosarcoma, patient populations, 507
colon and rectum involvement, 497
dedifferentiated liposarcoma
absence of well-differentiated component, 511
liposarcoma differ from, 511
EBV-associated smooth muscle tumors
characteristic histologic and immunohistochemical features, 506, 507
differential diagnosis, 507
patient populations, 506
esophagus, 496
familial adenomatous polyposis, 516, 517
fevers, 516
fibromatosis, demographic populations, 502, 503
gastrointestinal neuroectodermal tumor
and clear cell sarcoma of soft tissue, 501, 502
histologic findings, 501
immunohistochemical and molecular features, 501
genetic syndromes, 505
glomus tumor, hemangioma from, 508, 509
inflammatory myofibroblastic tumor
differential diagnosis, 500
histologic patterns, 500, 501
immunohistochemical findings, 500
molecular abnormalities, 499, 500
intestinal obstruction, 515, 516
intra-abdominal fibromatosis
growth patterns of, 503, 504
spindle cell neoplasms, 504, 505
leiomyosarcoma, characteristic histologic findings of, 505, 506
liposarcoma
angiomyolipoma distinguished from, 511, 512
immunohistochemical or molecular tests, 510, 511
malignant peripheral nerve sheath tumor, neurofibromas differentiated from, 498, 499
mesenchymal tumors, 496
neurofibromas, schwannomas from, 497, 498
plexiform fibromyxoma, characteristic location and features of, 499
retroperitoneum, liposarcoma of, 511
S100-positive GI tumors, 503
small bowel involvement, 496
stomach, characteristically involvement, 496
vascular neoplasms, 507, 508
Non-IBD noninfectious colitis
abdominal pain and bloody diarrhea, 163
acute ischemic injury, 153
Behçet disease
and Crohn disease, 161
clinicopathologic features of, 159
biopsy/resection specimen, histologic features in, 150, 152
chronic ischemic injury, diagnosis of, 154
chronic watery diarrhea, 161, 162
collagenous colitis, lymphocytic colitis distinguished from, 146
colon biopsies with intraepithelial lymphocytes, 148, 149
count intraepithelial lymphocytes, 146
Crohn disease, 163, 164
crypt abscesses and/or focal crypt architectural distortion, 147
diversion colitis, diagnosis of, 155
diversion colitis, histologic features, 154
diverticular disease, 150
diverticular-disease-associated colitis, diagnosis of, 150
fibromuscular dysplasia, histologic characteristics of, 153, 154
irritable bowel syndrome, histologic characteristics of, 161
ischemic bowel injury, etiologies for, 152
ischemic colitis and pseudomembranous colitis, 152, 153
low power features, 149, 150
masson trichrome stain, 148
microscopic colitis
diagnosis of, 146
histologic characteristics of, 146
nausea, vomiting, abdominal distention, abdominal pain and diarrhea, 164, 165
necrotizing enterocolitis
etiologies or risk factors for, 159
pathologic features of, 159
non-distorted biopsy, 149
patchy disease, microscopic colitis, 147
pneumatosis intestinalis/coli, histologic features of, 155, 156
radiation colitis, 156
radiation injury, changes in mucosa, 156
surface epithelial lymphocytes, biopsy with great increase, 149
Nonmucinous adenocarcinoma, 428
Nonneoplastic diseases of stomach
abdominal pain, 83
acute gastritis, 67, 68
autoimmune atrophic pangastritis, 83, 84
autoimmune gastritis, 77, 79, 80
chronic gastritis, 84, 85
collagenous gastritis, 80, 81
dyspepsia, 85
eosinophilic gastritis, 82
granulomatous gastritis, 81, 82
helicobacter heilmanni, 74
helicobacter pylori gastritis, 69–74
lymphocytic gastritis, 80
Menetrier disease, 86
peptic ulcer disease, 68, 69
reactive gastropathy, 74–77
Russel body gastritis, 82

Non-specific drug-induced gastrointestinal tract injury patterns, 268
chemical gastritis/reactive gastropathy, 269, 270
focal active colitis, 271
increased epithelial apoptosis, 271
ischemic colitis, 270, 271
microscopic colitis, 270
pill esophagitis, 268, 269
sloughing esophagitis, 269
Non-steroidal anti-inflammatory drugs (NSAIDs)-related GI tract mucosal injury, 271, 272
Non-syndromic epithelial polyps
ampullary adenomas, 348
appendiceal polyps, 359
Brunner gland hyperplasia, 345, 346
classic hyperplastic polyp, 351
colitis cystica profunda/polyposa, 345
colon polyps, 358
conventional adenomas, 355
cytologic dysplasia, 354
filiform polyposis, 350
gastric adenomas, 342
gastric foveolar metaplasia, 346
gastritis cystica profunda/polyposa, 345
gastritis/colitis cystica profunda/polyposa, 345
GCHP, 352
glycogenic acanthosis, diagnostic features and clinical significance of, 340
heterotopic pancreatic tissue, 347
high-grade dysplasia, 356
human papillomavirus, 340
hyperplastic polyps, 341, 342, 344
inflammatory cap polyps, 349
inflammatory cloacogenic polyp, 351
inflammatory myoglandular polyp, 351
inflammatory polyps, 348
intestinal-type gastric adenomas, 343
invasive adenocarcinoma, 358
morphologic progression, 354
mucosal prolapse, 350
multinucleated stromal cells, 348
muscularis mucosae, 356
MVHP, 352
non-syndromic epithelial polyps, foveolar-type gastric adenomas, 343
pancreatic acinar metaplasia, 348
Peutz-Jeghers polyposis, 359
Peutz–Jeghers polyposis, 359
pseudoinvasion, 356, 358
pyloric gland adenomas, 342, 344, 346
SPE, diagnostic features of, 340
squamous morule, 355
SSLs or SSA/Ps, 353
submucosal lymphoid follicles, 358
TSA, 353, 354
tubulovillous adenoma, 355
Nuclear pyknosis, 323

O
Odynophagia
esophagitis, 50, 51
Olmesartan, 98
Olmesartan-associated enteropathy, 276
Omphalomesenteric remnant
gastrointestinal disorders, developmental anomalies, 2, 3
Oxyntic gland adenomas, 344
Oxyntic mucosa, 466

P
Paget cells, 217
Paget disease, 209, 217
Pancreatic heterotopia, 7, 347
in stomach, 25
Pancreatic solid pseudopapillary neoplasm, 489
Paneth cell metaplasia, IBD, 115, 116
Paneth cells, 90
Papillary adenocarcinoma, 438
Paraganglioma, 487
Parasitic infections, 233
Paris staging system, diffuse large B-cell lymphoma and, 525
Patchy disease, microscopic colitis, 147
PD-1-associated colitis, 121
PDGFR mutations, 483
PD-L1 immunostaining, 464
Pediatric gastrointestinal polyp, 18, 19
Pediatric GIST, 477
Pediatric intussusceptions
malignancy associated with, 15
pathologic lead points, 15
Pediatric volvulus
vs. adult volvulus, 14
and intussusception, 14
Pembrolizumab, 121, 280
Pemphigus vulgaris, 46
diagnostic features of and differential diagnosis, 43, 44
tombstone pattern of, 51
Penicillium marneffei, 238
Peptic duodenitis, 90
Peptic erosion, 69
Peptic ulcer disease, 68
erosion and ulcer, 69
histological features of, 68
Perianal cancer, 201
Periappendiceal abscess, 171
Periappendicitis, 169, 171
Perineural invasion, 454
Perineuriomatous stromal cell proliferation, 353
period-acid Schiff (PAS), 57
Periodic acid-Schiff (PAS) stain, 443
Peutz–Jeghers polyps (PJP), 19, 359, 375, 376
Peutz–Jeghers syndrome (PJS), 375, 381, 382, 433
Peutz-Jeghers type hamartomatous polyp, 18
Peutz-Jeghers type polyp, 19
Phlegmonous gastritis, 68
Pill esophagitis, 269, 291
drug-induced gastrointestinal tract injury, 268, 269
Pill induced esophagitis, 40, 41
Pinworms, infections of gastrointestinal tract, 256, 257, 259
Plasma cell-rich lesion, differential diagnosis and workup for, 530
Plasma cells, gastrointestinal tract, 22
Plasma CMV PCR, infections of gastrointestinal tract, 229
Plasmablastic lymphoma, 533
Plasmacytic hyperplasia PTLD, 554
Plexiform angiomyxoid myofibroblastic tumor, 496
Plexiform fibromyxoma, 496, 500
characteristic location and features of, 499
Pneumatosis coli, 165
Pneumatosis intestinalis/coli, 160, 165
air-filled spaces of, 15
histologic features of, 155, 156
Pneumocystis carinii, 235, 238
infections of gastrointestinal tract, 238
Polymerase chain reaction (PCR) assays, 460
gastrointestinal tract, infections, 223, 224

Polymorphic PTLD, 554
Polyp, 15
Polypoid dysplasia, 467
Poorly differentiated adenocarcinoma, 428
Poorly differentiated carcinoma, 467, 491
Poorly differentiated neuroendocrine carcinoma, 212
Poorly differentiated squamous cell carcinoma, anal diseases, 208
Portal hypertensive gastropathy, 76, 77
Postinfectious intestinal pseudo-obstruction, 320, 321
Posttransplant complications, 544
Posttransplant lymphoproliferative disorder (PTLD), 544, 553, 555, 559
Pouchitis, 125
Programmed cell death protein 1 (PD-1) inhibitors, drug-induced gastrointestinal tract injury, 280, 281
Programmed death-ligand 1 (PD-L1) immunostaining, 464
Proton pump inhibitor (PPI)
  drug-induced gastrointestinal tract injury, 274, 275
  esophagitis, 36, 37
Proton pump inhibitor (PPI)-responsive EoE (PPI-REE), 293
Proton pump inhibitor effect, 274
Proton pump inhibitor-responsive eosinophilic esophagitis (PPI-REE), 36
Protozoa, 248
  infections of gastrointestinal tract, 248
    Coccidial infection, 252
    Cryptosporidium, 253
    Cyclospora cayetanensis, 253
    Cystoisospora spp., 253
    Entamoeba histolytica, 248–250
    Giardia lamblia, 251
    Leishmania, 252
    Leishmaniasis, 251, 252
    Microsporidia spp., 253
    Toxoplasma gondii, 254
Proximal margin, 10, 11
Proximal polyposis, 433
Psedomelanosis intestinalis, 272
Pseudo-goblet cells, 56, 64
  Barrett esophagus, 57
Pseudoinvasion, 356–358, 434, 435
Pseudomelanosis, 279
Pseudomelanosis enteri, 279, 280
Pseudomembranous colitis, 152, 153
Pseudomyxoma peritonei (PMP), 180
  PSOGI classification of, 182
Pseudopyloric metaplasia, 116
PTEN associated Bannayan Riley Ruvalcaba syndrome, 20
PTEN associated Cowden syndrome, 20
Pyloric gland adenomas, 342, 343
Pyloric gland metaplasia, 116
Pyloric metaplasia, 74

Q

Quiescent colitis, 110

R

Radiation colitis, 156
  histologic features of, 160
Radiation esophagitis, 291
Rapid plasma reagin (RPR), 244
Reactive atypia *vs*. dysplasia, 58
Reactive gastropathy, 74, 75, 269, 270
  clinical symptoms/endoscopic findings, 75
  diagnostic approach, 75
  from portal hypertensive gastropathy and from gastric antral vascular ectasia syndrome, 75–77
  types of patients, 74, 75
Reactive marginal zone hyperplasia, extranodal marginal zone lymphoma and, 524, 525
Reactive myofibroblastic proliferation, 505
Rectal adenocarcinoma, 462
Rectal bleeding, 187, 188
Rectal NETs, 419
Rectal sparing, in UC, 112
Rectal tonsil, 529, 530
Reflux esophagitis, 34, 38
Refractory celiac disease, 528
  clinical diagnosis of, 94
Regenerative epithelium, 130
Renal failure, hemodialysis for, 281, 282
Rendu-Osler-Weber disease, 152
Resection specimens, motility disorder, 314
Residual chronic inflammation, 72
Resins, 278
Restorative proctocolectomy, 125
Retention cyst, 182
Retroperitoneum, 514
  liposarcoma of, 511
Rheumatoid arthritis, 308
Rituximab, 120
Rosai-Dorfman disease, 304, 533
Ruptured diverticulum, 182
Russel body gastritis, 82

S

Salivary gland carcinomas, 442
Salmonella, 225
Salmonella enterocolitis, 226
Sarcina ventriculi, 82, 83
Sartan-related gastrointestinal injury, 98
Sartans, 95, 105
Schaumann bodies, 113
Schistosomiasis, 255
  infections of gastrointestinal tract, 255
Schwann cell hamartomas, 389, 390, 402
Schwannoma, 402, 496
  microcystic/reticular variant of, 497
  from neurofibromas of GI tract, 497, 498
Scleroderma, 318
  histopathologic features of, 319
Sclerosing mesenteritis, 505
SDHB-deficient gastrointestinal stromal tumor, 477, 490
SDHB-deficient tumors, 490
Secondary chronic intestinal pseudo-obstruction, 320
Seromuscular biopsies, 13
Serotonin secretion, 418
Serrated adenocarcinoma, 438, 439
Serrated dysplasia, 61
Serrated lesions, 182
Serrated polyposis, 433
Serrated polyposis syndrome (SPS), 378
Sessile serrated adenoma (SSA), 353
Sessile serrated lesion (SSL), 353, 361
Sessile serrated polyp (SSP), 353
Sevelamer, 41, 278, 279
Severe acute cellular rejection, 556, 557
Severe drug-induced injury, 556
Severe graft-*vs*.-host disease, 556

Sexually transmitted infectious, 243, 244
Shigella dysenteriae, 226
Shigellosis, 225
Shredded carrot, 498
Sigmoid colon, 331
Signet-ring cell carcinoma, 436
Skin adnexal tumors, 200
  hidradenoma papilliferum, 200
  stage in anal tumors, 200
    AJCC definition, 201
    clinical definition, 200, 201
  trichoepithelioma, 200
Sloughing esophagitis/esophagitis dissecans, 42, 43, 269
Small bowel, 238
  non-GIST primary mesenchymal tumors, GI tract, 496
Small bowel injury, malabsorptive pattern of, 91
  differential diagnosis for, 91
Small bowel transplant, 543, 544
Small cell carcinoma (SCC), 410
Small intestinal tumor, 424
Small intestine, 290, 294
  enteropathy-associated T-cell lymphoma, 539
  side by side tubular duplication of, 3
Small-medium-sized B-cell lymphoma, 522
Smudge cells, 230
Sodium polystyrene sulfonate, 278, 279
Solid gastric duplication, 3
Solitary fibrous tumor (SFT), 392
Solitary polypoid gangliomas, 392
Solitary polypoid ganglioneuroma, 392, 393
Solitary rectal ulcer, 360
Somatostatinomas, 416
Spindle cell carcinoma, 438
Spindle cell neoplasms, intra-abdominal fibromatosis, 504, 505
Spirochetosis, 245
Sporadic and SDHB-deficient GISTs, 478
Sporadic colorectal cancer, 381
Sporadic fundic gland polyps, 342
Sporadic gastric and intestinal adenomas, 433
Squamous cell carcinoma (SCC), 203–205, 428, 432, 456, 457
Squamous intraepithelial lesion (SIL), 219
Squamous intraepithelial neoplasia or lesion (AIN), 456
Squamous morules, 356
Squamous mucosa, 49, 335
Squamous papilloma, 387
Squamous papillomas of the esophagus (SPE), 340
Staphyloccus aureus, 246
Stomach, 290, 294
  extranodal marginal zone lymphoma of, 534
  gastrointestinal stromal tumor of, 18
  low-grade/small B-cell lymphomas of, 521–523
  mantle cell lymphoma in, 537
  non-GIST primary mesenchymal tumors, 496
  nonneoplastic diseases of
    acute gastritis, 67, 68
    autoimmune atrophic pangastritis, 83, 84
    autoimmune gastritis, 77, 79, 80
    chronic gastritis, 84, 85
    collagenous gastritis, 80, 81
    dyspepsia, 85
    eosinophilic gastritis, 82
    granulomatous gastritis, 81, 82
    Helicobacter heilmanni, 74
    Helicobacter pylori gastritis, 69–74
    lymphocytic gastritis, 80
    Menetrier disease, 86
    peptic ulcer disease, 68, 69
    reactive gastropathy, 74–77
    Russel body gastritis, 82
  tissue eosinophils, differential diagnosis of, 293
Stool PCR assay, 245, 246
Stricturing Crohn ileocolitis, 111
Stripped duodenal villi, 90
Strongyloides stercoralis, 257, 258, 294
Strongyloidiasis, 258
Submucosal cysts, 156
Submucosal plexuses, 315
Submucosally invasive adenocarcinoma, Barrett esophagus, 60, 61
Suction mucosal biopsies, 313
Suction rectal biopsy, Hirschsprung disease, 8, 9, 13, 14
Superficial Crohn colitis, 113
Superficial predominant pattern, 71
Suppurative appendicitis, 168
Surface epithelial injury, 285
Surface epithelial lymphocytes, biopsy with great increase, 149
Surface inflammation, IBD, 115
Sweet syndrome, 531
Switch/sucrose-nonfermenting (SWI/SNF), 439
Synaptophysin, 409, 416, 420, 422
Syndromic epithelial polyps
  Cowden/PTEN hamartoma syndrome, 377
  Cronkhite–Canada syndrome, 377
  FAP
    AFAP, 370
    Gardner syndrome, 369
    genetic and clinical features of, 367, 368
    gross and histologic features of, 368, 369
    prognostic and treatment implications, 370
    screening and treatment options, 370
    Turcot syndrome, 369
  GAPPS, 379
  Lynch syndrome
    clinical and histologic features of, 371, 373
    MMR gene mutations, 371
    molecular etiology, 370
    prognostic and treatment implications of, 374, 375
    sporadic mismatch repair deficiency form. hereditary, 373, 374
    sporadic MMR deficiency, 371
  MMR immunohistochemical patterns, 374
  MUTYH gene, 377
  Peutz–Jeghers syndrome
    GJP, 377
    JPC, 377
    juvenile polyp, 375
    prognostic implications in, 376
  SPS, 378
Syndromic GIST, 477
Syphilis, 118, 199, 243, 244
Syphilitic proctitis, 119, 243, 302
Systemic lupus erythematosus (SLE), 42
Systemic mastocytosis, 297, 305
  colonic involvement by, 300, 528
  diagnostic criteria for, 297, 528
  endoscopic and histologic features, 298, 299
  gastric involvement, 299
Systemic usual adult type follicular lymphoma (u-FL), 526

T

Talaromyces marneffei, 232
Tapeworms, 255
Taxane effect, 276, 284

Taxanes, 42, 275
Taenia saginata, 256
Thymic stromal lymphopoietin (TSLP), 293
Thymidine phosphorylase, 316
Tissue biopsy, 235
Tissue eosinophilia, 308
  clinical setting, 295
  colonic biopsies with inflammatory bowel disease, 294
  differential diagnosis of, 293, 294
  reporting, 295
Tombstone pattern of pemphigus vulgaris, 51
Toxoplasma gondii, 254
Traditional serrated adenoma (TSA), 353, 355
Traditional serrated adenoma-like dysplasia, 127
Transition zone, feature of, 10, 11
Transmural inflammation, in UC, 113
Transplant-related issues
  ACR grade, 545
  ACR, histologic features of, 544, 545
  acute GVHD, 551
  acute *vs.* chronic GVHD, 552
  allograft and native bowel, 546
  AMR, 548
  chronic rejection, 548
  crypt apoptotic body vs. intraepithelial lymphocyte, 545, 546
  epithelial apoptosis, 546
  GVHD, 551
  histologic features of ACR overlap, 547
  histologic features of infectious enteritis, 549, 550
  immunostains for adenovirus, 550
  increased apoptotic bodies, 552
  Lerner grading system, 552
  PTLD
    clinical features of, 553
    diagnosis of, 554
    lymphoid aggregates, 554
    types of, 553, 554
  small bowel transplant, 543, 544, 546, 549
  transplanted colon and stomach, 549
  tubular GI tract, 551
Treponema pallidum, 199, 243, 244
Trichoepithelioma, 200
Trichrome, 162
Trisomy 21, 11
Trophozoites, 251
Tropical sprue
  features, 100
Tuberculoma, 241
Tuberculosis, 242
Tuberculous colitis, 119
Tuberous sclerosis, 20
Tubular adenomas, 80
Tubular neuroendocrine tumor, 172, 173
Tubular NET, 418
Tubulovillous adenoma, 351, 362
Tufting enteropathy, 25, 26, 102
Tumor buds, 452
Tumor cells, 305, 510
Tumor deposit, 450, 451
Turcot syndrome, 369
Type 2 refractory sprue, 94
Typical angiomyolipoma, 512

U
Ulcer, 242
  from erosion, 69
Ulcerated colonic mucosa, 140
Ulcerated gastric mucosa, 466
Ulcerations, 33, 40, 42, 45, 109
Ulcerative appendicitis, 112
Ulcerative colitis (UC), 110, 112, 113, 133, 140
  anti-inflammatory therapy with mesalamine, 139
  backwash ileitis in, 113
  characteristic histologic features of, 116
  discontinuous inflammation in, 112
  granulomas in, 113
  histological features, 116, 117
  rectal sparing in, 112
  transmural inflammation in, 113
  upper GI manifestations, 124, 125
Ulcerative pancolitis, 110, 139–141
Ultrashort HD, 11
Umbilical polyp, with intestinal mucosa, 7
Undifferentiated carcinoma, 440
United States Multi-Society Task Force, 353
Unresectable dysplasia, 132
Upper gastrointestinal endoscopy
  Barrett esophagus, 62

V
Varices, 198
Varioliform gastritis, 80
Vascular neoplasms, GI tract, 507, 508
Venereal Disease Research Laboratory (VDRL) test, 244
Verrucous carcinoma (VC), 202–204, 456
Villi, 90
Villous blunting, 106
  malabsorption disorders, 104
Villous dysplasia, 128, 136
Villous flattening, 104
Villous shortening, 96
Viruses, infections of gastrointestinal tract, 229–232
Visceral myopathy, 317

W
Well differentiated adenocarcinoma, 428, 431, 468
Well differentiated colonic adenocarcinoma, 431
Well differentiated squamous cell carcinoma, 432
Well-differentiated liposarcoma (WDLPS), 400, 510
Whipple disease, 240, 241
Whipworm, 256

X
Xanthomata, 388

Y
Yersinia colitis, 226
Yttrium microspheres, 275

Z
Z-line, 55, 56
Zollinger-Ellison syndrome, 415, 416, 421